SENSATION & PERCEPTION

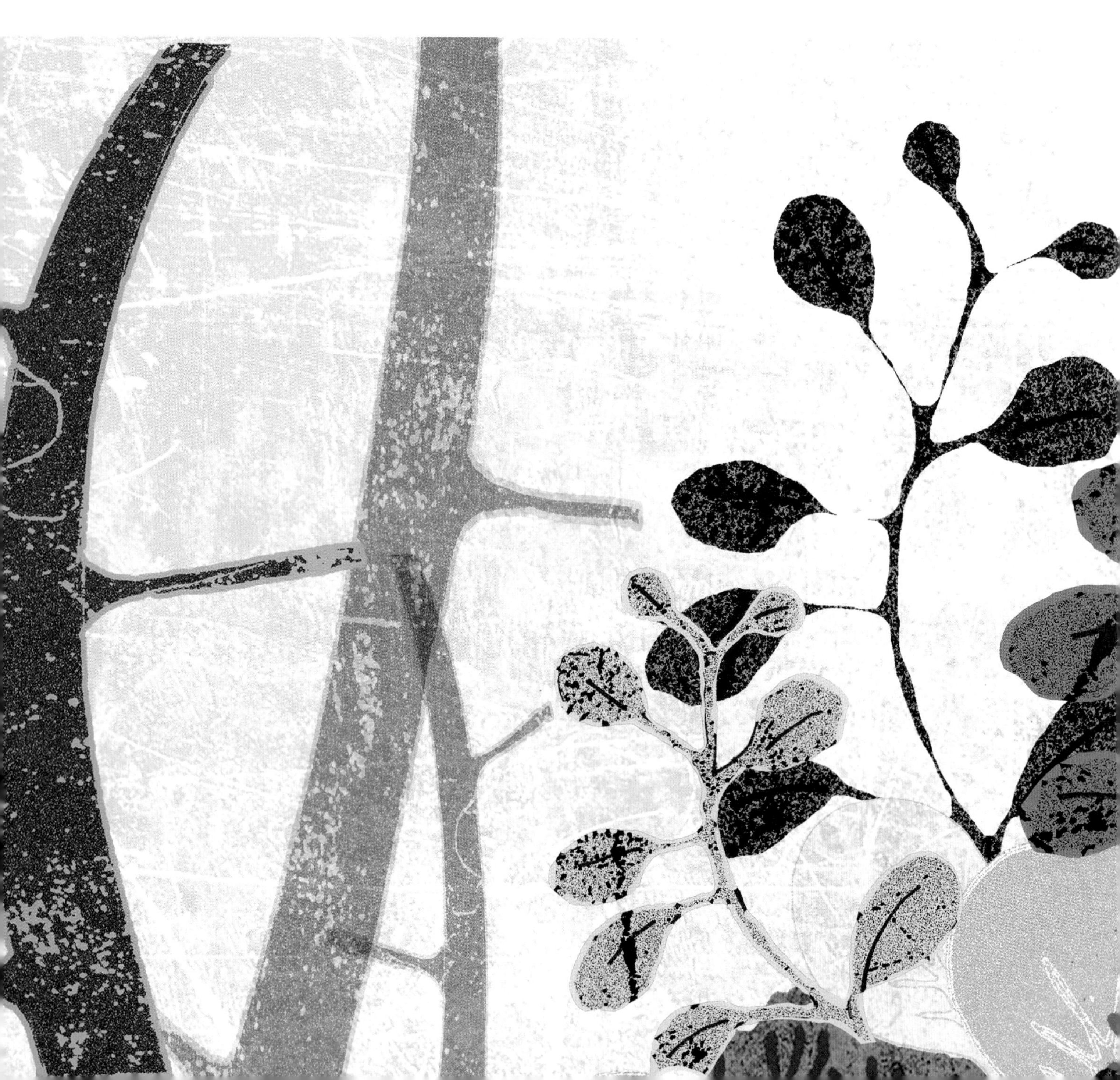

SENSATION & PERCEPTION

SEVENTH EDITION

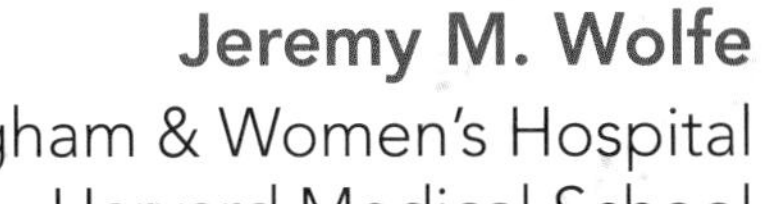

Jeremy M. Wolfe
Brigham & Women's Hospital
Harvard Medical School

Dennis M. Levi
University of California, Berkeley

Lori L. Holt
University of Texas, Austin

Linda M. Bartoshuk
University of Florida

Rachel S. Herz
Brown University

Roberta L. Klatzky
Carnegie Mellon University

Daniel M. Merfeld
The Ohio State University

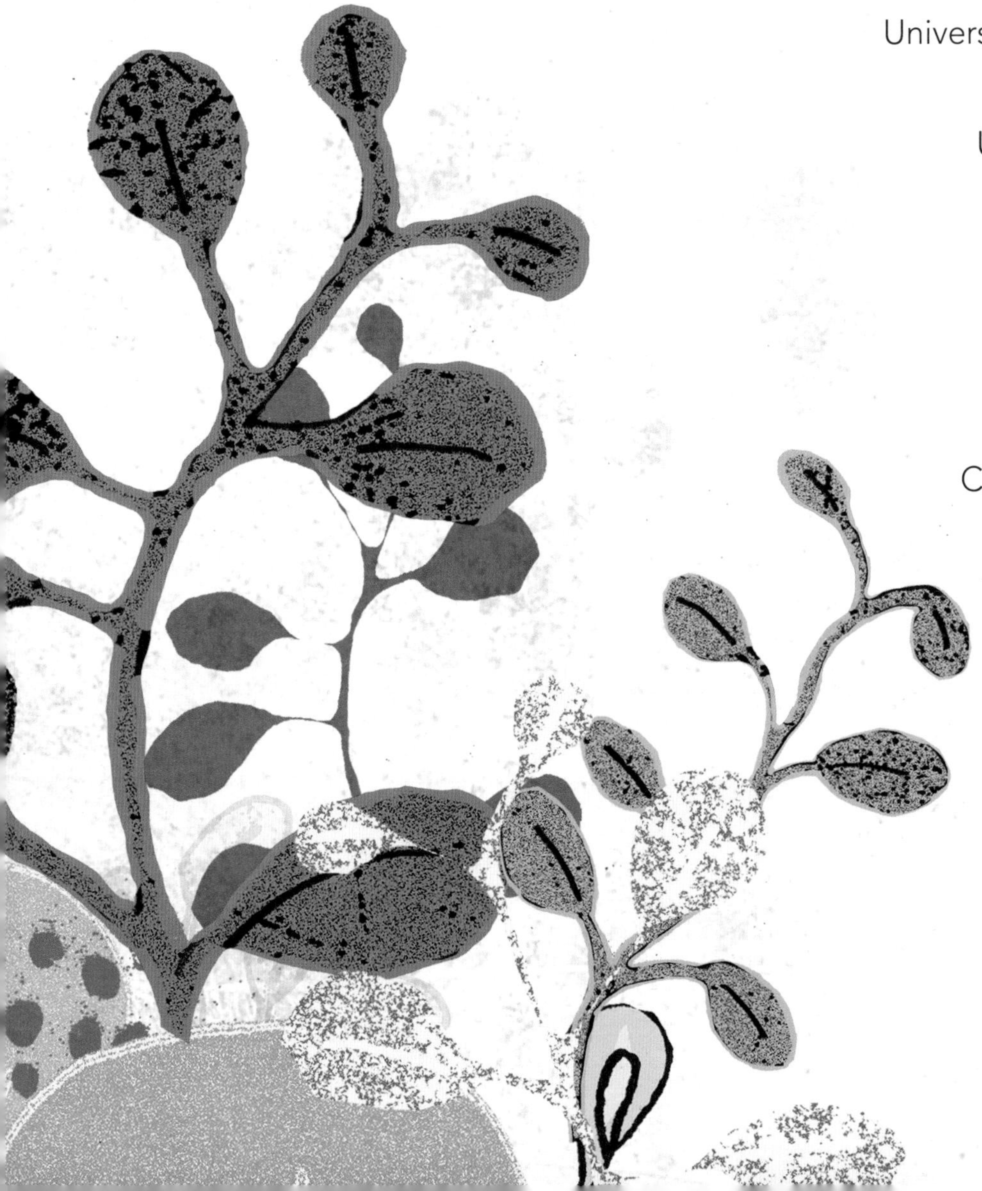

OXFORD
UNIVERSITY PRESS

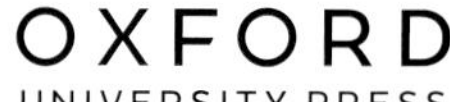

Oxford University Press is a department of the University of Oxford. It furthers the University's objective of excellence in research, scholarship, and education by publishing worldwide. Oxford is a registered trade mark of Oxford University Press in the UK and in certain other countries.

Published in the United States of America by Oxford University Press
198 Madison Avenue, New York, NY 10016, United States of America.

For titles covered by Section 112 of the US Higher Education Opportunity Act, please visit www.oup.com/us/he for the latest information about pricing and alternate formats.

Library of Congress Cataloging-in-Publication Data

Names: Wolfe, Jeremy M., author.
Title: Sensation and perception / Jeremy M. Wolfe Brigham & Women's Hospital Harvard Medical School [and six others].
Description: Seventh edition. | New York, NY, United States of America : Oxford University Press, [2025] | Includes bibliographical references and index.
Identifiers: LCCN 2023053741 (print) | LCCN 2023053742 (ebook) | ISBN 9780197663813 (paperback) | ISBN 9780197663844 (epub)
Subjects: LCSH: Senses and sensation. | Perception.
Classification: LCC QP431 .S445 2024 (print) | LCC QP431 (ebook) | DDC 612.8—dc23/eng20240307
LC record available at https://lccn.loc.gov/2023053741
LC ebook record available at https://lccn.loc.gov/2023053742

Printed by Sheridan Books, Inc., United States of America

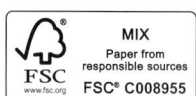

Brief Contents

CHAPTER 1 Introduction 3

CHAPTER 2 The First Steps in Vision: From Light to Neural Signals 33

CHAPTER 3 Spatial Vision: From Spots to Stripes 57

CHAPTER 4 Perceiving and Recognizing Objects 93

CHAPTER 5 The Perception of Color 131

CHAPTER 6 Space Perception and Binocular Vision 167

CHAPTER 7 Attention and Scene Perception 213

CHAPTER 8 Visual Motion Perception 249

CHAPTER 9 Hearing: Physiology and Psychoacoustics 273

CHAPTER 10 Hearing in the Environment 305

CHAPTER 11 Music and Speech Perception 335

CHAPTER 12 Vestibular Sensation 365

CHAPTER 13 Touch 409

CHAPTER 14 Olfaction 455

CHAPTER 15 Taste 507

About the Authors

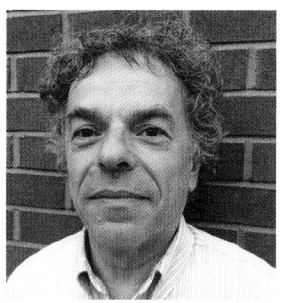

JEREMY M. WOLFE is a professor of ophthalmology and radiology at Harvard Medical School. Dr. Wolfe was trained as a vision researcher/experimental psychologist and remains one today. His early work includes papers on binocular vision, adaptation, and accommodation. The bulk of his recent work has dealt with visual search and visual attention in the lab and in real-world settings such as airport security and cancer screening. He taught Introductory Psychology for over 25 years at the Massachusetts Institute of Technology, where he won the Baker Memorial Prize for undergraduate teaching in 1989. He directs the Visual Attention Lab of Brigham and Women's Hospital.

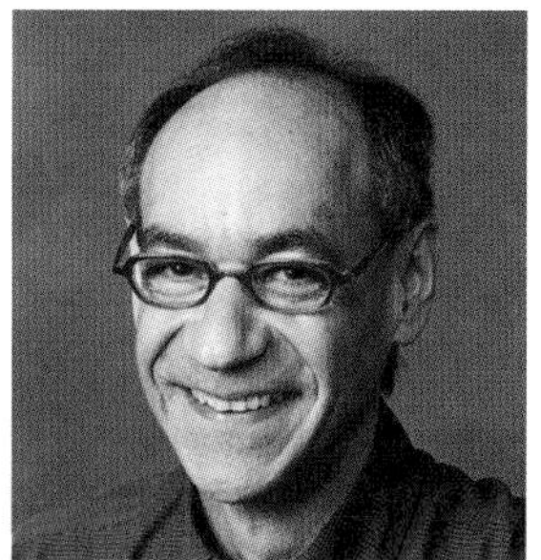

DENNIS M. LEVI is a professor of optometry, vision science, and neuroscience at the University of California, Berkeley. He served as dean of the School of Optometry from 2001 to 2014. In the lab, Dr. Levi and colleagues use psychophysics, computational modeling, and brain imaging (functional magnetic resonance imaging) to study the neural mechanisms of normal pattern vision in humans and to learn how they are degraded by abnormal visual experience (amblyopia).

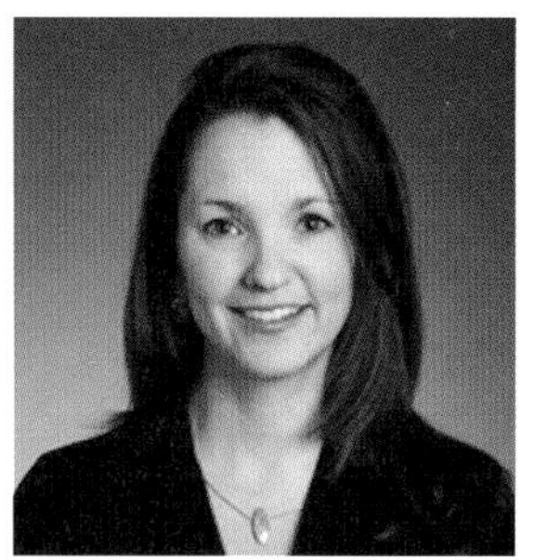

LORI L. HOLT is a professor of psychology at the University of Texas at Austin. Dr. Holt became captivated by perception as an undergraduate and continues to study the behavioral and biological mechanisms of auditory perception and cognition today. Her research has used behavioral and neurobiological methods to understand how learning, attention, and context influence what we hear, especially in the context of listening to speech. This work has had implications for how to better teach university students second languages and to better understand dyslexia.

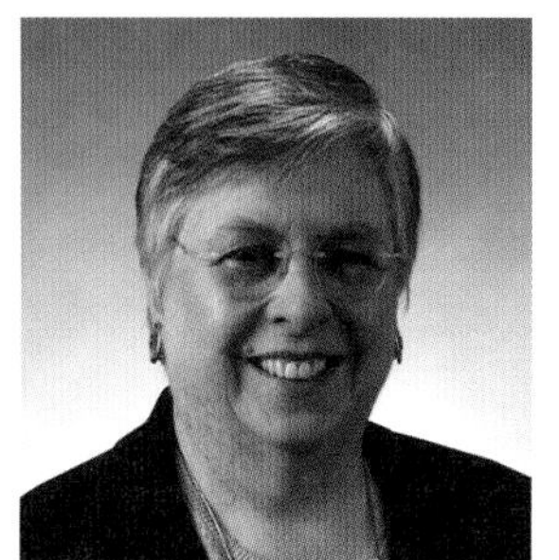

LINDA M. BARTOSHUK is Bushnell Professor, Department of Food Science and Human Nutrition, at the University of Florida. Her research on taste has opened broad new avenues for further study, establishing the impact of both genetic and pathological variation in taste on food preferences, diet, and health. She discovered that taste normally inhibits other oral sensations, such that damage to taste leads to unexpected consequences like weight gain and intensified oral pain. Most recently, working with colleagues in horticulture, her group found that a considerable amount of the sweetness in fruit is produced by interactions between taste and olfaction in the brain. This may lead to a new way to reduce sugar in foods and beverages.

RACHEL S. HERZ is an adjunct assistant professor in the Department of Psychiatry and Human Behavior at Brown University's Warren Alpert Medical School and part-time faculty in the Department of Psychology and Neuroscience at Boston College. Her research focuses on a number of facets of olfactory cognition and perception and on emotion, memory, and motivated behavior. Using an experimental approach grounded in evolutionary theory and incorporating both cognitive-behavioral and neuropsychological techniques, Dr. Herz aims to understand how biological mechanisms and cognitive processes interact to influence perception, cognition, and behavior.

ROBERTA L. KLATZKY is the Charles J. Queenan Jr. University Professor of Psychology at Carnegie Mellon University, where she also holds faculty appointments in the Human-Computer Interaction Institute and the Neuroscience Institute. She has done extensive research on haptic and visual object recognition, space perception and spatial thinking, and perceptually guided action. Her work has application to haptic interfaces, navigation aids for the blind, image-guided surgery, teleoperation, and virtual environments.

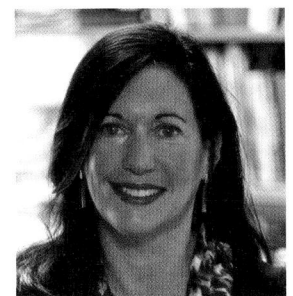

DANIEL M. MERFELD is a professor of otolaryngology/head and neck surgery at The Ohio State University College of Medicine and the senior vestibular scientist at the Naval Medical Research Unit, Dayton. Much of his research career has been spent studying how the brain combines information from multiple sources (i.e., multisensory integration), with a specific focus on how the brain processes ambiguous sensory information from the vestibular system in the presence of noise. Translational work includes research developing: (a) new methods to help identify people who are more likely to fall so we can intervene before a fall occurs, (b) new methods to diagnose patients experiencing vestibular symptoms, and (c) vestibular implants for patients who have severe problems with their vestibular labyrinth.

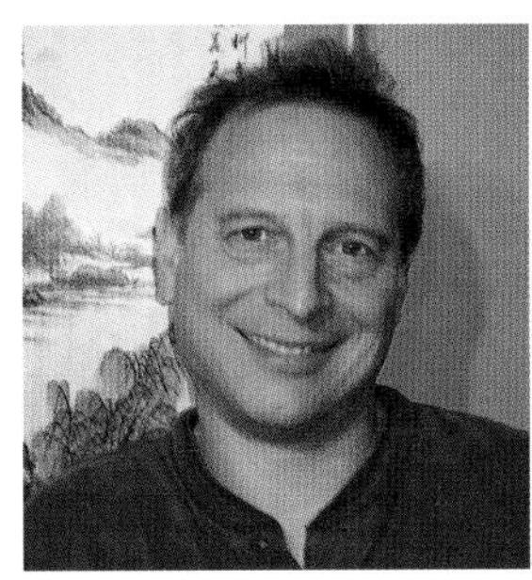

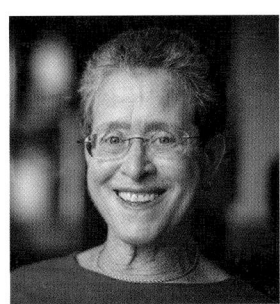

Contents

Preface xvi
Digital Resources for *Sensation & Perception*, Seventh Edition xx

1 Introduction 3

1.1 Sensation and Perception: Welcome to Your World through Our World 3
How Many Senses Do We Use to Perceive? 4
How Accurately Do We Perceive, and by What Method Would We Know? 5
1.2 Thresholds and Their Measurement by Psychophysics 7
Absolute Threshold 7
Difference Threshold 9
Scaling Methods 10
Measuring Discrimination: Signal Detection Theory 13
Measuring the Time Course of Perception 17
1.3 Sensory Neuroscience: What Do We Know About How the Nervous System Translates Physics into Experience? 18
Nerves and Specific Nerve Energies 18
Neuronal Connections 21
Acquiring Neuronal Data by Recording 22
Neuroimaging Methods 24
1.4 Computational Modeling as a Method to Understand Perceptual Processes 27
Computational Models: Probability, Statistics, and Networks 28
Deep Learning 30
Is Our Experience of Physical Properties Influenced by Prior Knowledge and Context? 30
Summary 31

2 The First Steps in Vision: From Light to Neural Signals 33

2.1 A Little Light Physics 33
2.2 Eyes That Capture Light 35
Focusing Light onto the Retina 37
The Retina 39
What the Doctor Saw 39
Retinal Geography and Function 41
2.3 Dark and Light Adaptation 44
Pupil Size 44
Photopigment Regeneration 45
The Duplex Retina 45
Neural Circuitry 46
- ***Sensation & Perception in Everyday Life*** *When Good Retina Goes Bad* 46

2.4 Retinal Information Processing 47
Light Transduction by Rod and Cone Photoreceptors 47
Lateral Inhibition through Horizontal and Amacrine Cells 49

Convergence and Divergence of Information via Bipolar Cells 49
Communicating to the Brain via Ganglion Cells 50
• *Scientists at Work* *Is One Photon Enough to See?* 54
Summary 54

3 Spatial Vision: From Spots to Stripes 57

3.1 Visual Acuity: Oh Say, Can You See? 58
A Visit to the Eye Doctor 62
More Types of Visual Acuity 62
Acuity for Low-Contrast Stripes 64
Why Sine Wave Gratings? 65
3.2 Retinal Ganglion Cells and Stripes 67
3.3 The Lateral Geniculate Nucleus 69
3.4 The Striate Cortex 70
The Topography of the Human Cortex 71
Some Perceptual Consequences of Cortical Magnification 72
3.5 Receptive Fields in Striate Cortex 73
Orientation Selectivity 74
Other Receptive-Field Properties 75
Simple and Complex Cells 75
Further Complications 76
3.6 Columns and Hypercolumns 77
3.7 Selective Adaptation: The Psychologist's Electrode 80
The Site of Selective Adaptation Effects 83
Spatial-Frequency-Tuned Pattern Analyzers in Human Vision 84
3.8 The Development of Vision 86
• *Sensation & Perception in Everyday Life* *The Girl Who Almost Couldn't See Stripes* 88
Development of the CSF 89
• *Scientists at Work* *Does the Duck's Left Eye Know What the Right Eye Saw?* 90
Summary 90

4 Perceiving and Recognizing Objects 93

4.1 From Simple Lines and Edges to Properties of Objects 93
4.2 *What* and *Where* Pathways 96
• *Scientists at Work* *Food on Your Mind* 99
4.3 The Problems of Perceiving and Recognizing Objects 101
4.4 Midlevel Vision 103
Finding Edges 104
Texture Segmentation and Grouping 109
Figure and Ground 114
Dealing with Occlusion 115
Parts and Wholes 116
Summarizing Midlevel Vision 116
From Metaphor to Formal Model 117
4.5 Object Recognition 118
Can We Build It? 120
Multiple Recognition Committees? 125
Faces: An Illustrative Special Case 126
Summary 128

5 The Perception of Color 131

5.1 Basic Principles of Color Perception 131

Three Steps to Color Perception 132

5.2 Step 1: Color Detection 132

5.3 Step 2: Color Discrimination 133

The Principle of Univariance 133

The Trichromatic Solution 134

Metamers 135

The History of Trichromatic Theory 137

A Brief Digression into Lights, Filters, and Finger Paints 138

From Retina to Brain: Repackaging the Information 138

Cone-Opponent Cells in the Retina and Lateral Geniculate Nucleus 139

5.4 Step 3: Color Appearance 141

Three Numbers, Three Dimensions, Many Colors 141

- ***Sensation & Perception in Everyday Life*** *Picking Colors* 142

The Limits of the Rainbow 143

Opponent Colors 144

Color in the Visual Cortex 146

5.5 Individual Differences in Color Perception 147

Language and Color 147

Genetic Differences in Color Vision 151

Does Everyone See the Same Colors? The Special Case of Synesthesia 152

5.6 From the Color of Lights to a World of Color 153

Adaptation and Afterimages 155

Color Constancy 157

The Problem with the Illuminant 158

Physical Constraints Make Constancy Possible 158

5.7 What Is Color Vision Good For? 159

- ***Scientists at Work*** *Filtering Colors 164*

Summary 164

6 Space Perception and Binocular Vision 167

6.1 Monocular Cues to Three-Dimensional Space 171

Pictorial Depth Cues 171

Occlusion 172

Size and Position Cues 172

Aerial Perspective 175

Linear Perspective 175

Seeing Depth in Pictures 177

6.2 Triangulation Cues to Three-Dimensional Space 178

Motion Cues 179

Accommodation and Convergence 180

6.3 Binocular Vision and Stereopsis 182

Stereoscopes and Stereograms 187

- ***Sensation & Perception in Everyday Life*** *Recovering Stereo Vision* 189

Random Dot Stereograms 190

Using Stereopsis 191

Stereoscopic Correspondence 192

The Physiological Basis of Stereopsis and Depth Perception 194

- ***Scientists at Work*** *Stereopsis in a Hunting Insect 198*

6.4 Combining Depth Cues 198

The Bayesian Approach Revisited 199

Illusions and the Construction of Space 200

Binocular Rivalry and Suppression 202
6.5 Development of Binocular Vision and Stereopsis 205
Abnormal Visual Experience Can Disrupt Binocular Vision 208
Summary 211

7 Attention and Scene Perception 213

7.1 Selection in Space 215
The "Spotlight" of Attention 217
7.2 Visual Search 217
Feature Searches Are Efficient 219
Many Searches Are Inefficient 219
Guided Searches in the Real World 220
• ***Scientists at Work*** *How Would You Study Visual Search by a Fish?* 221
The Binding Problem in Visual Search 225
Binding between the Senses 226
7.3 Attending in Time: Rapid Serial Visual Presentation and the Attentional Blink 226
7.4 The Physiological Basis of Attention 228
Attention Could Enhance Neural Activity 229
Attention Could Enhance the Processing of a Specific Type of Stimulus 229
Attention and Single Cells 230
Attention May Change the Way Neurons Talk to Each Other 232
7.5 Disorders of Visual Attention 233
Neglect 233
Extinction 234
• ***Sensation & Perception in Everyday Life*** *Selective Attention and Attention Deficit Hyperactivity Disorder* 235
7.6 Perceiving and Understanding Scenes 236
Two Pathways to Scene Perception 237
The Nonselective Pathway Computes Ensemble Statistics 238
The Nonselective Pathway Computes Scene Gist and Layout—Very Quickly 238
Memory for Objects and Scenes Is Amazingly Good 240
But . . . Memory for Objects and Scenes Can Be Amazingly Bad: Change Blindness 243
What Do We Actually See? 244
Summary 246

8 Visual Motion Perception 249

8.1 Motion Aftereffects 249
8.2 Computation of Visual Motion 251
Origins of Direction Selectivity 253
Apparent Motion 253
The Correspondence Problem: Viewing through an Aperture 253
Detection of Global Motion in Area MT 256
• ***Sensation & Perception in Everyday Life*** *The Man Who Couldn't See Motion* 258
Second-Order Motion 258
8.3 Using Motion Information 260
Going with the Flow: Using Motion Information to Navigate 260
Avoiding Imminent Collision: The Tao of Tau 261

Something in the Way You Move: Using Motion Information to Identify Objects 262
Motion-Induced Blindness 263
8.4 Eye Movements 263
Physiology and Types of Eye Movements 265
Eye Movements and Reading 267
Saccadic Suppression and the Comparator 267
Updating the Neural Mechanisms for Eye Movement Compensation 269
8.5 Development of Motion Perception 270
• ***Scientists at Work*** *Guess Who's Coming to Dinner 270*
Summary 271

9 Hearing: Physiology and Psychoacoustics 273

9.1 The Function of Hearing 273
9.2 What Is Sound? 274
Basic Qualities of Sound Waves: Frequency and Amplitude 274
Sine Waves and Complex Sounds 275
9.3 Basic Structure of the Mammalian Auditory System 277
Outer Ear 277
Middle Ear 277
Inner Ear 279
The Auditory Nerve 284
Auditory Brain Structures 290
9.4 Psychoacoustics 292
Intensity and Loudness 293
• ***Scientists at Work*** *Why Don't Manatees Get out of the Way When a Boat Is Coming? 294*
Frequency and Pitch 295
9.5 Hearing Loss 296
Types of Hearing Loss 297
Causes of Hearing Loss 298
Treating Hearing Loss 299
Using versus Detecting Sound 300
• ***Sensation & Perception in Everyday Life*** *Electronic Ears* 301
Summary 302

10 Hearing in the Environment 305

10.1 Sound Localization 305
Interaural Time Difference 306
Interaural Level Difference 309
Cones of Confusion 310
Pinnae and Head Cues 311
Auditory Distance Perception 314
• ***Scientists at Work*** *Vulcan Ears 315*
Spatial Hearing and Blindness 317
• ***Sensation & Perception in Everyday Life*** *Sounds from Wind Farms* 318
10.2 Complex Sounds 319
Harmonics 319
Timbre 320
Attack and Decay 321
10.3 Auditory Scene Analysis 322
Spatial, Spectral, and Temporal Segregation 324
Grouping by Onset 326
When Hearing Dominates Vision 326
When Sounds Become Familiar 327
10.4 Continuity and Restoration Effects 328
Restoration of Complex Sounds 329
10.5 Auditory Attention 330
Summary 332

11 Music and Speech Perception 335

11.1 Music 335

- ***Sensation & Perception in Everyday Life*** *Music and Emotion* 336

Musical Notes 336

Making Music 340

- ***Sensation & Perception in Everyday Life*** *Sonic Seasoning* 343

11.2 Speech 343

Speech Production 344

Speech Perception 348

- ***Scientists at Work*** *Tickling the Cochlea* 354

Learning to Listen 355

Speech in the Brain 358

Summary 362

12 Vestibular Sensation 365

12.1 Vestibular Contributions 367

12.2 Evolutionary Development and Vestibular Sensation 368

12.3 Modalities and Qualities of Spatial Orientation 369

Sensing Angular Motion ("Rotation"), Linear Motion ("Translation"), and Tilt 369

- ***Sensation & Perception in Everyday Life*** *The Vestibular System, Virtual Reality, and Motion Sickness* 370

Basic Qualities of Spatial Orientation: Amplitude and Direction 370

12.4 The Vestibular Organs 374

Hair Cells: Mechanical Transducers 374

Semicircular Canals 376

Otolith Organs 382

12.5 Spatial Orientation Perception 384

Rotation Perception 385

Translation Perception 386

Tilt Perception 387

Spatial Orientation Cognition 388

Spatial Cognition 389

Spatial Navigation 389

Nonspatial Cognition 389

12.6 Multisensory Integration 390

Visual-Vestibular Multisensory Integration 390

Vestibulo-interoceptive Multisensory Integration 391

12.7 Beyond Multisensory Integration: Active Sensing 392

12.8 Reflexive Vestibular Responses 392

Vestibulo-ocular Responses 393

Vestibulo-autonomic Responses 396

Vestibulospinal Responses 398

12.9 Multisensory Spatial Orientation Cortex 401

Vestibular Thalamocortical Pathways 402

Cortical Influences 402

12.10 When the Vestibular System Goes Bad 403

Falls and Vestibular Function 404

Mal de Debarquement Syndrome 404

- ***Scientists at Work*** *Vestibular Aging* 405

Ménière's Syndrome 405

- ***Sensation & Perception in Everyday Life*** *Amusement Park Rides—Vestibular Physics Is Fun* 406

Summary 407

13 Touch 409

13.1 Neural Pathways of Touch: From Physics to Brain 410
Neural Fibers, Receptors, and End Organs 410
Pathways from Skin to Brain 418
Neural Plasticity of Somatosensation 423

13.2 Submodalities of Touch 427
The Submodality of Discriminative Touch 427
The Submodality of Affective Touch 432
The Submodality of Pain and Itch 435
The Submodality of Interoception 439

13.3 Haptic Perception: Linking Touch with Action 440
Perception for Action 440
Action for Perception 441
• **Scientists at Work** *Haptic Exploratory Procedures Used by Sea Lions* 442
The *What* System of Touch: Perceiving Objects and Their Properties 444
The *Where* System of Touch: Locating Objects 448
• **Sensation & Perception in Everyday Life** *A Brain-Computer Interface with a Cortical Loop* 451

Summary 452

14 Olfaction 455

14.1 Olfactory Physiology 456
Odors and Odorants 456
The Human Olfactory Apparatus 456
How Well Do We Smell? 459
• **Sensation & Perception in Everyday Life** *Anosmia and the Effects of Olfactory Dysfunction* 460

14.2 Neurophysiology of Olfaction 464
The Genetic Basis of Olfactory Receptors 467
The "Feel" of Scent 469

14.3 From Chemicals to Smells 470
Theories of Olfactory Perception 470
The Importance of Patterns 474
Is Odor Perception Synthetic or Analytical? 475
Nasal Power 477
Odor Imagery 478

14.4 Olfactory Psychophysics, Identification, and Adaptation 478
Detection 478
Discrimination and Recognition 479
Psychophysical Methods for Detection, Discrimination, and Recognition 480
Identification: Olfaction and Language 480
Individual Differences 483
• **Scientists at Work** *A New Test to Diagnose Parkinson's Disease* 485
Adaptation 486
Cognitive Habituation and Odor Consciousness 489

14.5 Olfactory Hedonics 491
Pleasantness 491
Familiarity and Intensity 491
Nature or Nurture? 492
An Evolutionary Argument 494
The Importance of Emotional Associative Learning 495
Caveats 496

14.6 The Vomeronasal Organ, Human Pheromones, and Chemosignals 497

• ***Sensation & Perception in Everyday Life*** *Odor-Evoked Memory and the Truth behind Aromatherapy* 500

14.7 The Future of Scent 502

Digitizing Scent 502

Olfactory Virtual Reality 502

Summary 503

15 Taste 507

15.1 Taste versus Flavor 507

Localizing Flavor Sensations: The Role of Taste 509

• ***Sensation & Perception in Everyday Life*** *Volatile-Enhanced Taste: A New Way to Sweeten Foods* 510

Mixtures of Taste and Flavor 511

15.2 Anatomy and Physiology of the Gustatory System 512

Taste Myth: The Tongue Map 513

Taste Buds and Taste Receptor Cells 514

Nonoral Locations for Taste Receptors 515

Taste Processing in the Central Nervous System 515

15.3 The Four Basic Tastes? 517

Salty 518

Sour 518

Bitter 519

Sweet 520

15.4 Are There More Than Four Basic Tastes? Does It Matter? 521

Protein: The Umami Question 522

Fat 522

15.5 Genetic Variation in Bitter 523

Supertasters 524

Health Consequences of Variation in Taste Sensations 525

15.6 How Do Taste and Flavor Contribute to the Regulation of Nutrients? 526

Taste 527

• ***Scientists at Work*** *The Role of Food Preferences in Food Choices* 527

Flavor 528

Is All Olfactory Affect Learned? 530

15.7 The Nature of Taste Qualities 531

Taste Adaptation and Cross-adaptation 532

The Pleasure of the Burn of Chili Peppers 532

Summary 534

Glossary G-1

References R-1

Credits C-1

Index I-1

Preface

We wrote the sixth edition of this book during COVID. In a world that is returning to something like normal, we are happy to be writing the seventh edition of *Sensation & Perception* and are grateful to have the chance to update the book. The biggest change from the last edition is on the cover. Keith Kluender, our audition expert since the very first edition, has retired. His big academic shoes will be admirably filled by Lori L. Holt, who has been a professor at Carnegie Mellon University but will be a professor at the University of Texas, Austin, by the time you hold this textbook in your hands. We thank Keith for all the hard work over the years and we look forward to working with Lori.

Why We Wrote This Textbook

So, why did we write this textbook and why did we revise it for a seventh edition? Part of the answer is that the world keeps changing. Take anosmia, for example. Anosmia, an inability to smell, has always existed. It was an interesting topic of study, albeit to a relatively small crowd (including our author, Rachel S. Herz). Then COVID happened, and suddenly anosmia was important as a symptom of the disease. Interestingly, as we write this new edition, research is beginning to suggest that the newer mutations of COVID may not produce anosmia at the rate produced by the original COVID variants. For present purposes, the point is that the science keeps changing and circumstances around science keep changing as well, sometimes in quite dramatic ways. Our hope is to integrate the newest work with the older science of sensation and perception.

We wrote the original version and continue to revise it because we are fascinated by the human senses. We want to know the answers to fundamental questions about the senses: How does our brain create a three-dimensional perception of the world from two-dimensional images, formed on the back of each eye? Why do some substances taste "sweet"? Why does music sound "musical"? In our own labs, we study perceptual questions that arise from important problems in the world. How do radiologists find cancer in X-rays? Why is anosmia more than just a sign of a possible COVID infection? It is actually quite disabling. Individuals who are dealing with long COVID can find that anosmia has a major impact on diet and even on social interactions.

We also study the interactions of the senses. When you sit down to dinner, that is an experience with gustatory (taste) and olfactory (smell) components, of course, but it also involves vision, touch, and hearing (even if you are alone and hearing only the crunch of your carrot stick). If the carrot stick makes a squelchy sound and puts up no resistance to your bite, your experience of its "taste" will be quite different. And if you are dizzy (Chapter 12), well, the whole experience could be very different. We need to write about hearing as hearing and olfaction as olfaction, but, recognizing the multisensory nature of experience, we have tried to get out of our sensory silos and show you some of the interactions between the senses. In the seventh edition, these multisensory elements are called out in the text with this symbol: ✿ If you look in Chapter 11, for example, you will find a discussion of how music affects taste.

From its basic to its more applied aspects, we really love this material. We wrote this undergraduate textbook in the hope that we might spread some of our enthusiasm to you, our reader. In service of that goal, each of the 15 chapters of this book aims to tell a coherent and interesting story that will give the reader enough background and exposure to current research to understand why these topics are interesting and how they might be further investigated. The author of each chapter is an expert in the topic who is actively researching in the area. For every topic in the textbook, we are acutely aware that there is vastly more information than we can squeeze into a chapter. Moreover, we are not naive or immodest enough to believe that you will devour a chapter on "The Perception of Color" or "Perceiving and Recognizing Objects" in the way that you might devour a good novel. However, we do hope that you will find each chapter to be more than a compilation of facts. It is our hope that this book teaches enough to inspire the reader to want to know more. In service of these goals, chapters include "Scientists at Work" features that give a bit of detail about the way a specific topic has been studied, as well as sections on "Sensation & Perception in Everyday Life" that strive to bring the material out of the lab.

It is our intention to have produced a textbook that is reasonably comprehensive while still being digestible. It is possible that you, the student, may not think that a chapter on motion perception, for example, is particularly digestible at 3:00 a.m. the day before the final exam, but that was the goal. We want to present a coherent introduction to the important topics in our field. As noted, we can't cover *everything*. If you, the instructor, or you, the interested student, think we missed something that should be included, please feel encouraged to drop us an email. Indeed, drop us an email just because you actually read the preface. We always wonder if anyone looks at this bit of prose, so, since you are here, please send a note to jwolfe@bwh.harvard.edu. Whether you are a student or faculty, it is fun to hear from our "users." If you are reading this for a course, tell us who is teaching. Odds are that one of us knows your instructor. More important, please also feel encouraged to send us notes and comments as you read the text. Hearing from readers is an important way for us to make the textbook better. Thanks.

New to This Edition

Each time we revise the textbook, we add some new topics and we take some material out. We won't try to tell you everything that is new in the seventh edition, but here are a few things to look for:

- The are several places where we highlight "interoception" in this edition. We nearly gave it a chapter of its own. Interoception is a term for all the systems monitoring and reporting on what is going on inside your body, from stomachaches onward. It is beginning to be an important topic in the scientific literature.
- The chapter on touch has new material on "social touch," tickle, and itch.
- The color chapter has a revised discussion of "The Dress That Ate the Internet" (see Figure 5.14).
- "Olfaction" has a section on the role of smell in virtual reality.
- Both "Olfaction" and "Taste" talk about new research on COVID's effects.

Also new to this edition is Oxford Insight. Oxford Insight pairs best-in-class OUP content with curated media resources, activities, and gradable assessment in a guided learning environment that delivers performance analytics, drives student engagement, and improves student outcomes.

Accessible Content

Every opportunity has been taken to ensure that the content herein is fully accessible to those who have difficulty perceiving color. However, some of the figures and activities will be less accessible to some readers because of the intrinsic nature of the colors and activities.

Acknowledgments

With the seventh edition, we welcome our new editor, Chelsea Noack, who has successfully kept us on task and on time. We also thank our previous editor, Joan Kalkut, who oversaw the sixth edition and whose hand can still be seen in the new edition. Michele Laseau created our cover for the seventh edition. Karen Hunter researched new photos, including our new chapter openers. Johannah Walkowicz coordinated and oversaw the production process, as well as developed figures, helped clarify prose, and corrected any leftover inconsistencies or unclear writing. Mike Demaray and Craig Durant at Dragonfly Media Group created the stunning art program of this text. Many thanks are also due to Kathaleen McCormick, the marketing manager for *Sensation & Perception*.

Beyond the book, we would like to acknowledge Julia Wray, Sam Phillipart, and Rose Burrell for managing and overseeing the digital projects. Many of these digital resources have been designed by Evan Palmer of San Jose State University and Jennifer Corbett of the Massachusetts Institute of Technology. Both Evan and Jen have created and/or curated a host of great demonstrations of phenomena discussed in the text. Moreover, as noted earlier, with all that is new, we always need to prune out some old material to keep the book from growing too long. That often makes us sad, because we are deleting good material. When we get too sad, the material is included in the form of online essays. We would also like to thank Dr. Megan Kobel and Dr. Max Teaford for their assistance on Chapter 12, "Vestibular Sensation."

We are grateful to our colleagues who reviewed one or more of the chapters of this book. It is extremely helpful to have the wisdom of other experts in the field and of those who use the text in classroom.

Jessica Alexander, Centenary College of Louisiana
Susan Bachus, University of Maryland–Baltimore County
Sara Bagley, Lindenwood University
David Bennett, North Park University
Barbara Blatchley, Agnes Scott College
Cheryl Camenzuli, Molloy College
Yu-Chin Chiu, Purdue University–Main Campus
Kimberly Craig, University of New Haven
Carol Devolder, Saint Ambrose University
John Friedline, Piedmont College
Patrick Garrigan, Saint Joseph's University
Robbe Goris, University of Texas–Austin
Davidburton Hanbury, Averett University
Bryan Jones, Kent State University at Ashtabula
Jennifer Mailloux, University of Mary Washington
Karenna Malavanti, Baylor University
Frank Marchak, Montana State University
Sandra McFadden, Western Illinois University
Ryan Mears, University of Florida
Meredith Minear, University of Wyoming

Rolf Nelson, Wheaton College
Jamie Opper, Saint Cloud State University
Jennifer Peszka, Hendrix College
Kimberley Philips, Trinity University
Dmitri Poltavski, University of North Dakota
Mark Schmidt, Columbus State University
KatieAnn Skogsberg, Centre College
Laura Swain, University of South Carolina–Aiken
Nina Tarner, University of Maryland–Baltimore County
Jennifer Thomson, Messiah College
Ezra Wegbreit, Cazenovia College
Takashi Yamauchi, Texas A & M University–College Station
Christine Ziemer, Missouri Western State University

The following reviewers read and critiqued drafts and/or previous versions of the text, and we are grateful for their expert assistance:

Nicole D. Anderson, MacEwan University
Jeffrey Andre, James Madison University
Martin Arguin, University of Montreal
Benjamin Balas, North Dakota State University
Dirk Bernhardt-Walther, University of Toronto
Kent D. Bodily, Georgia Southern University
Simona Buetti, University of Illinois at Urbana–Champaign
Cheryl A. Camenzuli, Molloy College
Leslie Cameron, Carthage College
Amanda Carey, Simmons University
Linda C. Carson, University of Waterloo
Shao-Ying I. Cheng, University of Texas–Austin
Kathleen Cullen, McGill University
Thomas A. Daniel, Westfield State University
Nicolas Davidenko, University of California, Santa Cruz
Christopher DiMattina, Florida Gulf Coast University
Joshua Dobias, Rutgers, State University of New Jersey
Colin Ellard, University of Waterloo
Stephen Emrich, Brock University
Rhea Eskew, Northeastern University
Ahren Fitzroy, Mount Holyoke College
Danielle Gagne, Alfred University
Carmela Gottesman, University of South Carolina, Salkehatchie
Alexis Green, Charleston Southern University
Alexis Grosofsky, Beloit College
Laurence Harris, York University
Michael E. Hildebrand, Carleton University
Alan Ho, Ambrose University
Adam Hutcheson, Georgia Gwinnett College
Eric Jackson, University of New Mexico
Aaron Johnson, Concordia University
Ingrid S. Johnsrude, Western University
Jane Karwoski, University of Nevada, Las Vegas
Brock Kirwan, Brigham Young University
Timothy S. Klitz, Washington & Jefferson College
Roger Kreuz, University of Memphis
Leslie D. Kwakye, Oberlin College
Michael Landy, New York University
Michael Lantz, Concordia University at Loyola
Glenn Legault, Laurentian University
Max Levine, Siena College
Olga Lipatova, Christopher Newport University
Zili Liu, University of California, Los Angeles
Alejandro Lleras, University of Illinois at Urbana–Champaign
Stephen Lomber, McGill University
Justin A. MacDonald, New Mexico State University
Kristen L. Macuga, Oregon State University
Alexander Maier, Vanderbilt University
Frank M. Marchak, Montana State University
Janice C. McMurray, University of Nevada, Las Vegas
John Monahan, Central Michigan University
Katherine S. Moore, Arcadia University
Richard Murray, York University
Alexander O'Brien, University of Wisconsin–La Crosse
Gina O'Neal-Moffitt, Florida State University
Michael Owren, Emory University
Thanasis Panorgias, New England College of Optometry
Jennifer Peszka, Hendrix College
David Pittman, Wofford College
Steve Prime, University of Saskatchewan
Robert Remez, Barnard College, Columbia University
Adrián Rodríguez-Contreras, City College of New York
Lisa Sanders, University of Massachusetts, Amherst
Eriko Self, California State University, Fullerton
Kevin Seybold, Grove City College

Steve Shevell, University of Illinois at Chicago
Rachel Shoup, California State University, East Bay
T. C. Sim, Sam Houston State University
Joel Snyder, University of Nevada, Las Vegas
Miriam Spering, University of British Columbia
Kenneth Steele, Appalachian State University
William Stine, University of New Hampshire
Greg Stone, Arizona State University
Jeffrey Stowell, Eastern Illinois University
Julia Strand, Carleton College
Duje Tadin, University of Rochester
Jeroen van Boxtel, University of California, Los Angeles
D. Alexander Varakin, Eastern Kentucky University
Rachel Walker, Charleston Southern University
Dirk B. Walther, University of Toronto
Scott N. J. Watamaniuk, Wright State University
Nicholas Watier, Brandon University
Mareike Wieth, Albion College
Laurie Wilcox, York University
Meagan M. Wood, Valdosta State University

Many colleagues have sent us reprints and answered questions about points both specific and general. We gratefully acknowledge their help even if we cannot list all of their names (and even if we may still have failed to get things exactly right). We are also indebted to the students, faculty, and other users of the text who pointed out errors, typos, and other shortcomings in the first six editions. We hope we caught them all and we hope that the readers of this edition will continue to offer us assistance. As noted earlier in the preface, if you find a flaw or if you have any other comment—even a positive one—please feel encouraged to let us know. You can use jwolfe@bwh.harvard.edu as a point of contact for all of us.

Digital Resources for
Sensation & Perception, Seventh Edition

Sensation & Perception, Seventh Edition, is available in Oxford Insight. Oxford Insight delivers best-in-class content within a powerful, data-driven learning experience designed to increase student success. A guided and curated learning environment—delivered either via learning management system/virtual learning environment (LMS/VLE) integration or stand-alone—Oxford Insight provides access to the e-book, multimedia resources, assignable/gradable activities and exercises, and analytics on student achievement and progress. As students work through the course material, Oxford Insight automatically sets personalized learning paths for them, based on their specific performance.

Developed with applied social, motivational, and personalized learning research, Oxford Insight enables instructors to deliver an immersive experience that empowers students by actively engaging them with assigned reading. This approach, paired with real-time actionable data about student performance, helps instructors ensure that all students are best supported along their unique learning paths.

With Oxford Insight, instructors can:

- Assign autoscored multiple-choice, fill-in, and other machine-gradable questions;
- Score specific items (including open-ended questions) with feedback;
- Export grades and change grading points;
- Establish a course roster and add/drop students;
- Share courses and resources with students and faculty;
- Sync real-time assignments with LMS/VLE gradebooks; and
- Author new content and/or customize the publisher-provided content.

Contents include:

FOR THE STUDENT

- **Self-Assessment Quizzes** reinforce understanding of chapter material through end-of-section questions.
- **Chapter Overviews** give students an engaging entry point into the important concepts presented in each chapter.
- **Activities with quizzes** lead students through important processes, phenomena, and structures. These interactive exercises give students the opportunity to explore a variety of topics in an interactive, exploratory format, including perception experiments, illusions that illustrate key concepts, models of cognitive processes, and interactive diagrams of important structures.
- **Exam Prep Questions** help students prepare for end-of-chapter quizzes.
- **Essays** expand on selected topics from the textbook and provide additional coverage and examples.
- **Chapter quizzes** test students' understanding of each chapter.
- **Flashcards** help students master the hundreds of new terms introduced in the textbook.

FOR THE INSTRUCTOR

- **PowerPoint Presentations:** Two PowerPoint presentations are provided for each chapter of the textbook:
  - ***Figures & Tables***: All the figures and tables from the chapter, with titles on each slide, and complete captions in the Notes field.
  - ***Lecture***: A complete lecture presentation that consists of a detailed lecture outline with selected figures and tables.
- **Instructor's Manual**: The Instructor's Manual includes a variety of resources to aid in course development, lecture planning, and assessment. It includes the following resources for each textbook chapter: Chapter Introduction, Chapter Outline, Learning Objectives, Chapter Summary, References for Lecture Development, and Video and Image Resources.
- **Test Bank:** The Test Bank consists of a complete set of multiple-choice, short-answer, and essay questions for each chapter of the textbook. Questions cover the full range of material covered in each chapter, including both factual and conceptual questions. Questions are categorized by textbook section and Bloom's level and aligned to the section-level Learning Objectives.

For more information on how *Sensation & Perception,* Seventh Edition powered by Oxford Insight, can enrich the teaching and learning experience in your course, please visit oxfordinsight.oup.com or contact your Oxford University Press representative.

Instructors: This title can be integrated directly into learning management systems. To find out more about integration, or if you have any questions about the course content, please contact your OUP representative at (800) 280-0280 or http://learninglink.oup.com/support.

SENSATION & PERCEPTION

Chapter 1

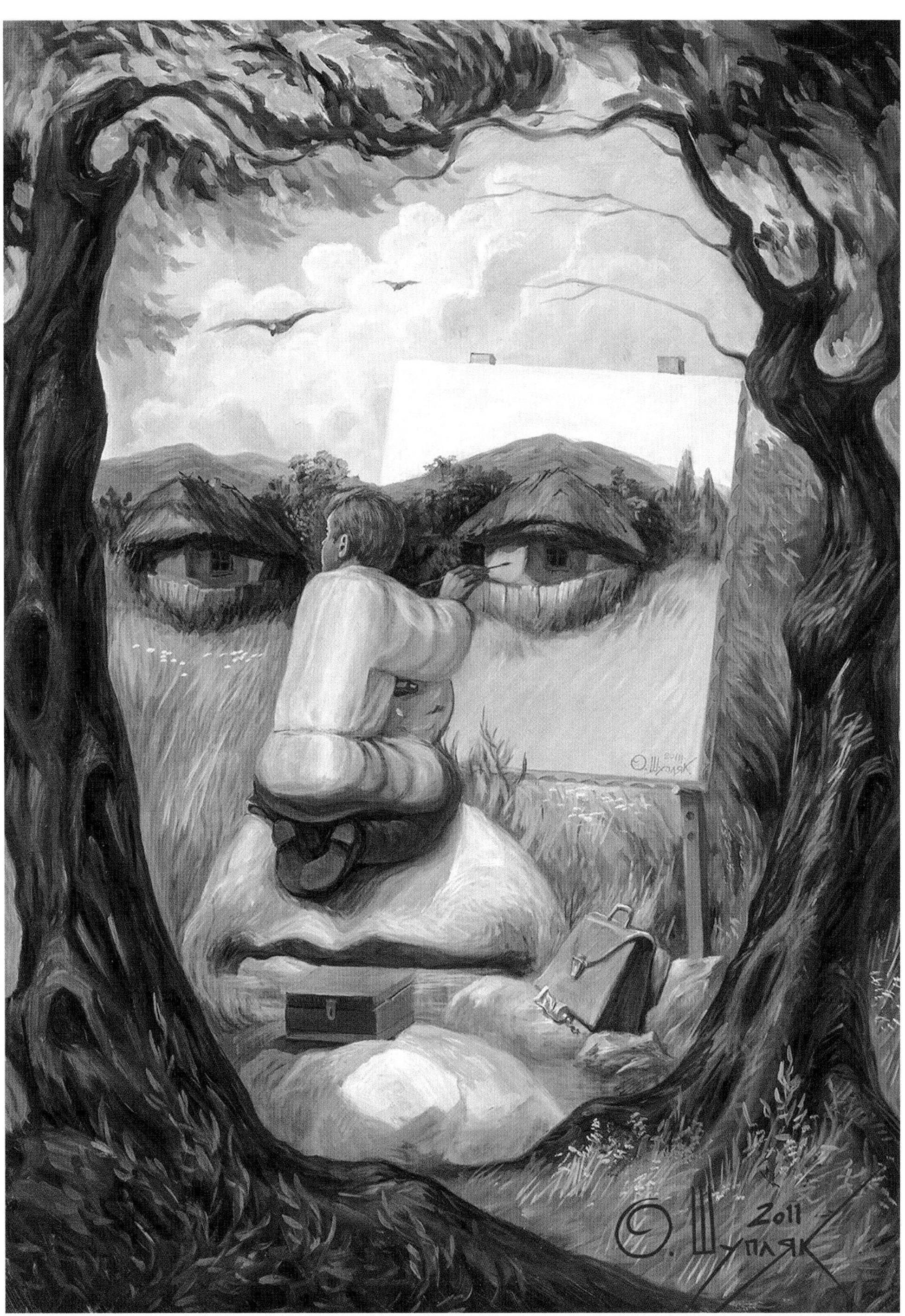

Oleg Shupliak, *Self-Portrait under the Lime Trees*, 2011

Introduction

Questions to Contemplate

Think about the following questions as you read this chapter.
By the chapter's end, you should be able to answer and discuss them.

- How many senses do we use to "perceive," that is, translate the physical world into subjective experience?
- How accurately and how quickly do we perceive?
- Are there "laws" that describe how physical stimuli become psychological experience?
- How does the nervous system accomplish this translation?
- Is our perceptual experience influenced by what we know or believe?

You've taken the plunge to read at least part of a textbook on "sensation and perception." You may be majoring in psychology or studying an allied field, such as neuroscience or biology, or you may be simply curious. No matter what interests you most, your understanding will be based on sensation and perception.

"Why?" you ask. Most everything you know or think you know about the world around you depends on how you sense and how you perceive. These foundational experiences began even before you were born. Your senses help you to keep upright, stay warm or cool, avoid pain and poisonous things, and avert danger. Your experiences of the rich tapestry of life through sensing and action inform most everything that you believe to be true.

It is no small wonder that the questions posed in this textbook have been front and center for big thinkers since the first written words, and probably earlier. Today, a small army of researchers continue to pursue answers. This first chapter provides an introduction to the sorts of questions that captivate the authors of this book and the sorts of methods that researchers have developed to answer those questions. These are only examples from the endless list of possibilities. The rest of the book will introduce you to the vast array of questions that must occupy the attention of anyone who really wants to know how we know what we think we know.

1.1 Sensation and Perception: Welcome to Your World through Our World

We live in a physical world. It's out there, but what do we know about it? Everything we know begins with sensors and ends with mental representations and/or actions. We cannot know exactly what is in the physical world. Perhaps more surprisingly, we don't know what other people experience about the physical world. Are your experiences the same as those of a friend? Only your own sensory experience is directly accessible to you. Nevertheless, this text can help you understand your own experiences and how they are likely to relate to those of others.

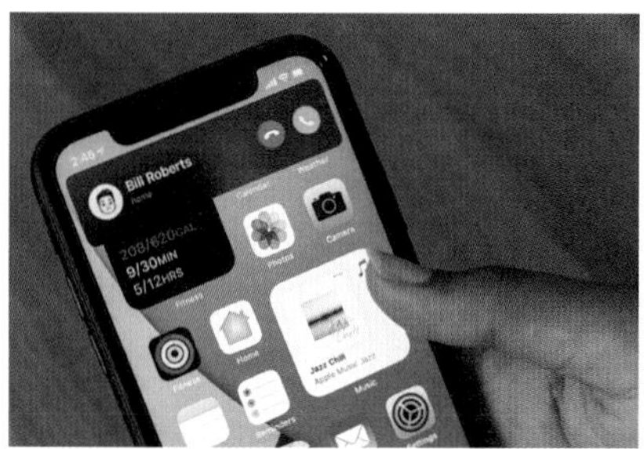

FIGURE 1.1 Cell phone senses? Both you and your phone can "sense" the contact of your finger and the screen. What is the difference?

This book is titled *Sensation & Perception*. The ability to detect the pressure of your finger as you turn a page or swipe a screen and turn that detection into your own private experience is an example of **sensation** (FIGURE 1.1). **Perception** can be thought of as the act of converting detected sensations into a representation that offers the ability to perform an action, derive meaning, or understand events in a broader social context. Suppose someone runs a finger down your back. Neurons within the skin respond to the pressure and send electrical signals farther into the nervous system. This elementary process of converting physical signals into neural responses is called **transduction**. What ensues is a sensation that might be perceived as a gesture of affection from a friend or something else from the officer at an airport security checkpoint. This book will trace the path from stimuli in the world, through your sense organs, to the representation and interpretation of the world you perceive.

Since everything we feel, think, and do depends on sensations and perceptions, it is not surprising that philosophers have thought, talked, and written about the topic for over two millennia. For instance, the eighteenth-century French philosopher Étienne Bonnot de Condillac (1715–1780) asked his readers to imagine the mental life of a statue with only a sense of smell. If the statue only smelled a rose, would it really know what a rose was? In a similar vein, the philosopher William Molyneux (1656–1698) wondered whether a person who had been blind since birth would be able to tell a cube from a sphere by sight, if suddenly given vision. Molyneux's intuition was that the sensations that are used by touch to tell cubes from spheres, like prickliness, may not directly translate to vision, and conversely, roundness and right-angle bends are not the neural language of touch. His question is answered in Chapter 13 on "Touch."

If our mental life depends on information from our senses, then it follows that the place for the study of the senses is within the science of human behavior and human mental life—that is, within psychology. Of course, psychologists do not have the topic entirely to themselves. Researchers studying topics in sensation and perception can be found in biology, computer science, medicine, neuroscience, and many other fields. Indeed, the authors of this book come from academic departments with different affiliations and identities. Critically, however, they approach the study of sensation and perception as a scientific pursuit. Let's return to the questions that opened this chapter and visit them from this scientific perspective.

How Many Senses Do We Use to Perceive?

No doubt, at some point in your education, you were told that you had five senses: seeing, hearing, smelling, tasting, and touching. It is true that you have visible sensory organs that meet this catalog description, but that's about where the accuracy of the description stops! How do you know that the elevator is starting to go up, or that you are lying flat rather than standing upright, or that you are about to get sick because the boat is rocking? That is the work of your vestibular system. Its sensory organs are not externally visible, but they allow you to perceive how you are physically oriented in the world (see Chapter 12).

The situation is further complicated by the perception of sensations that come from inside the body. This is called **interoception** and it is necessary for such basic functions as eating or knowing it's time to use the bathroom (S. L. Prescott and Liberles, 2022). Should interoception be considered another sense or are its signals just extensions of the classical senses? On the one hand, consider the fullness of your stomach that you feel after a meal. It is produced by a neural message of mechanical pressure, not unlike what happens when you touch the screen on a smartphone. You can experience an analogous "feeling" by puffing out your cheeks. So feeling

sensation The ability to detect a stimulus and, perhaps, to turn that detection into a private experience.

perception The act of giving meaning to a detected sensation.

transduction The conversion of a physical stimulus, such as light or sound, into a neural response through the activity of sensory receptors.

interoception The sense (or senses) of the internal state of the body.

full could be considered an aspect of a sense of touch. On the other hand, there are taste receptors in your gut very like the taste receptors in your mouth. They respond to chemical signals from food and influence behavior, but they do not seem to give rise to a conscious sensation like the sweet, sour, salty, or bitter of classical taste (Berntson and Khalsa, 2021).

Another difficulty with the five-senses story is that each external sense organ, be it the eyes, ears, nose, mouth, or skin, conveys information about multiple properties of the world. Should senses of temperature, itch, and tickle be separated, or are those all part of "touch"? We'll return to this topic in Chapter 13 on "Touch." For the present, it seems that trying to enumerate the senses is a pointless task.

How Accurately Do We Perceive, and by What Method Would We Know?

This question is one of the oldest to be studied by perceptual psychologists. It's long been known that perception is not a completely "accurate" description of the world. Bats and dogs hear sounds we humans can't. You think spinach is tasty and I don't, so who is right or wrong? As you will learn throughout your experience with this book, the data arriving at sensory receptors are inherently ambiguous. A tone perceived as "faint" might originate from a strong source far away or a weaker source nearby. If perception isn't simply an accurate, invariant measurement of the physical world, how can we quantify its properties? Are there regular "laws" that relate what we perceive to the physical properties of the world? Do those laws help us to understand where inaccuracies come from? This leads to a topic very dear to perceptual psychologists, namely, methods for measuring perception. The remainder of this section describes common assessments and the methods that are used to produce them. **TABLE 1.1** summarizes these methods.

TABLE 1.1 Methods for measuring perception

Method	Purpose	Techniques
Absolute threshold	Determine the minimum stimulus level required for perceptual detection	Constant stimuli: Measure accuracy for detecting each stimulus in a series; determine stimulus level needed to achieve a target accuracy
		Limits: Gradually adjust stimulus level from clearly perceived to not perceived or vice versa; determine the transition level
		Adjustment: Set a controller to present a stimulus level that is just perceived
Difference threshold	Determine the minimum stimulus difference required to perceive a change	Same as absolute threshold, but now comparing a changed stimulus to a standard level
Scaling	Characterize the perceptual response across a range of physical values	Magnitude estimation: Assign a number to a stimulus indicating its intensity, either freely or in comparison to a standard
		Cross-modal matching: Adjust a stimulus of one type to match the level of another
Signal detection	Measure the ability to make decisions about whether a stimulus falls into a category	Signal detection: Use accuracy of assignment to signal vs. noise to derive measures of discrimination (d') and the decision criterion
Time course of perception	Measure *when* perception occurs in relation to a stimulus event	Masking: Controlling stimulus duration by preceding or following with a competing event
		Simple reaction time: Measure the time from stimulus onset to response
Sensory neuroscience	Describe perception in terms of activity of sensory receptors, neurons, and brain regions	Recording from a neuron: Inserting an electrode to detect neural firing
		Neuroimaging: Noninvasively measuring brain activity by electrical, magnetic, or other signals
Computational models	Describe perception in the form of computer algorithms or mathematical equations	Statistical optimization, Bayesian, or neural net: Use past experience to direct processing of currently sensed information

METHOD 1: THRESHOLDS What is the faintest sound you can hear? How would you know? What is the loudest sound you can hear? This last question is not as silly as it may seem, though it could be rephrased like this: "What is the loudest sound you can hear safely or without pain?" If you listened to sounds above that limit, perhaps by blasting your music too enthusiastically, you would have changed the answer to the first question. You would have damaged your auditory system and now be unable to hear the faintest sound that you previously could hear. Your threshold would have changed (for the worse). How would you measure that threshold? As we'll learn in this chapter, a variety of methods are available for measuring just how sensitive your senses are.

METHOD 2: SCALING—MEASURING EXPERIENCE ACROSS A STIMULUS DIMENSION Scaling measures how a physical variable is perceived across a broad range. A physical stimulus may be experienced quite differently as the level goes from just above threshold to high intensities. Turning up the volume when sound is at the low level can lead to a pleasant improvement in our ability to hear, but upping the volume when the sound is loud can lead to discomfort. Scaling reveals variations in perception not only across the stimulus range, but also among perceivers themselves. When you say that you "hear" or "taste" something, are your experiences the same as those of the person you're talking to? You may think that the film is too loud, whereas I find it pleasant. Scaling allows us to demonstrate that different people do, in some cases, inhabit different sensory worlds. The discussion in this chapter will show how scaling methods can be used to perform this act of mind reading.

METHOD 3: SIGNAL DETECTION THEORY—MEASURING DIFFICULT DECISIONS A radiologist looks at a mammogram, the X-ray test used to screen for breast cancer. There's something on the X-ray that might be a sign of cancer, but it is not perfectly clear. What should the radiologist do? Suppose she decides to call it benign, not cancerous, and suppose she is wrong. Her patient might die. Suppose she decides to treat it as a sign of malignancy. Her patient will need more tests, perhaps involving surgery. The patient and her family will be terribly worried. If the radiologist is wrong and the spot on the mammogram is, in fact, benign, the consequences may be less dire than those of missing a cancer, but there will be consequences. This is a perceptual decision, made by an expert, that has real consequences. Our discussion of signal detection theory will show how decisions of this sort can be studied scientifically.

METHOD 4: MEASURING THE TIME COURSE OF PERCEPTION You start your computer and wait for the reassuring wake-up sound. The sound reaches your ears, but when can you be said to perceive it? And when it stops, when does your perception stop? We cannot assume that perception turns on and off precisely with the timing of physical events. These and other intriguing questions about the time course of perception are addressed in experiments that carefully control the onset and offset of stimulation and measure your response in terms of accuracy and/or how long it takes you to react.

METHOD 5: SENSORY NEUROSCIENCE Grilled peppers appear on your table as an appetizer. They have an appealing, smoky smell. When you bite into one, it has a complex flavor that includes some of that smokiness. Fairly quickly, you also experience a burning sensation. There is no actual change in the temperature in your mouth, and your tongue is no warmer than it was, but the "burn" is unmistakable.

How does the pepper fool your nervous system into thinking that your tongue is on fire? This chapter's exploration of sensory neuroscience will introduce the ways in which sensory receptors and nerves undergird your perceptual experience. One of the principal methods of sensory neuroscience is neuroimaging. Modern brain-imaging techniques enable us to see traces of experience as it takes place in the brain. Suppose, for example, you view completely different pictures with your two eyes. You might see a house with one eye and a face with the other (Tong et al., 1998). The result would be an interesting effect known as binocular rivalry (see Section 6.4). The two images would compete to dominate your perception: Sometimes you would see a house, and sometimes you would see a face. You would not see the two together. One reason binocular rivalry is interesting is that it represents a disconnect between the pictures simultaneously presented to your eyes and your private perceptual experience, which is typically limited to only one of them at a time. Data from your brain can invade your privacy and reveal which picture, face or house, you are aware of seeing at any point in time. Techniques for acquiring and analyzing data from the brain are rapidly advancing.

METHOD 6: COMPUTATIONAL MODELS Sensory receptors provide data about the physical world; perception arrives at a representation of that world. In between these two points, the data must be "processed," often over multiple interacting steps. Computational models offer details of processing and make precise quantitative predictions, allowing comparisons to be made with data from experiments that further test the model's validity. A computational model can predict the probability that perception will assign a stimulus to one category or another, for example, whether a speech sound is categorized as 'b' or 'p.' Models can incorporate the past experiences that shape perception and that might lead a native speaker of English to have a different b-to-p transition than someone who speaks Spanish.

1.2 Thresholds and Their Measurement by Psychophysics

Early on, study of the senses was a mix of experimental science and philosophy. A pioneer in more contemporary perceptual measurements was the nineteenth-century German scientist-philosopher Gustav Fechner (1801–1887). Although Fechner earned his degree in medicine, his interests turned from biological science to physics and mathematics. From his experience as a physicist, Fechner thought it should be possible to describe the relation between mind and body using mathematics. His goal was to formally describe the relationship between sensation (mind) and the energy (matter) that gave rise to that sensation. He called both his methods and his theory **psychophysics** (*psycho* for "mind" and *physics* for "matter"). Psychophysics has become a general term for the quantitative measurement of the relationship between physical events and their mental consequences. Fechner developed methods that are still in use today, albeit with variations made possible using computer-generated stimuli (Wixted, 2020).

psychophysics The science of defining quantitative relationships between physical and psychological (subjective) events.

absolute threshold The minimum amount of stimulation necessary for a person to detect a stimulus 50% of the time.

method of constant stimuli A psychophysical method in which many stimuli, ranging from rarely to almost always perceivable (or rarely to almost always perceivably different from a reference stimulus), are presented one at a time. Participants respond to each presentation: "yes/no," "same/different," and so on.

Absolute Threshold

One of the most basic psychophysical measures is the **absolute threshold**: the minimum intensity of a stimulus that can be detected (**FIGURE 1.2**).

As shown in Table 1.1, several techniques are used to measure an absolute threshold. One, known as the **method of constant stimuli**, requires creating many stimuli with different intensities to find the intensity that can be detected some proportion of the time (**FIGURE 1.3**). If you've had a hearing test, you had to report

	The weakest amount of a stimulus that a person can detect 50% of the time
Sight	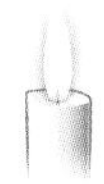 Seeing a candle flame thirty miles away on a clear night
Hearing	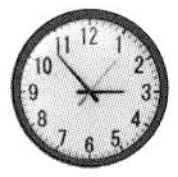 Hearing a watch ticking twenty feet away
Touch	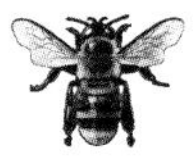 Feeling a bee's wing falling a distance of a half inch onto your cheek
Smell	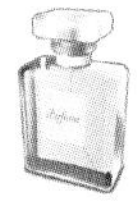 Smelling one drop of perfume in a three-room house
Taste	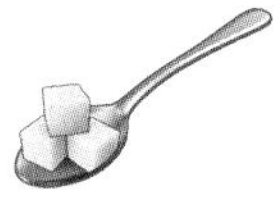 Tasting one teaspoon of sugar dissolved in two gallons of water

FIGURE 1.2 Absolute thresholds in the real world.

when you could and could not hear a tone that the audiologist played to you over headphones, usually in a very quiet room. In this test, the intensities of all of the tones were relatively low, not too far above or below the intensity where your threshold was expected to be. The tones, which varied in intensity, were presented randomly, and tones were presented multiple times at each intensity.

The "multiple times" piece is important. Subtle perceptual judgments such as threshold judgments are variable. The stimulus varies for physical reasons. The observer varies. Attention waivers and sensory systems fluctuate for all sorts of reasons. As a consequence, one measure is almost never enough. You need to repeat the measure over and over and then average the responses or otherwise describe the pattern of results. Some experiments require thousands of repetitions (thousands of "trials") to establish a sufficiently reliable data point.

Returning to our auditory example, as the listener, you would report whether you heard a tone or not. You would always report hearing a tone that was relatively far above threshold and almost never report hearing a tone that was well below threshold. In between, however, you would be more likely to hear some tone intensities than not to hear them, and you would hear other, lower intensities on only a few presentations. In general, the intensity at which a stimulus would be detected 50% of the time would be chosen as your threshold.

That 50% definition of absolute threshold is rather interesting. Weren't we looking for a way to measure the *weakest* detectable stimulus? Using the hearing example, shouldn't that be a value below which we just can't hear anything

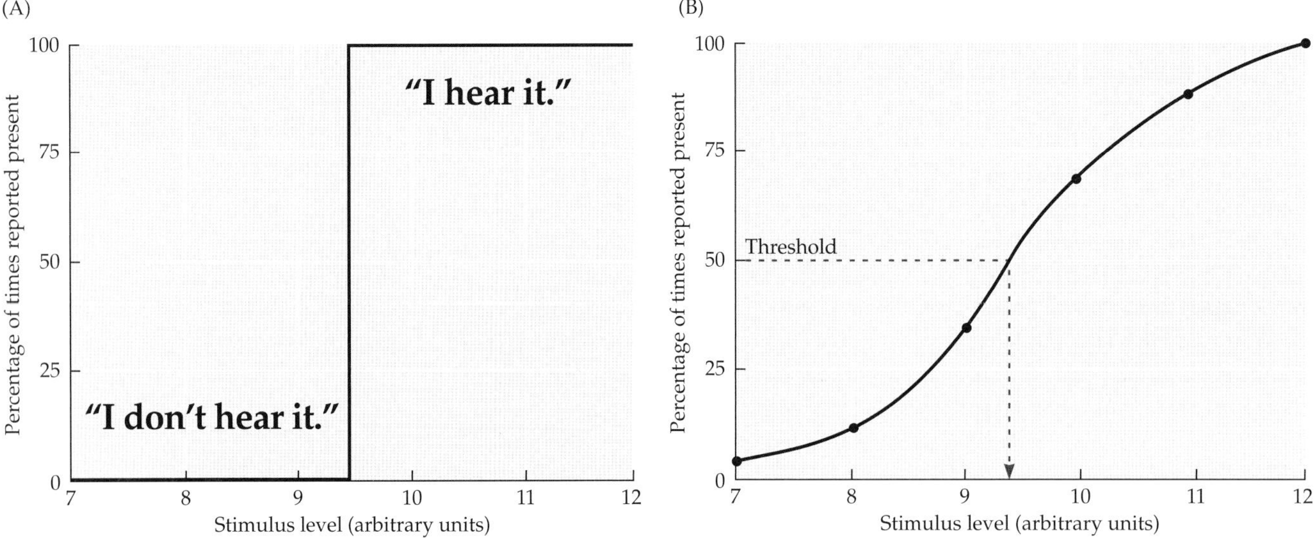

FIGURE 1.3 The method of constant stimuli (A) You might expect the threshold to be a sharp change in detection from never reported to always reported, as depicted here, but this is not so. (B) In reality, experiments measuring absolute threshold produce shallower functions relating stimulus to response. A somewhat arbitrary point on the curve, often 50% detection, is designated as the threshold (dashed line).

(see Figure 1.3A)? It turns out that no such hard boundary exists. Because of variability in the nervous system, stimuli near threshold will be detected sometimes and missed at other times. As a result, the function relating the probability of detection with the stimulus level will be gradual (see Figure 1.3B), and we must settle for a somewhat arbitrary definition of an absolute threshold. We will return to this issue when we talk about signal detection theory.

The method of constant stimuli is simple to use, but it is an inefficient way to conduct an experiment, because much of the listener's time is spent with stimuli that are well above or below threshold. A more efficient approach is the **method of limits** (**FIGURE 1.4**). With this method, the experimenter again begins an ordered set of stimuli—again, suppose that they are tones that vary in intensity. Instead of random presentations, the stimuli are presented in order of increasing or decreasing intensity. When tones are presented in ascending order, from faintest to loudest, listeners are asked to report when they first hear the tone. With descending order, the task is to report when the tone is no longer audible. Data from an experiment such as this show that there is some "overshoot" in judgments. It usually takes more intensity to report hearing the tone when intensity is increasing, and it takes more decreases in intensity before a listener reports that the tone cannot be heard. The average of these crossover points—when listeners shift from reporting hearing the tone to not hearing the tone, and vice versa—is taken to be the threshold. An important consideration in the method of limits is to avoid stimuli that differ by too large a step size, in which case the jump between unperceived and perceived will be so large that we can only say, "The threshold is in there somewhere" (and the data will look something like Figure 1.3A). Adaptive methods can be used to adjust the step size as the threshold is approached, allowing greater precision in the estimate.

The third and final of these classic measures of absolute thresholds is the **method of adjustment**. This method is similar to the method of limits, except that there is essentially continuous control over the level of the stimulus, and the person being tested is allowed to steadily increase or decrease the intensity of the stimulus. The method of adjustment may be the easiest method to understand, because it is much like day-to-day activities such as adjusting the volume dial on a stereo or the dimmer switch for a light. As with the method of limits, care must be taken to avoid big steps in the adjustment knob, and even then, some variability in a person's response from trial to trial must be expected.

Trial series

Intensity (arbitrary units)	↓1	↑2	↓3	↑4	↓5	↑6	↓7	↑8
20	Y						Y	
19	Y		Y		Y		Y	
18	Y		Y		Y		Y	
17	Y		Y		Y		Y	
16	Y		Y		Y		Y	Y
15	Y	Y	Y	Y	Y	Y	Y	Y
14	Y	N	Y	N	Y	N	Y	Y
13	N	N	Y	N	Y	N	N	Y
12		N	N	N	N	N		N
11		N		N		N		N
10		N		N		N		N
	13.5	14.5	12.5	14.5	12.5	14.5	13.5	12.5

Crossover values (average = 13.5)

FIGURE 1.4 The method of limits Here the listener attends to multiple series of trials. For each series, the intensity of the stimulus is gradually increased or decreased until the listener detects (Y) or fails to detect (N), respectively, the stimulus. For each series, an estimate of the threshold (red dashed line) is taken to be the average of the stimulus level just before and after the change in perception (i.e., the average "crossover value").

Difference Threshold

Whereas the absolute threshold assesses our ability to tell something from nothing, the difference threshold measures how well we can tell something from something else. It was introduced by Ernst Weber (1795–1878), an anatomist and physiologist who was Fechner's colleague and inspiration. For Fechner, Weber's most important findings involved judgments of lifted weights. Weber would ask people to lift one standard weight (that is, a weight that stayed the same over a series of experimental trials) and one comparison weight that differed from the standard. Weber increased the comparison weight in incremental amounts over the series of trials. He found that the ability of a person to detect the difference between the standard and comparison weights depended greatly on the weight of the standard. When the standard was relatively light, people were much better at detecting a small difference when they lifted a comparison weight. When the standard was heavier, people needed a greater difference before they could detect a change. He called the difference required for detecting a change in weight the **just noticeable difference**, or **JND**. Another term for JND, the smallest change in a stimulus that can be detected, is the **difference threshold**.

method of limits A psychophysical method in which the particular dimension of a stimulus, or the difference between two stimuli, is varied incrementally until the participant responds differently.

method of adjustment A method of limits in which the participant controls the change in the stimulus.

just noticeable difference (JND) or **difference threshold** The smallest detectable difference between two stimuli, or the minimum change in a stimulus that enables it to be correctly judged as different from a reference stimulus.

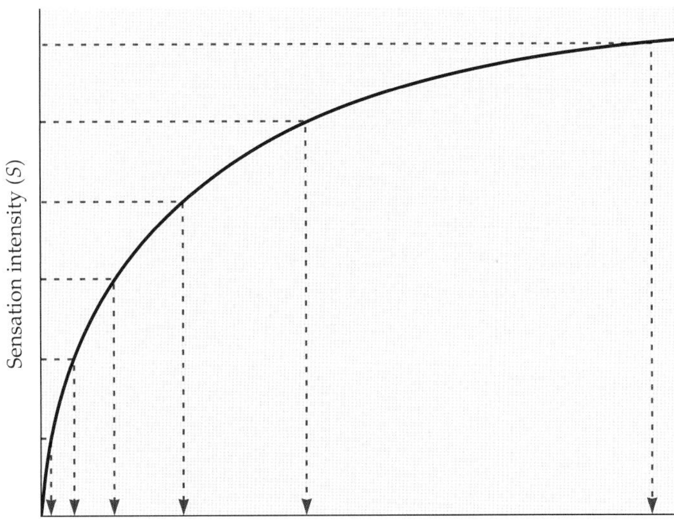

FIGURE 1.5 Fechner's law As the intensity of a physical stimulus increases (*x*-axis), a larger change in that physical stimulus is required to produce a just noticeable difference in sensation (*y*-axis). This is seen graphically in the increasing amount of space between the dashed lines on the *x*-axis required to produce evenly spaced dashed lines on the *y*-axis. The relationship between *X* and *Y* values is logarithmic.

Weber noticed that JNDs change in a systematic way. The smallest change in weight that could be detected was always close to 1/40 of the standard weight. Thus, a 1-gram change could be detected when the standard weighed 40 grams, but a 10-gram change was required when the standard weighed 400 grams. Weber went on to test JNDs for a few other kinds of stimuli, such as the lengths of two lines (for which the detectable change ratio was 1:100). For virtually every measure—whether brightness, pitch, or time—a constant ratio between the change and the standard could describe the threshold of detectable change quite well. This ratio rule holds true except for extreme stimuli—stimuli so small or large that they approach the minimum or maximum of our senses. In recognition of Weber's discovery, Fechner called these ratios, or proportions, **Weber fractions**, and he called the mathematical formula that described the general rule **Weber's law**. Weber's law states that the size of the JND (ΔI) is a constant proportion (K) of the level of the stimulus (I).

In Weber's observations, Fechner found what he was looking for: a way to describe the relationship between mind and matter. Fechner assumed that the smallest detectable change in a stimulus (ΔI) could be considered a unit of the mind because this is the smallest bit of change that is perceived. He then mathematically extended Weber's law to create what became known as **Fechner's law** (**FIGURE 1.5**):

$$S = k \log R$$

where S is the psychological sensation, which is equal to the logarithm of the physical stimulus level ($\log R$) multiplied by a constant, k. This equation describes the fact that our psychological experience of the intensity of light, sound, smell, taste, or touch increases less quickly than the actual physical stimulus increases.

Scaling Methods

Fechner's law underscores a very fundamental principle of perception: Mind and matter are related, but mental representations are not direct copies of physical properties. Transformations take place that can fundamentally change the scale between physical properties and their perceptual counterparts. Accordingly, perceptual scientists take care to distinguish between units of measurement for physical entities (such as light or sound) and measures of people's perception ("brightness," "loudness"). For example, the physical intensity of a sound—the sound pressure level—is a physical entity that can be measured in decibels, whereas a person's perception of "loudness" is psychophysical and subjective (see Section 9.2). Similarly, frequency is a measure of the rate of fluctuations of the physical sound pressure, while the "pitch" of a musical note describes a psychophysical response to that physical phenomenon. Frequency and pitch are not the same thing, although they are closely correlated. Over a wide range, as frequency increases, so does pitch, though it is unclear whether there is a perception of pitch for the highest audible frequencies (B. G. Green, 2005).

These observations point to the need for techniques that describe the scale of mental experience in relation to physical variation. A surprisingly straightforward

Weber fraction The constant of proportionality in Weber's law.

Weber's law The principle describing the relationship between stimulus and resulting sensation that says the just noticeable difference is a constant fraction of the comparison stimulus.

Fechner's law A principle describing the relationship between stimulus and resulting sensation that says the magnitude of subjective sensation increases proportionally to the logarithm of the stimulus intensity.

way to address the question of the strength or size of a sensation is to simply ask observers to rate the experience. For example, we could give observers a series of sugar solutions and ask them to assign numbers to each sample. We would just tell our observers that sweeter solutions should get bigger numbers, and if solution A seems twice as sweet as solution B, the number assigned to A should be twice the number assigned to B. This method is called **magnitude estimation**, and the approach works well, even when observers are free to choose their own range of numbers. Alternatively, we might begin the experiment by presenting one solution at an intermediate level and telling the taster to label that level as a specific value—10, for instance. All of the responses should then be scaled sensibly above or below this standard of 10. If you do this for sugar solutions, you will get data that look like the blue "sweetness" line in **FIGURE 1.6**.

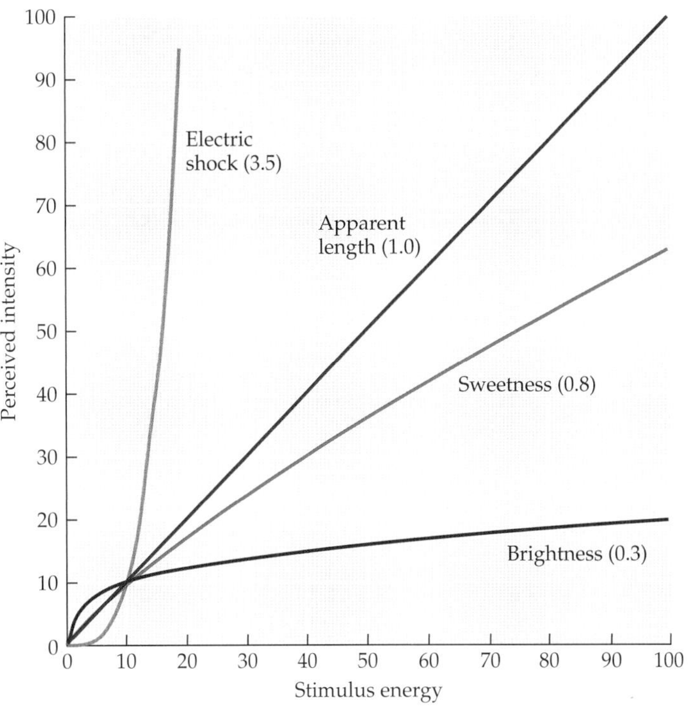

FIGURE 1.6 Magnitude estimation The lines on this graph represent data from magnitude estimation experiments using electric shocks of different currents, lines of different lengths, solutions of different sweetness levels, and lights of different brightness levels. The exponents for the "power functions" that describe these lines are 3.5, 1.0, 0.8, and 0.3, respectively. For exponents greater than 1, such as for electric shock, Fechner's law does not hold, and Stevens's power law must be used instead.

Inspired by his student Richard Held, a distinguished vision researcher whose work you will learn about in Sections 6.4 and 13.1, Harvard psychologist S. S. Stevens (1962, 1975) developed magnitude estimation. Stevens, his students, and their successors measured functions like the one in Figure 1.5 for many different sensations. Even though observers were asked to assign numbers to private experience, the results were orderly and lawful. However, they were not the same for every type of sensation. That relationship between stimulus intensity and sensation is described by what is now known as **Stevens's power law**:

$$S = aI^b$$

which states that the sensation (S) is related to the stimulus intensity (I) by an exponent (b). (The letter a is a constant that corrects for the units you are using. For example, if you measured your stimulus in meters and then switched to measuring it in centimeters, you would need to multiply by 0.01 [= divide by 100] to keep your sensation numbers the same.) So, for example, experienced sensation might rise with intensity squared ($I \times I$). That would be an exponent of 2.0. If the exponent is less than 1, it means that the sensation grows less rapidly than the stimulus—which is what Fechner's law and Weber's law would predict.

Suppose you have some lit candles and you light 10 more. If you start with 1 candle, the change from 1 to 11 candles must be quite dramatic. If you start with 100 and add 10, the change will be modest. Adding 10 to 10,000 won't even be noticeable. In fact, the exponent for brightness is about 0.3. The exponent for sweetness is about 0.8 (Bartoshuk, 1979). Properties like length have exponents near 1. As a result, reasonably enough, a 12-inch-long stick looks twice as long as a 6-inch-long stick (S. S. Stevens and Galanter, 1957). Note that this length relationship is true over only a moderate range of sizes. An inch added to the size of a spider changes your sensory experience much more than an inch added to the height of a giraffe. Some stimuli have exponents greater than 1. In the painful case of electric shock, the pain grows with $I^{3.5}$ (S. S. Stevens, Carton, and Shickman, 1958), so a 4-fold increase in the electrical current is experienced as a 128-fold increase in pain!

Weber's and Fechner's laws have rather broad implications beyond questions of apparent brightness or loudness. Some plants, for example, will respond to the

magnitude estimation A psychophysical method in which the participant assigns values according to perceived magnitudes of the stimuli.

Stevens's power law A principle describing the relationship between stimulus and resulting sensation that says the magnitude of subjective sensation is proportional to the stimulus magnitude raised to an exponent.

psychophysical experience of the bees that pollinate them (Nachev et al., 2017). Suppose you are a plant pollinated by bees that are attracted to your flowers because those flowers have sweet nectar. How much sugar do you need to put into that nectar? After all, it's going to cost you energy to produce sugar. If your nectar has 2 units of sugar and the neighbor flower only has 1, you probably have a competitive advantage over the neighbor. However, if yours has 12 units and the neighbor's has 11, that difference of 1 unit might fall below the bee's Weber fraction for sweetness. Thus, there will be greater evolutionary pressure to go from 1 to 2 than from 11 to 12. Similarly, a peacock with 51 feathers in his tail probably does not have much of a reproductive advantage over a 50-feather peacock. The peahen might not notice the difference, putting an evolutionary brake on tail inflation (Farris, 2017).

At this point in our discussion of psychophysics, it is worth taking a moment to compare Weber's, Fechner's, and Stevens's laws:

1. *Weber's law* involves a clear objective measurement. We know how much we varied the stimulus, and either the observers can tell that the stimulus changed or they cannot.
2. *Fechner's law* begins with the same sort of objective measurements as Weber's, but the law is actually a calculation based on some assumptions about how sensation works. In particular, Fechner's law assumes that all JNDs are perceptually equivalent. In fact, this assumption turns out sometimes to be incorrect and leads to instances where the "law" is violated, such as in the electric shock example just given.
3. *Stevens's power law* describes rating data quite well, but notice that rating data are qualitatively different from the data that support Weber's law. We can record the observer's ratings and we can check whether those ratings are reasonable and consistent, but there is no way to know whether they are objectively right or wrong.

A useful variant of the scaling method shows us that different individuals can live in different sensory worlds, even if they are exposed to the same stimuli. This method is called **cross-modality matching**. In cross-modality matching, an observer adjusts a stimulus of one sort to match the perceived magnitude of a stimulus of a completely different sort (J. C. Stevens, 1959). For example, we might ask a listener to adjust the brightness of a light until it matches the loudness of a particular tone. Again, though the task might sound odd, people can do this, and for the most part, everyone with "normal" vision and hearing will produce a similar pattern of matches of a sound to a light. We still can't examine someone else's private experience, but at least the relationship of visual experience and auditory experience appears to be similar across individuals.

This similarity does not hold when it comes to the sense of taste. There is a molecule called propylthiouracil (PROP) that some people experience as very bitter, while others experience it as almost tasteless. Still others fall in between. This relationship between a chemical and bitter taste can be examined formally with cross-modality matching (Marks et al., 1988). When observers are asked to match the bitterness of PROP to other sensations completely unrelated to taste, we do not find the sort of agreement that is found when observers match sounds and lights (**FIGURE 1.7**). Some people—we'll call them nontasters—match the taste of PROP to very weak sensations, like the sound of a watch or a whisper. A group of "supertasters" assert that the bitterness of PROP is similar in intensity to the brightness of the sun or the most intense pain ever experienced. Medium tasters match PROP to weaker stimuli, such as the smell of frying bacon or the pain of a mild headache (Bartoshuk, Fast, and Snyder, 2005). As we will see in Section 15.5,

cross-modality matching The ability to match the intensities of sensations that come from different sensory modalities. This ability allows insight into sensory differences. For example, a listener might adjust the brightness of a light until it matches the loudness of a tone.

signal detection theory A psychophysical theory that quantifies the response of an observer to the presentation of a signal in the presence of noise. Measures obtained from a series of presentations are sensitivity (d') and criterion of the observer.

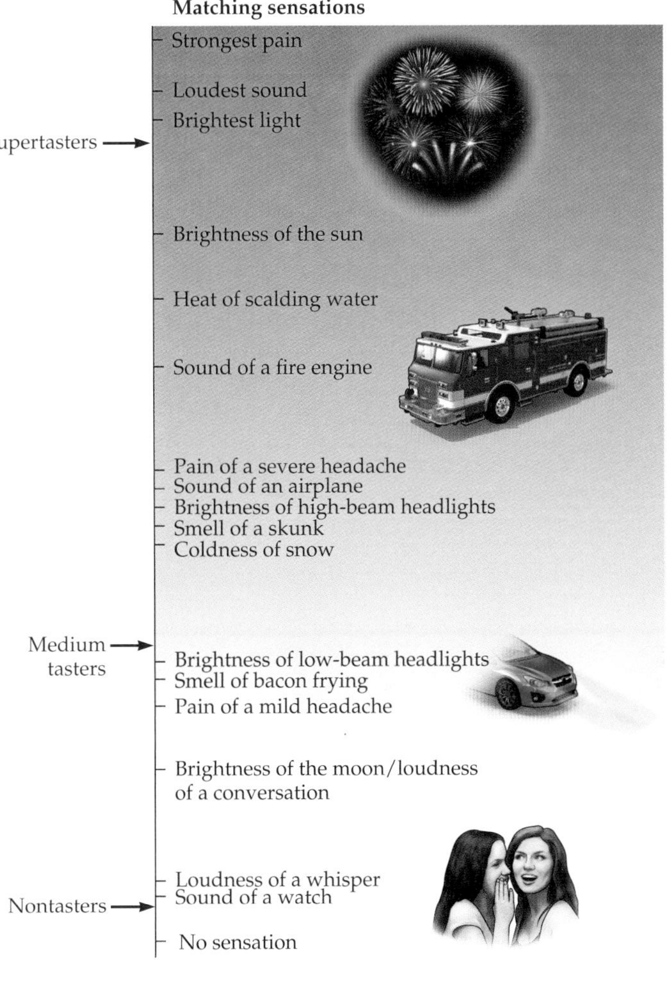

FIGURE 1.7 Cross-modality matching The levels of bitterness of concentrated propylthiouracil (PROP) perceived by nontasters, medium tasters, and supertasters of PROP are shown on the left. The perceived intensities of a variety of everyday sensations are shown on the right. The arrow from each taster type indicates the level of sensation to which those tasters matched the taste of PROP.

there is a genetic basis for this variation, and it has wide implications for our food preferences and, consequently, for health. For the present discussion, this example shows that we can use scaling methods to quantify what appear to be real differences in individuals' taste experiences.

Measuring Discrimination: Signal Detection Theory

Let's return to thresholds—particularly to the fact that they are not absolute. An important way to think about this fact and to deal with it experimentally is known as **signal detection theory** (D. M. Green and Swets, 1966). Like so much of modern psychophysics, even signal detection theory was anticipated by Fechner over a hundred years earlier (Wixted, 2020). Signal detection theory begins with the fact that the stimulus you're trying to detect (the "signal") is always being detected in the presence of "noise." If you sit in the quietest place you can find and put on your best noise-canceling headphones, you will find that you can still hear *something*. Similarly, if you close your eyes in a dark room, you still see something—a mottled pattern of gray with occasional brighter flashes. This is internal noise, the static in your nervous system. Many neurons in the brain are firing all the time, even when nothing is happening. For example, many neurons in the auditory system fire up to 50 times per second when there is no sound at all, and you will learn in Chapter 12 that neurons in the vestibular system fire 100 times per second even when you're perfectly motionless. When you're trying to detect a faint sound or flash of light, you must be able to detect it in the presence of such internal noise. Near your threshold, it will be hard to tell a real stimulus from a random surge of internal noise.

There is external noise, too. Consider again that radiologist reading a mammogram looking for signs of breast cancer. As you can see in **FIGURE 1.8**, the mammogram contains lots of similar regions; the marked white region is the danger sign. We can think of the cancer as the signal. Viewed in the context of an X-ray, the cancer generates a signal in noise. Elsewhere in the image, and in other images, are regions

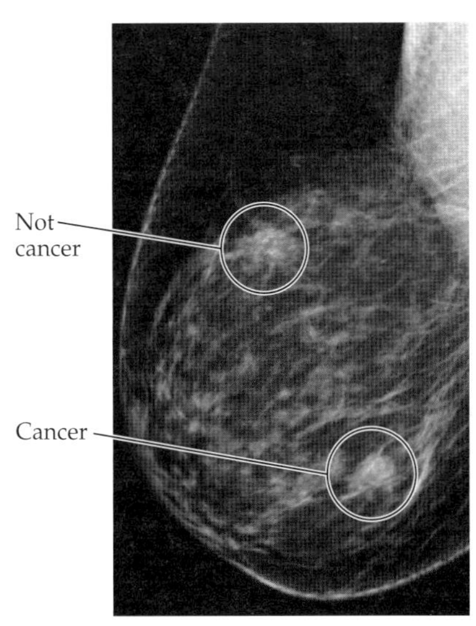

FIGURE 1.8 Differentiating signal from noise Mammograms—X-rays of the breast—are used to screen women for breast cancer. The solid white region is the signal of a cancerous growth; however, the mammogram contains many similar regions ("noise"). Reading such images is a difficult perceptual task. Even for a radiologist trained to discriminate and identify particular signals, there is always uncertainty because of internal and external noise.

that are just noise but look similar to the cancer signal plus noise. The radiologist is a visual expert, trained to find these particular signals, but sometimes the signal will be lost in the noise and missed, and sometimes some noise will look enough like cancer to generate a false alarm (Nodine et al., 2002). Thus, the radiologist will be faced with uncertainty, introduced both as external and as internal noise.

Of course, sometimes neither internal nor external noise is much of a problem. When you see this dot, •, you are seeing it in the presence of internal noise, but the magnitude of that noise is so much smaller than the signal generated by the dot that the noise has no real impact. Similarly, the dot may not be exactly the same as other dots, but that variation—the external noise—is also too small to have an impact. If asked about the presence of a dot on the page here, •, and its absence here, , you will be correct in your answer essentially every time. Signal detection theory exists to help us understand what's going on when we make decisions under conditions of uncertainty.

Because we are not expert mammographers, let's introduce a different example to illustrate the workings of signal detection theory. You're in the shower. The water is making a noise that we will imaginatively call "noise." Sometimes the noise sounds louder to you; sometimes it seems softer. We can plot the distribution of your perception of noise as shown in **FIGURE 1.9A**. On the x-axis, we have the magnitude of your sensation from "less" to "more." Imagine that you were asked, over and over again, about your sensation. Or imagine many repeated measures were made of the response in your nervous system to the sound. For some instances,

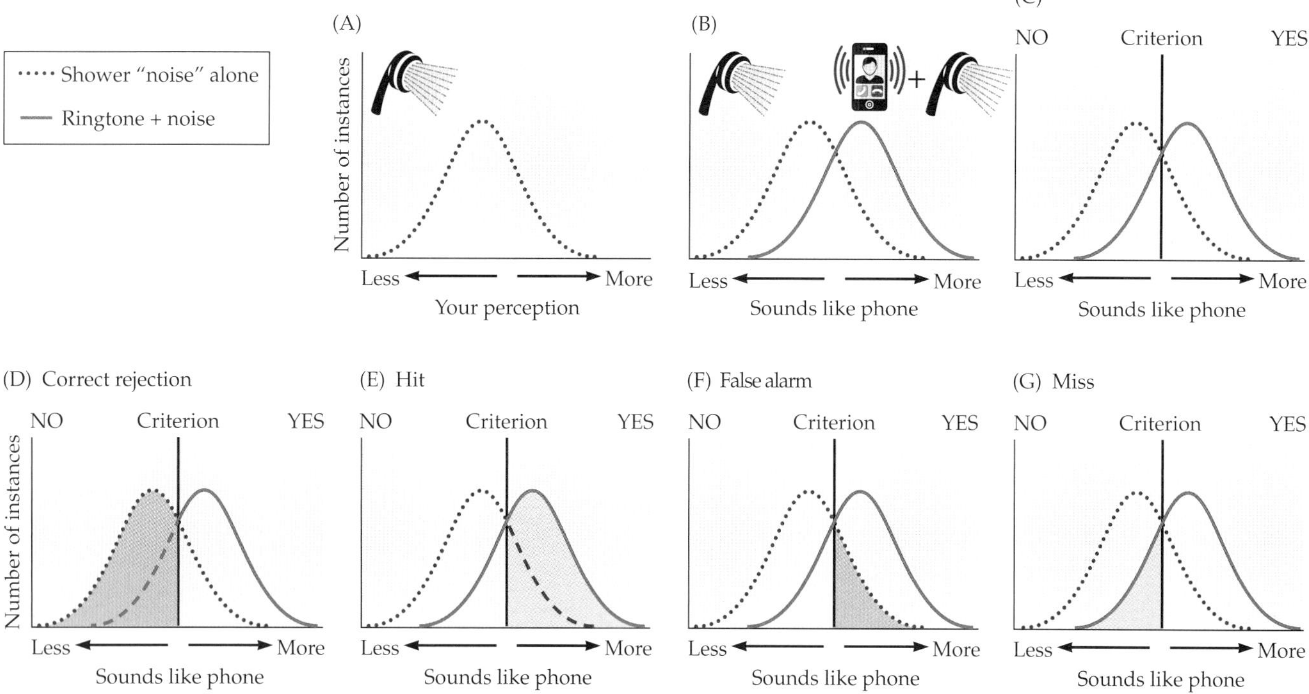

FIGURE 1.9 Detecting a stimulus using signal detection theory (A) Signal detection theory assumes that all perceptual decisions are made against a background of noise (the red curve) generated both in the world and in the nervous system. (B) Your job is to distinguish nervous system responses resulting from noise alone (dotted red curve) or from signal plus noise (solid blue curve). (C) The best you can do is establish a criterion (solid black line) and declare that you detect something if the response is above that criterion. (D–G) Signal detection theory includes four classes of responses. (D) "Correct rejection" (you say "no" and there is, indeed, no signal). (E) "Hits" (you say "yes" and there is a signal). (F) "False-alarm errors" (you say "yes" to no signal). (G) "Miss errors" (you say "no" to a real signal).

the response would be "less." For some, it would be "more." On average, it would lie somewhere in between. If we tabulated all of the responses, we would get a bell-shaped (or "normal") distribution of answers, with the peak of that distribution showing the average answer that you gave.

Now a ringtone plays. That will be our "signal." Your perceptual task is to detect the signal in the presence of the noise. What you hear is a combination of the ringtone and the shower. That is, the signal is added to the noise, so we can imagine that now we have two distributions of responses in your nervous system: a noise-alone distribution and a signal-plus-noise distribution (**FIGURE 1.9B**).

For the sake of simplicity, let's suppose that "more" response means that it sounds more like the phone is ringing. So now your job is to decide whether it's time to jump out of the shower and answer what might be the phone. The problem is that you have no way of knowing at any given moment whether you're hearing noise alone or signal plus noise. The best you can do is to decide on a **criterion** level of response (**FIGURE 1.9C**). If the response in your nervous system exceeds that criterion, you will jump out of the shower and run naked and dripping to find the phone. If the level is below the criterion, you will decide that it is not a ringtone and stay in the shower. Note that this "decision" is made automatically; it's not that you sit down to make a conscious (soggy) choice. Thus, in signal detection theory, a criterion is a value that is somehow determined by the observer. Within the observer, a response above the criterion will be taken as evidence that a signal is present. A response below that level will be treated as noise.

There are four possible outcomes in this situation: You might say "no" when there is no ringtone; that's a correct rejection or true negative (**FIGURE 1.9D**). You might say "yes" when there is a ringtone; that's known as a hit or true-positive response (**FIGURE 1.9E**). Then there are the errors. If you jump out of the shower when there's no ringtone, that's a false alarm or false positive (**FIGURE 1.9F**). If you miss the call, that's a miss or false negative (**FIGURE 1.9G**).

How sensitive are you to the ringtone? In **FIGURE 1.10**, the sensitivity is graphed as the separation between the noise-alone and signal-plus-noise distributions. If the distributions are on top of each other (Figure 1.10A), you can't tell noise alone from signal plus noise. A false alarm is just as likely as a hit. By knowing the relationship of hits to false alarms, you can calculate a **sensitivity** measure known as d' (d-prime), which would be about zero in Figure 1.10A. In Figure 1.10C we see the case of a large d'. Here you could detect essentially all the ringtones and never make a false alarm error. The situation we've been discussing is in between (Figure 1.10B).

criterion In reference to signal detection theory, an internal threshold that is set by the observer. If the internal response is above criterion, the observer gives one response (e.g., "Yes, I hear that"). Below criterion, the observer gives another response (e.g., "No, I hear nothing").

sensitivity In reference to signal detection theory, a measure that defines the ease with which an observer can tell the difference between the presence and absence of a stimulus or the difference between stimulus 1 and stimulus 2.

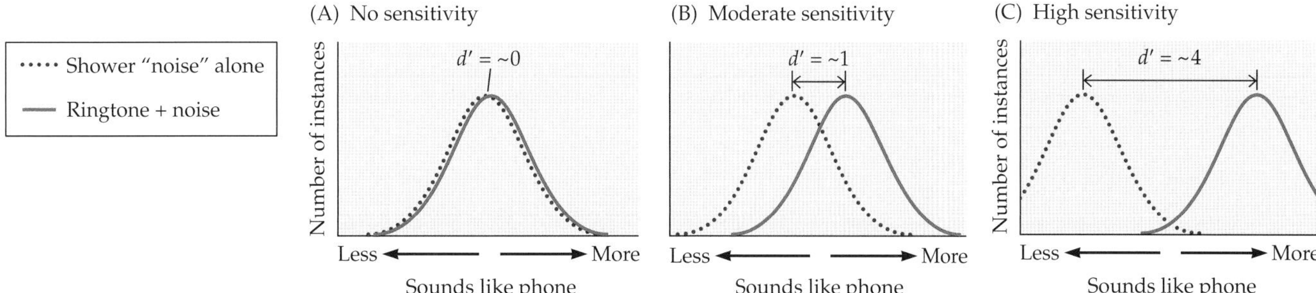

FIGURE 1.10 Sensitivity (d') in signal detection theory Your sensitivity to a stimulus is illustrated by the separation between the distributions of your response to noise alone (dotted red curve) and to signal plus noise (solid blue curve). This separation is captured by the measure d' (d-prime). (A) If the distributions completely overlap, d' is almost 0 and you have no ability to detect the signal. (B) If d' is intermediate, you have some sensitivity, but your performance will be imperfect. (C) If d' is big, then distinguishing signal from noise is easy.

receiver operating characteristic (ROC) curve In reference to studies of signal detection, the graphical plot of the hit rate as a function of the false-alarm rate. If these are the same, points fall on the diagonal, indicating that the observer cannot tell the difference between the presence and absence of the signal. As the observer's sensitivity increases, the curve bows upward toward the upper left corner. That point represents a perfect ability to distinguish signal from noise (100% hits, 0% false alarms).

Now suppose you're waiting for an important call. Even though you really don't want to miss the call, you can't magically make yourself more sensitive. All you can do is move the criterion level of response, as shown in **FIGURE 1.11**. If you shift your criterion to the left, you won't miss many calls, but you will have lots of false alarms (Figure 1.11A). That's annoying. You're running around naked, dripping on the floor, and traumatizing the cat for no good reason. If you shift your criterion to the right, you won't have those annoying false alarms, but you will miss most of the calls (Figure 1.11C). For a fixed value of d', changing the criterion changes the hits and false alarms in predictable ways. If you plot false alarms on the x-axis of a graph against hits on the y-axis for different criterion values, you get a curve known as a **receiver operating characteristic (ROC) curve** (**FIGURE 1.12**).

Suppose you were guessing (the Figure 1.10A situation). You might guess "yes" on 40% of the occasions when the phone rang, but you would also guess "yes" on 40% of the occasions when the phone did not ring. If you moved your criterion and guessed "yes" on 80% of phone-present occasions, you would also guess "yes" on 80% of phone-absent occasions. Your data would fall on that "chance performance" diagonal in Figure 1.11. If you were perfect (the Figure 1.10C situation), you would have 100% hits and 0% false alarms, and your data point would lie at the upper left corner in Figure 1.12. Situations in between (Figure 1.10B) produce curves between guessing and perfection (the green, purple, and blue curves in Figure 1.12). If your data lie below the chance line, you did the experiment wrong!

Let's return to our radiologist. She will have an ROC curve whose closeness to perfection reflects her expertise. On that ROC, her criterion can slide up and to the right, in which case she will make more hits but also more false alarms, or down and to the left, in which case she will have fewer false alarms but more misses. Where she places her criterion (consciously or unconsciously) will depend on many factors. Does the patient have factors that make her more or less likely to have cancer? What is the perceived cost of a missed cancer? What is the perceived cost of a false alarm? You can see that what started out as a query about the lack of absolute thresholds can become, quite literally, a matter of life and death.

Signal detection theory can become a rather complicated topic in detail (e.g., what happens if those noise and signal + noise curves are not exactly the same shape?). To learn about how to calculate d' and about ROC curves, you can take advantage of many useful websites and several texts (e.g., Hautus, Macmillan, and Creelman, 2021; see Burgess, 2018a, 2018b, if you're interested in the application to radiology).

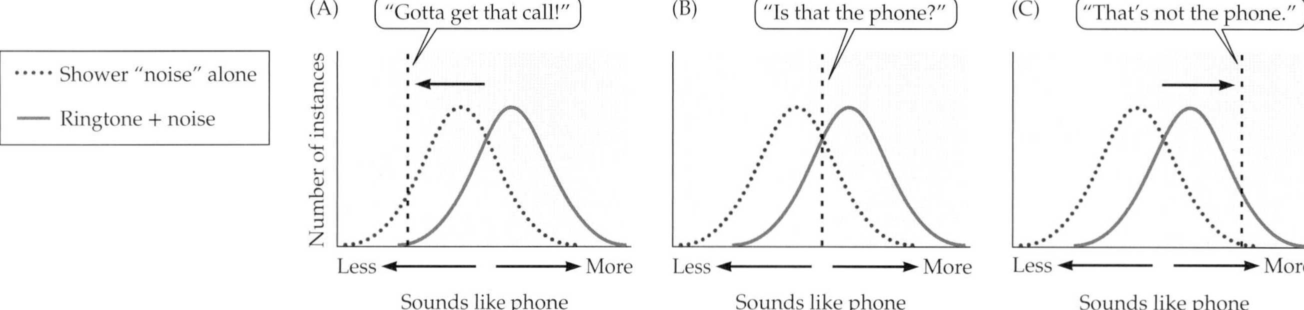

FIGURE 1.11 Criterion in signal detection theory For a fixed d', all you can do is change the pattern of your errors by shifting the response criterion. If you don't want to miss any signals, you move your criterion to the left (A), but then you have more false alarms. If you don't like false alarms, you move the response criterion to the right (C), but then you make more miss errors. In all these cases (A–C), your sensitivity, d', remains the same.

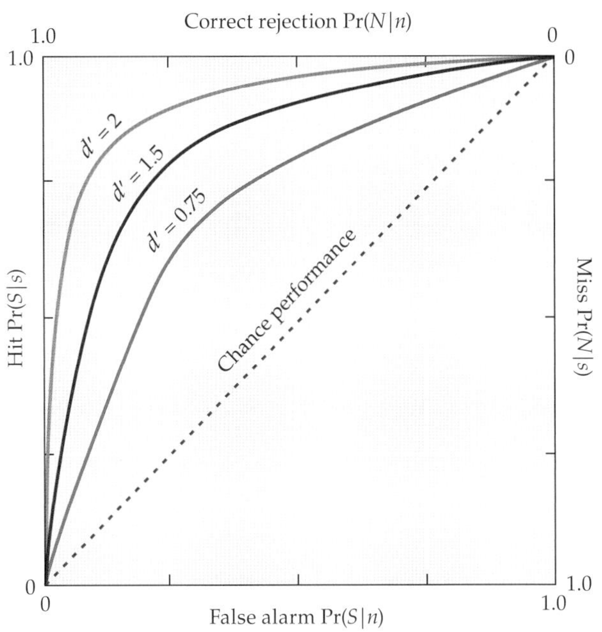

FIGURE 1.12 Receiver operating characteristic (ROC) curves Theoretical ROC curves for different values of *d′*. Note that *d′* = 0 when performance is at the chance level. Higher values of *d′* indicate that the probability of hits and correct rejections increases and the probability of misses and false alarms decreases. Pr(*N*|*n*) = probability of the response "no signal present" when no signal is present (correct rejection); Pr(*N*|*s*) = probability of the response "no signal present" when signal is present (miss); Pr(*S*|*n*) = probability of the response "signal present" when no signal is present (false alarm); Pr(*S*|*s*) = probability of the response "signal present" when signal is present (hit).

Measuring the Time Course of Perception

We have been discussing if a stimulus can be detected. Let's think about when it is detected. There are several questions here. How long does a stimulus need to be present to be detected? If the stimulus is sufficiently strong, its presentation can be arbitrarily short ("**Bloch's law**," Gorea, 2015). Thus, a very bright light can be seen, even if it is presented for a tiny fraction of a second (**FIGURE 1.13A**). That very bright light will not be fully processed in that tiny fraction of a second. Processing will continue well after the physical stimulus ends. That means that using the stimulus duration as the measure of the time course of active perception would be misleading. For this reason, researchers often measure the time required to detect a target stimulus by adding a following "masking" stimulus

(A) Bloch's Law

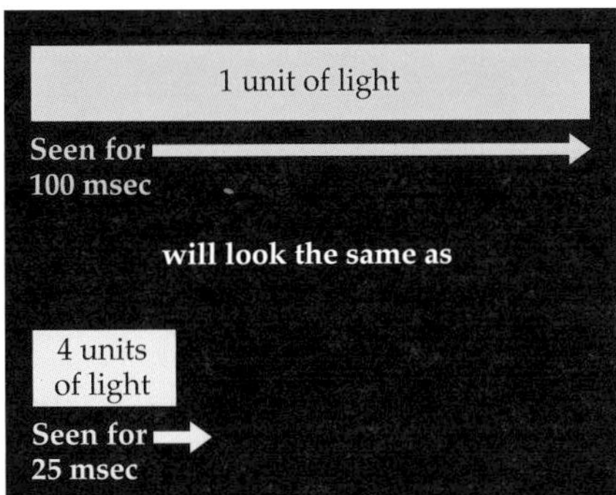

(B) Stimulus onset asynchrony (SOA)

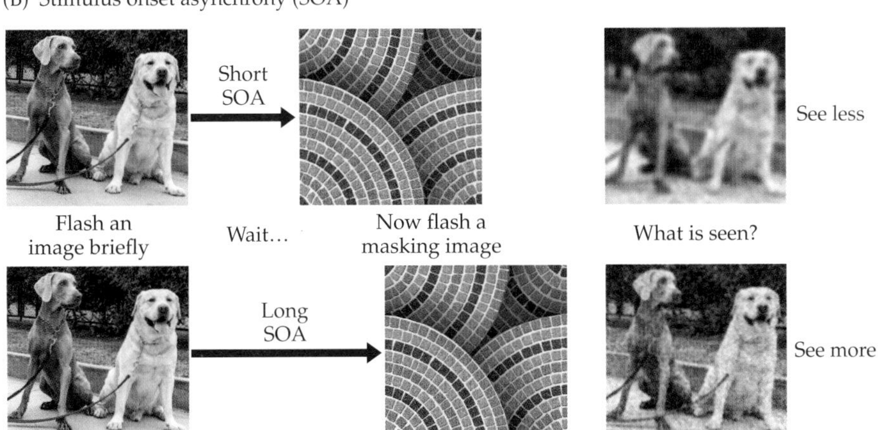

FIGURE 1.13 Bloch's law (A) Bloch's law says that, for very short flashes, visibility is the product of luminance and time. (B) If you show one stimulus and follow it with another, masking stimulus, you get more from the same first stimulus if the delay—the stimulus onset asynchrony (SOA)—is longer.

Bloch's law The detection threshold for a brief flash of light (<0.1 second) is the product of the luminance of the light and its duration.

that is assumed to terminate perceptual analysis of the target. Now the time course measure would be the time from the start of the stimulus to the start of the mask (the **stimulus onset asynchrony—SOA**) (**FIGURE 1.13B**). How long does that SOA need to be in order to perceive the target stimulus? This will depend on what we are trying to perceive. For example, we can perceive the category of a familiar object, like a chair, with SOAs on the order of 50 milliseconds (ms; 1 ms = 1/1000 second). Surprisingly, we can extract the "gist" or general content of a scene, like knowing that it is in the seashore or desert category, in about the same amount of time (see Chapter 7). For a different task, like knowing that a member of the bird category is a pigeon, we will need a longer exposure (Grill-Spector and Kanwisher, 2005).

We could also ask how long it takes to respond to a stimulus, called the simple reaction time. How long does it take to get a signal from the world through a sensor to the relevant part of the brain and then back out in the form of some overt response, like pressing a button? This can vary with the sensory system. Suppose we compare the speed with which observers can respond to stimulation in the visual system, the auditory system, touch (specifically vibration), and vestibular (the sense that the head is moving). Barnett-Cowan and Harris (2009) found that reaction times to sound, touch, and light all occurred within about 200–250 ms, whereas the vestibular response (e.g., Is my head tilted?) was considerably more sluggish, at over 400 ms. Reaction times can vary considerably within a sensory system. While people can respond to vibration on their skin within 250 ms, it might take a full second to judge that the same skin is encountering a stimulus that is warmer or cooler than the ambient temperature. That's because detecting a thermal stimulus relies on a relatively slow physical process of heat flow between the skin and the surface being touched (see Chapter 13). More subtle or difficult acts of perception can take markedly longer.

Thus far, we have been considering the time for simple detection. Perceptual discriminations like those typically measured in a signal detection task will typically be slower and will depend on the magnitude of the difference between stimuli.

1.3 Sensory Neuroscience: What Do We Know About How the Nervous System Translates Physics into Experience?

Many of you reading this book will have had some introduction to neuroscience. Here, a brief review is provided of some of the neuroscience that is relevant to the study of sensation and perception. If this is your first encounter with neuroscience, you will want to consult a neuroscience text or website to give yourself a more detailed background.

Nerves and Specific Nerve Energies

How does information from the world get into our brains and how do our brains know what kind of information it is? After all, there are no lights or tastes in the brain. There are nerve signals that we experience as light, taste, and so forth. Back in the 1830s, the German physiologist Johannes Müller (1801–1858) formulated the **doctrine of specific nerve energies** as an answer. The central idea is that, since we are only aware of the activity in our nerves, what is most important must be *which* nerves are stimulated, and not *how* they are stimulated. For example, we experience vision when the optic nerve leading from the eye to the brain is stimulated. It does not matter whether light, or something else, stimulates the nerve. To prove to yourself that this is true, close your eyes and press very gently on the outside corner of one eye through the lid. (This works better in a darkened room.) You will see a

stimulus onset asynchrony (SOA) The time from the start of a stimulus to the start of the next stimulus.

doctrine of specific nerve energies A doctrine, formulated by Johannes Müller, stating that the nature of a sensation depends on *which* sensory fibers are stimulated, rather than *how* they are stimulated.

spot of light toward the inside of your visual field by your nose. Your gentle poke stimulates your optic nerve and your brain interprets any input from your optic nerve as informing you about something visual (even if it is mistaken, in this case).

cranial nerves Twelve pairs of nerves (one set for each side of the body) that originate in the brainstem and reach sense organs and muscles through openings in the skull.

Many of the paths from the world to the brain are shown in **FIGURE 1.14**. These are the **cranial nerves**. The two optic nerves form one of 12 pairs of cranial nerves that pass through small openings in the bone at the base of the skull. In neuroscience and medicine, the cranial nerves are given names and Roman numerals. Three pairs of nerves are exclusively dedicated to sensory information:

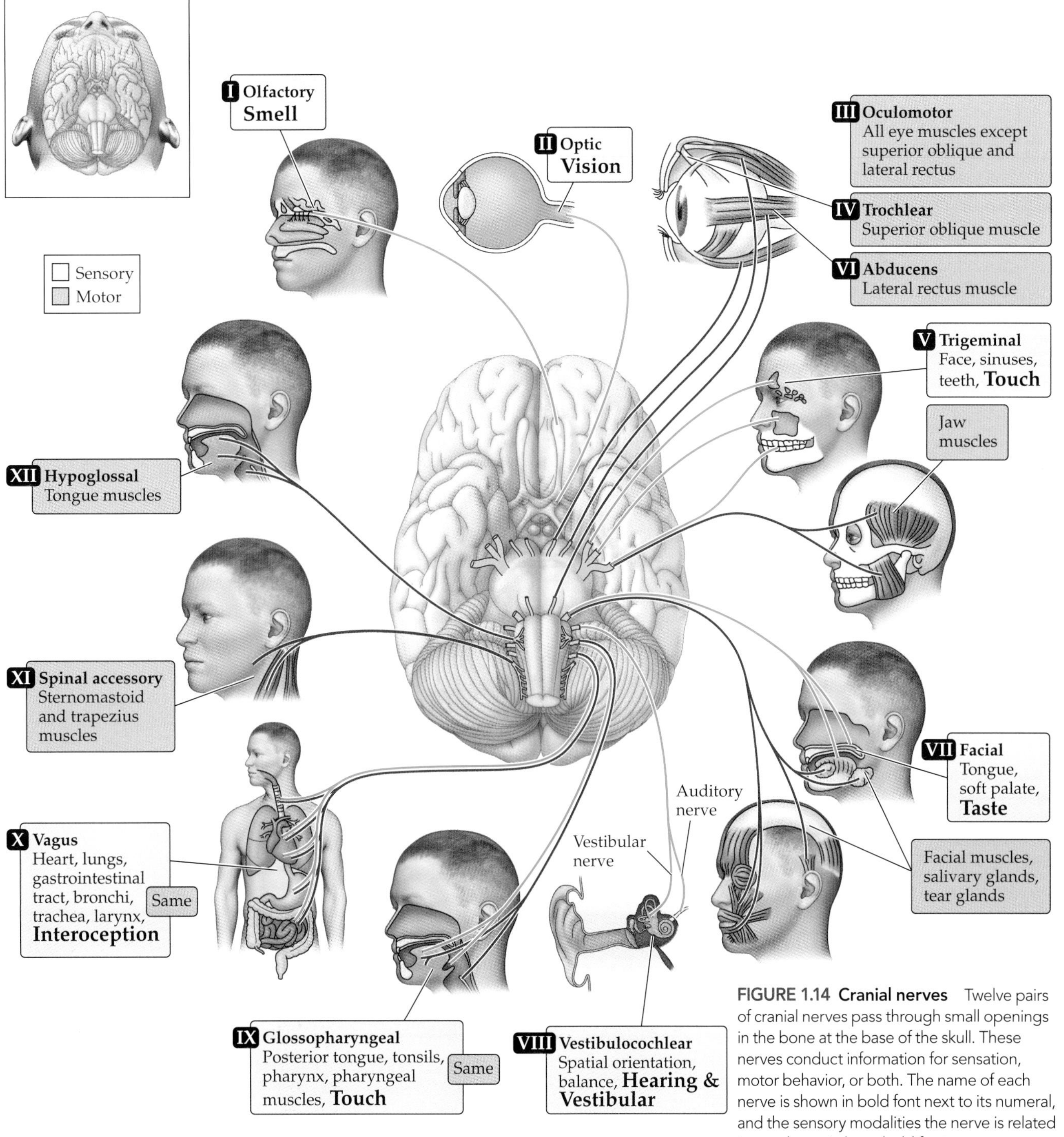

FIGURE 1.14 Cranial nerves Twelve pairs of cranial nerves pass through small openings in the bone at the base of the skull. These nerves conduct information for sensation, motor behavior, or both. The name of each nerve is shown in bold font next to its numeral, and the sensory modalities the nerve is related to are shown in large bold font.

olfactory (I), optic (II), and **vestibulocochlear (VIII)**. The vestibulocochlear nerve serves two sensory modalities: the vestibular sensations that support our sense of equilibrium (see Chapter 12) and hearing (discussed in Section 9.3). Three more pairs are dedicated to muscles that move the eyes: **oculomotor (III)**, **trochlear (IV)**, and **abducens (VI)** (see Section 8.4). Some senses use more than one set of cranial nerves. Taste input comes through three: **facial (VII)**, **glossopharyngeal (IX)**, and **vagus (X)**, and multiple pairs of nerves convey sensations of touch, pain, and temperature. Three cranial nerves are exclusively motor (spinal accessory [XI] and hypoglossal [XII]). Three others convey both sensory and motor signals (trigeminal [V], facial [VII], glossopharyngeal [IX], and vagus [X]). The vagus nerve is particularly important for interoception (see Section 1.1).

The effects of chili peppers and menthol turn out to be interesting illustrations of the doctrine of specific nerve energies. There are warmth and cold nerve fibers that respond to increases and decreases in temperature on the skin (see Section 13.1). On the one hand, capsaicin, a chemical that occurs naturally in chili peppers, causes warmth fibers to fire, creating a sense of increasing heat even though the temperature has not changed. On the other hand, menthol stimulates cold fibers (Bautista et al., 2007), so skin feels cooler without getting physically colder. In sufficiently high amounts, both capsaicin and menthol stimulate pain receptors in the skin, as will very hot or cold stimuli. The result is that you can consume stupidly powerful hot sauce and know that, as you writhe in pain, you are not damaging tissues. Note, however, that this is not true of all spicy heat. Don't try this with mustard, for example. The mechanism is different and it can produce very real blisters.

Just as different nerves are dedicated to individual sensory and motor tasks, areas of the brainstem and cerebral cortex are similarly dedicated to particular tasks. The areas depicted in **FIGURE 1.15** are "primary" sensory areas. Areas of the cortex dedicated to perception are actually much larger than the areas shown in darker, more intense color in the figure. More complex sensory processing involves cortical regions that spread well beyond these primary areas. For example, visual perception uses cortex that extends both anteriorly (forward) into parietal cortex

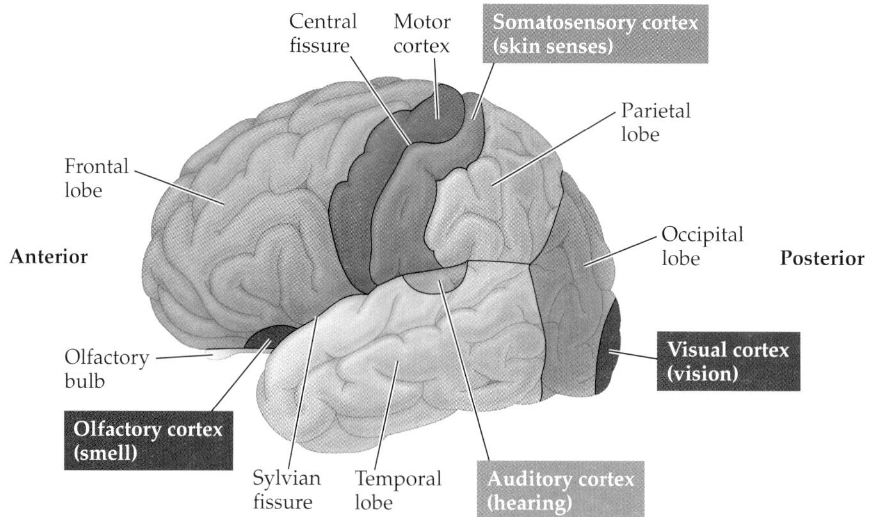

FIGURE 1.15 Cortex of the human brain The cortex is the outer layer of the cerebral hemispheres. This lateral view shows the left hemisphere. The anterior (front of head) is on the left and the posterior (back of the head) is on the right. The darkened areas show where information from four of our sensory modalities first reaches the cortex. Also shown is the motor cortex, which is engaged in balance, touch, and some auditory processing.

olfactory (I) nerves The first pair of cranial nerves. The axons of the olfactory sensory neurons bundle together after passing through the cribriform plate to form the olfactory nerve, which conducts impulses from the olfactory epithelia in the nose to the olfactory bulb.

optic (II) nerves The second pair of cranial nerves, which arise from the retina and carry visual information to the thalamus and other parts of the brain.

vestibulocochlear (VIII) nerves The eighth pair of cranial nerves, which connect the inner ear with the brain, transmitting impulses concerned with hearing and spatial orientation. The vestibulocochlear nerve is composed of the cochlear nerve branch and the vestibular nerve branch.

oculomotor (III) nerves The third pair of cranial nerves, which innervate all the extrinsic muscles of the eye except the lateral rectus and the superior oblique muscles, and which innervate the elevator muscle of the upper eyelid, the ciliary muscle, and the sphincter muscle of the pupil.

trochlear (IV) nerves The fourth pair of cranial nerves, which innervate the superior oblique muscles of the eyeballs.

abducens (VI) nerves The sixth pair of cranial nerves, which innervate the lateral rectus muscle of the eyeballs.

facial (VII) nerves The seventh pair of cranial nerves, which innervate the tongue, soft palate, facial muscles, salivary glands, and tear glands.

glossopharyngeal (IX) nerves The ninth pair of cranial nerves, which innervate the tongue, tonsils, pharynx, and pharyngeal muscles.

vagus (X) nerves The tenth pair of cranial nerves, which innervate the heart, lungs, gastrointestinal tract, bronchi, trachea, and larynx.

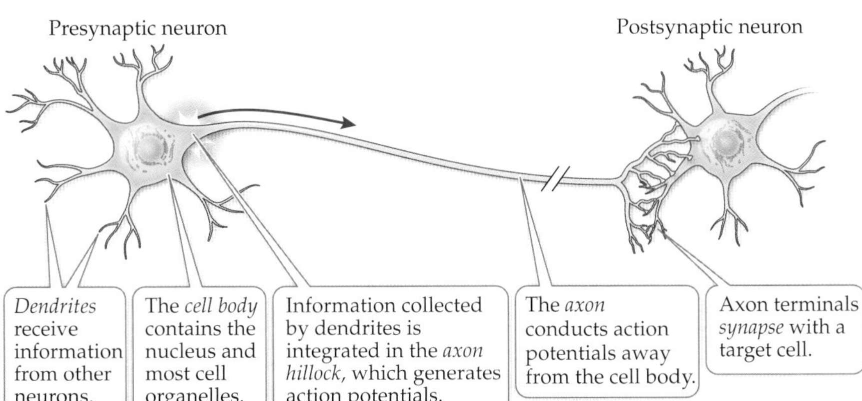
Presynaptic neuron
Postsynaptic neuron
Dendrites receive information from other neurons.
The *cell body* contains the nucleus and most cell organelles.
Information collected by dendrites is integrated in the *axon hillock,* which generates action potentials.
The *axon* conducts action potentials away from the cell body.
Axon terminals *synapse* with a target cell.

FIGURE 1.16 A typical neuron Features of a typical neuron and their functions are described. Axon length and dendrite branching patterns vary greatly across the different types of neurons.

and ventrally (lower) into regions of the temporal lobe (see Figures 4.2 and 4.4). In addition, as processing extends beyond primary areas, cortex often becomes **polysensory**, meaning that information from more than one sense is being combined in some manner. While this textbook is organized into sense-specific chapters, we always want to remember that we live in a multisensory world. Researchers specifically study what is called **sensory integration** or **multisensory integration**.

polysensory Referring to blending multiple sensory systems.

sensory integration or **multisensory integration** The process of combining different sensory signals. The senses typically work together to learn about the world and to guide behavior. This is not the same as the mathematical process of integration learned in calculus (e.g., the integral of acceleration is velocity).

Neuronal Connections

If you prod something with your toe to see if it moves, the signal generated by that stimulus will stimulate a **neuron** (**FIGURE 1.16** on the left). That neuron will produce an action potential that will propagate up the neuron's axon from your toe to the base of your spine (one very long neuron!). The action potential is a traveling electrochemical signal (**FIGURE 1.17**). The action potential reaches the axon

neuron The fundamental type of cell in the nervous system, collecting signals from sense organs, transmitting signals to muscles, and performing the mental operations in between.

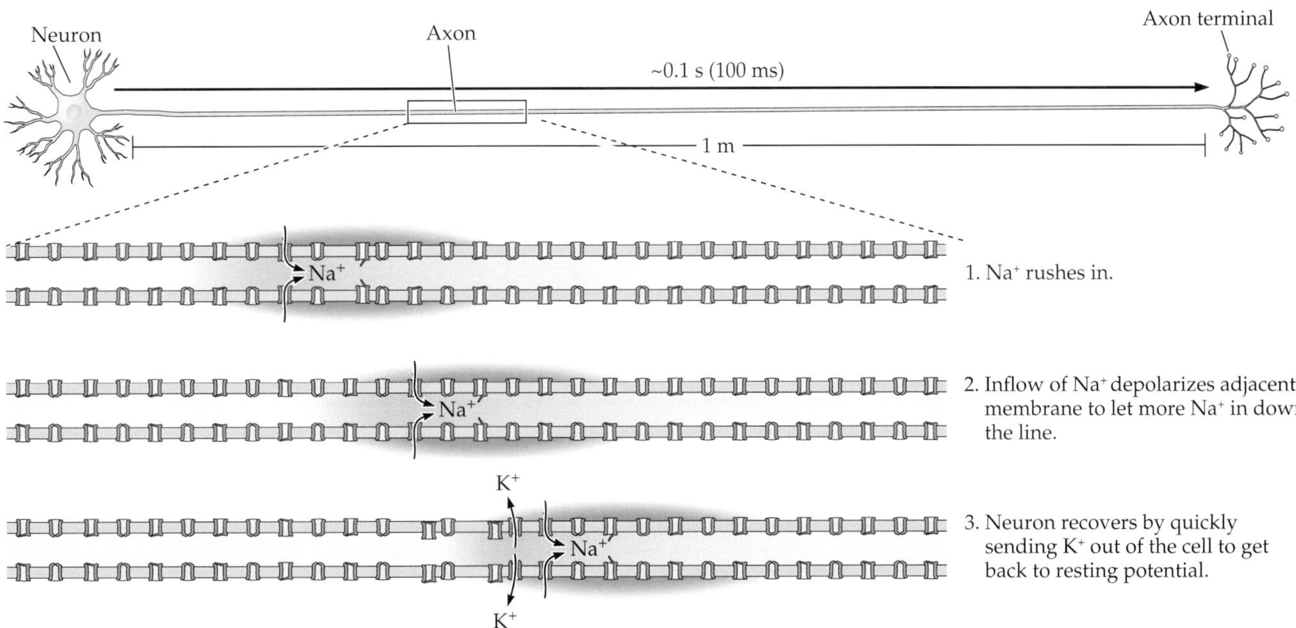
Neuron
Axon
Axon terminal
~0.1 s (100 ms)
1 m
Na^+
1. Na^+ rushes in.
Na^+
2. Inflow of Na^+ depolarizes adjacent membrane to let more Na^+ in down the line.
K^+
Na^+
K^+
3. Neuron recovers by quickly sending K^+ out of the cell to get back to resting potential.

FIGURE 1.17 Generating an action potential A neuron "fires" when a stimulus makes the voltage across a piece of the cell membrane a bit more positive than its negative "resting potential." This is called depolarization. Depolarization permits sodium ions (Na^+) to rush into the cell, thus increasing the voltage and generating an action potential. Very quickly afterward, potassium ions (K^+) flow out of the cell, bringing the voltage back to the resting voltage. An action potential is analogous to a wave, sweeping across the ocean or around a football stadium. Here, the action potential sweeps along the length of the axon until it reaches the axon terminal.

synapse The junction between neurons that permits information transfer.

neurotransmitter A chemical substance used in neuronal communication at synapses.

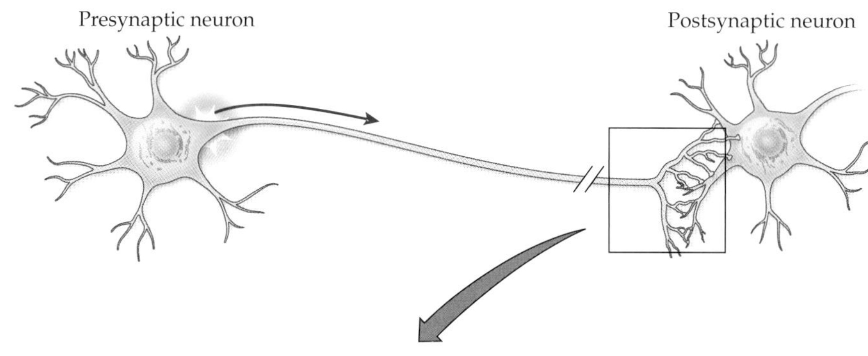

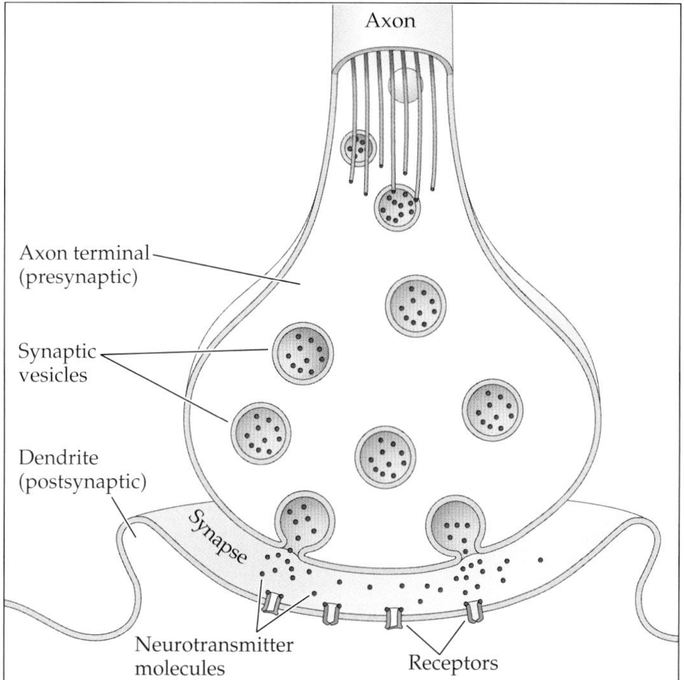

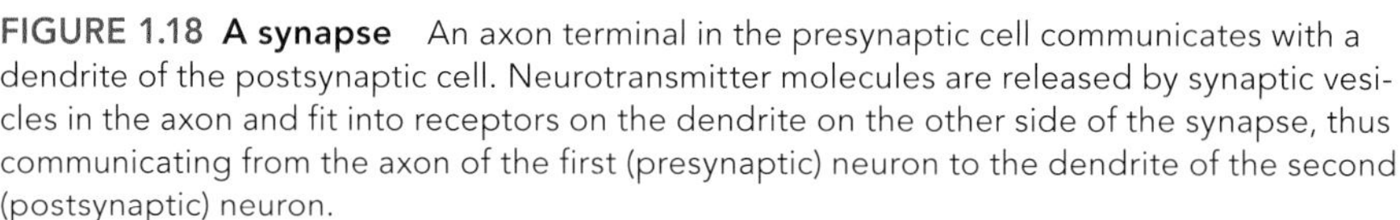

FIGURE 1.18 A synapse An axon terminal in the presynaptic cell communicates with a dendrite of the postsynaptic cell. Neurotransmitter molecules are released by synaptic vesicles in the axon and fit into receptors on the dendrite on the other side of the synapse, thus communicating from the axon of the first (presynaptic) neuron to the dendrite of the second (postsynaptic) neuron.

terminals of the neuron, where the neuron will make contact with other neurons by way of a **synapse** (the term comes from the Greek word meaning "to fasten together"). The most canonical type of synapse (illustrated in **FIGURE 1.18**) is a tiny gap between one neuron and the next. The arrival of the action potential releases **neurotransmitter** chemicals from the presynaptic neuron. Those molecules bind to receptors on the postsynaptic neuron and, depending on the neurotransmitter, that will make that postsynaptic neuron either more or less likely to "fire," sending its action potential onward, in this case up the spinal cord to the brain. Again, if this is all news to you, you will likely want to learn a bit more about basic neuroscience in preparation for the chapters to come. Fortunately, introductions at the level needed to understand this book are widely available through public resources.

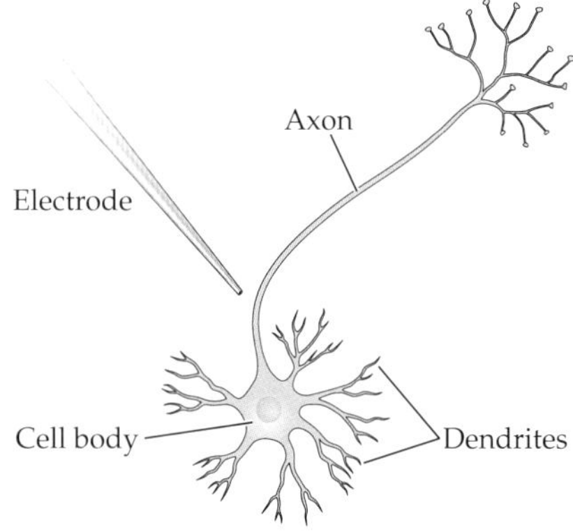

FIGURE 1.19 Recording from a neuron Neuroscientists record the activity of single neurons with electrodes placed close to the axons. Modern techniques permit the insertion of multiple electrodes to measure activity in multiple neurons so that we can better understand how neurons work in concert when encoding sensory information.

Acquiring Neuronal Data by Recording

Neuroscientists can "listen" in on neurons by placing very fine electrodes in or near neurons (**FIGURE 1.19**). In this way, they can record action potentials as well as other electrical and chemical signals. By measuring different aspects of neurons firing, it is possible to learn about how individual neurons encode and transmit information from sense organs through higher levels of the brain.

One way to investigate what a neuron encodes is to try to identify the stimulus that makes it fire the most vigorously. For example, a neuron in the primary visual cortex (see Section 3.4) might respond best to lines that are vertical, less to lines tilted to the left or right, and not at all to horizontal lines. The response of a neuron can be measured by summing the number of times it fires in some interval. This approach, called rate coding, does not take into account the timing between individual action potentials, or "spikes" (**FIGURE 1.20A**). Some neural systems, however, respond to the temporal variations in a stimulus with the temporal pattern of their spiking (**FIGURE 1.20B**). For example, as you will learn when studying the auditory system in Chapter 9, the pitch of a sound is determined by pressure variations reaching the ear. Chapter 13 will describe how rubbing a texture like corduroy gives rise to regularly spaced vibrations on the skin. In each of these systems, neurons can be found that produce spikes that vary rhythmically with the input signal, a form of coding called spike timing. You should keep in mind that although the activity of a single neuron can induce a sensory experience, complex perception is generally achieved by combining the responses of many interacting neurons, called population coding.

Sometimes we learn a lot by simply finding the threshold that gets a neuron to fire at all. For example, **FIGURE 1.20C** shows data obtained by measuring the responses of six different neurons to sounds of different frequencies (tones that sound "low" are low-frequency stimuli). The datapoints show the intensity of the stimulus in decibels (dB) at different frequencies required to get a response from the cell. The resulting functions are called *tuning curves* because they show how patterns of neuronal firing are selectively "tuned" to different frequencies that vary from 0 to 50 kilohertz (kHz = 1000 hertz, or 1000 cycles per second; plotted on the

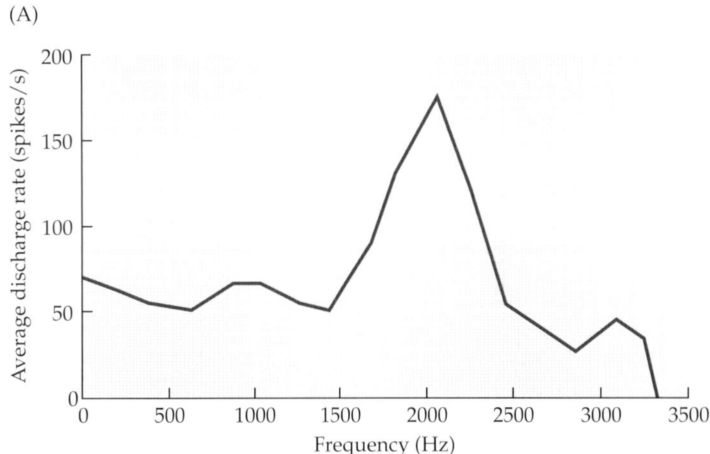

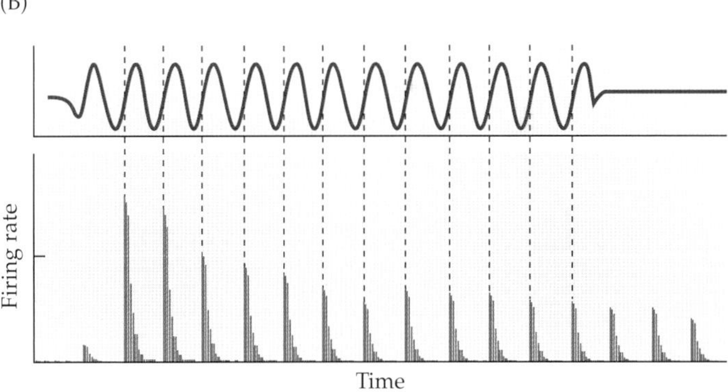

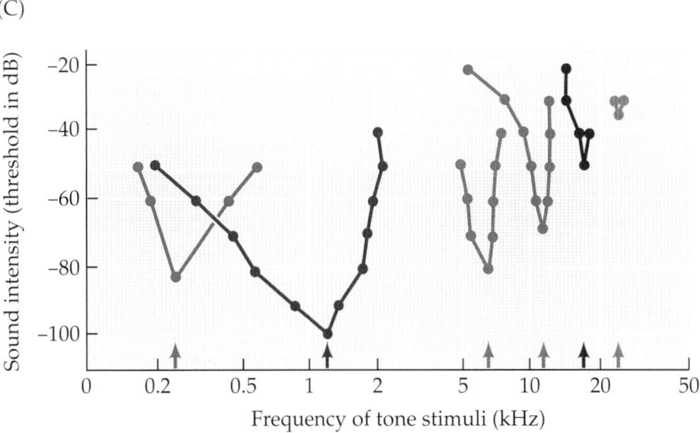

FIGURE 1.20 Tuning curves of auditory neurons (A) Rate coding: Firing rate of an auditory neuron presented with a tone of constant intensity at different frequencies. The neuron has peak response to a tone with a frequency near 2000 Hz (cycles/second). (B) Spike timing: Firing rate of an auditory neuron to a low-frequency tone over a period of time; note that the neuron is most likely to fire at one point in the cycling of the tone, a phenomenon called phase locking. (C) Graph of the threshold (intensity needed to make the neuron fire) of six different neurons (shown in different colors) to sounds of different frequencies and intensities. Arrows along the x-axis indicate the frequency that generated the best response from that neuron in terms of the lowest threshold. Note that this is essentially an inversion of rate coding shown in (A): Neurons tend to give peak responses where their threshold is lowest.

x-axis). Thus, the best frequency for the neuron whose responses are plotted in red in Figure 1.20C is about 1.3 kHz. To get that cell to respond to another frequency, the sound will need to be louder. As another example, the purple line shows a different cell whose best frequency is about 6 kHz.

Neuroimaging Methods

Recording the activity of single neurons continues to be very informative, but it will never be possible to record from more than a tiny fraction of neurons and, even then, almost never in humans (but see Section 4.2). Fortunately, modern perception researchers can now use other tools to understand how thousands or millions of neurons work together within the human brain. In many cases, we look at the results of these methods by making pictures of the brain that reveal its structure and functions. These methods can be collectively referred to as **neuroimaging** methods. Neuroanatomists have long described the structure of the human brain, and neuropsychological studies of individuals with brain damage have taught us much about the functions of different parts of the brain. However, the great advance in recent decades has been the invention of neuroimaging methods that allow us to look at the structure and function of the human brain in healthy, very much living human observers.

For example, **electroencephalography (EEG)** measures electrical activity through dozens of electrodes placed on the scalp (**FIGURE 1.21A**). EEG does not allow researchers to learn what individual neurons are doing or to pinpoint the exact area of neural activity. However, EEG can be used to roughly localize whole populations of neurons (**FIGURE 1.21D**) and to measure their activities with excellent temporal accuracy.

Like a single behavioral measurement, a single EEG signal recorded for a single event is usually not terribly informative. If you want to know the brain's response to a prick of the skin or a flash of light against a background of millions of neurons firing for other reasons or for no reason at all, you will want to repeat the measurement many, many times. Three hypothetical responses to the onset of a light are shown in **FIGURE 1.21B**. You then average all the responses aligned to the moment that the stimulus was present. The resulting averaged waveform is known as an **event-related potential (ERP)**. **FIGURE 1.21C** shows the typical ERP from an experiment in which observers saw brief flashes of light. The EEGs for the 600 ms after each flash were averaged together to produce the waveform. On average, nothing much happens for the first 50 ms or so. Then there is a small positive deflection of the signal, followed by a larger negative deflection. These signals can tell us quite a bit about the temporal processing of a stimulus. **FIGURE 1.21D** shows the signal as a function of time and space: where on the scalp are electrodes picking up a signal? In this case, the response to a light first appears at the back of the head, the home of "primary visual cortex," before flowing forward in the brain to later stages of visual processing (see Section 3.4).

A related method known as **magnetoencephalography (MEG)** (**FIGURE 1.22**) also provides good measures of neuronal timing while providing a better idea of where in the brain neurons are most active. MEG takes advantage of the fact that very small changes in local magnetic fields accompany the small electrical changes that take place when a neuron fires. MEG researchers use extremely sensitive devices to measure these tiny magnetic field changes. Why use EEG if you can have MEG's better spatial resolution? EEG recording is relatively simple, relatively cheap, and relatively portable. MEG devices like that shown in Figure 1.22A use superconducting quantum interference devices. These devices are much more expensive and much less portable than EEG.

neuroimaging A set of methods that generate images of the structure and/or function of the brain. In many cases, these methods allow us to examine the brain in living, behaving humans.

electroencephalography (EEG) A technique that, using many electrodes on the scalp, measures electrical activity from populations of many neurons in the brain.

event-related potential (ERP) A measure of electrical activity from a subpopulation of neurons in response to particular stimuli that requires averaging many electroencephalography recordings.

magnetoencephalography (MEG) A technique, similar to electroencephalography, that measures changes in magnetic activity across populations of many neurons in the brain.

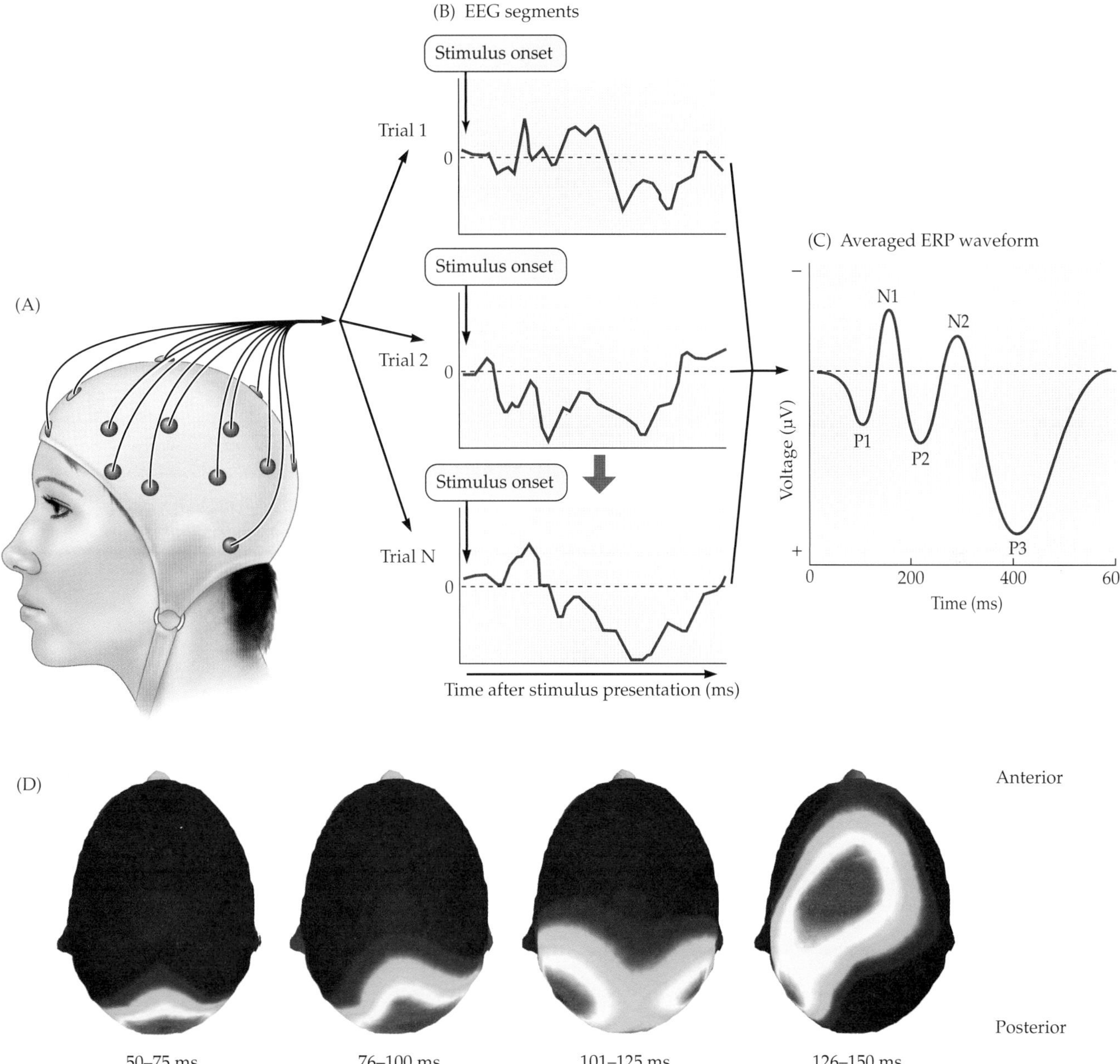

FIGURE 1.21 Electroencephalography (EEG) (A) Electrical activity from the brain can be recorded from the scalp using an array of electrodes. (B) The activity from one electrode is quite variable, even if the same stimulus (perhaps a flash of light) is presented multiple times. (C) However, if many such signals are averaged, a regular pattern of electrically positive (P) and negative (N) waves can be seen. Electrical activity (voltage) is measured in microvolts (μV). (D) Different signals from different electrodes can be used to create a rough map of scalp topography of the activity elicited by a stimulus. These views, looking down at the brain from above, illustrate the typical changes one might see from 50 to 150 ms after the onset of a visual stimulus. Notice that the signal is initially focused over early visual cortex (50–100 ms), then shifts to more anterior areas of visual cortex (101–125 ms), and then begins to activate frontal cortex (126–150 ms).

As noted above, one of the most exciting and important changes in neuroscience in the past generation has been the advent of methods that enable us to see the brain while it is still in its living owner's head. **FIGURE 1.23A** shows an actor viewing what used to be the best we had—a standard X-ray of a skull; **FIGURE 1.23B** shows an example of the much richer images that **magnetic resonance imaging (MRI)** can produce. You can easily imagine the improvements in medical care that

magnetic resonance imaging (MRI) An imaging technology that uses the responses of atoms to strong magnetic fields to form images of structures like the brain. The method can be adapted to measure activity in the brain as well.

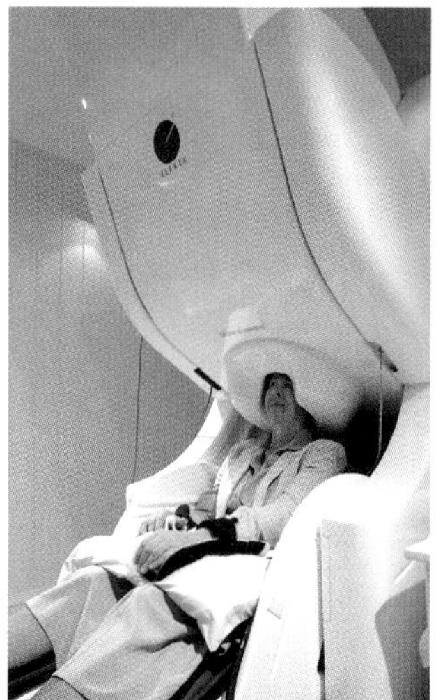

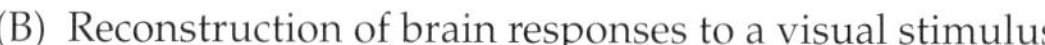

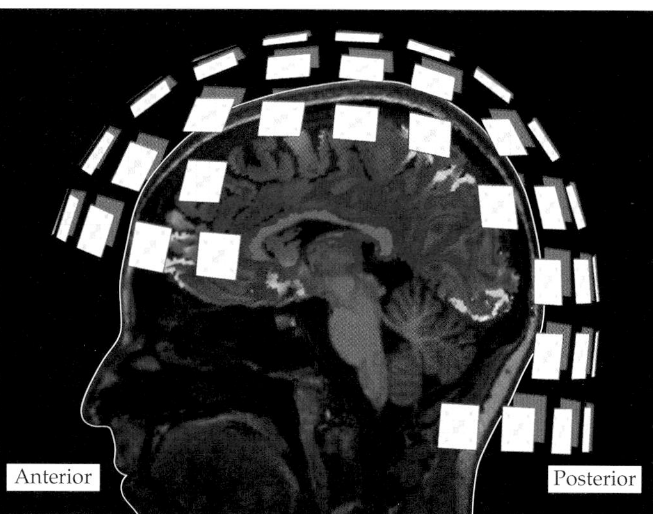

FIGURE 1.22 Magnetoencephalography (MEG) (A) What looks like a huge helmet contains superconducting magnets. (B) The output of MEG recording can be used to visualize activity in the brain. In this case, the individual saw pictures of objects. In this lateral view, "hotter" colors (yellows and reds) indicate more activity, and the "hot spot" at the back of the brain is the primary visual cortex. The superimposed floating squares represent the array of MEG detectors.

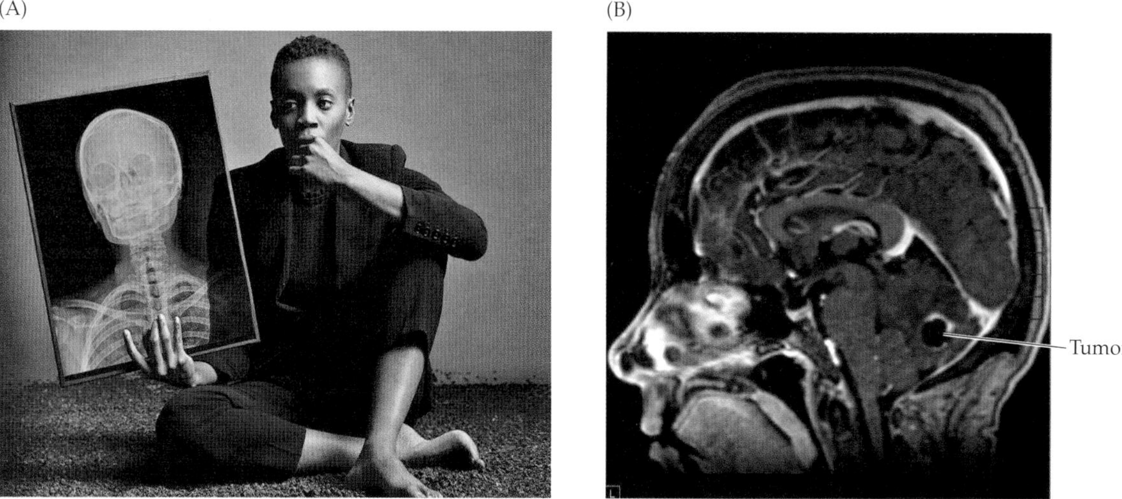

FIGURE 1.23 Magnetic resonance imaging (MRI) Standard X-rays of the head do not reveal much about the brain. (A) Here, actor Amaka Umeh, portraying Hamlet at Stratford, Canada, contemplates an X-ray of the skull of Yorick (You remember: "Alas, poor Yorick, I knew him ..."). (B) A magnetic resonance image, or MRI, shows considerably more detail than an X-ray, including a cancer in the cerebellum (dense black circle at lower right).

became possible once doctors could see a tumor or a blood clot without having to open the skull (see Figure 1.23B).

To produce MRI images of the brain, that brain and its owner are placed in a magnetic field powerful enough to influence the way the atoms spin. The physics is complicated and beyond the scope of our text, but by pulsing the magnetic field, it is possible to measure a signal that indicates the presence of specific elements in the tissue. If you ask about hydrogen in the brain, you are (mostly) asking about

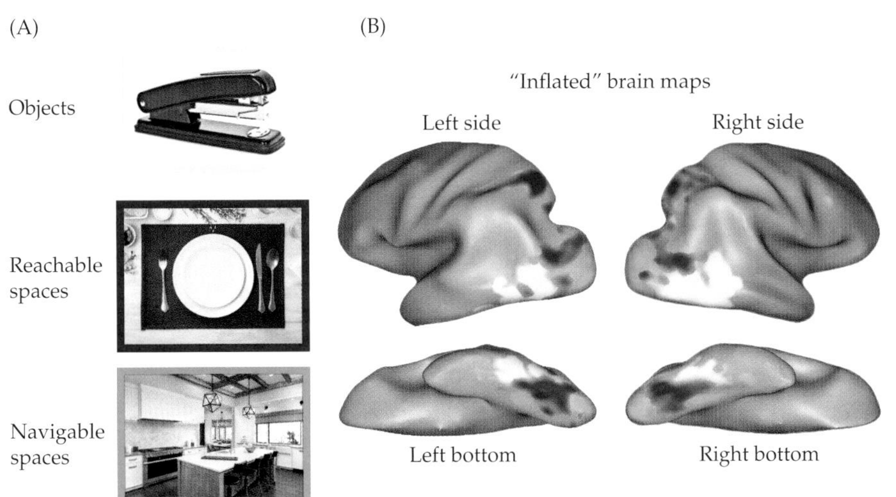

FIGURE 1.24 Functional magnetic resonance imaging (fMRI) (A) Objects and scenes of different kinds are shown to an observer. (B) The blood oxygen level–dependent signal, recorded by magnetic resonance imaging, can be used to gain insight into what the brain is doing, not just its structure. Here we see the regions of the cortex that are particularly responsive to different types of scenes, from single objects to scenes you could walk through.

water, and your computer can use the hydrogen signal to reconstruct the structure of the water-rich tissue inside your head.

For the study of the senses and, indeed, for the study of many topics in psychology, the most remarkable use of MRI technology is **functional magnetic resonance imaging**, or **fMRI**. With fMRI, we can see the activity of the living brain. Here the critical factor is that active brain tissue is hungry brain tissue. It needs oxygen. Oxygen and other supplies are delivered by the blood, so an active brain demands more blood. The result is that there is a **blood oxygen level–dependent (BOLD) signal** that can be measured by the MRI device. Instead of indicating the presence of water, the magnetic pulses and recording are used to pick up evidence of the demand for more oxygenated blood. There are some drawbacks. It takes a few seconds for the BOLD signal to rise after a bit of brain becomes more active, so the temporal resolution of the method is slow compared with EEG/ERP and MEG. The machines are noisy, making auditory experiments difficult. Moreover, acquiring and running these machines is expensive. Still, none of these drawbacks has prevented the method from revolutionizing the study of the brain. In particular, fMRI has essentially replaced, for research purposes, an earlier approach called **positron emission tomography**, which required introduction of a radioactive tracer into the bloodstream.

FIGURE 1.24 shows some of the results from one fMRI experiment. The observer was looking at images like those shown in Figure 1.24A. Those could be isolated objects, scenes where the observer could imagine reaching the objects, or scenes where she could imagine walking around. All of these images would activate large portions of the brain, but if we compare levels of activation, we see that there are some regions of the brain that prefer one type of image, while other regions prefer other types of images. In these fMRI images, shown in Figure 1.24B, the brain has been "inflated" by the computer so you can see into the sulci (the folds) in the cortical surface.

functional magnetic resonance imaging (fMRI) A variant of magnetic resonance imaging that makes it possible to measure localized patterns of activity in the brain. Activated neurons provoke increased blood flow, which can be quantified by measuring changes in the response of oxygenated and deoxygenated blood to strong magnetic fields.

blood oxygen level–dependent (BOLD) signal The ratio of oxygenated to deoxygenated hemoglobin that permits the localization of brain neurons that are most involved in a task.

positron emission tomography (PET) An imaging technology that enables us to define locations in the brain where neurons are especially active by measuring the metabolism of brain cells using safe radioactive isotopes.

mathematical model The use of mathematical language and equations to describe psychological and/or neural processes.

1.4 Computational Modeling as a Method to Understand Perceptual Processes

Mathematics and computer programs have been used for a long time to better understand sensation and perception. Based on their research with giant squid axons in the 1950s, Hodgkin and Huxley went on to develop a **mathematical model** to

computational model The use of mathematical language and equations to describe steps in psychological and/or neural processes (often implemented on a computer).

describe how action potentials in neurons are initiated and propagated (Hodgkin, 1964; Huxley, 1964). Weber's, Fechner's, and Stevens's laws can also be considered mathematical models. Mathematical models use mathematical language, concepts, and equations to closely mimic psychological and neural processes with mathematical precision.

In principle, mathematical models could be (and often were) worked out with pencil and paper. Modern computational technology has allowed us to expand such models into a new class of **computational models** that can take advantage of ever faster and more powerful computers to describe and understand sensation and perception in ways that would be impossible using manual techniques. Perhaps most significant, modern computational models are often learning models that change as a function of their experience. You were not born knowing what a fruit salad looks like. You learned from experience. Modern models learn, too, though they may not be learning in exactly the same way we do.

Computational Models: Probability, Statistics, and Networks

To begin, imagine for a moment what the visual world would look like if it was just noise, something like **FIGURE 1.25A, TOP**. Or, imagine that all your ears heard was the hiss of a white noise machine that some people use to sleep better. Of course, the real world does not deliver only random noise to your senses (**FIGURE 1.25A, BOTTOM**). The real world is structured and predictable—not completely predictable, but, for instance, in the bottom part of Figure 1.25A, if you know that pixel X is white, you could guess that the pixel next to it is white, too. You might not always be right, but you won't be guessing either. An effective perceptual system learns about predictability and structure through experience.

What brightness is a pixel hidden here?
Or here?

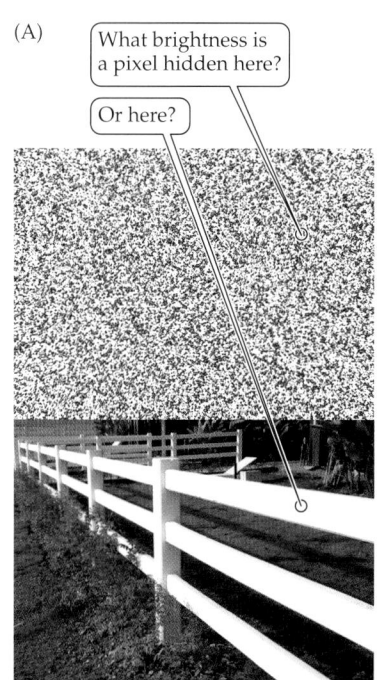

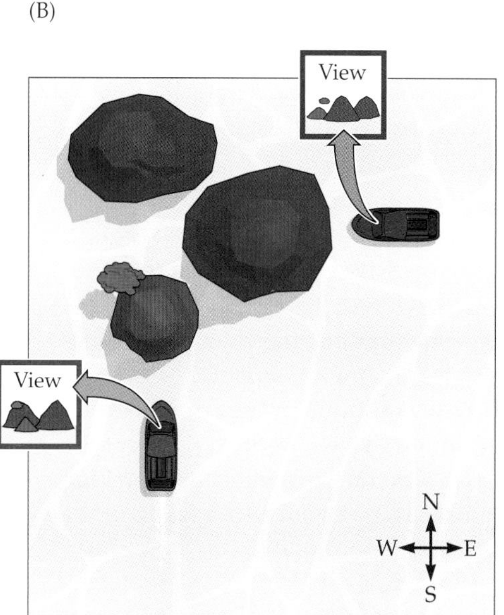

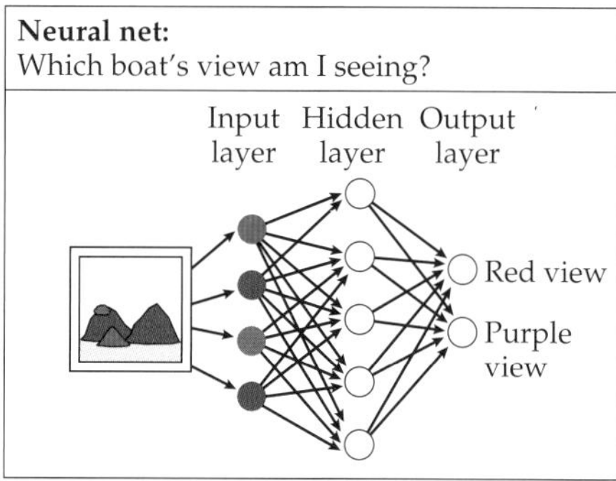

Maxium likelihood: Which boat's view gives a more reliable estimate of the distance from Green Island to Blue Island?
Bayesian: If the red boat drifts west, what will it see?
Efficient coding: Do I need to code this pixel in the view from the purple boat?

Neural net:
Which boat's view am I seeing?
Input layer
Hidden layer
Output layer
Red view
Purple view

FIGURE 1.25 **Pixel predictability** (A) A pixel in the top image, random visual noise, cannot be predicted. In contrast, the real-world image at bottom illustrates how predictable pixels can be from context. (B) Goals of computational models. Left: The "Oval Islands" depicted from above, along with the direct views of the islands as seen by the two boats. Right: Computational models use the data from the images to answer different questions, as shown.

Statistical optimization models begin with the statistics we have amassed through perceptual experiences, like the experience of holding a pencil or listening to someone speak. These statistics are used to make some aspect of perception function at its best. But what does "best" mean? One type of model, called an **efficient coding model**, attempts to maximize the amount of information that is transmitted by a perceptual source, where information is mathematically defined (by a measure you may recognize from computers, the *bit*) (Shannon, 1948). This approach puts less emphasis on signals that are predictable or redundant, because they offer little new information (Attneave, 1954; Barlow, 1961, 2001). So, if pixels 1, 2, 4, and 5 are green, an efficient system would not spend a lot of effort encoding the greenness of pixel 3. Another form of optimization, maximum likelihood estimation, makes the best use of multiple sources of information about the same physical property of the world in order to estimate its quantity (Ernst and Banks, 2002). If we test for the ripeness of a tomato by squeezing, the observable change in its shape provides one estimate of its compliance, while the feeling of pressure on our fingers may offer a different one. To optimize the outcome, a maximum-likelihood estimator takes both senses into account, but favors the one that has proved more reliable when making such estimates in the past. Because the world is generally predictable, the use of the past to evaluate the present turns out to be advantageous (Geisler, 2011).

Bayesian models build on the assumption behind maximum-likelihood estimation, in that they use the statistics of past experience to interpret the energy currently arriving at the senses. Unlike the statistical assumptions behind the *t*-tests and analyses of variance of your statistics course, these models do not treat each perceptual experience as an independent observation; to the contrary, they assume that earlier observations should bias expectations for future events. If pixels 1, 2, 3, 4, and 5 are green, there is a pretty good case for predicting that pixel 6 will be green as well. Based on prior as well as current observations, a Bayesian model makes a "best guess," or prediction, about inputs at each point in time and then evaluates whether the predicted input corresponds with the input that was received. If not, the system will attempt to reduce this mismatch, or *prediction error*, by adjusting its prediction about the state of the environment and adapting the model accordingly (Van de Cruys, Van der Hallen, and Wagemans, 2017). Through this iterative process, Bayesian statistics can be useful in understanding how perceptual systems adapt with experience.

Artificial neural networks, inspired by biological neural networks, provide another computational framework to better understand how sensory systems develop based on experience. Sometimes called *connectionist models*, artificial neural networks are composed of layers of heavily interconnected computational units. These units are analogous to neurons massively connected to one another through their axons, dendrites, and synapses. Each neuron receives activation through its connections to others, and collectively, the network performs population coding. The strength of the connections between units can increase or decrease, depending on how they contribute to the network's success (Rumelhart, McClelland, and PDP Research Group, 1986). This is akin to the strength of a synapse changing with experience. Some neural network models "learn" based on feedback—that is, being told whether or not they are correct—while others function without feedback. If a model is given feedback when it is right or wrong, it is a "supervised" model; models without this feedback are "unsupervised." Neural network models typically require multiple cycles of taking inputs and producing outputs before they settle into a best solution.

Is one computational model better than another? Each approach is useful for its purpose, as illustrated in Figure 1.25B.

statistical optimization model A computational account describing how a perceptual system uses the statistics of past experience to improve its current performance, for example, by minimizing the processing load or making the best use of multiple sources of information.

efficient coding models Theoretical and/or computational models that explain neural processing by assuming that sensory systems become tuned to predictability in natural environments in ways that economically encode predictable sensory inputs while highlighting inputs that are less predictable.

Bayesian models Theoretical and/or computational models that employ Bayesian statistical methods to generate an internal model of the source of sensory inputs based on prior experience.

artificial neural networks Also referred to as *connectionist models*, these are computational methods that consist of networks of nodes with weighted connections between them. Connection weights increase and decrease following experience in ways that resemble the organization of biological neural networks.

deep neural networks (DNNs) Artificial neural networks that have a very large number of layers of nodes with millions of connections.

Deep Learning

These days, the most important forms of neural network models are **deep neural networks (DNNs)**, also called deep neural learning models or, simply, deep learning. Deep learning models can have many layers of units (or nodes) with millions of connections (that is the "deep" part), harnessing the speed and massive memory capacities of modern computers. Such networked models are particularly good at taking vast amounts of information and classifying it into categories. One huge success has been in the field of object recognition. As Section 4.5 will discuss, DNNs now routinely take as input millions of images and learn to identify all the dogs, cats, tomatoes, and so on, accurately labeling thousands of different types of objects (Krizhevsky, Sutskever, and Hinton, 2012; Kriegeskorte, 2015). This is the technology behind the artificial intelligence boom that has brought you (for better or worse) devices like Apple's Siri and the facial recognition software used by many police and security agencies. If we ever have fully autonomous cars, DNNs will be an important part of their "brains." Deep learning technology is on the verge of transforming tasks like those performed by expert radiologists, because a network that can be trained to find cat videos can be trained to find cancer, too (Mendelson, 2018; Borstelmann, 2020).

The ability of DNNs to perform like humans leads us to wonder if they are in fact models of how humans perform the task. They might be, or the DNN might be doing the task quite differently. A jet plane, for example, is not a great model of how a sparrow or a bumblebee flies. The difficulty is that, like the brain, these models are very complex and, like the brain, it is not a trivial task to figure out how they do what they do (Kriegeskorte and Douglas, 2018). This can be a problem when DNNs are used in the real world. For example, if a DNN was really going to be the "expert" looking for cancer in an X-ray, we would want that expert to be able to explain how and why it made a particular decision (Handelman et al., 2018). At present, that is not something that DNNs are good at. Still, these computational tools are making rapid progress and it safe to predict that future sensation and perception texts will have more to say on this topic.

Is Our Experience of Physical Properties Influenced by Prior Knowledge and Context?

This last question moves the study of perception from the direct relation of matter to mind into the realm of how the mind affects the mind! As you go through the chapters of this book, you will discover that although perception may be triggered by stimulation of sensory receptors and may progress though neural connections to the brain, the ultimate representation that we form of our physical surroundings is profoundly influenced by what we know and the totality of our past and current experience. The question of "What color is the dress?" (see Chapter 5) captivated the internet because it seemed impossible that two people's minds could reach such different conclusions. These mental variations are an inevitable consequence of the fact that sensory inputs are, in general, inadequate to fully represent the world. Perception fills in by a hodgepodge of statistical guesses, rules of thumb, and expectations. In this book, you will see these under the names of Bayesian priors, heuristics, committees, and top-down processes. Such mental guesswork creates perceptual illusions, individual differences, and failures to see what is in front of our eyes. As you continue to read this book, keep your own mind open to the possibilities of how representation is not simply determined by the physics of the world.

Summary

1. Sensation and perception are central to, and often precede, almost all aspects of human behavior and thought. There are many practical applications of our increased understanding of sensation and perception.
2. Gustav Fechner invented several clever methods for measuring the relationship between physical changes in the world and consequent psychological changes in observers. These methods remain in use today. Using Fechner's methods, researchers can measure the smallest levels of a stimulus that can be detected (absolute threshold) and the smallest differences that can be detected (difference thresholds, or just noticeable differences).
3. A more recent development for understanding performance—signal detection theory—permits us to simulate changes in the perceiver (e.g., internal noise and biases) to understand perceptual performance better.
4. We learn a great deal about perception by understanding the biological structures and processes involved. One early observation—the doctrine of specific nerve energies—expresses the fact that people are aware only of the activity of their nervous systems. For this reason, what matters is *which* nerves are stimulated, not *how* they are stimulated. The central nervous system reflects specializations for the senses, from cranial nerves to areas of the cerebral cortex involved in perception.
5. The essential activities of all neurons, including those involved in sensory processes, are chemical and electrochemical. Neurons communicate with each other through neurotransmitters, molecules that cross the synapse from the axon of one neuron to the dendrite of the next. Nerve impulses are electrochemical; voltages change along the axon as electrically charged sodium and potassium ions pass in and out of the membranes of nerve cells.
6. Recordings from individual neurons enable us to measure how different stimuli activate different neurons.
7. Neuroimaging methods have revolutionized the study of sensation and perception by allowing us to study the brain in healthy, living human observers. Useful methods include electroencephalography, magnetoencephalography, and functional magnetic resonance imaging. Each comes with its own combination of temporal and spatial properties, making one method suitable for researching some questions and other methods more suitable for other questions.
8. Computational methods have become increasingly useful in the study of the senses. Many computational models are able to learn the regularities in the world after being exposed to many samples from the world.
9. Deep learning algorithms, in particular, are powerful tools that can take in vast amounts of data (e.g., pictures) and categorize them ("That's a cat."). Such tools may become important in applications like autonomous driving or detecting cancer in medical images.

Chapter 2

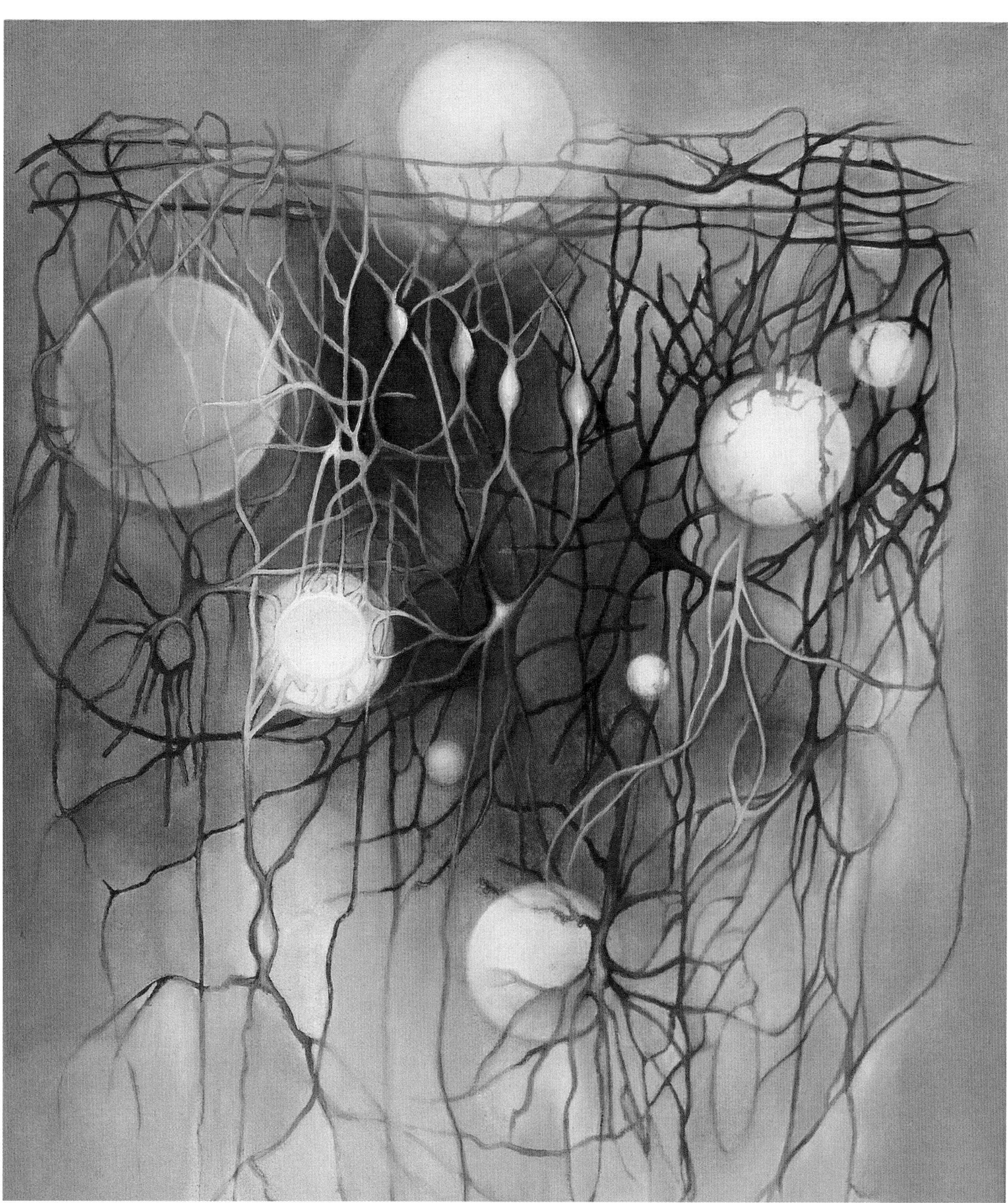

Alicia Hunsicker, *Thought Forms*, 2011

The First Steps in Vision: From Light to Neural Signals

Questions to Contemplate

Think about the following questions as you read this chapter.By the chapter's end, you should be able to answer and discuss them.

- How are images of the world formed on the retina?
- How is energy from light converted into the electrical neural signals that lead to "seeing"?
- When the eye doctor says you have 20/20 vision, what does she mean?
- How is it that you are able to see over a huge range of brightness levels?

Imagine looking into the night sky at your favorite star. The light coming from that star reaches your eye after traveling as far as 2000 light-years (almost 12 quadrillion miles in round numbers). Remarkably, in a dark winter sky far from city lights, the neighboring galaxy, Andromeda, is visible at over 2 *million* light-years away! This chapter describes the first steps in seeing. To understand how we see, we must first consider a little physics and optics, and then we'll look at how the eye is built to capture light and how specialized cells in the retina act to change physical light energy into electrical neural energy.

In Chapters 3–8, we'll see how light information gleaned by the eyes travels back through the head to the brain, as well as how the brain transforms this information into a meaningful interpretation of the outside world.

2.1 A Little Light Physics

Light is a form of electromagnetic radiation—energy produced by vibrations of electrically charged material. There are two ways to conceptualize light: as a **wave** or as a stream of **photons**, tiny particles that each consist of one quantum of energy. This dual nature of light can be confusing to physics and psychology students alike. In this discussion, we'll try to avoid confusion as much as possible by treating light as being made up of waves when it moves around the world and being made up of photons when it is absorbed.

The electromagnetic spectrum is made up of energy that varies over a very wide range of wavelengths (that is, the distances between successive points in the wave), and light makes up only a tiny portion of this spectrum. FIGURE 2.1A illustrates the electromagnetic spectrum, from gamma rays (which have very short wavelengths) to radio and television waves (which have very long wavelengths). Visible light waves have wavelengths between 400 and 700 nanometers (nm; 1 nm = 10^{-9} meter), as illustrated on the bottom of Figure 2.1A. Note that as the wavelength varies in the visible spectrum, the **hue** we observe changes, from violet at about 400 nm, through the whole spectrum of the rainbow, up to red at about 650 nm. (As we'll discuss in Chapter 5, however, the light waves themselves are not colored; it is only after our visual system interprets an incoming wave that we perceive the light as a specific color.)

wave An oscillation that travels through a medium by transferring energy from one particle or point to another without causing any permanent displacement of the medium.

photon A quantum of visible light or other form of electromagnetic radiation demonstrating both particle and wave properties.

hue The perceptual attribute of colors that enables them to be classed as similar to red, green, or blue, or something in between.

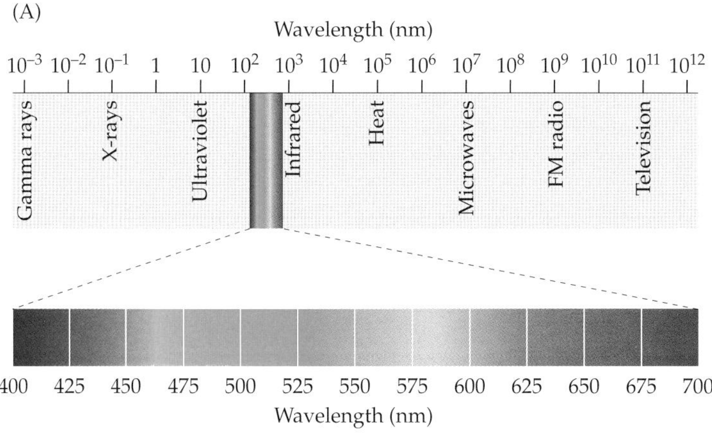

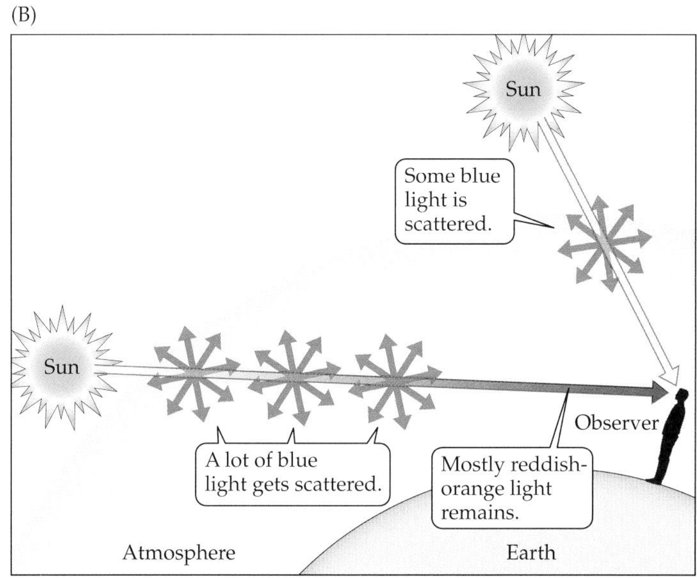

FIGURE 2.1 The electromagnetic energy spectrum (A) The spectrum of electromagnetic energy (specified in nanometers, nm), with the visible spectrum (400–700 nm) expanded. Note that 1 nm = 10^{-9} meter. (B) Rayleigh scattering. Scattering of light causes the sky to look blue when the sun is high and to look red when the sun is low.

Note that the electromagnetic wavelength spectrum in Figure 2.1A is on a logarithmic scale. To quote Tom Cornsweet, "If, instead, we consider actual lengths or distances, not their logarithms, and we represent the range between AM radio and X-ray wavelengths as the distance from New York to Los Angeles, then the wavelengths we are able to see would be represented on that scale as a distance of less than an eighth of an inch. Science had to invent instruments to detect wavelengths represented by the rest of that distance" (Cornsweet, 2017, p. 2).

Let's consider what happens to light on its way from a star to an eye. In empty space, the electromagnetic radiation from a star travels in a straight line at the speed of light (about 186,000 miles per second). Once it reaches the atmosphere, some of the starlight's photons are **absorbed** by encounters with dust, vaporized water, and so on; and some of the light is **scattered** (sometimes called diffracted) by these particles. Scattering of sunlight by small particles (Rayleigh scattering, named after Lord Rayleigh) gives the sky its color: blue when the sun is high, because short-wavelength (blue) light is scattered more strongly than other wavelengths; red at sunset, when the sun is near the horizon, because the sunlight must pass through more atmosphere near the Earth's surface, scattering more of the short-wavelength (blue) light (**FIGURE 2.1B**), allowing the longer-wavelength light (red and yellow)

absorb To take up something—such as light, noise, or energy—and not transmit it at all.

scatter To disperse something—such as light—in an irregular fashion.

to reach your eyes. Most of the photons, however, make it through the atmosphere and eventually hit the surface of an object.

If a ray of starlight were to strike a light-colored surface, most of the light would be **reflected**. Indeed, the fact that most of the light bounces off the surface accounts for that surface's "light" appearance. However, most of the light striking a dark surface is absorbed. Light that is neither reflected nor absorbed by the surface is **transmitted** through the surface. If we are gazing at our star through a window as the light travels from air into the glass, some of the rays will be bent, or **refracted**, as light is transmitted.

Refraction also occurs when light passes from air into water or into the eyeball. In fact, the part of an eye exam in which the eye doctor checks the patient's prescription is often called a refraction because the doctor determines how much the light must be bent by eyeglasses for it to be properly focused on the retina. In the next section, we'll see how the optic system of our eyes performs this same kind of focusing.

reflect To redirect something that strikes a surface—especially light, sound, or heat—usually back toward its point of origin.

transmit To convey something (e.g., light) from one place or thing to another.

refract 1. To alter the course of a wave of energy that passes into something from another medium, as water does to light entering it from the air. 2. To measure the degree of refraction in a lens or eye.

image A picture or likeness.

cornea The transparent "window" into the eyeball.

transparent Referring to the characteristic of a material that allows light to pass through it with no interruption such that objects on the other side can be clearly seen.

2.2 Eyes That Capture Light

To see stars or anything else, we need some type of physiological mechanism for sensing light. Even single-celled organisms such as amoebas respond to light, changing their direction of motion to avoid bright light when it is detected. But eyes go well beyond mere light detection. An eye can form an **image** of the outside world, enabling animals that possess eyes to use light to recognize objects, not just to determine whether light is present and what direction it's coming from.

Before explaining how eyes form images, let's take a tour through the human eye to become familiar with its important parts. **FIGURE 2.2** shows a front-to-back slice through a human eye, with the most important structures labeled.

The first tissue that light from the star will encounter is the **cornea**. The cornea provides a window to the world because it is **transparent** (that is, most light

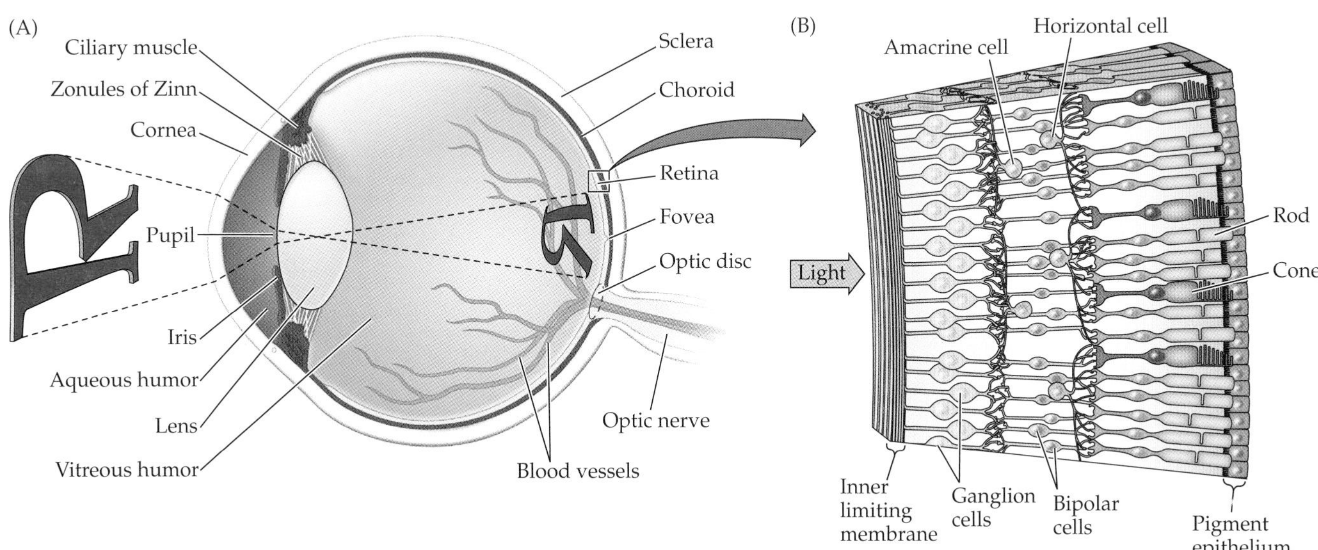

FIGURE 2.2 The human right eye in cross section (viewed from above) (A) Note that the *R* on the retina is reversed right to left, and it is upside down. The "hole" in the retina where the optic nerve leaves the eyeball is the optic disc (where the absence of photoreceptors results in a blind spot). (B) This enlargement of a cross section through the retina shows the main cell types. These will be discussed in Section 2.3.

photons are transmitted through it, rather than being reflected or absorbed). It is transparent because it is made of a highly ordered arrangement of fibers and because it contains no blood vessels or blood, which would absorb light. The cornea does, however, have a rich supply of transparent sensory nerve endings, which are there to force the eyes to close and produce tears if the cornea is scratched, to preserve its transparency. If you have ever scratched your cornea or worn contact lenses too long, you know exactly how painful this can be! Fortunately, the external layers of the cornea regenerate very quickly, so even when a cornea is scratched, it usually heals within 24 hours.

If you wear contact lenses, you will know that they sit on a thin film of tears in front of the cornea. The tear film is important because it provides the eyes with a smooth, clear surface, helps to protect and lubricate the eyes, and washes away dust and particles. Tears also help to reduce the risk of eye infections. Besides, without tears, crying just wouldn't be the same.

You might be wondering how the cells of the cornea get their oxygen and nutrients if it has no blood supply. The **aqueous humor**, a fluid derived from blood, fills the space immediately behind the cornea and supplies oxygen and nutrients to, and removes waste from, both the cornea and the **lens**. Like the cornea, the lens has no blood supply, so it can be completely transparent. As we'll see later, the shape of the lens is controlled by the ciliary muscles.

To get to the lens, the light from our star must pass through the **pupil**, which is simply a hole in a muscular structure called the **iris**. The iris gives the eye its distinctive color and controls the size of the pupil, and thus the amount of light that reaches the retina, via the pupillary light reflex. When the level of light increases or decreases, the iris automatically expands or contracts to allow more or less light into the eye, respectively. Interestingly, like the aperture of a camera, the pupil of the iris plays an important role in the image quality. Under low illumination, when the pupil is large, the depth of focus (the range of distances over which the image is sharply focused) is reduced, resulting in poor image quality.

After passing through the lens, our starlight will enter the vitreous chamber (the space between the lens and the retina), where it will be refracted for the fourth and final time by the **vitreous humor**. This is the longest part of the journey through the eyeball; this chamber comprises 80% of the internal volume of the eye. The vitreous is gel-like and viscous (a bit like egg white), and it is generally transparent. While staring up at the bright blue sky on a lazy sunny day, however, you may have noticed "floaters," small bits of debris (biodebris) that drift around in the vitreous. Floaters are quite common, and they are usually not a cause for concern.

Finally, after traveling through the vitreous chamber, the light emitted by our favorite star will (hopefully) be brought into focus at the **retina**. To be a bit more precise, only some of the light will actually reach the retina. Much of the light energy will have been lost in space or the atmosphere, because of absorption and scattering, as described already. In addition, a good deal of light will have become lost in the eyeball, so only about half of the starlight that arrives at the cornea will reach the retina. The role of the retina is to detect light and "tell the brain about aspects of light that are related to objects in the world" (Oyster, 1999). In other words, the retina is where seeing really begins, because it is here that light energy is turned into electrical neural signals—a process known as transduction.

Interestingly, our ability to detect a briefly presented dim light (and many other visual stimuli) is limited not only by the retinal transduction processes and the neural signals that it generates, but also by the noise in the visual pathways, and by other factors too. For example, detection thresholds can be enhanced by providing a sound at precisely the same time as the dim light (Spence and Ngo, 2012).

aqueous humor The watery fluid in the anterior chamber of the eye.

lens The structure inside the eye that enables the changing of focus.

pupil The dark, circular opening at the center of the iris in the eye, where light enters the eye.

iris The colored part of the eye, consisting of a muscular diaphragm surrounding the pupil and regulating the light entering the eye by expanding and contracting the pupil.

vitreous humor The transparent fluid that fills the vitreous chamber in the posterior part of the eye.

retina A light-sensitive membrane in the back of the eye that contains photoreceptors and other cell types that transduce light into electrochemical signals and transmit them to the brain through the optic nerve.

accommodation The process by which the eye changes its focus (in which the lens gets fatter as gaze is directed toward nearer objects).

focal distance The distance between the lens (or mirror) and the viewed object, in meters.

diopter A unit of measurement of the optical power of a lens. It is equal to the reciprocal of the focal length, in meters. A 2-diopter lens will bring parallel rays of light into focus at 0.5 meter (50 centimeters).

This "cross modal facilitation" may be caused by the sound reducing uncertainty about when precisely the visual stimulus will appear (see Chapter 1) or by the top-down focusing of attention at precisely the time that the visual stimulus appears (see Chapter 7). ●

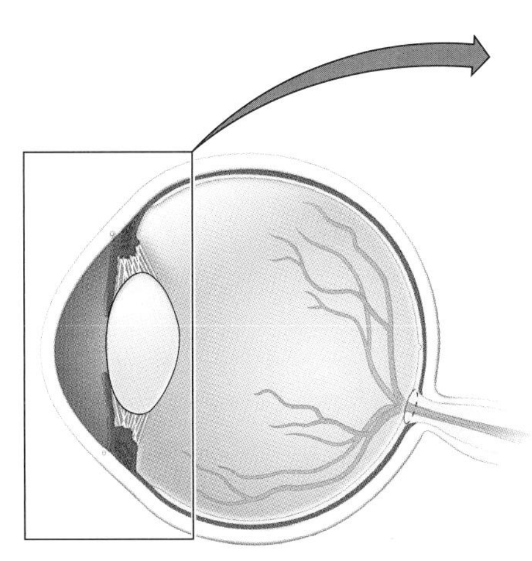

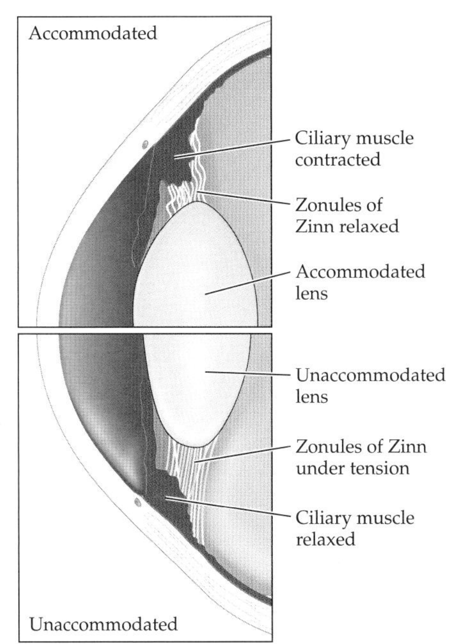

FIGURE 2.3 Accommodation changes the power of the lens The left side of this cross section shows the relaxed (unaccommodated) lens. The right side (top) shows the bulging accommodated lens, resulting from decreased tension of the zonules when the ciliary muscle contracts.

Focusing Light onto the Retina

To focus a distant star onto the retina, the refractive power of the four optical components of the eye—cornea, aqueous humor, lens, and vitreous humor—must be perfectly matched to the length of the eyeball. Because the cornea is highly curved and has a higher refractive index than air (1.376 versus 1), it forms the most powerful refractive surface in the eye. The aqueous and vitreous humors also help refract light. However, the refractive power of each of these three structures is fixed, so they cannot be used to bring close objects into focus. This job is performed by the lens, which can alter the refractive power by changing its shape—a process called **accommodation**.

Accommodation (change in focus) is accomplished through contraction of the ciliary muscle. The lens is attached to the ciliary muscle through tiny fibers (suspensory ligaments known as the zonules of Zinn) (**FIGURE 2.3**). When the ciliary muscle is relaxed, the zonules are stretched and the lens is relatively flat. In this state, the eye will be focused on very distant objects (like our star). But to focus on something closer—say, a wristwatch or smartphone—the ciliary muscle must contract. This contraction reduces the tension on the zonules and enables the lens to bulge. The fatter the lens is, the more power it has, and the closer you can focus.

presbyopia Literally "old sight"; the age-related loss of accommodation, which makes it difficult to focus on near objects.

Accommodation enables the power of the lens to vary. Lens power (P) = $1/f$, where f is the **focal distance** in meters. So, if your unaccommodated eyes were perfectly corrected for distant vision, 15 **diopters** of accommodation would enable you to read your watch at a distance of about 0.067 meter (1/15) or 6.7 centimeters (cm; to convert meters to centimeters, simply multiply by 100). If you can read your watch at 6.7 cm (while wearing your distance correction), you are either very lucky or very young. Our ability to accommodate declines with age, starting from about 8 years old, and we lose about 1 diopter of accommodation every 5 years up to age 30 (and even more after age 30). By the time most people are between 40 and 50 years old, they find that their arms are too short because they can no longer easily accommodate the 2.5 diopters or so needed to see clearly at 40 cm (1/0.4 = 2.5). This condition is called **presbyopia** (meaning "old sight"), and it is, like death and taxes, inevitable! **FIGURE 2.4** illustrates the precipitous drop in accommodation with age.

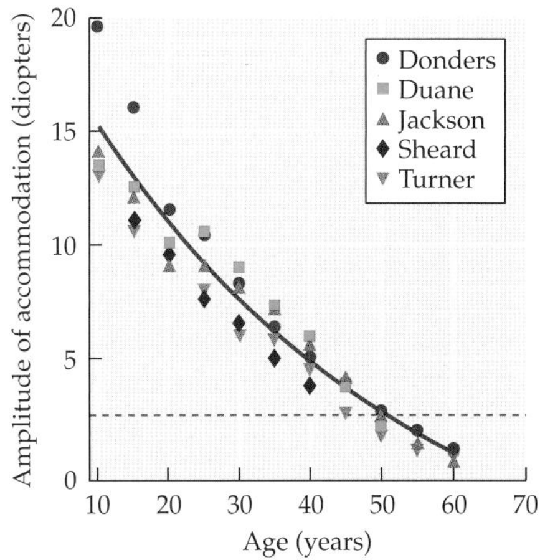

FIGURE 2.4 The precipitous drop in amplitude of accommodation with age The dashed line indicates the amplitude of accommodation required to focus at a distance of 40 cm. Each colored symbol represents data from a different classical study.

Why do we all have presbyopia to look forward to? The main reason is that the lens becomes harder, and the capsule that encircles the lens, enabling it to change shape, loses its elasticity. Lucky for us, Benjamin Franklin (1706–1790) invented bifocals—lenses that have one power at the top (permitting us to see distant objects) and a different power at the bottom (allowing us to focus on objects at a comfortable reading distance).

Like the other optical components of the eye, the lens is normally transparent. It is transparent because the crystallins (a class of proteins that make up the lens) are packed together very densely and therefore are very regular. Anything that interferes with the regularity of the crystallins will result in loss of transparency (that is, result

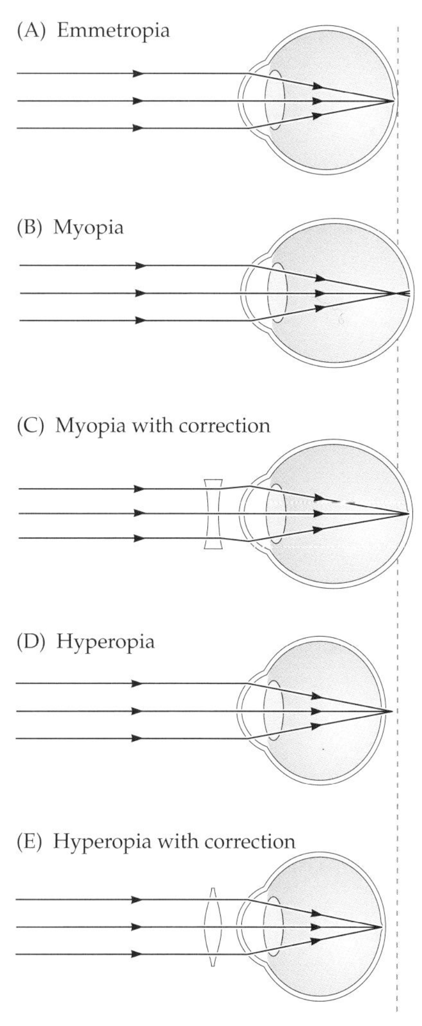

FIGURE 2.5 Optics of the human eye Examples of an eye with no visual defects (emmetropia) (A), nearsightedness (myopia) (B), myopia with correction (C), farsightedness (hyperopia) (D), and hyperopia with correction (E).

in areas that are opaque, or opacities). Opacities of the lens are known as **cataracts**. Cataracts can occur at different ages and take many different forms. Congenital cataracts (present at birth) are relatively rare, but if they are dense (and therefore interfere with retinal image quality), they can have devastating effects on normal visual development if not treated promptly. Most cataracts are discovered after age 50, and the prevalence of cataracts increases with age, so by 70 almost everyone has some loss of transparency. Cataracts can interfere with vision because they absorb and scatter more light than the normal lens does. Fortunately, treatment of cataracts (in which the opacified lens is extracted and replaced with a plastic or silicone implant) has become quite routine—often just a 30-minute procedure in the eye doctor's office. There is much ongoing effort to develop new types of lens implants that can change focus. Hopefully these will be perfected before you need cataract surgery!

When the refractive power of the four optical components of the eye (cornea, aqueous humor, lens, and vitreous humor) are perfectly matched to the length of the eyeball, this is known as **emmetropia** (**FIGURE 2.5A**). A person who is emmetropic does not need corrective lenses to see distant objects. On average, the adult human eye is 24 millimeters (mm) long, about the diameter of a quarter. However, eyeballs can be quite a bit longer or shorter and still be emmetropic because eyes generally grow to match the power of the optical components we're born with. (Most newborns are hyperopic because the optical components of their eyes are relatively well developed at birth compared with the length of their eyeballs.)

Refractive errors occur when the eyeball is too long or too short relative to the power of the four optical components. If the eyeball is too long for the optics (**FIGURE 2.5B**), the image of our star will be focused *in front* of the retina, and the star will thus be seen as a blur rather than a spot of light. This condition is called **myopia** (or nearsightedness). Individuals with myopia cannot see distant objects clearly; luckily, myopia can be corrected with negative (minus) lenses, which diverge the rays of starlight before they enter the eye (**FIGURE 2.5C**). If the eyeball is too short for the optics (**FIGURE 2.5D**), the image of our star will be focused *behind* the retina—a condition called **hyperopia** (or farsightedness). If the hyperopia is not too severe, a young hyperope can compensate and see clearly by accommodating, thereby increasing the power of the eye. If accommodation fails to correct the hyperopia, the star's image will again be blurred. Hyperopia can be corrected with positive (plus) lenses, which converge the rays of starlight before they enter the eye (**FIGURE 2.5E**).

As noted earlier, the most powerful refracting surface in the eye is the cornea, which contributes about two-thirds of the eye's focusing power. In an emmetrope, the cornea is spherical, like a basketball or soccer ball (**FIGURE 2.6A**). However, if the cornea is not spherical, but rather shaped like a football (that is, the curvature is different in the horizontal and vertical meridians; **FIGURE 2.6B**), the result is

cataract An opacity of the crystalline lens.

emmetropia The condition in which there is no refractive error, because the refractive power of the eye is perfectly matched to the length of the eyeball.

refractive error A very common disorder in which the image of the world is not clearly focused on the retina. The most common refractive errors are myopia, hyperopia, astigmatism, and presbyopia.

myopia Nearsightedness, a common condition in which light entering the eye is focused in front of the retina and distant objects cannot be seen sharply.

(A)

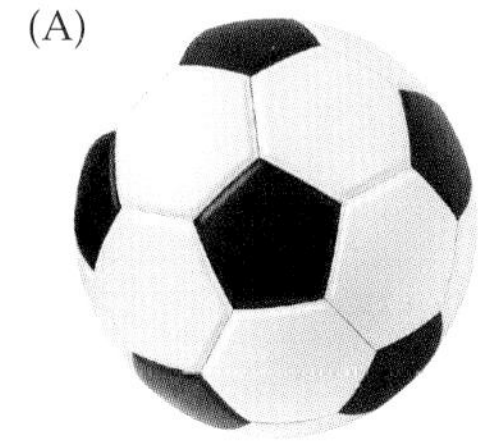

(B)

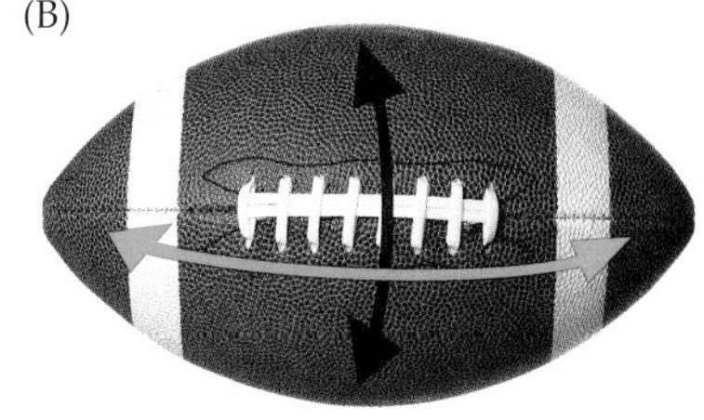

FIGURE 2.6 Two balls, two shapes (A) Basketballs and soccer balls are spherical. (B) Rugby and American football balls are elliptical. If the cornea is shaped like a football, with different curvatures in the horizontal and vertical meridians, it will result in astigmatism.

astigmatism. With astigmatism, vertical lines may be focused slightly in front of the retina, while horizontal lines may be focused slightly behind it (or vice versa). If you have a reasonable degree of uncorrected astigmatism, one or more of the lines in **FIGURE 2.7** may appear to be out of focus while other lines appear sharp. Lenses that have two focal points (that is, lenses that provide different amounts of focusing power in the horizontal and vertical planes) can correct astigmatism. The development of refractive surgery such as LASIK (laser-assisted in situ keratomileusis) as an alternative to glasses or contact lenses is based on the cornea's refractive power.

If you are a college student (and if you are reading this, the odds are that you are), there's a high probability that you are myopic. While the causes of myopia are complex, involving both genes and environment (see Harb and Wildsoet, 2019, for a review), it has long been suggested that there is a link between the level of education and the development of myopia. Moreover, the prevalence of myopia is increasing, and myopia is predicted to affect more than half of the world's population in the next 30 years. One potentially important player in this increase may be related to the amount of time we now spend on our devices (smartphones, tablets, and computers). This is an area of active research.

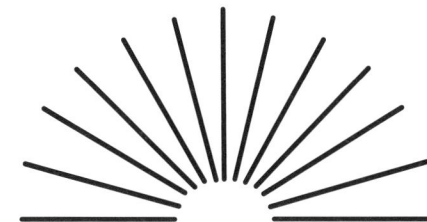

FIGURE 2.7 Fan chart for astigmatism Take off your glasses (if you wear glasses) and view this "fan." If you have a significant degree of astigmatism, one or more of the lines will appear to have lower contrast.

hyperopia Farsightedness, a common condition in which light entering the eye is focused behind the retina and accommodation is required to see near objects clearly.

astigmatism A visual defect caused by the unequal curving of one or more of the refractive surfaces of the eye, usually the cornea.

transduce To convert from one form of energy to another (e.g., from light to neural electrical energy, or from mechanical movement to neural electrical energy). Neurons use electrical signals in their communication.

fundus The back layer of the retina: what the eye doctor sees through an ophthalmoscope.

photoreceptor A light-sensitive receptor in the retina.

The Retina

The preceding discussion covered how the human visual system delivers a focused image of our favorite star onto the retina, which is spread across the back of the eyeball. The optics involved (see Figure 2.2) include a mechanism for regulating the amount of light (the iris) and a lens for adjusting focal length (see Figure 2.3) so that both near and distant objects can be focused on the retina. However, unlike a camera, the human visual system has the job of interpreting this image. This is the difference between taking a picture and seeing a picture. And the process of seeing begins with the retina, where the light energy from our star is **transduced** into neural energy that can be interpreted by the brain.

What the Doctor Saw

Eye doctors use an instrument called an ophthalmoscope to look at the back surface of their patients' eyes, which is called the **fundus** (plural *fundi*). (You probably remember all too well having that bright light shining into your eye while the doctor examined your fundus.) **FIGURE 2.8** shows a photograph of a normal fundus. The white circle is known as the optic disc. This is the point where the arteries and veins that feed the retina enter the eye and where the axons of ganglion cells (which we will get to shortly) leave the eye via the optic nerve. This portion of the retina contains no **photoreceptors**, and consequently it is blind. For that reason, it is referred to as the blind spot or physiological blind spot. You can experience your own blind spot, corresponding to the optic disc, by closing your left eye, fixating on the *F* in **FIGURE 2.9A** with your right eye, and adjusting the distance of the book from your eyes until the red circle disappears. You don't normally notice this large blind spot in your visual field because you have two eyes, and objects whose images

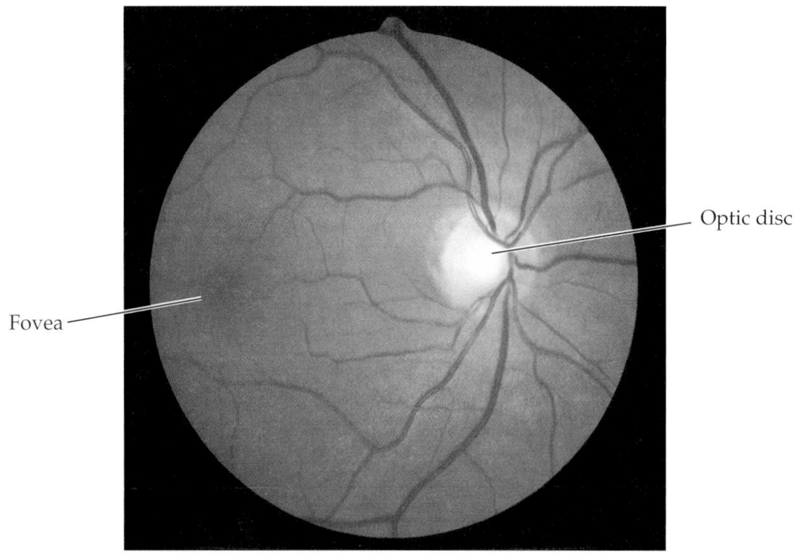

FIGURE 2.8 Fundus of the right eye of a human The branching blood vessels are called the vascular tree.

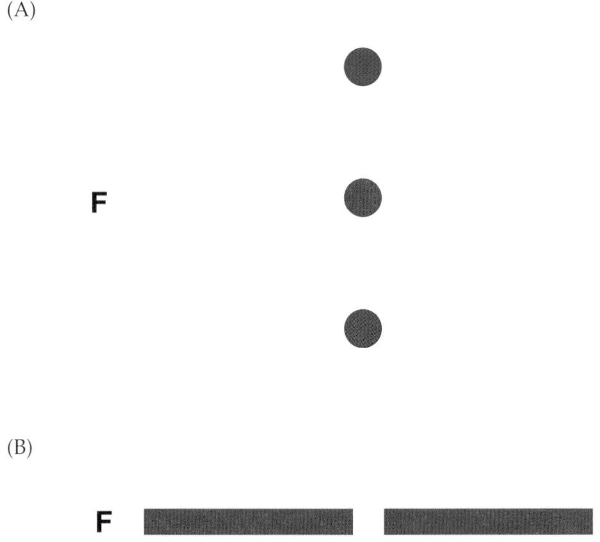

FIGURE 2.9 Your blind spot To experience your blind spot, close your left eye, fixating on the *F* in (A) with your right eye. Hold the book about 15 cm away from your eye to begin and adjust the distance of the book from your eyes until the red circle disappears. This is your blind spot. Ordinarily you are not aware of it, because the visual system "fills in" the blind spot with information from the surrounding area. If you fixate on the *F* in (B) with your right eye and again adjust the distance, when the gap in the line falls in your blind spot, it will be filled in and you will see a continuous red line.

fall into the blind spot of one eye can be seen by the other eye (see Chapter 6). However, even with the other eye closed, the visual system "fills in" the blind spot with information from the surrounding area (**FIGURE 2.9B**).

Another prominent feature of the fundus is the **fovea** (the 1.5-mm brownish spot in Figure 2.8), which is located near the center of the **macula**. The central ~0.5 mm of the fovea has no blood vessels, thus allowing all of the light to pass through. This anatomy is responsible for the depression in the center of the fovea (this depression can be seen more clearly in Figure 2.10). Note that the fovea is in the approximate center of the retina; however, it appears to be off to the side in Figure 2.8 because of the limited view of the fundus photo. The fundus is the only place in the body where one can see the arteries and veins directly, so it provides doctors with an important window on the well-being of the body's vascular system. The vascular "tree" (that is, the branched blood vessels) spreads out across the retina in a characteristic way, but stops short of the fovea.

You can see your own vascular tree by using a simple trick that requires only a penlight. In a dark room, close your eyes and place the penlight against the outside corner of one eye. Holding the penlight against the eye, gently move the light around (up and down, and back and forth). Within a few seconds you should see the shadows cast by your blood vessels looking like the branches of a tree. We don't normally see them, because the blood vessels move with our eyes, so their shadows are stabilized retinal images and, as with the blind spot, the visual system fills in behind them. The motion of the penlight makes the shadows move, enabling us to see them.

Even when viewed through an ophthalmoscope with a lot of magnification, the fundus does not provide a detailed view of the retina. The retina is the neural structure of the eye where transduction takes place. To get a good look at the structure of the retina, we need a cross section, which reveals that the retina is a layered sheet of clear neurons, about half the thickness of a credit card (Rodieck, 1998), with another layer of darker cells, the pigment epithelium, lying behind the final layer. While your eye doctor can't see this level of detail, she may use optical coherence tomography to see each layer of your retina in cross section (**FIGURE 2.10**). Optical coherence tomography is a noninvasive imaging technique that uses low-coherence light to capture high-resolution images from within light-scattering media (like the retina).

As we'll see in the next section, together these neurons constitute a minicomputer that begins the process of interpreting the information contained in visual images. The transduction of light energy into neural energy begins in the backmost layer of the retina, which is made up of photoreceptors. When photoreceptors sense light, they can stimulate neurons in the intermediate layers, including bipolar cells, horizontal cells, and amacrine cells. These neurons then connect with the frontmost layer of the retina, made up of ganglion cells, whose axons pass through the optic nerve to the brain.

Before we describe the function of these layers, we should address an obvious question regarding the structure of the retina: Why are the photoreceptors at the back—that is, in the last layer? This arrangement requires light to pass through the

fovea A small pit located near the center of the macula and containing the highest concentration of cones and no rods. It is the portion of the retina that produces the highest visual acuity and serves as the point of fixation.

macula The pigmented region with a diameter of about 5.5 millimeters near the center of the retina. It is sometimes referred to as the macula lutea (from the Latin) because of its yellow appearance.

rod A photoreceptor specialized for night vision.

cone A photoreceptor specialized for daylight vision, fine visual acuity, and color.

eccentricity The distance between the retinal image and the fovea.

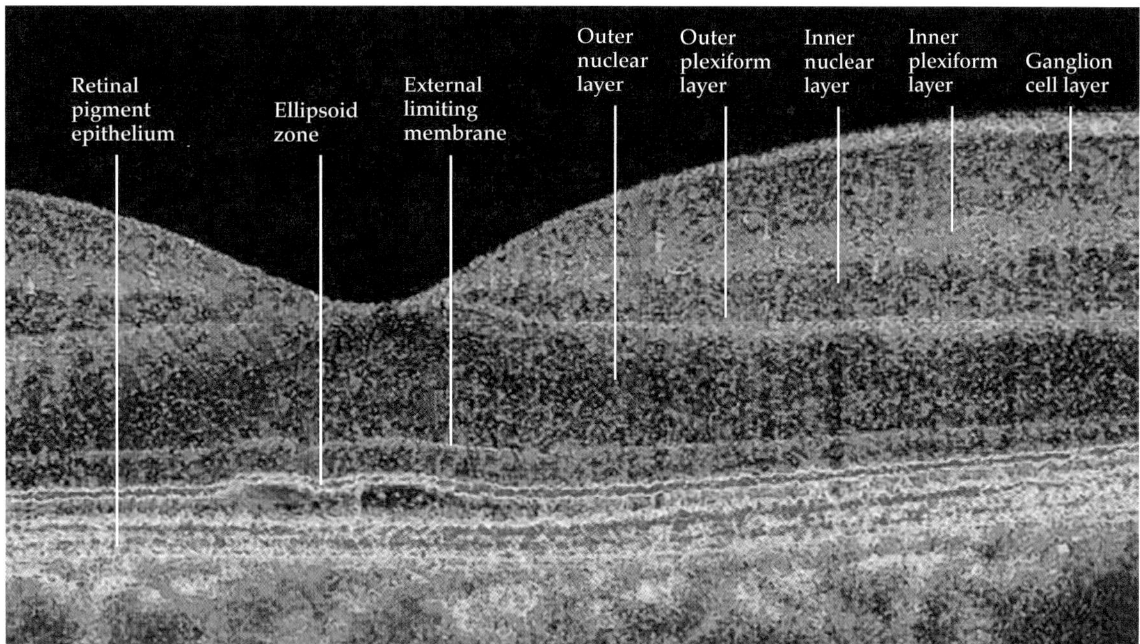

FIGURE 2.10 **Optical coherence tomography of the retina** A high-resolution cross section of the retina and pigment epithelium showing the different layers (as labeled). Note the foveal depression where the ganglion cell layer thins.

ganglion, horizontal, and amacrine cells before making contact with the photoreceptors. However, these neurons are mostly transparent, whereas cells in the pigment epithelium, which provide vital nutrients and recycling (or housekeeping) functions to the photoreceptors, are opaque. Once we see that the photoreceptors must be next to both the pigment epithelium, for nutrition and recycling, and the other neurons, in order to pass along their signals, the layering order makes much more sense.

duplex In reference to the retina, consisting of two parts: the rods and cones, which operate under different conditions.

visual angle The angle that an object subtends at the eye.

Retinal Geography and Function

Each retina contains roughly 100 million photoreceptors. These are the neurons that capture light and initiate the act of seeing by producing chemical signals. The human retina contains at least two types of photoreceptors: **rods** and **cones**. These two types not only have different shapes (which is how they earned their names; FIGURE 2.11), but also have different distributions across the retina and serve different functions.

Humans have many more rods (about 90 million in each eye) than cones (about 4–5 million in each eye), and the two types of cells have very different geographic distributions on the retina (FIGURE 2.12). Rods are completely absent from the center of the fovea, and their density increases to a peak at about 20 degrees and then declines again. The cones are most concentrated in the center of the fovea, and their density drops off dramatically with retinal **eccentricity** (distance from the fovea). The fovea is the "pit" in the inner retina that is specialized for seeing fine detail. Because human retinas have both rods and cones, they are considered **duplex** retinas. Some animals, such as rats and owls, have mostly rod retinas; others (e.g., certain lizards) have mostly cone retinas.

As the photographs of photoreceptors at different eccentricities in Figure 2.12 illustrate, in the foveal center (0.0 mm) the cones are smaller and more tightly packed than in other areas of the retina. This rod-free area (about 300 square micrometers [μm] on the retina) is directly behind the center of the pupil and subtends a **visual angle** (the angle at the eye) of about 1 degree. How big is 1 degree? Here's a rule

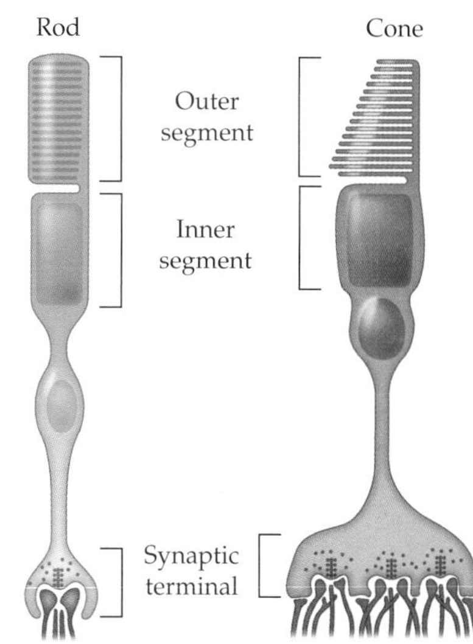

FIGURE 2.11 **Photoreceptors** Rod and cone.

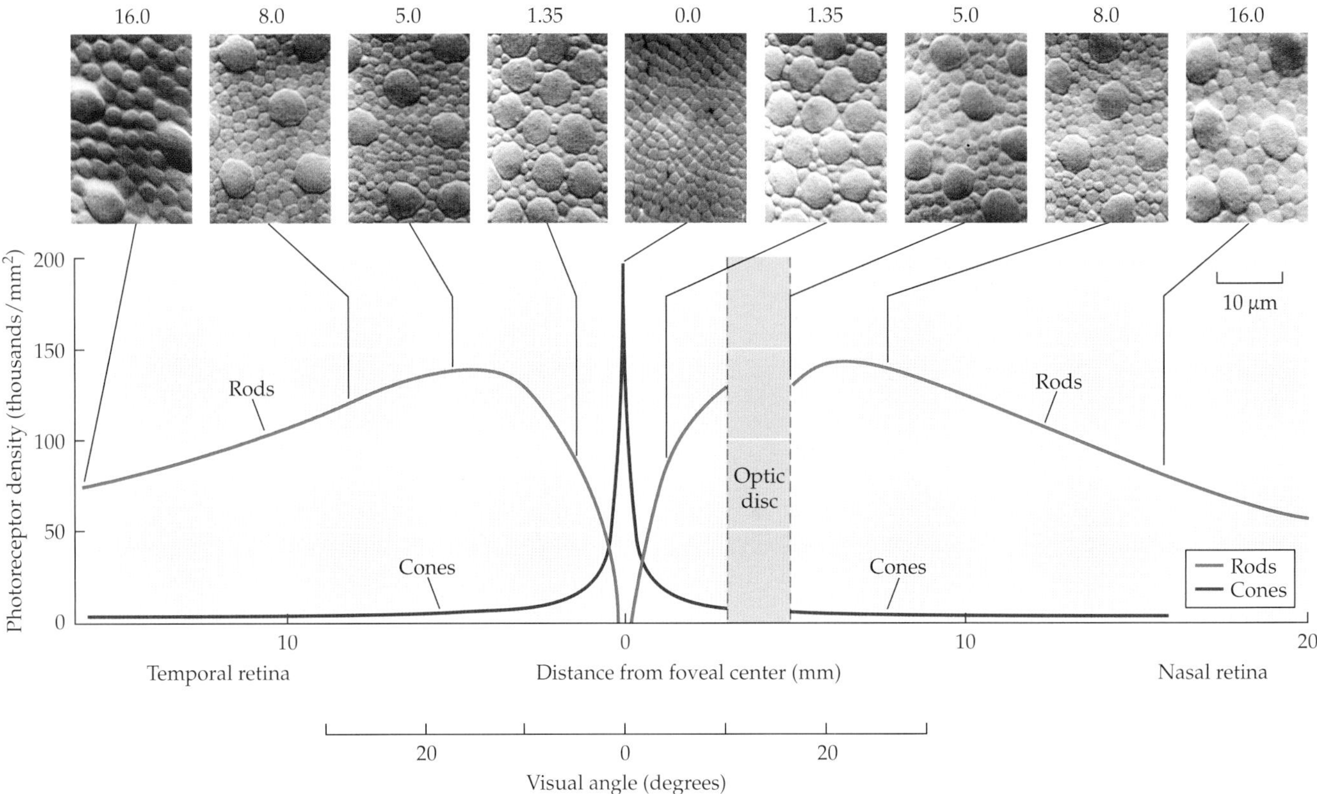

FIGURE 2.12 Photoreceptor density across the retina The top panels show slices through the photoreceptor inner segments at different eccentricities (distances from the fovea). The graph shows the density of rods and cones plotted as a function of distance from the fovea. Note that in the peripheral slices, the cones are always the larger cells.

of thumb, illustrated in **FIGURE 2.13**: your thumb, when viewed at arm's length, subtends an angle of about 2 degrees on the retina (assuming your thumb is about 2 cm across and your outstretched arm extends about 57 cm from your eye). So if we look directly at an object whose image is smaller than 1 degree, the image will land on a region of the retina that has only cones. You may have noticed that when you wake up in the middle of the night and head to the bathroom without turning on the lights, you don't have any problem moving around. That's because our rods provide us with sufficient information for navigation. However, we don't see a hole or a gap when we try to look directly at a small object with our rod-free fovea,

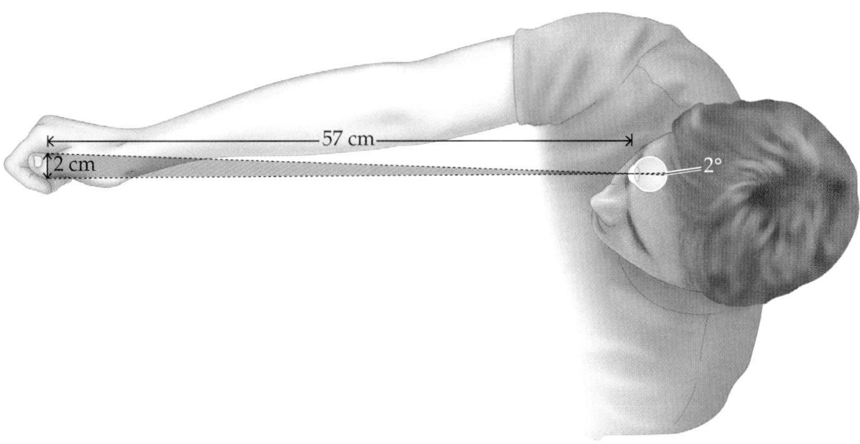

FIGURE 2.13 The "rule of thumb" When viewed at arm's length, your thumb subtends an angle of about 2 degrees on the retina.

even though the object itself may "disappear." Rather, the visual field appears to be seamlessly filled in by the surrounding retina. Interestingly, despite the absence of rods in the central 1 degree, a recent study shows that we place more trust in central vision than in peripheral vision, even in the dark (Gloriani and Schütz, 2019). Specifically, the study showed that when observers were asked to select either the central or the peripheral part of a stimulus for making perceptual judgments about the stimulus orientation, they typically chose the central part, despite the fact that what they saw in the central region (with their rod-free fovea) was an illusion, filled in from the peripheral part of the stimulus! **TABLE 2.1** illustrates some of the fundamental differences in the properties of the fovea compared with the peripheral retina. Most important for us, the fovea has high acuity and we use it to identify objects, to read, and to inspect fine detail. We use the periphery when detecting and localizing stimuli that we aren't looking at directly (e.g., seeing a moving truck out of the "corner of the eye").

The cones become larger and more sparse away from the foveal center, so the small cells that appear outside the fovea at 1.35 mm in Figure 2.12 are rods (they are about the same size as the cones are in the fovea, at 0.0 mm). In all of the micrographs except for the one at 0.0, the large cells are always the cones.

Rods and cones operate best under different lighting conditions: Rods function relatively well under conditions of dim (scotopic) illumination (which is why animals such as opossums with all-rod retinas are nocturnal), but cones require brighter (photopic) illumination (e.g., sunlight or room lights) to operate efficiently. Having an area at the center of the fovea with no rods means that under dim illumination the central 1 degree or so around the fovea is effectively blind! Indeed, practiced stargazers know that it is often easier to spot a dim star by looking out of the corner of one's eye than by looking directly at it. We will revisit photopic and scotopic vision again in Chapter 5.

Rods and cones differ functionally in another important way. Because all rods have the same type of photopigment, they cannot signal differences in color. Each cone, however, has one of three different photopigments that differ in the wavelengths at which they absorb light most efficiently. Therefore, cones can signal information about wavelength, and thus they provide the basis for our color vision.

You may wonder why we have both rods and cones and why 95% of our photoreceptors are rods, given that for city dwellers in this day and age, our vision is almost entirely mediated by cones. The answer is that roughly 400–500 million years ago, a particular fishy ancestor of ours developed rods (they already had cones), and this provided an advantage in survival at very low light levels at the bottom of the ocean. That advantage has survived till now (Lamb, 2016).

Rods and cones use a great deal of energy, which they get from the retinal pigment epithelium, which lies below the retina. Recent work suggests that the rods and cones burn glucose, converting the leftovers into lactate, which they

● TABLE 2.1 Properties of the fovea and periphery in human vision

Property	Fovea	Periphery
Photoreceptor type	Mostly cones	Mostly rods
Bipolar cell type	Midget	Diffuse
Convergence	Low	High
Receptive-field size	Small	Large
Acuity (detail)	High	Low
Light sensitivity	Low	High

feed back to the retinal pigment epithelium, which in turn uses the lactate for its energy (Kanow et al., 2017).

FURTHER DISCUSSION of cones and color detection can be found in Section 5.2.

2.3 Dark and Light Adaptation

When you enter a dark room from bright sunlight, the number of photons of light entering your eye might be reduced by a factor of several billion (more than 12 log units) (**FIGURE 2.14**). Initially you will have trouble seeing anything, but after about 30 minutes in the dark, you will be able to detect even just a few photons. The solid purple curve in **FIGURE 2.15** illustrates the change in the threshold light intensity, or the least light needed, to detect a peripheral spot (see Chapter 1 for a discussion of thresholds). Initially the threshold is very high, indicating low sensitivity. But over 20 minutes or so, the threshold is greatly reduced (meaning sensitivity is increased). And when you emerge from the dark and return to the sunlight, you will be able to see almost instantly. How does the visual system alter its sensitivity over such a large operating range?

There are four primary ways in which the visual system adjusts to changes in illumination: pupil size, photopigment regeneration, the duplex retina, and neural circuitry.

Pupil Size

When a flashlight is shone in someone's eye in a dimly lit room, the pupil quickly constricts. The diameter of the pupil can vary by about a factor of 4, from about 2 mm in bright illumination to about 8 mm in the dark (**FIGURE 2.16**). Because the amount of light entering the eye is proportional to the area of the pupil, the 4-fold increase in diameter accounts for a 16-fold improvement in sensitivity. In other words, 16 times as many quanta can enter the eye when the pupil is completely dilated, compared with when it is constricted. Although this adaptive ability certainly helps, pupil dilation has a time course of a few seconds, while dark adaptation takes many minutes. Thus, pupil size accounts for only a small part of the visual system's overall ability to adapt to light and dark conditions.

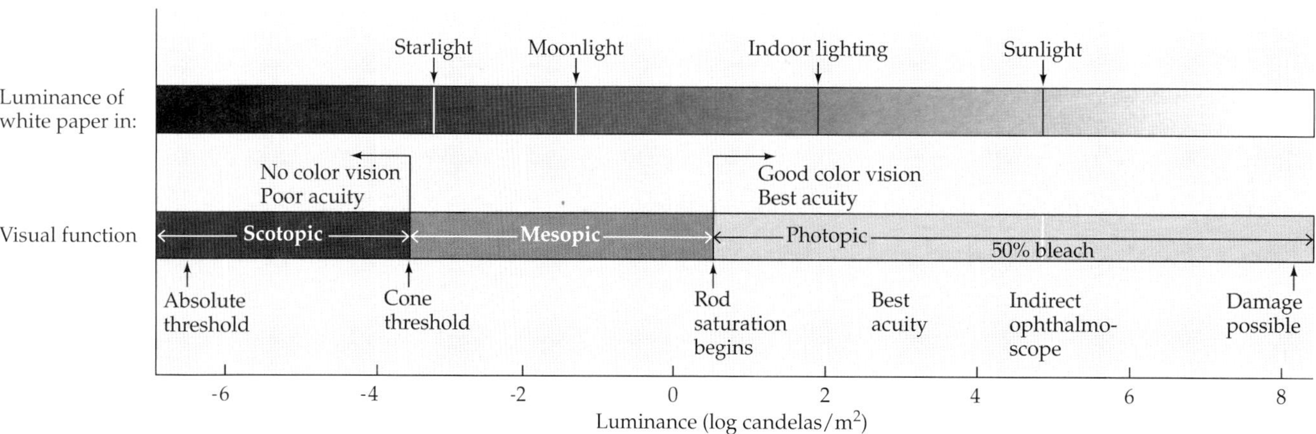

FIGURE 2.14 Luminance levels The visual system operates over a huge range of luminance levels, from just a few photons to very bright sunshine.

Photopigment Regeneration

A second mechanism for achieving a large sensitivity range is provided by the way photopigments are used up and replaced in receptor cells. In dim lighting conditions, plenty of photopigment is available, and rods and cones absorb and respond to as many photons as they can. As already noted, rods provide better sensitivity in such situations than do cones. Indeed, the rod system is capable of detecting a single quantum of light! After a photopigment molecule is bleached (used to detect a photon), the molecule must be regenerated before it can be used again to absorb another photon.

As the overall light level increases, the number of photons starts to overwhelm the system: photopigment molecules cannot be regenerated fast enough to detect all the photons hitting the photoreceptors. This slow regeneration is a good thing for increasing our sensitivity range. If photons are scarce, we use them all to see; if we have an overabundance, we simply throw some of them away and use the leftovers.

Interestingly, at very low light levels, we are about a factor of 2 more sensitive to a *decrease* in light levels (as might occur if there were a shadow) than to an increase (Patel and Jones, 1968). This might be important for survival if you are a mouse foraging for food in dim light trying to avoid being eaten by a cat! Recent work suggests that near threshold, decreases in illumination in dim light are detected via OFF retinal ganglion cells (Westö et al., 2022; Fain, 2022).

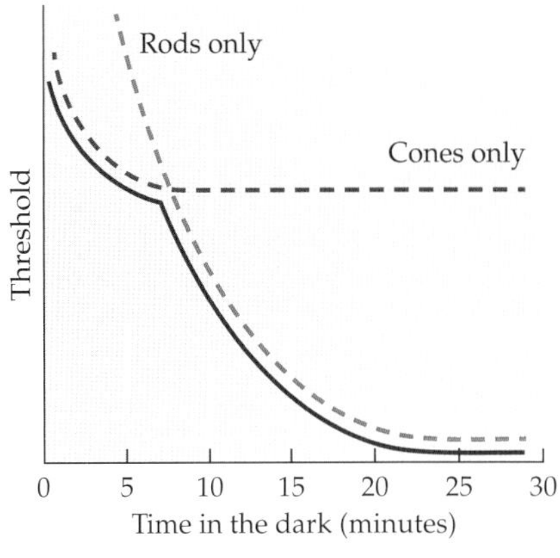

FIGURE 2.15 Dark adaptation The solid purple curve shows the threshold light intensity required to detect a peripheral spot following several minutes of adaptation to a bright light. The dashed red curve illustrates the rapid adaptation of the cones. The dashed blue curve shows the slower recovery of the rods to much lower threshold intensities (that is, greater sensitivity). The solid purple curve represents the more sensitive of the two at any given time.

The Duplex Retina

The light compensation mechanism is enhanced by humans' duplex retinas. Rods provide exquisite sensitivity at low light levels, but they become overwhelmed when the background light becomes moderately bright, leading to a loss in information quality. Cones are much less sensitive than rods (they function poorly under very dim light), but their operating range is much larger, stretching from about ten photons per second (just enough light to see color) to hundreds of thousands of photons per second (e.g., a snowcapped mountain in bright sunlight). So we use rods to see when the light is low, and the cones take over when there is too much light for the rods to function well. After adapting to a bright light, cones recover sensitivity quickly (dashed red curve in Figure 2.15) and then saturate. They are not very sensitive to very dim light. Rods recover more slowly (dashed blue curve in Figure 2.15), but after 20 minutes or so they are very sensitive to dim light. When our eyes are fully dark adapted, lights that are close to the detection threshold appear colorless.

(A) Darkness

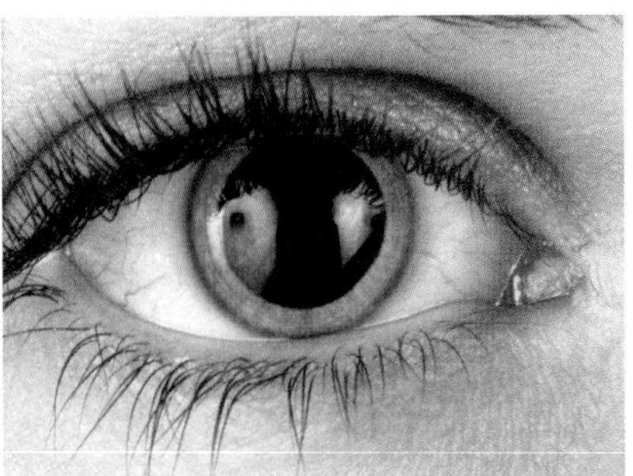

8-mm pupil

(B) Bright illumination

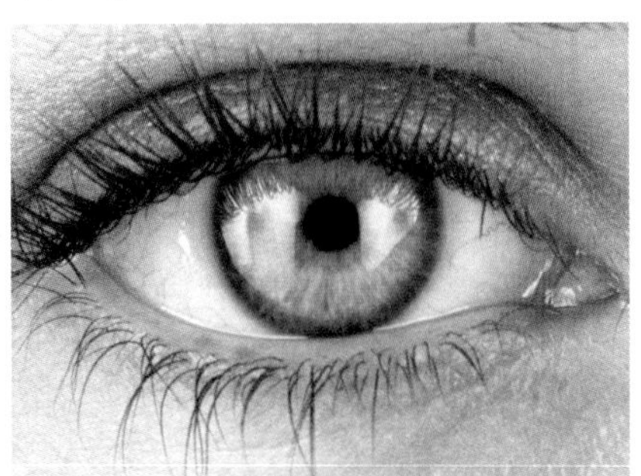

2-mm pupil

FIGURE 2.16 Two pupils The black spots in the middle of these two irises show the possible range of pupil sizes as we go from darkness (A) into bright illumination (B).

receptive field The region on the retina in which visual stimuli influence a neuron's firing rate.

age-related macular degeneration A disease associated with aging that affects the macula. It gradually destroys sharp central vision, making it difficult to read, drive, and recognize faces. There are two forms: wet and dry.

retinitis pigmentosa A progressive degeneration of the retina that affects night vision and peripheral vision. It commonly runs in families and can be caused by defects in a number of different genes that have recently been identified.

Neural Circuitry

Although pupil size, photopigment regeneration rates, and the rod/cone dichotomy all play a role in dark and light adaptation, the most important reason we are not bothered by variations in overall light levels has to do with the neural circuitry of the retina. As we will see below, a ganglion cell is most sensitive to *differences* in the intensity of the light in the center and in the surround of its **receptive field**, the region on the retina (and the corresponding region in visual space) in which visual stimuli influence the neuron's firing rate. Ganglion cells are less affected by the average intensity of the light. But they will still fire at an above-spontaneous rate when light falls on the entire receptive field, as long as the photoreceptors feeding the ganglion cells are not completely saturated. Thus, the ganglion cells will encode the pattern of relatively light and relatively dark areas in the retinal image. And the pattern of illumination, not the overall light level, is the primary concern of the rest of the visual system.

To sum up, the answer to the question of how the visual system deals with such large variations in overall light levels has two parts. First, we reduce the scale of the problem by regulating the amount of light entering the eyeball, by using different types of photoreceptors in different situations, and by effectively throwing away photons we don't need. Second, by responding to the contrast between adjacent retinal regions, the ganglion cells do their best to ignore whatever variation in overall light level is left over.

Sensation & Perception in Everyday Life

When Good Retina Goes Bad

Millions of people around the world suffer from blinding diseases in which the rods and/or cones degenerate. These include **age-related macular degeneration** and **retinitis pigmentosa**. At present, there are no effective cures to prevent the progressive degeneration of the photoreceptors that occurs in these diseases. For people with age-related macular degeneration, this may lead to an inability to read or recognize faces. For people with long-standing retinitis pigmentosa, this leads inevitably to irreversible blindness.

Early attempts to assist the blind were based on "sensory substitution"—the idea that the sense of touch could act as a substitute for the loss of vision. Bach-y-Rita and his colleagues (Bach-y-Rita et al., 1969) connected a TV camera to an array of 400 tactile stimulators that vibrated against the skin of the backs of blind study participants. Following extensive training, these individuals were able to discriminate the orientation of lines and recognize some geometric shapes. Unfortunately, the skin has very poor resolution compared with vision, and this approach was largely abandoned. A more recent attempt to substitute another sense for vision uses auditory substitution—a device that converts visual signals to auditory signals (J. Ward and Meijer, 2010). Like the earlier attempts at sensory substitution, this approach has limitations. ●

Fortunately, there are several exciting technological developments that provide hope for people who are blind. These are all based on the notion that while the photoreceptors are dead or dying, postreceptoral neurons and their connections are largely intact. One approach is to substitute an electronic prosthesis (an artificial device to replace or augment a missing or impaired part of the body) into the retina. Typically, the prosthesis uses a camera to convert light into energy; an array of electrodes implanted in the retina generates an electrical stimulation pattern based on the light pattern on the camera and delivers this stimulation pattern to the intact postreceptoral neurons (**FIGURE 2.17**). Unfortunately, while these retinal prostheses can restore some sight, there are technical challenges to implanting them, and they suffer low spatial resolution (Weiland, Cho, and Humayun, 2011), allowing only perception of spots of light and very-high-contrast edges.

Another approach that has had some early success in animal models is to use gene therapy to express light-activated channels in surviving photoreceptors

Sensation & Perception in Everyday Life *(continued)*

using adeno-associated viral vectors. This approach has been successfully used in several clinical trials in patients.

A third strategy is to chemically modify endogenous channels in retinal ganglion cells to make them light-sensitive. This approach essentially adds a synthetic small molecule "photoswitch" to confer light sensitivity onto retinal ganglion cells, and it has been shown to reinstate light sensitivity in blind mice (Tochitsky et al., 2014). One limitation of this approach is their low light sensitivity and inability to adapt to changes in ambient lighting. However, recent work (Berry et al., 2019) suggests that medium-wavelength cone opsin overcomes these limitations, enabling blind mice with retinitis pigmentosa to function well in low-light conditions and to adapt to changes in ambient lighting.

Each of these approaches provides promise for new treatments for people with blinding retinal disorders.

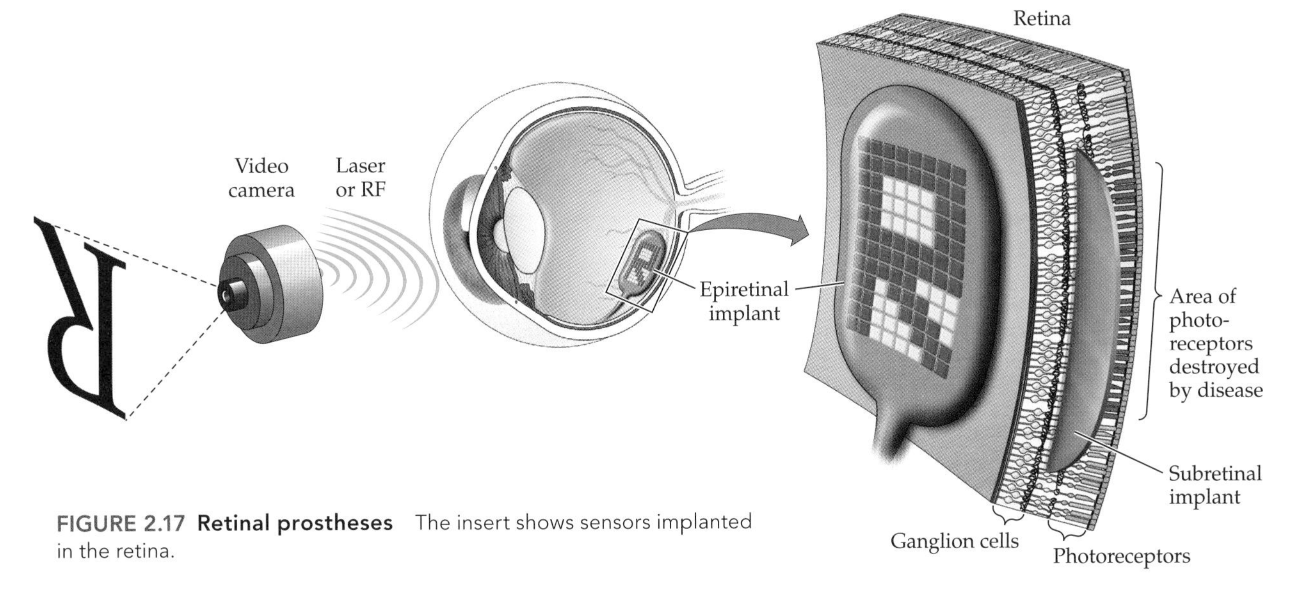

FIGURE 2.17 **Retinal prostheses** The insert shows sensors implanted in the retina.

2.4 Retinal Information Processing

The retina contains five major classes of neurons: photoreceptors, horizontal cells, bipolar cells, amacrine cells, and ganglion cells mentioned earlier in this chapter. Let's take a closer look at the functions of each of these cell types.

Light Transduction by Rod and Cone Photoreceptors

When photoreceptors capture light, they produce chemical changes that start a cascade of neural events ending in a visual sensation. Photoreceptors send their signals by way of the synaptic terminals, specialized structures for contacting other retinal neurons. Figure 2.11 shows examples of rod and cone synaptic terminals. The synaptic terminals contain connections from the neurons that photoreceptors "talk to": the horizontal and bipolar cells.

Both types of photoreceptors consist of an **outer segment** (which is adjacent to the pigment epithelium), an **inner segment**, and a **synaptic terminal**. Molecules called visual pigments are made in the inner segment (which is like a little factory, filled with mitochondria) and stored in the outer segment, where they are incorporated into the membrane. Each visual pigment molecule consists of a protein (an opsin),

outer segment The part of a photoreceptor that contains photopigment molecules.

inner segment The part of a photoreceptor that lies between the outer segment and the cell nucleus.

synaptic terminal The location where axons terminate at the synapse for transmission of information by the release of a chemical transmitter.

chromophore The light-catching part of the visual pigments of the retina.

rhodopsin The visual pigment found in rods.

melanopsin A photopigment that is sensitive to ambient light.

photoactivation Activation by light.

hyperpolarization A change in membrane potential such that the inner membrane surface becomes more negative than the outer membrane surface.

graded potential An electrical potential that can vary continuously in amplitude.

the structure of which determines which wavelengths of light the pigment molecule absorbs, and a **chromophore**, which captures light photons. The chromophore is the part of the pigment molecule that determines its color by selectively absorbing specific wavelengths of light. The chromophore, known as Retinal, is derived from vitamin A, which is in turn manufactured from beta-carotene, which is why your mother told you to eat your carrots! The opsin and chromophore are connected. Each photoreceptor has only one of the four types of visual pigments found in the human retina. The pigment **rhodopsin** is found in the rods, concentrated mainly in the stack of membranous discs in the outer segment. Each cone has one of the other three pigments, each of which responds to long, medium, or short wavelengths only. Figure 5.1 shows the absorption spectra of the four photoreceptor types.

Evidence suggests that there may be another type of photoreceptor—one that "lives" among the ganglion cells and that is involved in adjusting our biological rhythms to match the day and night of the external world (Baringa, 2002). These photoreceptors are sensitive to the ambient light level and contain the photopigment **melanopsin**, and they send their signals to the suprachiasmatic nucleus, the home of the brain's circadian clock, which regulates 24-hour patterns of behavior and physiology. They are known as melanopsin-containing retinal ganglion cells or intrinsically photosensitive retinal ganglion cells (ipRGCs). The melanopsin signals may also influence pupil responses (Spitschan et al., 2014).

When a photon from our favorite star makes its way into the outer segment of a rod and is absorbed by a molecule of rhodopsin, it transfers its energy to the chromophore portion of the visual pigment molecule. This process, known as **photoactivation** (also referred to as bleaching), initiates a biochemical cascade of events eventually resulting in the closing of cell membrane channels that normally allow ions to flow into the rod's outer segment. Closing these channels alters the balance of electrical current between the inside and outside of the rod's outer segment, making the inside of the cell more negatively charged. This process is known as **hyperpolarization**. Hyperpolarization closes voltage-gated calcium channels at the synaptic terminal, thereby reducing the concentration of free calcium inside the cells. The lowering of the calcium concentration, in turn, reduces the concentration of neurotransmitter (glutamate) molecules released in the synapse, and this change signals to the bipolar cell that the rod has captured a photon. The entire sequence of events takes only a matter of milliseconds. While we have focused this discussion on rhodopsin, cone visual pigment molecules act in a qualitatively similar fashion.

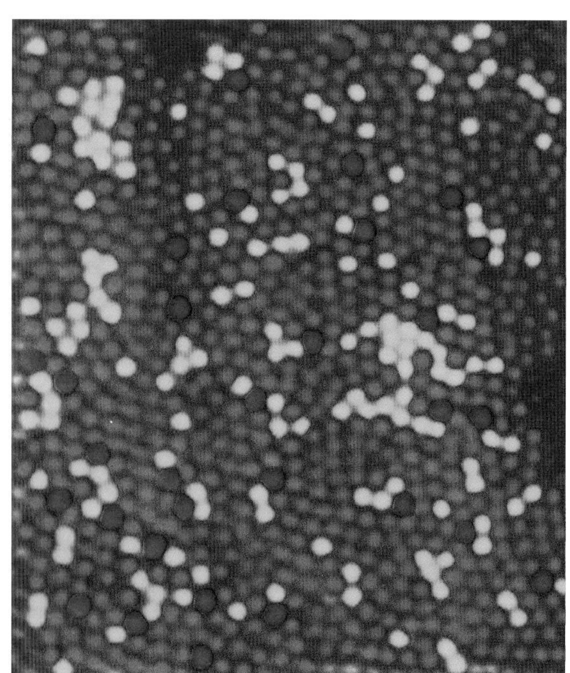

FIGURE 2.18 **Cones in a live human** Blue, green, and red represent the S-, M-, and L-cones, respectively, of a living human being in a patch of retina at 1 degree from the fovea. This pseudocolor image was made by the use of adaptive optics, to measure and bypass the aberrations of the eye, and of selective bleaching, to isolate the different photopigments.

The amount of glutamate present in the photoreceptor–bipolar cell synapse at any one time is inversely proportional to the number of photons being absorbed by the photoreceptor. Thus, unlike most other types of neurons, photoreceptors do not respond in an all-or-nothing fashion. They pass their information on to bipolar cells via **graded potentials**, which vary in size, instead of all-or-none action potentials or spikes, which are found throughout the nervous system (see Chapter 1).

The three cone photopigments are not distributed equally among the cones (**FIGURE 2.18**). Short wavelength–sensitive cones (S-cones) constitute only about 5–10% of the total cone population, and they are essentially missing from the center of the fovea. Thus, the foveal center is dichromatic (it has only two color-sensitive cone types). We also know that there are more long wavelength–sensitive cones (L-cones)

● **TABLE 2.2** Properties of human photopic and scotopic vision

Property	Photopic system	Scotopic system
Photoreceptor	4–5 million cones	90 million rods
Location in retina	Throughout retina, with highest concentration close to fovea	Outside fovea
Spatial acuity (detail)	High	Low
Light sensitivity	Low	High
Response speed	Fast	Slow
Saturation	No saturation	Saturate at ~twilight levels
Dark adaptation	Recovery in ~5 minutes	Recovery in ~40 minutes
Light adaptation	Fast (Weber's law)	Slow (square root law)
Color vision	Trichromatic	None

than medium wavelength–sensitive cones (M-cones); it has been estimated that there are, on average, about twice as many L-cones as M-cones, although the ratio of L- to M-cones varies enormously among individuals. **TABLE 2.2** illustrates some of the fundamental differences in the properties of the photopic (high-illumination) and scotopic (low-illumination) visual systems.

Lateral Inhibition through Horizontal and Amacrine Cells

As the name implies, **horizontal cells** run perpendicular to the photoreceptors, making contacts between nearby photoreceptors. These lateral connections play an important functional role in the form of **lateral inhibition**, which enables the signals that reach retinal ganglion cells to be based on differences in activation between nearby photoreceptors. Lateral inhibition plays an important role in visual perception, as well as in several visual illusions (e.g., Mach bands and the Hermann grid). We will have more to say about lateral inhibition in the "Center-Surround Receptive Fields" section.

Amacrine cells are also part of the lateral pathway. Like horizontal cells, amacrine cells run perpendicular to the photoreceptors in the inner layers of the retina, where they receive inputs from bipolar cells and other amacrine cells and send signals to bipolar, amacrine, and retinal ganglion cells. Amacrine cells come in many flavors, by some estimates as many as 40 (Rodieck, 1998). Although amacrine cells have been implicated in both contrast enhancement and temporal sensitivity (the detection of changes in light patterns over time), their precise function remains unclear.

Convergence and Divergence of Information via Bipolar Cells

If horizontal and amacrine cells form a lateral pathway in the retina, then photoreceptors, bipolar cells, and ganglion cells can be considered to form a vertical pathway. Bipolar cells are the intermediaries. There are various types of bipolar cells, and their wiring determines the information that is passed from the photoreceptors to the ganglion cells. For example, in peripheral vision a **bipolar cell** receives input from as many as 50 photoreceptors, pools this information, and passes it on to a ganglion cell. This convergence of information from many photoreceptors to a **diffuse bipolar cell** (a single bipolar cell) is a characteristic of the rod pathway, and the same sort of convergence also occurs in the cone pathway in the peripheral retina.

Pooling of information from many photoreceptors is a very important mechanism for increasing visual **sensitivity**. Indeed, the fact that most rods communicate with ganglion cells through diffuse bipolar cells largely accounts for the ability of the

horizontal cell A specialized retinal cell that contacts both photoreceptor and bipolar cells.

lateral inhibition Antagonistic neural interaction between adjacent regions of the retina.

amacrine cell A retinal cell found in the inner nuclear layer that makes synaptic contacts with bipolar cells, ganglion cells, and other amacrine cells.

bipolar cell A retinal cell that synapses with either rods or cones (not both) and with horizontal cells and then passes the signals on to ganglion cells.

diffuse bipolar cell A bipolar retinal cell whose processes are spread out to receive input from multiple cones.

sensitivity 1. The ability to perceive via the sense organs. 2. Extreme responsiveness to radiation, especially to light of a specific wavelength. 3. The ability to respond to transmitted signals.

visual acuity A measure of the finest detail that can be resolved by the eyes.

midget bipolar cell A small bipolar cell in the central retina that receives input from a single cone.

ON bipolar cell A bipolar cell that depolarizes in response to an increase in light captured by the cones.

OFF bipolar cell A bipolar cell that hyperpolarizes in response to an increase in light captured by the cones.

ganglion cell A retinal cell that receives visual information from photoreceptors via two intermediate neuron types (bipolar cells and amacrine cells) and transmits information to the brain and midbrain.

P ganglion cell A small ganglion cell that receives excitatory input from single midget bipolar cells in the central retina and feeds the parvocellular layer of the lateral geniculate nucleus.

M ganglion cell A ganglion cell resembling a little umbrella that receives excitatory input from diffuse bipolar cells and feeds the magnocellular layer of the lateral geniculate nucleus.

koniocellular cell A neuron located between the magnocellular and parvocellular layers of the lateral geniculate nucleus. This layer is known as the koniocellular layer.

rod system to function well in dim lighting conditions. A diffuse bipolar cell may respond at the same rate in response to a single point of bright light or several spots of dim light, since multiple photoreceptors synapse on each diffuse bipolar cell, and a ganglion cell listening to the diffuse bipolar cell will be unable to tell which pattern of light is present. The high degree of neural convergence in peripheral vision has important consequences for **visual acuity**, which falls off rapidly with eccentricity (see Table 2.1).

FURTHER DISCUSSION of visual acuity can be found in Section 3.1.

In contrast, in the fovea, **midget bipolar cells** receive input from single cones and pass this information on to single ganglion cells. The fact that one-to-one pathways between cones and ganglion cells exist only in the fovea accounts for why images are seen most clearly when they fall on this part of the retina. The high degree of convergence in the retinal periphery ensures high sensitivity to light but poor acuity. The low degree of convergence in the fovea ensures high acuity but poor sensitivity to light (see Table 2.2).

Each foveal cone contacts two bipolar cells (representing a divergence of information): one depolarizes in response to an increase in light captured by the cone and is called an **ON bipolar cell**; the other hyperpolarizes and is called an **OFF bipolar cell**. ON and OFF bipolar cells respond differently to the same photoreceptor input because they express different types of postsynaptic glutamate receptors that ultimately lead to changes in membrane potential in opposite directions.

The existence of both ON and OFF bipolar cells provides information about whether the retinal illumination increased or decreased, and as we will see, the ON/OFF distinction built into the anatomical structure of the retina is present at many levels of the visual pathway.

Communicating to the Brain via Ganglion Cells

By the time signals arrive at the **ganglion cells**, the final layer of the retina, there has already been a lot of information processing. Some information has been pooled through convergence; some has been enhanced or inhibited by lateral pathways.

By now you are probably getting the idea that each cell type comes in many varieties, and ganglion cells are no exception. The human retina contains about 1,250,000 ganglion cells, about 1% of the number of photoreceptors. Midget bipolar cells send their signals to small ganglion cells, which are widely referred to as **P ganglion cells** because they feed the parvocellular ("small cell") layer of the lateral geniculate nucleus (discussed in Chapter 3). P ganglion cells constitute about 70% of the ganglion cells in the human retina. Diffuse bipolar cells project to ganglion cells that are known as **M ganglion cells** (FIGURE 2.19) because they feed the magnocellular ("large cell") layer of the lateral geniculate nucleus. The dendrites of the M ganglion cells spread out much more than those of the P ganglion cells, giving them an umbrellalike appearance. About 8–10% of ganglion cells in the human retina are of the M variety. The dendrites of both P and M ganglion cells increase in size with retinal eccentricity, but at all eccentricities the P ganglion cells have much smaller dendritic trees than do the M ganglion cells.

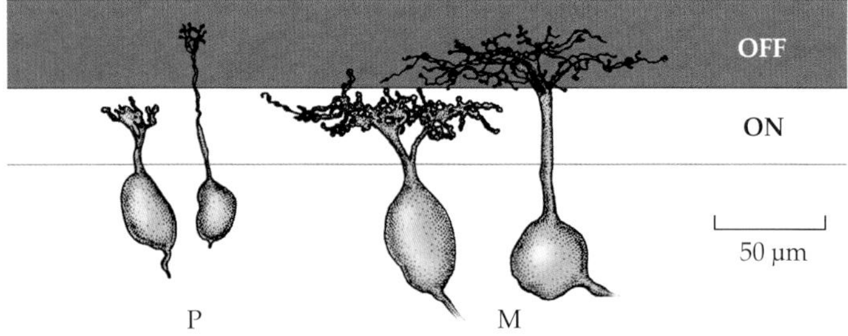

FIGURE 2.19 **Retinal ganglion cells** Different types of retinal P and M ganglion cells. Shown are ganglion cells in section.

The astute reader may have noticed that M and P ganglion cells together constitute about 80% of all ganglion cells. Other ganglion cells, the bistratified ganglion cells also known as **koniocellular cells**, project to koniocellular layers in the lateral geniculate nucleus. Some of these, with input from S-cones, may be part of a "primordial" blue-yellow pathway, while yet other ganglion cells that project to the koniocellular layers are thought to correspond to "nonblue" koniocellular cells. For a functional classification of the many (and often confusing) types of retinal cells, see Vlasits, Euler, and Franke (2019).

CENTER-SURROUND RECEPTIVE FIELDS Much of what we know about how retinal ganglion cells work comes from painstaking physiological studies in which tiny electrodes are used to study the electrical changes in individual ganglion cells. Ganglion cells fire action potentials spontaneously, at about one spike per second, even in the absence of visual stimulation. However, each ganglion cell has a small window on the world known as its receptive field. As noted earlier, the receptive field is the region on the retina (and the corresponding region in visual space) in which visual stimuli influence the neuron's firing rate. This influence can be either excitatory, increasing the ganglion's firing rate, or inhibitory, decreasing the ganglion's firing rate.

FURTHER DISCUSSION of receptive fields can be found in Section 3.5.

Work on horseshoe crabs and frogs provided some of our earliest information on the receptive fields of retinal neurons (Hartline, 1940). But it was Stephen Kuffler who first mapped out the receptive fields of individual retinal ganglion cells in the cat, using small spots of light (Kuffler, 1953). **FIGURE 2.20** illustrates Kuffler's main

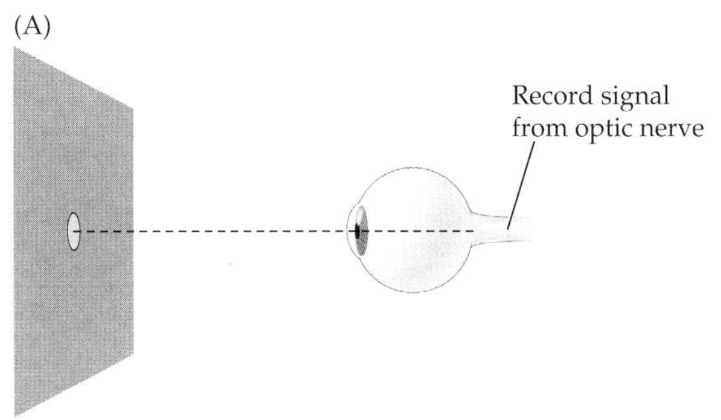

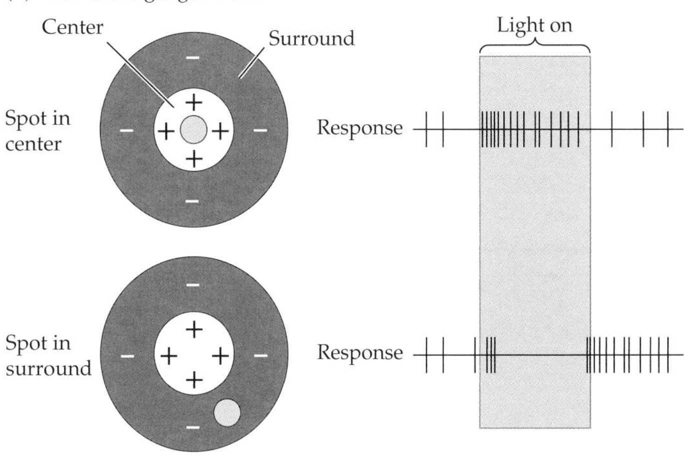

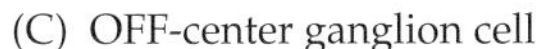

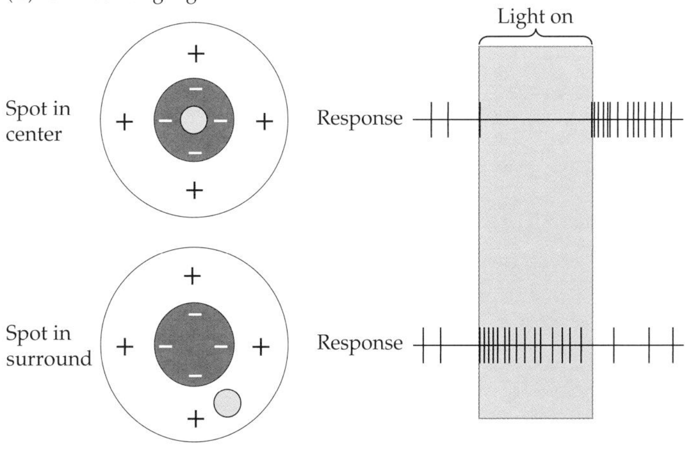

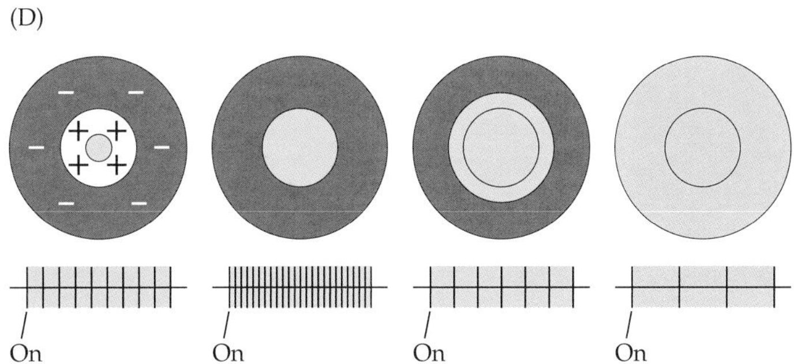

FIGURE 2.20 Retinal ganglion cell receptive fields
(A) Mapping retinal receptive fields. (B) ON-center field. In each image on the left, the small white circle illustrates the region on the retina where the retinal ganglion cell increased its firing rate when the spot (small yellow circle) was turned on. The large gray circle illustrates the region on the retina where the retinal ganglion cell decreased its firing rate when the spot was turned on and increased its rate when the spot was turned off. The plots on the right illustrate the spikes fired by the associated retinal ganglion cell. (C) OFF-center field. In each image on the left, the large white circle illustrates the region on the retina where the retinal ganglion cell increased its firing rate when the spot was turned on. The small gray circle illustrates the region on the retina where the retinal ganglion cell decreased its firing rate when the spot was turned on and increased its rate when the spot was turned off. The plots on the right illustrate the spikes fired by the associated retinal ganglion cell. (D) The effect of varying the spot size. Note that firing is fastest when the spot just fills the receptive-field center. Increasing the spot size further results in reduced firing because of lateral inhibition from the surround.

ON-center cell A cell that increases firing in response to an increase in light intensity in its receptive-field center.

OFF-center cell A cell that increases firing in response to a decrease in light intensity in its receptive-field center.

filter An acoustic, electrical, electronic, or optical device, instrument, computer program, or neuron that allows the passage of some frequencies or digital elements and blocks the passage of others.

contrast The difference in luminance between an object and the background or between lighter and darker parts of the same object.

findings, which also apply to the retina in primates, and provides some important insights into how the retina processes visual information.

Let's consider Figure 2.20B. Kuffler's visual stimulus was a small spot of light on a projector screen, which moved about on the retina, turning on and off while he recorded impulses from a single retinal ganglion cell. When the spot was placed on a specific small region of the retina, the ganglion cell *increased* its firing rate when the light was turned on (this response is indicated by a plus sign in the figure). This area of the retina is called the "center" of the ganglion cell's receptive field. When the spot was moved to an adjacent area of the retina, the ganglion cell *decreased* its firing rate when the light was turned on (indicated by a minus sign). It is interesting that turning the light *off* in this area surrounding the receptive-field center led to a brief surge in the cell's firing rate, after which the cell settled down to its spontaneous rate.

The cell just described is known as an **ON-center cell**. It increases its firing rate when a light is turned on in the center of its receptive field, and it decreases its firing rate when the light is turned on in the surround. However, nearly as many ganglion cells do exactly the opposite: their firing rates decrease when a light is turned on in a spot in the center of the receptive field and increase when a light is turned on in a spot in the surround. These are known as **OFF-center cells** (Figure 2.20C). Most retinal ganglion cells have one of these two types of concentric center-surround organization.

An important finding of Kuffler's was that the spatial layout of the ganglion cell's receptive field is essentially concentric; that is, a small circular area in the center responds to an increase in illumination, and a surrounding ring responds to a decrease in illumination, and size matters! The ganglion cell fires fastest when the size of the spot of light matches the size of the excitatory center. (The size of the receptive-field center reflects the convergence discussed above, that is, the number of photoreceptors and bipolar cells that feed into the retinal ganglion cell center.) The ganglion cell reduces its firing rate when the spot of light begins to encroach on its inhibitory surround (Figure 2.20D). This antagonistic interaction between the center and surround is known as lateral inhibition and is mediated in part by horizontal cells.

The center-surround organization has two important functional consequences. First, as noted above, each ganglion cell will respond best to spots of a particular size (and will respond less to spots that are either bigger or smaller). In this way, retinal ganglion cells act as a **filter** by responding best to stimuli that are just the right size and less to stimuli that are larger or smaller. Second, ganglion cells are most sensitive to *differences* in the intensity of the light in the center and in the surround, and they are less affected by the average intensity of the light. This is a useful quality because the average intensity of the light falling on the retina varies a lot, depending on whether you are indoors or outdoors, whether it is daytime or nighttime, how far away you and the objects you're looking at are from the source of illumination, and so on. But the **contrast**—the difference in luminance or brightness between adjacent bits of the scene—will be roughly the same regardless of lighting conditions.

The center-surround antagonism, or lateral inhibition, also has other important perceptual consequences, resulting in the illusions of stripes and spots (**FIGURE 2.21**).

Phenomenologically, we have the impression that our eyes work like video cameras, capturing faithful snapshots of the world around us. Note, though, that the rest of the visual system sees only what the retinal ganglion cells show it, and the ganglion cells are not content simply to pass along the raw images encoded by the photoreceptors. Instead, the ganglion cells, together with the bipolar, amacrine, and horizontal cells, act as an image filter, transforming the raw image into a new representation. This new representation highlights certain important information, such as contrast, and largely discounts other types of less useful information, such as ambient light intensity. In fact, the whole visual system can be considered a long series of filters, with each stage in the system responsible for extracting a particular aspect of the visual world and passing this aspect on to the next stage.

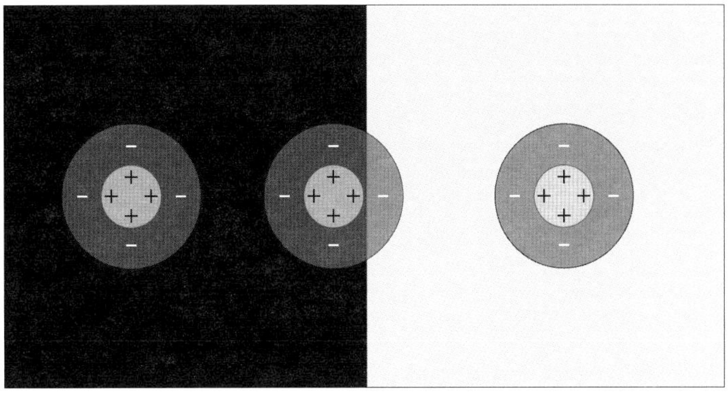

FIGURE 2.21 Mach bands Diagram showing a classic neuronal explanation for the optical illusion of stripes where none actually appears (known as Mach bands). See the text for details on center-surround organization and antagonism.

P AND M GANGLION CELLS REVISITED As already mentioned, retinal ganglion cells come in several types; for human visual perception, the most important of these are the P and M cells. The receptive fields of these two types of ganglion cells differ in some important ways. First, at all eccentricities, P cells have smaller receptive fields than M cells have. This isn't too surprising, because the size of the receptive field is determined by the size of its dendritic field and the type of bipolar cells it is connected to (see Figure 2.19); since M cells listen to more photoreceptors (via mainly diffuse bipolar, horizontal, and amacrine cells) than P cells do, M cells respond to a larger portion of the visual field.

An additional consequence of the differing sizes of M and P receptive fields is that M cells are much more sensitive—better able to detect visual stimuli—than are P cells under low-light conditions (e.g., at night). However, the smaller receptive fields of P cells enable them to provide finer resolution (greater acuity) than M cells can, if there is enough light for the P cells to operate.

P and M ganglion cells also differ in their temporal responses. P cells tend to respond with changes in sustained firing while light shines on their excitatory regions. M cells tend to respond more transiently: an M cell will respond with a brief burst of impulses when the spot is turned on, and then it will quickly return to its spontaneous rate, even if the spot remains lit. Thus, M and P ganglion cells signal different information to the brain. P cells provide information mainly about the contrast in the retinal image, and M cells signal information about how the image changes over time.

Finally, P and M cells differ in what they say to the brain about the color of the light they detect (see Chapter 5).

INTRINSICALLY PHOTOSENSITIVE RETINAL GANGLION CELLS (ipRGCs) IN THE DEVELOPING RETINA As noted earlier, ipRGCs respond to light, but they receive no input from rods or cones. These are the first photoreceptors that mature in the retina and therefore are the first to send light-driven signals to the developing brain, as early as the second trimester. So, babies in the womb can detect light long before they can see images. UC Berkeley graduate student Franklin Caval-Holme and her mentor, Marla Feller, recently discovered that different types of ipRGCs and other retinal ganglion cells in the newborn mouse retina form a network that detects light and encodes light intensity (Caval-Holme, Zhang, and Feller, 2019).

Scientists at Work

Is One Photon Enough to See?

Question The seminal experiments of Hecht, Schlaer, and Pirenne (1942) and others suggest that under ideal conditions, humans are able to detect as few as five to seven photons. However, the long-standing question is, Can the human visual system detect a single photon?

Hypothesis Evolution has optimized the visual system and post-processing performed by the human retina and brain to detect a single photon.

Test All previous studies were hampered by light sources that were intrinsically and irreducibly variable in the number of photons emitted. In this ingenious work, the researchers built a special single-photon quantum light source that produced correlated pairs of photons. With this, the researchers could detect one of the photons and send the other to a human observer's eye, enabling them to identify trials in which it was clear that only one photon was sent to the observer's eye (Tinsley et al., 2016).

Results Human observers can detect a single-photon incident on the cornea with a probability well above chance.

Conclusion Evolution has optimized the visual system and post-processing performed by the retina and brain to detect a single photon.

Future work The single-photon quantum light source may provide a new method for directly measuring and understanding the visual system's internal noise.

Summary

1. This chapter provided some insight into the complex journey light must take for us to see stars and other spots of light. The path of the light was traced from a distant star through the eyeball and to its absorption by photoreceptors and its transduction into neural signals. In subsequent chapters, we'll learn how those signals are transmitted to the brain and translated into the experience of perception.
2. Light, on its way to becoming a sensation (a visual sensation, that is), can be absorbed, scattered, reflected, transmitted, or refracted. It can become a sensation only when it's absorbed by a photoreceptor in the retina.
3. Vision begins in the retina, when light is absorbed by rods or cones. The retina is like a minicomputer that transduces light energy into neural energy.
4. The high degree of convergence in the retinal periphery ensures high sensitivity to light but poor acuity.
5. The low degree of convergence in the fovea ensures high acuity but poor sensitivity to light.
6. The one-to-one pathways between cones and ganglions exist only in the fovea and account for why images are seen most clearly when they fall on this part of the retina.
7. The visual system deals with large variations in overall light intensity by (a) regulating the amount of light entering the eyeball, (b) using different types of photoreceptors in different situations, and (c) effectively throwing away photons we don't need.
8. The retina sends information to the brain via ganglion cells, neurons whose axons make up the optic nerves. Retinal ganglion cells have center-surround receptive fields and are concerned with changes in contrast (the difference in intensity between adjacent bits of the scene).

9. Age-related macular degeneration is a disease associated with aging that affects the macula. The leading cause of visual loss among the elderly in the United States, it gradually destroys sharp central vision, making it difficult to read, drive, and recognize faces.
10. Retinitis pigmentosa is a family of hereditary diseases characterized by the progressive death of photoreceptors and degeneration of the pigment epithelium. In the most common form of the disease, patients first notice vision problems in their peripheral vision and under low-light conditions—situations in which rods play the dominant role in collecting light.
11. Several exciting developments are aimed at restoring sight in individuals with blinding retinal diseases.

Chapter 3

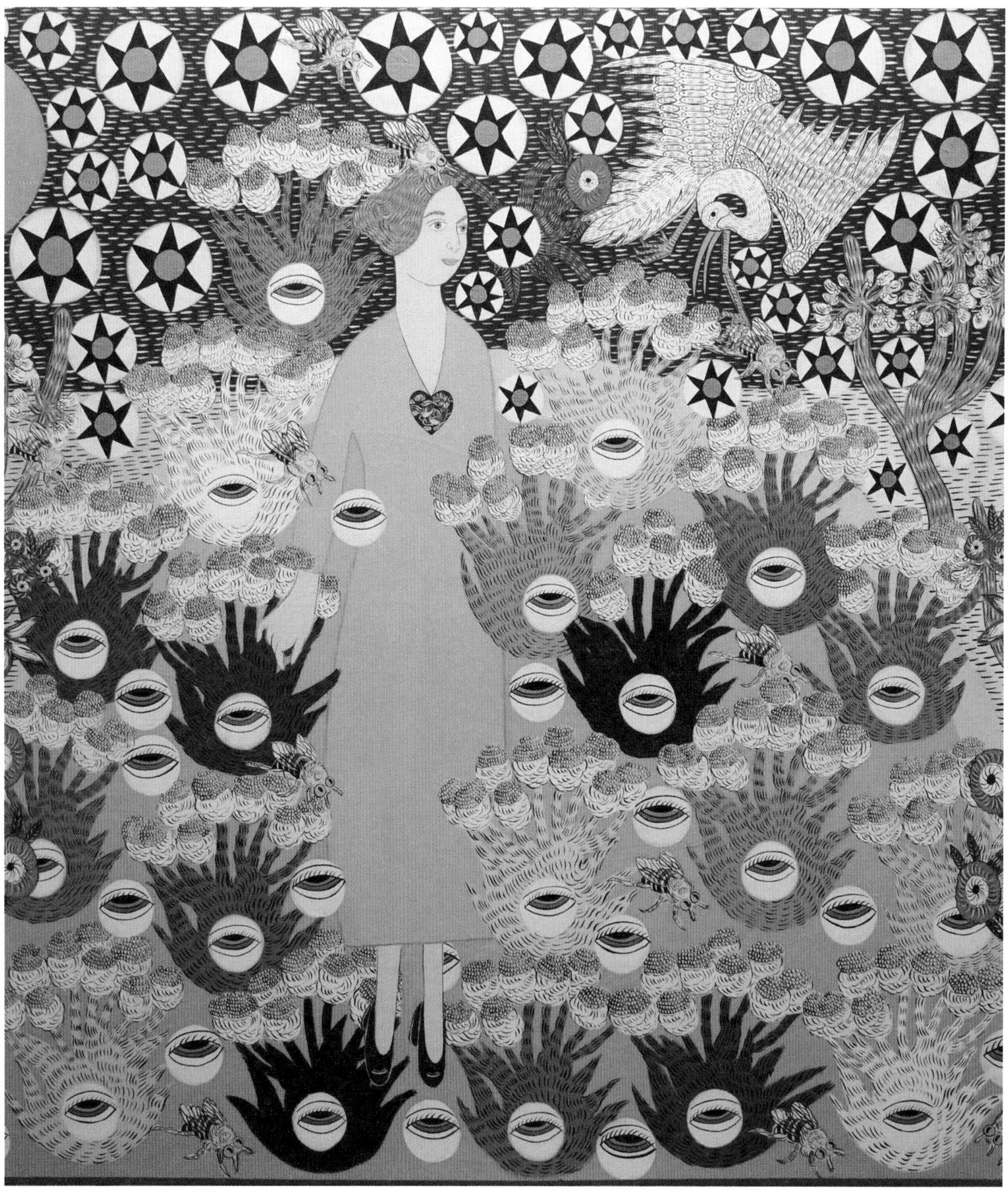

Iruka Maria Toro, *Your Soul Has Become an Invisible Bee*, 2014

Spatial Vision: From Spots to Stripes

Questions to Contemplate

Think about the following questions as you read this chapter.
By the chapter's end, you should be able to answer and discuss them.

- How do the images formed on the retina reach the brain and enable us to see the world?
- How do we see things "right side up" when the image on our retina is upside down?
- What can a baby see?

In Chapter 2 we learned that the macroscopic structures of the human eye function essentially as a biological camera: The iris regulates the amount of light entering the eyeball. The cornea, lens, and aqueous and vitreous humors focus the light rays so that a clear image is formed on the retina. The rod and cone photoreceptors capture this image in a way that is roughly analogous to the way the film in a camera captures photographic images.

It is here, however, that the analogy between visual system and camera ends. Cameras take pictures. Visual systems see, and seeing leads to actions. How do we get from an image of the world in front of us to an interpretation of that world—what is out there, where it is, and what we can do with it? The process starts in the eyeball itself, where the postreceptoral layers of the retina translate the raw light array captured by the photoreceptors into the patterns of spots surrounded by darkness, or vice versa, detected by the ganglion cells (see Figure 2.20). As we discussed in Chapter 2, this retinal translation helps us perceive the pattern of light and dark areas in the visual field, regardless of the overall light level (e.g., it enables us to see almost as well at dusk as we can at noon).

In this chapter, we follow the path of image processing from the eyeball to the brain (**FIGURE 3.1**). Ganglion cells in the retina respond preferentially to spots of light (Figure 3.1C, top). As we will see, neurons in the cerebral cortex prefer lines, edges, bars, and stripes (Figure 3.1C, bottom). Furthermore, this portion of visual cortex is organized into thousands of tiny microprocessors, each responsible for determining the orientation, width, color, and other characteristics of the scene in one small portion of the visual field. In Chapter 4, we will continue this story by examining how other parts of the brain assemble the outputs from these minicomputers to produce a coherent representation of the objects whose reflected light started the photoreceptors firing in the first place.

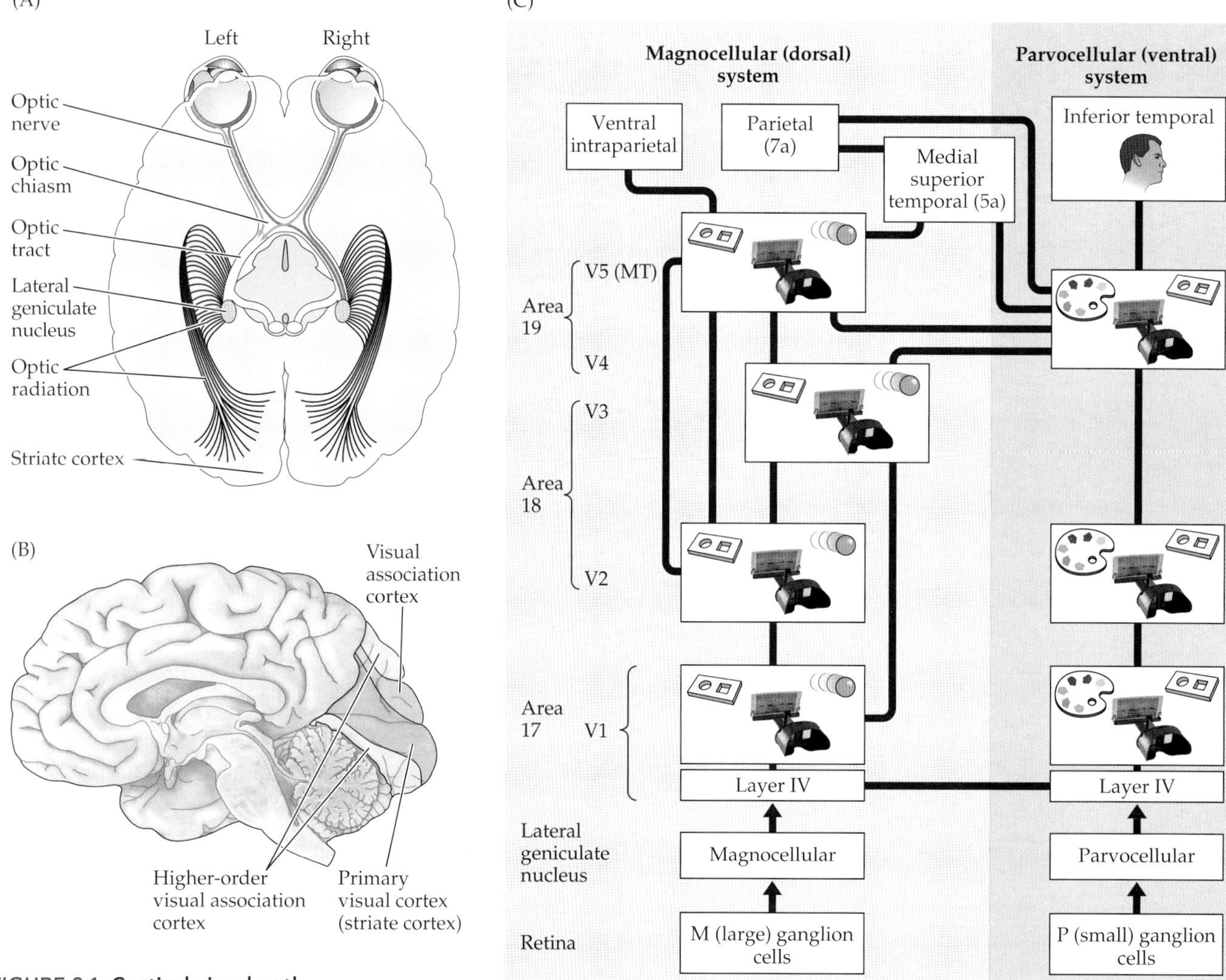

FIGURE 3.1 Cortical visual pathways (A) The basic organization of the primary visual pathway from eyeball to striate cortex, in transverse section. (B) A lateral view of the brain, illustrating primary visual cortex, visual association cortex, and higher-order visual association cortex. (C) The transformation of optimal visual stimuli from retinal ganglion cells (bottom), which respond best to small spots of light, to primary visual cortex (third from the bottom), which respond best to appropriately oriented bars and edges, and beyond (upper rows).

3.1 Visual Acuity: Oh Say, Can You See?

The King said, "I haven't sent the two Messengers, either. They're both gone to the town. Just look along the road, and tell me if you can see either of them."

"I see nobody on the road," said Alice.

"I only wish I had such eyes," the King remarked in a fretful tone. "To be able to see Nobody! And at that distance, too!"

—Lewis Carroll, *Through the Looking Glass*

contrast The difference in luminance between an object and the background, or between lighter and darker parts of the same object.

Since we'll be talking in this chapter about how the visual system codes images in terms of oriented stripes, let's start by determining just how well we see stripes when they are very close together and/or when the **contrast**—the difference in illumination between the stripes and the background—is very low. In addition to

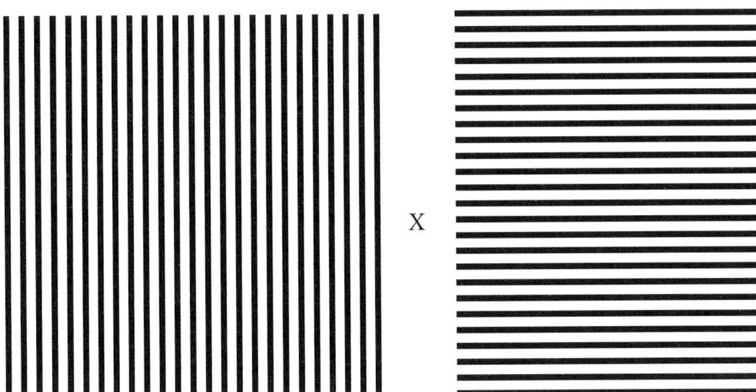

FIGURE 3.2 A visual acuity self-test Focusing on the central *X* at different distances reveals the farthest point at which you can distinguish the orientation (horizontal versus vertical) of the lines. The steps for this simple test of your visual resolution acuity are detailed in the text.

setting the boundary conditions for how well we should expect the visual system to be able to perform, we will use this section to introduce some important jargon that we'll need in the rest of the chapter.

acuity The smallest spatial detail that can be resolved at 100% contrast.

visual angle The angle subtended by an object at the retina.

cycle For a grating, a pair consisting of one dark bar and one bright bar.

Get a tape measure, prop your textbook up, and, while looking at the *X* in the middle of **FIGURE 3.2**, back up until you cannot tell the orientation of the black and white stripes. Measure how far your eye is from the page. Now walk forward a bit until you're sure you can see which grating includes vertical stripes and which horizontal stripes, and again measure your distance from the page. Congratulations! You just completed a fast (but not terribly accurate) measurement of your own visual resolution acuity, or simply **acuity**.

Eye doctors specify acuity in terms like *20/20* (more about this in a moment), but vision scientists prefer to talk about the smallest visual angle we can resolve—that is, the visual angle subtended by the stripes when they can no longer be resolved (**FIGURE 3.3**). **Visual angle**, which we mentioned briefly in Chapter 2, is the angle that would be formed by lines going from top and bottom (or left and right, depending on the orientation of the stripes) of a cycle on the page, passing through the center of the lens, and ending on the retina. Vision scientists generally express the resolution limit in terms of the number of grating cycles per degree of visual angle. A **cycle** is simply one repetition of a black stripe and a white stripe (each of the two gratings in Figure 3.2 has 25 total cycles).

To calculate the visual angle of your resolution acuity (Figure 3.3), divide the size of the cycle in Figure 3.2 (which is 2 millimeters [mm]) by the viewing distance at which you could just barely make out the orientation of the gratings (average your first and second measurements to get a rough estimate of this distance), and then take the arctangent of this ratio. Under ideal conditions, humans with very good vision can resolve gratings like those in Figure 3.2 when one cycle subtends an angle of approximately 1 minute of arc (1 arc minute, or 0.017 degree). As a rough rule of thumb (see Figure 2.13), 1 centimeter (cm) ≈ 1 degree (60 arc minutes) at a viewing distance of 57 cm. If the size of the just resolvable cycle were 1 cm, you would need to back up to about 3.42 meters (57 cm × 60 = 3420 cm) to be at the acuity limit.

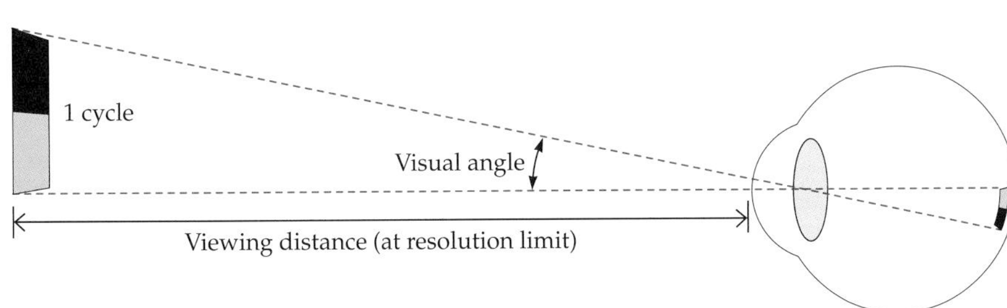

FIGURE 3.3 Visual angle Shown here is the angle size of one cycle of a grating at the retina.

sine wave grating A grating with a sinusoidal luminance profile, as shown in Figure 3.4A.

This resolution acuity represents one of the fundamental limits of spatial vision: it is the finest high-contrast detail that can be resolved. The limit is determined primarily by the spacing of photoreceptors in the retina. To see why, imagine that we're projecting the **sine wave gratings** shown in FIGURE 3.4A onto the retina. The light intensity in such gratings varies smoothly and continuously across each cycle (unlike the gratings in Figure 3.2 and FIGURE 3.4B, in which intensity changes abruptly from black to white and then back to black). However, the visual system "samples" the grating discretely, through the array of receptors at the back of the retina (in this respect, the eye is more like a digital camera than like a traditional camera that uses film). If the receptors are spaced such that the whitest and blackest parts of the grating fall on separate cones (FIGURE 3.4C), we should be able to make out the grating. But if the entire cycle falls on a single cone (FIGURE 3.4D), we will see nothing but a gray field.

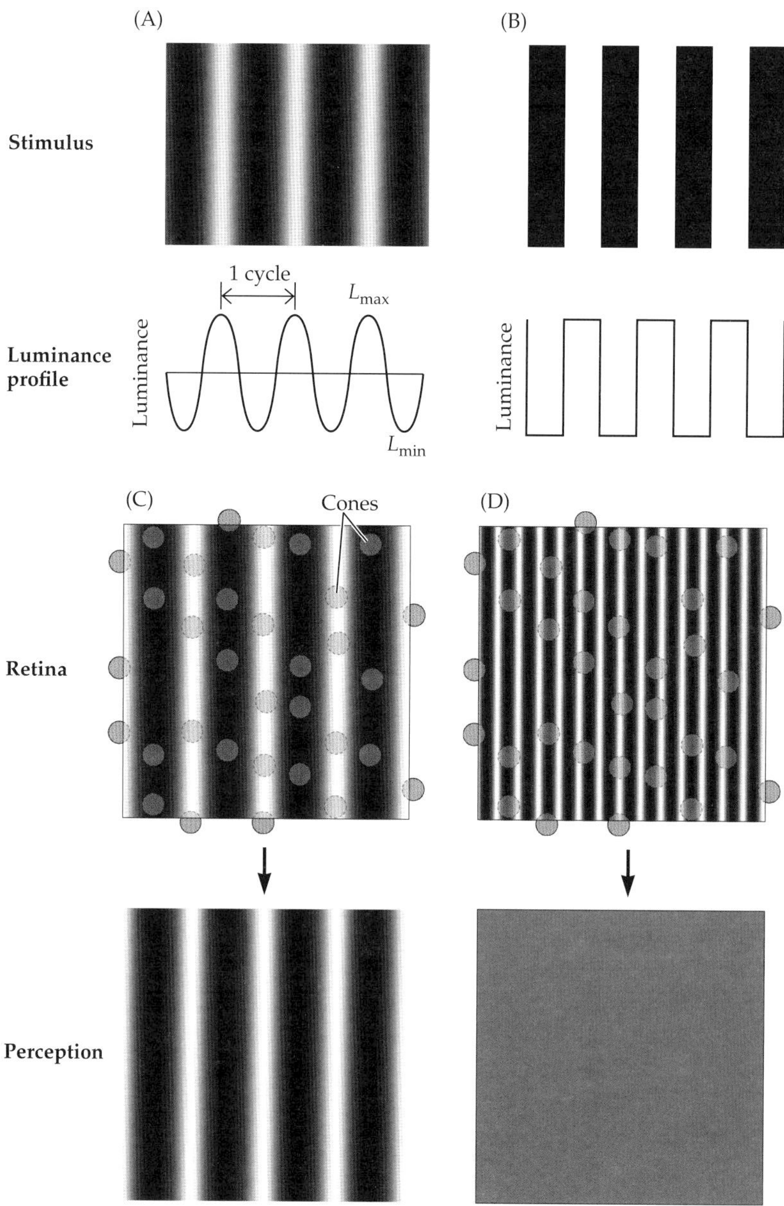

FIGURE 3.4 **Grating patterns** (A) A sine wave grating. (B) A square wave grating. (C) The stripes of the sine wave grating are wider than the photoreceptors (pink circles in the top panel), and the grating can be reconstructed vertically. (D) The stripes of the sine wave grating are narrower than the photoreceptors, so both black and white bars will fall inside a single receptor (top panel), resulting in a uniform gray field (bottom panel).

Cones in the fovea have a center-to-center separation of about 0.5 minute of arc (0.008 degree), which fits nicely with the observed acuity limit of 1 minute of arc (remember that we need two cones per cycle, one for the dark bar and one for the bright bar, to be able to perceive the grating accurately). Rods and cones in the periphery are packed together less tightly (recall that in the periphery, rods are physically more tightly packed [denser] than cones, as shown in Figure 2.12), and here many receptors converge on each ganglion cell. As a result, visual acuity is much poorer in the periphery than in the fovea.

Visual acuity in peripheral vision is not uniform—it falls off more rapidly along the vertical midline of the visual field than along the horizontal midline. This is known as horizontal and vertical asymmetry. Thus, if you fix your eyes on one point, you have (slightly but measurably) better acuity 5 degrees left or right than you do 5 degrees up or down. We also have better acuity a fixed distance below the midline of the visual field than above. This is known as vertical meridian asymmetry (Abrams, Nizam, and Carrasco, 2012).

Interestingly, although visual acuity falls off rapidly in the visual periphery, it is not the major obstacle to reading or object recognition. The real problem in the periphery is known as **visual crowding**—the deleterious effect of clutter on peripheral object recognition (Levi, 2008; Whitney and Levi, 2011). Objects that can be easily identified in isolation seem indistinct and jumbled when surrounded by other objects (**FIGURE 3.5**).

Luckily, we are able to make eye movements in order to foveate and scrutinize individual objects in clutter.

There is another surprising difference between central vision and peripheral vision: central vision is considerably slower than peripheral vision. Recent work (Sinha et al., 2017) suggests that peripheral cones respond about twice as quickly to light as do foveal cones (30 versus 60 ms). Foveal cones have longer axons than peripheral cones in order to allow dense packing in the central fovea, and the longer axons transmit slow signals better than fast ones (Masland, 2017). The slow

visual crowding The deleterious effect of clutter on peripheral object recognition.

(A)

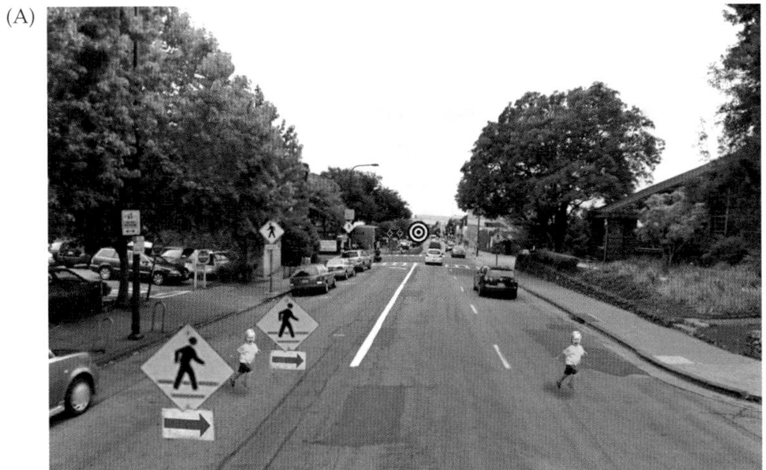

(B)

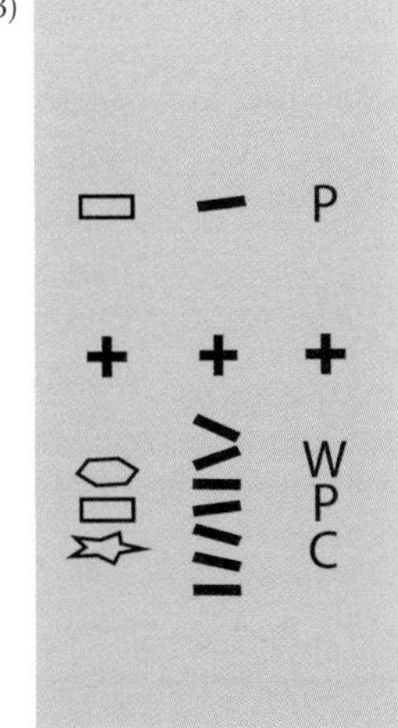

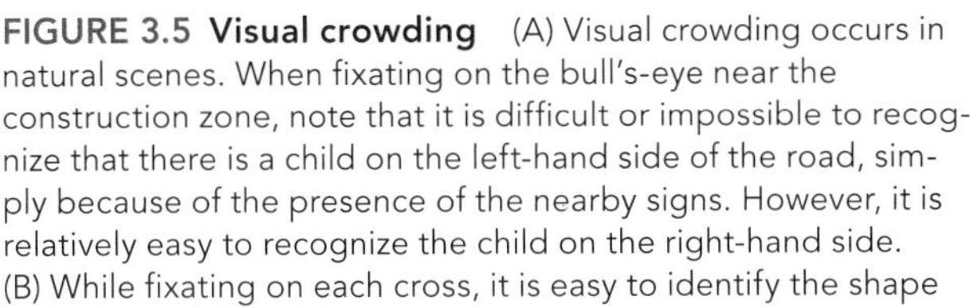

FIGURE 3.5 Visual crowding (A) Visual crowding occurs in natural scenes. When fixating on the bull's-eye near the construction zone, note that it is difficult or impossible to recognize that there is a child on the left-hand side of the road, simply because of the presence of the nearby signs. However, it is relatively easy to recognize the child on the right-hand side. (B) While fixating on each cross, it is easy to identify the shape (left cross), line orientation (middle cross), or letter (right cross) above it, but it is difficult or impossible to identify the same shape, line orientation, or letter when it is in the middle of a group below the cross. However, it is easy to do when looking at the patterns directly. Crowding in peripheral vision impairs the ability to recognize objects, but it does not make them disappear.

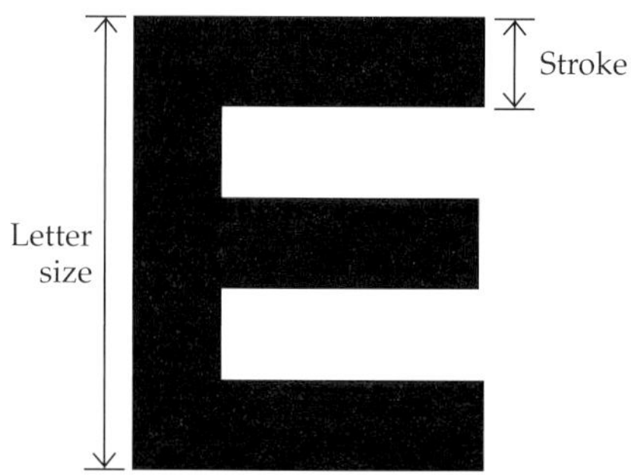

FIGURE 3.6 Snellen Visual Acuity Chart This chart is a familiar test for visual acuity used since the late 1800s. The letter size is five times the stroke size. Letters get progressively smaller down the lines of a Snellen chart, but this ratio remains the same.

response may allow foveal cones to increase their reliability by integrating their inputs over a longer time.

A Visit to the Eye Doctor

Eye doctors don't describe acuity in terms of visual angles and cycles. The last time you visited your eye doctor, she may have asked you to read letters, decreasing the size of the letters until you made several errors. Then she may have told you that your visual acuity was 20/20 if your vision was good, or 20/40 if you needed glasses, or possibly 20/10 if you could read the smallest letters on the eye chart. This method for designating visual acuity was invented in 1862 by a Dutch eye doctor, Herman Snellen (1834–1908). Snellen constructed a set of block letters for which the letter as a whole was five times as large as the strokes that formed the letter (**FIGURE 3.6**). Note that the resulting patterns are reminiscent of the gratings in Figure 3.2. He then defined visual acuity as follows:

$$\frac{\textit{(distance at which a person can just identify the letters)}}{\textit{(distance at which a person with ``normal'' vision can just identify the letters)}}$$

In later adaptations of the Snellen test, the viewer was positioned at a constant distance of 20 feet, and the size of the letters, rather than the position of the viewer, was altered. So normal vision came to be defined as 20/20. To relate this measure back to visual angle, a 20/20 letter is designed to subtend an angle of 5 arc minutes (0.083 degree) at the eye, and each stroke of a 20/20 letter subtends an angle of 1 arc minute (the familiar 0.017 degree). Thus, if you can read a 20/20 letter, you can discern detail that subtends 1 minute of arc. If you have to be at 20 feet to read a letter that someone with normal vision can read at 40 feet, you have 20/40 vision (worse than normal). Although 20/20 is often considered the gold standard, most healthy young adults have an acuity level closer to 20/15. Note that while the acuity for stripes and letters is quite similar for individuals, the two types of stimuli provide different cues and are subject to different constraints. Indeed, in some patients with **amblyopia**, acuity with Snellen letters may be much more affected than acuity with gratings.

amblyopia A developmental disorder characterized by reduced spatial vision in an otherwise healthy eye, even with proper correction for refractive error. Also known as *lazy eye*.

More Types of Visual Acuity

How should we define the keenness of sight? The term *visual acuity* specifies a spatial limit. So far, we've discussed two forms of visual acuity: (1) the finest stripes that can be resolved (sometimes referred to as the *minimum resolvable acuity*) and (2) the smallest letter that can be recognized (the *minimum recognizable acuity*). Over the centuries, there have emerged various ideas about how to define, measure, and specify visual acuity. **TABLE 3.1** lists four of the most common definitions and we briefly discuss them next.

TABLE 3.1 Summary of the different forms of acuity and their limits

Type of acuity	Measured	Acuity (degrees)
Minimum visible	Detection of a feature	0.00014
Minimum resolvable	Resolution of two features	0.017
Minimum recognizable	Identification of a feature	0.017
Minimum discriminable	Discrimination of a change in a feature	0.00024

MINIMUM VISIBLE ACUITY Minimum visible acuity refers to the smallest object that one can detect. Under ideal conditions, humans can detect a long, dark wire (like a cable of the Golden Gate Bridge) against a very bright background (like the sky on a bright, sunny day) when they subtend an angle of just 0.5 arc second (about 0.00014 degree). Minimum visible acuity is so small for two reasons. First, the optics of the eye (described in Chapter 2) spread the image of the thin line, making it much wider on the retina; and second, the fuzzy retinal image of the line casts a shadow that reduces the light on a row of cones to a level that is just detectably less than the light on the row of cones on either side. Although we specify the minimum visible acuity in terms of the angular size of the target at the retina, it is limited by our ability to discriminate the intensity of the target relative to its background; that is, *minimum visible acuity* is a limit in the ability to discern small changes in contrast, rather than a spatial limit per se, and is not used clinically.

MINIMUM RESOLVABLE ACUITY Minimum resolvable acuity is what you just measured! It refers to the smallest angular separation between neighboring objects that one can resolve. Ancient Egyptians assessed visual acuity by the ability of an observer to resolve double stars. However, today the minimum resolvable acuity is much more likely to be assessed by determining the finest black and white stripes that can be resolved. Under ideal conditions (e.g., high contrast and luminance), humans with very good vision can resolve black and white stripes when one cycle subtends an angle of approximately 1 minute of arc (0.017 degree). This minimum resolvable acuity represents one of the fundamental limits of spatial vision: it is the finest high-contrast detail that can be resolved. In foveal vision, the limit is determined primarily by the spacing of photoreceptors in the retina.

MINIMUM RECOGNIZABLE ACUITY Minimum recognizable acuity refers to the angular size of the smallest feature that one can recognize or identify. This approach, still used by eye doctors today, was introduced more than a century ago by Herman Snellen and his colleagues, as discussed earlier.

MINIMUM DISCRIMINABLE ACUITY Minimum discriminable acuity refers to the angular size of the smallest *change* in a feature (e.g., a change in size, position, or orientation) that one can discriminate. Perhaps the most studied example of minimum discriminable acuity is our ability to discern a difference in the relative positions of two features. Our visual system is very good at telling where things are relative to each other. Consider two abutting horizontal lines, one slightly higher than the other. The smallest misalignment that we can reliably discern is known as Vernier acuity, named after the Frenchman Pierre Vernier (1580–1637). Vernier's scale was based on the fact that humans are very adept at judging whether nearby lines are lined up or not. Vernier alignment is still widely used in precision machines and even in the dial switches in modern ovens. Under ideal conditions, Vernier acuity may be just 3 arc seconds (about 0.0008 degree)! This performance is even more remarkable when you consider that it is about ten times smaller than even the smallest foveal cones. Consider that the optics of the eye spread the image of a thin line over a number of retinal cones and that the eyes are in constant motion, and this performance appears even more remarkable.

Vernier acuity is not the most remarkable form of hyperacuity. *Guinness World Records* (2005) describes the "highest hyperacuity" as follows: "In April 1984, Dr. Dennis M. Levi [yes, that's one of the authors of this book] repeatedly identified the relative position of a thin, bright green line within 0.8 seconds of arc (0.00024 degree). This is equivalent to a displacement of some 0.25 inches (6 mm) at a distance of 1 mile (1.6 km)."

Acuity for Low-Contrast Stripes

Up to now, we've been discussing the tiniest high-contrast details that we can resolve. We learned that high-contrast sine wave gratings can be distinguished from a uniform gray field, as long as adjacent pairs of light or dark stripes are separated by at least 1 arc minute of visual angle. But what happens if the contrast of the stripes is reduced—that is, if the light stripes are made darker and the dark stripes lighter?

This was the question asked by Otto Schade in 1956, when he was working for the RCA Corporation. Schade showed people sine wave gratings with different spatial frequencies and had them adjust the contrast of the gratings until they could just be detected. **Spatial frequency** refers to the number of times a pattern, such as a sine wave grating, repeats (a cycle) in a given unit of space (degree of visual angle). Thus, it is measured as number of **cycles per degree** of visual angle. For example, if you view your book from about 120 cm away, the visual angle between each pair of white stripes in FIGURE 3.7A shows a grating with a relatively low spatial frequency—about 2 cycles per degree. FIGURE 3.7B is about 0.25 degree, so the spatial frequency of this grating is 1/0.25 = 4 cycles per degree, and FIGURE 3.7C illustrates a relatively higher spatial frequency (about 8 cycles per degree).

spatial frequency The number of grating cycles (e.g., changes in light and dark) per unit of visual angle (usually specified in degrees) in a given unit of space.

cycles per degree The number of grating cycles per degree of visual angle.

contrast sensitivity function (CSF) A function describing how the sensitivity to contrast (defined as the reciprocal of the contrast threshold) depends on the spatial frequency (size) of the stimulus.

contrast threshold The smallest amount of contrast required to detect a pattern.

Intuitively, you might think that the wider the stripes (that is, the lower the spatial frequency), the easier it would be to distinguish the light stripes from the dark stripes. But this is not what Schade found. He, and later Fergus Campbell and Dan Green (1965), demonstrated that the human **contrast sensitivity function (CSF)** is shaped like an upside-down *U*, as shown in FIGURE 3.8. We obtain the units for the left side of the *y*-axis—the observer's contrast sensitivity—by taking the reciprocal of the **contrast threshold**, graphed on the *y*-axis on the right. For example, for a 1 cycle/degree grating (the *x*-axis) to be just distinguishable from uniform gray, the stripes must have a contrast of about 1.0% (that is, if the mean luminance is 1000 photons, then a tiny patch of a light stripe reflects 1010 photons and a patch of a dark stripe should reflect 990 photons). The contrast, *C*, of a grating is generally specified according to the definition described by the first American to win the Nobel Prize, the physicist Albert Michelson. (He won the Nobel Prize in 1907 for

(A) Low

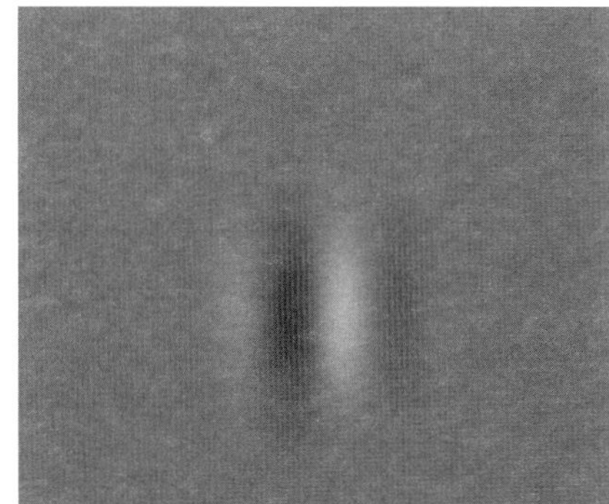

(B) Medium

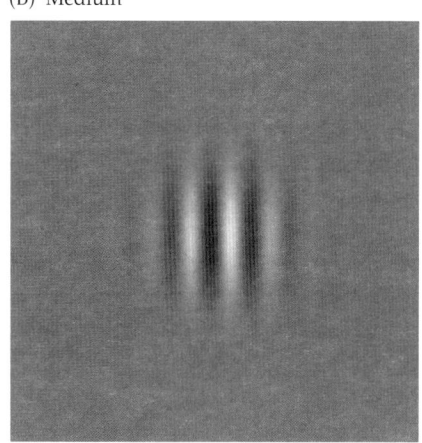

(C) High

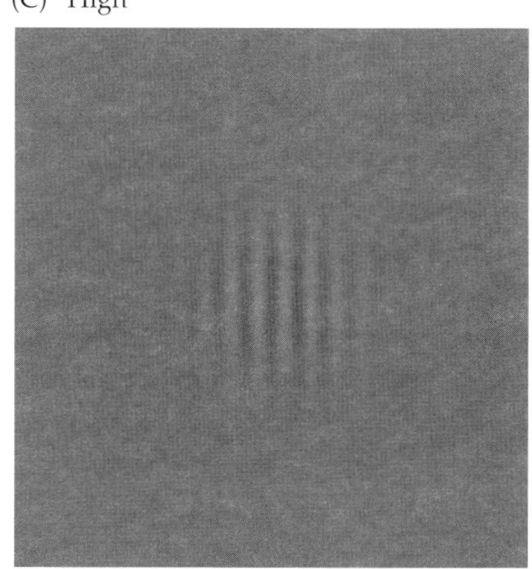

FIGURE 3.7 **Different spatial frequencies** Sine wave gratings illustrating low, medium, and high spatial frequencies.

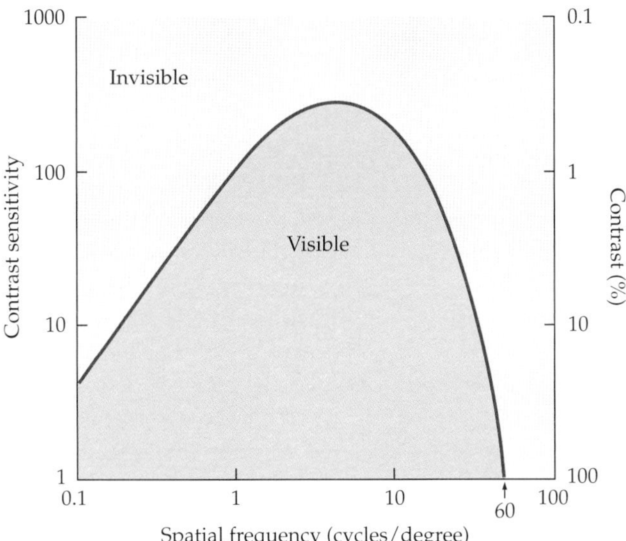

FIGURE 3.8 **The contrast sensitivity function and the window of visibility** The *y*-axis on the left is the observer's contrast sensitivity; its units are obtained by taking the reciprocal of the object's contrast at threshold (the *y*-axis on the right), determined using the Michelson equation described in the text. Any objects whose spatial frequencies (*x*-axis) and contrast thresholds (right *y*-axis) fall within the yellow region will be visible. Those outside the yellow region are outside the window of visibility. The red line delimits the contrast sensitivity function—the threshold between seeing and not seeing.

his work on the measurement of the speed of light.) According to the Michelson definition, $C = (L_{max} - L_{min})/(L_{max} + L_{min})$, where L_{max} and L_{min} are the maximum and minimum luminance, respectively. In our example, $C = (1010 - 990)/(1010 + 990) = 0.01$ or 1% (0.01×100). The reciprocal of this threshold is $1/0.01 = 100$, so this is the point plotted on the red CSF line in Figure 3.8 for this spatial frequency.

Note that a contrast of 100% corresponds to a contrast sensitivity value of 1. The CSF reaches this value on the far-right side of the curve in Figure 3.8, at about 60 cycles/degree. Sixty cycles/degree corresponds to a cycle width of 1 minute of arc, the resolution limit we measured previously for high-contrast stripes, which, recall, is determined primarily by cone spacing. The falloff in the CSF on the other side of the curve cannot be explained by cone spacing or by limitations in the optics of the eye. Instead, this part of the function must be a result of neural factors, which we will discuss later in the chapter.

You can visualize your own CSF using **FIGURE 3.9**. Here we see a sinusoidal grating whose contrast increases continuously from the top of the figure to the bottom and whose spatial frequency increases continuously from the left side of the graph to the right. If you view the figure from a distance of about 2 meters, you will notice the inverted *U* shape where the grating fades from visibility to invisibility. If you bring the book closer to your eye, you should be able to see the stripes on the right side of the figure going farther up, whereas the tops of the stripes on the left side will become less distinct.

There are many factors that influence the exact form of the CSF. These include the adaptation level of the eye (**FIGURE 3.10A**), the temporal modulation of the targets (i.e., how it varies over time; **FIGURE 3.10B**), and the age (**FIGURE 3.10C**) and refractive state (e.g., nearsightedness) of the individual.

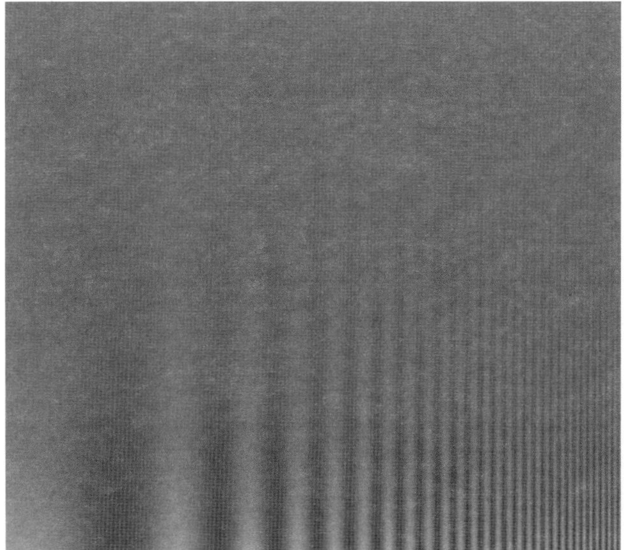

FIGURE 3.9 **Visualizing your contrast sensitivity function (CSF)** When viewed from a distance of about 2 meters, a grating modulated by contrast (vertically) and by spatial frequency (horizontally) appears in the inverted *U* shape of the CSF.

Why Sine Wave Gratings?

One answer to this question is that, although "pure" sine wave gratings may be rare in the real world, patterns of stripes with more or less fuzzy boundaries are quite common: think of trees in a forest, books on a bookshelf, and a map of Manhattan

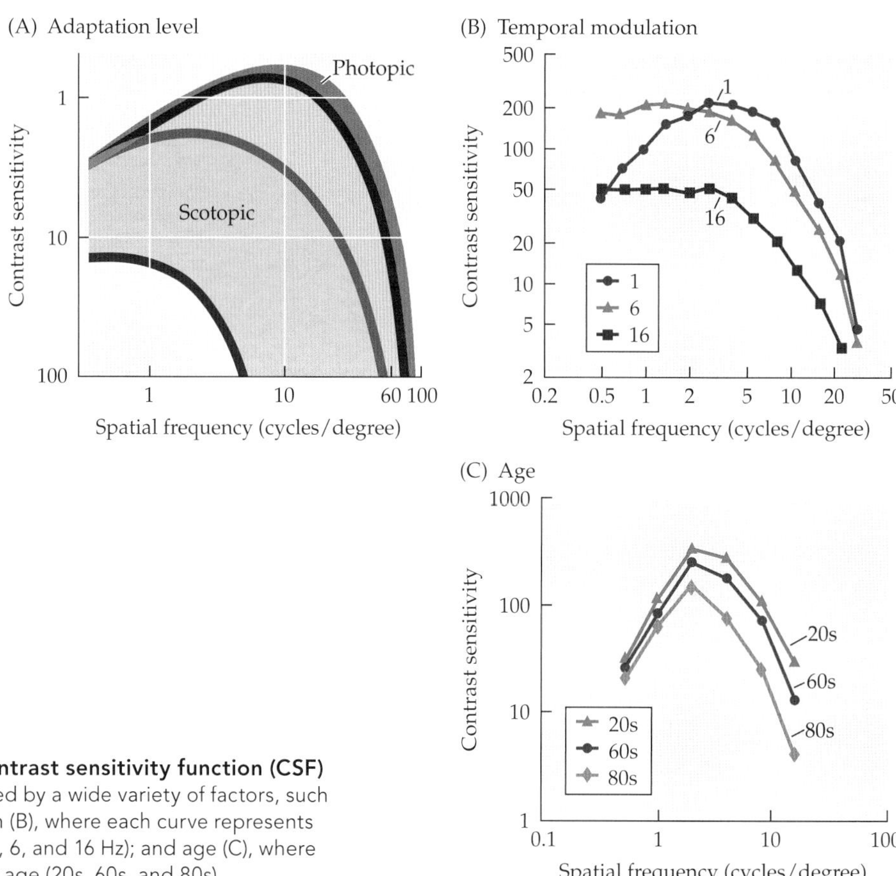

FIGURE 3.10 Factors influencing the contrast sensitivity function (CSF) The shape and height of the CSF is influenced by a wide variety of factors, such as adaptation level (A); temporal modulation (B), where each curve represents the CSF at a different temporal frequency (1, 6, and 16 Hz); and age (C), where each curve represents the CSF at a different age (20s, 60s, and 80s).

(the latter includes a pattern of horizontal stripes superimposed on a pattern of vertical stripes). Furthermore, the edge of any object produces a single stripe, often blurred by a shadow, in the retinal image.

On a larger scale, the visual system appears to break down real-world images into a vast number of components, each of which is, essentially, a sine wave grating with a particular spatial frequency. This method of processing is analogous to the way in which the auditory system deals with sound. French mathematician Joseph Fourier (1768–1830) developed analyses that help modern perception scientists to better describe how complex sounds such as music and speech, complex head motions, and complex images can be decomposed into a set of simpler components—that is, sine waves. Any complex sound can be broken down into individual sine wave components through this process, which is called **Fourier analysis**. Fourier analysis is a powerful mathematical tool that is used in many research fields. As we will see in Section 12.4, Fourier analysis is used extensively by vestibular and spatial orientation researchers. Vision researchers use Fourier analysis to describe images in terms of their spatial frequencies—that is, as the cycle of changes from light and dark across space (**FIGURE 3.11**, left column). Images can be broken down into components that capture how often changes from light to dark occur over a particular region in space, called spatial frequencies. Spatial frequencies are defined as the number of these light/dark changes across 1 degree of a person's visual field. Thus, in vision, the units of spatial frequency are cycles per degree of visual angle. Similarly, a complex sound can be broken down into a set of sine wave pure tones. Conversely, complex images can be constructed by adding together sine waves of different amplitudes and phases (*Fourier synthesis*). The **phase** of the sine wave is its position relative to

Fourier analysis A mathematical procedure by which any signal can be separated into component sine waves at different frequencies. Combining the sine waves (Fourier synthesis) will reproduce the original signal.

phase The position of a grating relative to a fixed position measured in degrees, where one complete cycle is 360 degrees.

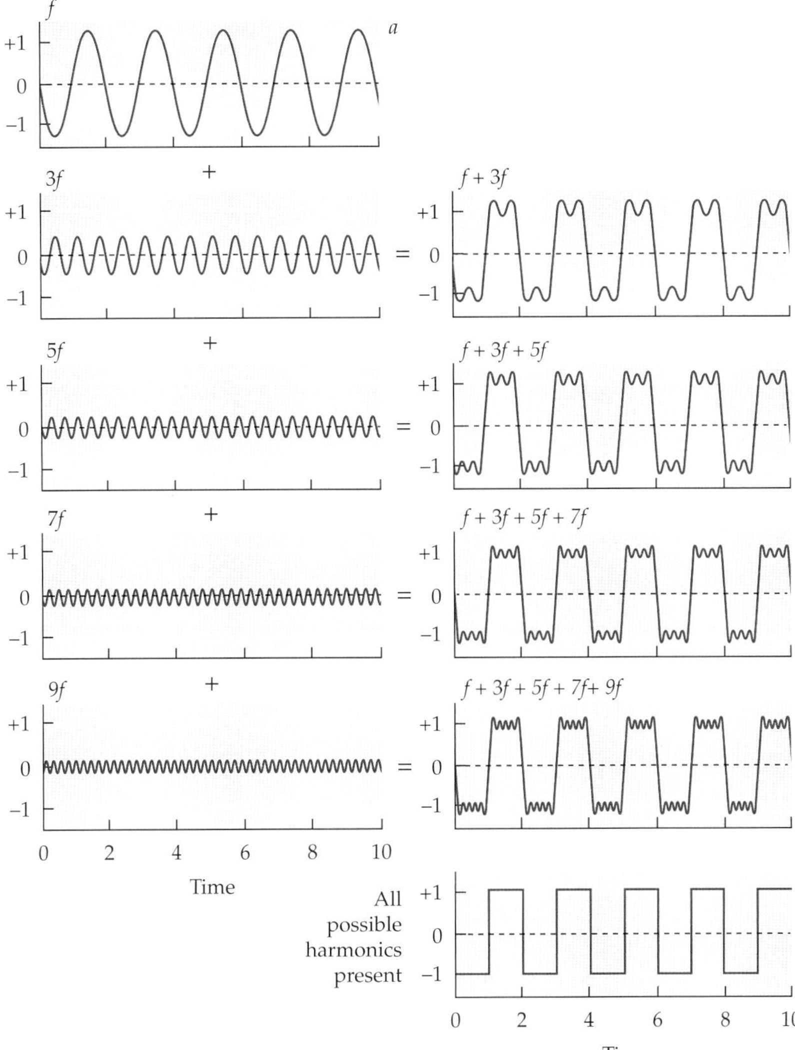

FIGURE 3.11 Fourier analysis (Left column) Sine waves of different spatial frequencies and amplitudes. From top to bottom: First row, the "fundamental" spatial frequency (f) with amplitude a; amplitude decreases as frequency increases (second row, $3f$, $a = 1/3$; third row, $5f$, $a = 1/5$; fourth row, $7f$, $a = 1/7$; fifth row, $9f$, $a = 1/9$). (Right column) Illustration of how a square wave can be constructed by adding a series of sine waves with the appropriate amplitudes and phases.

a fixed marker. Phase is measured in degrees, with 360 degrees of phase across one period, like the 360 degrees around a circle. For example, Figure 3.11, right column, illustrates how a simple square wave can be constructed by adding a series of sine waves with the appropriate amplitudes and phases. We'll return to this idea later in the chapter. Of course, most visual images consist of features with different sizes and orientations; that is, they are two-dimensional. Just how this is done is beyond the scope of this chapter. For now, rest assured that scientists don't use sine wave gratings just because they're convenient to manipulate in experiments (although they do make very nice stimuli).

3.2 Retinal Ganglion Cells and Stripes

In Section 2.4, we learned that retinal ganglion cells respond vigorously to spots of light. As it turns out, each ganglion cell also responds well to certain types of gratings, or stripes. **FIGURE 3.12** shows how an ON-center retinal ganglion cell responds to gratings of different spatial frequencies. When the spatial frequency of the grating is too low, the ganglion cell responds weakly because part of the

(A) Low frequency yields weak response.

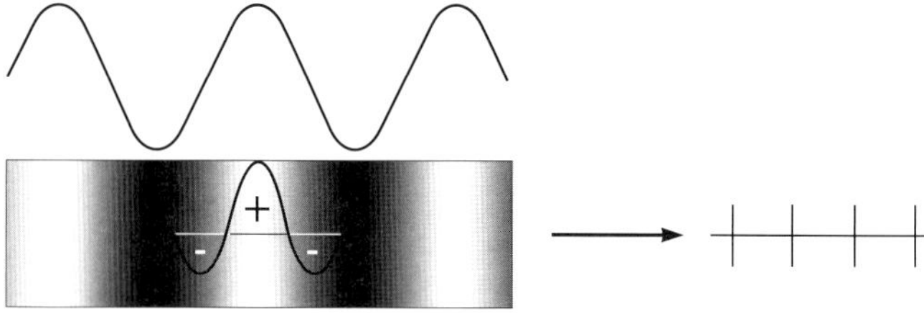

(B) Medium frequency yields strong response.

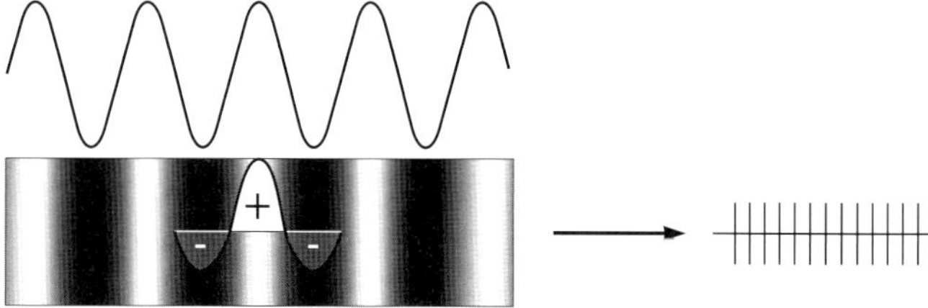

(C) High frequency yields weak response.

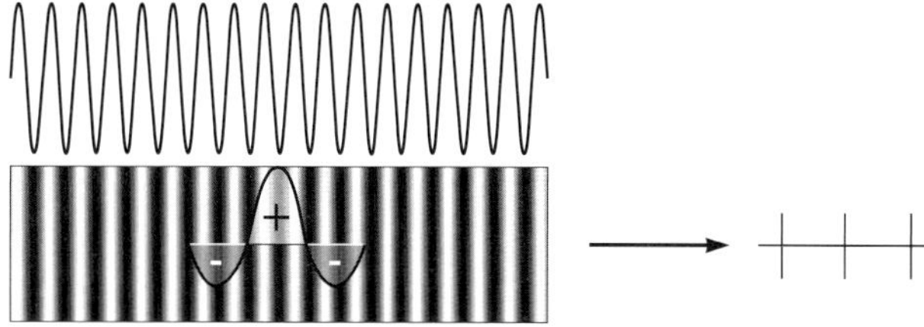

FIGURE 3.12 ON-center ganglion cell response to gratings The response (right) of an ON-center retinal ganglion cell to gratings of different spatial frequencies (left). (A) Too low: The ganglion cell responds weakly because part of the stimulus (bright white) lands in the inhibitory surround. (B) "Just right": The cell responds vigorously when a bright bar fills the field's center and dark bars fill the surround. (C) Too high: Bright and dark stripes both fall within the center of the field, washing out the cell's response.

fat, bright bar of the grating lands in the inhibitory surround, damping the cell's response. Similarly, when the spatial frequency is too high, the ganglion cell responds weakly because both dark and bright stripes fall within the receptive-field center, washing out the response. But when the spatial frequency is just right, with a bright bar filling the center and dark bars filling the surround, the cell responds vigorously. Thus, these retinal ganglion cells are "tuned" to spatial frequency: each cell acts like a **filter**, responding best to a specific spatial frequency that matches its receptive-field size and responding less to both higher and lower spatial frequencies.

Christina Enroth-Cugell and John Robson (1984) were the first to record the responses of retinal ganglion cells to sine wave gratings. In addition to showing that these cells respond vigorously to gratings of just the right size, the investigators discovered that responses depend on the *phase* of the grating—its position within the receptive field. **FIGURE 3.13** illustrates how an ON-center retinal ganglion cell might respond to a grating of just the right spatial frequency (that is, a bar width about the size of the receptive-field center) in four different phases. Note, however, that ganglion cells located to the left or right of the target cell shown in Figure 3.13 might respond to the 90-degree and 270-degree phases (Figures 3.13B and 3.13D), but not to the 0-degree and 180-degree (Figures 3.13A and 3.13C) phases, which is why the visual system as a whole is able to see all four phases equally well.

FURTHER DISCUSSION of ON- and OFF-center ganglion cells can be found in Section 2.4.

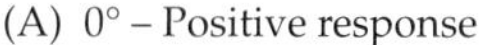

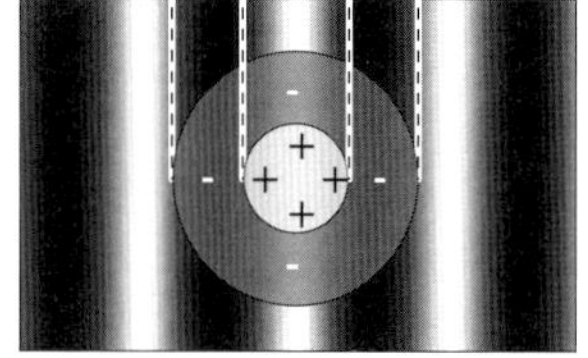

(B) 90° – No response

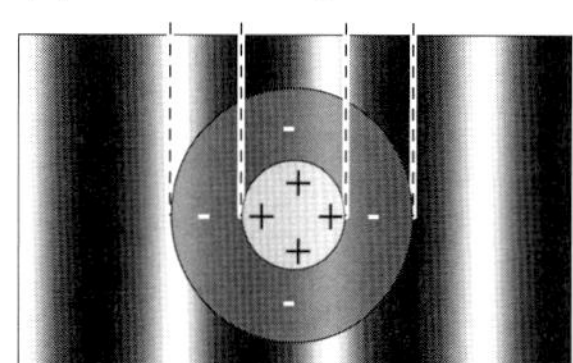

(C) 180° – Negative response

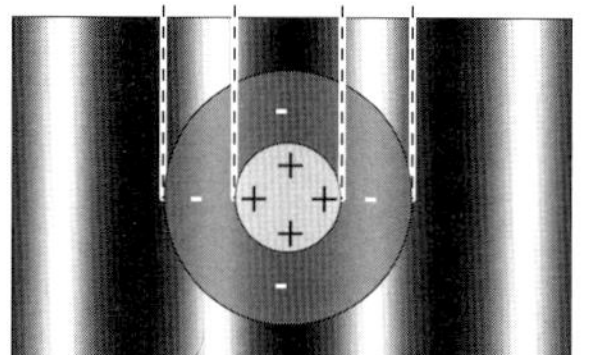

(D) 270° – No response

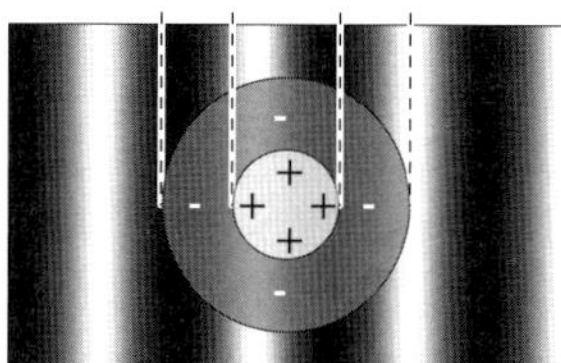

FIGURE 3.13 The response of a ganglion cell depends on phase The image depicts the response of an ON-center retinal ganglion cell to four different phases of an optimally sized grating. (A) When grating size and phase are optimal (i.e., a light bar fills the receptive-field center and dark bars fill the surround), this ON-center ganglion cell responds vigorously, increasing its firing rate. (B) If the grating phase is shifted by 90 degrees, half the receptive-field center is filled by a light bar and half by a dark bar, and similarly for the surround. There is thus no net difference between the light intensity in the center and surround, and the cell's response rate will not change from its resting rate. (C) A second 90-degree phase shift puts the dark bar in the center and the light bars in the surround, producing a negative response. (D) A third 90-degree shift returns us to the situation after the first shift, with the overall intensities in the center and surround equivalent and the cell therefore blind to the grating.

3.3 The Lateral Geniculate Nucleus

The axons of retinal ganglion cells synapse in the two **lateral geniculate nuclei (LGNs)**, one in each cerebral hemisphere. These nuclei (clusters of similar neurons) act as relay stations on the way from the retina to the cortex (see Figure 3.1). **FIGURE 3.14** shows that the LGN of primates is a six-layered structure, a bit like a stack of pancakes that has been bent in the middle (*geniculate* means "bent"). The neurons in the bottom two layers are physically larger than those in the top four layers; for this reason, the bottom two are called **magnocellular layers**, and the top four are called **parvocellular layers** (*magno-* and *parvo-* are Latin for "large" and "small," respectively). The two types of layers also differ in another, more important, way: the magnocellular layers receive input from M ganglion cells in the retina, and the parvocellular layers receive input from P ganglion cells (see Section 2.4). The layers differ in more than the size of the cells. Studies in which magnocellular and parvocellular layers are chemically lesioned indicate that the magnocellular pathway responds to large, fast-moving objects, and the parvocellular pathway is responsible for processing details of stationary targets. This distinction is interesting because it shows that the visual system splits input from the image into different types of information.

Even more splitting takes place *between* the layers. There, we find the layers consisting of **koniocellular cells** (*konio* is Greek for "dust"; these little cells were ignored for many years). The koniocellular layers are in the spaces between the magno and parvo layer (Figure 3.14) (Casagrande et al., 2007; Nassi and Callaway, 2009; Szmajda, Grünert, and Martin, 2008). Each koniocellular layer seems to be involved in a different aspect of processing. For example, one layer is specialized for relaying signals from the S-cones and may be part of a "primordial" blue-yellow pathway (Hendry and Reid, 2000).

The organization of the retinal inputs to the LGNs, diagrammed in **FIGURE 3.15**, provides some important insights into how our visual world is mapped to the brain. First, the left LGN receives projections from the left side of the retina in both eyes, and the right LGN receives projections from the right side of both retinas. Second,

filter An acoustic, electrical, electronic, or optical device, instrument, computer program, or neuron that allows the passage of some range of parameters (e.g., orientations, frequencies) and blocks the passage of others.

lateral geniculate nucleus (LGN) A structure in the thalamus, part of the midbrain, that receives input from the retinal ganglion cells and has input and output connections to the visual cortex.

magnocellular layer Either of the bottom two neuron-containing layers of the lateral geniculate nucleus, the cells of which are physically larger than those in the top four layers.

parvocellular layer Any of the top four neuron-containing layers of the lateral geniculate nucleus, the cells of which are physically smaller than those in the bottom two layers.

koniocellular cell A neuron located between the magnocellular and parvocellular layers of the lateral geniculate nucleus. This layer is known as the koniocellular layer.

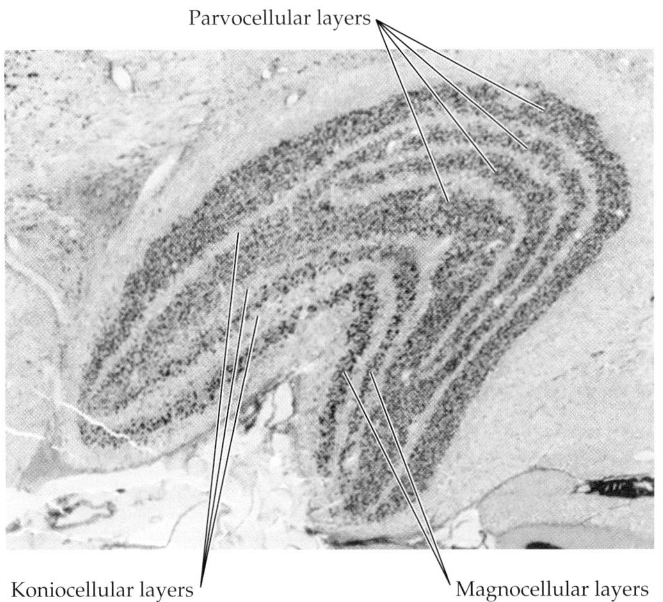

FIGURE 3.14 **The lateral geniculate nucleus (LGN)** This cross section shows the six-layered structure of a primate LGN. Layers 1 and 2 are the magnocellular layers; these larger neurons receive input from the M ganglion cells of the retina. Layers 3–6 are the parvocellular layers, whose smaller cells receive input from the retina's P ganglion cells. The magno- and parvocellular layers are separated by dustlike koniocellular cells. There is an LGN in each of the brain's two hemispheres.

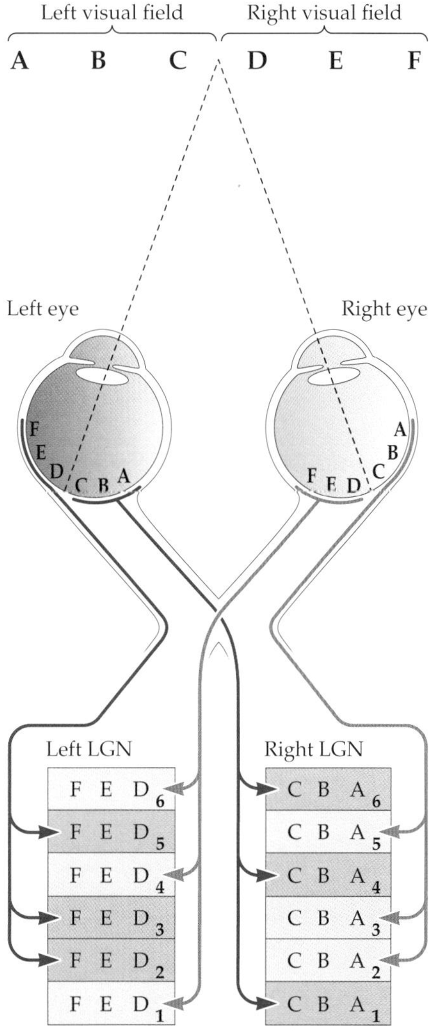

FIGURE 3.15 Topographic mapping of two eyes into the brain Input (in this case the letters ABCDEF) from the right visual field is mapped in an orderly fashion onto the different layers of the left lateral geniculate nucleus (LGN), and input from the left visual field is mapped to the right LGN. Information from the two eyes is segregated into separate layers.

each layer of the LGN receives input from one or the other eye. From bottom to top, layers 1, 4, and 6 of the right LGN receive input from the left (**contralateral**) eye, while layers 2, 3, and 5 get their input from the right (**ipsilateral**) eye. Thus, information from the two eyes is segregated in different layers in the LGN.

Each LGN layer contains a highly organized map of a complete half of the visual field. Figure 3.15 shows schematically how objects in the right visual field (objects to the right of where our gaze is fixated) are mapped onto the different layers of the left LGN (the right side of the world falls on the left side of the retina, whose ganglion cells project to the left LGN). This ordered mapping of the world onto the visual nervous system, known as **topographical mapping**, provides us with a neural basis for knowing where things are in space (we will return to this point a little later).

LGN neurons have concentric receptive fields that are very similar to those of retinal ganglion cells: they respond well to spots and gratings. Given that the LGN cells respond to the same patterns as the ganglion cells that provide their input, you might wonder why the visual system bothers with the LGN. Why don't the ganglion cell axons simply travel directly back to the cerebral cortex? One important reason is that the LGN is not merely a stop on the line from retina to cortex. There are many connections between other parts of the brain and the LGN (Babadi et al., 2010; Dubin and Cleland, 1977). Moreover, there are more feedback connections from the visual cortex to the LGN than feed-forward connections from the LGN to the cortex. Indeed, a recent brain imaging study (Poltoratski et al., 2019) shows that BOLD activity in human LGN can be modified by figure ground organization, even when the figure is presented to one eye and the background to the other eye. Since information from the two eyes is segregated in different layers in the LGN, this BOLD modulation must be a result of feedback from the cortex.

It seems that the LGN is a location where various parts of the brain can modulate input from the eyes. For example, the LGN is part of a larger brain structure called the thalamus (the medial geniculate nucleus, part of the auditory pathway, is another portion of the thalamus; see Section 9.3). When you go to sleep, the entire thalamus is inhibited by circuitry elsewhere in the brain that works to keep you asleep. Thus, even if your eyelids were open while you were sleeping at night, you would not see anything in your dimly lit room. Input would travel from your retinas to your LGNs, but the neural signals would stop there before reaching the cortex, so they would never be registered. The thalamic inhibition is not complete, which is why loud noises (e.g., the alarm clock) or bright lights will be perceived, waking you up.

3.4 The Striate Cortex

If you place one hand at the back of your head, about an inch or two above the top of your neck, you should be able to feel a small bump known as the inion. The receiving area for LGN inputs in the cerebral cortex lies below the inion. This area has several names: **primary visual cortex (V1)**, **area 17**, and **striate cortex**. *Striate* means "striped," for the striped pattern V1 develops following a certain type of staining procedure. By now you're probably getting the idea that layers are an important property of neural structures in the visual pathway. The striate cortex consists of six major layers, some of which have sublayers (**FIGURE 3.16**). Fibers from the LGN project mainly (but not exclusively) to layer 4C, with magnocellular axons coming into the upper part of layer 4C (known as 4Cα) and parvocellular axons projecting to the lower part of layer 4C (known as 4Cβ) (Yabuta and Callaway, 1998).

contralateral Referring to the opposite side of the body or brain.

ipsilateral Referring to the same side of the body or brain.

topographical mapping The orderly mapping of the world in the lateral geniculate nucleus and the visual cortex.

primary visual cortex (V1), area 17, or striate cortex The area of the cerebral cortex of the brain that receives direct inputs from the lateral geniculate nucleus, as well as feedback from other brain areas.

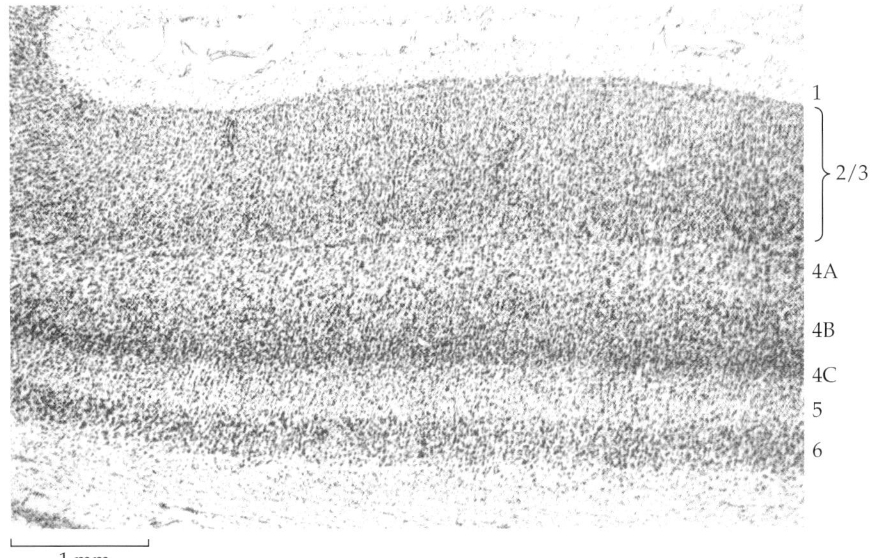

FIGURE 3.16 Striate cortex Like the lateral geniculate nucleus (LGN), striate cortex consists of six layers. Fibers from the LGN project mainly (but not exclusively) to layer 4C.

Like the LGN, the striate cortex has a systematic topographical mapping of the visual field. But the striate cortex is not simply a larger version of the LGN. A major and complex transformation of visual information takes place in the striate cortex. For starters, striate cortex contains on the order of 200 million cells—more than 100 times as many as the LGN has! This massive expansion of the number of neurons in V1 may be important for representing our complex natural visual world.

FIGURE 3.17 illustrates two important features of the visual cortex: topography and magnification. First, the fact that the image of the woman's right eyebrow (*her* right; it appears on the left in Figure 3.17) is mapped onto regions corresponding to the numbers 3 and 4 in the striate cortex tells the visual system that the eyebrow must be in positions 3 and 4 of the visual field. This is topographical mapping. Second, information is dramatically scaled from different parts of the visual field. In Figure 3.17, the fovea is represented by number 5 on the retina. Objects imaged on or near the fovea are processed by neurons in a large part of the striate cortex, but objects imaged in the far-right or -left periphery are allocated only a tiny portion of the striate cortex. This distortion of the visual-field map on the cortex is known as **cortical magnification** because the cortical representation of the fovea is greatly magnified compared with the cortical representation of peripheral vision.

To gain a sense of the extent of this cortical magnification factor, hold your arms out in front of you, put up your index fingers, hold them about 10 cm (4 inches) apart, close your left eye, and fixate on your right finger. In this position, your right fingernail, which is taking up about 1 degree of visual angle on the fovea, is being processed by neurons in about 20 mm of striate cortex. Your left fingernail, which is covering the same amount of visual angle but is falling 10 degrees to the left of the fovea, is being processed by only 1.5 mm of cortex.

The Topography of the Human Cortex

Much of what we know about cortical topography and magnification comes from anatomical and physiological studies in animals. The earliest studies in humans were based on correlating visual-field defects with cortical lesions. That is, someone with damage to this part of visual cortex would be blind in that part of the visual field. **FIGURE 3.18A** illustrates how **eccentricity** (distance from the fovea, position 5

cortical magnification The amount of cortical area (usually specified in millimeters) devoted to a specific region (e.g., 1 degree) in the visual field.

eccentricity The angular distance from the fovea (the region of highest visual acuity).

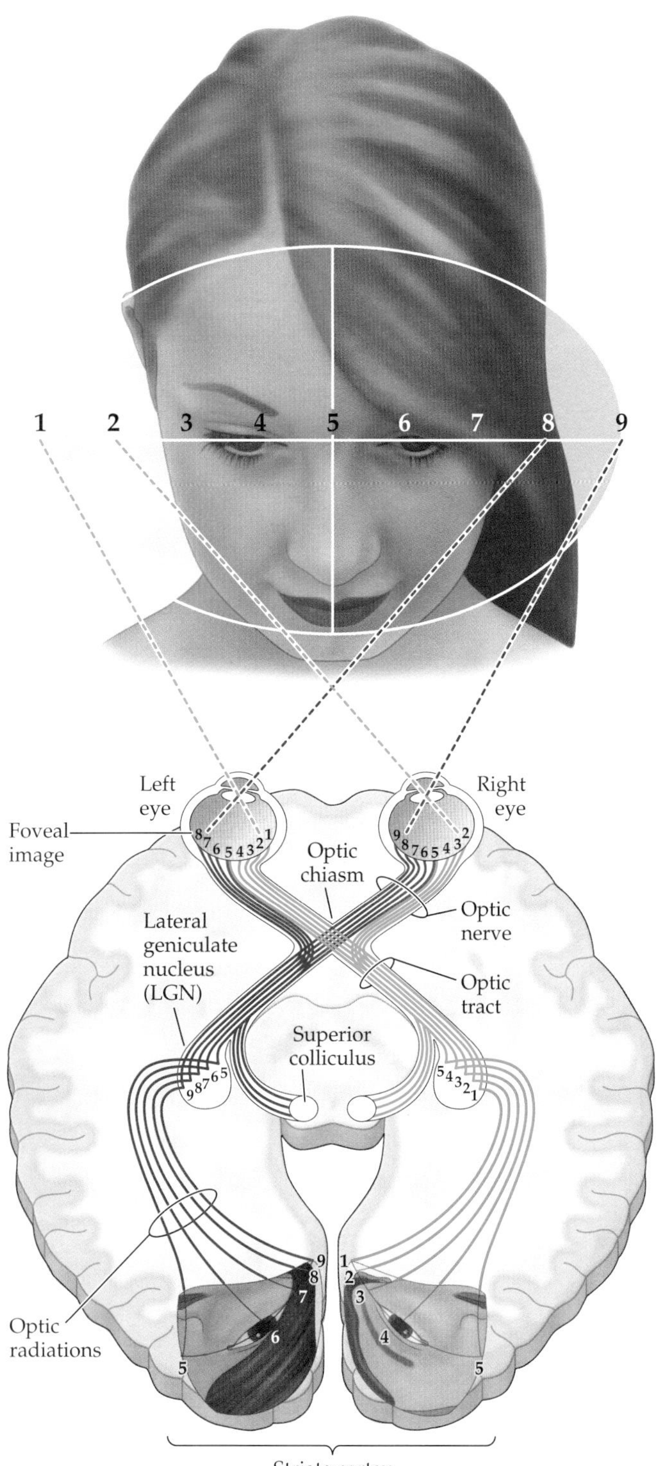

FIGURE 3.17 The mapping of objects in space onto the visual cortex This image illustrates both topographical mapping (represented by the positions of numerals 1–9) and the dramatic magnification of the foveal representation in the cortex. In the striate cortex, representation of the fovea (position 5) is greatly magnified compared to that of peripheral vision.

in Figure 3.18A) maps onto visual cortex, as deduced from studying lesions. However, in the past 20 years or so there have been major advances in our knowledge of human visual cortex—in large part through developments in brain-imaging techniques. If you've ever injured your knee or back, you may be familiar with magnetic resonance imaging. MRI is very useful for anatomical imaging of soft tissues, including thc brain.

MRI lets us see the structure of the brain. *Functional* magnetic resonance imaging is a noninvasive technique for measuring and localizing brain activity. As discussed in Section 1.3, fMRI does not measure neural activity directly. Rather, it measures changes in blood oxygen level that reflect neural activity. Blood oxygen level–dependent (BOLD) signals reflect a range of metabolically demanding neural signals (Wandell and Winawer, 2011). If you compare blood flow when visual stimuli are presented in one portion of the visual field to blood flow when the field is blank, you can find portions of the brain that respond specifically to that stimulation of that portion of the field. In this way, it is possible to map the topography of V1 in the living human brain (**FIGURE 3.18B**). Different parts of the visual field are mapped onto Figure 3.18 with a color code. Notice that the red area is just the central few degrees. The blue areas cover vast parts of the more peripheral field, from 20 to 40 degrees. Because of cortical magnification of the central field, these red and blue regions are similar in size.

Some Perceptual Consequences of Cortical Magnification

Visual acuity declines in an orderly fashion with eccentricity (Levi, Klein, and Aitsebaomo, 1985), a phenomenon demonstrated by Hermann Rudolf Aubert well over a century ago (Aubert, 1886). **FIGURE 3.19** allows you to demonstrate this phenomenon yourself; the letters are scaled in size such that each one covers an approximately equal cortical area. Why is the foveal representation in the cortex so highly magnified? The visual system must make a trade-off. High resolution requires a great number of resources: a dense array of photoreceptors, one-to-one lines from photoreceptors to retinal ganglion cells, and a large chunk of striate cortex (not to mention the real estate in other areas of cortex necessary to do something with the visual information coming out of V1). To see the entire visual field with such high resolution, we might need eyes

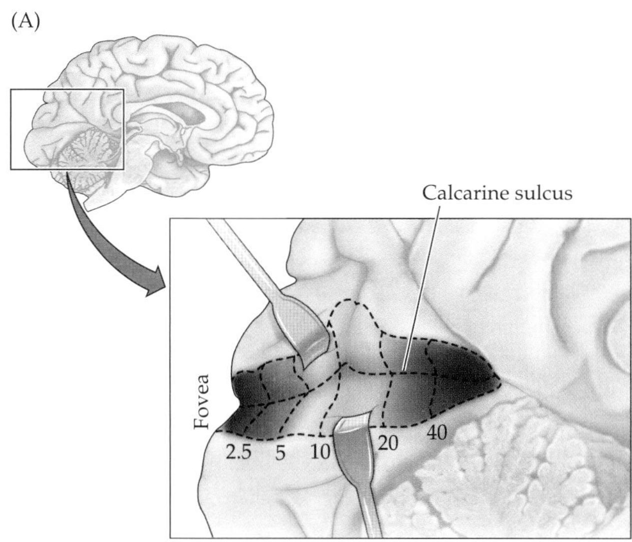

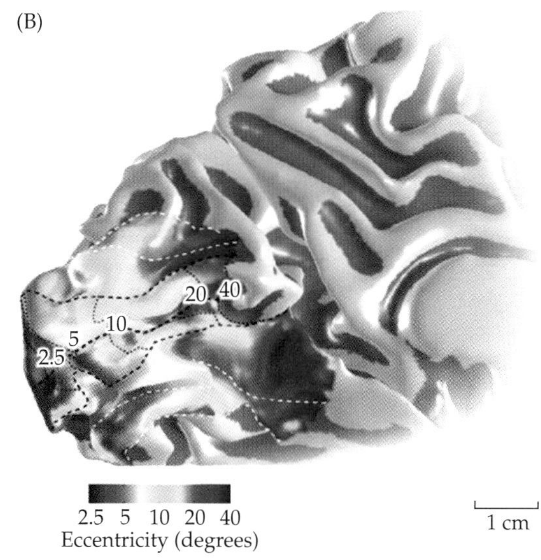

FIGURE 3.18 Cortical mapping Mapping the visual field onto the cortex as deduced from studying lesions (A) and from functional magnetic resonance imaging (B). Different parts of the visual field are mapped onto the cortex according to the color code shown in (B). The red area is just the central few degrees adjacent to the fovea, while the blue areas cover substantially more of the peripheral field, from 20 to 40 degrees.

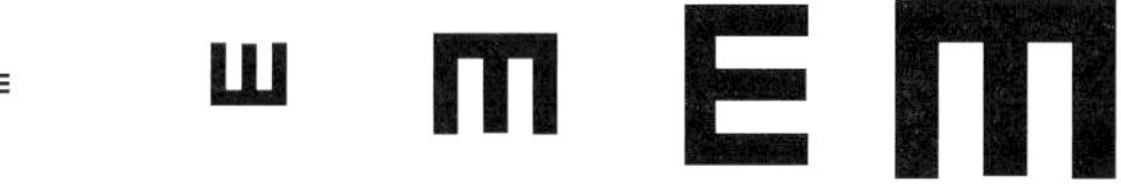

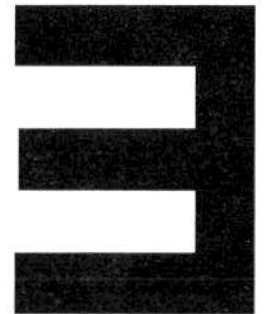

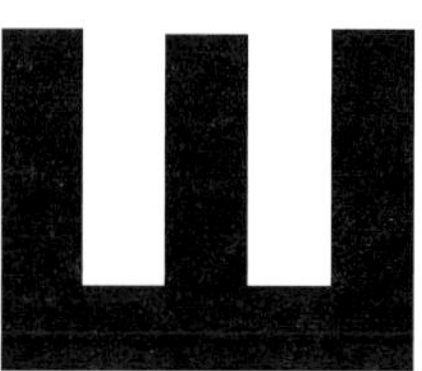

FIGURE 3.19 A cortically scaled letter chart A letter chart in which the letter size increases with eccentricity in proportion to the inverse cortical magnification factor. If you fixate your gaze on the far-left side of the figure, all seven letters should be equally easy to see because those on the right, which are in the periphery, are so much larger.

and brains too large to fit in our heads! Thus, we have evolved a visual system that provides high resolution in the center and lower resolution in the periphery. If you need to process the details of an object that appears in the corner of your eye, you can simply turn your eye or head so that the object falls on the fovea instead.

FURTHER DISCUSSION of eye movements can be found in Section 8.4.

3.5 Receptive Fields in Striate Cortex

In 1958, David Hubel and Torsten Wiesel began work as postdoctoral students in Stephen Kuffler's laboratory. Their goal was to extend Kuffler's groundbreaking work on retinal ganglion cells and to apply it to the cortex. So they began trying to map the receptive fields of neurons in striate cortex of cats using spots of light, much as Kuffler (1953) had done earlier (see Section 2.4).

Recall from Chapter 2 that the receptive field of a neuron is the region in space in which the presence of a stimulus alters the neuron's firing rate. To Hubel and Wiesel's dismay, they found that a cat's cortical cells hardly responded at all to the same spots that made its ganglion cells fire like crazy. To project their stimuli onto

orientation tuning The tendency of neurons in striate cortex to respond optimally to certain orientations and less to others.

ocular dominance The property of the receptive fields of striate cortex neurons by which they demonstrate a preference, responding somewhat more rapidly when a stimulus is presented in one eye than when it is presented in the other.

simple cell A cortical neuron whose receptive field has clearly defined excitatory and inhibitory regions.

the retina, Hubel and Wiesel inserted a glass slide with a black spot into a slot in a special ophthalmoscope (that's the instrument the doctor uses when she shines a bright light into your eye to see your retina). One day, they had been recording from a neuron without much luck, when suddenly the cell emitted a strong burst of firing as they inserted the glass slide into the slot. Eventually, they realized that the response had nothing to do with the spot itself; instead, the cell had been responding to the shadow cast by the *edge* of the glass slide as it swept across the ophthalmoscope's light path. And the rest, as they say, is history. Hubel related this story when he and Wiesel received the 1981 Nobel Prize in Physiology or Medicine for uncovering many of the remarkable properties of the visual cortex (Hubel, 1982) (**FIGURE 3.20A**).

Hubel and Wiesel's most fundamental discovery was that the receptive fields of striate cortex neurons are not circular, as they are in the retina and LGN. Rather, they are elongated. As a result, they respond much more vigorously to bars, lines, edges, and gratings than to round spots of light.

Orientation Selectivity

Further investigation by Hubel and Wiesel (1962) uncovered a number of other important properties of the receptive fields of neurons in striate cortex. First, an individual neuron will not respond equivalently to just any old stripe in its receptive field. It responds best when the line or edge is at just the right orientation and hardly at all when the line is tilted more than 30 degrees away from the optimal orientation (a change equivalent to movement of the minute hand of a clock from 12 to 1). Scientists call this selective responsiveness **orientation tuning**: the cell is tuned to detect lines in a specific orientation.

A typical orientation tuning function looks like the plot in **FIGURE 3.20B**. The neuron featured here fires vigorously when the line is oriented vertically, but the response tapers off rapidly as the line is tilted one way or another, diminishing to close to the cell's resting rate when the line is tilted about 30 degrees in either direction. Other cells in striate cortex are selective for horizontal lines and lines at 45 degrees, 20 degrees, 62 degrees, and so on, so the population of neurons as a whole detects all possible orientations. However, more cells are responsive to horizontal and vertical orientations than to obliques (De Valois, Yund, and Hepler, 1982; B. Li, Peterson, and Freeman, 2003). This physiological finding meshes well with the psychophysical finding that humans have somewhat lower visual acuity and contrast sensitivity for oblique targets than for horizontal and vertical targets.

(A)

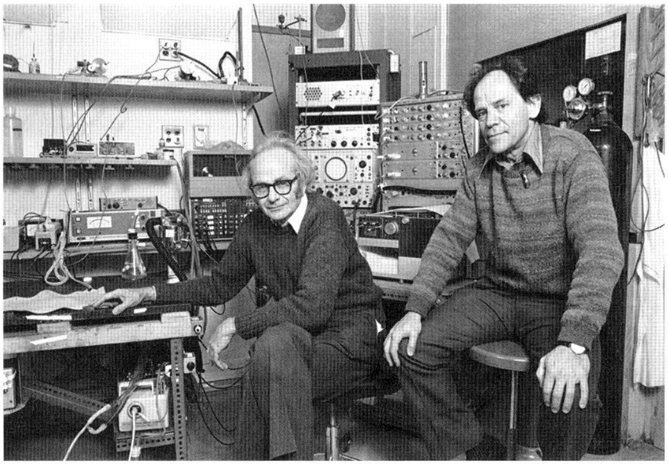

(B)

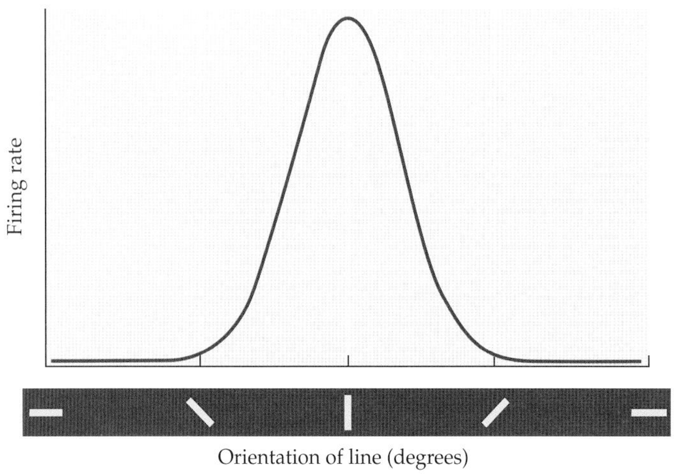

Firing rate

Orientation of line (degrees)

FIGURE 3.20 Nobel men (A) David Hubel (left) and Torsten Wiesel, shown here in their lab, received the 1981 Nobel Prize for discoveries that furthered understanding of information processing in the visual system. (B) Orientation tuning function of a cortical cell. The neuron fires vigorously when the line is oriented vertically, but hardly at all when the line orientation is changed by 30 degrees. While this example is for a cell tuned to vertical lines, other cells are tuned to different orientations.

How are the circular receptive fields in the LGN transformed into the elongated receptive fields in striate cortex? Hubel and Wiesel (Hubel and Wiesel, 1979) suggested a very simple scheme to explain this transformation. Simply put, their idea was that the concentric LGN cells that feed into a cortical cell are all in a row (**FIGURE 3.21**). Later studies (e.g., J. S. Anderson et al., 2000) have shown that the arrangement of LGN inputs is indeed crucial for establishing the orientation selectivity of striate cortex cells. However, other evidence suggests that neural interactions (e.g., lateral inhibition; see Section 2.4) within the cortex also play an important role in the dynamics of orientation tuning (Pugh et al., 2000).

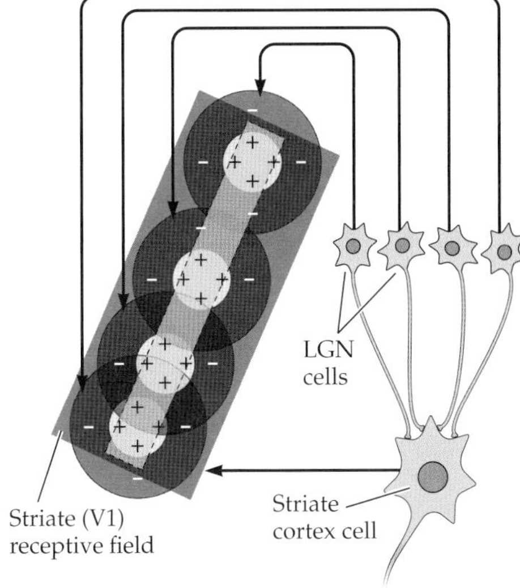

FIGURE 3.21 How striate cortex cells get tuned This simple model illustrates Hubel and Wiesel's hypothesis that lateral geniculate nucleus (LGN) cells are lined up in a row, feeding into the elongated, linear arrangement of the striate cortex receptive fields.

Other Receptive-Field Properties

Cortical cells don't just respond to bars, lines, and edges. Like retinal ganglion cells, they also respond well to gratings (which are, after all, collections of lines). And, like ganglion cells, they respond best to gratings that have just the right spatial frequency to fill the receptive-field center. That is, each striate cortex cell is tuned to a particular spatial frequency, which corresponds to a particular line width. Indeed, cortical cells are much more narrowly tuned (that is, they respond to a smaller range of spatial frequencies) than retinal ganglion cells (De Valois, Albrecht, and Thorell, 1982). These narrow tuning functions mean that each striate cortex neuron functions as a filter for the portion of the image that excites the cell. We will return to the idea of striate cortex as a collection of filters later in the chapter.

Another important discovery made by Hubel and Wiesel (1979) was that many cortical cells respond especially well to *moving* lines, bars, edges, and gratings. Moreover, many neurons respond strongly when a line moves in one direction—say, from left to right—but not at all when the same line moves, say, from right to left.

As noted earlier, information from the two eyes is kept separate in the LGN: each LGN cell responds to one eye or the other, but never to both eyes. This arrangement changes dramatically in striate cortex, where a majority of cells can be influenced by input from both the left eye and the right eye. In other words, if a striate cortex neuron responds best to a 5 cycle/degree grating oriented at 45 degrees, it will respond to such a stimulus whether that stimulus is presented in the right eye or the left eye. However, striate cortex neurons often have a preference, responding somewhat more strongly when a stimulus is presented in one eye than when it is presented in the other. Hubel and Wiesel (1979) called this property of striate receptive fields **ocular dominance**.

Given that we see a single, unified world, intuitively it makes sense that information from the two eyes should be brought together at some point. Until Hubel and Wiesel's discovery, however, there were heated arguments about whether the information converged at all and, if so, whether it was in a specialized "fusion center" in the brain—a notion that dates back to Descartes (1664) (see I. P. Howard and Rogers, 2001). We'll describe some of these issues in Chapter 6, when we discuss binocular vision.

(A) Edge detector

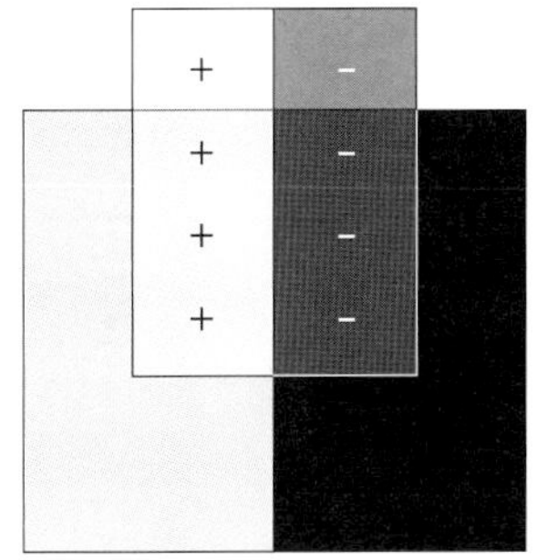

(B) Stripe detector

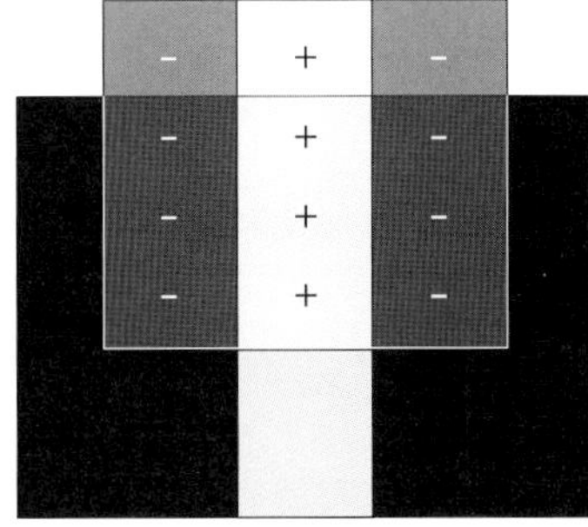

FIGURE 3.22 Two flavors of simple cells Simple cells of the striate cortex have distinct excitatory (+) and inhibitory (–) regions and respond primarily to specifically oriented bars and gratings. Diagrammed here are the firing patterns of (A) an edge detector cell and (B) a stripe detector cell.

Simple and Complex Cells

Like precortical neurons, cortical neurons come in a wide variety of types. Hubel and Wiesel characterized some neurons as **simple cells**. Simple cells are cortical neurons whose receptive fields have clearly defined excitatory and inhibitory regions. **FIGURE 3.22** shows two varieties of simple-cell receptive fields and their preferred stimuli. An edge detector (Figure 3.22A) is most highly excited when there is light on one side of its receptive field and darkness on the other side. A stripe detector

complex cell A cortical neuron whose receptive field does not have clearly defined excitatory and inhibitory regions.

end stopping The process by which a cell in the cortex increases its firing rate as the length of a bar increases until the bar fills up its receptive field, and then it decreases its firing rate as the bar is lengthened further.

(Figure 3.22B) responds best to a line of light that has a particular width, surrounded on both sides by darkness. If a grating with the appropriate spatial frequency drifts across the receptive field of this cell, the cell's response will be modulated as dark and bright bars drift across the receptive-field center, in exactly the same way the response of the retinal ganglion cell shown in Figure 3.13 is modulated.

Other neurons show responses that cannot be predicted simply from their responses to stationary bars of light. Hubel and Wiesel called these **complex cells**. Complex cells are cortical neurons whose receptive fields do not have clearly defined excitatory and inhibitory regions. Like simple cells, each complex cell is tuned to a particular orientation and spatial frequency and shows an ocular preference. However, whereas a simple cell might respond only if a stripe is presented in the center of its receptive field, a complex cell will respond regardless of where the stripe is presented, so long as it is somewhere within the cell's receptive field (**FIGURE 3.23**). Another way of stating this difference is to say that simple cells are "phase-sensitive" and complex cells are "phase-insensitive." When tested with a drifting grating, the complex cell gives a robust response, with little or none of the modulation shown by simple cells (as well as retinal ganglion and LGN cells).

As with all other neurons in the visual system (with the exception of retinal photoreceptors), the receptive fields of complex cells represent a pooling of the responses of several subunits. The subunits give the complex cell its spatial frequency and orientation tuning, but the complex pooling operation makes the complex cell insensitive to the precise position of the stimulus within its receptive field. Hubel and Wiesel (1979) hypothesized a hierarchy in which LGN cells fed into simple cells, which in turn provided excitatory inputs to complex cells. However, substantial evidence now suggests that complex cells represent a separate parallel pathway (that is, that both simple and complex cells get direct input from LGN neurons).

Further Complications

Hubel and Wiesel described another property of some cells in striate cortex that they called **end stopping**. When they tested an end-stopped cell with bars of increasing lengths, the response rate first increased as the bar filled up the cell's receptive field and then decreased markedly as the bar was lengthened further (**FIGURE 3.24**). Hubel and Wiesel called these cells "hypercomplex" cells, although they now appear to be subclasses of the simple and complex cells already discussed (that is, there are simple end-stopped cells and complex end-stopped cells). End stopping is thought to play an important role in our ability to detect luminance boundaries and discontinuities.

Research has revealed additional idiosyncrasies in the receptive fields of striate cortex neurons. For example, the size of a particular cell's receptive field appears to vary with target contrast; for instance, the cell might respond to a smaller portion of the visual field when the grating stimulus has a high contrast than it will when

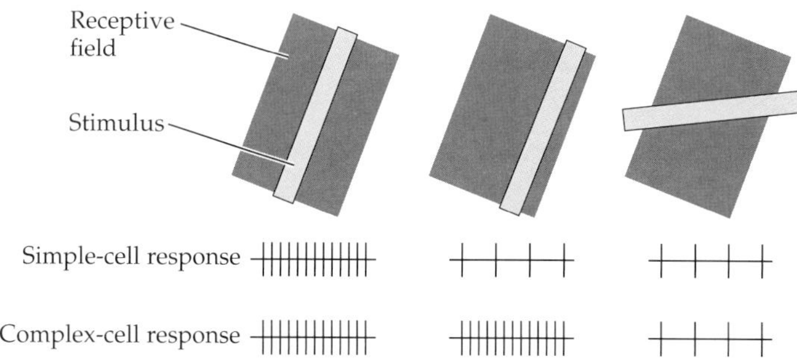

FIGURE 3.23 Simple and complex cells A simple cell and a complex cell might both be tuned to a stimulus of the same orientation and stripe width (spatial frequency), but the complex cell will respond to that stripe presented anywhere within its receptive field, whereas the simple cell might respond to the stripe in only one position.

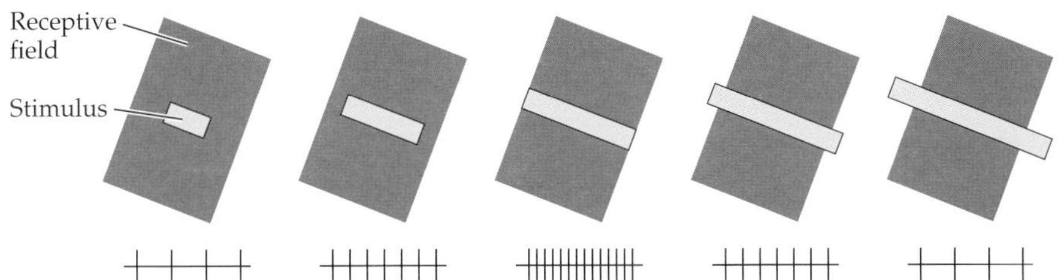

FIGURE 3.24 End stopping When the stimulus (bar) does not reach the outside edge of the receptive field of an end-stopped cortical neuron or if it extends beyond the receptive field, the neuron fires less than when the stimulus is just the right length. Both simple and complex cells can display this property.

the difference between light and dark bars is more subtle (Sceniak et al., 1999). Additionally, neurons can be influenced by stimuli that fall outside the classic receptive field, via short- or long-range lateral connections and/or via feedback from neurons in other layers (Zipser, Lamme, and Schiller, 1996).

As is the case for most of the visual system, what we don't know about the workings of striate cortex neurons almost certainly dwarfs what we do know.

3.6 Columns and Hypercolumns

As we've discussed, each of the approximately 200 million neurons in striate cortex responds to a distinctive set of stimulus properties: stripes, edges, and/or gratings that are oriented at a particular angle, with a particular width or spatial frequency, possibly moving in a particular direction. Some neurons are simple cells and some are complex cells, and each one can be end-stopped or not. Most neurons also respond preferentially to stimuli presented in one eye or another. And each neuron responds only when its preferred stimulus is presented in one particular part of the visual field.

Hubel and Wiesel noticed very early on that these various receptive-field properties are not scattered haphazardly around striate cortex. Once they had figured out what the cells were looking for (i.e., stripes rather than spots), they discovered that if they pushed the recording electrode down through the layers of the cortex in a direction perpendicular to the cortical surface, all the cells they encountered showed similar orientation preferences. If they shifted the electrode position over a tiny distance and made another perpendicular penetration, all the cells then responded best to a slightly different orientation, perhaps 10 or 15 degrees from the original orientation. Based on these observations, Hubel and Wiesel (1979) concluded that neurons with similar orientation preferences are arranged in **columns** that extend vertically through the cortex.

When Hubel and Wiesel made tangential penetrations into striate cortex (inserting an electrode in a direction parallel to the cortical surface, rather than perpendicular), they found a systematic and progressive change in preferred orientation and encountered essentially all the orientations in a distance of about 0.5 mm. This finding has been confirmed via alternative physiological techniques. **FIGURE 3.25A** shows a small portion of a monkey's striate cortex prepared so that neurons responding to vertically oriented lines are stained black, while other neurons remain white. The distance between the vertical orientation columns revealed by this technique is, sure enough, just about 0.5 mm (LeVay, Hubel, and Wiesel, 1975).

Orientation is not the only property arranged in columns in the visual cortex. Neurons that share the same eye preference (exhibiting ocular dominance) also have a columnar arrangement (**FIGURE 3.25B**). Furthermore, single-cell recording

column A vertical arrangement of neurons. Neurons within a single column tend to have similar receptive fields and similar orientation preferences.

(A) Orientation columns

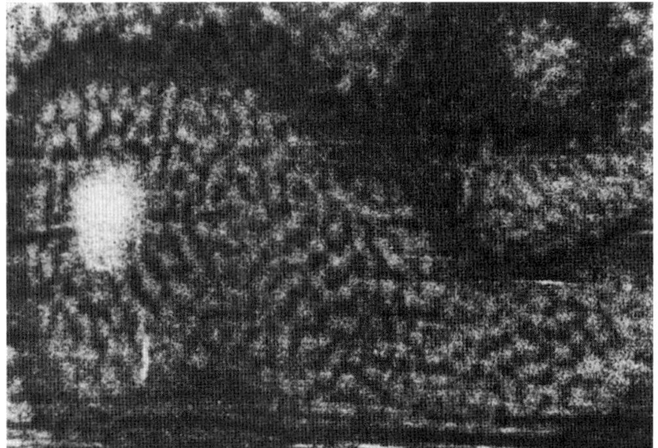

(B) Ocular dominance columns

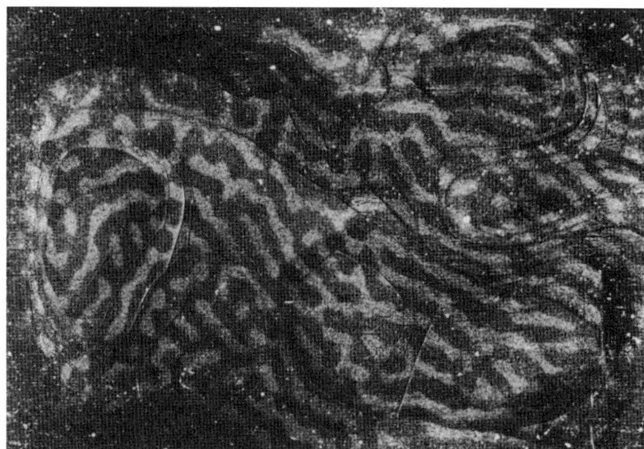

(C) Orientation maps

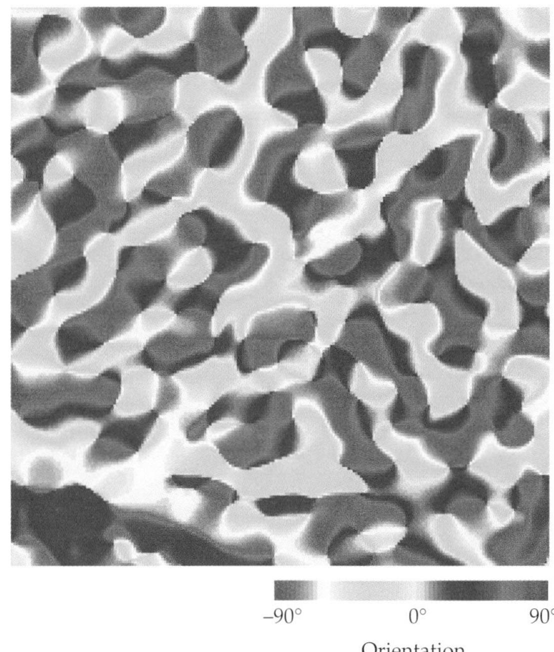

FIGURE 3.25 Cortical columns Orientation (A) and ocular dominance (B) columns revealed by staining a small portion of a monkey's striate cortex. (C) Optical imaging of the orientation maps in monkey cortex. Light reflected from the surface of the exposed brain reflects the activity of underlying neurons; each different color defines a set of neurons activated by the same given orientation.

experiments, as well as staining experiments, indicate that eye preference switches (you guessed it) every 0.5 mm or so.

Roughly 30 years ago, optical imaging techniques made it possible to create detailed maps of the orientation tuning of cells in the cortex, such as the one in FIGURE 3.25C. Here you can see the complex, yet orderly organization of orientation tuning in the cortex (Blasdel and Salama, 1986). More recent work (Paik and Ringach, 2011) suggests that this beautiful arrangement arises during early development as a consequence of statistical wiring mechanisms combined with evenly spaced mosaics of ON- and OFF-center retinal ganglion cells.

Through their studies, Hubel and Wiesel arrived at the model of striate cortical architecture illustrated in FIGURE 3.26. They proposed that a 1-mm block of striate cortex contains "all the machinery necessary to look after everything the visual cortex is responsible for, in a certain small part of the visual world" (Hubel, 1982).

FIGURE 3.26 A model of a hypercolumn This model consists of two ocular dominance columns (one for each eye) and many orientation columns, and it illustrates the locations of the cytochrome oxidase (CO) blobs.

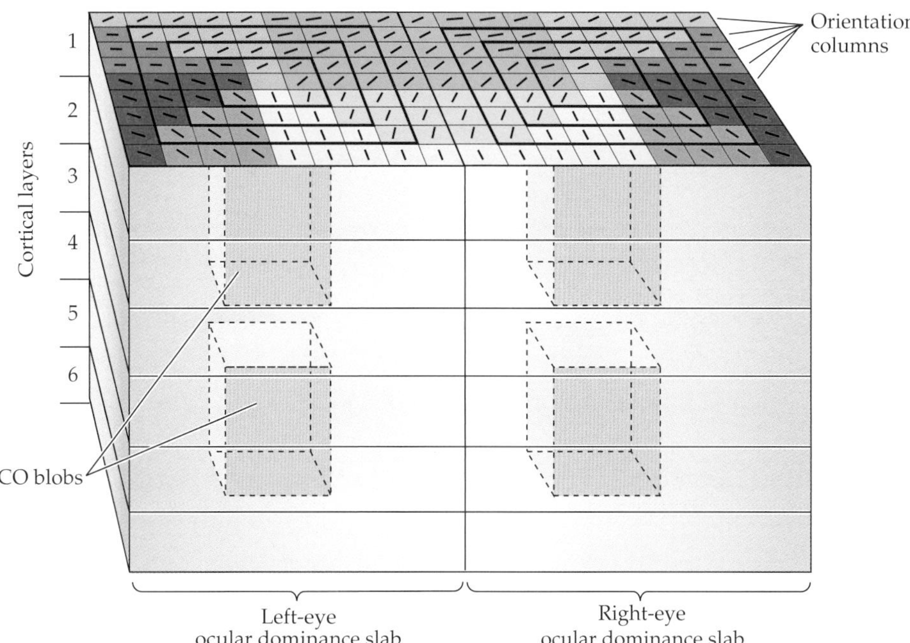

Each of these sections of cortex is called a **hypercolumn**. It contains at least two sets of columns, each covering every possible orientation (0–180 degrees), with one set preferring input from the left eye and one set preferring input from the right eye.

Hypercolumns are roughly 1 mm across throughout the striate cortex, but because of the cortical magnification factor discussed earlier, not all hypercolumns see the world at the same level of detail. A hypercolumn in the part of the cortex that represents the fovea may "see" a portion of the visual field that is 0.05 degrees of visual angle across; a hypercolumn responding to input 10 degrees to the right of the fovea should cover about 14 times as large an area (0.7 degrees across).

Orientation and ocular dominance are probably not the only stimulus dimensions that have a systematic columnar arrangement in the visual cortex. For example, another staining technique, which takes advantage of an enzyme called cytochrome oxidase (CO), has revealed a regular array of **CO blobs** (shown in section in **FIGURE 3.27**), spaced that magical distance of about 0.5 mm apart (see Figure 3.26). The functional role of these blobs remains unclear, but CO blob columns have

hypercolumn A 1-millimeter block of striate cortex containing two sets of columns, each covering every possible orientation (0–180 degrees), with one set preferring input from the left eye and one set preferring input from the right eye.

CO blobs Regular arrays of "blobs" spaced about 0.5 millimeter apart in the striate cortex (V1), so named because their presence is visualized by staining with the enzyme cytochrome oxidase. They may function in color perception.

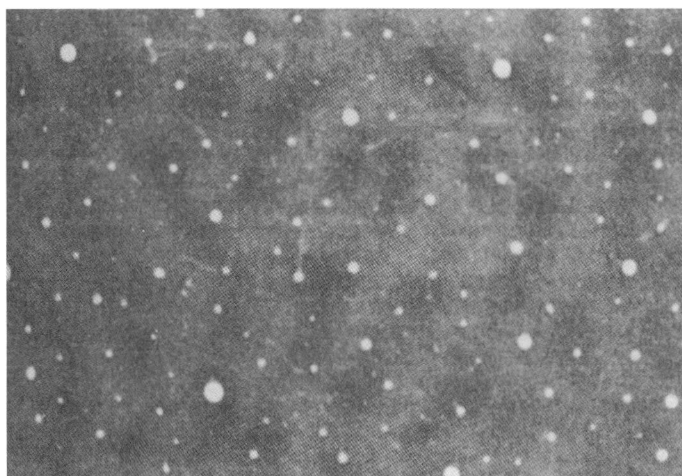

FIGURE 3.27 Cytochrome oxidase blobs Staining with the enzyme cytochrome oxidase (CO) reveals regularly arrayed "blobs" within the striate cortex. Although their exact function is not yet clear, CO blobs are believed to play a role in color processing, while the regions surrounding them process movement and orientation.

been implicated in processing color, with the interblob regions (note the elegant scientific jargon that has developed around this field of study) processing motion and spatial structure (Livingstone and Hubel, 1988). This view is probably too simplistic, but the blob array does suggest some kind of additional organizational layer on top of the orientation and ocular dominance arrays.

FURTHER DISCUSSION of CO blobs, which are implicated in processing color, can be found in Section 5.4.

In sum, the current state of understanding is that striate cortex is concerned with analyzing the orientation, size, shape, speed, and direction of motion of objects in the world and that it does so using modular groups of neurons—hypercolumns—each of which receives input from and processes a small piece of the visual world. We can think of this arrangement as a big bank of filters. Combining information from multiple hypercolumns is presumably the job of other portions of cortex farther downstream in the visual system. We will consider some of these portions in Section 4.3, when we discuss the representation and recognition of whole objects.

3.7 Selective Adaptation: The Psychologist's Electrode

Most of the physiological research reported up to this point in the chapter was done using cats, monkeys, or other animals as subjects. Does the human visual system also include neurons selective for orientation, line width, direction of motion, and so on? The difficult thing about answering this question is that we can't normally poke electrodes into a human's brain (which is why Hubel, Wiesel, and their peers had to use cats and monkeys), so indirect methods of learning about brain function had to be devised. One such method is based on **adaptation**, the diminished response that follows previous exposure to a stimulus. The technique gives psychologists a noninvasive "electrode" they can use to probe the human brain. (Although often attributed to John Frisby [1980], the term "the psychologist's electrode" was actually coined by Sir Colin Blakemore in the 1970s.)

Selective adaptation (i.e., adaptation to a limited set of stimuli) can provide insights into the properties of cortical neurons, as illustrated in **FIGURE 3.28**. The bars in Figure 3.28A illustrate the normal firing rates of cells tuned to various orientations (degrees of 0, 10, –10, 20, –20, and so on) relative to a vertical grating. By definition, gratings oriented at 0 degrees (vertical) elicit the strongest response from the 0-degree selective cells, followed closely by the 10-degree and –10-degree selective cells, followed by the 20-degree and –20-degree selective cells, and so on. Now suppose we expose the visual system that contains these cells to a 20-degree grating for an extended period. This adapting stimulus causes the 20-degree selective cells to be most active, and the extended activity will fatigue these cells (that is, their maximum firing rate will be reduced for a short period following adaptation). The adaptation procedure will also affect the other cells to some extent: the 10-degree and 30-degree cells will be the next most fatigued, followed by the 0-degree and 40-degree cells, and so on.

adaptation A reduction in response caused by prior or continuing stimulation.

Figure 3.28B shows what should happen when we present the vertical grating again after adaptation to the 20-degree grating, assuming that our orientation perception is really caused by populations of orientation-selective cells like those

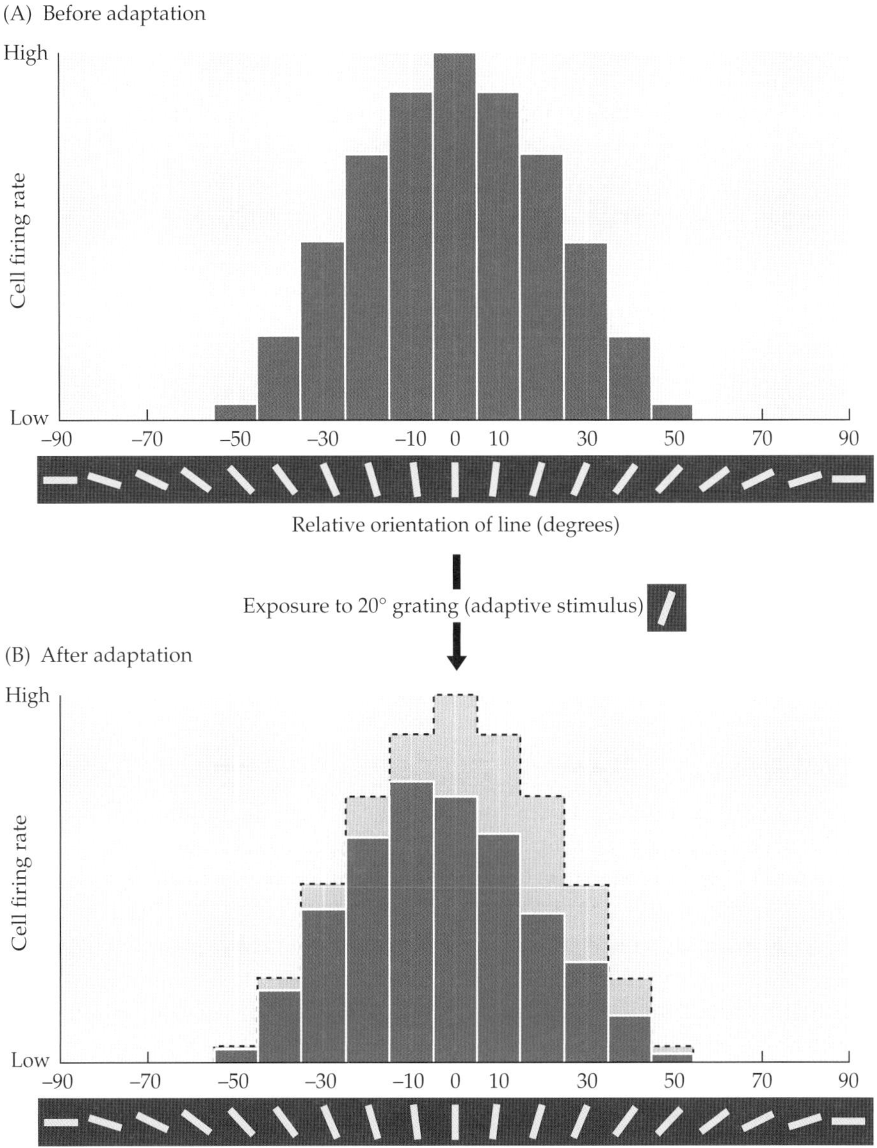

FIGURE 3.28 "The psychologist's electrode" This schematic diagram shows how selective adaptation may alter the distribution of neural responses and therefore perception. (A) Firing rates of cells tuned to various orientations in a grating. (B) Firing rates of the same cells after being exposed for a time to a 20-degree grating (yellow bar). The lighter bars reproduce the amount of firing before adaptation; the difference between the lighter and darker bars corresponds to the degree of fatigue for each type of cell.

that Hubel and Wiesel found in the cat cortex. As the darker bars show, because the 0-degree cells have been fatigued more than the –10-degree cells, the –10-degree cells are now firing fastest. As a result, we should perceive the vertical test stimulus as being oriented 10 degrees to the left. Thus, adaptation results in both a decrease in firing rate and a change in the tuning curve.

You can test the validity of this technique yourself using the stimuli in **FIGURE 3.29**. First, look at the middle of Figure 3.29A and notice that the top and bottom stripes are vertical and the same. Next, look at Figure 3.29C and notice that the top and bottom are both tilted, forming an arrowhead of sorts, pointing left. Now we will make Figure 3.29A look like Figure 3.29C. Look at the white bar in the middle of Figure 3.29B (the "adapting" stimulus). Notice it points to the right. Look at this pattern for about 20 seconds, keeping your eyes pointed at the white horizontal bar. Now quickly look at the middle of Figure 3.29A. It should look like

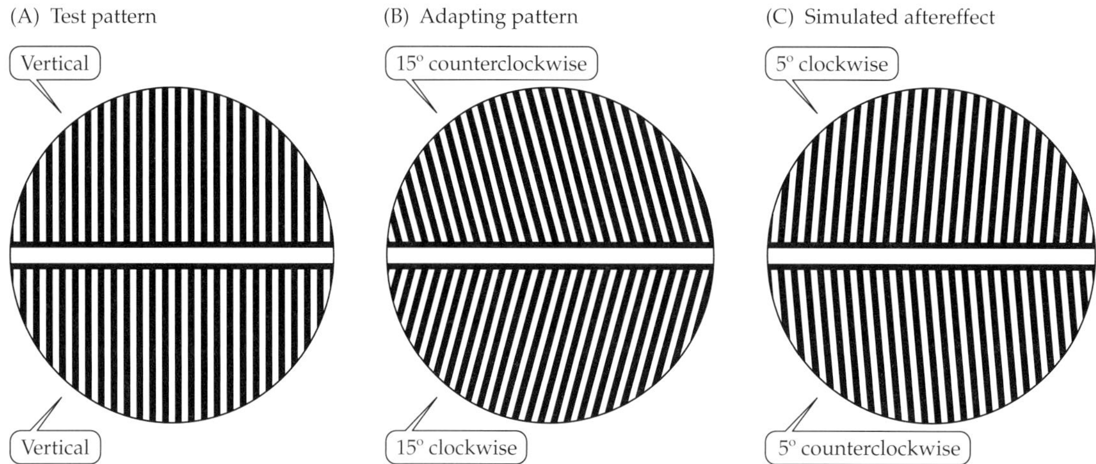

FIGURE 3.29 Demonstrating selective adaptation: The tilt aftereffect (A) The top and bottom halves have the same vertical orientation. (B) In the adapting pattern, the top lines are tilted left and the bottom lines are tilted right. The whole patterns look like an arrowhead pointing right. If you look at the bar between top and bottom in (B) for about 20 seconds and then look back at the vertical lines in (A), they will appear to point left, like what you see in (C), though probably less strongly and certainly more fleetingly.

tilt aftereffect The perceptual illusion of tilt, produced by adaptation to a pattern of a given orientation.

it is pointed a bit to the left. The effect may grow a bit stronger if you alternate a few seconds of Figure 3.29B with a brief glance at Figure 3.29A. That is the **tilt aftereffect**, just as predicted by the model of the human visual system based on the cat research and diagrammed in Figure 3.29. The tilt aftereffect strongly supports the idea that the human visual system contains individual neurons selective for different orientations.

Selective adaptation also provides evidence that the human visual system contains neurons selective for spatial frequency. You can check this with the gratings shown in **FIGURE 3.30**. First, look at Figure 3.30B and make a mental note of your CSF (the inverted *U*-shaped area where the gratings fade into the gray background; see Figure 3.9. Next, adapt for about 10–20 seconds to the grating in Figure 3.30A, and then quickly shift your gaze back to Figure 3.30B and make a mental note of your CSF now. After you repeat this procedure a few times, the outline of your CSF in Figure 3.30B should look something like the red curve in Figure 3.30C. It should have a notch (indicating reduced contrast sensitivity for spatial frequencies that are close to the adapting spatial frequency in Figure 3.30A). This demonstration shows that adaptation to the high-contrast top panel (Figure 3.30A) is selective—it results in a loss of sensitivity for spatial frequencies close to the adapting frequency, but no loss for spatial frequencies that are much higher or lower than the adapting frequency. Note that adaptation to the bottom panel (Figure 3.30D) does not result in a similar notch, since spatial-frequency adaptation is orientation-selective. Thus, there is little or no effect on sensitivity to vertical gratings following adaptation to a horizontal grating.

As noted earlier, selective adaptation causes the neurons most sensitive to the adapting stimulus to become fatigued. In this demonstration, neurons sensitive to the spatial frequency of the adapting stimulus have their contrast sensitivity reduced. That is, higher contrast is needed after adaptation for a test grating to stimulate these neurons. Neurons responsive to much higher or much lower spatial frequencies are not fatigued by the adaptation procedure, so contrast sensitivity for these spatial frequencies is not affected.

(A)

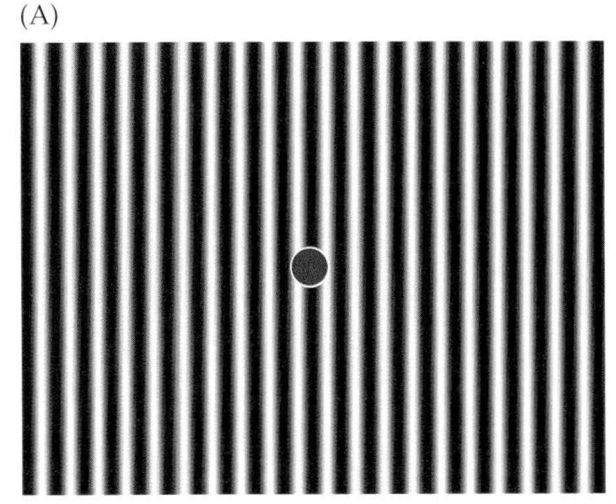

(B)

(C)

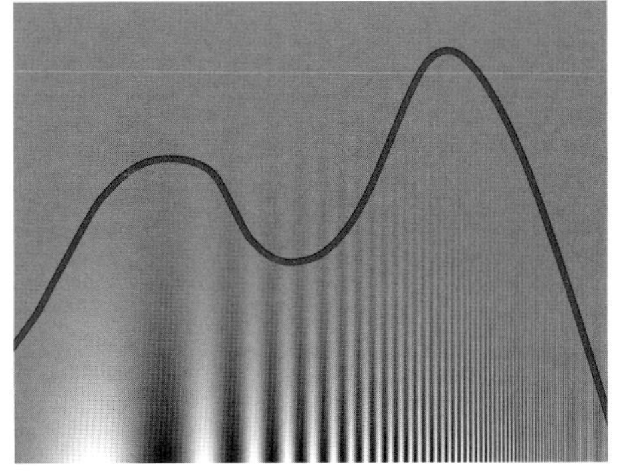

(D)

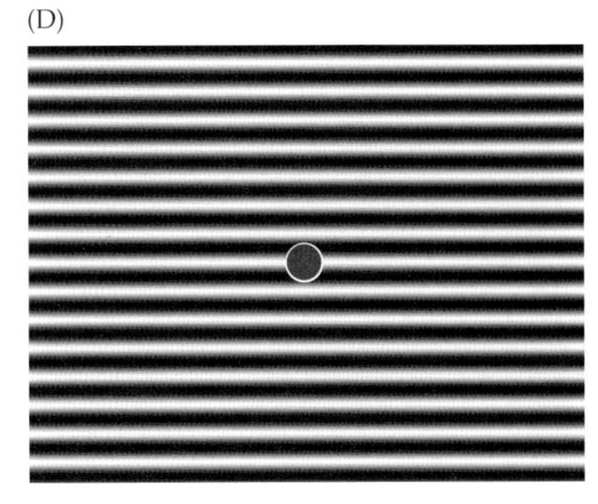

FIGURE 3.30 A demonstration of adaptation to specific spatial frequency Detailed instructions for this exercise are given in the text. (A) The adapting grating. (B) A grating modulated in contrast (vertically) and spatial frequency (horizontally). This pattern lets you visualize your own contrast sensitivity function (CSF; see Figure 3.9). Before adaptation, your CSF should have the appearance of an inverted *U*. After adaptation to (A), your CSF should look something like the red curve in (C). The red curve illustrates the effect of adaptation. The notch indicates reduced contrast sensitivity for spatial frequencies that are close to the adapting spatial frequency. Adapting to the horizontal grating in (D) results in little or no reduction in sensitivity.

FIGURE 3.31A shows more precisely how selective adaptation to a 7 cycle/degree grating produces a selective loss of contrast sensitivity at spatial frequencies of about 7 cycles/degree, with little or no loss at, for example, 1 cycle/degree or 15 cycles/degree. After adaptation, the CSF has a "notch," as if the detectors sensitive to spatial frequencies near 7 cycles/degree were selectively desensitized (luckily, the effects of spatial-frequency adaptation are reversible).

From these measurements of contrast sensitivity before and after adaptation, we can construct the spatial-frequency tuning function shown in **FIGURE 3.31B**. This function represents the change in contrast threshold (contrast threshold after adaptation divided by contrast threshold before adaptation) plotted against the spatial frequency of the test grating. This curve represents the spatial-frequency tuning function for a "channel" that is most sensitive to a grating of 7 cycles/degree. The shape and selectivity of this channel are very similar to the spatial-frequency tuning functions for striate cortex neurons of cats and monkeys. **FIGURE 3.31C** illustrates that the CSF represents the "upper envelope" of the sensitivities of many spatial-frequency channels, each tuned to a different spatial frequency. The key idea here is that you can see the pattern when at least one mechanism (one channel) detects it.

The Site of Selective Adaptation Effects

The adaptation experiments replicated here provide strong evidence that orientation and spatial frequency are coded by neurons somewhere in the human visual system. In cats and monkeys, we know that these neurons are located in striate cortex, not in the retina or LGN. Can we localize the orientation-selective and spatial frequency–selective neurons in humans?

As it turns out, we can do just that with a clever variation on the adaptation experiments. Repeat the orientation (Figure 3.29) and spatial-frequency (Figure 3.30) adaptation demonstrations, but this time view the adapting stimuli with your left eye only, keeping your right eye closed during the adaptation period. Then view the test stimuli with your right eye (close your left eye and open your right eye as you shift your gaze to the test stimuli). You should find that the tilt aftereffect and the decreased contrast sensitivity transfer from one eye to the other, although the effect may be somewhat less pronounced than when you did the demonstrations with both eyes open. This transfer of adaptation from the adapted to the nonadapted eye is known as interocular transfer (C. Blakemore and Campbell, 1969).

Now recall that information from the two eyes is kept completely separate in the retinas and in the two LGNs: no single neuron receives input from both eyes until the striate cortex. The transfer of adaptation effects from one eye to the other thus implies that selective adaptation occurs in cortical neurons, just as we would predict from animal physiology studies.

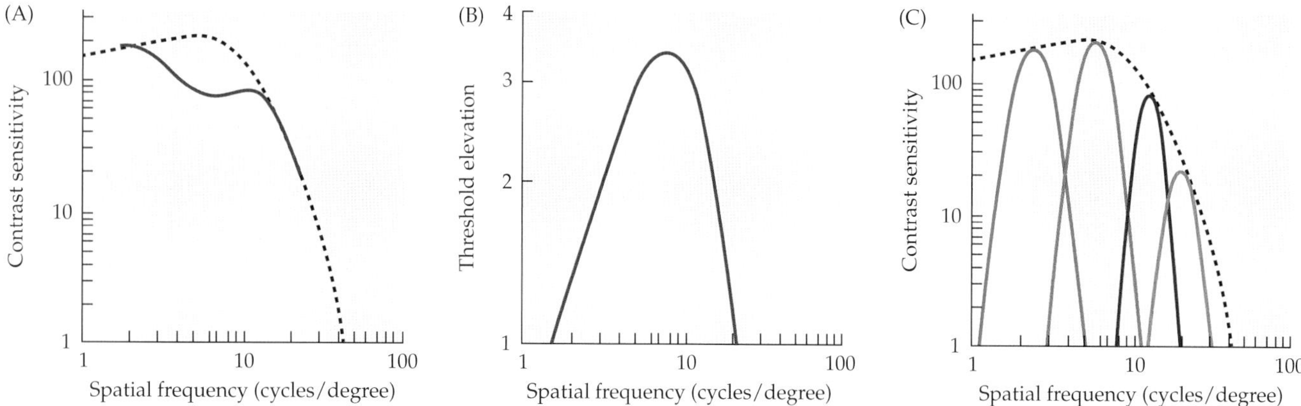

FIGURE 3.31 Spatial-frequency adaptation (A) Selective adaptation to a 7 cycle/degree grating produces a selective loss of contrast sensitivity at spatial frequencies of about 7 cycles/degree, leaving a notch (solid red line) in the contrast sensitivity function (CSF; black dashed curve). (B) Threshold elevation (the change in contrast threshold) following adaptation. (C) Physiologically measured spatial-frequency tuning functions for striate cortex neurons in monkeys (solid, colored curves represent different neurons). The dashed black curve—the CSF—represents the "upper envelope" of the sensitivities of the underlying channels.

spatial-frequency channel A pattern analyzer, implemented by an ensemble of cortical neurons, in which each set of neurons is tuned to a limited range of spatial frequencies.

Spatial-Frequency-Tuned Pattern Analyzers in Human Vision

Selective adaptation to spatial frequency, as well as other evidence, provides strong support for the notion, first suggested by Fergus Campbell and John Robson (1968), that the human CSF actually reflects the sensitivity of multiple individual pattern analyzers. These pattern analyzers are implemented by ensembles of cortical neurons, with each set of cells tuned to a limited range of spatial frequencies and orientations, and these cell sets are often referred to as **spatial-frequency channels**. Remember the unexplained falloff in the contrast sensitivity function at very low spatial frequencies (the left side of the CSF curve in Figure 3.9)? Although a number of explanations have been suggested (e.g., lateral inhibition), the most likely explanation is that we simply have fewer neurons tuned to low spatial frequencies (De Valois, Albrecht, and Thorell, 1982) to compensate for the overrepresentation of energy in the lower spatial frequencies in natural scenes (Field, 1987).

The multiple-spatial-frequency model of vision implies that spatial frequencies that stimulate different pattern analyzers will be detected independently, even if the different frequencies are combined in the same image. Consider the compound grating pattern in **FIGURE 3.32**, made by adding a sine wave with frequency f to a sine wave with frequency $3f$. Graham and Nachmias (1971) found that the contrast sensitivity for this compound pattern was almost the same as the contrast sensitivity for detecting the individual components of the pattern separately. If the two component sine waves had stimulated

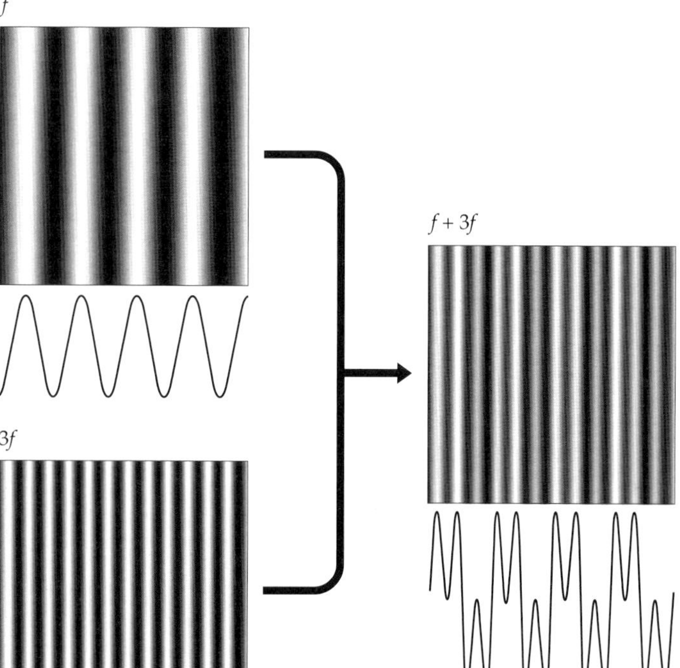

FIGURE 3.32 Multiple-spatial-frequency model Contrast sensitivity for the compound grating pattern on the right, made by the addition of a sine wave of frequency f (top left) to one of frequency $3f$ (bottom left), is almost the same as the contrast sensitivity function for detecting each of the component patterns separately.

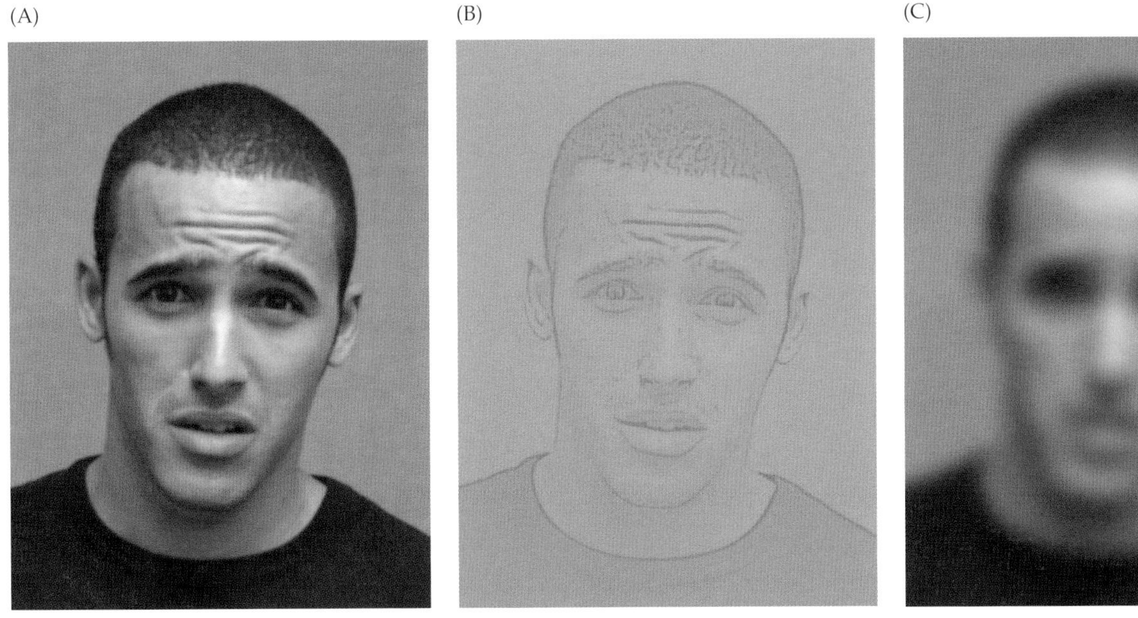

FIGURE 3.33 Different spatial frequencies emphasize different information (A) A complete facial image. (B) Reconstruction of (A) with the low spatial frequencies removed, leaving only the high-frequency components of the image. (C) Analogous reconstruction with the high spatial frequencies removed, leaving only the low-frequency components.

a common pattern analyzer, then their effects on the analyzer should have been added, so contrast sensitivity should have been greatly improved. This may sound a bit like the Fourier analysis idea discussed early in this chapter. However, it's now pretty clear that the visual system doesn't carry out an actual Fourier analysis, analyzing the world into very narrow bands of spatial frequencies. Rather, it filters the image into spatially localized receptive fields that have a limited range of spatial frequencies. (Something like a Fourier analysis may be important in quickly appreciating the gist of a scene; see Section 7.6.)

Why would the visual system use spatial-frequency filters to analyze images? One important reason may be that different spatial frequencies emphasize different types of information. **FIGURE 3.33** breaks down a facial image (Figure 3.33A) into versions that show only its high-frequency or low-frequency components (Figures 3.33B and 3.33C, respectively). These images show that low frequencies emphasize the broad outlines of the face, and high frequencies carry information about fine details. If we want to know how many people are in a scene, it is most efficient to consult our low-frequency channels. But if we want to know about the fine details—for example, whether a person is frowning or smiling—we must rely on our high-frequency channels.

Note that high spatial frequencies can mask low spatial frequencies. You can experience this for yourself in **FIGURE 3.34**, where the high spatial frequencies introduced by the small blocks mask the low spatial frequencies that convey the underlying portrait of a famous American. Squinting your eyes will blur the blocks, minimizing the effect of the mask

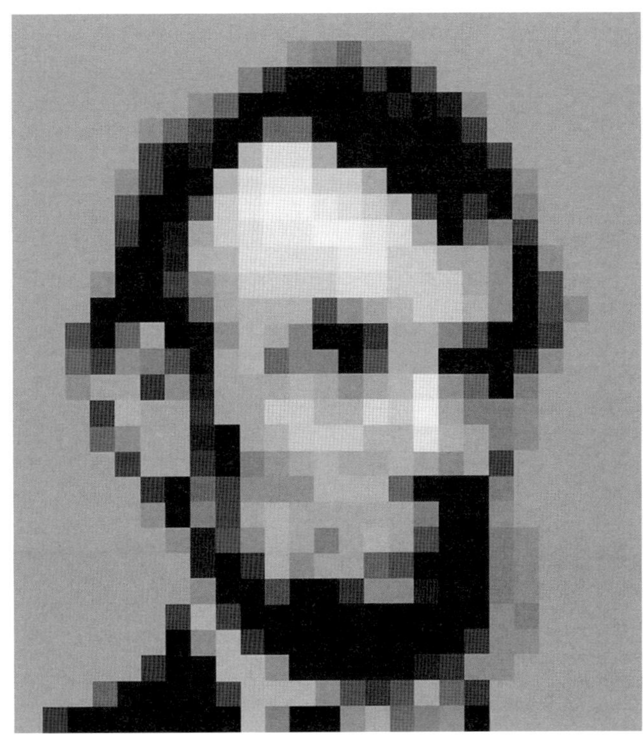

FIGURE 3.34 Who is that masked man? Who is hidden behind the high-spatial-frequency mask in this image?

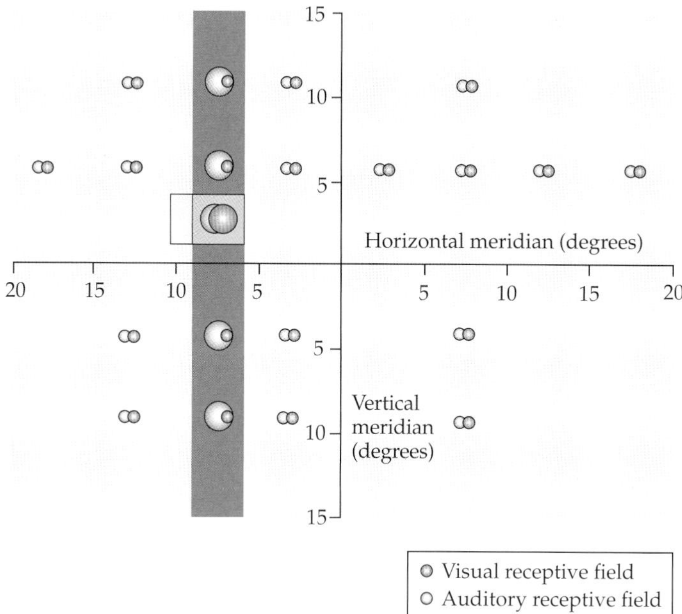

FIGURE 3.35 **Spatial specificity of bimodal (visual and acoustic) receptive fields in V1** Larger circles represent greater response. The dark-gray area represents the region where the auditory and visual receptive fields are aligned. The yellow box highlights the visual receptive field with the largest response.

to a point where the face you've seen countless times on the five-dollar bill will show through.

Although we've described the neurons in the striate cortex as "visual," a significant portion of them also respond to auditory stimuli (at least in cats) (Fishman and Michael, 1973; Morrell, 1972). Importantly, the auditory and visual receptive fields of these neurons have similar directional tuning and are spatially aligned in the horizontal meridian (**FIGURE 3.35**). Interestingly, while visual receptive fields are localized both horizontally and vertically, auditory receptive fields are very elongated in the vertical dimension. The similar locations of auditory and visual receptive fields may be helpful in accurate spatial localization, at least in the horizontal direction. Indeed, in the brain's superior colliculus (discussed in Section 8.4), when auditory and visual cues are close in space and time, they often enhance the responses of multisensory neurons, while competing cues (i.e., stimuli that are spatially or temporally dissimilar) result in no enhancement or even reduced responses (B. E. Stein, Stanford, and Rowland, 2014). ●

3.8 The Development of Vision

William James (1890) described the infant's world as "a blooming, buzzing confusion." However, studies over the past several decades have shown that the human visual system is much more developed at birth than we used to think. One of the difficulties in assessing vision in infants is that we can't simply ask them what they see. Rather, we have to think of tricky ways to coax that information from them.

The most widely used method for studying infant vision is based on an observation that Robert Fantz made in the early 1960s: he noticed that when infants are shown two scenes, they invariably stare at the more complex scene (the scene with the most contours) (Fantz, 1963). So, if an infant is shown two patches, one containing stripes and the other uniform gray, the infant will prefer to look at the stripes. Because an infant who couldn't see the stripes would be equally likely to stare at the gray patch as at the striped patch, preferential looking is one important method used by infant researchers (grown psychologists studying infant vision, not babies in lab coats) to learn what infants can see and respond to behaviorally (**FIGURE 3.36A**).

The success of preferential looking depends on the willingness of babies to stare at stimuli near threshold level. An alternative approach, used with considerable success in more recent years, is to measure visually evoked electrical potentials—that is, electrical signals from the brain that are evoked by visual stimuli—by attaching electrodes to the infant's scalp and measuring the changes in electrical activity that are elicited by the changing visual stimulus (**FIGURES 3.36B** and **3.36C**). Using this technique, we can measure an entire CSF in as little as 10 seconds in a nonverbal infant.

These techniques have provided a great deal of insight into the development of visual mechanisms and sensitivities. One insight is that different visual functions may emerge at different times and may develop at different rates. Thus, for example, the rod system appears to be functional in early infancy (Brown, 1990; Fulton, 1988; Powers et al., 1981; Teller and Bornstein, 1986; Werner, 1982). While rods and rhodopsin are functional early on, postreceptoral mechanisms may mature later, since dark-adapted spatial summation areas of infants are considerably enlarged

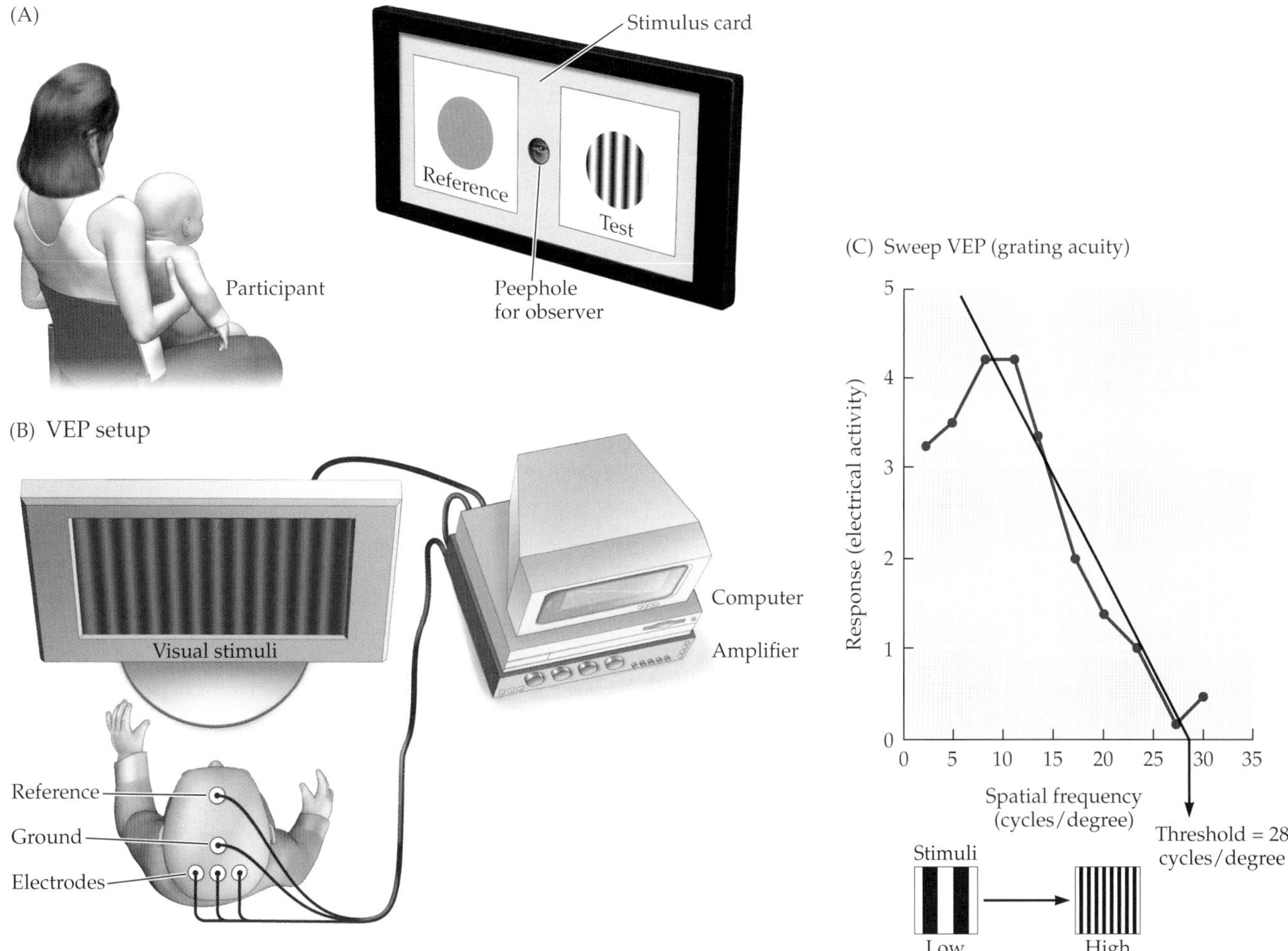

FIGURE 3.36 Assessing vision in infants (A) The experimental setup for a forced-choice preferential-looking study. (B) Setup for a visually evoked electrical potential (VEP) experiment. VEP studies measure changes in brain electrical activity elicited by a changing stimulus image. (C) Results of a VEP experiment in which the spatial frequency of the stimulus is swept (i.e., continuously varied from low to high spatial frequency), illustrating the extrapolated CSF and associated acuity threshold (in this case, 27.6 cycles/degree).

Sensation & Perception in Everyday Life

The Girl Who Almost Couldn't See Stripes

Normal visual development requires normal visual experience. Abnormal early visual experience can have serious and often permanent consequences for seeing patterns, as illustrated by the story of a girl named Jane. Jane was born with a dense cataract (an opacity of the lens) in her left eye, which prevented clear patterns from forming on her left retina. In addition to causing form deprivation in the left eye, the cataract prevented Jane's two eyes from seeing the same images at the same time.

Studies in cats and monkeys dating back to Hubel and Wiesel in the early 1960s have shown that monocular form deprivation can cause massive changes in cortical physiology that result in a devastating and permanent loss of spatial vision (Wiesel, 1982). Hubel and Wiesel, and many other workers since, demonstrated that there is a **critical period** of early visual development when normal binocular visual stimulation is required for normal cortical development. In cats and monkeys, this critical period covers the first 3–4 months of life; in humans it is extended to something on the order of the first 3–8 years. During the critical period, cortical neurons are still being wired to their inputs from the two eyes. This is a period of neural plasticity, when abnormal visual experience can alter the normal neural wiring process. If one eye is not receiving normal stimulation, the neurons that should be destined to respond to that eye do not become properly connected. In fact, some evidence suggests that these neurons are actually co-opted by inputs from the other, normally functioning eye.

If cataracts are left untreated during the critical period, the misplaced cortical connections can never be repaired. The result is often amblyopia: reduced visual acuity in one eye because of abnormal early visual experience (commonly known as lazy eye) and a lack of binocular depth perception, or stereopsis (see Section 6.3). Correcting the cataract later in life will thus have little effect, because the information from the now-functioning eye can never be properly conveyed to or processed by the cortex.

Luckily for Jane, her pediatrician found the cataract early, and the cataractous lens was surgically replaced by an artificial lens when she was 3 months old. The visual acuity in Jane's left eye just after the replacement lens was inserted was 20/1200, about four times worse than the normal value for a 3-month-old. But when she was tested again 1 month later, acuity in her left eye had already begun to catch up with the acuity in her right eye. In fact, a study of 28 infants (Maurer et al., 1999) found significant acuity improvements only an hour after corrective measures had been taken.

Not all individuals with congenital cataracts are as lucky as Jane. For example, in much of the third world, because of poverty, children born with congenital cataracts (often in both eyes) go untreated and grow up essentially blind. According to the World Health Organization, India is home to the largest population of blind children in the world. Recently, Pawan Sinha and his collaborators initiated an undertaking (Project Prakash) to perform free corrective cataract surgeries and track how these "blind" children learn to see. These studies are providing important new insights into brain plasticity. One such insight is that while spatial vision is severely compromised in newly sighted children, their temporal processing is relatively spared (Ji et. al., 2021).

Congenital cataracts are not the only cause of amblyopia. Early in life, two other disorders—**strabismus** (in which one eye is turned so that it is receiving a view of the world from an abnormal angle) and **anisometropia** (in which the two eyes have very different refractive errors; e.g., one eye is farsighted and the other is not)—may also cause amblyopia. These forms of amblyopia are typically less severe, and often they have a later onset than congenital cataracts.

For over 250 years, the standard clinical treatment for amblyopia has been to put a patch over the good eye and "force" the amblyopic eye to work. This treatment is ordinarily performed only in young children (typically younger than 8 years). However, several recent studies suggest that there may be hope for recovery of vision in older children, and even in adults, through "perceptual learning"—repeated practice of a demanding visual task (Levi and Li, 2009) or playing action video games (R. W. Li et al., 2011).

compared with those of adults (Hamer and Schneck, 1984). Many investigations of cone-mediated vision have focused on the development of mechanisms of color vision, visual acuity, and contrast sensitivity. It is now reasonably well established that by 2–3 months after birth, infants must have three functioning cone types. The question of when each of the three cone types functions normally is less clear. Infants less than 1 month old fail to make chromatic discriminations; however, what remains unclear is whether these failures reflect immature cones or postreceptoral mechanisms (Teller and Bornstein, 1986; Teller and Movshon, 1986) or lack of attention. Uniform field flicker sensitivity appears to be adultlike by 3 months of age (Regal, 1981), while acuity and contrast sensitivity for high spatial frequencies develop slowly and may not reach adult levels until several years of age.

critical period A phase in the life span during which abnormal early experience can alter normal neuronal development.

strabismus A misalignment of the two eyes such that a single object in space is imaged on the fovea of one eye and on a nonfoveal area of the other (turned) eye.

anisometropia A condition in which the two eyes have different refractive errors (e.g., one eye is farsighted and the other is not).

Development of the CSF

The emerging picture suggests that sensitivity to low spatial frequencies develops much more rapidly than sensitivity to high spatial frequencies. Thus, at low spatial frequencies, contrast sensitivity may reach nearly adult levels as early as about 9 weeks of age, whereas sensitivity at higher spatial frequencies continues to develop dramatically (**FIGURE 3.37**). There remains a substantial difference in the contrast sensitivity of adults and 33-week-olds at high spatial frequencies (Norcia, Tyler, and Hamer, 1990).

What limits the development of acuity and contrast sensitivity? The primary postnatal changes in the retina concern differentiation of the macular region (Boothe, Dobson, and Teller, 1985). After birth, foveal receptor density and cone outer segment length both increase, as foveal cones become thinner and more elongated. There is a dramatic migration of ganglion cells and inner nuclear layers from the foveal region as the foveal pit develops during the first 4 months of life, and not until about 4 years of age is the fovea fully adultlike (interestingly, the peripheral retina appears to develop much more rapidly than the fovea) (Yuodelis and Hendrickson, 1986).

From birth to beyond 4 years of age, cone density increases in the central region because of both the migration of receptors and the decreases in their

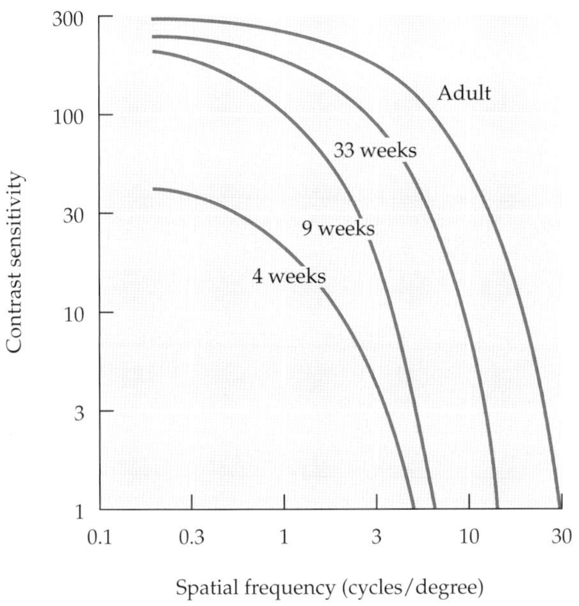

FIGURE 3.37 The development of contrast sensitivity Note that the shape of the contrast sensitivity function is "lowpass" (that is, there is no drop in sensitivity at low spatial frequencies) because the gratings were temporally modulated.

Scientists at Work

Does the Duck's Left Eye Know What the Right Eye Saw?

Question The question that two zoologists from Oxford University (Martinho and Kacelnik, 2016) asked was, If a duckling imprinted on its mother with one eye, would it recognize her with the other eye?

Hypothesis The corpus callosum is the bundle of fibers that enables the left and right brain hemispheres to communicate with each other in humans. However, birds don't have a corpus callosum (although that's not why we refer to bird brains). Therefore, in ducklings, information obtained through the left eye might not be recognized when viewed through the right eye.

Test One eye of each of 64 ducklings was covered with a blindfold, and then they were presented with a fake adult duck colored either red or blue. The ducklings imprinted on the colored fake duck, which became "mom," and the ducklings followed it around.

Results When the blindfold was switched to the previously open eye, the ducklings no longer recognized their mom and were equally likely to follow red or blue fake ducks.

Conclusion Each side of the avian brain seems to have a separate record of memory.

Future work Given that ducks do not have a corpus callosum, it will be important to understand how they integrate the separate information streams from the two eyes in order to make decisions.

dimensions. Both factors result in finer cone sampling (by decreasing the distance between neighboring cones). Alterations in cone spacing and the light-gathering properties of the cones during early development probably contribute a great deal to the improvements in acuity and contrast sensitivity during the first months of life. The massive migration of retinal cells, as well as the alterations in the size of retina and eyeball (along with changes in interpupillary distance), may necessitate the plasticity of cortical connections early in life.

Summary

1. In this chapter, we followed the path of image processing from the eyeball to the brain. Neurons in the cerebral cortex translate the array of activity signaled by retinal ganglion cells into the beginnings of forms and patterns. The primary visual cortex is organized into thousands of tiny computers, each responsible for determining the orientation, width, color, and other characteristics of the stripes in one small portion of the visual field. In Chapter 4, we will continue this story by seeing how other parts of the brain combine the outputs from these minicomputers to produce a coherent representation.
2. Perhaps the most important feature of image processing is the remarkable transformation of information from the circular receptive fields of retinal ganglion cells to the elongated receptive fields of the cortex.

3. Cortical neurons are highly selective along a number of dimensions, including stimulus orientation, size, direction of motion, and eye of origin.
4. Neurons with similar preferences are often arranged in columns in the primary visual cortex.
5. Selective adaptation provides a powerful, noninvasive tool for learning about stimulus specificity in human vision.
6. The human visual cortex contains pattern analyzers that are specific to spatial frequency and orientation.

Chapter 4

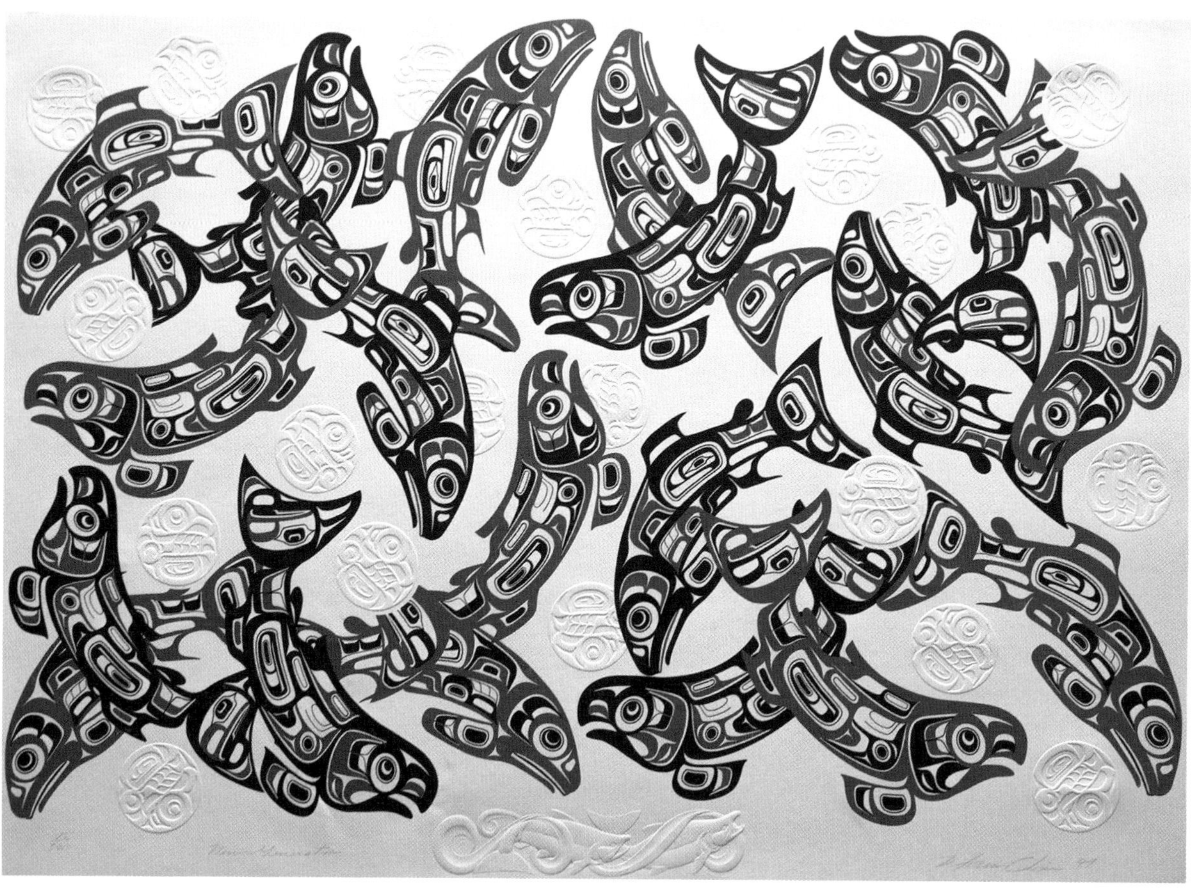

Marvin Oliver, *Next Generation*, 1997

Perceiving and Recognizing Objects

Questions to Contemplate

Think about the following questions as you read this chapter.
By the chapter's end, you should be able to answer and discuss them.

- Can the identity and location of an object be processed separately by the brain?
- How do we know what object (if any) an edge belongs to?
- How do we know if an object continues behind another, occluding object?
- How do we know what an object is made of?
- When do two bits of a visual image belong together in the same group or object?
- How do we recognize objects?
- Does the brain use just one way to represent a shape or an object?
- How could a computer recognize an object?

We have been traveling up the visual system from the eyes into the brain. By the end of Chapter 3, we had reached primary visual cortex (= V1, striate cortex), where we encountered cells that were optimally stimulated by bars and gratings of different orientations. Of course, when you look at the world, you do not see an array of bars and gratings; you see coherent objects and extended surfaces. Moreover, you recognize specific objects, even if they are odd objects, as in **FIGURE 4.1**. This chapter continues our journey through the visual system and considers how that visual system manages the task of perceiving and recognizing objects.

4.1 From Simple Lines and Edges to Properties of Objects

To begin, let's extend the visual pathways beyond V1 and beyond what was shown in Figure 3.1. Recall that cells in V1 are interested in the basic features of the visual image, responding to edges or lines of specific orientation, motion, size, and so forth. These neurons have relatively small and precise receptive fields. That is, a cell will respond to its preferred stimulus only if that stimulus is presented in a very specific location relative to the point where the observer (whether monkey, cat, or human) is fixating their gaze. Beyond V1 is the **extrastriate cortex**, a set of visual areas so called because they lie just outside the primary visual (striate) cortex. In the monkey, these areas are named V2, V3, and so on, though they are not a simple chain of processing areas, and the

extrastriate cortex The region of cortex bordering the primary visual cortex and containing multiple areas involved in visual processing.

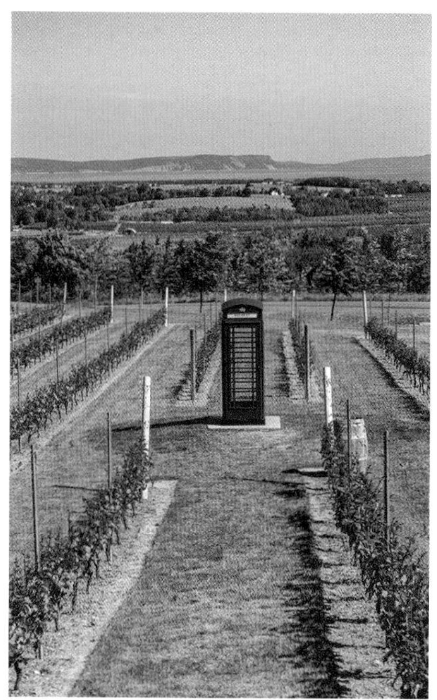

FIGURE 4.1 **Novelty is usually comprehensible** We see a world full of identifiable objects, even if we have never seen them in this particular arrangement before.

naming convention breaks down pretty rapidly. **FIGURE 4.2** shows the main visual areas of the macaque monkey brain, and **FIGURE 4.3** shows one "wiring" diagram of these and a few other visual areas. The human visual system is not identical to that of a macaque. However, the basic plan, mapped out in **FIGURE 4.4**, is similar. Basic, local properties are pulled out of the image by early stages of visual cortex, but sophisticated tasks like object recognition require a great deal of subsequent processing involving a large number of apparently distinct visual-processing areas.

We can sketch a broad structure of the visual areas beyond V1. In the extrastriate regions just beyond V1 (such as V2), receptive fields begin to show an interest in properties that will be important for object perception. As we saw in Chapter 3, cells in V1 have preferences for lines and edges of specific orientations in specific locations in the visual field. Imagine a cell tuned to edges tilted to the left of vertical with the darker side on the right. Such a cell would be activated if its receptive field lined up with the red ovals in any of the panels of **FIGURE 4.5**.

The hypothetical V1 cell would not care that the edge in Figure 4.5B is the edge of a black square, while the edge in Figure 4.5C is the edge of a gray square. You, the perceiver, do care about this. You care about what H. Zhou, Friedman, and von der Heydt (2000) called **border ownership**. When an object like the black square in Figure 4.5B is sitting on a background, the edges defining the border between object and background "belong" to the object. When Zhou and colleagues recorded from area V2, they found many cells that cared about border ownership. Suppose that a cell was activated by a dark edge on the right side of its receptive field

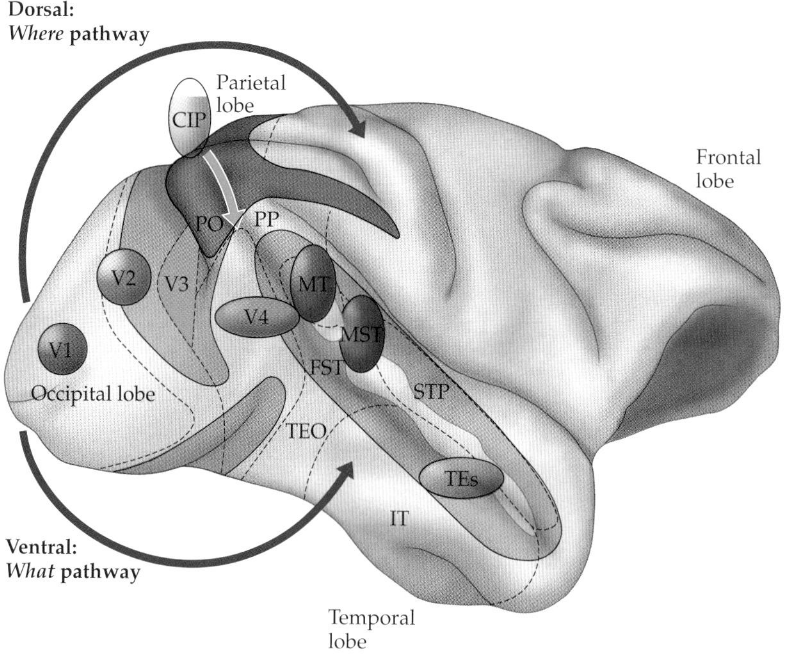

FIGURE 4.2 **The main visual areas of the macaque monkey cortex** Humans have comparable visual areas (see Figure 4.4). The drawing of the brain has been distorted to show areas that lie deep in the folds (sulci) of the cortex. Each abbreviation refers to a different visual area, not all of which will be discussed here. Visual cortical processing can be divided into two broad streams. One, heading for the parietal lobe, can be thought of as being interested in *where* things are. The other, heading down into the temporal lobe, is concerned with *what* things are.

border ownership When one object is in front of another, there will be a visual border formed between the object and the background. That border is "owned" by the object. It is the edge of the object, not a property of the background.

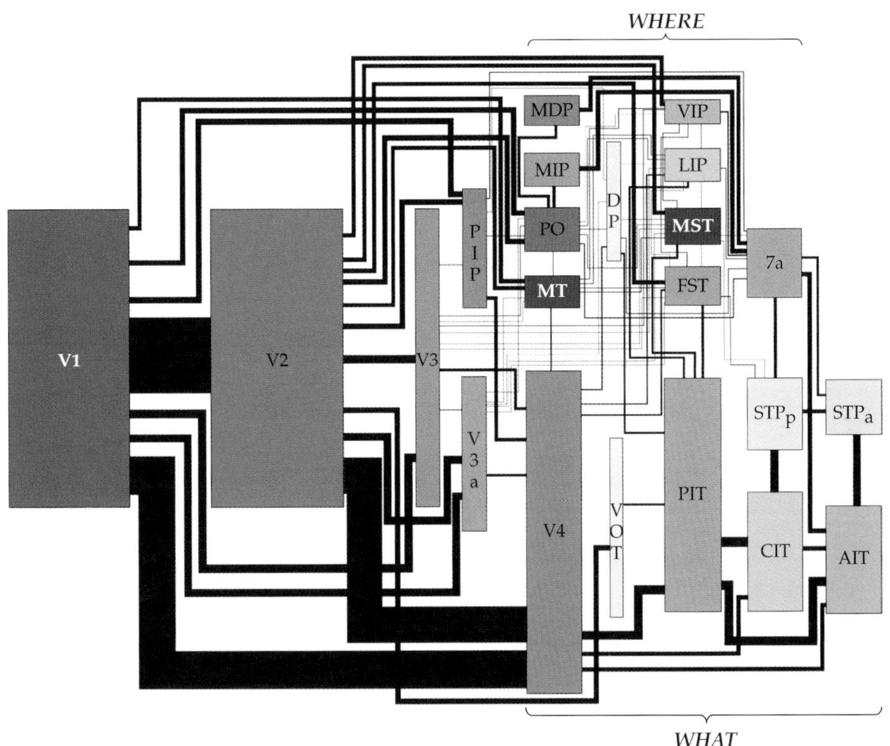

FIGURE 4.3 A "wiring" diagram for the monkey visual system In this schematic diagram, the relative size of the rectangles reflects the size of the area in the brain of the macaque monkey (we don't have these data for humans). The thickness of the wires (black lines) reflects the number of nerve fibers connecting areas. As in Figure 4.2, abbreviations refer to the different visual areas. The main message is that (1) the visual pathways are very complex, and (2) there are many visual areas. In addition, visual processing is a two-way street: there are both feed-forward and feedback connections between areas. For a bit of orientation, visual information from the eyes and the lateral geniculate nucleus enters at the left of the diagram. The *where* pathway of Figure 4.2 is shown in browns, golds, and reds at the upper right. The *what* pathway is shown in blues and greens at the lower right.

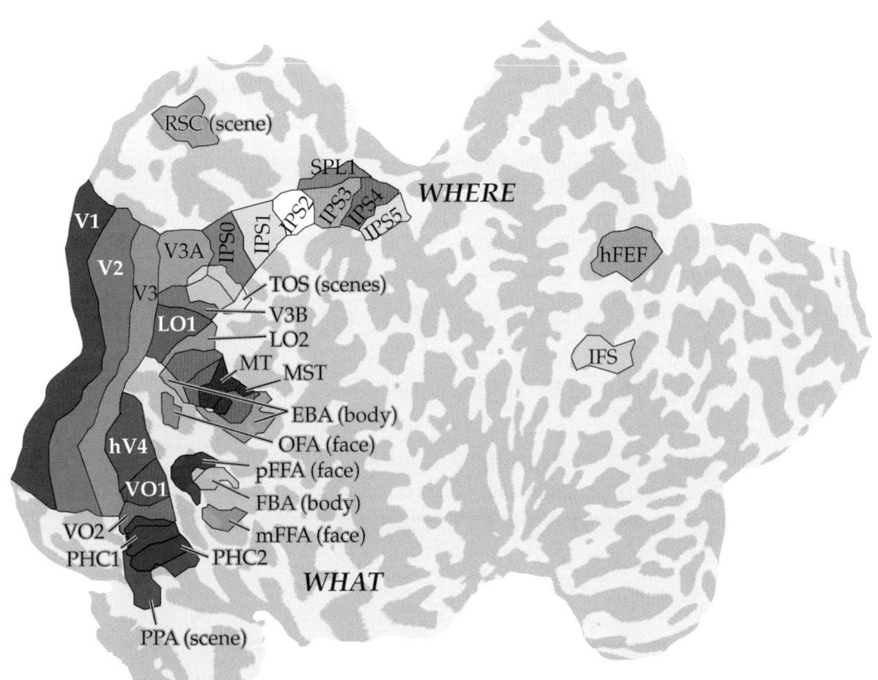

FIGURE 4.4 The main visual areas of the human cortex Compare with Figure 4.2 and Figure 3.1. Here the convoluted, wrinkled surface of the brain has been flattened. Each abbreviation refers to a different visual area. The color scheme is intended to roughly match that used in Figure 4.3. If you are curious, a little surfing on the internet will yield the definitions of all the acronyms as well as other maps that will give you an idea of the complexities of mapping human visual processing. Here you should notice the *what* and *where* pathways and the areas specialized for faces (FFA), bodies (FBA), and scenes (PPA).

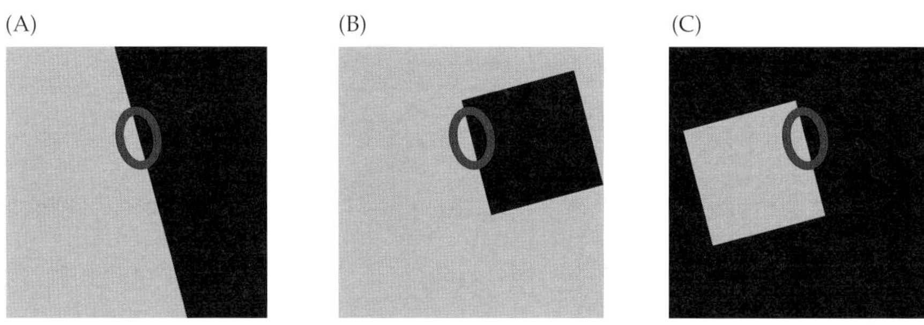

FIGURE 4.5 Edges and the receptive field All the edges inside the receptive field, marked by the red ovals, are the same (i.e., gray on the left, black on the right) and would present the same stimulus to a V1 cell. However, V2 cells distinguish a phenomenon termed "border ownership" and would differentiate between (B) the edge of a black square on a gray background and (C) the edge of a gray square on a black background.

(as in Figure 4.5A). In V2, a border ownership cell would respond more strongly to Figure 4.5B, the edge of a black square, than to Figure 4.5C, the locally identical edge of a gray square.

4.2 *What* and *Where* Pathways

From the extrastriate regions of the occipital lobe of the brain, visual information moves out along two main pathways (see Figure 4.2). One pathway, sometimes known as the *where* pathway, heads up (or dorsally) into the parietal lobe. Visual areas in this pathway seem to be important for processing information relating to the location of objects in space and the actions required to interact with them (moving the hands, the eyes, and so on). As we will see in Chapter 7, the *where* pathway plays an important role in the deployment of attention. The other pathway heads down (ventrally) into the temporal lobe and is known as the *what* pathway. This pathway appears to be the locus for the explicit acts of object recognition that are of particular importance in this chapter (Ungerleider and Mishkin, 1982). As we move into the temporal lobe, receptive fields get much bigger and, as the pathway's name implies, *what* the object is seems more important than *where* it is. However, though it is a useful organizing principle, one should not become too addicted to this *what* and *where* distinction (de Haan and Cowey, 2011). For instance, some basic object information is represented simultaneously in both pathways (Konen and Kastner, 2008), and some *where* information is encoded in the temporal lobe *what* pathway.

If we go back to the monkey brain in Figure 4.2, you will find an area labeled "IT" down at the end of the *what* pathway. IT stands for **inferotemporal cortex**. In the 1970s, Charlie Gross and his colleagues began to record the activity of single cells in this area. What they found was quite striking. We have seen that neurons in striate cortex are activated by simple stimuli and respond only if their preferred stimuli are presented in very restricted portions of the visual field. In contrast, cells in the IT cortex were discovered to have receptive fields that could spread over half or more of the monkey's field of view. Even more striking were the sorts of stimuli that activated IT cells. The usual spots and lines didn't work well at all, but the silhouette of a monkey hand worked fantastically for some cells. Monkey faces excited other cells. There was even a cell with a distinct preference for a toilet brush shape (Gross, Rocha-Miranda, and Bender, 1972).

Findings like this led Horace Barlow (1972) and others to suggest a hierarchical model of visual perception in which the small receptive fields and simple features of visual cortex are combined with ever-greater complexity as one moves from striate cortex to IT cortex, eventually culminating in small networks of cells that might fire when you see your grandmother or a fork or some other highly specific object or type of object. Indeed, the term *grandmother cell*, coined by Jerry Lettvin,

inferotemporal (IT) cortex Part of the cerebral cortex in the lower portion of the temporal lobe, important in object recognition.

has entered the jargon of the field to stand for any cell that seems to be selectively responsive to one specific object (Barlow, 1995). It would be a mistake, however, to think of a single cell in your brain as *the* cell that recognizes your grandmother in all of the ways she might appear in your visual field. Think what would happen if that particular cell (or small group of cells) died. Grandmother recognition is more likely to involve quite a large network of cells, with individual cells participating in recognition of more than one stimulus, even if they do respond vigorously to grandma. We don't know exactly what brain activity gives rise to the experience of grandmother. However, when scientists monitored the activity of 100 randomly chosen cells in IT cortex, they were able to identify the object that the monkey was viewing from a long list of possible objects (Hung et al., 2005). Later, we will discuss how this process can be modeled.

The IT cortex maintains close connections with parts of the brain involved in memory formation, notably the hippocampus. This is important because those IT cells need to *learn* their receptive-field properties. The receptive-field properties of primary visual cortex could be written into the genetic code in some manner, but neurons that respond to "grandmothers" clearly cannot be hardwired, since everyone's grandmother is different. Nikos Logothetis and his coworkers demonstrated that cells in IT cortex have precisely this type of plasticity (Logothetis, Pauls, and Poggio, 1995). After training monkeys to recognize novel objects, these researchers found IT neurons that responded with high firing rates to those objects—but only when the objects were seen from viewpoints similar to those from which they had been learned.

The anatomy of human and macaque monkey brains is not identical. When areas in the human and monkey appear to have similar roles, we call those **homologous regions**. Human cortex has areas that appear to be homologous with monkey IT cortex and hippocampus. One of the more amazing demonstrations of this fact comes from a 2005 study by Quiroga et al. They made recordings from single cells in the temporal lobe (hippocampus and its neighbors) of human observers. Normally, we do not put electrodes into the human brain, but these observers were patients being prepared for brain surgery to treat epilepsy. Implanting electrodes was part of the treatment plan, and recording visual responses from these cells involved no extra risk to the patient or interference with treatment. In the experiment, the observer just looked at a collection of images while the activity of a cell was monitored. As **FIGURE 4.6** shows, some of these cells turned out to have very specific tastes. The cell shown in Figure 4.6 responded strongly only to the actress Jennifer Aniston and to nothing else presented to the observer. Other cells had preferences for different people, such as former president Bill Clinton. One cell responded to the Sydney Opera House; another responded to the Eiffel Tower and the Leaning Tower of Pisa, but not to other landmarks (Quiroga et al., 2005).

While we do not have a lot of systematic data on the responses of single cells in the human visual system, we have a growing volume of functional imaging data that documents areas in the human brain that appear be specialized for different sorts of stimuli. Conveniently, as shown in Figure 4.4, many of these have been given names that make that proposed specialization clear. Thus, cells in the **fusiform face area (FFA)** are interested in faces (Kanwisher, McDermott, and Chun, 1997), while those in the **extrastriate body area (EBA)** are activated by body structures other than the face. The **parahippocampal place area (PPA)** has cells that respond to spaces in the world, like rooms with furniture in them (Epstein and Kanwisher, 1998). The visual system has many different problems to solve—like the problem of face processing—and it appears to have modules that are specialized for working on different problems (Kanwisher, 2017).

homologous regions Brain regions that appear to have the same function in different species.

fusiform face area (FFA) A region of extrastriate visual cortex in humans that is specifically and reliably activated by human faces.

extrastriate body area (EBA) A region of extrastriate visual cortex in humans that is specifically and reliably activated by images of the body other than the face.

parahippocampal place area (PPA) A region of extrastriate visual cortex in humans that is specifically and reliably activated more by images of places than by other stimuli.

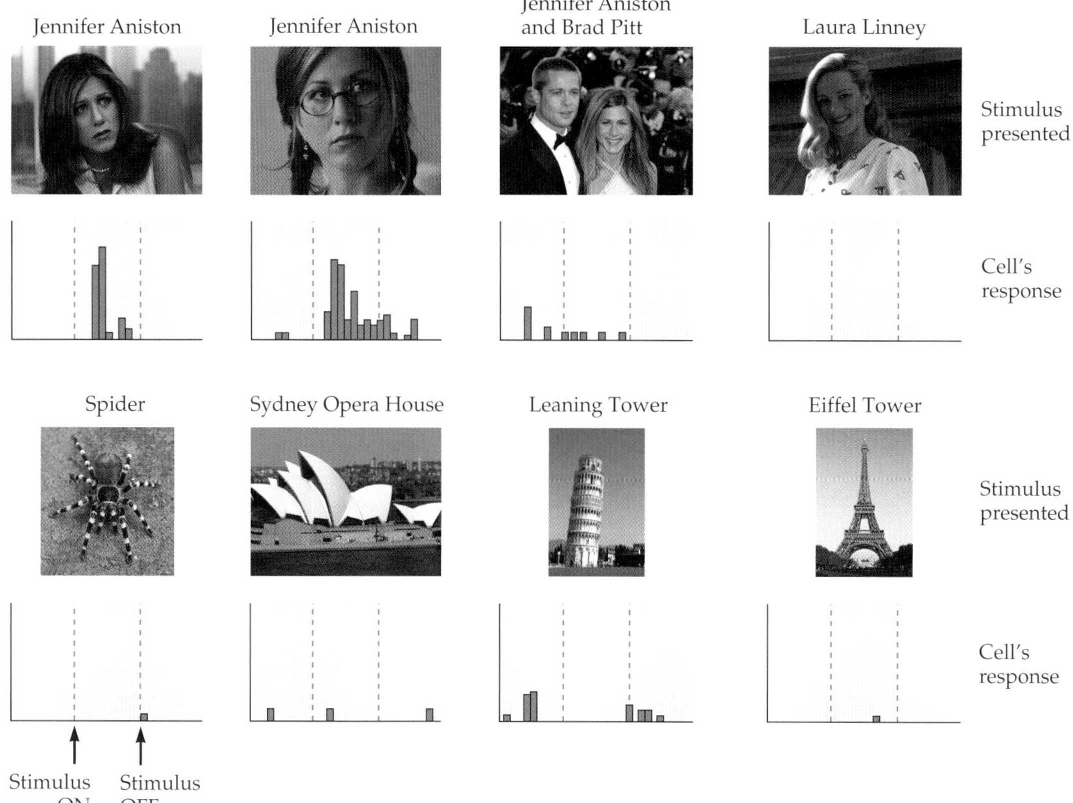

FIGURE 4.6 A Jennifer Aniston cell Results of recording the activity of one cell in the temporal lobe (hippocampus and its neighbors) of a human patient. This cell responded to pictures of the actress Jennifer Aniston. The cell did not respond to pictures of anything else, including a similar photograph of a different actress.

Interestingly, there is a **visual word form area (VWFA)** (McCandliss, Cohen, and Dehaene, 2003). This is interesting because for all but the most recent few moments of evolutionary time, humans have been illiterate. Yet, we have a piece of brain that becomes specialized for recognizing visual (written) words, but only when an individual learns to read (He et al., 2009). In right-handed humans, other language abilities (e.g., speaking, recognizing spoken words) are concentrated in the left cerebral hemisphere. It turns out that, when the visual word area emerges, it occupies nearby space in that hemisphere. It seems to use cortical real estate that might otherwise have been interested in faces. As a result, face areas in literate individuals are found more prominently in the right hemisphere (Behrmann and Plaut, 2020).

More recently, new evidence has appeared for a food area. This is discussed in the "Scientists at Work" box.

Other evidence for specific recognition areas comes from brain **lesions** caused by strokes or other accidents. Humans with lesions in the temporal lobe often show symptoms of **agnosia**, the ability to see without the ability to know what is being seen. Sometimes these agnosias can be quite specific. **Prosopagnosia**, an inability to recognize faces, is one example that has received a lot of study and that will be discussed at the end of this chapter (Damasio, Damasio, and Van Hoesen, 1982). There are other interesting subdivisions of agnosia as well, such as the ability to recognize animate objects (e.g., animals) but not inanimate objects (e.g., tools) (Newcombe and de Haan, 1994). The implications of specific agnosias in specific

visual word form area (VWFA) A region of extrastriate visual cortex in humans that is specifically and reliably activated more by images of written words than by other stimuli.

lesion In reference to neurophysiology, 1. (n) A region of damaged brain. 2. (v) To destroy a section of the brain.

agnosia A failure to recognize objects despite the ability to see them. Agnosia is typically a result of brain damage.

prosopagnosia An inability to recognize faces.

individuals should not be taken too far, however. Although areas specialized for faces or places seem to be readily documented in humans, and you might have areas specialized for some other categories of objects (e.g., tools; see Hutchison et al., 2014), you probably do not have a separate area for each and every category of object that you can recognize (Kanwisher and Dilks, 2013).

Scientists at Work

Food on Your Mind

Question Nancy Kanwisher spent many years using functional magnetic resonance imaging (usually abbreviated as fMRI) to explore the *what* pathway as it flows from the occipital cortex into the temporal cortex. She had a major role in establishing the face (FFA), place (PPA), and other stimulus-specific areas that you can find on the cortical map in Figure 4.4. What other cortical specializations might contribute to the perception of different types of objects? Most previous work had attacked this problem by asking the brain, "Are you interested in tools or animals or some other category of item?" Kanwisher and her colleagues Khosla and Ratan Murty decided to try a different method where the brain could reveal its interests. As they say, "We need a more complete inventory of human cortical specializations, one that reflects not just the idiosyncratic hypotheses scientists have already thought to test but also the actual functional organization of the cortex itself" (Khosla, Ratan Murty, and Kanwisher, 2022, p. 4159). They wanted to be "hypothesis neutral." This is interesting, in part, because usually scientists are supposed to have a hypothesis and not just go off on what is sometimes derisively referred to as a "fishing expedition." So, the authors decided to ask the brain to tell them what it was doing.

Test Khosla, Ratan Murty, and Kanwisher were not just fishing. They had a clear plan. They would show observers 5000 to 10,000 images from a huge database of scenes while the activity of the brains of those observers were monitored using fMRI methods. All manner of different objects could be found in these thousands of images, and the brain responds differently to each picture. In their analysis, the authors asked what factors explained the greatest amount of variability in those brain responses. The details of the analysis go beyond what we can describe here, so if you want more, have a look at the paper.

Results FIGURE 4.7 is one way of illustrating the top five components that they found. Each column shows

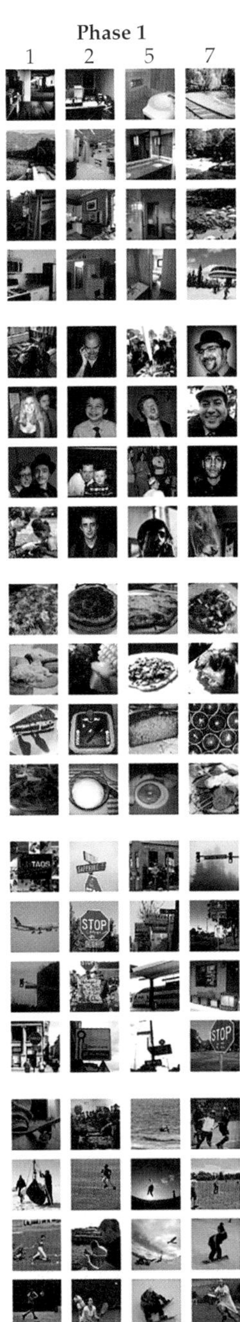

FIGURE 4.7 Objects in cortex The authors found five areas in the cortex, specialized for different kinds of objects. This figure shows the images that most interested each area for each of four observers. From top to bottom, these were scenes, faces, food, text, and bodies.

(Continued)

Scientists at Work *(continued)*

results for one observer. Each square shows one of the components. Each image is one of the top four images for that component for that observer. Obviously, this method has not generated a random selection of images. Component 1 favors scenes. Component 2 favors faces. Component 4 wants to see text and all the Component 5 images contain bodies or parts of bodies.

This is good. Temporal lobe regions for faces, places, bodies, and text have been reported before, and it is encouraging that this method finds them again. But what about component 3? All of those pictures contain food. Is there a food area? Kanwisher had argued against the existence of such an area over 20 years previously (Downing and Kanwisher, 1999), but this new method seemed to be showing that distinct patches of cortex were very interested in food images. Is this really about food? Could there be some other stimulus factor that could explain the results? Good scientists will do their best to check out other explanations for their results. When they submit the paper for publication, other scientists will review the manuscript ("peer review") and may have still more possible explanations, and the editor of the journal may send the submission back to the authors, asking for more analysis.

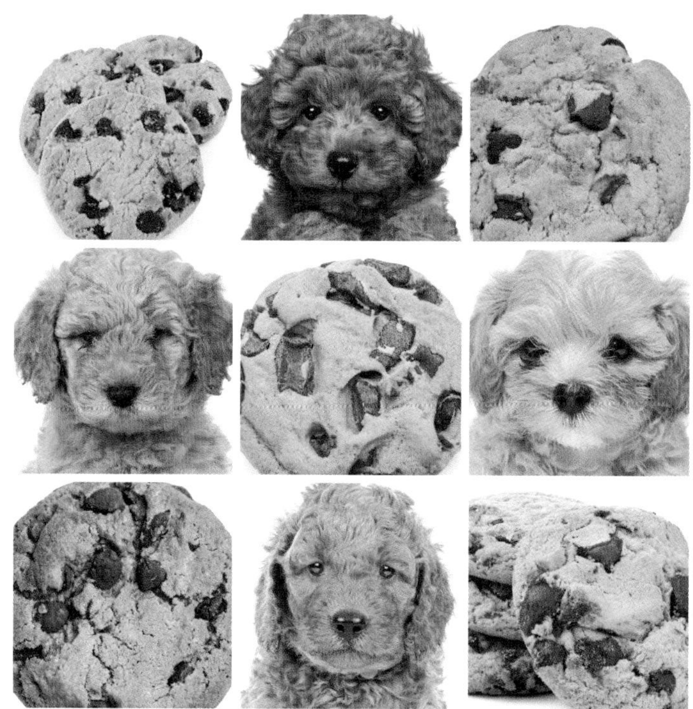

FIGURE 4.8 **Puppies look like cookies?** As the internet knows, very different objects can be composed of rather similar visual features. Here, labradoodles look surprisingly like chocolate chip cookies, at least at first glance.

What else might explain these results? Figure 4.7 hints at one possibility. That third block of food images is "warmer" in its colors than the other blocks. This turns out to be true of the food images in general. They have more "warm" yellow and red shades than other categories of object. Maybe these neurons just like warm colors? There is a connection in the brain between color selectivity and food (Pennock et al., 2023). For one test of this hypothesis, Khosla, Ratan Murty, and Kanwisher compared cool (bluish and greenish) food images with warmer nonfood images. Color makes a difference, but the cool food images are better than warm nonfood images in component 3. Well, maybe the pattern in the data is produced by some set of more basic visual features. Maybe food stimuli have more of some specific curves or texture. One way to test this is to try to match food and nonfood stimuli for these lower-level visual stimuli. Such matches have generated a host of internet memes, as shown in **FIGURE 4.8**.

Who knew that chihuahuas look like blueberry muffins while labradoodles look like fried chicken? The authors carefully curated food images and nonfood images that matched the food in the manner shown in Figure 4.8. When they repeated their analysis with those stimuli, component 3 still preferred food to nonfood stimuli.

Conclusion After a host of other control experiments, Khosla, Ratan Murty, and Kanwisher came away convinced that there really was a specialization for food in the ventral pathway.

Future work Is that the end of the story? Are there only specializations for faces, places, bodies, text, and food? A bit of caution is required. Other researchers have reported on areas that seem to be interested in animals (Mahon et al., 2009) or tools and whether an object is likely to be picked up and manipulated (e.g., Magri, Konkle, and Caramazza, 2021). Kanwisher's group didn't find these categories using their methods. Discrepancies like this will drive more research.

Some processing that leads to the categorization of objects and scenes can be very fast. Electrical activity from the brain can be recorded from electrodes placed on the scalp. If we flash a picture to an observer and ask whether it contains an animal, we can record a signal in the observer that reliably differentiates animal from nonanimal scenes within 150 milliseconds (ms) from the onset of the stimulus (Thorpe, Fize, and Marlot, 1996). That's fast enough to mean that there cannot be a lot of feedback from higher visual or memory processes, suggesting that it must be possible to do some rough object recognition on the basis of the first wave of activity as it moves, cell by cell, synapse by synapse, from retina to striate cortex to extrastriate cortex and beyond. That **feed-forward process** must be able to generate an "animal" signal from a wide range of animals in different positions, sizes, and so on (Serre, 2019). At the same time, it is important to remember that all those many areas in Figure 4.3 have feedback connections as well as those that feed forward. More complex acts of recognition ("That is my cat, Cardinal Wolsey. He is looking plump.") rely on this feedback. Hochstein and Ahissar (2002) proposed a **reverse-hierarchy theory**. It argues that the feed-forward processes give you a general, categorical impression of the world, but that you don't become aware of the details until "re-entrant" feedback (Di Lollo, 2012) goes back down the visual pathway. This "re-entrant processing" will become important in Chapter 7, when we discuss what it means to "pay attention" to one part of the visual input.

feed-forward process A process that carries out a computation (e.g., object recognition) one neural step after another, without need for feedback from a later stage to an earlier stage.

reverse-hierarchy theory A theory that fast, feed-forward processes can give you crude information about objects and scenes based on activity in high-level parts of the visual cortex. You become aware of details when activity flows back down the hierarchy of visual areas to lower-level areas where the detailed information is preserved.

To summarize, two pathways emerge from visual cortex. The *where* pathway will be taken up in later chapters. The *what* pathway moves through a succession of stages (backward as well as forward), building a representation of your grandmother or your dinner or the Eiffel Tower out of the very specific, very localized spots, lines, and bars that interest the cells in the retina, lateral geniculate nucleus, and primary visual (striate) cortex. That's a start, but don't be lulled into thinking we fully understand the process of object recognition simply because we have some notion of the neural pathways involved. It is a really difficult problem, and in the rest of the chapter we will illustrate why object recognition is so complicated and how the visual system attempts to solve different parts of it.

4.3 The Problems of Perceiving and Recognizing Objects

FIGURE 4.9 shows four images of elephants. Figure 4.9A is a photograph of a living elephant. Figure 4.9B looks quite realistic but, with a bit of scrutiny, turns out to be made of LEGO blocks. Figure 4.9C is a sculpture that we might call "realistic," even though it isn't, really, and Figure 4.9D is another sculpture that is a long way from the real thing but is still clearly an elephant. Not only do you recognize all these elephants, but also you can tell that they are made of different materials. Just by looking at them, you can guess how they would feel.

These seemingly simple acts of object identification require a lot from the *what* pathway, and they constitute the main topic of the rest of this chapter. Like many seemingly simple acts, object perception is a collection of complex and remarkable accomplishments.

There is a famous story about a group of blind men (they always seem to be men, sorry) who encounter an elephant. Each man touches only one part of the elephant, and each has a very different idea about what the object they are touching is (**FIGURE 4.10A**). It is a snake, says the one holding its trunk; it is a boulder, says the man climbing its back; it is a tree trunk, says the man groping a leg. And so on. The beginnings of the object perception problem are somewhat like this.

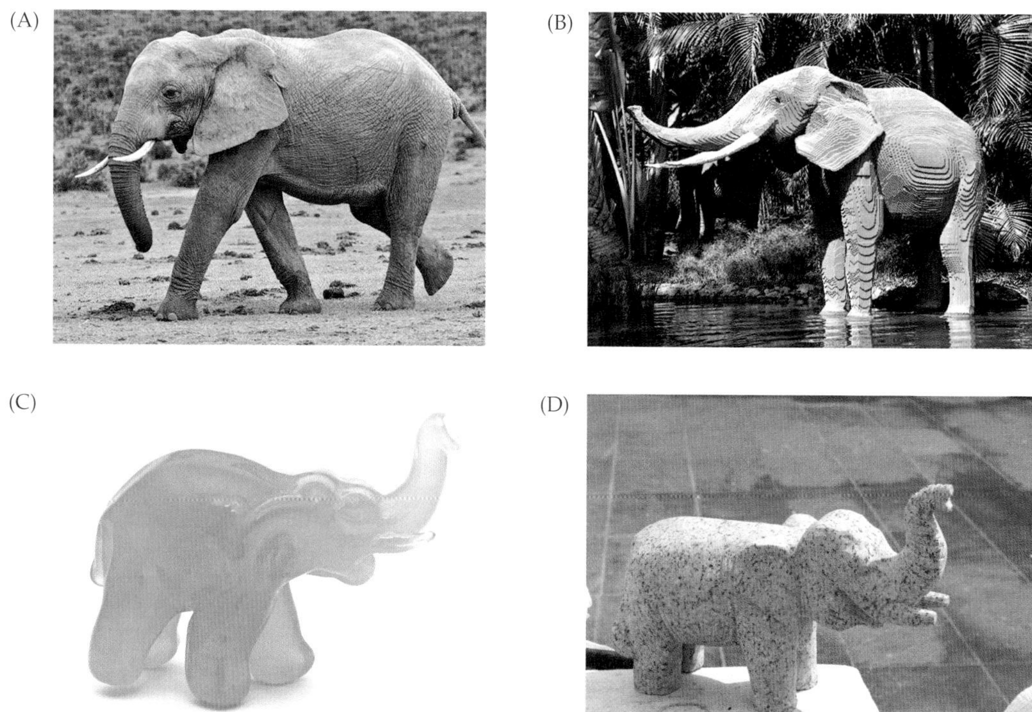

FIGURE 4.9 The problem of object recognition These are all recognizable as elephants even though (A) is a photograph of a real elephant, (B) is a LEGO elephant, (C) is a jade sculpture, and (D) is a quite schematic stone sculpture.

The preceding chapters showed us how single cells in the early visual system respond to stimuli such as simple lines. In **FIGURE 4.10B**, think of each circle as representing the receptive field of a simple cortical cell. An "end-stopped" cortical cell like (a) would be like the end of the tusk. Cell (b) would be a good stimulus for edge-detecting cells like those shown in Figure 4.5. Cells (c) and (d) have corners in their receptive fields. How does the visual system figure out that (c) is responding to the intersection of two parts of the elephant, while (d) is responding to the occlusion of a bit of the elephant by the zebra? And how do we figure out that the contours in (e) are surface markings and not edges like those in (a) and (b)? Each limited receptive field is like a window that allows the cell to "see" only a small part of the world. None of these simple cells sees an elephant; they just collect local features.

At the very least, the local features will need to be assembled into an object that can then be recognized as "elephant." This process could be imagined as the natural extension of a process we have already discussed. One way to "construct" the lines detected by simple cells is to imagine combining a row of dots detected by retinal ganglion cells (Figure 3.22). Dots could be grouped together into lines. A pair of lines, each collected by a different cell, could be combined by another cell that would sense a corner. This process could go on and on until we had an elephant. However, it is clear that this process would not be easy. How do we know which edges go with which objects? In receptive field (f), where does the elephant end and the rock begin? Clearly, we must have processes that successfully combine features into objects.

midlevel (or middle) vision A loosely defined stage of visual processing that comes after basic features have been extracted from the image (low-level, or early, vision) and before object recognition and scene understanding (high-level vision).

Before we embark on the detailed discussion of object recognition, however, it is worth asking how to define an object and to recognize that this is not a simple question. Is your cat an object? Presumably, yes. Is the cat's tail an object? Clearly, it would be some sort of object if it were detached from the cat. In its normal position, it is certainly a part of an object, and perhaps an object in its own right. What about a spoken sentence or a smell? Even though this chapter is about visible objects, we shouldn't limit objecthood to visual things. In the dark, we can feel a thing that we cannot see. A smell and a sentence are things that are perceived and can be described as perceptual objects (O'Callaghan, 2016). Moreover, a perceptual object can have attributes from more than one sense. If you imagine a steel ball hitting a hard floor, the perceptual experience will include its visual motion and the sound as the ball bounces (or splinters the floor). The precise timing of sound and visual contact is important to the perception of an audiovisual object, and such an object will be easier to detect if the sound and sight properly merge in time (B. E. Stein and Meredith, 1993). Interestingly, the timing becomes less critical as we age (Laurienti et al., 2006), perhaps to make up for a decline in the precision of our senses as we age. ●

4.4 Midlevel Vision

The crucial processes that make it possible to recognize objects define the work of **midlevel (or middle) vision** (as opposed to low-level vision, which was the topic of Chapters 2 and 3). Light bounces off surfaces in the world, and we need to understand what that reflected light is telling us about the shape and composition of a surface. Chapter 5 will deal in detail with the analysis that gives us the perceived color of surfaces, but we want to know about more than the color of a surface. We also want to differentiate between the many substances that surround us. Look again at the jade elephant in Figure 4.9C. Why does it look like that? You are seeing the result of light interacting with that object in several different ways, as shown in **FIGURE 4.11**. Some light bounces directly off the smooth surface and into your eye (or into the camera taking the picture). The surface behaves like a mirror and produces **specular reflections**. The white patches on the surface of the grapes in Figure 4.11A are specular reflections. They are white because you are seeing a white light source being reflected. Specularities tell you that the surface is smooth and shiny. Their position provides some good information about the shape of the surface (A. Blake and Bulthoff, 1990).

(A)

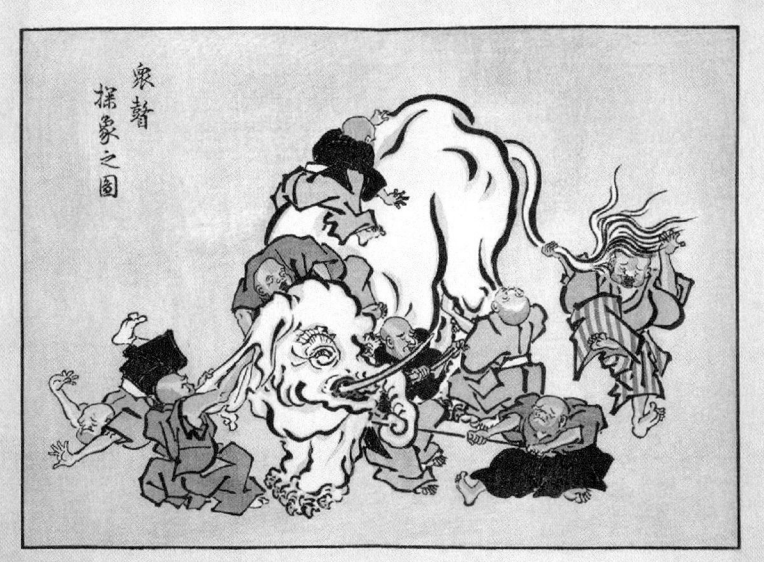

(B)

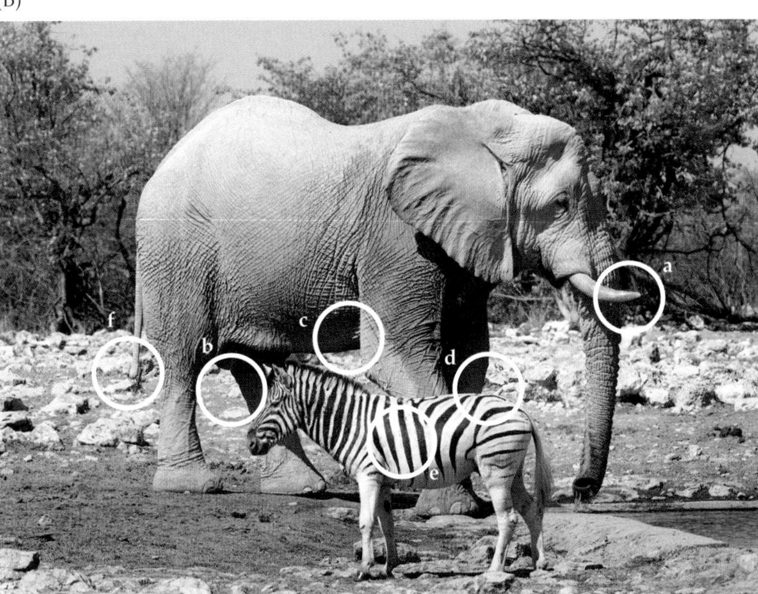

FIGURE 4.10 Local elements, global elephants (A) Hanabusa Itchō (1652–1724) illustrates the classic Indian fable that imagines what would happen if several blind people tried to describe an elephant after touching only one body part. (B) The visual system faces a similar problem: the receptive fields (white circles a–f) of individual cells early in visual processing respond to only a small patch of the elephant. How does our brain put it all together?

Most of the rest of what you see arises when light penetrates some distance into the surface and some light scatters back out. If shallow scatter dominates, the surface will look matte (like in Figures 4.9D and 4.11B). When light gets a little way into the surface, it encounters materials that absorb some of the photons and scatter other photons back out of the surface. As we will see in Chapter 5, light of some wavelengths is absorbed while other light is scattered back, and the surface

specular reflections Bright spots produced by some light bouncing off an object.

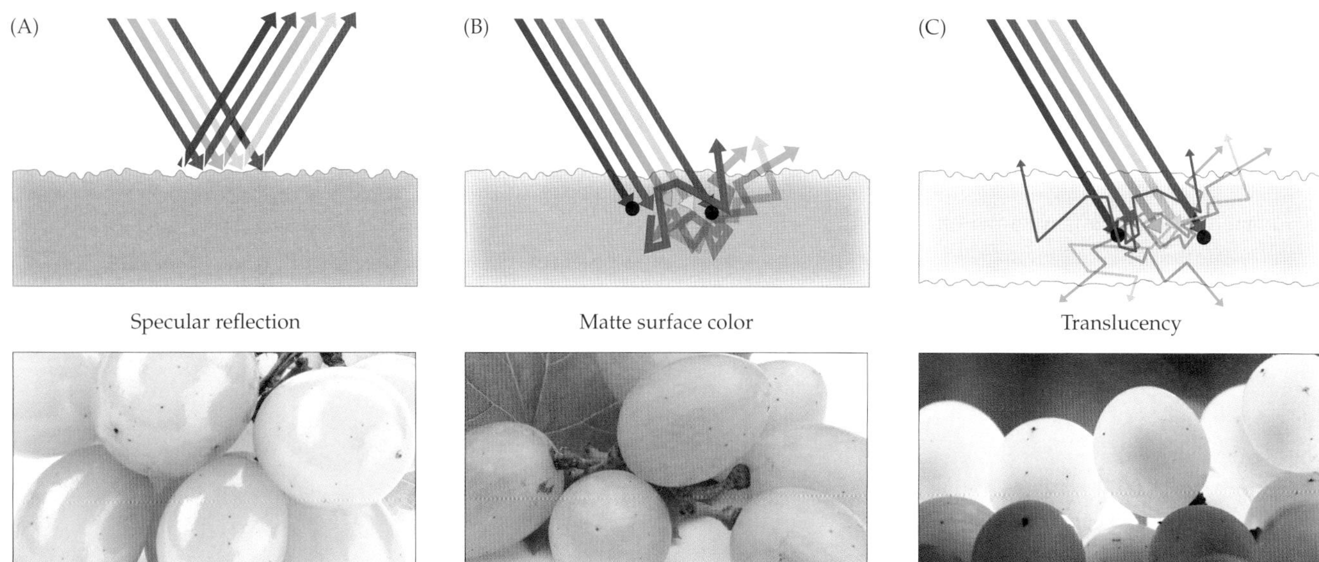

FIGURE 4.11 Light scattering from surfaces (A) Light bounces off smooth surfaces like it does off a mirror. This produces bright spots, "specular reflections" of the same color as the light source. (B) Some light penetrates a little way into a surface. Some of that light is absorbed. Other light scatters around and emerges back out of the surface, letting us see it and giving the object its color. (C) Some materials allow light to penetrate farther and scatter more widely. This can give the impression of a translucent object.

subsurface scatter An event that occurs when some light gets into an object and bounces around before escaping, thus causing the object to appear translucent.

synthesis An ability to put local bits of information together into recognizable objects.

will appear colored (pale green in Figure 4.11B). Some light gets farther into the object before bouncing around inside the material and then escaping (Figure 4.11C). This **subsurface scatter** gives rise to the appearance of *translucence*, the impression that the material is semitransparent. If the light goes straight through a material, that material is transparent.

The relative contributions of each of these factors to what you are seeing depends on the material that is being illuminated. It also depends on the shape of the surface. For instance, some parts of the object block light from reaching other parts of the object. This leads to the patterns of shading on the elephants in Figure 4.9. The rules governing shading are important cues to shape (V. S. Ramachandran, 1988). Making the roles of these cues explicit is complex because all the cues interact with each other. The translucency of a material changes its color, for example (Fleming, 2022; Marlow, Gegenfurtner, and Anderson, 2022). Nevertheless, as perceivers, we are very good at the *analysis* that allows us to use reflected and transmitted light to infer a great deal about the shape and composition of objects.

We can think of two types of problems that need to be solved by midlevel vision: analysis and synthesis (B. L. Anderson, 2020). We have been talking about the analysis of the optical structure of light, scattered and reflected from objects. **Synthesis** refers to the ability to put local bits of information together into recognizable objects. Let's begin with the simplest case of an object isolated on a simple background. Finding the edges of this object will be a good starting place on the road to assembling and recognizing the object.

Finding Edges

In Chapter 3, we discussed how neurons in striate cortex can detect bits of lines. But how do we decide which bits belong to which objects? We have already established that we can't just group all the edges that touch each other into an object. Because objects abut and overlap other objects, simple connectedness will not work. Worse yet, before we can concern ourselves with grouping edges, we need to worry about the quality of the raw edge information. **FIGURE 4.12A** shows a simple, arrow-shaped outline. It is easy to see that arrow. Notice, however, that in some places the object is lighter than the background, while in other places it is darker. This means that if we trace the edge of the object with a finger, we will pass through locations where there is no difference between the luminance of the object and the luminance of the background. In other words, at these points the shape has no edge at all, as shown in **FIGURE 4.12B**.

Interestingly, this occasional lack of an edge doesn't seem to bother our visual system at all. In fact, it may be hard to see the gap in Figure 4.12A. Asking simple computer graphics software to find the edges in Figure 4.12A would yield something like Figure 4.12B. The computer program would also find many very convincing edges in the zebra in Figure 4.10B, while the human visual system is able to figure out which edges mark the boundaries of different objects and which represent surface features like a zebra's stripes. All these different bits of information are then combined to make the visual system's best guess about the presence and meaning of a contour.

The inferential nature of contour perception can be appreciated in the more extreme demonstration shown in **FIGURE 4.13**. This is an example of a Kanizsa figure, named after the Italian psychologist Gaetano Kanizsa (1913–1993), who spent many years investigating such stimuli. Here it is still easy to see the arrow outline, even though most of the outline is missing. Check it yourself. There really is no border between the white figure and the white background. These apparent edges, called **illusory contours**, are perceived because they are the visual system's best guess about what is happening in the world at that location.

OCCLUSION Why is an illusory contour a good guess about the world? We can imagine the visual system asking why the vertical line in **FIGURE 4.14A** suddenly stops. One reasonable guess might be that it stops because something else gets in the way, hiding it from our view. The visual system seems to come up with the hypothesis that there is another contour *occluding* the vertical line. The notches in the circles seem to support the idea that a horizontal contour marks the edge of an otherwise invisible occluder (**FIGURE 4.14B**).

FIGURES 4.14C and **4.14D** illustrate another example of this inference of occlusion. If each black line in Figure 4.14C generated weak illusory contours at right angles to its end point, then this figure would contain a set of inferred line segments that could imply the illusory circle we see in Figure 4.14D. In the early twentieth

(A)

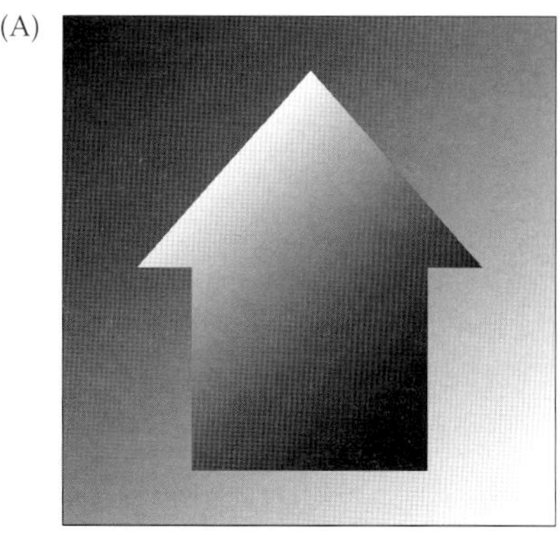

(B)

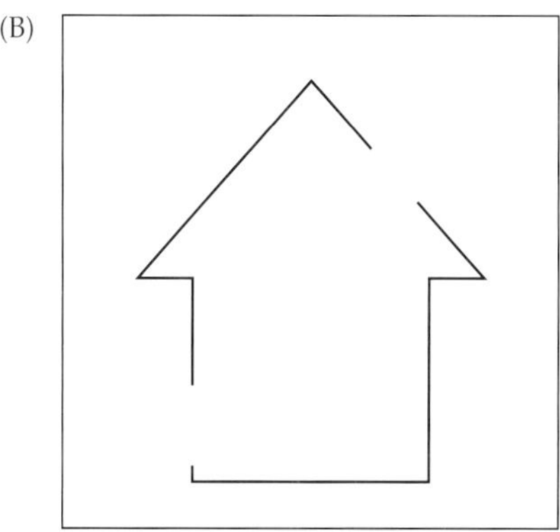

FIGURE 4.12 Seeing invisible contours (A) In some places this object is darker than the background. In other places it is lighter. If the changes are continuous, it follows that there must be places where the edge of this shape simply disappears, even if you see the edges as continuous. (B) The "find edges" function in a popular graphics program finds gaps in the borders of the image in (A)—gaps that we do not see.

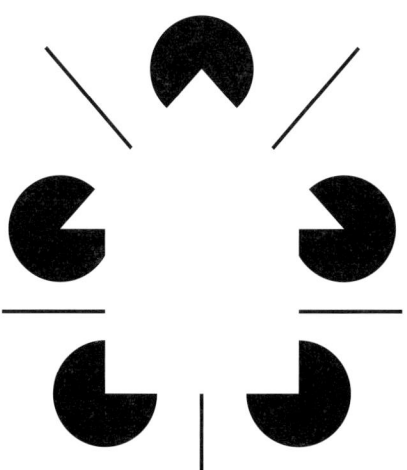

FIGURE 4.13 Illusory contours This "arrow" outline is constructed from illusory contours. Even though the contour is clearly visible, there is no physical difference between the white background and the white arrow in the center.

illusory contour A contour that is perceived even though nothing changes from one side of it to the other in an image.

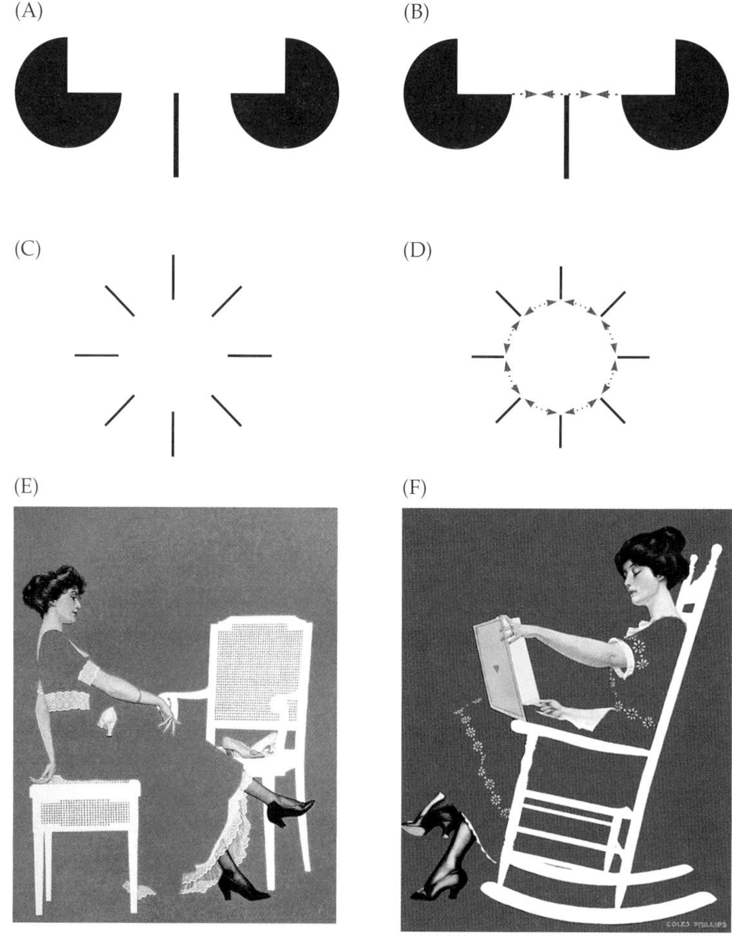

FIGURE 4.14 The making of illusory contours The gray arrows in (B) and (D) represent the visual system's best guess about what is going on in (A) and (C). The illusory disk in (C) arises when the visual system combines a whole collection of guesses about the line terminations, as shown in (D). Images (E) and (F) show very sophisticated use of subjective contours by American graphic artist C. Coles Phillips (1880–1927).

century, the artist C. Coles Phillips (1880–1927) made clever use of the rules of subjective contours to generate some very striking images (**FIGURES 4.14E** and **4.14F**). Notice how his subjective contours are really subjective three-dimensional volumes with rounded arms and legs under a seemingly visible dress (Tse, 1999).

RULES OF EVIDENCE This tendency of the visual system to make inferential leaps like those that form the illusory contours of Figures 4.13 and 4.14 was problematic for one of the earliest groups of perceptual psychologists, the **structuralists**. Structuralists such as Wilhelm Wundt (1832–1920) and Edward Bradford Titchener (1867–1927) argued that perceptions are the sum of atoms of sensation—bits of color, orientation, and so forth. In the structuralist view, perception is built up of local sensations the way a crystal might be built up of an array of atoms. An illusory contour challenges this view because an extended edge is seen bridging a gap where no local atom of "edgeness" can be found.

Over time, it became clear that there are many examples where the structuralist argument seems to fail. Inspired by these examples, a second group of psychologists, led by Max Wertheimer (1880–1943), Wolfgang Köhler (1887–1967), and Kurt Koffka (1886–1941), formed the **Gestalt** school (Wagemans et al., 2012). Gestalt theory held that the perceptual whole is more than the sum of its sensory parts. Perhaps the most enduring contribution of this school was to begin the description of a set of organizing principles, sometimes known as **Gestalt grouping rules**, that describe the visual system's interpretation of the raw retinal image. In the following

structuralism In reference to perception, a school of thought that believed that complex objects or perceptions could be understood by analysis of the components.

Gestalt In German, literally "form." In reference to perception, a school of thought stressing that the perceptual whole can be greater than the apparent sum of the parts.

Gestalt grouping rules A set of rules describing which elements in an image will appear to group together. The original list was assembled by members of the Gestalt school of thought.

sections, we will discuss some of those rules. More than the specific rules, however, it is important to remember the overarching goal: The visual system is trying to make sense of the vast and often ambiguous and noisy inputs from the early stage of visual processing. Gestalt grouping rules are useful parts of that effort because they reflect regularities in the world. They allow the visual system to say, "If the input looks like that, I can infer that this is the state of the visual world."

With that in mind, consider **FIGURE 4.15A**, where we have a collection of randomly oriented short line segments. Some segments may appear to be connected to neighbors, but nothing very clear emerges. In **FIGURE 4.15B**, each little line in Figure 4.15A has been rotated by 45 degrees, revealing one subset of segments that seem to form a contour—an irregular, circular loop with a dent in the lower right quadrant. The "rule," illustrated in **FIGURE 4.15C**, is that we tend to see similarly oriented lines as part of the same contour (Field, Hayes, and Hess, 1992). Polat and Sagi (1993) measured how pieces of similar contour support each other. The effect is hard to see in print, but the fainter lines in the middle of the triplets of lines in **FIGURE 4.15D** would be easier to see on the left, when they are collinear with the lines that flank them above and below. Those "flankers" provide evidence for lines of the same orientation in between. When a set of lines forms a closed

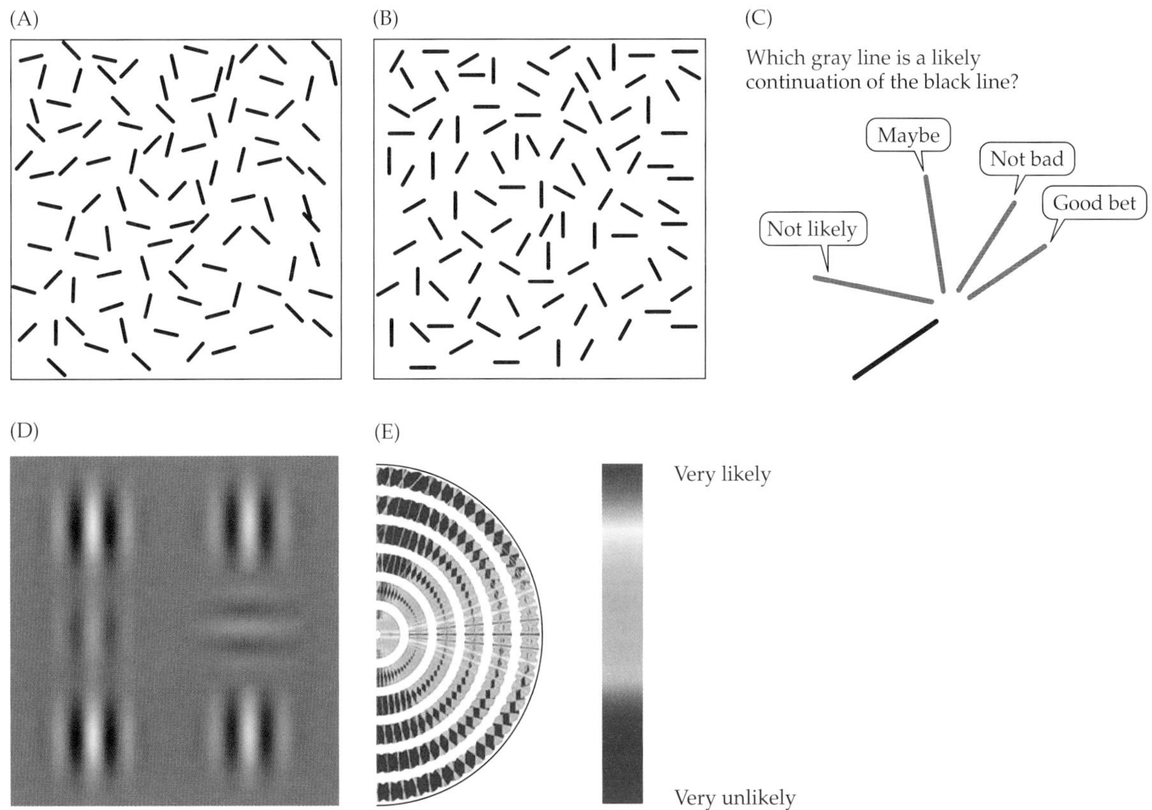

FIGURE 4.15 Contour completion (A) These line segments are randomly oriented, though some will seem to be related to their neighbors. (B) If each line in (A) is rotated by 45 degrees, one set of segments lines up to form the roughly circular contour seen in the center of this diagram. This results from the visual system's application of the rule shown in (C): that we see similarly oriented lines as part of the same contour. (D) Polat and Sagi (1993) found that it was easier to see a faint set of bars if they were flanked by bars of the same (left) rather than different (right) orientation. (E) Geisler and Perry (2009) measured the relationships between nearby line segments in natural scenes. This figure shows the probability that a horizontal line segment would co-occur with other line segments in the image at different distances and orientations. The most likely pairs are colinear, or nearly so.

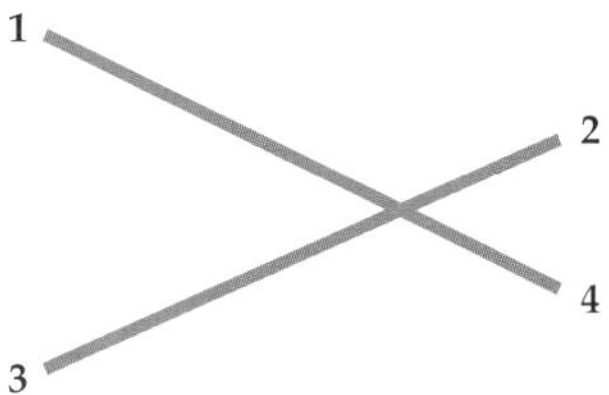

FIGURE 4.16 The principle of good continuation This rule states that 1 connects most strongly with 4, while 2 connects preferentially with 3. You are unlikely to see 1 and 3, or 2 and 4, connected via a sharp turn in the contour.

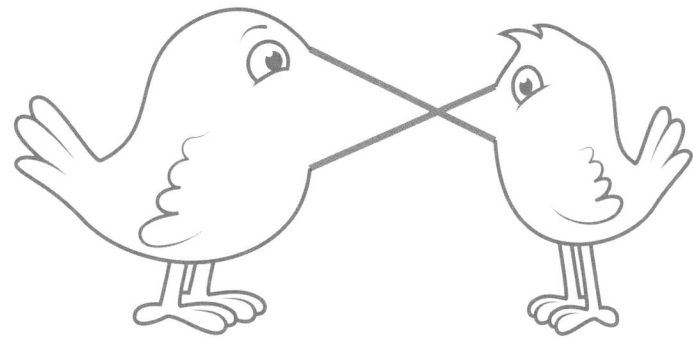

FIGURE 4.17 Good continuation isn't everything Now the sharp turns connecting 1 and 3 and 2 and 4 make sense; you can see these connections, even in Figure 4.16.

good continuation A Gestalt grouping rule stating that two elements will tend to group together if they seem to lie on the same contour.

shape like the roughly circular contour in Figure 4.15B, the short segments support each other even more strongly (Kovacs and Julesz, 1993). Geisler and Perry (2009) documented the regularity in the world that supports the rule shown in Figure 4.15C. They labeled many, many contours in natural scenes. Then they examined pairs of contour pieces and asked, "What is the chance that *this* piece of contour of *this* orientation at *this* location is part of the same larger contour as *that* piece of contour at *that* orientation at *that* location?" These likelihoods are color-coded in **FIGURE 4.15E**, showing that in the real world, if two contour elements are close to colinear, they are likely to come from the same contour. Sharp turns are much rarer. The Gestaltists called this the principle of **good continuation**.

A very simple example of the good continuation principle is shown in **FIGURE 4.16**. We tend to see this figure as a pair of intersecting lines, so it is most likely that you would see point 1 as connected to point 4. Point 1 could be connected to point 2, but a connection from points 2 to 3 seems more likely. These rules are not absolute. **FIGURE 4.17** shows that identical set of lines can be interpreted quite differently.

Are these rules based on our experience or do they trump our experience? We discussed Figures 4.13 and 4.14 as if we were reasoning about the contours, based on what we know about the world. However, in **FIGURE 4.18A**, you can see that good continuation is strong enough to violate common sense and create an apparently transparent child, and in **FIGURE 4.18B**, the same rules that created very plausible

(A)

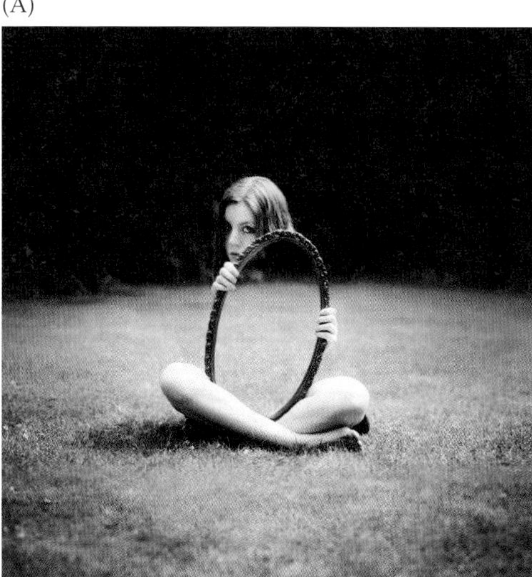

(B)

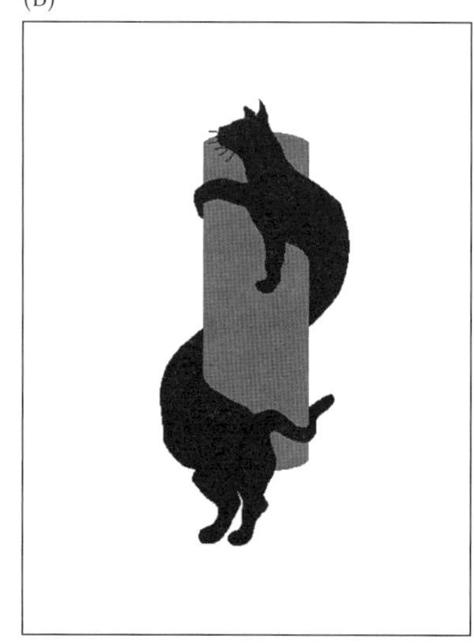

FIGURE 4.18 How "sensible" are these rules? (A) Photographer Laura Williams cleverly exploits good continuation by lining up the edge of the field with the reflected edge in the mirror. This allows the good continuation cue to trump the occlusion cue (see "Dealing with Occlusion" later in this section) to produce this striking image. (B) Psychologist Peter Tse shows that rules that allow us to see vivid three-dimensional volume in this two-dimensional image do not care very much about what we know about the shape of cats.

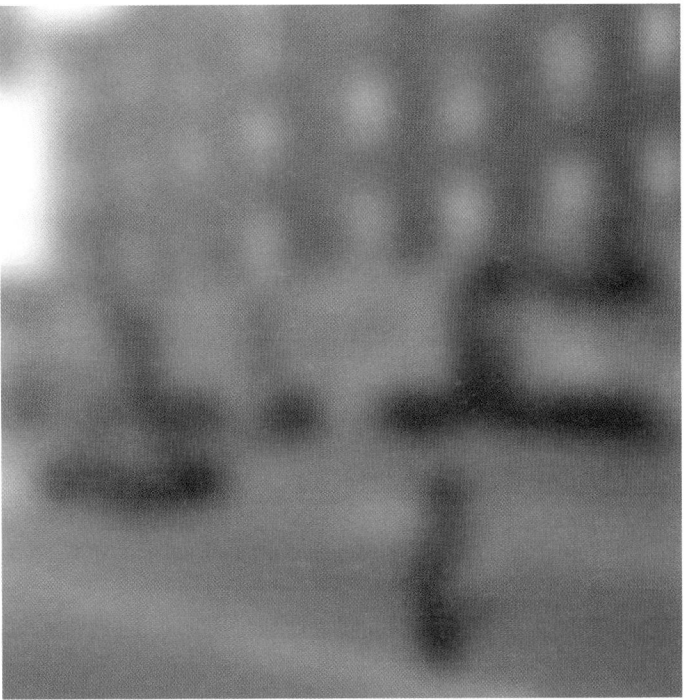

FIGURE 4.19 Context counts The "car" and the "pedestrian" in this blurred image are exactly the same set of pixels, just rotated from vertical to horizontal. Context provides the meaning in this case.

dresses in Figures 4.14E and 4.14F can create a very implausible cat wrapped around a very plausible cylinder (Tse, 1999). So Gestalt rules can shape how we see the world and, at the same time, the world can shape what we see (Gerbino, 2020). Oliva and Torralba (2007) provide a compelling example of the effects of context. **FIGURE 4.19** is blurred, but you can make out a car and a pedestrian on the street. What is less obvious is that those two objects are identical, except for a 90-degree rotation. It is the context that supplies all the meaning to those blobs.

Interestingly, there seem to be differences between individuals in their application of these sorts of rules, especially with regard to meaningless patterns like that in Figure 4.15A. Some people are more likely than others to see apparently meaningful shapes and objects in such stimuli. This could reflect a broader tendency to make connections where real connections may not exist. For instance, there seems to be a correlation between a tendency to see objects in noise and a willingness to endorse conspiracy theories about COVID-19 (Hartmann and Müller, 2023). Of course, an inability to see connections, visually or cognitively, would be very disabling. The trick is to find the "right" connections.

Texture Segmentation and Grouping

Connecting short line segments, as in Figure 4.15, will get us only so far in dividing the raw image into objects. If you look at **FIGURE 4.20**, you will immediately see a border dividing the left from the right side, even though an edge-detecting cell or algorithm would not find an edge. In this case, the border is found by the visual system's sophisticated mechanisms for **texture segmentation** (Beck, 1982; Bergen and Adelson, 1988; Malik and Perona, 1990). One way the visual system decides that two regions are different is by looking at the statistics of all the features in one region and determining that those statistics differ from the statistics in the

texture segmentation Carving an image into regions of common texture properties.

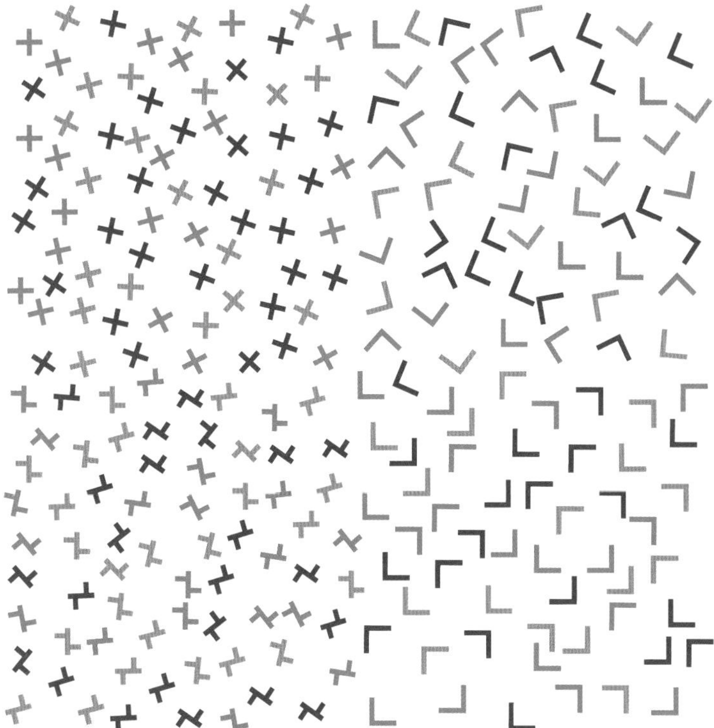

FIGURE 4.20 **Regions defined by texture** Differences between types of local elements like *L*s and +s create a vertical border dividing the image in half. The horizontal division is harder to see, but notice that there are four distinct quadrants here.

neighboring region (Alvarez, 2011; Whitney and Yamanashi Leib, 2018). However, not every statistic works for this purpose. Thus, the difference between left and right in Figure 4.20 is based on something like "number of line terminations" (Gurnsey and Browse, 1987). The distinction between the plusses in the top left and the very different shape in the lower left is much less obvious because the nature of line intersections does not seem to support texture segmentation (Wolfe and DiMase, 2003).

Figuring out the properties of a group of items is not a matter of scrutinizing each one. In FIGURE 4.21, for example, it is immediately obvious that the average of the blue lines on the left is near vertical. However, you will have to search to determine whether any individual blue line is perfectly vertical. The green lines in the middle have the same average orientation, but you can tell that there is more variability, and it is easy to notice that the purple items on the right differ in *average* size and *average* orientation from the other items.

Texture segmentation is closely related to the Gestalt grouping principles that we've been discussing. FIGURE 4.22A illustrates two of the strongest principles of texture segmentation: similarity and proximity. **Similarity** means that image chunks that are similar to each other will be more likely to group together. Similar in what ways? Grouping of elements can be based on similarity in a limited number of features such as color, size, orientation, and, as illustrated in Figure 4.22A, aspects of form. Notice that these are similar to (maybe the same as) the features that can be used for the averaging shown in Figure 4.21. Combinations ("conjunctions") of features do not support grouping or segmentation (A. Treisman, 1986b). Thus, the texture segmentation between the left and right sides of FIGURE 4.22B is not clear, even though the left side contains orange diamonds and green squares and the right side contains green diamonds and orange squares.

similarity A Gestalt grouping rule stating that the tendency of two features to group together will increase as the similarity between them increases.

proximity A Gestalt grouping rule stating that the tendency of two features to group together will increase as the distance between them decreases.

The principle of **proximity** holds that items near each other are more likely to group together than are items that are more widely separated. Proximity grouping gives Figure 4.22A its horizontally striped appearance because horizontal items are closer to each other than vertical items. Gestalt principles like those of proximity and similarity can be put into conflict with each other, as seen in FIGURE 4.22C.

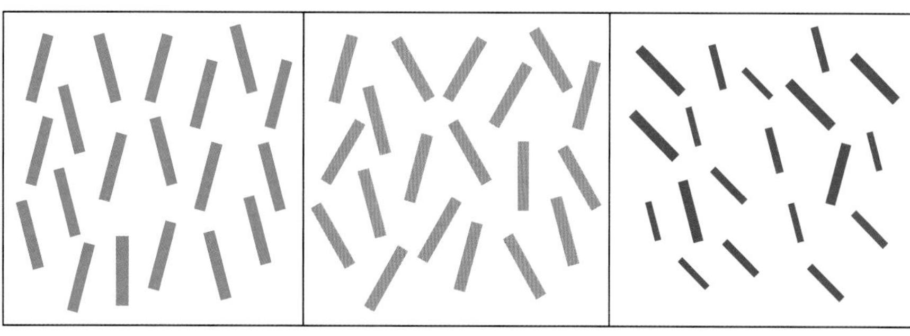

FIGURE 4.21 **Image statistics** It is easy to see the approximate average orientation and size of the lines in the three regions of this figure. It will take more work to determine whether any one line is vertical.

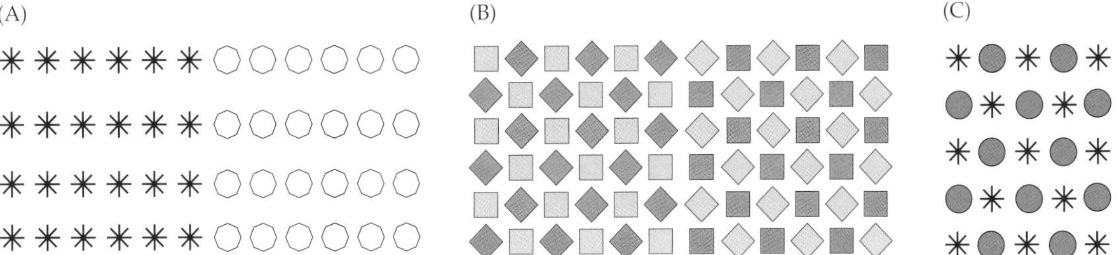

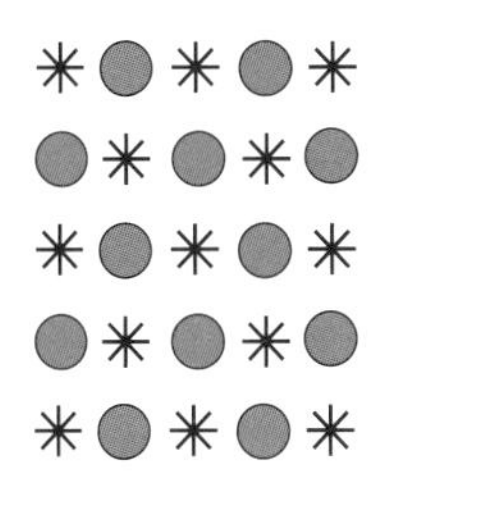

FIGURE 4.22 Similarity and proximity (A) Grouping by similarity and by proximity is useful. (B) Grouping by a conjunction of color and form does not work. (C) Similarity (diagonals) and proximity (rows) in conflict.

CAMOUFLAGE The same principles that are normally used to help us find objects in the world can be exploited to hide them. The art of camouflage is, to a great extent, the art of getting your features to group with the features of the environment so as to persuade an observer that your features do not form a perceptual group of their own. **FIGURE 4.23** shows two examples from the animal kingdom. The exercise for you is to determine which principles of grouping are at work hiding the camouflaged animals in Figures 4.23A and 4.23C. Camouflage does not need to be entirely about hiding things. In World War I, navies painted some of their ships with very dramatic patterns (Figure 4.23D); this "dazzle camouflage" was designed to make a clearly visible object hard to understand.

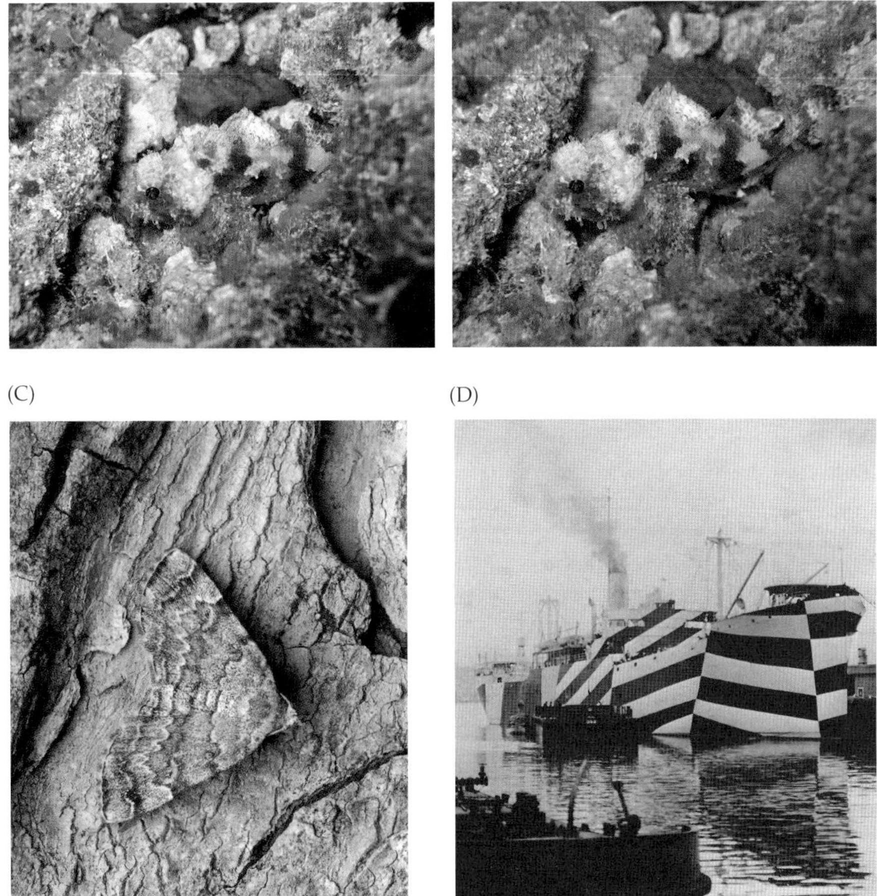

FIGURE 4.23 Camouflage (B) shows the hidden animal in (A). We leave (C) as an exercise for the reader. (D) Sometimes camouflage is meant to confuse the viewer rather than to hide the object.

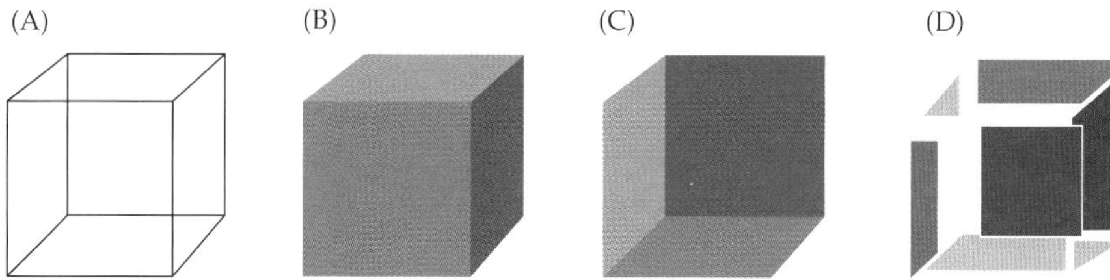

FIGURE 4.24 The Necker cube The wire-frame cube (A) can easily be perceived as either of the solids shown in (B) or (C). It is much less likely to be seen as a collection of flat regions on the page (D), even though that's really what it is!

AMBIGUITY AND PERCEPTUAL "COMMITTEES" How do we put all these grouping rules together into a single percept of the world? As the Gestalt psychologists knew, and as we will see, a host of rules, principles, and good guesses contribute to our organized perception of the world, and they seem to operate according to a sort of committee model. Everyone gets together and voices opinions about how the stimulus ought to be understood. In Figure 4.22C, it is the "good similarity" and "proximity" committee members who are arguing. You might see horizontal lines or a diagonal structure, or perhaps the image is ambiguous. Ambiguity is rare in normal, everyday vision. A consensus view almost always quickly emerges as our perceptual committees settle on a single interpretation of the visual scene. This committee metaphor is very useful and will recur throughout this chapter.

ambiguous figure A visual stimulus that gives rise to two or more interpretations of its identity or structure.

Necker cube An outline that is perceptually bi-stable. Unlike the situation with most stimuli, two interpretations continually battle for perceptual dominance.

accidental viewpoint A viewing position that produces some regularity in the visual image that is not present in the world (e.g., the sides of two independent objects lining up perfectly).

COMMITTEE RULES: HONOR PHYSICS AND AVOID ACCIDENTS Though we usually come to a single coherent interpretation of the current contents of the sensory world, the decisions made by perceptual committees need not be final. We saw that Figure 4.22C is an **ambiguous figure**—a figure that generates two or more plausible interpretations. **FIGURE 4.24A** shows another example, the famous **Necker cube**. Midlevel-vision committees of the visual system are willing to entertain either of the two solids shown in **FIGURES 4.24B** and **4.24C** as interpretations of the wire frame pictured in Figure 4.24A. However, the system is unwilling to readily consider any of the infinite number of other possible interpretations of the wire image—for example, the flat collection of polygons in **FIGURE 4.24D**.

When Paul Philippon moved from academia to the brewing of beer, he brought another classic ambiguous figure with him, as seen in **FIGURE 4.25**.

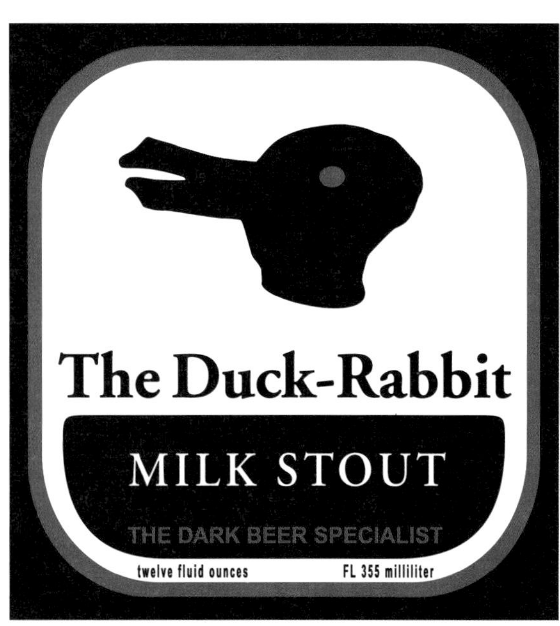

FIGURE 4.25 Ambiguity in advertising A classic ambiguous figure gets a new role.

Necker cubes and duck-rabbits are really the exceptions that prove the rule. *Every* image is, in theory, ambiguous, but the perceptual committees almost always agree on a single interpretation. Consider, for example, **FIGURE 4.26**. If you saw Figure 4.26A, that could be the retinal image projected by the scene depicted in **FIGURE 4.26C**: four surfaces with different shapes, arranged in different orientations, and at different distances. However, for Figure 4.26C to produce Figure 4.26A, your eye (**FIGURE 4.26B**) would need to be at exactly one, very precise location—what object recognition researchers call an **accidental viewpoint**. Any slight shift in viewpoint—say, moving just slightly to the left—would destroy the illusion of the four identically shaped, abutting, square regions.

The perceptual committees know about accidental viewpoints. More specifically, they know enough not to bet on them. The chances that Figure 4.26A is the two-dimensional representation of the three-dimensional scene in Figure 4.26C are so slim that the visual system refuses even to consider this possibility. Nevertheless,

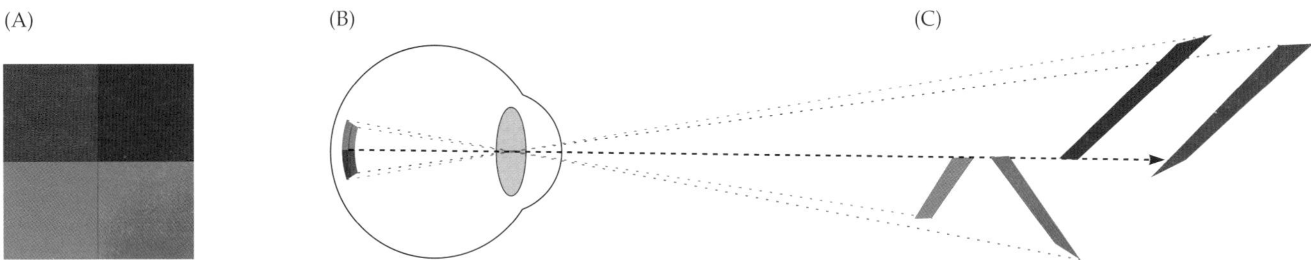

FIGURE 4.26 **Accidental viewpoint** (A) Suppose you see these four squares: you would typically infer that you were looking at a large square, divided into four quadrants, *but* maybe the eye (B) just happens to be in exactly the right position to see these four arbitrary shapes (C) at four arbitrary depths so that they line up to form the pattern in (A). That would be quite a coincidence and would be what is called an accidental viewpoint.

FIGURE 4.27 shows us that sometimes the visual system can be fooled (in whole or in part) by an accidental viewpoint. At some level, you know that these people are not holding the Leaning Tower of Pisa, but it looks quite convincing. If the camera was moved, just a little, the illusion would vanish.

The visual system also makes some assumptions based on an implicit understanding of some aspects of the physics of the world. For example, returning to the Kanizsa image in Figure 4.13, we infer the arrow-shaped object in part because of our *implicit* understanding that solid objects block light. This understanding of opacity causes us to infer that the lines disappear because something is blocking our view of them. Calling this understanding "implicit" means that we need not be able to verbalize the rule in order to use it. Monkeys seem to see the subjective contours without benefit of instruction in physics (von der Heydt, Peterhans, and Baumgartner, 1984), and we may assume that similar abilities extend far into the animal kingdom. We and our visual systems "know" this and other physical principles in the same way that a ball "knows" about gravity.

These principles and assumptions may seem so obvious as to be meaningless. But remember that an image has no meaning whatsoever until mid- and high-level visual processes dig into it. One committee uses the knowledge that opaque objects occlude other objects behind them to generate plausible interpretations of image elements like the notched circles and dead-end edges in Figures 4.13 and 4.14. Another committee considers all the possibilities and devalues any that involve accidental viewpoints, reducing what is initially a theoretically unsolvable problem (finding the one correct interpretation in an infinite number of possible ones) to a potentially solvable one. Other committees make implicit guesses about the materials in the work (Figure 4.9). And so we proceed further and further into the visual system, until a single, generally correct interpretation emerges.

FIGURE 4.27 **Accidental tourist** In this case, the view from an accidental viewpoint is accepted.

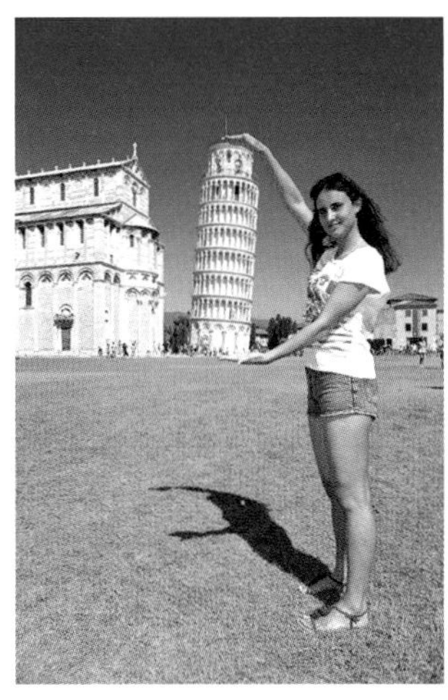

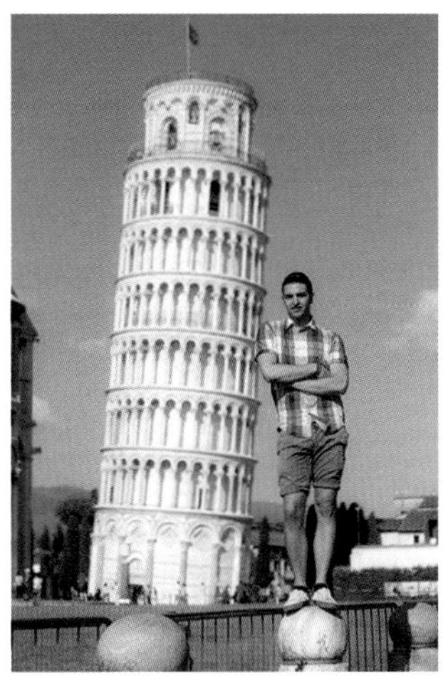

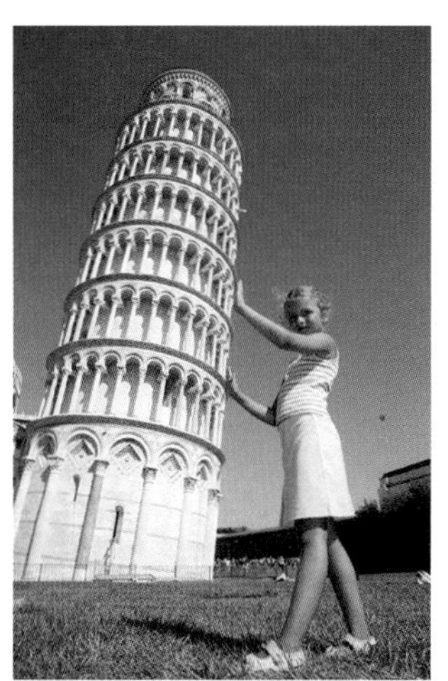

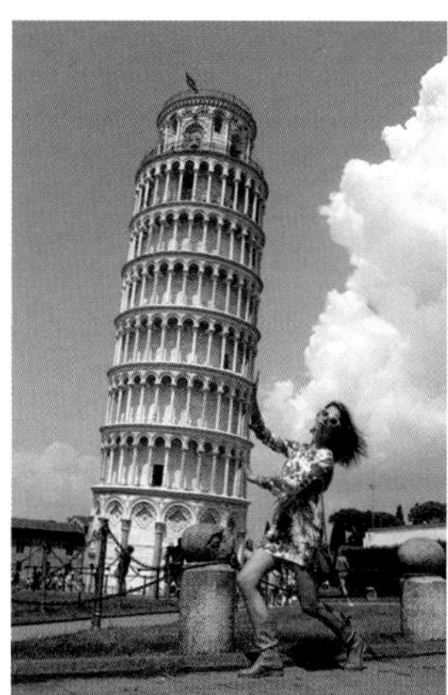

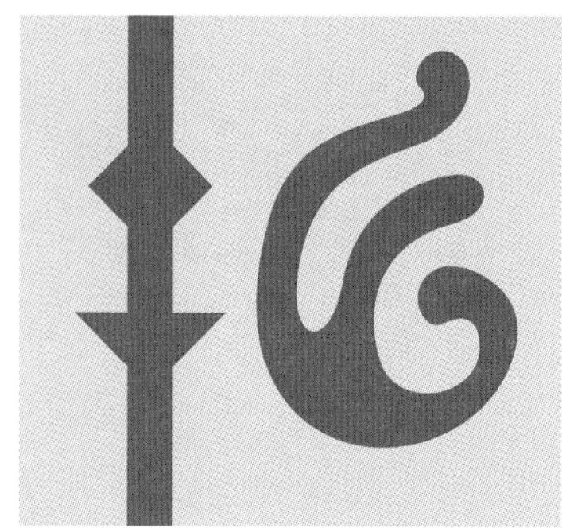

FIGURE 4.28 **Figure-ground segmentation** What is figure and what is ground, and why?

figure-ground assignment The process of determining that some regions of an image belong to a foreground object (figure) and other regions are part of the background (ground).

surroundedness A rule for figure-ground assignment stating that if one region is entirely surrounded by another, it is likely that the surrounded region is the figure.

Figure and Ground

Armed with this understanding of the ground rules of committee deliberation, we can continue with the effort to go from simple features to recognizable objects. The edge- and region-finding mechanisms discussed earlier would divide FIGURE 4.28 into yellow and red regions without much difficulty. But how should those regions be understood? It is extremely likely that we would interpret the illustration as two red figures on a yellow background. That is, we would infer that the yellow would continue behind the red objects if we could lift them up to check. That need not be the case, however. We could be looking at yellow and red puzzle pieces, cut to fit each other perfectly. Or we could be looking at two yellow objects, a smaller one on the left and a larger one with a squiggly hole on the right, both sitting on top of a red background.

The ability to distinguish figures (objects in the foreground) from ground (surfaces or objects lying behind the figures) is a critical step on the path from image to object recognition. Like the finding of edges and regions, this is the work of another one (?) of these perceptual committees that weigh different factors to decide how the visual world should be understood. As before, the governing goal is to determine the most likely reality behind the image on the retina.

Like the grouping principles, the topic of **figure-ground assignment** became important in visual perception because of the work of the Gestalt psychologists. FIGURE 4.29 shows the classic vase/face figure introduced in the 1920s by the Danish psychologist Edgar Rubin (1886–1951). It must be the best-known illustration from the Gestalt school, and it is analogous to the Necker cube in that it illustrates one of those rare cases in which a perceptual committee has a difficult time reaching consensus. Though all visual stimuli are inherently ambiguous, the processes that determine figure and ground almost always manage to come to a single conclusion about the world that produced the stimuli (as in Figure 4.28). We are surprised when the process fails and delivers two or more interpretations. The surprise we register when Figure 4.29 "flips" between a vase and a pair of faces reminds us of the perceptual stability that we usually take for granted.

What principles are at work in the assignment of regions to figure or ground? We can list some of them:

- *Surroundedness.* If one region is entirely surrounded by another, it is likely that the surrounded region is the figure. This **surroundedness** is a factor in labeling the red region on the right in Figure 4.28 as the figure.
- *Size.* The smaller region is likely to be the figure. A cow is smaller than the field in which she stands, so she is the figure.
- *Symmetry.* A symmetrical region is more likely to be seen as the figure. How likely is it that the two yellow regions in Figure 4.28 just happen to have the symmetrical contours facing each other over what would be the red gap on the left?
- *Parallelism.* Regions with parallel contours are more likely to be seen as the figure (does light blue or dark blue "win" as figure in FIGURE 4.30?). Again, how likely is it that two contours would be parallel with one another if they did not belong to the same object?
- *Relative motion.* How surface details move relative to an edge can also determine which portion of a display is the foreground figure and which is the background (Yonas, Craton, and Thompson, 1987).

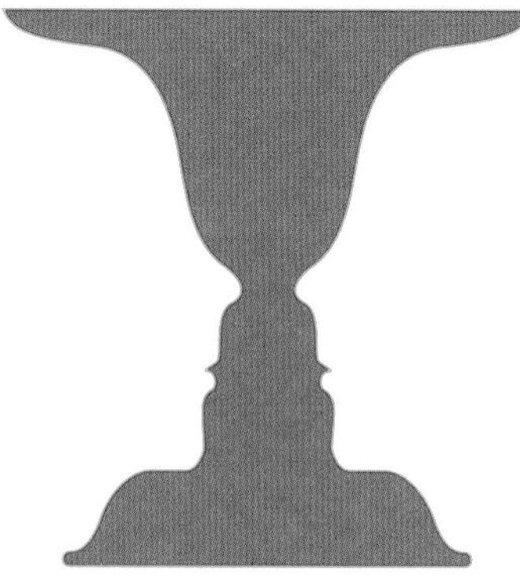

FIGURE 4.29 **The ambiguous Rubin vase/face figure** Notice that the boundary, marked by the green line, changes its allegiance when the figure flips interpretation from a vase to two faces. The boundary is "owned" by the currently perceived figure.

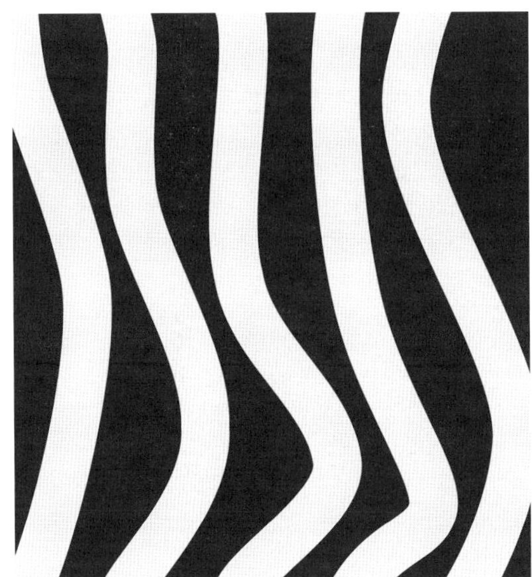

FIGURE 4.30 Parallel contours Why do the pale-blue stripes appear to be the figure when the pale-blue and dark-blue regions are about equal in size? Parallel contours are often taken to belong to the figure.

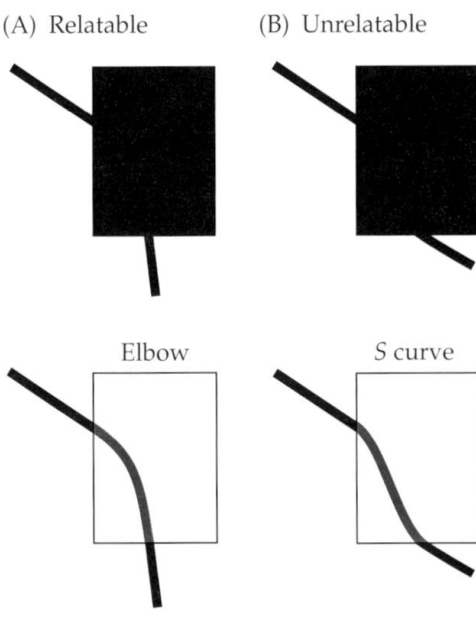

FIGURE 4.31 Relatability Two edges are relatable if they can be connected with a smooth convex or smooth concave curve (A), but not if the connection requires an *S* curve (B).

Dealing with Occlusion

Objects are rarely kind enough to present themselves to us in splendid isolation on blank backgrounds. In the real world, objects are often partially hidden by other objects. Indeed, three-dimensional objects always hide parts of themselves (you don't see the back of a ball, for example). We've already discussed how edge-finding processes can fabricate illusory contours on the basis of the physics of occlusion. Now let's think about the work required to connect the visible pieces of occluded objects by inferring the presence of hidden pieces of the object when necessary.

The Gestalt principle of good continuation comes into play here (see Figures 4.16–4.18). How do we understand the continuation of a contour when it disappears from view, behind an occluder? Philip Kellman and Thomas Shipley (1991) speak about the **relatability** of two contour segments, illustrated in **FIGURE 4.31**. Do the two black line segments in each part look like they belong to the same curve, occluded by the black square? For Figure 4.31A, the answer is "yes." For Figure 4.31B, the answer is "maybe not." Kellman and his colleagues argue that the critical difference is that the lines in Figure 4.31A can be related by a simple curve, like an elbow or a bend in the road. The lines in Figure 4.31B require a more complex *S* curve to make a smooth connection between them. The visual system is unwilling to propose such an elaborate relationship, so it concludes that the lines are not related (that is, they are not parts of the same object). Like the figure-ground rules, this **heuristic** (mental shortcut) is not infallible—after all, some objects really do have *S*-shaped contours. The occlusion committee is apparently willing to accept a few missed completions to reduce the vast number of possible completions we would have to consider if we tried to connect every pair of occluded edges.

Additional heuristics emerge when we move from two dimensions to three, as **FIGURE 4.32** shows. Here we see a pair of box-shaped objects, one partially occluding the other. The overlap of the boxes produces a variety of different line junctions, all of which can be classified as *Y*, *T*, or arrow junctions. *T* junctions

relatability The degree to which two line segments appear to be part of the same contour.

heuristic A mental shortcut.

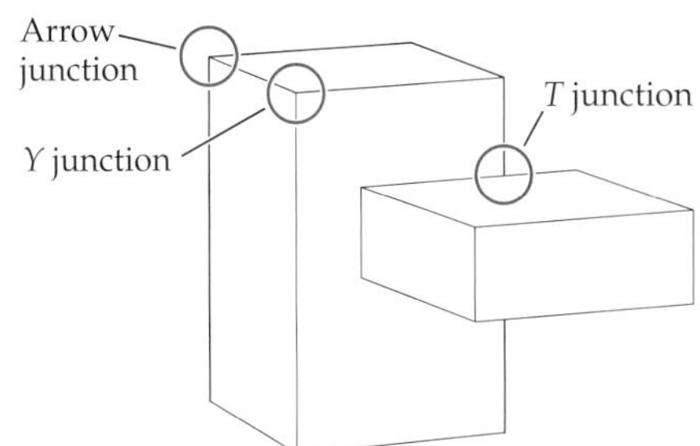

FIGURE 4.32 Line junctions are non-accidental features Except in rare instances of accidental viewpoint (see Figure 4.26), *T* junctions indicate occlusion of one region by another. *Y* and arrow junctions indicate the object's corners.

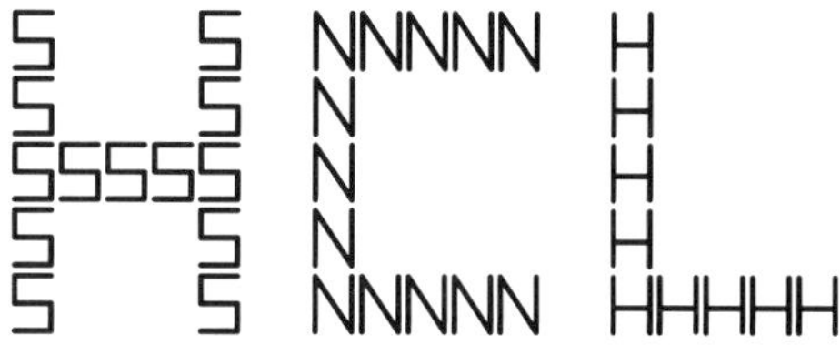

FIGURE 4.33 The global superiority effect You will see the large (global) *H* much more quickly than you identify the small (local) *H*s.

nonaccidental feature A feature of an object that is not dependent on the exact (or accidental) viewing position of the observer.

global superiority effect The finding in various experiments that the properties of the whole object take precedence over the properties of parts of the object.

almost always occur when one surface occludes another; *Y* and arrow junctions almost always correspond to corners and thus don't signal occlusions. These rules fail to hold true only when we're viewing the scene from an accidental viewpoint. Hence, the various junction types are known as **nonaccidental features** (Lowe, 1985), and they provide another potential tool for use by the perceptual committees charged with dividing the scene into objects and deciding whether one object is occluding another.

Parts and Wholes

Objects in the world tend to have parts. Indeed, it is not obvious how to define a visual object. Look at yourself in the mirror. In some sense, you are an object, but your nose, eyes, shirt, and so on can each be thought of as objects in their own right. In the lab, stimuli like those in **FIGURE 4.33** have been used to investigate the relationship of visual objects to their component parts. Look for *H*s in Figure 4.33. Did you find the big (global) *H* more quickly than the little (local) *H*s? Using stimuli like these, David Navon (1977) found that the global letters interfered with naming of the local letters more than the local letters interfered with recognition of the global letters. This **global superiority effect** is consistent with an implicit assumption we've been making throughout our discussion of midlevel vision: that the first goal of midlevel vision is to carve the retinal image into large-scale objects.

In the Navon letters, the division into parts and wholes—local and global—is easy. It is not so easy to ask how we "carve" a human form into parts like legs and arms. One heuristic is illustrated in **FIGURE 4.34**. Don D. Hoffman and Whitman Richards (1984) noted that when one blob is pushed into another, a pair of concavities is created in the silhouette of the resulting two-part object (Figure 4.34A). A process that embodied this bit of physics would conclude that valleys, rather than bumps, should be used to mark part boundaries. Thus, we are inclined to parse the object into the two parts shown in Figure 4.34B, not into three parts as in Figure 4.34C.

The global superiority effect and Hoffmann and Richard's point about concavities should be thought of as examples of the ways that we figure out the shape of an object. As J. T. Todd and Petrov (2022) make clear, there are "many facets of shape." We are just illustrating the work of a couple of the members of the brain's shape committee.

Summarizing Midlevel Vision

Before moving on, it is worth briefly reviewing how we got here. Early-vision processes gave us the local features in the visual world. Midlevel-vision processes began the work of understanding what those local features might be telling us about

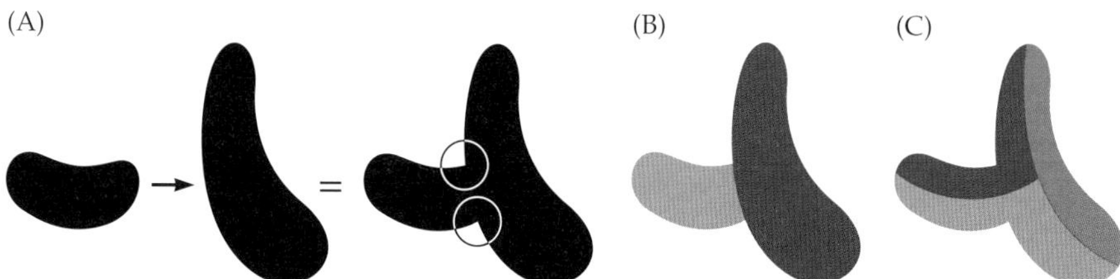

FIGURE 4.34 Finding parts from object boundaries (A) When one blob is pushed into another, a pair of concavities is created. We know this implicitly, and we work backward from this fact to carve this figure into the two parts shown in (B) rather than according to a different scheme, such as the three-part figure shown in (C).

the state of the world. The work of the midlevel processes discussed so far in this chapter might be summarized in five principles:

1. *Bring together that which should be brought together.* We have the Gestalt grouping principles (similarity, proximity, parallelism, symmetry, and so forth), and we have the processes that complete contours and objects even when they are partially hidden behind occluders (e.g., the relatability heuristic).
2. *Split asunder that which should be split asunder.* Complementing the grouping principles are the edge-finding processes that divide regions from one another. Figure-ground mechanisms separate objects from the background. Texture segmentation processes divide one region from the next on the basis of image statistics.
3. *Use what you know.* Two-dimensional edge configurations can tell us about three-dimensional corners or occlusion borders or how objects are divided into parts because we have implicit knowledge of the physics of image formation.
4. *Avoid accidents.* Avoid interpretations that require assumptions of highly specific, accidental combinations of features or accidental viewpoints.
5. *Seek consensus and avoid ambiguity.* Every image is ambiguous. There are always multiple, even infinite, physical situations that could generate a given image. Using the first four principles, the "committees" of midlevel vision must try to eliminate all but one of the possibilities, thereby resolving the ambiguity and delivering a single solution to the perceptual problem at hand.

Bayesian approach A way of formalizing the idea that our perception is a combination of the current stimulus and our knowledge about the conditions of the world—what is and is not likely to occur. The Bayesian approach is stated mathematically as Bayes' theorem: $P(A|O) = P(A) \times P(O|A)/P(O)$, which enables us to calculate the probability (P) that the world is in a particular state (A) given a particular observation (O).

From Metaphor to Formal Model

We have been talking about perceptual committees in midlevel vision. While we hope that is a useful way to think about what's going on, it is just a metaphor. There are formal, mathematical ways to model the way in which knowledge about regularities in the world can constrain the interpretation of ambiguous sensory input. One of the most fruitful approaches is known as the **Bayesian approach** (see Yuille and Kersten, 2006; W. J. Ma, Kording, and Goldreich, 2023), which we discussed briefly in Section 1.4. Thomas Bayes (1702–1761), an eighteenth-century Presbyterian minister, was the first to describe the relevant mathematics.

Look at **FIGURE 4.35**. Our visual system looks at the stimulus and makes some observations. Where are the edges and surfaces? What are the colors? What is this made of? As noted earlier, there is an infinite set of hypotheses that could be based on these observations. How does our visual system decide that one of these is the best hypothesis? The Bayesian approach asks us to think about two factors. First, before you look at anything, how likely is what you are proposing? This is known as the *prior probability*. The prior probability of a unicorn is much lower than the prior probability of a cow. Thus, if you make an observation that seems consistent with either unicorn or cow, you should be more inclined to accept the cow hypothesis. Second, how consistent is each hypothesis with the observations? Suppose you had the hypothesis that you were looking at a red square in Figure 4.35. The prior probability of a red square is no lower than the prior probability of a green square, but the observations will not support the red square hypothesis.

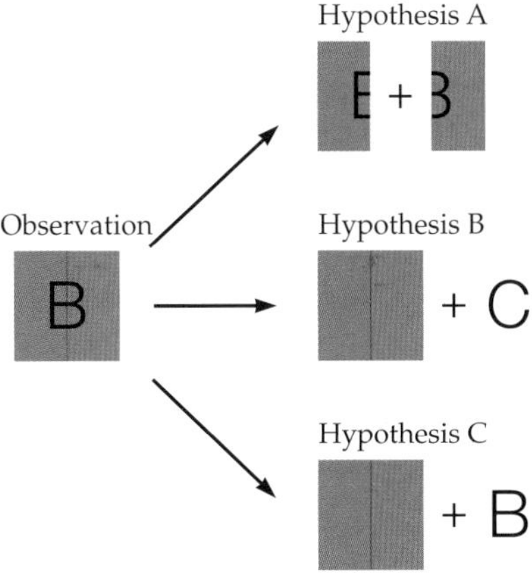

FIGURE 4.35 Bayesian perception When the visual system is faced with a stimulus, it tries to figure out the most likely real-world situation that has produced the particular pattern of activity observed by the low-level processes.

Let's consider just three hypotheses for the stimulus on the left of Figure 4.35. Hypothesis A proposes that we're looking at two green rectangles. The light one has a narrow letter *E* on it, and the dark one has a narrow numeral 3. Hypothesis A would require that the two halves just happen to precisely line up to produce the stimulus that we observe. That is consistent with the observation, but its prior probability is low because the *E* and 3 would need to line up very precisely—an accidental viewpoint. Hypothesis B suggests that this is a green square with a *C* on it. That is not particularly unlikely, but it is not consistent with the sensory data. Hypothesis C proposes that this is a square, half green and half purple, with the letter *B* on it. That does not require anything very unlikely in the world, and it is consistent with the observation.

What is really powerful about the Bayesian approach is that these sorts of ideas can be reduced to formal, mathematical equations.

FURTHER DISCUSSION of the Bayesian approach can be found in Section 6.4.

4.5 Object Recognition

Now, armed with tools that should be useful for object recognition, let's return to Quiroga's discovery of cells that respond to highly specific objects (Quiroga et al., 2005). Traveling the *what* pathway from V1 into the temporal lobe, we can see a progressive change in the responses of cells in different visual areas. In V1, cells respond best to lines and edges in very specific areas of the visual field. In V2, we get early steps from local features to objects. These cells have a sensitivity to "border ownership." They are also sensitive to illusory contours (Peterhans et al., 1986; von der Heydt, Peterhans, and Baumgartner, 1984). By area V4, cells appear to be interested in much more complex attributes, like those shown in **FIGURE 4.36**. No one has ever definitively determined the perfect set of stimuli for V4 cells. Figure 4.36A shows some older geometric ideas from Gallant, Braun, and Van Essen (1993); Figure 4.36B shows a small subset of a collection of bumpy, 3D blobs from the work of Srinath et al. (2021). In both cases, you can see from Figure 4.36 that one specific cell will show more response to some stimuli and less to others.

(A)

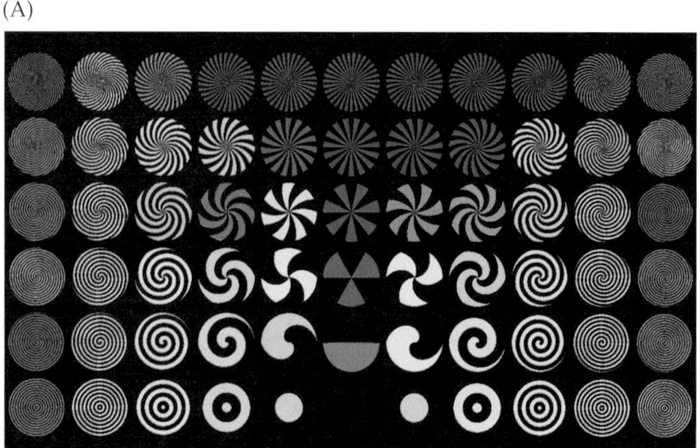

(B)

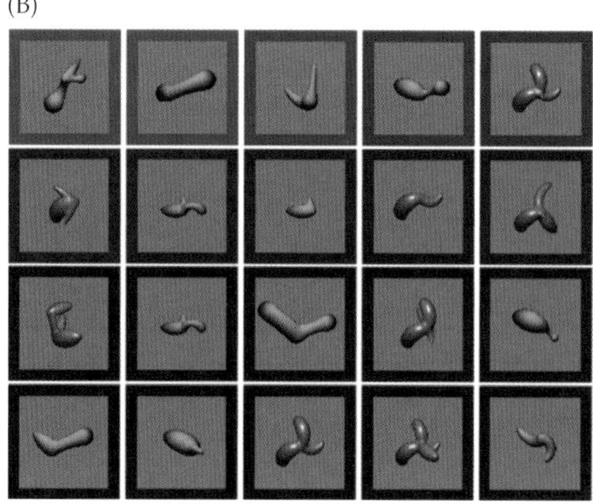

FIGURE 4.36 Response of V4 cells to different shapes (A) Gallant, Braun, and Van Essen (1993) tried this set of stimuli. Warm colors (red, orange, yellow) indicate more response from one particular cell in area V4. (B) Srinath et al. (2021) presented shapes like these to V4 neurons. Here, redder outlines indicate more response from one particular cell.

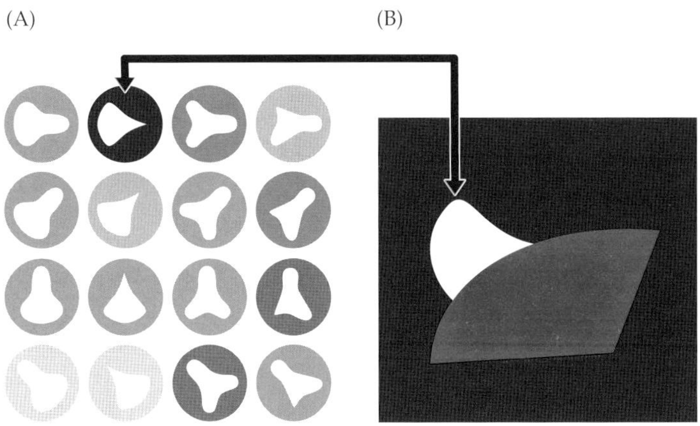

FIGURE 4.37 **Occluded shapes** (A) One cell in V4 responds best to the shape in the dark circle (darkness indicates the strength of the response). The cell responds well to sharp features pointing to the right but (B) the same shape might not produce the same response when the sharp point in (B) is the "accidental" result of occlusion.

The images in Figure 4.36 illustrate a fact about objects: while you can vary orientation or color or other basic features in a systematic way, it is much harder to imagine how you vary object shape. What are the dimensions of shape? We really don't know. In FIGURE 4.37A, the darkness of the circles indicates how well a specific cell responded to a variety of two-dimensional shapes. (Many more were used. Just a few are shown here.) As you can see, this particular cell seems to have a taste for stimuli with a feature pointing to the right. The connection to object perception is illustrated in FIGURE 4.37B. This V4 cell might respond to a stimulus like the one in Figure 4.37A, but it will not respond well to a stimulus like the one in Figure 4.37B, because that white object probably doesn't really have a feature pointing right. Its sharp point is an accident of occlusion. The border ownership rules, established in V2, now become part of the process of understanding object shape (Bushnell et al., 2011).

Things get more complex as we move deeper into the temporal lobe. FIGURE 4.38 illustrates the hopeful hypothesis that a vast family of shapes like those in Figure 4.36A and/or B might be a basis for object perception, just as letters and syllables can be the basis for words (Ungerleider and Bell, 2011). We may not know exactly what optimally activates individual cells as we progress along the *what* pathway into the temporal lobe. However, as mentioned before, functional imaging studies such as fMRI can show us that different regions of the cortex are activated better by some categories of stimuli than by others. One way to show this is a so-called **subtraction method**. If you show a human observer a series of pictures of spaces like rooms and fields and city streets, lots of pieces of the brain will be activated by these places. Now show the observer other pictures with similar properties that do not happen to be places—maybe scrambled versions of the places, maybe objects or abstract designs. Again, large areas of brain will be active. However, if you subtract the two patterns of activation, there will be at least one region—the PPA, discussed in Section 4.2—that is specifically and reliably activated more by places than by other stimuli (Epstein and

subtraction method In functional magnetic resonance imaging (fMRI), comparison of brain activity measured in two conditions: one with and one without the involvement of the mental process of interest. The difference between the images for the two conditions may show regions of brain specifically activated by that mental process.

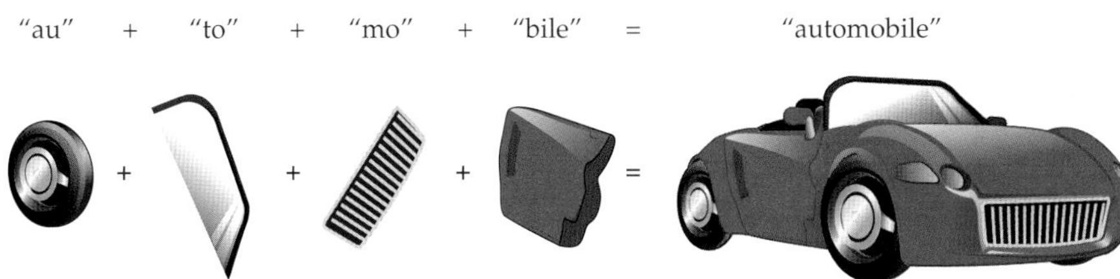

FIGURE 4.38 **From meaningless to meaningful** Just as letters and syllables form words, individual neurons might be sensitive to shapes that can be put together into a recognizable object, even if no single cell's preferred shape looks like any object we have seen.

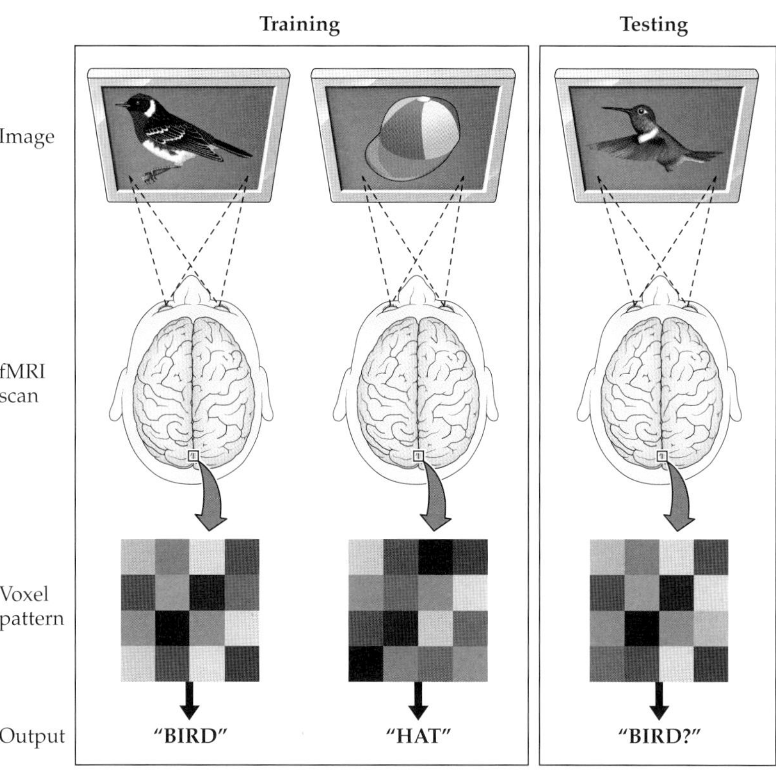

FIGURE 4.39 Object-decoding methods in functional magnetic resonance imaging (fMRI) First, researchers train a computer system by showing a large set of images to an observer in a scanner. Then, they attempt to decode the observer's brain activity produced by a new image. By finding the best match to the previously recorded brain activity, researchers can often guess the identity of the new image and can map the parts of the brain that contain that information.

decoding The process of determining the nature of a stimulus from the pattern of responses measured in the brain or, potentially, in an artificial system like a computer network. The stimulus could be a sensory stimulus or it could be an internal state (e.g., the contents of a dream).

Kanwisher, 1998). (We also mentioned two other well-established specialized areas, the fusiform face area and the extrastriate body area; see Figure 4.4.)

More modern functional imaging studies make use of **decoding** methods, as shown in FIGURE 4.39. First, an observer in a magnetic resonance imaging scanner is presented with a range of images of a vast series of objects, each in many different sizes, positions, and so forth. Researchers then catalog the responses of the brain to each of these "training" images. Next, the observer sees a new image of a randomly selected object, and researchers use the patterns of the observer's brain activity to try to guess the identity of the object. Perhaps there is some part of the brain that generates patterns that allow your visual system to correctly determine that this stimulus was a cat and that stimulus was a shoe. This does not prove that this specific piece of brain was the locus of recognition, but it does show that information about object identity is present in that region (K. N. Kay et al., 2008). Eventually, decoding could take us to some rather interesting places. If you knew the patterns of activity associated with a wide set of objects presented while someone was awake, could you decode that person's dreams if you let her sleep in the scanner? We are not there yet, but a start has been made (Horikawa et al., 2013).

Can We Build It?

Chapters 2, 3, and 4 have described a story in which more and more complex attributes of the visual input are processed as we move from the eyes to the lateral geniculate nucleus to early visual cortex and beyond. Advances in computer science over the past decade have shown that models, built on an approximation of this architecture, can do a good job in classifying objects in scenes. Oliver Selfridge (1959) suggested a version of such a model more than 50 years ago. His

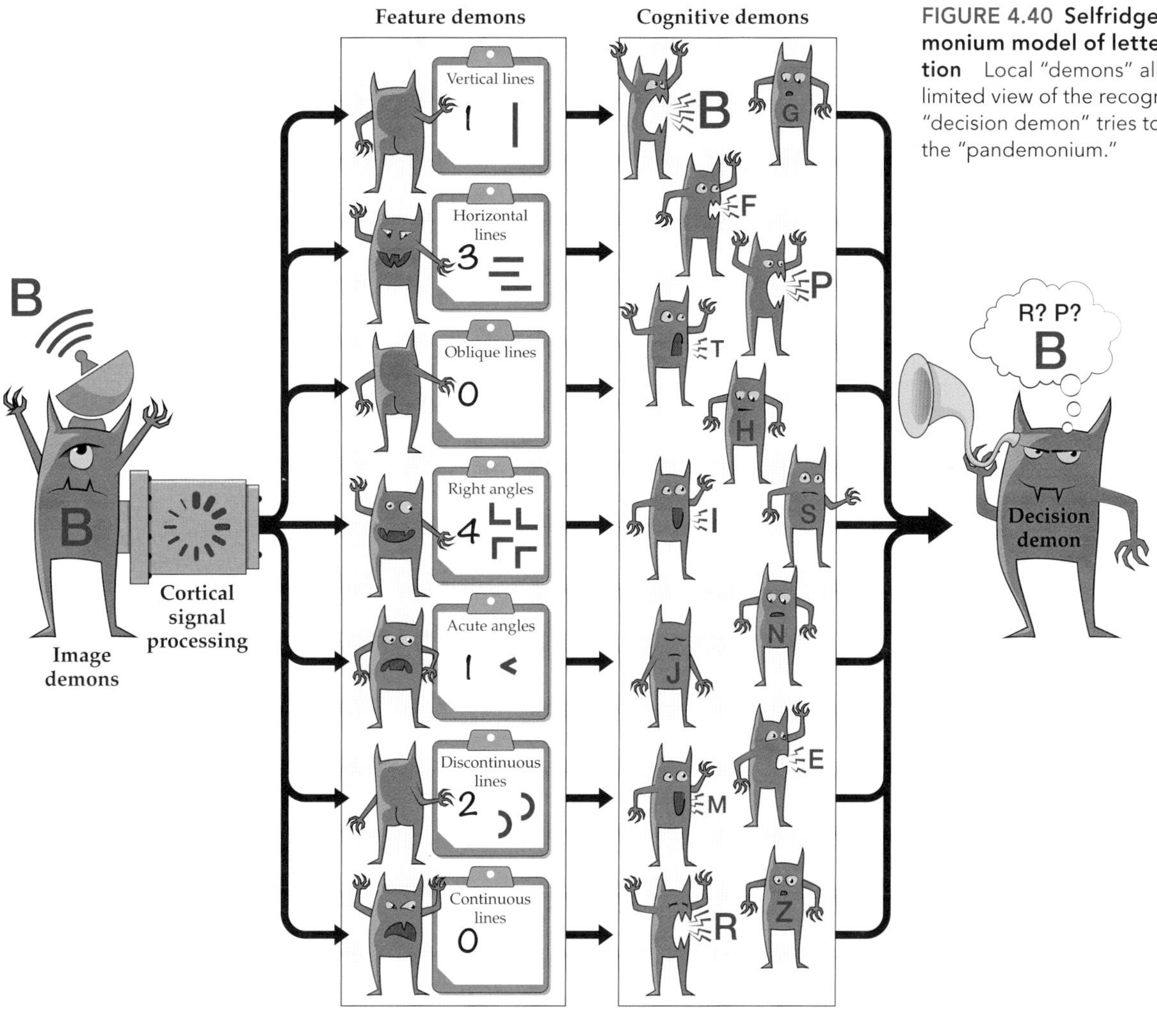

FIGURE 4.40 Selfridge's pandemonium model of letter recognition Local "demons" all yell about their limited view of the recognition problem. A "decision demon" tries to make sense of the "pandemonium."

"pandemonium model" was an account of letter recognition, a relatively simple subset of the object recognition problem (**FIGURE 4.40**). Selfridge used "demons" as a metaphor for processes that we would discuss in neural terms today. Indeed, the word *pandemonium*, which we define as "noise and chaos," was originally coined by the poet John Milton (1608–1674) as the name of the home of all demons in *Paradise Lost*. Selfridge had an initial early-vision signal-processing stage. Next, features were extracted: oriented lines, curves, and so on. In his third step, a set of "cognitive demons" each looked for the features of one letter. Finally, the "decision demon" pooled information across all the third-layer demons and chose the loudest demon as the answer.

That is not a bad start, but of course the real network will be more complicated than Selfridge's fairly simple network of demons. Even for a constrained task like letter recognition, the network needs to accept all the letter *A*s in **FIGURE 4.41** as *A*s. It needs to recognize *A*s in many locations, many sizes, and many orientations. And an *A* is a simple case. The object recognition network needs to be able to categorize each object in **FIGURE 4.42** as a cow. No simple cow **template** will do that . . . and think about how you might recognize members of the category "animal" or, if you were an airport security officer, how you would recognize a member of the category "threat." The basic idea of a template is rather like a lock and key. As we will see

template The internal representation of a stimulus that is used to recognize the stimulus in the world. Unlike its use in, for example, making a key, a mental template is not expected to look like the stimulus that it matches.

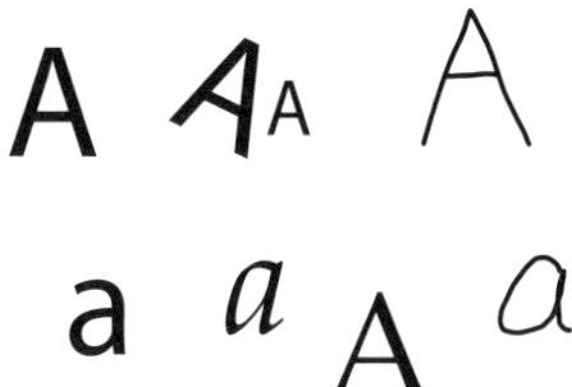

FIGURE 4.41 Templates The problem with templates is that we would need a lot of them to recognize the same object in all its aspects and orientations.

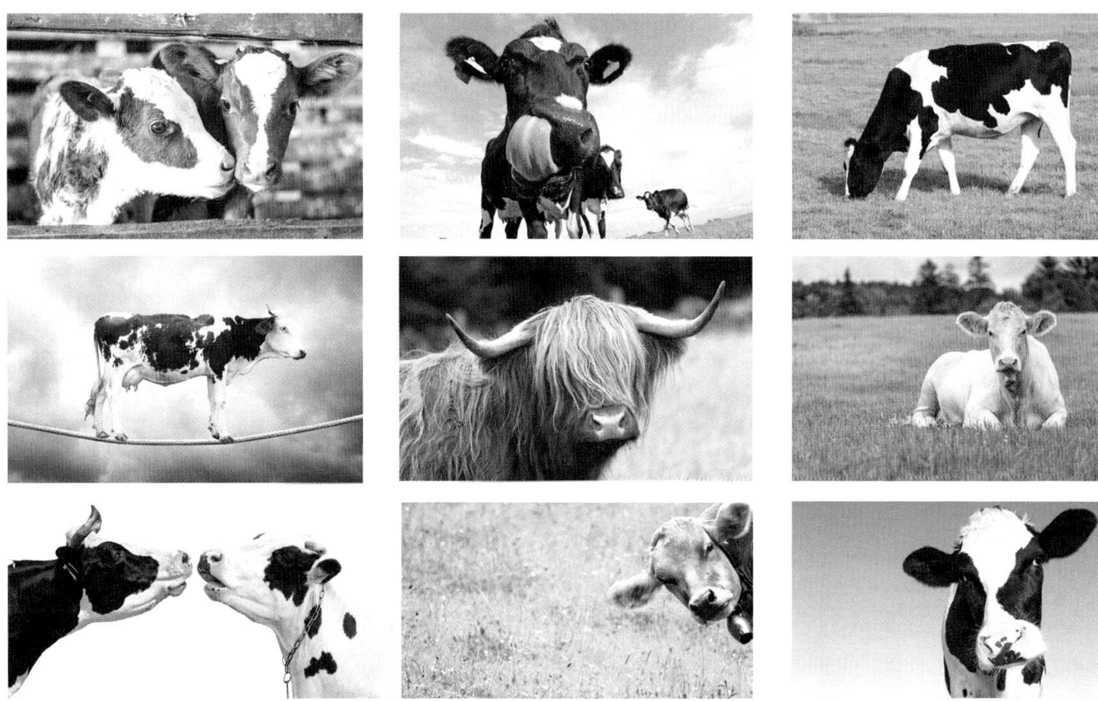

FIGURE 4.42 Cow templates What would a cow template look like?

in Chapters 14 and 15, the lock-and-key metaphor is quite apt in smell and taste, where the "key" to be recognized is a molecule like a specific odorant and where that molecular key presents itself in more or less the same shape every time (see, for instance, the "shape-pattern" theory of olfaction in Section 14.3). Objects, however, are not like molecules: the same category of object can present itself in infinite ways.

One way out of this problem is to notice that all the *A*s—or, at least, all the capital *A*s—in Figure 4.41 share a basic structure. Instead of matching each point in the image to a point in a template, perhaps we perform a more conceptual match. Just about any capital *A* can be described by the relationship of its three lines: the two flanking lines meet, and the third line spans the angle created by those two lines. Now the image of the *A* is being matched to a **structural description** of a capital *A*, a specification of an object in terms of its parts and the relationships between the parts.

Biederman (1987), in his **recognition-by-components model**, proposed something like this for objects more generally. He suggested that a set of **geons** ("geometric ions") could be the basic building blocks of the perception of objects in the world. **FIGURE 4.43** shows a few geons in isolation and a few simple objects composed of two geons. The idea is that the visual system should be able to recognize an object on the basis of the relationship of its geons, regardless of how the geon is oriented in space (as long as it's not an accidental view). But there are problems with structural description models. Real-object recognition is not as viewpoint-independent as the model would propose. Moreover, no one has ever come up with a set of geon-like primitives that would work over all objects. Would the geon description of a book differ from the description of a box containing that book? Or look at the "potatoes" in **FIGURE 4.44**. It is hard to imagine a geon account that usefully describes their family similarity and their individual differences.

structural description A description of an object in terms of the nature of its constituent parts and the relationships between those parts.

recognition-by-components model Biederman's model of object recognition, which holds that objects are recognized by the identities and relationships of their component parts.

geon In Biederman's recognition-by-components model, any of the "geometric ions" out of which perceptual objects are built.

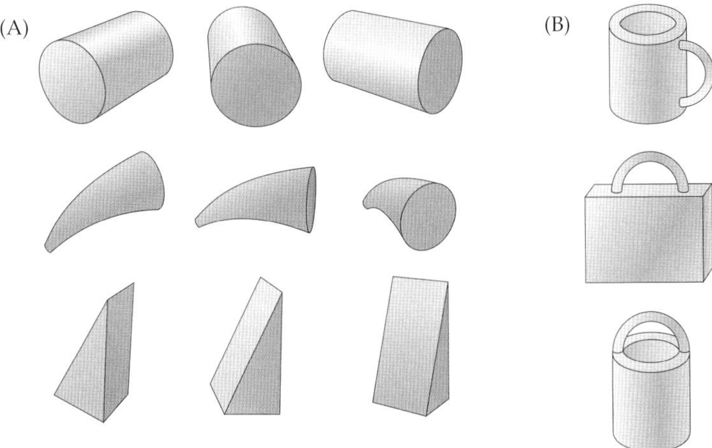

FIGURE 4.43 Building objects from geons (A) Cylinders, cones, and triangles are 3 of the 36 or so geons in Biederman's recognition-by-components model of object recognition. (B) Three of the many objects that could be made from just 2 geons.

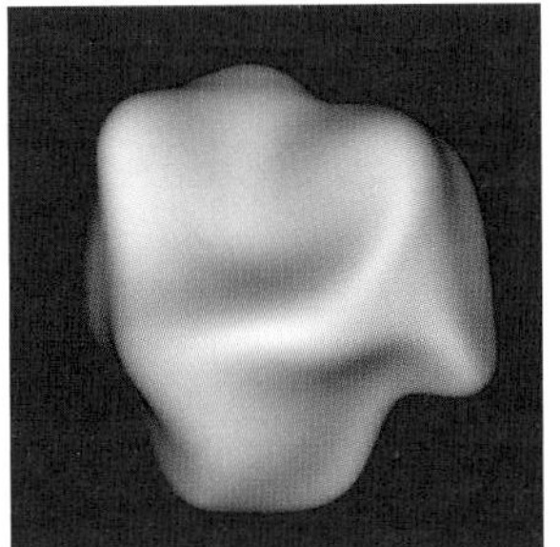
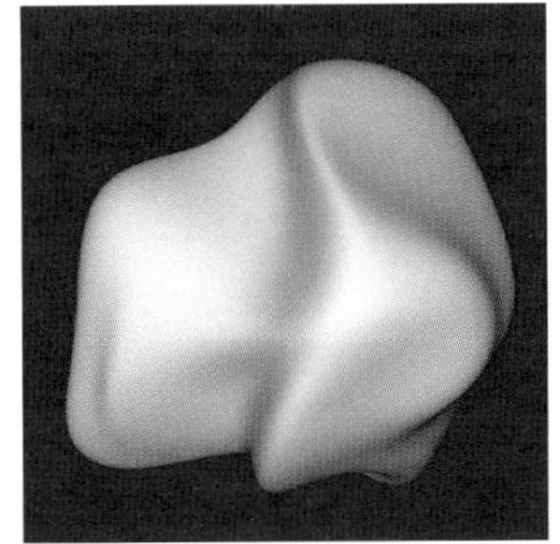
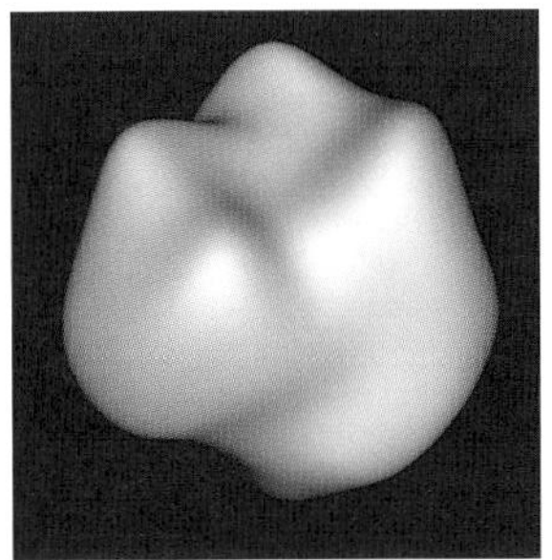
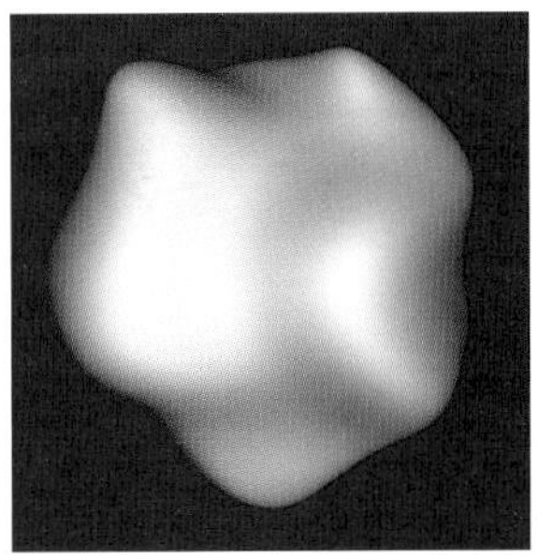

FIGURE 4.44 What are the geons here? These objects differ from each other, but it would be hard to capture either their shape or their differences with geons.

These objections don't mean that geon theory is wrong. They merely point out that a structural description would have to be only a part of the answer to the problem of object recognition. Again, remember those "many facets of shape" from J. T. Todd and Petrov (2022). Other parts of the answer would include information about materials and surface markings. Those factors, for instance, would tend to differentiate a box and a book. In addition, it is important to remember that object identities are learned and that learning may be influenced by the viewpoint(s) at which the object is seen (Gauthier et al., 1998).

As hinted at the start of this section, the real breakthrough in the area of object recognition has come from computer science. The advent of faster computers with more and more memory has allowed researchers to build **deep neural network (DNN)** models (see Section 1.4) with many more layers than Selfridge's and with a set of rules that let the model learn to categorize objects (Kriegeskorte, 2015; Serre, 2019; Rust and Jannuzi, 2022). In broad outline, the ideas behind DNNs should sound familiar. A set of features is extracted from the image (**FIGURES 4.45A** and **4.45B**). In the first layer of a DNN, this is quite like what *simple cells* in visual cortex are doing (see Section 3.5). Then that information is pooled in a manner that is something like what *complex cells* are doing (**FIGURE 4.45C**). You can think of these operations as creating a new image that the next layer of the DNN will take as its input for feature extraction and pooling (**FIGURES 4.45D** and **4.45E**). These processes of feature extraction and pooling are repeated for a number of layers (**FIGURE 4.45F**). Then, at the top of this stack of layers, you have what amounts to a set of "grandmother cells," one for each category of object that you

deep neural network (DNN) A type of "machine learning" in artificial intelligence in which a computer is programmed to learn something (here, object recognition). These are artificial neural networks that have a large number of layers of nodes with millions of connections. First, the network is "trained" using input for which the answer is known ("That is a cow"). Subsequently, the network can provide answers from input that it has never seen before.

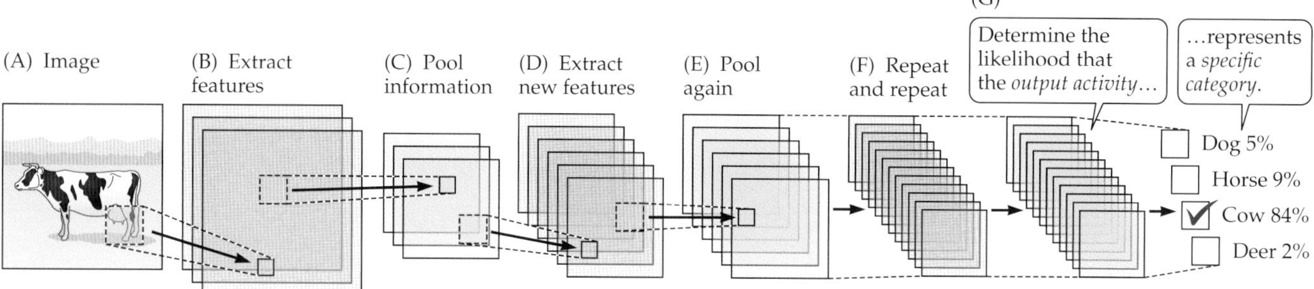

FIGURE 4.45 A deep neural network recognizes a cow The network has been trained using images of a wide range of animals. Now, faced with an image it has never seen before, the network can declare that "cow" is the most likely category.

are trying to identify. If the set of object categories included "grandmother," then one of these cells really would be a grandmother cell. It would be looking at the pattern of activity across the top layer of the network to determine how likely it was that the pattern indicated the presence of "grandmother" (**FIGURE 4.45G**). A different cell would look for "cat," or "egg beater," or whatever categories you cared to ask about.

All of the myriad connections between bits of this big network are governed by weights that say, "This is a strong connection, while that is a weak connection." It is not possible to set all these weights by hand. Instead, the network learns its weights. Initially, the weights are random and the network produces random results. Show it a grandmother, and perhaps it says that the most likely answer is "cat." If you show the network a set of images whose identities you know, you can calculate the size of the error the network is making. Now you can change the weights a bit and repeat. If the error gets smaller, that is good. If it gets larger, you made the wrong changes. Repeat this process many times (with some good rules for how to change weights), and you find a set of weights that minimizes the network's error—you have a "trained" network. If you feed a properly trained network new images that it has never seen before, it will categorize most of those images successfully (this is the basis of the decoding research illustrated in Figure 4.39).

Notice that this has a quite natural feel to it. Once upon a time, you were a child with a good network but not much training. You might not have known much about animals. Over time, you were shown examples of cats, dogs, kangaroos, and wombats. We can imagine that the weights in your network were adjusted appropriately and then, one day, faced with a specific cat you had never seen before, you were likely to correctly categorize it. Learning the weights is how the specific features in a network are created. Interestingly, these object recognition networks learn features that seem to make some physiological sense. The first layer tends to grow features that look like oriented line and edge detectors with various color combinations. Intermediate layers become more complex, responding to textures and shapes, while the features in the final layers can look quite specific, reminiscent of cells in inferotemporal cortex that might respond to something face-like, for example.

DNNs have a lot of potential for real-world applications, from self-driving cars to medical diagnosis (see Section 1.4). In radiology, a very important part of medicine, hardly a week passes without a new paper describing an algorithm that matches or beats human experts (e.g., Ardila et al., 2019; Lotter, et al., 2021). At the same time, it would be a mistake to think that DNNs have "solved" vision. DNNs can be surprisingly easy to fool. If you have a clever DNN, it is possible to train another, "adversarial" network to design images that will fool that DNN (Serre, 2019). In some cases, the original DNN can make errors that no child would make, like thinking a picture of a sock with a bit of "noise" added was really an elephant (Serre, 2019). A different problem concerns networks' abilities to generalize. A human radiologist, trained to detect breast cancer in the mammograms from one hospital, will not have much trouble adapting to the images at another hospital. This is not always true for a DNN. Trained on one set of images, it may perform less impressively on a different set of apparently similar images (X. Wang et al., 2020).

entry-level category For an object, the label that comes to mind most quickly when we identify it (e.g., "bird"). At the subordinate level, the object might be more specifically named (e.g., "eagle"); at the superordinate level, it might be more generally named (e.g., "animal").

Multiple Recognition Committees?

If this chapter has had one theme, it is that no step on the road from image to recognition is taken by a single process acting alone. From the grouping of similar pieces of the image to the segregation of figure and ground, every step is based on consensus—a committee decision. It seems likely that the act of recognition is similar. Indeed, recognition may not be a single act. We can recognize an object in multiple ways, perhaps simultaneously. As an example, **FIGURE 4.46** shows three birds. In the terminology of Pierre Jolicoeur and his colleagues (Jolicoeur, Gluck, and Kosslyn, 1984), "bird" is the **entry-level category** for these objects—the first word that comes to mind when we're asked to name them. But these objects are also quite clearly different. At a subordinate level—a more specific level beneath the entry level—Figure 4.46A shows a fox sparrow, Figure 4.46B shows a cardinal, and

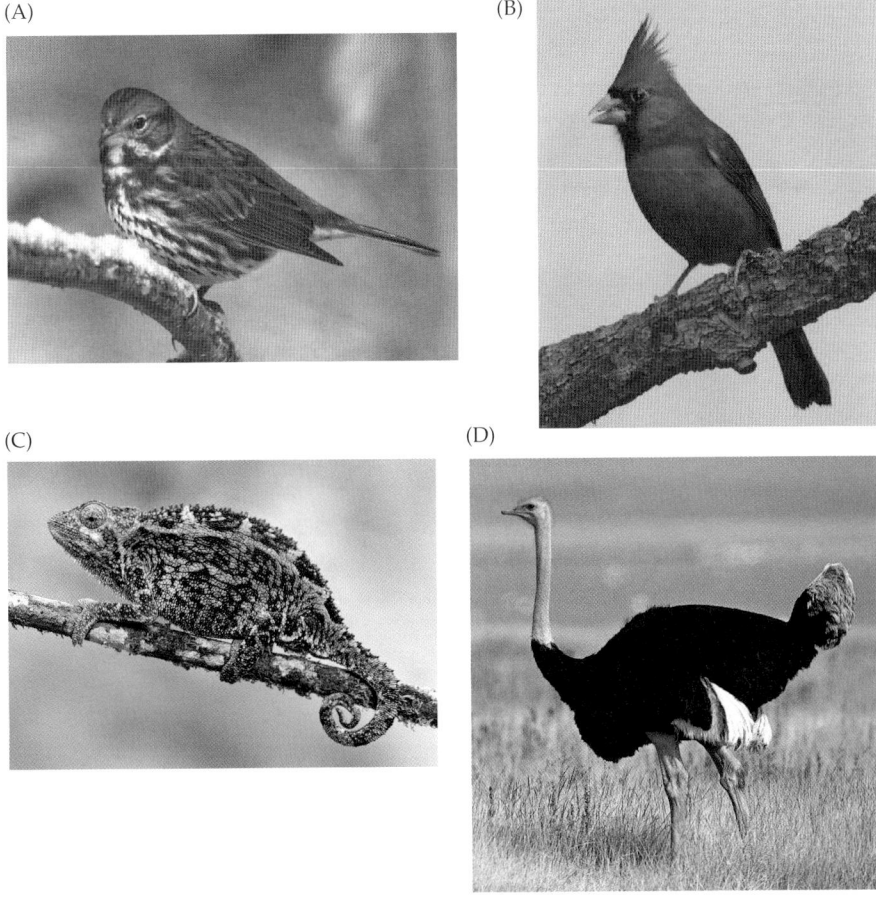

FIGURE 4.46 Is it a bird? Four images, all readily recognized as "animals." (A and B) Two quite different but easily recognizable "birds." (C and D) Would visual system input alone be enough to instantly classify either of these images as "bird" or "not bird"?

holistic processing Processing based on analysis of the entire object or scene and not on adding together a set of smaller parts or features.

Figure 4.46D shows an ostrich. At a superordinate level—a broader level above the entry level—these three objects, as well as the one in Figure 4.46C, are all animals.

We can imagine that each of these acts of recognition ("fox sparrow," "bird," "animal") might rely on different stored representations and different analyses of the visual stimulus. This is one reason to think that DNNs have not "solved" vision yet. A good DNN might identify a fox sparrow, the cardinal, and the ostrich as birds, but you and what might be your vast collection of DNNs can answer many questions about that bird as a visual stimulus. You could explain why the ostrich is an unusual bird. The DNN probably could not. Despite amazing progress, it will be a while before artificial vision systems approach the visual world with the flexibility of the human system.

Faces: An Illustrative Special Case

Faces are an interesting special case of object recognition. Take, for example, the images in **FIGURE 4.47A**. You should have little difficulty recognizing these as faces, but you will probably have some difficulty quickly identifying which one has been modified. If you turn the faces right side up, however, one of the pictures will look quite strikingly wrong (Thompson, 1980). You can see this in **FIGURE 4.47A**. Effects like these are taken as evidence for **holistic processing** of faces. That is, you don't recognize your friend's face by recognizing her specific eye and nose and mouth and then combining those features into a face. Instead, you seem to process the complex face as a single thing, although your face-analyzing processes seem to be very concerned with the precise configuration of eyes, nose, and mouth. However, it is not clear how that configuration is specified. For example, if you look at **FIGURE 4.47B**, you will see that recognition seems to survive stretching the face even though that changes the relative distances between different features (Burton, 2013).

In recent years, there has been significant progress in understanding the neural basis of face perception. In Section 4.2, we mentioned the FFA as a patch of brain

(A)

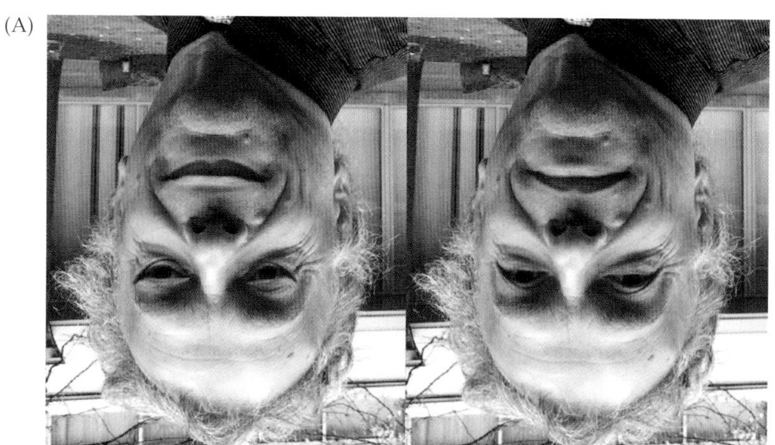

(B)

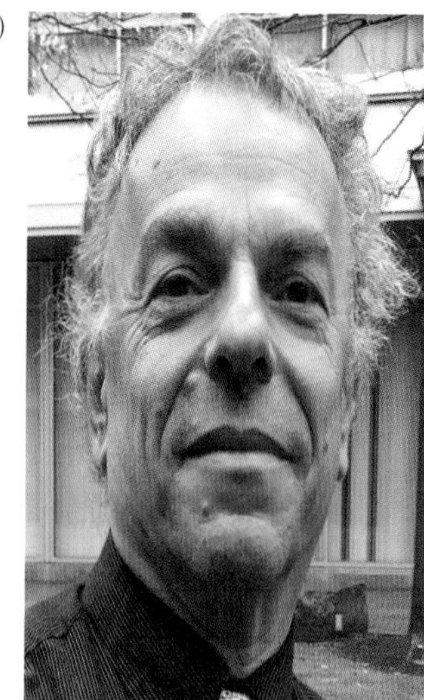

FIGURE 4.47 Faces (A) Which of these two photos has been altered? You can see for yourself that both of these images of one of the authors look quite normal upside down, but one of them looks strikingly "wrong" when turned right-side up (see Figure 4.48). (B) The "wholistic" interpretation of this face does not seem to be greatly disturbed by stretching the image.

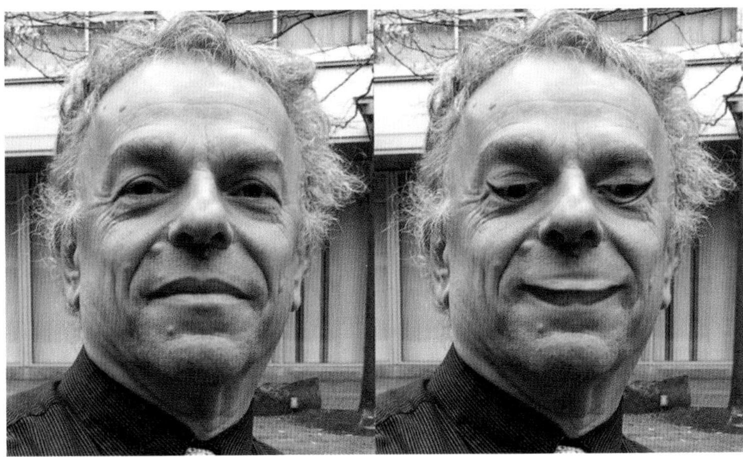

FIGURE 4.48 That is obvious When we turn Figure 4.47A to an upright position, it is very obvious which face is distorted.

that is very interested in faces. Actually, there are quite a few "face patches" in the brain—the monkey brain as well as the human brain (Grimaldi, Saleem, and Tsao, 2016). L. Chang and Tsao (2017) have an idea about how those patches make it possible to recognize your grandmother, regardless of how she is posed. Interestingly, that idea provides a link to the chapter on color perception that follows this one. If you open the "color picker" in one of your computer's apps, you will be able to define a color with three numbers. One common version is RGB: this much *R*ed, this much *G*reen, and this much *B*lue. If you know those numbers, you know the color, at least of an isolated patch (see Figure 5.15). L. Chang and Tsao (2017) found "face space" to be quite similar to "color space": different cells respond to different axes in the space and, if you know responses on several axes, you can identify the face.

Identifying a face is a good start, but in addition to this *invariant* property (your friend's face is recognizably the same as their face yesterday or last year), you also want to process the *dynamic* aspects of face processing (What is she saying? Is she happy?). Haxby, Hoffman, and Gobbini (2000) proposed two pathways through the FFA, one dealing with invariant identity and a second dealing with more dynamic facial expressions. Like the *what* and *where* pathways described in Section 4.2, these FFA pathways are not completely separate, but interact and support each other (Duchaine and Yovel, 2015).

Neuropsychology provides further evidence that face processing can be separated into different functions. Damage to specific areas in the temporal lobe of the brain can produce prosopagnosia, a disorder in which someone cannot identify faces. He may be able to recognize an object as a face, and he may know that the face looks angry. However, he will not know who the person is, even if it is someone he interacts with every day. If the person speaks, then auditory information, processed elsewhere in the brain, might provide identity information. You may think you're experiencing prosopagnosia yourself when you fail to match a name to a face. However, that is a much more common failure of memory. You can recognize the face; you just can't remember the name that goes with it. Someone with prosopagnosia would not know that this particular face was familiar while another one was not.

congenital prosopagnosia A form of face blindness apparently present from birth, as opposed to acquired prosopagnosia, which would typically be the result of an injury to the nervous system.

It is possible to be born with a specific impairment in the ability to recognize faces. The existence of this **congenital prosopagnosia** is a good indication that there is indeed a specific neural module for face recognition (Behrmann and Avidan, 2005). If you can be born without this face-recognizing ability, it seems likely that you are born with some ability. One study even suggests that some face-processing ability is present *before* birth. Reid et al. (2017) projected very schematic faces onto the abdomens of pregnant women. The abdominal wall is not much of a screen, so these were just triangles of dots mimicking two eyes and a nose or mouth. Nevertheless, Reid et al. reported that there were more fetal head turns toward the "upright face." Once the baby is born, it is much easier to show that very young infants have a preference for faces (Mondloch et al., 1999).

Summary

1. A series of extrastriate visual areas continue the work of visual processing. Emerging from V1 (primary visual cortex, striate cortex) are two broad streams of processing: one going into the temporal lobe and the other into the parietal lobe. The temporal pathway seems specifically concerned with *what* a stimulus might be. This chapter follows that pathway. (The parietal *where* pathway will be considered in later chapters.)
2. After early visual processes extract basic features from the visual input, it is the job of midlevel vision to organize these features into the regions, surfaces, and objects that can, in turn, serve as input to object recognition and scene-understanding processes.
3. Perceptual "committees" serve as an important metaphor in this chapter. The idea is that many semi-independent processes are working on the input at the same time. Different processes may come to different conclusions about the presence of an edge or the relationship between two elements in the input. Under most circumstances, we see the single conclusion that the committees settle on. Bayesian models are one way to formalize this process of finding the most likely explanation for input. Deep neural networks may be a way to build members/parts of the committee.
4. Multiple processes seek to carve the input into regions and to define the edges of those regions, and many rules are involved in this parsing of the image. For example, image elements are likely to group together if they are similar in color or shape, if they are near each other, or if they are connected. Many of these grouping principles were first articulated by members of the Gestalt school.
5. Other, related processes seek to determine whether a region is part of a foreground figure (like this black *O*) or part of the background (like the white area around the *O*). These rules of grouping and figure-ground assignment are driven by an implicit understanding of the physics of the world. Thus, events that are very unlikely to happen by chance (e.g., two contours parallel to each other) are taken to have meaning. (Those parallel contours are likely to be part of the same figure.)
6. The processes that divide visual input into objects and background have to deal with many complexities. Among these are the fact that parts of objects may be hidden behind other objects (occlusion) and the fact that objects

themselves have structure. Is your nose an object or a part of a larger whole? What about glasses or hair or a wig?

7. In addition to perceiving the shapes of objects and their parts, we are also adept at categorizing the material that an object seems to be made of—glass, stone, cloth, and so on. We use material perception to estimate physical properties. What would the object feel like? Can it be grasped like a bottle, or would it slip through our fingers like sand?
8. It is common to talk about the role of "templates" in object recognition. The idea is that an object in the world is recognized when its image fits a particular representation in the brain in the way that a key fits a lock. It has always been hard to see how naive template models could work, because of the astronomical number of templates required: we might need one "lock" for every object in every orientation in every position in the visual field.
9. Deep neural networks are modern efforts to create computer algorithms that can categorize objects very well. Unlike a literal, lock-and-key template, a deep neural network tries to match an image with a complex pattern of activity in a network that arises when the network encounters an object in a specific category. This allows the network to categorize an infinite set of images as "cat," "coffee cup," and so on.
10. Faces are a special case of object processing. Viewpoint is very important. Upright faces are much easier to recognize than inverted faces. Moreover, some regions of the brain seem to be specifically interested in faces. Different regions may be important for different aspects of face processing ("Who is it?" versus "How is he feeling?").

Chapter 5

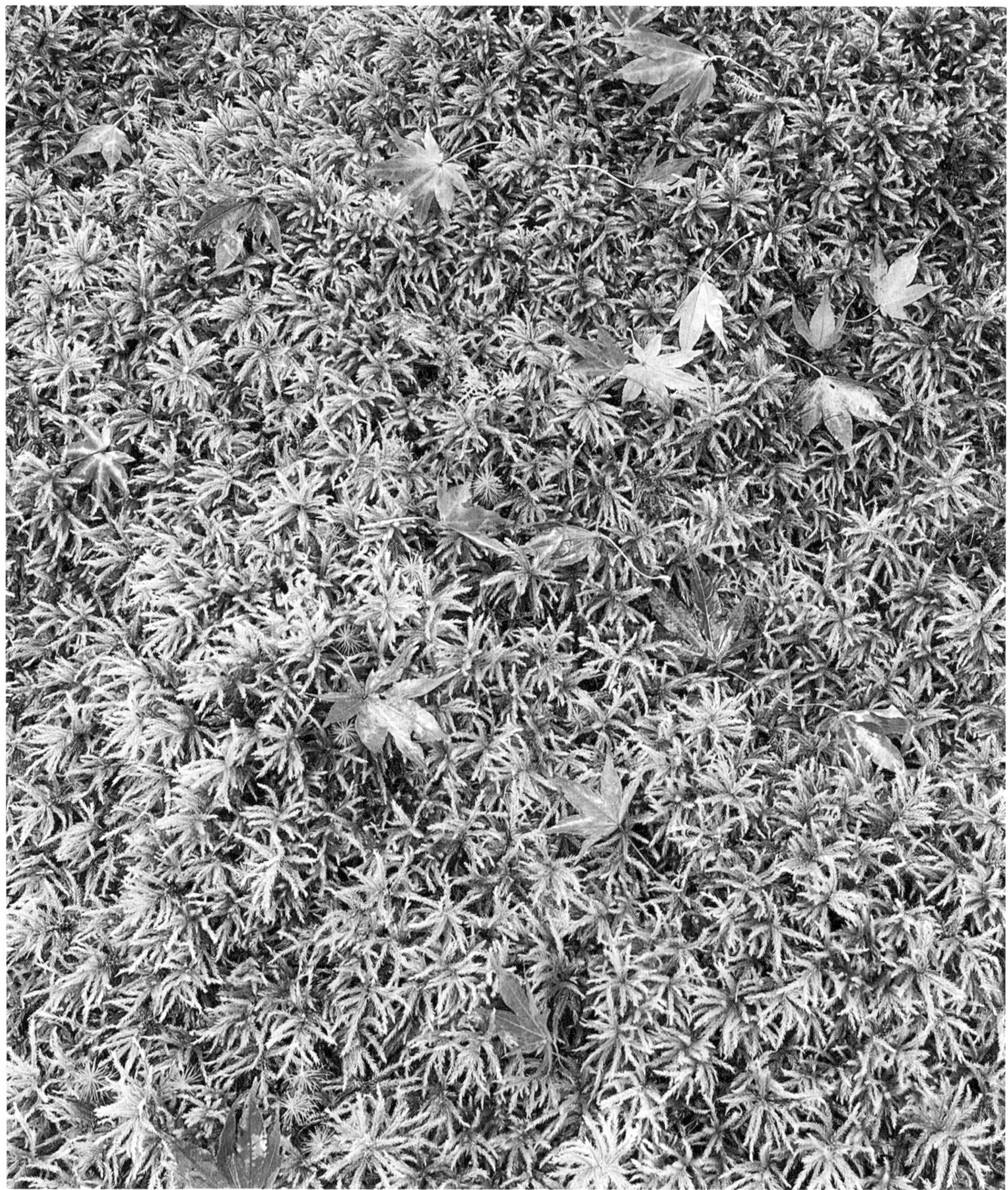

Philip Wolfe, *Fall Leaves*, 2022

The Perception of Color

Questions to Contemplate

Think about the following questions as you read this chapter.
By the chapter's end, you should be able to answer and discuss them.

- What is color for?
- Does everyone see the same colors?
- Suppose you have an orange on your plate for lunch. It looks orange. If you send a photo of that orange, the photo will look orange too. The physical bases of those two orange experiences are very different. How does that work?
- Suppose that the orange looks a bit green. Will it taste different?

Imagine that you could turn off your color vision the way you can when editing a cell phone photo (**FIGURE 5.1**). Your perceptual world would be diminished, but vision works quite well without color. Television thrived in black and white, for example. You would be much more impaired if you somehow lost orientation perception or motion perception (see Chapter 8). That said, an ability to use color has evolved multiple times in multiple ways in the animal kingdom, and it seems very central to your perceptual life. You have probably been asked about your favorite color. When was the last time anyone asked you to name your favorite orientation? The goal of this chapter is to explain how we see color and to speculate about why.

5.1 Basic Principles of Color Perception

Although color itself is not a physical property of things in the world, it is related to a physical property. As discussed in Chapter 2, humans see a narrow range of the electromagnetic spectrum between the wavelengths of about 400 and 700

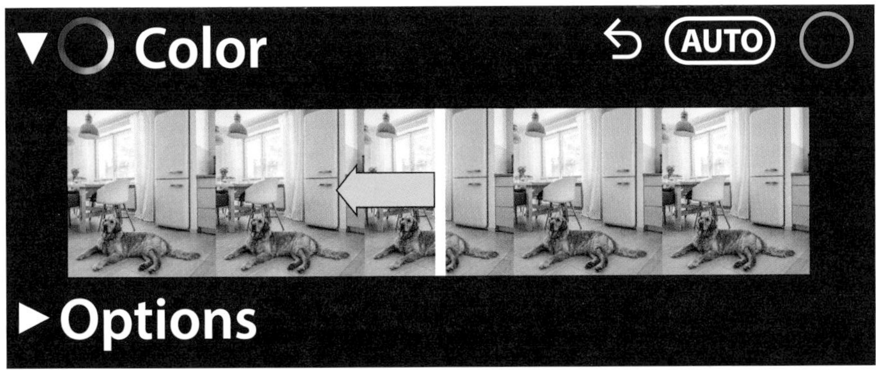

FIGURE 5.1 Photo editing software lets you turn off color as can be seen in the leftmost panel.

nanometers (nm). Recall that 1 nm is 10^{-9} or 0.000000001 meters. The apparent color of a piece of the visible world is correlated with the wavelengths of the light rays reaching the eye from that piece of the world.

Most of the light that we see is reflected light. Typical light sources, like the sun or a light bulb, emit a broad spectrum of wavelengths that hit surfaces in the world around us. Some wavelengths are absorbed by the surfaces they hit. The more light a surface absorbs, the darker it appears. Other wavelengths are reflected, and some of that reflected light reaches the eyes. The color of a surface depends on the mix of wavelengths that reach the eye from the surface (and, as we will see later, from the other surfaces and lights that are present in the scene). In the case of red roses, for instance, more of the longer-wavelength light (>600 nm) is reflected into the eyes of the observer. Even though (almost) all humans would declare this collection of wavelengths to appear red, it would be a big mistake to think of specific wavelengths of light as being specific colors. As Steven Shevell (2003) puts it, "There is no red in a 700 nm light, just as there is no pain in the hooves of a kicking horse." Like pain, color is the result of the interaction of a physical stimulus with a particular nervous system.

Three Steps to Color Perception

Several problems must be solved to go from physical wavelengths to the perception of color. We will organize our discussion around three steps (Stockman and Brainard, 2010):

1. *Detection.* Wavelengths must be detected. For this, we need photoreceptors to convert light into signals in the nervous system.
2. *Discrimination.* We must be able to tell the difference between different mixtures of wavelengths. To do this, we need neurons that compare inputs from different kinds of photoreceptors.
3. *Appearance.* We want to assign perceived colors to lights and surfaces in the world. Moreover, we want those perceived colors to go with the object (that rose looks red) and not to change dramatically as the viewing conditions change (that rose should remain red in sun and shadow, for example). For this, we need some very clever processing that we do not fully understand yet.

S-cone A cone that is preferentially sensitive to short wavelengths, colloquially (but not entirely accurately) known as a "blue cone."

M-cone A cone that is preferentially sensitive to middle wavelengths, colloquially (but not entirely accurately) known as a "green cone."

L-cone A cone that is preferentially sensitive to long wavelengths, colloquially (but not entirely accurately) known as a "red cone."

spectral sensitivity The sensitivity of a cell or a device to different wavelengths on the electromagnetic spectrum.

photopic Referring to light intensities that are bright enough to stimulate the cone receptors and bright enough to "saturate" the rod receptors, that is, drive them to their maximum responses.

scotopic Referring to light intensities that are bright enough to stimulate the rod receptors but too dim to stimulate the cone receptors.

5.2 Step 1: Color Detection

Detection was largely covered in Chapter 2. To briefly review, we have three types of cone photoreceptors. These cones differ in the photopigment they carry, and as a result, they differ in their sensitivity to light of different wavelengths. FIGURE 5.2 shows those sensitivities as a function of wavelength. Each cone type is named for the location of the peak of its sensitivity on the spectrum: The cones that have a peak at about 420 nm are known as short-wavelength cones, or **S-cones**. The medium-wavelength cones, or **M-cones**, peak at about 535 nm. Long-wavelength cones, or **L-cones**, peak at about 565 nm. As you can see from Figure 5.2, there is a lot of overlap between the sensitivities of different cones. That is, even though the L-cone is maximally sensitive at about 565 nm, the M-cone can detect that wavelength as well. Their **spectral sensitivities** overlap. As mentioned in Chapter 2, S-cones are relatively rare, and they are less sensitive than M- and L-cones. The combination of sensitivities of the three types

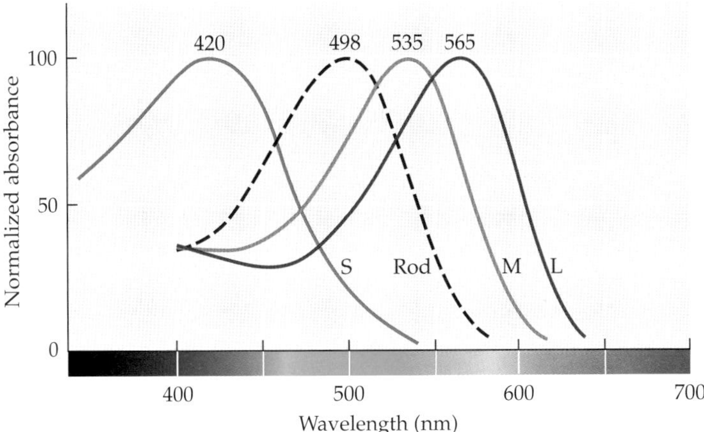

FIGURE 5.2 **Photoreceptor types** The retina contains four types of photoreceptors. These differ in their sensitivity to the wavelengths of light. Three cone types are maximally sensitive at short (S), medium (M), and long (L) wavelengths. The single type of rod photoreceptor (dashed line) has its peak sensitivity between those of the S- and M-cones.

of cones gives us our overall ability to detect wavelengths from about 400 nm to about 700 nm (see Figure 5.2). Remember also that cones work at **photopic** light levels (bright light, like daylight). We have one type of rod photoreceptor; it works in **scotopic** (dimmer) light and has a somewhat different sensitivity profile, peaking at about 500 nm.

5.3 Step 2: Color Discrimination

We can detect wavelengths between 400 and 700 nm, but how do we distinguish between lights whose energy is narrowly concentrated around 450, 550, and 625 nm, for example? With a little oversimplification, we will talk about these lights as if they contained just one wavelength. To see how discrimination differs from detection, let's examine the response of a single photoreceptor to a single wavelength of light. FIGURE 5.3 shows how one kind of human photoreceptor responds to light of a specific wavelength while the intensity of the light is held constant. Because of the properties of the photopigment in the photoreceptor cell, 400 nm light produces only a small response in each cell of this type, 500 nm light produces a greater response, and 550 nm light produces even more. However, 600 nm light produces less than the maximal response, and 650 nm light produces a minimal response. Light of 625 nm produces a response of moderate strength.

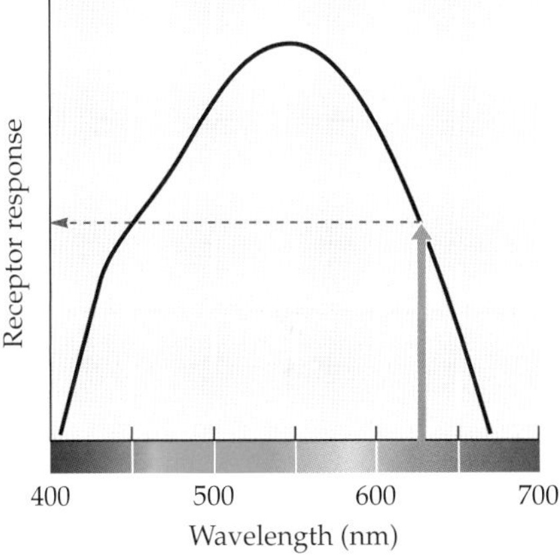

FIGURE 5.3 **Responding to one wavelength** A single photoreceptor shows different responses to lights of different wavelengths but the same intensity. A 625 nm light of this intensity, indicated by the arrow, produces a response midway between the maximum and minimum responses.

The Principle of Univariance

So far, so good. We know that different wavelengths of light give rise to different experiences of color, and the varying responses of this photoreceptor to different wavelengths could provide a basis for color vision. But there is a problem, as illustrated in FIGURE 5.4. Suppose we change the wavelength from 625 nm to 450 nm. Figure 5.4 shows that an equal amount of 450 nm light will produce the same response from this photoreceptor that 625 nm light does. If we were looking at the output of the photoreceptor, we would have no way of distinguishing between the two lights. But when we look with a normal human color vision system, the 625 nm light looks orange and the 450 nm light looks bluish.

Actually, the problem is much worse. Remember that Figures 5.3 and 5.4 represent the photoreceptor's response rate when all wavelengths are presented at the same intensity. Under these conditions, as the graphs indicate, light at either

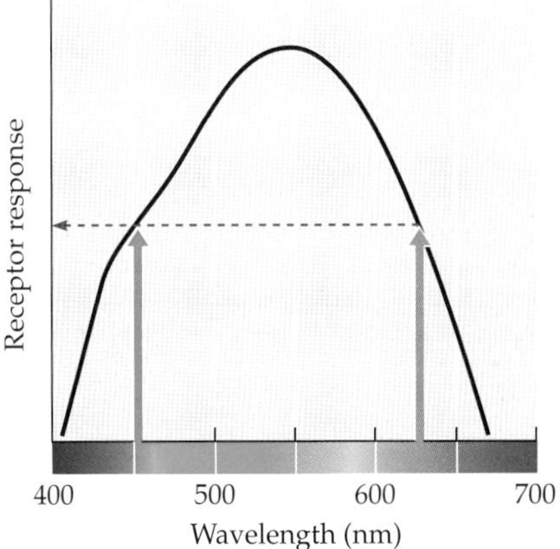

FIGURE 5.4 **Univariance** Lights of 450 and 625 nm both elicit the same response from the photoreceptor whose responses are shown here and in Figure 5.3. This situation illustrates the principle of univariance.

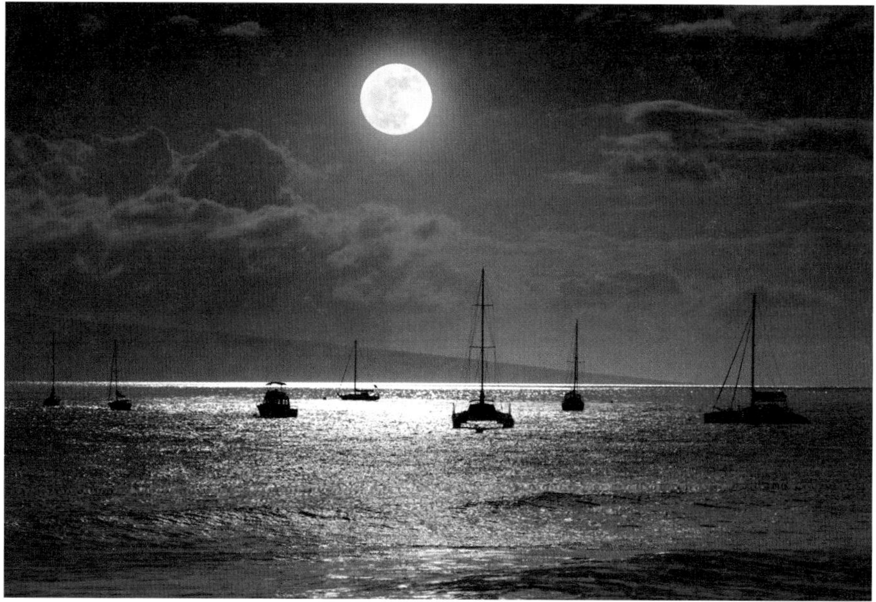

FIGURE 5.5 Rod vision The moonlit world appears drained of color because we have only one type of rod photoreceptor transducing light under these scotopic conditions. With just one type of photoreceptor, we cannot make discriminations based on wavelength, so we cannot see color.

450 or 625 nm produces a response lower than the peak response obtained at about 535 nm. If we had a 535 nm light, we could reduce its intensity until it produced exactly the same level of response from our photoreceptor as the 450 or 625 nm light did at the higher intensity. Indeed, we could take a "white light" or any mix of wavelengths and, by properly adjusting the intensity, get exactly the same response out of the photoreceptor.

Thus, when it comes to seeing color, the output of a single photoreceptor is completely ambiguous. An infinite set of different combinations of wavelength and intensity can elicit exactly the same response, so the output of a single photoreceptor cannot by itself tell us anything about the wavelengths stimulating it. This constraint is known as the **principle of univariance** (Rushton, 1972).

Obviously, the human visual system has solved the problem, but not under all circumstances. Univariance explains the lack of color in dimly lit scenes. Remember that there is only one type of rod photoreceptor. All rods contain the same type of photopigment molecule: rhodopsin. Thus, they all have the same sensitivity to wavelength. As a consequence, although it is possible to tell light from dark under scotopic conditions, the problem of univariance makes it impossible to discriminate colors. Our nighttime color-blindness is one hint that color is psychophysical and not physical. The world seen under a bright moon (FIGURE 5.5) has not been physically drained of color. The same mix of wavelengths that produces color perception during the day remains present on that moonlit night, but we fail to see colors under dim light sources like moonlight, because dim light stimulates only the rods, and the output of that single variety of photoreceptor does not permit color vision.

The Trichromatic Solution

principle of univariance The fact that an infinite set of different wavelength-intensity combinations can elicit exactly the same response from a single type of photoreceptor. One photoreceptor type cannot make color discriminations based on wavelength.

We can detect differences between wavelengths or mixtures of wavelengths precisely because we have more than one kind of cone photoreceptor. FIGURE 5.6 shows how our three cone types give us the foundation on which to build a color vision system to tell the difference between lights of different wavelengths. Look at the three cones' responses to the two wavelengths—450 and 625 nm—that produced the same response from the single cone in Figure 5.4. The two wavelengths

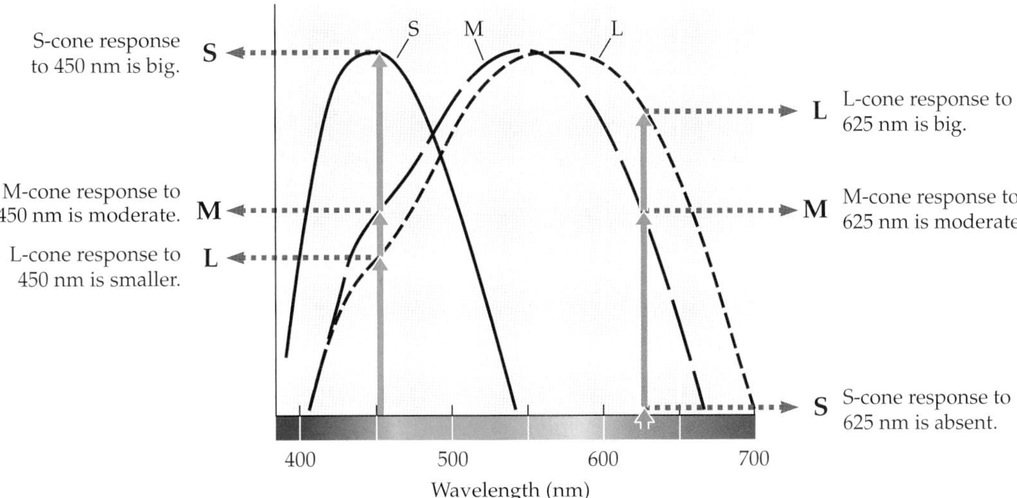

FIGURE 5.6 Solving univariance The two wavelengths that produce the same response from one type of cone (M) produce different patterns of responses across the three types of cones (S, M, and L).

of light still produce the same response from that type of cone, now revealed to be the M-cone. However, these two wavelengths produce different outputs from the L-cones and S-cones. This combined signal, a triplet of numbers for each "pixel" in the visual field, can be used as the basis for color vision. (We can see from about 400 to 700 nm, but the very long and very short wavelengths each stimulate only one type of cone.)

In our discussion of the univariance problem, we noted that we can make any wavelength produce the same response as any other from a single cone type by adjusting the intensity of the light. That is not a problem in the three-cone world of human color vision. A specific light produces a specific set of three responses from the three cone types. Suppose that the light produces twice as much M response as S response and twice as much S response as L response. If we increase the intensity of the light, the response sizes will change but the relationships will not. There will still be twice as much M response as S response and twice as much S response as L response, and those relationships will define our response to the light and, eventually, the color that we see. (Think what might happen if the lights were really bright.) The ability to discriminate one light from another is based not just on measuring three numbers from a patch of light, but also on the ability of our visual system to respond to the relationships among those three numbers. This is the heart of **trichromacy**, or more elaborately, the **trichromatic theory of color vision**.

Metamers

The examples presented thus far involve the responses of the visual system to single wavelengths. However, you may have noticed that we have been referring to "wavelengths or mixtures of wavelengths." That's because we are not typically exposed to single wavelengths. Almost every light and every surface that we see is emitting or reflecting a wide range of wavelengths. A laser pointer would emit a very narrow range of wavelengths, but a more normal situation is shown in **FIGURE 5.7**. It shows the relative amounts of light reflected from groups of Granny Smith apples exposed to different amounts of sunlight during growth. How can we discriminate the "sunburned" from the "unsunburned" apples? When we're studying color vision,

trichromacy or **trichromatic theory of color vision** The theory that the color of any light is defined in our visual system by the relationships of three numbers—the outputs of three receptor types now known to be the three cones. Also called the Young-Helmholtz theory.

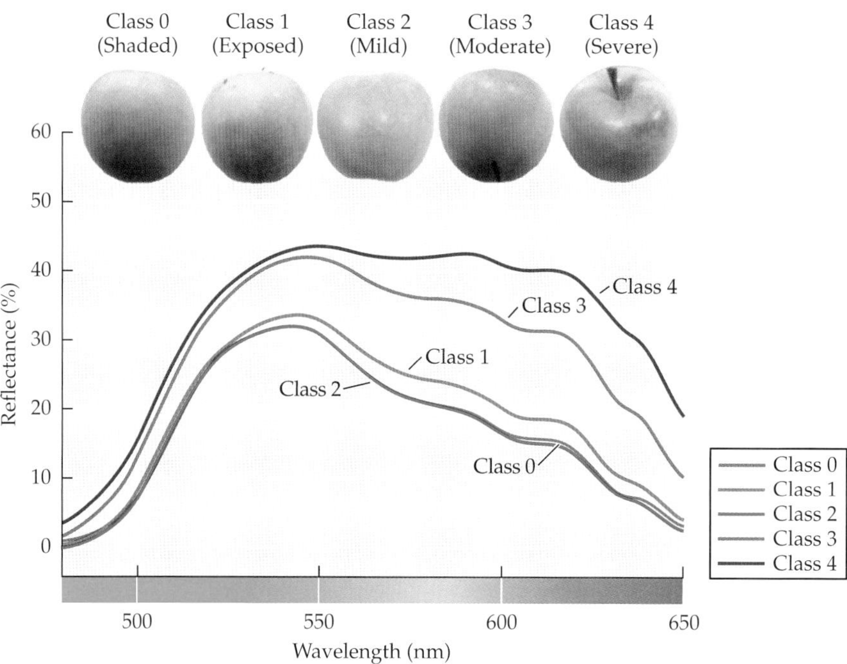

FIGURE 5.7 Real-world reflectance functions Objects in the real world reflect light across the spectrum in different amounts. This graph plots the **reflectances** of sun injury development in Granny Smith apples. You can see how the appearance changes as the amount of reflected long-wavelength light changes.

this real-world concern gets reduced to a different question: How do our cones respond to combinations of wavelengths of light?

To answer this question, consider what happens if we mix just two wavelengths. For the sake of this example, we will oversimplify by ignoring the S-cones and redrawing the M- and L-cones to make the numbers simpler. Imagine that we shine a wavelength that looks red and a wavelength that looks green onto a white piece of paper so that a mixture of both is reflected back to the eyes (FIGURE 5.8A). Suppose that the light that looks green produces 80 units of activity in the M-cones and 40 in the L-cones (remember, we are ignoring the S-cones for now). In addition, suppose that the light that looks red produces 40 units of activity in the M-cones and 80 in the L-cones. If we assume that we can add the cone responses together, then summing the "red" and "green" lights produces a response of 120 units in each cone. The absolute value is not important, because it could change if the intensity of the light changed. What is important is that these two lights, mixed together, produce a mixture that excites the L- and M-cones equally.

The key point is that the rest of the nervous system knows *only* what the cones tell it. If the mixture of lights that, individually, look red and green produces the same cone output as the single wavelength of light that looks yellow (FIGURE 5.8B), then the mixture and the single wavelength *must look identical.* Mixtures of different wavelengths that look identical are called **metamers**. The single wavelength that produces equal M- and L-cone activity will look yellow, and the correct mixture of longer- and shorter-wavelength lights will also look yellow. Two quick warnings:

reflectance The percentage of light hitting a surface that is reflected and not absorbed into the surface. Typically, reflectance is given as a function of wavelength.

metamers Different mixtures of wavelengths that look identical, or more generally, any pair of stimuli that are perceived as identical despite physical differences.

1. Mixing wavelengths does not change the physical wavelengths. If we mix 500 and 600 nm lights, the physical stimulus contains wavelengths of 500 and 600 nm. It does not contain the average (550 nm). It does not contain the sum (1100 nm)

(which we would not be able to see anyway). Color mixture is happening in the visual system. It is not a change in the physics of light.

2. For a mixture of a red and green to look perfectly yellow, we would have to have just the right red and just the right green. Other mixes might look a bit reddish or a bit greenish.

   This example generalizes to *any* mixture of lights. All the light reaching the retina from one isolated patch in the visual field will be converted into three numbers by the three cone types. If those numbers are sufficiently different from the numbers in another isolated patch, you will be able to discriminate those patches. If not, those patches will be metamers: they will look identical, even if the wavelengths are physically different.

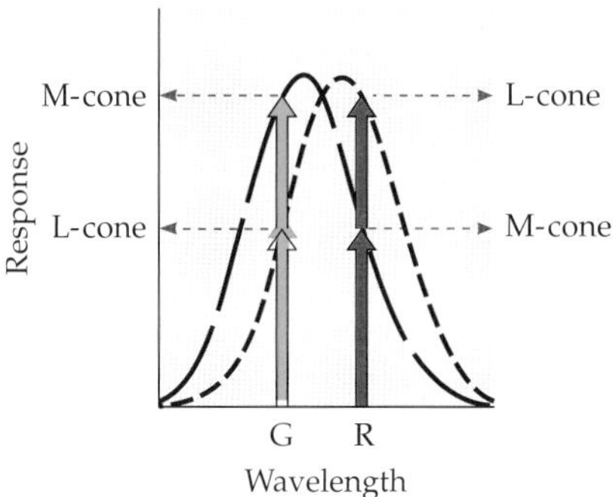

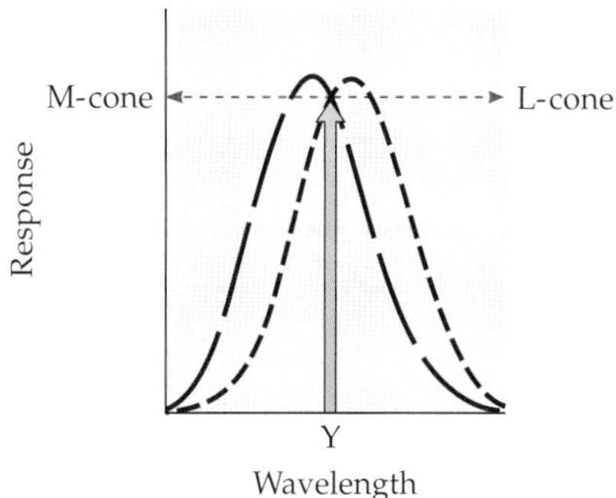

FIGURE 5.8 Metamers In (A), the long-wavelength light that looks red and the shorter-wavelength light that looks green mix together to produce the same response from the cones as does the medium-wavelength light that looks yellow in (B). If two sets of lights produce the same responses, they are metamers and must look identical, so the red plus the green will look yellow.

The History of Trichromatic Theory

From what you've read so far in this book, you would be forgiven for supposing that clever anatomists and physiologists identified the three cone types and built the trichromatic theory of color vision from there. Indeed, there have been beautiful experiments of this sort: For instance, Schnapf, Kraft, and Baylor (1987) managed to record the activity of single photoreceptors. Nathans, Thomas, and Hogness (1986) found the genes that code for the different photopigments. Austin Roorda & David Williams (1999) even developed a method for photographing and identifying different cone types in the living human eye (see Figure 2.18).

Such research has cemented our understanding of the physical basis of trichromacy, but the basic theory was established by psychophysical experimentation. The theorizing started with Isaac Newton's great discovery that a prism would break up sunlight into the spectrum of hues, and a second prism would put the spectrum back together into light that looked white. In 1666, Newton understood that the prism was separating light into different components but that "the rays to speak properly are not coloured" (from *Opticks*, published originally in 1704). Newton knew that perceived color is a mental event.

The three-dimensional nature of the experience of color was worked out in the nineteenth century by Thomas Young (1773–1829) and subsequently by Hermann von Helmholtz (1821–1894). In their honor, trichromatic theory is often called the Young-Helmholtz theory. James Clerk Maxwell (1831–1879) developed a color-matching technique that was central to Helmholtz's work on this topic. (Somehow Maxwell missed having his name attached, or we would have the Young-Maxwell-Helmholtz theory.) Maxwell's technique is illustrated in **FIGURE 5.9**. The observer in a modern version of Maxwell's experiments would try

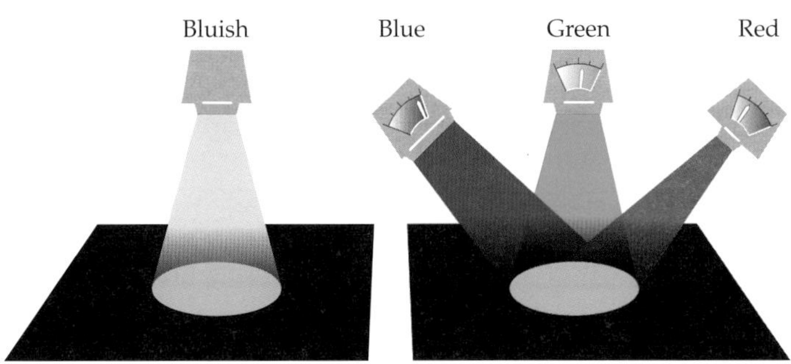

FIGURE 5.9 Maxwell's color-matching experiment A color is presented on the left. On the right, the observer adjusts a mixture of the three lights to match the color on the left.

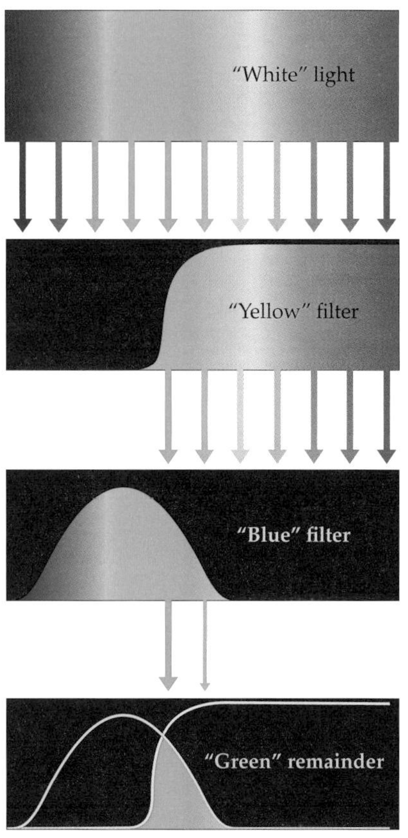
1. Take "white" light that contains a broad mixture of wavelengths.
"White" light
2. Pass it through a filter that absorbs shorter wavelengths. The result will look yellowish.
"Yellow" filter
3. Pass that through a bluish filter that absorbs all but a middle range of wavelengths.
"Blue" filter
4. The wavelengths that make it through both filters will be a mix that looks greenish.
"Green" remainder

FIGURE 5.10 Subtractive color mixture In this example, "white"—broadband—light is passed through two filters. The first one absorbs ("subtracts") shorter wavelengths, transmitting a mix of wavelengths that looks yellow. The second absorbs longer wavelengths and the shortest wavelengths, transmitting a mix that looks blue. The wavelengths that can pass through both filters without being subtracted are a middle range of wavelengths that appear green.

to use different amounts of "primary" colored lights (e.g., the lights looking red, green, and blue on the right side of the figure) to exactly match another reference color (e.g., the light looking cyan, or bluish, on the left side).

The central observation from these experiments was that only three mixing lights are needed to match any reference light. Two primaries are not enough, and four are more than are needed. Long before physiology could prove it, these results led Young and Helmholtz to deduce that three different color mechanisms must limit the human experience of color.

A Brief Digression into Lights, Filters, and Finger Paints

The ubiquity of video screens in the twenty-first century may make color mixing and metamers reasonably intuitive. If you've never done so, find a magnifying glass and take a very close look at a yellow patch on your computer screen. You'll find that the patch is composed of thousands of intermixed red and green dots, though with new monitors, it is getting harder and harder to see the tiny pixels. The "red + green = yellow" formula is an example of **additive color mixture** because we are taking one wavelength or set of wavelengths and *adding* it to another.

For most of us, color mixture begins in kindergarten or earlier, with paints. In that world, red plus green doesn't make yellow; that mixture typically looks brown. A finger paint, or any other pigment, looks a particular color because it absorbs some wavelengths, subtracting them from the broadband ("white") light falling on a surface covered with the pigment. When a toddler smears together red and green, almost all wavelengths are absorbed by one pigment or the other, so we perceive the **subtractive color mixture** as a dark color like brown.

Actually, the physics of finger paint mixtures are rather complicated, with some particles of different pigments sitting next to each other and effectively adding their different reflected lights to the result that you see. Other particles occlude each other, and others are engaged in still other complex interactions. Colored filters, like those you might put over stage lights, are a cleaner example of subtractive color mixture. FIGURE 5.10 shows how a subtractive mixture of yellow and blue filters would subtract wavelengths, leaving only wavelengths in a middle range, which typically appear green. An additive mixture of lights that look blue and yellow will look white (if you have exactly the right blue and yellow) (FIGURE 5.11) because that combination produces a mix of wavelengths that stimulate the three cone types roughly equally.

additive color mixture A mixture of lights. If light A and light B are both reflected from a surface to the eye, in the perception of color the effects of those two lights add together.

subtractive color mixture A mixture of pigments. If pigments A and B mix, some of the light shining on the surface will be subtracted by A and some by B. Only the remainder will contribute to the perception of color.

From Retina to Brain: Repackaging the Information

The cones in the retina are the neural substrate for detection of lights. What is the neural basis for discriminating between lights with different wavelength composition? To tell the difference between different lights, the nervous system will look at differences in the activities of the three cone types. This work begins in the retina. We could send separate L, M, and S signals to the brain, but that approach would be less useful than one might think. For example, the L- and M-cones have very similar sensitivities (see Figure 5.2), so most of the time they are in close agreement: L says, "Lots of light coming from location X." "Yes, lots of light coming from location X," M agrees.

Computing differences between cone responses turns out to be a much more useful way to transmit information to the brain. The nervous system computes two differences, the difference between long and medium (L – M) and the difference between short, on one side, and the combination of long and medium on the other ((L + M) – S). Why these two? Comparisons across species suggest that the comparison between S-cones and an LM-cone happened first, perhaps 500 million years ago (Mollon, 1989). Then, about 40 million years ago, the LM-cone split into very similar L- and M-cones (Nathans et al., 1986), and the difference between those cone types turned out to be useful. We don't know exactly why the L-M comparison became important in color vision, but there are theories. For example, blushing and turning pale are useful signals to observe, and our specific photopigments may have evolved to help us see those signals by making it possible to discriminate different amounts of blood in skin (Changizi, Zhang, and Shimojo, 2006). That is not the only possibility. The L – M difference may also be very useful if you want to tell the difference between fruit and leaves, different shades of green in the foliage, or the ripeness of a berry (B. C. Regan et al., 2001). In either case, being sensitive to subtle differences in the relative amounts of medium and long wavelengths would be important.

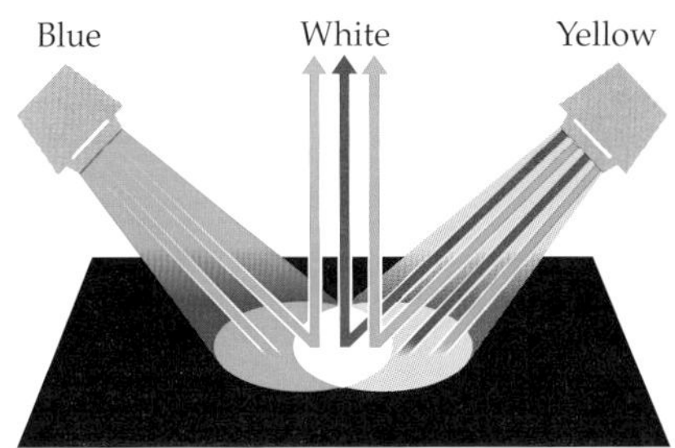

FIGURE 5.11 Additive color mixture If we shine a light that looks blue and a light that looks yellow on the same patch of paper, the wavelengths will add, producing an additive color mixture. Remember that the light that looks yellow is equivalent to a mix of a long wavelength and a medium wavelength, so blue plus yellow results in a mix of short, medium, and long wavelengths. The mixture looks white (or gray, if it is not the brightest patch in view).

In addition to L – M, we could create L – S and M – S signals. However, because L and M are so similar, a single comparison between S and (L + M) can capture almost the same information that would be found in (L – S) and (M – S) signals. Finally, combining L and M signals is a pretty good measure of the intensity of the light. (It happens that S-cones make a rather small contribution to our perception of brightness.) Thus, on theoretical grounds, it might be wise to convert the three cone signals into three new signals: L – M, (L + M) – S, and L + M (Buchsbaum and Gottschalk, 1983; Zaidi, 1997)—and the visual system does something reasonably close to this.

Cone-Opponent Cells in the Retina and Lateral Geniculate Nucleus

The earliest work on the combination of cone signals was done with fish (Svaetichin and Macnichol, 1959). By the 1960s, Russell de Valois and others had begun to show that these sorts of signals exist in the **lateral geniculate nucleus (LGN)** of macaque monkeys (de Valois, Abramov, and Jacobs, 1966). As described in Chapter 3, many ganglion cells in the retina and the LGN of the thalamus are maximally stimulated by spots of light. These cells have receptive fields with a characteristic center-surround organization. For example, some cells are excited when a light turns on in the central part of their receptive fields and inhibited when a light turns on in the surround (see Figure 2.20).

A similar antagonistic relationship characterizes color. Some of these retinal and LGN ganglion cells can be excited by an L-cone onset in their center and inhibited by surround-dominated by M-cone inputs. These L – M cells are one type of **cone-opponent cell**, so named because different sources of chromatic information are pitted against each other. There are also M – L, (M + L) – S, and S – (M + L) cells—just the sorts of cells we would like to have to support

lateral geniculate nucleus (LGN) A structure in the thalamus, part of the midbrain, that receives input from the retinal ganglion cells and has input and output connections to the visual cortex.

cone-opponent cell A cell type—found in the retina, lateral geniculate nucleus, and visual cortex—that, in effect, subtracts one type of cone input from another.

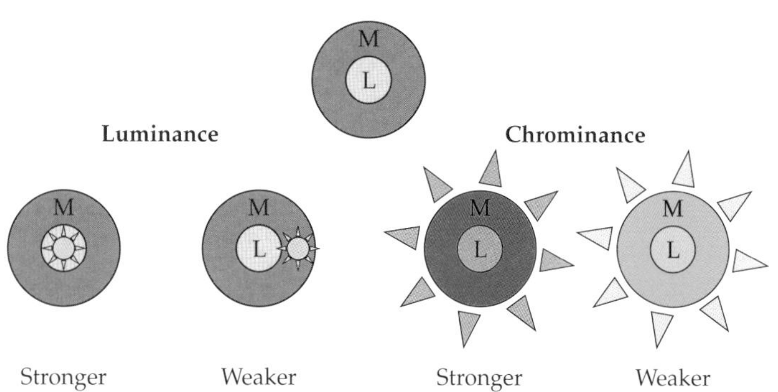

FIGURE 5.12 **Receptive fields for color and space** This cell (perhaps in the retina or the lateral geniculate nucleus) has an excitatory center dominated by L-cone input and an inhibitory surround dominated by M-cone input. Its output can be modulated by the spatial position of a small spot of light and/or the wavelength composition of a big spot.

the repackaging of cone signals, as described in the previous section. The cells that were excited by light onset could be thought of as L + M cells. Thus, we have the three signals that we wanted on theoretical grounds. The actual physiology is quite complicated. As mentioned in Chapters 2 and 3, for example, the S-cone signals go through the **koniocellular** layers in the LGN, while the M- and L-cone opponent signals are mostly found in the **parvocellular** layers (Xiao, 2014).

koniocellular Referring to cells in the koniocellular layer of the lateral geniculate nucleus of the thalamus. *Konio*, from the Greek for "dust," refers to the appearance of the cells.

parvocellular Referring to cells in the parvocellular layers of the lateral geniculate nucleus of the thalamus. *Parvo*, from the Greek for "small," refers to the size of the cells.

FIGURE 5.12 shows an interesting complication of this arrangement. Suppose we have a cell in the retina or LGN that has a receptive field with a center-surround organization. Let's have the center dominated by L-cone input. Indeed, if the receptive field is in the fovea, that center could receive input from just one L-cone. This inhibitory surround is dominated by M-cone input. If you shine a small spot of light on the center of the receptive field, you will get more response from the cell than if you shine the same spot on the surround. Thus, the cell could tell you something about where a spot of light was located. At the same time, if you shine a big patch of light, dominated by longer wavelengths, you will get more of a response than if the big patch is dominated by medium or shorter wavelengths. Thus, the cell could tell you something about the color of the light. What is it telling you? Like a single, univariant cone (see Figure 5.3), this cell, by itself, is ambiguous. It will take more comparisons, later in the visual system, to sort out color and spatial luminance information (and there are illusions that arise when the two types of information get confused (Brainard, 2019).

One interesting way to illustrate the complicated relationship between cones and color is to stimulate one single cone at a time. You may recall from Figure 2.12 that Roorda and Williams (1999) figured out how to use some very sophisticated optics to allow them to see and classify individual cones in the retina of a human observer. More recently, Roorda and his colleagues (Sabesan et al., 2016) managed to focus tiny spots of light onto individual cones and ask those observers what they saw (FIGURE 5.13). Amazingly, the researcher could test the same cone in sessions many days apart. The results are summarized by the little white circles on top of cones in Figure 5.13. (Note: The red, green, and blue colors are just to label L-, M-, and S-cones. Cones themselves are not colored.) The more complete the ring, the more often a little spot of light was labeled "white." Many of the responses are "white"; others are usually some version of red and green. The experiment is showing us that, as illustrated in Figure 5.12, single cones and single center-surround cells can contribute to many different sensations.

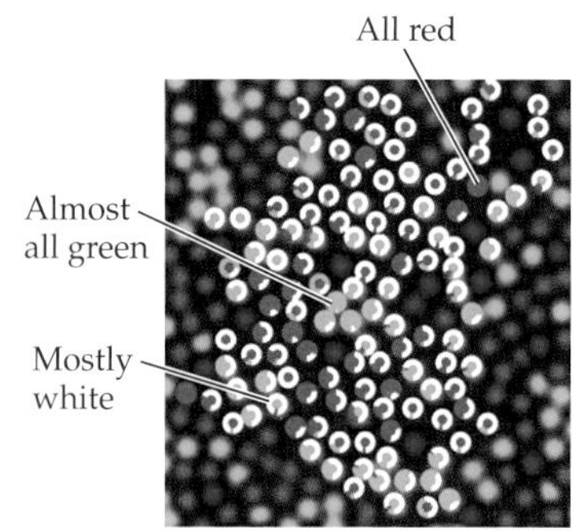

FIGURE 5.13 **The retinal mosaic** A piece of the retina with the L-, M-, and S-cones colored red, green, and blue. On top of many cones are white rings of varying degrees of completion. Each shows the responses of that cone to tiny spots of light. A full white ring, for example, means the observer always said the spot looked white.

5.4 Step 3: Color Appearance

So far, we have described a color vision system with three cone types whose outputs are used to produce cone-opponent difference signals: (L – M) and ((L + M) – S). How do we go from those basics to the world of perceived color? The short answer is that, while we know a great deal about color appearance, there are a surprising number of fundamental mysteries. This can be illustrated by The Dress. In 2015, a fairly ordinary picture of a dress swept the internet. The picture that caused all the fuss is shown in FIGURE 5.14. Some people asserted that the stripes appeared to be black and blue. Others insisted they were white and gold. If you saw someone wearing this dress out on the street, you would likely agree with almost everyone that the dress looks black and blue. Why don't people agree on what color the dress appears in the picture? This is not a problem of detection or discrimination of wavelength information. It is a color appearance problem.

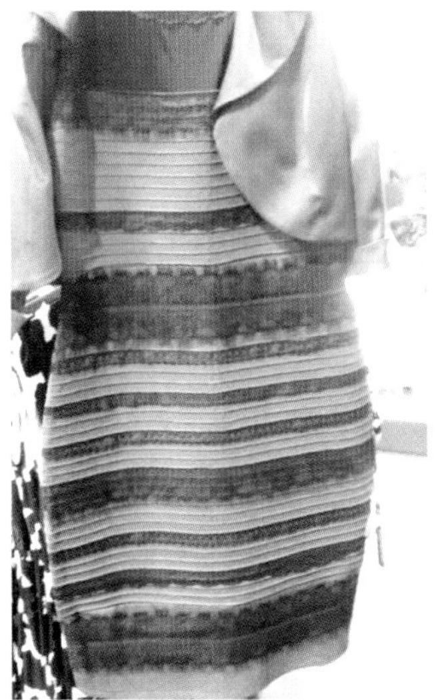

FIGURE 5.14 The Dress Is it blue and black or white and gold (or something else), and why?

Three Numbers, Three Dimensions, Many Colors

To begin, if we are going to talk about color appearance, it is useful to have a system for talking about all the colors we can see. Because we have exactly three different types of cone photoreceptors and the neural hardware for comparing their outputs, the light reaching any part of the retina will be translated into three responses, one for each local population of cones. After that translation, the rest of the nervous system cannot glean anything more about the physical wavelengths of the light. If the light rays reflecting off two surfaces in the same surroundings produce the same set of cone responses, the two surfaces must and will appear to be exactly the same color. They will be metamers, even if their physical characteristics are quite different. Thus, it is possible to produce a bloodred color on a page without mimicking the physical properties of blood.

Working with just three numbers might not sound very promising, but it has been estimated that, with this system, we can discriminate the surfaces of more than 2 million different colors (Pointer and Attridge, 1998; Linhares, Pinto, and Nascimento, 2008). A lot of these colors are lightness variations of what we would colloquially consider the same color: bloodred in dim light, bloodred in brighter light, and so on. But even if we ignore lightness, we can still distinguish about 26,000 colors (Foster, 2011). Unless you're in paint sales, you don't know this many distinctive color *names*, but you could tell two different colors apart even if they were both named "pea green" or "sky blue."

We need some way to talk about all those colors in an orderly way. We can describe each of the colors in the spectrum with a single number—for example, the light's wavelength. Going beyond the spectrum, we have a three-dimensional **color space** analogous to a three-dimensional physical space. It doesn't make much sense to talk about height, length, and width in color space, but the space that contains the set of all perceptible colors has three dimensions based on the three numbers that come from the outputs of the three cone types.

color space The three-dimensional space, established because color perception is based on the outputs of three cone types, that describes the set of all colors.

Sensation & Perception in Everyday Life

Picking Colors

Representing the three-dimensional color space becomes a practical problem when you are using your computer. Many applications let you pick the colors of fonts, objects, and so on, and the app developers needed to devise an interface that would make that practical. One solution has been simply to present a fixed set of options (e.g., the crayon-box color-picking tool in many applications). However, if the developers want to provide access to all the possible colors, then they can present one or more color pickers that represent a three-dimensional color space. For example, look at **FIGURE 5.15**. It shows two different ways of using three "sliders" to define colors (here, borrowed from PowerPoint). In Figure 5.15A are three sliders for red, green, and blue. These RGB sliders are useful because computer monitors have red, green, and blue elements in each pixel, and using RGB values is a good way to specify the signal to send to each of those elements. Thus, the green shown in Figure 5.15A is what you get from 62 units (out of 255) delivered by the red elements, 180 from the green, and 60 from the blue. These RGB sliders define a three-dimensional space that can be represented by the cube shown in Figure 5.15C. Notice that white is in the upper corner closest to you on the cube. Black is hidden in the back corner, farthest from you.

In Figure 5.15B, we see the same shade of green defined by a different set of three numbers. This time, the variables are hue (H), saturation (S), and brightness (B). Part of the resulting HSB color space is shown in Figure 5.15D. These variables are very different concepts from red, green, and blue, but notice that again the system is three-dimensional. Look at the circular, top surface of the HSB space. Hue is the chromatic aspect of a light. It changes as you move around the circumference of the circle. Each point on the spectrum defines a different hue. As you can see from the HSB sliders, the whole family of colors with a hue of 120 (out of 360 degrees around the circle) will look like some version of green. The saturation dimension corresponds to the amount of hue present in a light. In the HSB space (Figure 5.15D), it is shown as the distance from the center of the circle. At the center, where saturation is 0, the resulting color would appear somewhere on the achromatic axis from black to white. Here, 67 (out of 100) describes a fairly saturated green. Finally, brightness describes that black-to-white achromatic axis. The black bottom of the HSB cone has a brightness of 0 (out of 100). The space tapers to a point because when brightness

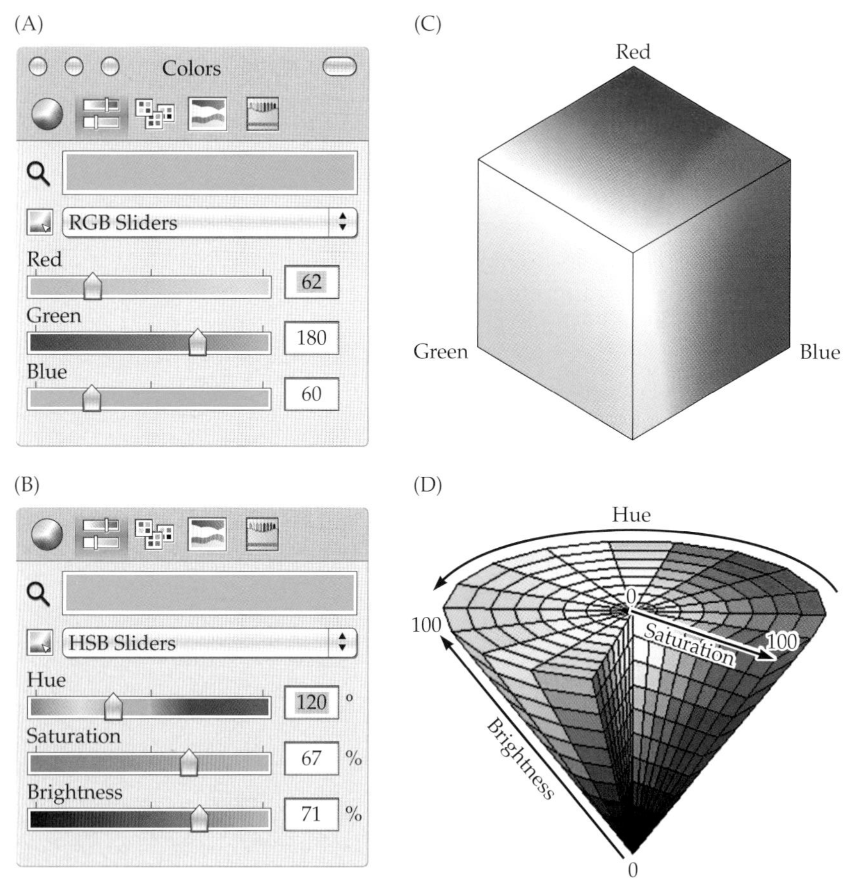

FIGURE 5.15 Computer color pickers may offer several ways to specify a color in a three-dimensional color space These "sliders" from Microsoft PowerPoint are based on an RGB (red, green, blue) set of primaries in (A) and (C) and on HSB (hue, saturation, brightness) in (B) and (D). See the text for details.

Sensation & Perception in Everyday Life *(continued)*

is 0, hue and saturation no longer have meaning. The full three-dimensional space, in this case, includes a cone, rising from a black point to a multicolored surface at a brightness of 100 and then climbing to a white peak (not shown). Brightness is the perceptual consequence of the physical intensity of a light. For instance, the physically intense light of the sun looks brighter than the less intense moon.

Thus, when you use your color picker to find just the right color, you are illustrating the fundamental nature of trichromacy. There is one interesting exception. Along with RGB and HSB color pickers, many applications will also give you CMYK. This is a four-dimensional system, with sliders for cyan (C), magenta (M), yellow (Y), and black (K because B might be thought to stand for blue). You might notice that these are the colors of the ink cartridges in your color printer. Color printing is a subtractive process, and CMYK is designed for printing. The black slider is a convenience because using black ink is a better way to get to the black point in your color space than mixing cyan, magenta, and yellow inks. We will leave it as an exercise for the reader to figure out why CMYK uses C, M, and Y rather than R, G, and B inks.

The Limits of the Rainbow

The spectrum that you can see in the hue slider in Figure 5.15B looks similar to the rainbow/wavelength spectrum that you can see at the bottom of **FIGURE 5.16A**, but it is not identical. There are hues that you can see that do not exist on the wavelength spectrum. Figure 5.16 illustrates how this can come to be. For example, suppose we combined a pure 420 nm light with a pure 680 nm light. This combination would strongly stimulate the L- and S-cones and produce minimal stimulation in the M-cones. No single wavelength of light could do that, but such a mixture is visible and must look like *something*. In fact, such mixtures will produce purplish magentas that seem to us to lie naturally between red and blue on a color circle (**FIGURE 5.16B**). When we wrap the

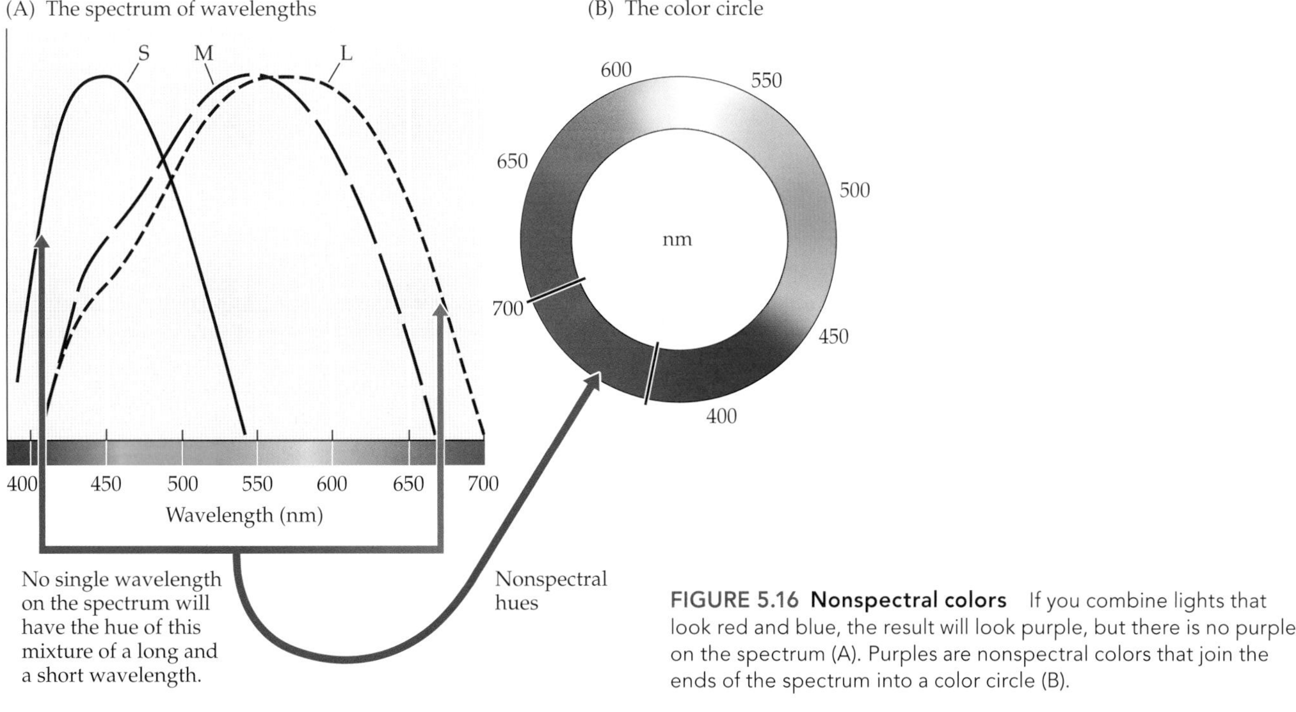

FIGURE 5.16 Nonspectral colors If you combine lights that look red and blue, the result will look purple, but there is no purple on the spectrum (A). Purples are nonspectral colors that join the ends of the spectrum into a color circle (B).

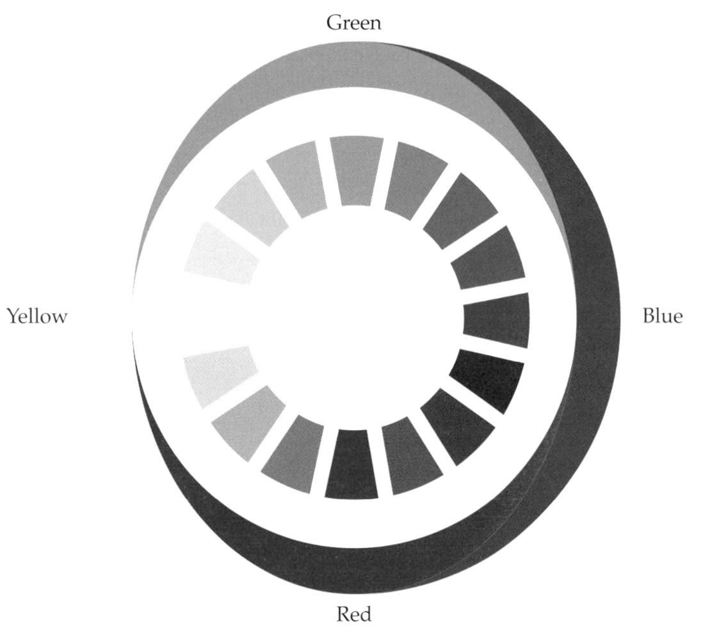

FIGURE 5.17 Opponent colors Ewald Hering noted that all the colors on the "color circle" (the center ring) could be represented by two pairs of opposing colors: blue versus yellow and red versus green (shown in the outer ring). Thus, a color could be a reddish yellow or a bluish green, but not a reddish green or a bluish yellow.

wavelength spectrum into a color circle, we join the red and blue ends with a set of colors that are called nonspectral hues—hues that can arise only from mixtures of wavelengths. While we are on the topic, it is worth noting that there are other commonly perceived colors that are not included in the spectrum's "all the colors of the rainbow." Brown is one such color. There are no brown lights. Brown is seen when a mixture of wavelengths that would look yellow, greenish yellow, or orange is seen in the company of other, brighter patches of color. You cannot see an isolated brown light in the dark (S. Buck, 2015).

Opponent Colors

In the nineteenth century, Ewald Hering (1834–1918) described a curious feature of color vision: some combinations of colors seem to be perceptually "illegal." We can have a bluish green, a reddish yellow (which we would call "orange"), or a bluish red (which we would call "purple"), but reddish green and bluish yellow don't exist. Red and green are, in some fashion, opposed to each other, as are blue and yellow (Hering, 1878). Young and Helmholtz described a trichromatic theory with three basic colors (red, green, and blue); Hering's **opponent color theory** had four basic colors in two opponent pairs: red versus green and blue versus yellow. A black-versus-white component formed a third opponent pair.

FIGURE 5.17 illustrates this idea. The center ring shows the hue dimension of HSB space, wrapped into the color circle as in Figure 5.16B. The outer ring offers a cartoon of four color mechanisms in two pairs. The inner patch on the center left looks yellow, in opponent color theory, because it stimulates the yellow pole of the yellow-blue opponency and does not stimulate either red or green. Move a bit counterclockwise, and the orange patches add increasing red to the decreasing yellow.

Leo Hurvich and Dorothea Jameson (1957) revived Hering's ideas and developed one way to quantify this opponency. The method, called hue cancelation, is shown in **FIGURE 5.18**. Let's start with the blue-yellow mechanism. For every wavelength, we will find out how much blue or yellow we need to cancel the yellow or blue in a light of that color. So, in Example 1, we start with a wavelength, say, 430 nm, that looks blue. Those yellow circles indicate that we are adding increasing amounts of yellow and asking if the mixture still looks at all bluish. It takes quite a lot of yellow to cancel that blue, leaving a pale green. This tells us that this wavelength strongly stimulates the blue part of the blue-yellow mechanism. The blue in the bluish green of Example 2 can be canceled with less yellow. For the orange color in Example 3, we would need to add blue to cancel the yellow component in orange. A color that is neither blue nor yellow occurs when the blue-yellow function crosses zero (see graph in Figure 5.18A). The color is "unique green." No one wavelength is "unique red." Everything above ~650 nm will look red.

The orange spot in Example 4 has both yellow and red in it. If we cancel the red with green, we are plotting the red-green mechanism (see Figure 5.18B). The spots where the function crosses zero are the wavelengths that are "unique blue" and "unique yellow." If you cancel both red-green and blue-yellow opponent processes, you would get a gray that you could call "unique gray" (Webster, 2017).

opponent color theory The theory that perception of color is based on the output of three mechanisms, each of them resulting from an opponency between two colors: red-green, blue-yellow, and black-white.

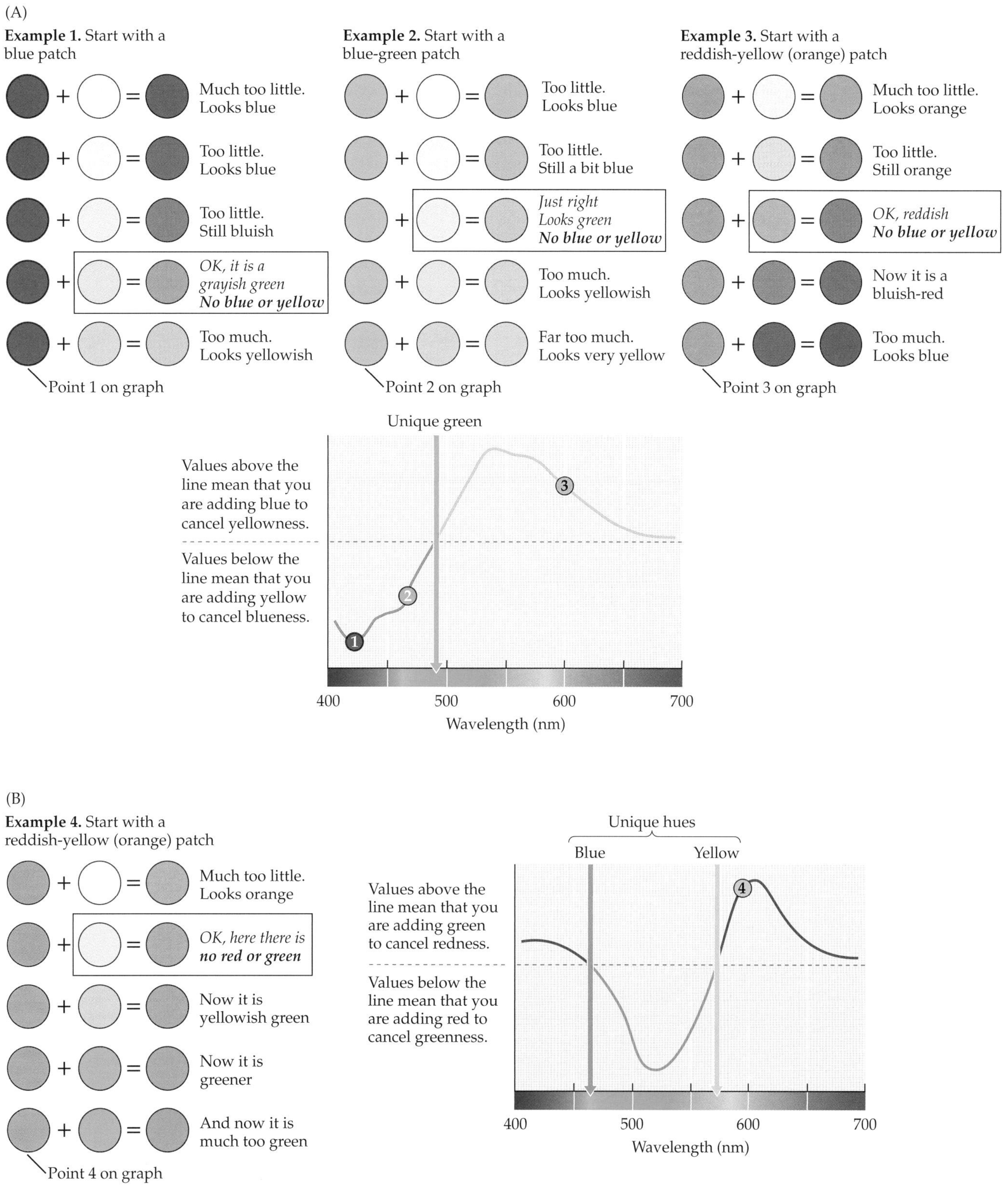

(A)
Example 1. Start with a blue patch
Much too little. Looks blue
Too little. Looks blue
Too little. Still bluish
OK, it is a grayish green No blue or yellow
Too much. Looks yellowish
Point 1 on graph
Example 2. Start with a blue-green patch
Too little. Looks blue
Too little. Still a bit blue
Just right Looks green No blue or yellow
Too much. Looks yellowish
Far too much. Looks very yellow
Point 2 on graph
Example 3. Start with a reddish-yellow (orange) patch
Much too little. Looks orange
Too little. Still orange
OK, reddish No blue or yellow
Now it is a bluish-red
Too much. Looks blue
Point 3 on graph
Unique green
Values above the line mean that you are adding blue to cancel yellowness.
Values below the line mean that you are adding yellow to cancel blueness.
1
2
3
400
500
600
700
Wavelength (nm)
(B)
Example 4. Start with a reddish-yellow (orange) patch
Much too little. Looks orange
OK, here there is no red or green
Now it is yellowish green
Now it is greener
And now it is much too green
Point 4 on graph
Unique hues
Blue
Yellow
4
Values above the line mean that you are adding green to cancel redness.
Values below the line mean that you are adding red to cancel greenness.
400
500
600
700
Wavelength (nm)

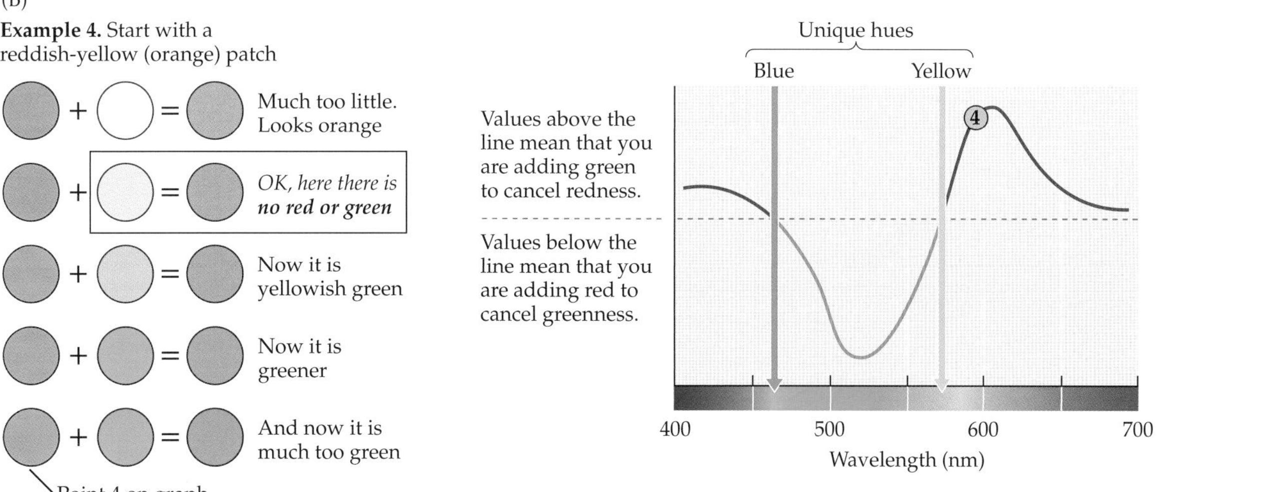

FIGURE 5.18 Color cancelation method Using color cancelation to measure opponent processes and unique hues in a blue-yellow (A) and a red-green (B) process. The locations where the hue cancelations cross the neutral midpoint are the neutral point locations of the unique green (A) and blue and yellow (B) hues—for example, the green hue with no hint of blue or yellow in it.

unique hue In the context of opponent color theory, any of four colors that can be described with only a single color term: red, yellow, green, blue. Other colors (e.g., purple or orange) can also be described as compounds (reddish blue, reddish yellow).

This opponent-process, color-appearance story sounds rather similar to the L – M and (L + M) – S story. However, L – M is not the same as red versus green, and (L + M) – S is not the same as yellow versus blue. If this were the case, an (L + M) – S cell should be a yellow-blue cell: a cell that would be maximally excited by unique yellow and maximally inhibited by unique blue. However, that (L + M) – S cell would actually be stimulated most strongly by a yellowish-greenish hue and least by a purple hue (Siuda-Krzywicka et al., 2019).

The L – M cells aren't in quite the right place either. The L-cone end of the axis is near perceptual red, but the M-cone end is very near the border between blue and green (Eskew, 2008). Krauskopf, Williams, and Heeley (1982) call these endpoints the "cardinal directions" in color space, but they are not perceptual red, green, yellow, and blue. We need at least three steps to get to color appearance. These are shown in FIGURE 5.19. First, three cones detect light in different ranges of wavelengths. Then, opponent processes measure the differences in activity between cone types. Finally, some further transformations are needed to create the color opponency described by Hering (Stockman and Brainard, 2010), but we are not really sure what those are. If it were just another calculation, like (L + M) – S, we would expect that everyone would have the same **unique hues**, but, in fact, there is quite a range of variation across individuals (Webster, 2020). For example, unique green can range from at least 495 to 530 nm between observers (Nerger, Volbrecht, and Ayde, 1995).

Color in the Visual Cortex

We know that transformations that produce perceived color take place in the visual cortex; it is not clear how the physiology gives rise to perception (Webster, 2017).

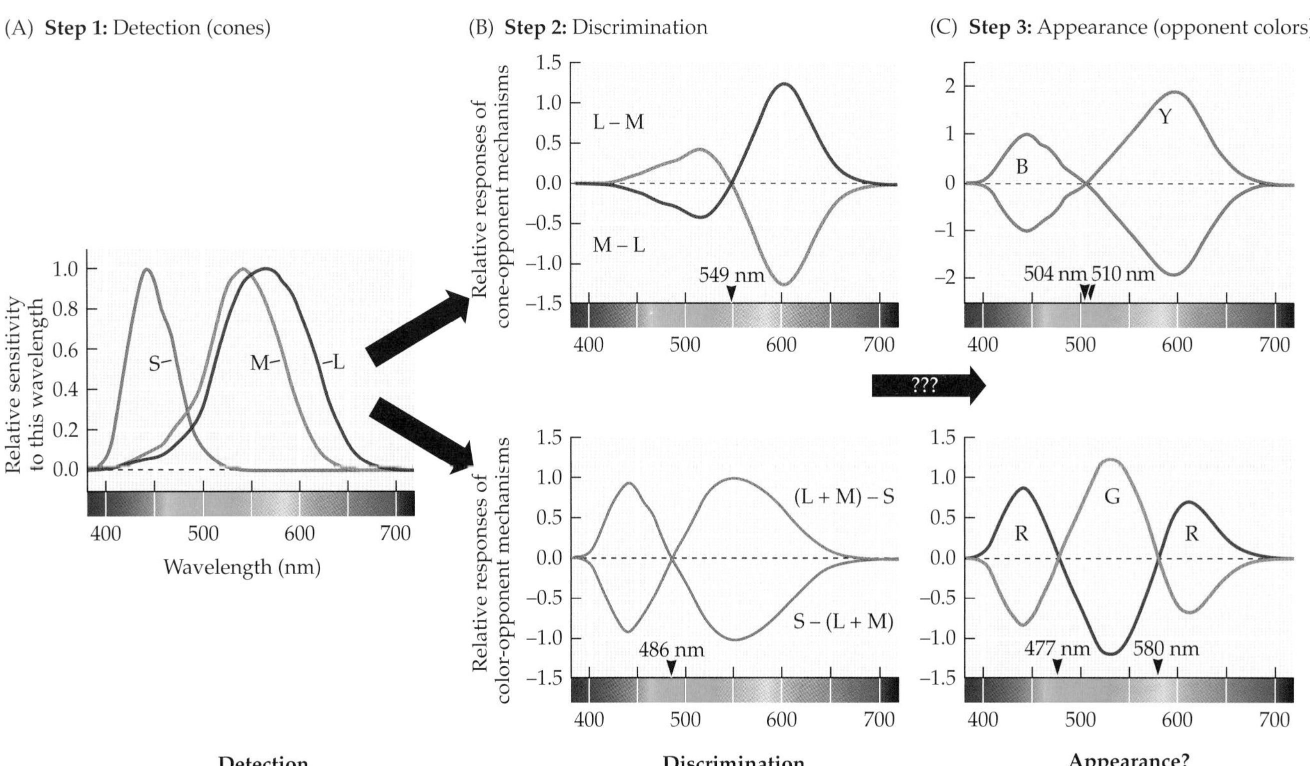

FIGURE 5.19 Three steps to color perception Three steps may lead from detection by the cones to discrimination by comparison between cones to color appearance, but we aren't sure how to get from step 2 to step 3.

Many cells in cortex are interested in color but do not seem to linearly add and subtract inputs from different cone types, as in Figure 5.19B. For now, we may have to agree with Conway (2014, p. 201): "There is still no good neural explanation for Hering's psychologically important colors . . . or . . . the unique hues often associated with them."

Even if the responses of single neurons are not telling a clear story about cortical color processing, neuroscience can offer answers to some questions about the processing of color appearance. For instance, is there a specific area or are there areas in the brains of monkeys and humans specialized for color vision? In the 1980s, evidence favored a separate pathway for color. If you recall the maps of the visual areas in Chapter 4 (Figures 4.2–4.4), in the 1980s researchers found "blobs" in V1 where cells did not seem interested in orientation but seemed very interested in color. The blobs sent output to "thin stripe" regions in V2 (Livingstone and Hubel, 1988) and from there to V4, an area that Semir Zeki argued was specialized for color, with cells that responded not to wavelength, but to perceived color (Zeki, 1983a, 1983b). More recently, functional imaging in monkeys has been used to uncover color hot spots in visual cortex. These have been named "globs" (really!) (Conway, Moeller, and Tsao, 2007), and cells in these regions also seem more interested in color than do cells outside. However, although these anatomical pathways are there (Federer et al., 2009), it has become less clear that we can separate color processing from other perceptual processes in cortical anatomy (Shapley and Hawken, 2011). Indeed, you may remember from Chapter 4 that V4 is a popular candidate for a "shape" area. This doesn't mean that it is uninterested in color, but merely that it is probably not *only* interested in color (Roe et al., 2012).

FURTHER DISCUSSION of the elegantly named "blobs" can be found in Section 3.6.

Modern imaging studies show some areas of the human visual cortex that seem particularly interested in color (Grill-Spector and Malach, 2004), but what about color *appearance?* L. Kim et al. (2020) did an experiment using a form of binocular rivalry (see Section 6.4). The observer received purple in one eye and green in the other, alternating back and forth so both colors were always present. The observer saw just one at a time: sometimes green, sometimes purple. Using functional magnetic resonance imaging methods, L. Kim et al. found that early cortical areas (V1) saw both colors, while later areas like V4 saw just one, like the observer.

5.5 Individual Differences in Color Perception

Thus far, with a little caution, we have been talking about color as if we all see colors the same way, but do we? This is one of those questions that everyone asks at one point or another, often as a child. Like many "childish" questions, this has been the topic of much decidedly unchildlike philosophical and psychophysical work. The fact that there is substantial variation in unique hues is one hint that this might not be a simple topic.

Language and Color

Putting aside the finer points of philosophy, suppose you are in a clothing store and you find a shirt you like, but you want a different color. You might go to the clerk and ask, "Do you have this in blue?" You simply assume that you and that clerk agree about the meaning of *blue*. You can discriminate on the order of millions of different colors (Linhares, Pinto, and Nascimento, 2008), but you don't have a separate word for each of them. There is a vast range of color words, but in looking for that shirt, you would not typically ask for "azuline" or "cerulean" (both varieties of blue). You would use

basic color terms Color words that are single words (like *blue*, not *sky blue*), are used with high frequency, and have meanings that are agreed on by speakers of a language.

cultural relativism In sensation and perception, the idea that basic perceptual experiences (e.g., color perception) may be determined in part by the cultural environment.

a word like *blue* that almost every speaker of your language would use quickly and consistently in naming colors. These color names are the **basic color terms** of the language. What makes a color term basic? Berlin and Kay (1969) asserted that it must be common (like *red* and not like *beige*), not an object or substance name (excluding *bronze* and *olive*), and not a compound word (no *blue green* or *light purple*). It could not be a subset of another basic color (excluding *crimson*, a type of red.) Under these rules, Berlin and Kay argued that, in English, the rules yield a list of 11 terms: *red, green, blue, yellow, black, white, gray, orange, purple, brown*, and *pink*.

Defined in this way, the numbers of "basic" color terms differ dramatically across cultures, down to as few as 2 or 3. At one time, it was thought that the differing numbers of basic color terms in different languages meant that color categorization was arbitrary. This notion was called **cultural relativism**, meaning that each group was free to create its own linguistic map of color space. Berlin and Kay's (1969) important discovery was that the various maps used in different cultures are actually rather similar (Lindsey and Brown, 2006). After surveying many languages, they claimed that the 11 basic color terms in English are about as many as any group possesses. That might not be quite right. For example, Korean might have as many as 15 (Witzel, 2019). Of course, the words themselves differ. Red becomes *rouge* in French or *adom* in Hebrew. Moreover, languages do not select randomly among the possible color terms. If a language has only two basic color terms, speakers of the language divide colors into "light" and "dark." If a language has three color terms (one chromatic term beyond *light* and *dark*), what do you think the third usually is? If you guessed *red*, you are correct. Typically, the fourth color term would be *yellow*, then *green* and *blue*. This ordering is not absolute, but you won't find a language with, for example, just *purple, green*, and *gray* as its basic color terms.

Could you really have a language with just two color terms? Since that claim was made, it has been suggested that this conclusion might depend on the precise definition of a basic color term. The Dani of New Guinea, who seemed to have just two terms, may have a much more complete set if we allow terms related to the colors of specific objects (Groh, 2016). Some of the English color terms have roots that go back to object names, too. Orange is a pretty clear example. Still, there does seem to be a set of color terms that are basic. Those terms do vary across cultures, but not randomly.

How do new basic color terms emerge? Berlin and Kay (1969) argued that a big color term can be partitioned into two smaller terms. Levinson (2000) suggested that new basic terms tend to emerge at the boundary between two existing color terms, in the area where neither existing term works well. In fact, both processes may be at work. Lindsey and Brown (2014) looked at the use of color words in American English by asking 51 Americans to name the color of each of 330 color patches (like paint chips). These observers were told to use a single word. That word had to be a word that could be used for anything of that color (you can't have a "blond" car, can you?). Lindsey and Brown were looking for the sort of word you might use in everyday speech to name the color of a car or a shirt. Those 51 Americans used 122 terms for 330 colors. Everyone used the basic 11, but there was evidence that American English might be moving beyond the 11 basics. The color term *teal* may become basic. It emerges in the no-man's-land of colors that are neither blue nor green. A term like *purple* may eventually be partitioned, with a term like *lavender* or *lilac* taking over some of the purple real estate in color space (**FIGURE 5.20**).

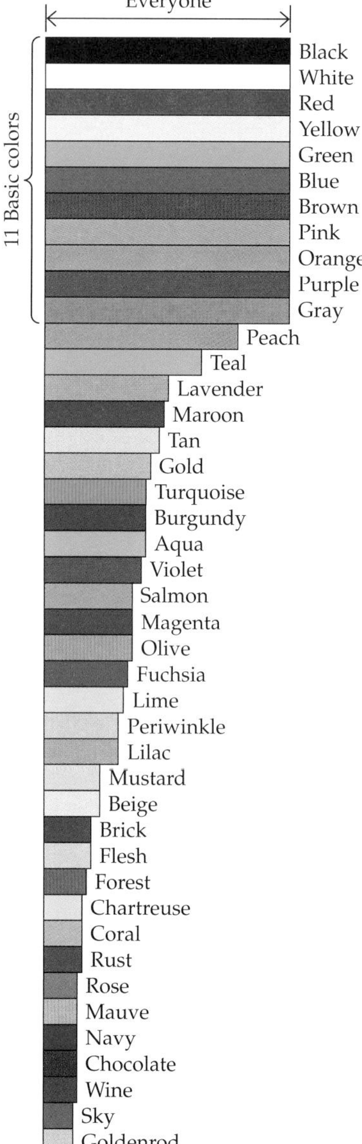

FIGURE 5.20 Basic color names When Lindsey and Brown (2014) asked Americans to name color patches, everyone used the 11 "basic" color names. The other color terms were used by fewer and fewer people, going toward the bottom of the graph. A few of these other terms, like *peach* and *teal*, may come to be considered basic color names over time.

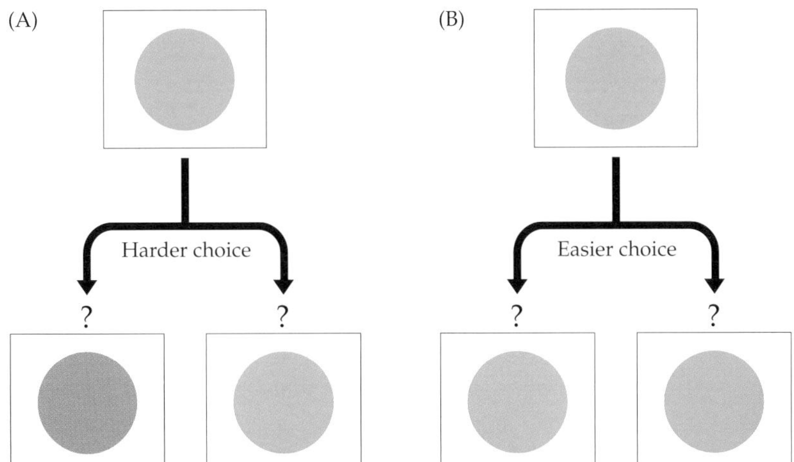

FIGURE 5.21 Color category boundaries It is easier to remember which of two colors you have seen if the choices are categorically different. For example, suppose you had to remember the blue patch shown at the top of each part of the figure. Picking between two blues, as in (A), would be rather hard. The task would be easier if one of the choices were blue and the other green, as in (B), even if the distances in color space were the same in the two cases.

If our set of basic color terms increased, would that change the way we *see* color? If a language has fewer basic color terms, do its speakers *see* colors differently than we do with our 11 basic terms? Eleanor Rosch (Heider, 1972) studied this question among the Dani of New Guinea, a tribe whose language has only two basic color terms: *mola* for light-warm colors and *mili* for dark-cool colors. Now, it is hard enough to ask your neighbor to define the experience of "blue" and then ask if that is the same as your experience of "blue." It is much more difficult to ask these questions across a great cultural divide. But there are tricks, as the experiment illustrated in **FIGURE 5.21** demonstrates. Suppose you are shown a bluish color chip and asked to remember it. Then you are shown two test chips and asked to pick the color you saw before. Obviously, the less similar the two test colors are, the easier this task is. But more important, you will do better if the wrong choice is on the other side of a color categorical boundary. Color boundaries are sharper than you might think. If you show people a collection of colors and ask, "Which are blue and which are green?" people do the task without much difficulty. If you have to remember a color, as in the task shown in Figure 5.21, you are likely to give it a label like "green" or "blue." If the next color has the same label, you are more likely to be confused than if it has a different label.

Rosch found that the Danis' performance on such tasks reflected the same color boundaries, even when their language did not recognize the distinction between the two colors (a Dani might use the term *mili* for all the colors in Figure 5.21, but would still do better with the task in Figure 5.21B). This finding leads to the conclusion that color perception is not especially influenced by culture and language; blue and green are *seen* as categorically different, even if one's language does not employ color terms to express this difference. If you want some convincing evidence that color categorization isn't just a function of language, consider a study by Caves et al. (2018). They did a version of the experiment illustrated in Figure 5.21 with songbirds as the observers and obtained evidence that they, too, seem to group colors into categories.

However, there is some evidence that language and color naming can influence color discrimination. In the late 1990s, Debi Roberson went up the Sepik River in New Guinea to study the Berinmo, whose language, like the Danis', has a limited set of basic color terms. Unlike previously studied groups, the Berinmo have terms that form novel boundaries in color space that we do not have. For example, their *nol/wor* distinction lies in the middle of colors we categorize as green. *Nol* and *wor* may roughly distinguish live from dead or dying foliage. When Roberson asked

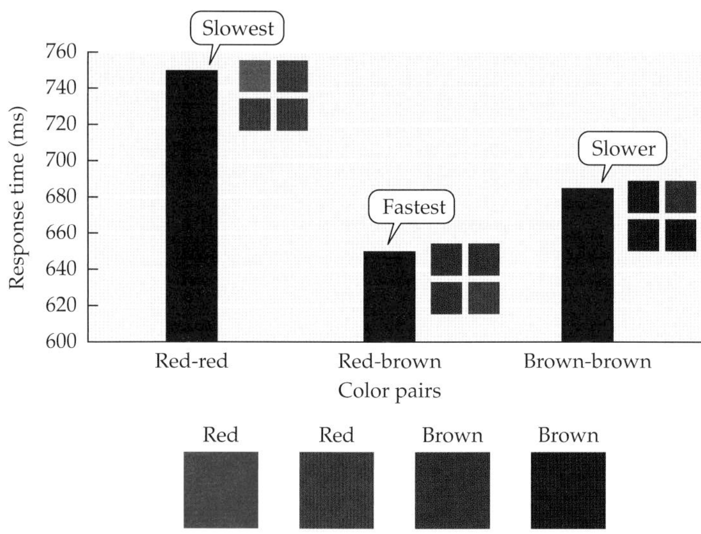

FIGURE 5.22 A color category experiment Observers see four color patches and simply locate the one patch that is different from the other three. Responses are faster and more accurate when the two colors cross a color boundary—in this case, between red and brown.

the Berinmo to do the color memory task, they performed better across their *nol-wor* boundary than across the blue-green boundary. English speakers showed the opposite result (Davidoff, Davies, and Roberson, 1999).

You might think that this was just about the role of language in memory. Suppose you call a spot "green" when you see it first. Then, when you see one spot that looks green and another that looks blue, you know which one you have seen. If you see two different green spots, the word *green* won't help. Of course, that would not explain what the Caves et al. (2018) birds were doing. Moreover, color boundaries have an influence, even if the task doesn't have a memory component. As you can see in **FIGURE 5.22**, Witzel and Gegenfurtner (2016) measured how long it took to say which one of four patches was a different color. They used four different pairs of colors selected from red and brown patches. Each patch was separated from the next patch by two just noticeable differences. (If you don't remember *just noticeable differences*, revisit Section 1.2). They found that people were faster to identify the different one and more accurate when the patches were separated by the border between red and brown than when all patches were within the "red" or "brown" category. So the color names matter, even when you compare two colors side by side.

So, is color appearance essentially universal, with different languages simply providing different ways to talk about color, or do the color terms of the language shape color *perception* and not just color *talk*? We aren't really sure (Lindsey and Brown, 2021). Nevertheless:

1. It is clear that different languages have different sets of color terms.
2. It is also clear that those terms are not random. There are patterns across languages.
3. But the very definition of a "basic color term" may work better for English than for other languages.
4. Those clever color border experiments rely on having a very clear idea of the "distance" between two colors and a very precise way of producing those colors (in the mountains of New Guinea!). Problems with the stimuli call into question some of the results about discrimination within and between categories (Witzel, 2019).

5. We once thought that the basic colors grew out of the Hering opponent colors, red-green and blue-yellow, but now it seems that they might start with objects in the world (oranges on a tree, purple dyes from shellfish, etc.) (Lindsey and Brown, 2021).

Perhaps we can say that languages are all constrained by the same world of red blood and green plants. The color terms of a language may or may not tweak perception, but they probably do influence how we pay attention to color. We will return to this topic in Chapter 7.

Genetic Differences in Color Vision

The individual differences described in the previous two sections are small. Under most circumstances, if you declare two lights to be metamerically matched, those around you will generally agree, even if we can't make definitive statements about the **qualia** (singular *quale*) that each individual experiences. *Qualia* is a term that refers to the conscious experience (in this case of a color). We can talk about your qualia—your experiences, but only you can actually experience them.

There is a significant exception to this universality of color matching. Some 8% of the male population and 0.5% of the female population have a form of color vision deficiency commonly known as "color-blindness," in which there is a variation in one or more of the genes coding the three cone photopigments. It's a "guy thing" because the genes that code for the M- and L-cone photopigments are on the X chromosome (Nathans, 1986). Males have only one copy of the X chromosome, so if one is defective, the male in question will have a problem. Females have two copies and can have normal color vision even if one copy is abnormal. In fact, some women can end up with four different cone pigments, and in very rare cases, that produces **tetrachromatic** color vision—color vision based on four numbers per patch of light (Jordan and Mollon, 2019). Such individuals may see colors that trichromats cannot see. The S-cone photopigment is coded elsewhere, so everyone has two copies, and therefore S-cone color deficiencies are rare (Alpern, Kitahara, and Krantz, 1983).

There are several types of color-blindness. One determining factor is the type of cone affected. A second factor is the type of defect; either the photopigment for that cone type is anomalous (different from the norm) or the cone type is missing altogether. Although we call people who are missing one cone type "color-blind," it is a mistake to think that this means they cannot see colors at all. As you will recall, if you have all three cones with their standard photopigments, you need three primary colors to make a metameric match with an arbitrary patch of color. If you have two cone types rather than three, the normally three-dimensional color space becomes a two-dimensional space. The world will still be seen in color, but you will have a "flatter" color experience, different from that of people with normal color vision.

Because M- and L-cone defects are the most common, most color-blind individuals have difficulty discriminating lights in the middle- to long-wavelength range. For example, consider the wavelengths 560 and 610 nm. Neither of these lights activates S-cones very much, and the L-cones fire at about the same rate for both. But most of us can distinguish the lights on the basis of the M-cone outputs they elicit, which will be higher for the 560 nm light than for the 610 nm light (you can confirm these assertions by consulting Figure 5.6). English-speaking trichromats would label the colors of these two lights "green" and "reddish orange," respectively.

Now consider a **deuteranope**, someone who has no M-cones. His photoreceptor output to these two lights will be identical. Following our maxim that the rest of the visual system knows only what the photoreceptors tell it, 560 and 610 nm lights must and will be classified as the same color by our deuteranopic individual.

qualia In philosophy, private conscious experiences of sensation or perception.

tetrachromatic Referring to the rare situation (in humans, at least) where the color of any light is defined by the relationships of four numbers—the outputs of those four receptor types.

deuteranope An individual who suffers from color-blindness that is caused by the absence of M-cones.

protanope An individual who suffers from color-blindness that is caused by the absence of L-cones.

tritanope An individual who suffers from color-blindness that is caused by the absence of S-cones.

color-anomalous A better term for the commonly used term *color-blind*. Most "color-blind" individuals can still make discriminations based on wavelength. Those discriminations are different from the norm—that is, anomalous.

cone monochromat An individual with only one cone type. Cone monochromats are truly color-blind.

rod monochromat An individual with no cones of any type. In addition to being truly color-blind, rod monochromats are badly visually impaired in bright light.

achromatopsia An inability to perceive colors that is caused by damage to the central nervous system.

agnosia A failure to recognize objects despite the ability to see them. Agnosia is typically a result of brain damage.

anomia An inability to name objects despite the ability to see and recognize them (as shown by usage). Anomia is typically a result of brain damage.

synesthesia The perceptual experience (e.g., a color) elicited by a stimulus (e.g., a letter) that does not typically produce that experience, while the stimulus (e.g., wavelength information) that does normally produce the experience is absent.

A **protanope**—someone who has no L-cones—will have a different set of color matches based on the outputs of his two cone types (M and S). And a **tritanope**—with no S-cones—will be different again. Genetic factors can also make people **color-anomalous.** Color-anomalous individuals typically have three cone photopigments, but two of them are so similar that these individuals experience the world in much the same way as individuals with only two cone types.

We have some notion of exactly what the world looks like to color-deficient individuals, because there are a few very rare cases of individuals who are color-blind in only one eye. They can compare what they see through the color-blind eye with what they see through the normal eye, enabling us to reconstruct the appearance of the color-blind world (MacLeod and Lennie, 1976).

True color-blindness does occur, but it is very unusual. It is possible to be a **cone monochromat**, with only one type of cone in the retina. Cone monochromats (who also have rods) live in a one-dimensional color space, seeing the world only in shades of gray. Even more visually impaired are **rod monochromats**, who are missing cones altogether. Because the rods work well only in dim light and are generally absent in the fovea, these individuals not only fail to discriminate colors, but also have very poor acuity and serious difficulties seeing under normal daylight conditions.

There have been various clever efforts to improve the color vision of individuals with abnormal color vision. For example, if you have L- and M-cones that are anomalously similar to each other, the right filter, placed in front of the eyes, can more effectively separate the two cone types. This will change what you would see and, to judge by testimonials, some "color-blind" individuals experience a richer world of color. Unfortunately, these filters, worn as glasses, do not give people normal color vision (Gómez-Robledo et al., 2018; Martínez-Domingo et al., 2019), though they might allow you to "learn" to see more colors (Webster, 2020; Werner, Marsh-Armstrong, and Knoblauch, 2020).

We already mentioned one other very interesting class of color-blindness, coming not from photoreceptor problems, but from damage to the visual cortex. Lesions of specific parts of the visual cortex beyond primary visual cortex can cause **achromatopsia**. An achromatopsic individual sees the world as drained of color, even while showing evidence that wavelength information is processed at earlier stages in the visual pathway. Brain lesions can also produce various forms of color agnosia or anomia (Oxbury, Oxbury, and Humphrey, 1969). In **agnosia**, the patient can *see* something, but fails to know what it is. **Anomia** is an inability to name—in this case, an inability to name colors. A patient with anomia might be able to pick the banana that "looks right," but unable to report that the banana is or should be yellow.

Does Everyone See the Same Colors? The Special Case of Synesthesia

In 1885, the artist Van Gogh was taking piano lessons. He would tell his music teacher that, for him, the sounds made by different keys on the piano were associated with different colors. The music teacher found this strange enough that he decided that Van Gogh was insane, and that ended the lessons (Voskuil, 2013). Now, Van Gogh might not have been the most emotionally stable of men. (There is that time where he cut off an ear.) However, in associating specific colors with specific sounds or even in *seeing* colors in response to sounds, he was not insane or even particularly unusual. He was experiencing **synesthesia**. Synesthesia is a phenomenon where one stimulus evokes the experience of a different stimulus. The prevalence of synesthesia in the general population is estimated at around 4–5% (Safran and Sanda, 2015). It is hard to know exactly, because experiences like Van

Gogh's, even today, discourage people from reporting the phenomenon (Safran and Sanda, 2015). The most common form is so-called grapheme-color synesthesia, experienced by about two-thirds of synesthetes. For these individuals, letters, numbers, or sometimes words have specific and idiosyncratic colors. So, the letter *A* might always look red for one synesthete. Next comes colored time units (e.g., Blue Monday) and then colored music. We are talking about this phenomenon in this chapter, which is about color, but many other types of synesthesia have been described (sounds with specific smells, for instance; Zellner, 2013).

We are all synesthetes to some extent. If you were asked about the color of a slow, sad piece of music, you would probably have an answer that would be different than if we asked you about a fast, happy dance tune. These colors might be associations that you have between emotions and colors (S. E. Palmer et al., 2013; Curwen, 2018). ("I feel blue" is a nice multisensory statement.) Most of us would not say that we actually see those colors, however. They simply come to mind. In contrast, a "projective" synesthete would see those colors out in the world.

How do we know this is a real phenomenon and not just a story that a would-be synesthete is telling us? We can't directly interrogate someone else's conscious experience (qualia again), but there are methods. For example, a grapheme-color synesthete will give a specific color name to each of the 26 letters of the alphabet. Yes, anyone can do that, but the synesthete will give the same answer next week—something a nonsynesthete could do only with practice by memorizing the pairs. Synesthetes can do this because they just need to look at the letter and report what they always see (Rich, Bradshaw, and Mattingley, 2005).

What is going on here? We don't really know. One hypothesis is that synesthetes have different, more extensive connections between sensory areas of the brain (V. S. Ramachandran and Hubbard, 2001), but neural evidence for this is rather thin. Others would argue that there is a continuum between those who project synesthetic colors into the world and those who internally associate one stimulus with another, but mapping a specific color to every letter seems qualitatively different from associating sadness with blue. We do know that synesthesia is acquired, not entirely innate, because people have to learn letters (for example) before they can develop color-letter associations (Witthoft and Winawer, 2013). Perhaps the most important point to be made is that, whatever Van Gogh's piano teacher thought, synesthesia is an interesting and normal multisensory experience. ●

5.6 From the Color of Lights to a World of Color

The material presented so far in this chapter about color is quite complex, but the fact is that it has only addressed the relatively simple problems related to the detection, discrimination, and appearance of isolated lights. We pointed to the limits of this approach to color when we noted that there are no "brown" lights. A surface looks brown when there are other, typically brighter surfaces in the neighborhood. A nonspectral color like brown just scratches the surface of the puzzles that must be solved if we want to understand color in the world. Think about this. **FIGURE 5.23** shows a black-and-white zebra on grass. Let's assume that you are looking at this in print (the story would be different on a screen, but the principles would be similar). The black, white, and green are products of reflection from paper, covered with specific inks. Let's suppose you are reading this deep in the bowels of the library, by the light of a yellowish light bulb. You take the book outside and continue to read in sunlight. The number of photons coming from the page to your eye is now thousands of times greater

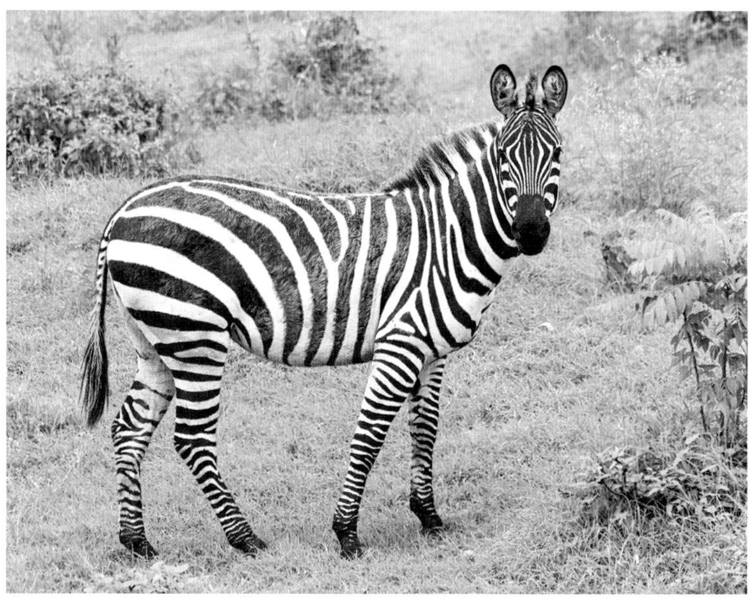

FIGURE 5.23 Color constancy This zebra looks like a black-and-white beast in a green field whether you are looking at this book under a dim yellow bulb inside, under the bright sky outside, or, for that matter, on your computer screen. How does that work?

than it was inside. Outside, a piece of a "black" stripe is now sending much more energy to your photoreceptors than did a similar piece of a "white" stripe when viewed inside. Moreover, the mix of wavelengths reflected from the grass will be very different if the light source is the sun rather than a dim bulb. Nevertheless, the grass looks green and the zebra looks black and white in both locations. How (and why) do you do experience this **color constancy**?

Let's start by just putting colors next to each other. We live in a world where regions of one color abut regions of another, and this proximity changes the appearance of colors. FIGURE 5.24 shows **color contrast** effects. The color of one region induces the opponent color in a neighboring region. Thus, the yellow surround weakens the yellow of a central square and strengthens the blue. FIGURE 5.25 shows a vivid version of a **color assimilation** effect where adjacent colors bleed into each other. Underneath the red, green, or blue stripes, those spheres on the left are all the same color, just as they are on the right (Shevell and Kingdom, 2008).

Not only can other colors in the scene alter the color of a target region, but also scenes can contain colors that cannot be experienced in isolation. Though it may be hard to believe unless you try it, you cannot sit in complete darkness and see a gray light, all by itself. That light will look white if seen as an isolated or **unrelated color**. To be seen as gray, it must be seen in relation to other patches of color.

color constancy The tendency of a surface to appear the same color under a fairly wide range of illuminants.

color contrast A color perception effect in which the color of one region induces the opponent color in a neighboring region.

color assimilation A color perception effect in which two colors bleed into each other, each taking on some of the chromatic quality of the other.

unrelated color A color that can be experienced in isolation.

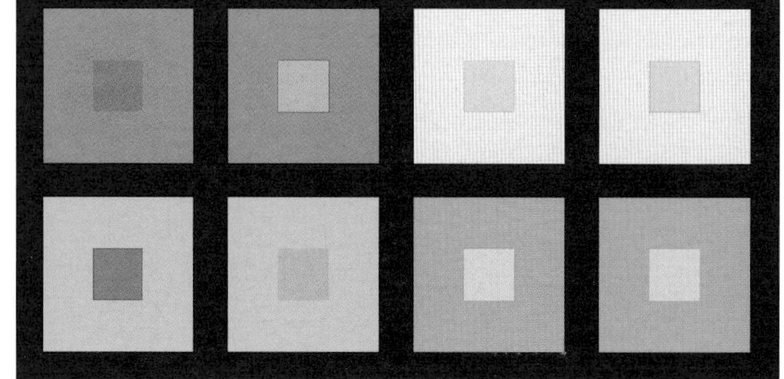

FIGURE 5.24 Color contrast The central square takes on chromatic attributes that are opposite those of the surround. For instance, the green central square in column 2 looks greener on the red background than on the green background.

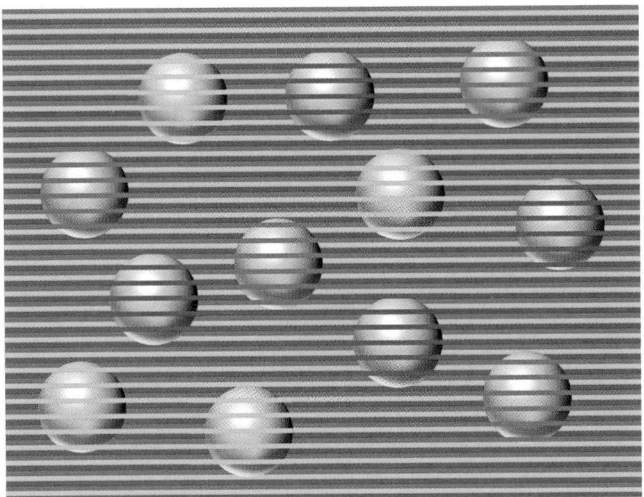
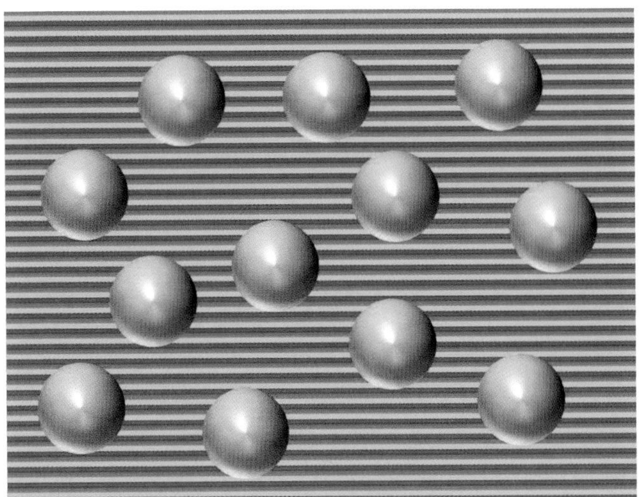

FIGURE 5.25 Color assimilation Here, colors blend together locally. The apparent color of each sphere comes from stripes that lie on top of it in the group on the left. Remove the stripes, as on the right, and the spheres are all the same color.

Thus, it is a **related color**. Brown is another related color. As discussed earlier, we can distinguish a few thousand unrelated colors by just their hue and saturation. Allowing for context effects such as the relative level of other nearby patches of light is what boosts the number of distinguishable colors to the millions (Shevell, 2003; Linhares, Pinto, and Nascimento, 2008).

Adaptation and Afterimages

Color contrast effects show how the spatial relations between colors can influence color appearance. Temporal relations matter too: what you saw before has an influence on the color you see now. You already know this from the discussion of light adaptation in Chapter 2. Adapting to a bright light makes a moderate light look darker. Adapting to darkness would make that same moderate light appear brighter.

FURTHER DISCUSSION of the time course of dark adaptation can be found in Section 2.3.

Now let's extend that principle to color. Adaptation can be color-specific, as we see in the phenomenon of **negative afterimages**. If you look at one color for a few seconds, a subsequently viewed achromatic region will appear to take on a color roughly opposite the original color. We can call the first colored stimulus the **adapting stimulus**. The illusory color that is seen afterward is the negative afterimage.

The principle is illustrated in **FIGURE 5.26**. Figure 5.26A consists of a circle of gray spots. Stare at the black dot at the center of Figure 5.26B and consider what happens as you expose one bit of your retina and visual system to the red dot at the top of Figure 5.26B. The L-cones will be more stimulated than the M- or S-cones. L+/M– opponent processes will be stimulated. You will see "red." When you move your eyes back to fixate on the black dot at the center of Figure 5.26A, the red is withdrawn from that area of the visual field. The L-cones will be more adapted than M- or S-cones, as will the later processes in the retina and brain that were more stimulated by the red spot. Adapted processes behave as though they are somewhat

related color A color, such as brown or gray, that is seen only in relation to other colors. For example, a "gray" patch in complete darkness appears white.

negative afterimage An afterimage whose polarity is the opposite of the original stimulus. Light stimuli produce dark negative afterimages. Colors are roughly complementary; for example, red produces green afterimages, and yellow produces purplish afterimages.

adapting stimulus A stimulus whose removal produces a change in visual perception or sensitivity.

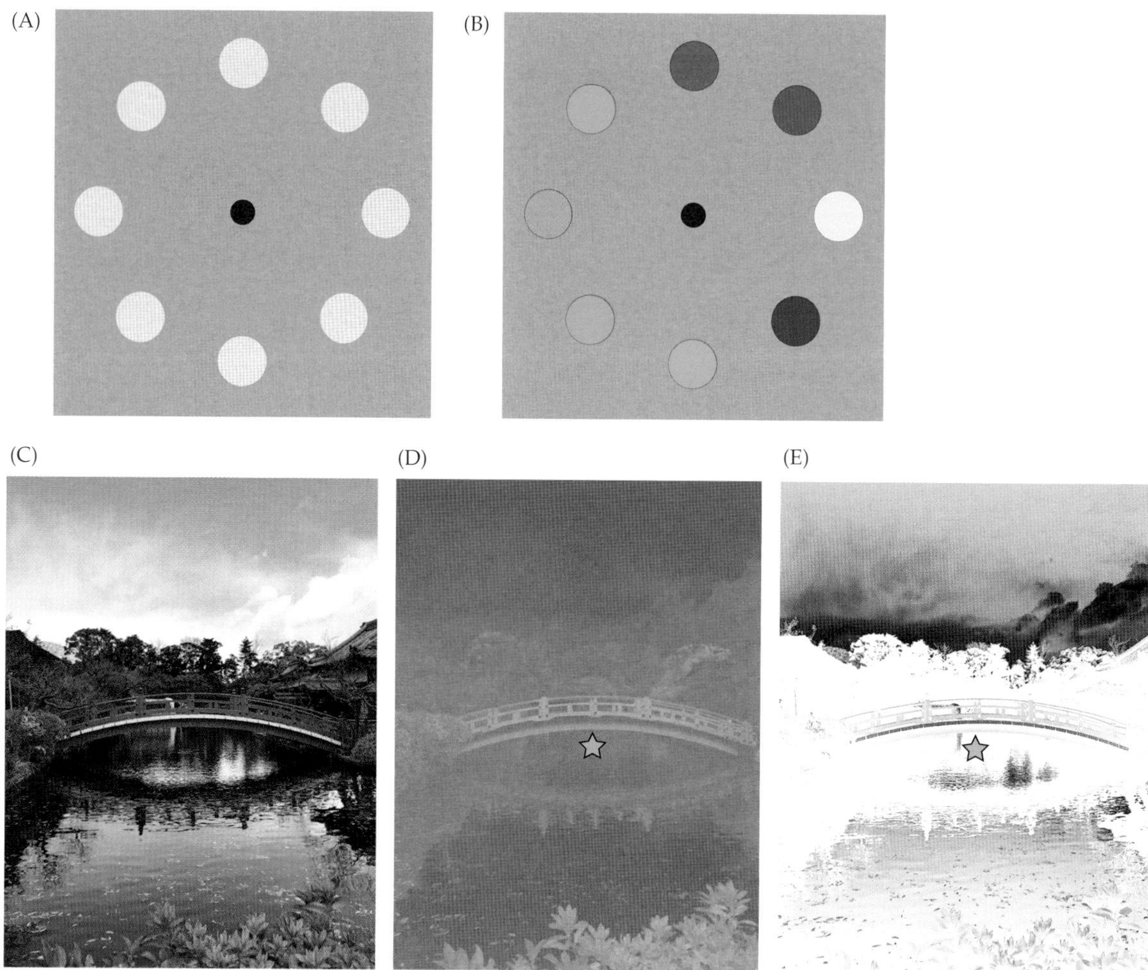

FIGURE 5.26 Negative afterimages Study the image in (A) and convince yourself that the ring of circles is gray. Now stare at the black dot in (B). After 10 seconds or so, shift your fixation to the black dot in (A). The circles should now look colored. This is a negative afterimage. Why does it happen? (If it didn't happen, try fixating more rigorously. Really look at the black dot.) Now try with a real scene. Fixate on the star in (E), and then flick your eyes to the same spot in (D). Looking back and forth helps. You should see a washed-out version of the colors in (C).

tired. As a consequence, if processes that signal "red" are a bit tired, the gray spot appears greenish until they recover.

If you look at the green dot at the bottom of Figure 5.26B and then look back at the gray image (Figure 5.26A), you will see the result of pushing the red-green mechanism in the other direction. Other colors will produce other results. An adapting color from one side of the circle in Figure 5.17 will produce an afterimage of a color in the vicinity of the other side of the circle, near the opponent color, but not exactly there (Koenderink et al., 2020). In Figures 5.26C–5.26E, you can try this with a real scene. If you stare at the star in Figure 5.26E and then quickly move your eyes to the same spot in Figure 5.26D, you will see a pale, tinted version of the real photograph (Figure 5.26C). Notice that we are not attributing negative afterimages to *just* the cones or *just* one set of cone- or color-opponent processes. Adaptation occurs at multiple sites in the nervous system, though the primary generators are in the retina (Zaidi et al., 2012).

Color Constancy

Let's return to the zebra. The fact that the picture looks black, white, and green whether viewed inside or outside is an illustration of color constancy, the tendency for the colors of objects to appear relatively unchanged despite substantial changes in the lighting conditions. All the color figures in this book will seem to have more or less the same colors wherever you read the book (though there is an entire research area hidden in what we might mean by "more or less"; Foster, 2011).

FIGURE 5.27 illustrates why color constancy is yet another difficult problem for the visual system to solve. In fact, we don't fully understand the apparent lightness of a surface (Soranzo and Gilchrist, 2019). For instance, why does this paper look white inside the library or outside in the sunlight? The heart of the problem is that the **illuminant**, the light that illuminates a surface, is not constant. Lighting changes

illuminant The light that illuminates a surface.

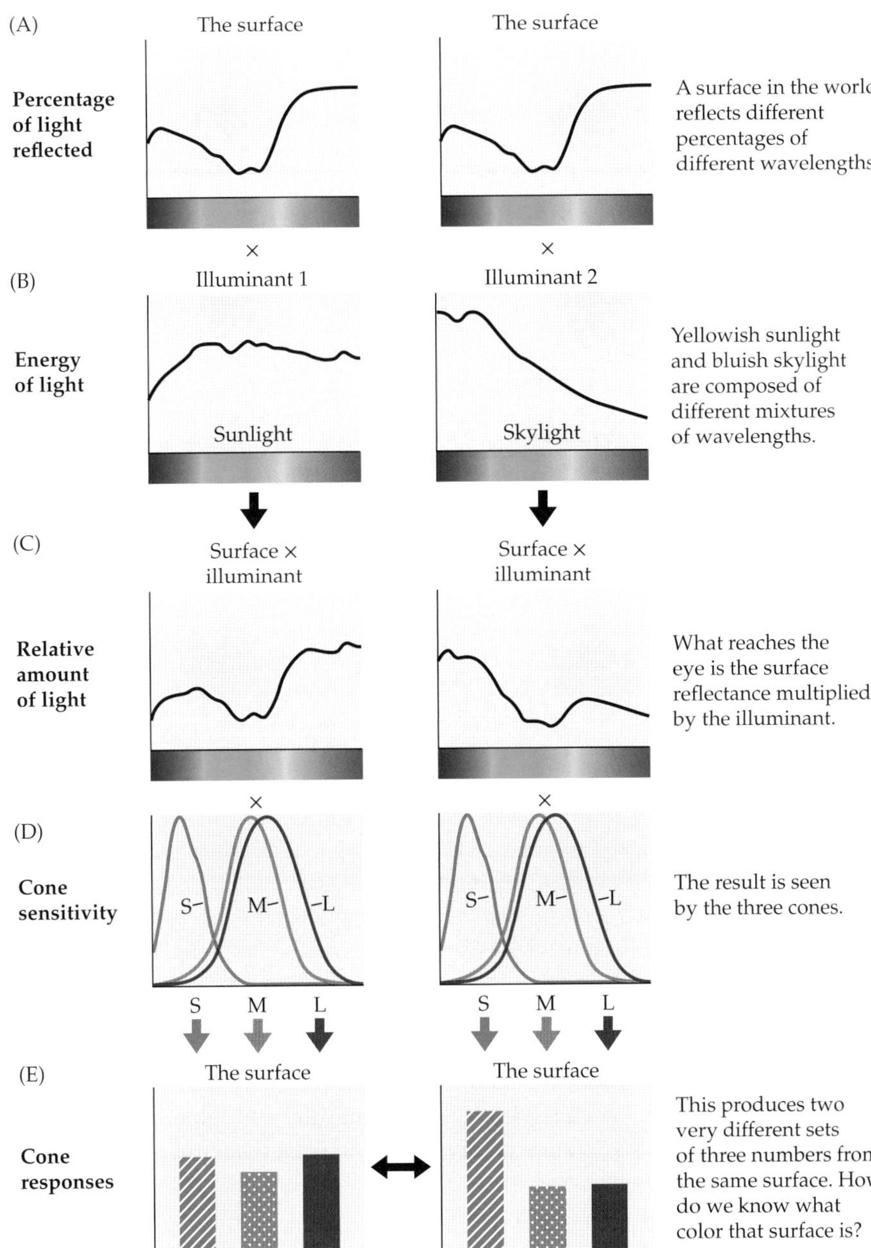

FIGURE 5.27 Color constancy The same surface (A) illuminated by two different lights (B) will generate two different patterns of activity in the S-, M-, and L-cones (C–E). However, the surface will appear to be the same color under both illuminants. This phenomenon is known as color constancy.

spectral reflectance function The percentage of a particular wavelength that is reflected from a surface.

spectral power distribution The physical energy in a light as a function of wavelength.

as we go from indoors to outdoors or as the sun moves from the horizon to high in the sky. Figure 5.27A shows the **spectral reflectance function** for a surface—the percentage of each wavelength that is reflected from a particular surface. With its preponderance of long and short wavelengths and that dip in the middle wavelengths, this surface probably looks purplish. Let's call it "lilac." Figure 5.27B shows the **spectral power distribution**—the relative amount of light at different visible wavelengths—of two different types of "daylight": sunlight and skylight. Sunlight is a yellowish light, richer in middle and long wavelengths; skylight is more bluish, with more short-wavelength energy. Figure 5.27C shows that the light reflected to our eyes is the product of the surface and the illumination. For example, a surface might reflect 90% of any 650 nm light, but no 650 nm light would reach the eye unless there was some in the original illumination. Figures 5.27D and 5.27E show that those two different products of surface and illumination are converted into two different sets of three numbers by the L-, M-, and S-cones.

Here's the problem: Even though the three numbers from the three cones are different in the two conditions, that lilac-colored surface will look lilac under both illuminants. White paper will look white. A banana will look yellow. This color constancy is beneficial because we want to know the color of the object. Under normal circumstances, we don't care about the spectral composition of the lights.

The Problem with the Illuminant

Let's think about color constancy as a math problem. In simple terms, we have an illuminant (call it I) and a surface (S). As shown in Figure 5.27C, what we can sense is a result—the product of $I \times S$—but what we want to know is S. We say that we want to "recover" the surface, S, from the mixture, $I \times S$. It is as if we were given a number (say, 48), told that it is the product of two other numbers, and asked to guess what those two numbers might be. The answer could be 12 and 4. Or it could be 16 and 3. Or 6 and 8. Given just the number 48, we cannot solve the problem. Nevertheless, given the result of $I \times S$, the visual system does a pretty good job of figuring out S.

We sometimes talk about "discounting" the illuminant as if our whole goal were to throw away the I term and just see the surface color. However, this is not quite right. For instance, you can get different answers if you point to two patches under two different illuminants and ask if the patches were "cut from the same cloth" or if they are the "same color" (Arend and Reeves, 1986). If you just discarded the illuminant information, these answers would be the same—but they are not. Similarly, you can tell the difference between a scene lit by the morning sun and a scene illuminated by the sun at high noon. Thus, not only can you recover the color of the surface, but also you know something about the illuminant. How do you do this?

Physical Constraints Make Constancy Possible

As noted in the previous section, it is impossible to know which two integers are multiplied to produce 48. However, if you are told that the first number is between 9 and 14, you're saved. The first number must be 12, and the second, then, must be 4. In an analogous way, color constancy must be based on some information or assumptions that constrain the possible answers. There are many possible assumptions that could help. Suppose we assumed that, in a complex scene, the brightest region was white (Land and McCann, 1971) or that the average color across the whole scene was gray (Buchsbaum, 1980). We could scale the other colors relative to these white or gray anchors. However, this can't be entirely right. Think what would happen if you were in a dark room with two spots of light on the wall: a red one and a blue one. Under a simple version of a bright-is-white theory, the brighter spot should look white and the other spot should change color. That can't be right (and theorists knew this, so the actual theories are more subtle, but they still do not work perfectly).

If you have read Chapter 4, you have encountered the Bayesian approach to dealing with an ambiguous stimulus by combining the stimulus with an inference about what is likely in the world. In the nineteenth century, Helmholtz wrote about "unconscious inference" (Helmholtz, 1924, in the English translation). Our guesses about the world may make an important contribution to color constancy. **FIGURE 5.28** illustrates something of an exception that may help to make this point. The photos on the right have either a blue (top) or a yellow (bottom) filter placed over the view through this Roman arch. You may make the inference that outdoor light is bluish. On the one hand, making it a bit more bluish might change the quality of the light (top). If there is more yellow through the arch, on the other hand, you may infer that the surfaces are more yellow. The stone might look different. If you find that the objects in the world have a golden glow at sunset, that may be because you are seeing the shift in the light of the setting sun to longer wavelengths but attributing that change to the surfaces illuminated by that sun.

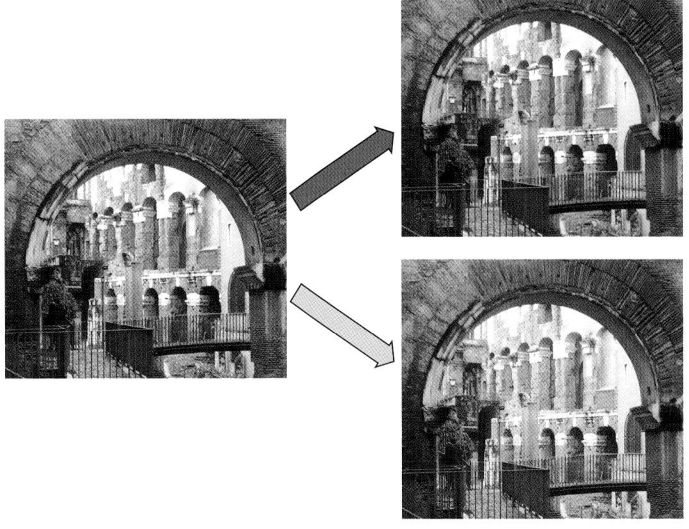

FIGURE 5.28 Changing the color of the illuminant When the view through the arch is made more bluish, we tend to see a change in the lighting. When the view is made more yellow, we may see an apparent change in the surface color. Is that railing now golden?

Or . . . it is possible that you do not see things that way. For the most part, we seem to make similar inferences about colors and illuminants, but not always. Differences in inferences are at the heart of the ambiguous picture of #TheDress that swept the internet in 2015. It also attracted the attention of many color researchers who were professionally interested in why people disagreed about the colors of the dress (Brainard and Hurlbert, 2015; Gegenfurtner, Bloj, and Toscani, 2015; Lafer-Sousa, Hermann, and Conway, 2015; Wallisch, 2017; Witzel, O'Regan, and Hansmann-Roth, 2017). Why did some argue for gold and white, while others insisted that the dress was dark blue and black? In all probability, people are differing in their unconscious inferences about the lighting. On the one hand, if the dress is being lit from the front, then the darker blue and black inferences are a better guess about the colors of the surfaces. If, on the other hand, the dress is in deep shadow, with the light behind, then inferring white and gold makes more sense. Typically, we would all make similar inferences about the lighting, but if we don't, odd things can happen (Witzel and Gegenfurtner, 2018).

5.7 What Is Color Vision Good For?

Having introduced some of the basics and some of the complications of color vision, we will wrap up this chapter by returning to our opening question about the usefulness of color vision. The ability to use wavelength information has evolved several times in several ways over the course of time. Evolutionary theory tells us that, for this to be true, color vision must provide an advantage that makes it worth the trouble. Color is not an absolute requirement. If we could not make wavelength discriminations, we could still identify a lion (**FIGURE 5.29A**), and we could still find our way through the forest (**FIGURE 5.29B**). Although color vision might make the lion stand out a bit better from the background, we would be much more impaired if we lacked "orientation vision" or "motion vision." Across the animal kingdom, however, there seem to be at least two realms of behavior where color

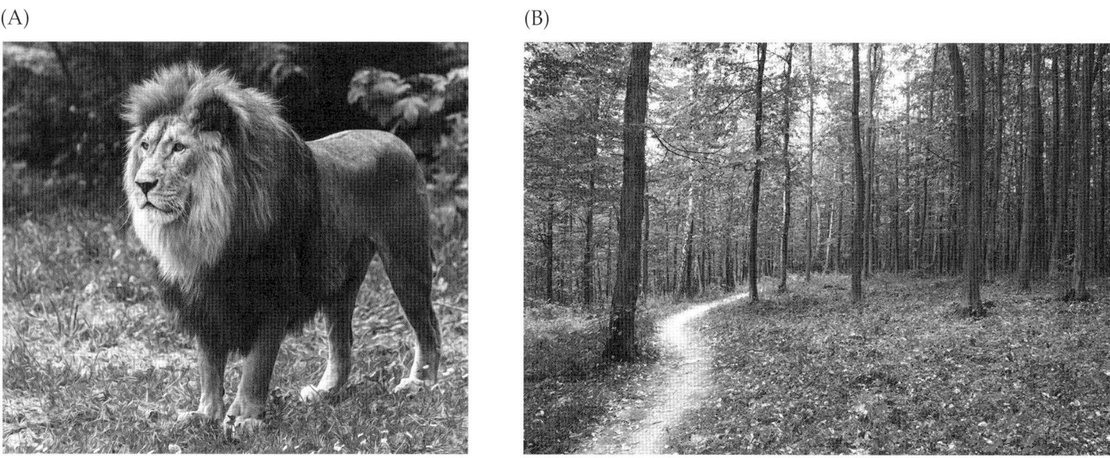

FIGURE 5.29 **Do humans need color vision?** (A) A black-and-white lion is still a lion, and (B) you could still find a path in the woods without color vision.

vision is especially useful: eating and sex. More generally, color vision seems to be particularly helpful in visual search tasks (see Chapter 7).

Having color vision does seem to make it easier to find candidate foods and to discriminate good food from bad food. Comparing the two versions of FIGURE 5.30 shows that finding berries is easier with color vision, though it could still be done in the achromatic world (Bompas, Kendall, and Sumner, 2013). Perhaps of more importance, color tells you which berries are ripe and good to eat. You may recall that we mentioned this as a possible use for the L- and M-cone difference earlier in the chapter. Most diurnal animals (animals who are active in daytime) have two photopigments: roughly an S-cone and an LM-cone. Some primates have evolved separate L and M photopigments and the neural circuitry to exploit the rather small differences between the responses of those cone types. There has been considerable debate regarding whether this really conveys an advantage in telling ripe from unripe fruit or distinguishing subtle differences among green leaves (B. C. Regan et al., 2001; Troscianko et al., 2003). Some have argued that shape and texture information, along with dichromatic color vision, are good enough for these purposes. How can we find out? In some monkey species (e.g., capuchins), there is a mix of dichromats and trichromats (as in the human species). Do the

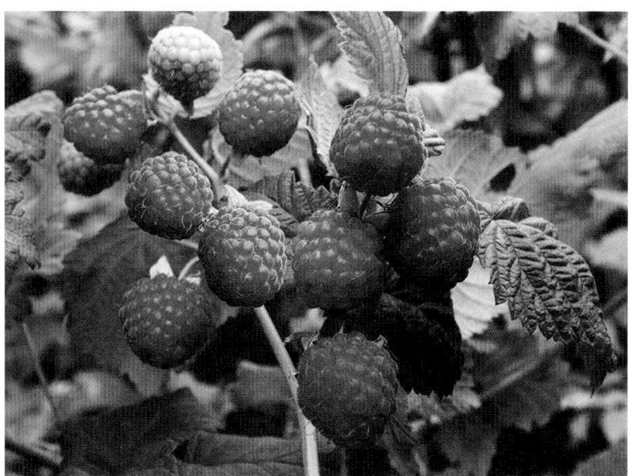

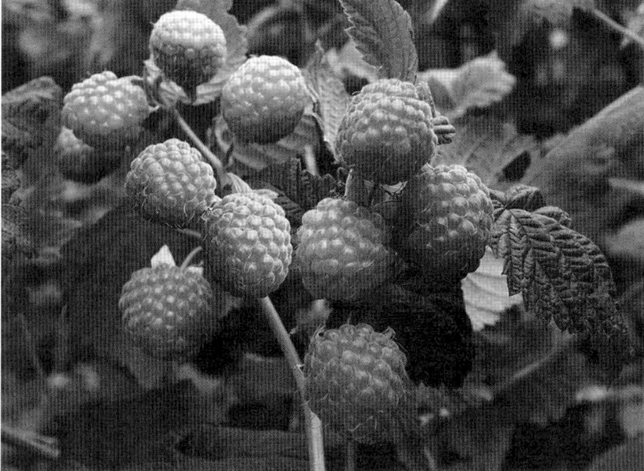

FIGURE 5.30 **Using color vision** Finding a raspberry is easier if you have color vision, as is deciding if that berry is ripe.

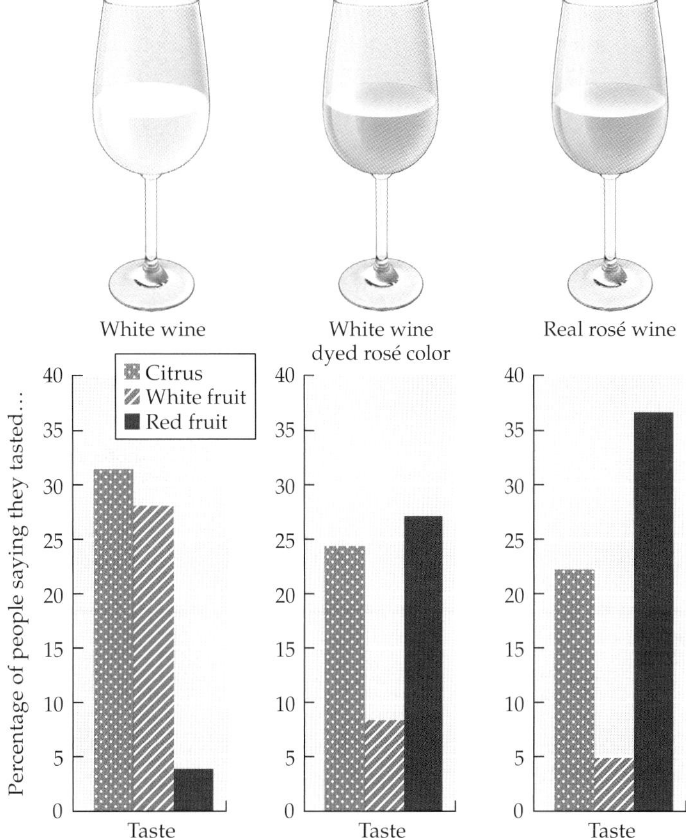

FIGURE 5.31 **Color and flavor** The color of a food can change its reported flavor. Here, white wine is reported to taste like rosé when it is colored pink.

trichromats have an advantage in hunting for food? Rather than test this in capuchins, Melin et al. (2013) carefully simulated six varieties of capuchin color vision in human observers and had those observers search for capuchin food in photographs of those fruits as they would appear in the Costa Rican forests where the monkeys live. The result was a clear advantage for trichromatic vision.

Not only does color help you find something to eat, but also it can have a significant impact on your experience of the flavor of a food. One nice example comes from the world of wine tasting. Q. Wang and Spence (2019) had participants taste a white wine, a rosé wine, and more of the same white wine that had been colored to look like the rosé. For each wine, participants picked terms referring to smells and flavors that they detected in each wine. As you can see in **FIGURE 5.31**, white wine was judged to have "notes" of white fruits (like pears), while rosé produced reports of red fruit (strawberries, raspberries, etc.). Interestingly, the fake rosé was reported to have a flavor profile like the real rosé even though it was the white wine in disguise.

Did the color change the flavor of the wine, or did it change the answers in a difficult, subjective taste test? It would be interesting to know what the participants would have reported if they had not seen the wine. Does the real rosé still taste of red fruit if you can't see the red? That condition was not part of this experiment. We do know that there are limits on the effects of color on flavor. Shankar et al. (2010) did an experiment where participants tasted a purple drink designed to inspire thoughts of grape juice. If the real flavor was cranberry, they got grape reports. However, if the real flavor was vanilla, mere color was not enough to affect the reported flavor. ●

In addition to searching for and assessing food, animals spend significant time and effort searching for and assessing potential mates. Here, too, color plays a central role. Colorful displays—from the dramatic patterns on tropical fish (**FIGURE 5.32A**) to the tail of a peacock (**FIGURE 5.32B**) to the face of the mandrill (**FIGURE 5.32C**)—are all sexual signals. Why is the male peacock with the most colorful tail the most desirable mate for a female peacock? We can't ask the female, of course, but a colorful tail might somehow indicate that this male's genes are better than his competitors'. A peahen who could only see the world in black and white wouldn't be able to perceive this information and would be at an evolutionary disadvantage. In another example that we mentioned earlier, the development of separate L- and M-cones may have made primate color vision particularly well suited to detecting the amount of blood in a blushing or blanched cheek (Changizi, Zhang, and Shimojo, 2006).

Color vision is accomplished in different ways in different species. We are trichromats, with 3 different types of cone photoreceptors. Dogs appear to be

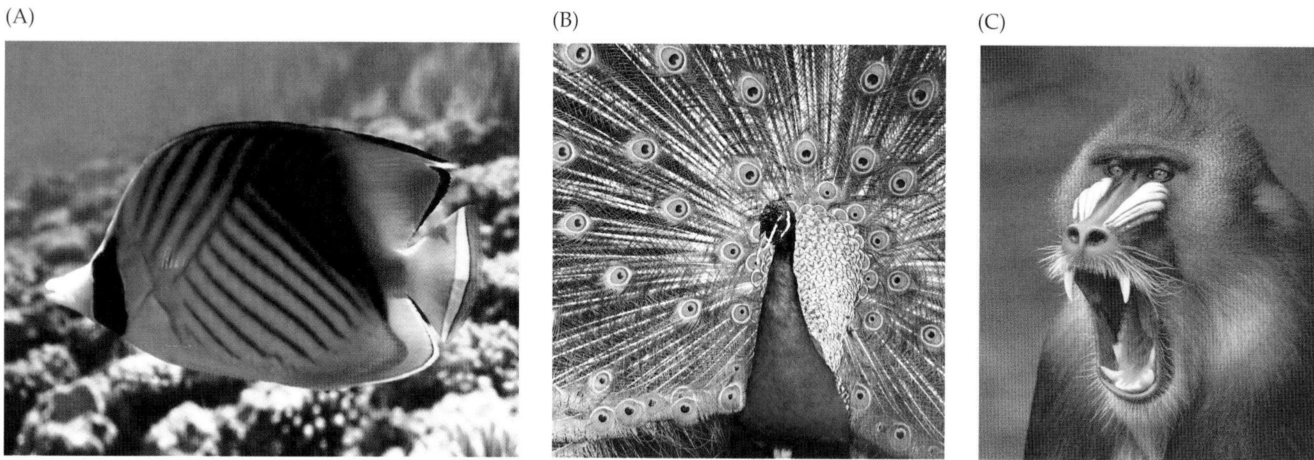

FIGURE 5.32 **Color and sex** The colors of animals—from (A) tropical fish to (B) peacocks to (C) mandrills—are often advertisements to potential mates.

dichromats, with 2 types of cone photoreceptors (Neitz, Geist, and Jacobs, 1989). Chickens, surprisingly enough, turn out to be tetrachromats, with 4 (Okano, Fukada, and Yoshizawa, 1995). There is not much gain in information if the number of cone types is increased beyond 3 or 4 (Maloney, 1986), which probably explains why octachromats or dodecachromats—individuals with 8 or 12 types of cones—are very rare. They are rare, but not nonexistent. If you have some time, look into the case of the mantis shrimp, a wonderfully eccentric beast with at least 12 types of photoreceptors (Marshall and Arikawa, 2014). Note that the shrimp might not have the neural hardware for 12-dimensional vision, but they do have a lot of photoreceptor types. Amazingly, the current record for the greatest number of photopigments for a vertebrate may lie with a deep-sea fish, the silver spinyfin (*Diretmus argenteus*), which has 2 cone photopigments and 38 rod photopigments (Musilova et al., 2019). The spinyfin is just one of a group of frightening-looking fish (**FIGURE 5.33**) that live where there is very little light and may have evolved a rich set of photopigments in an effort to catch every photon that they can.

FIGURE 5.33 **Extreme color vision** (A) The absorption spectra of the 38 (!) different rod photopigments of the silver spinyfin (*Diretmus argenteus*). Notice that these pigments have peak sensitivity in the short-wavelength (blue) end of the spectrum. These fish and other occupants of the deep sea emit their own light (a bit like fireflies), and that bioluminescence is in the short wavelengths. (B) The threadfin dragonfish (*Echiostoma barbatum*), another deep-sea fish with many photopigments.

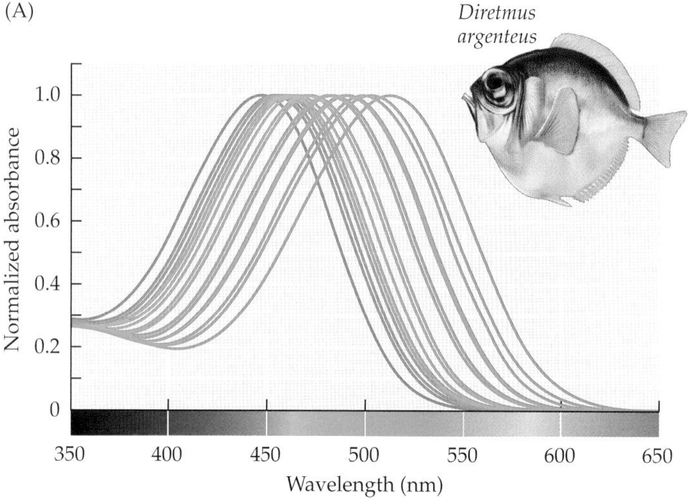

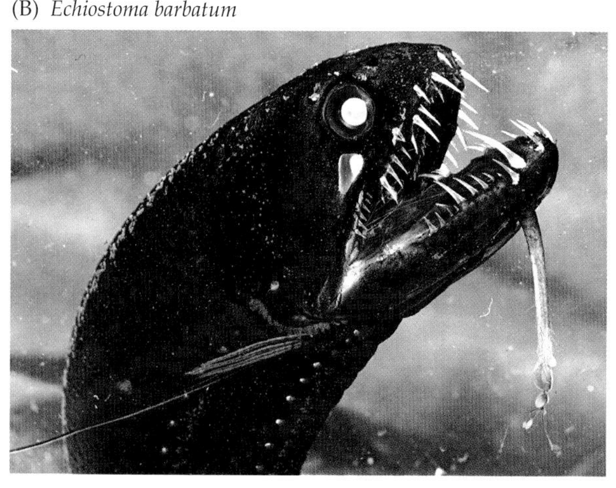

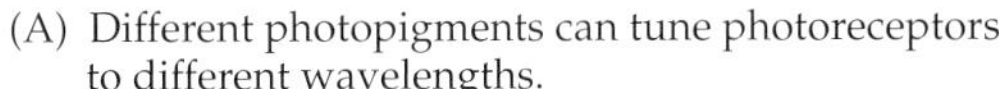

(A) Different photopigments can tune photoreceptors to different wavelengths.

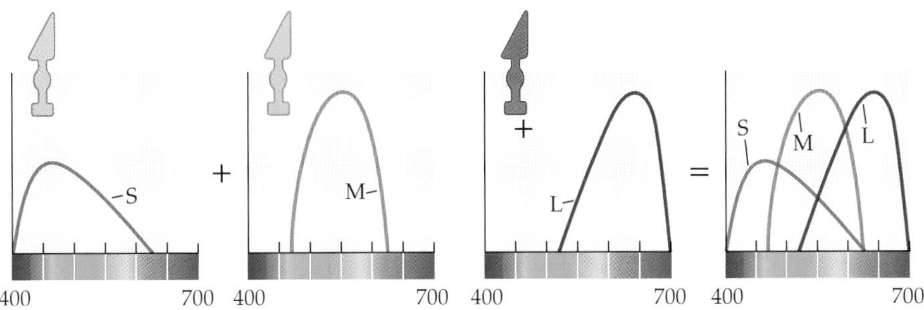

(B) Colored oil droplets can also tune photoreceptors to different wavelengths.

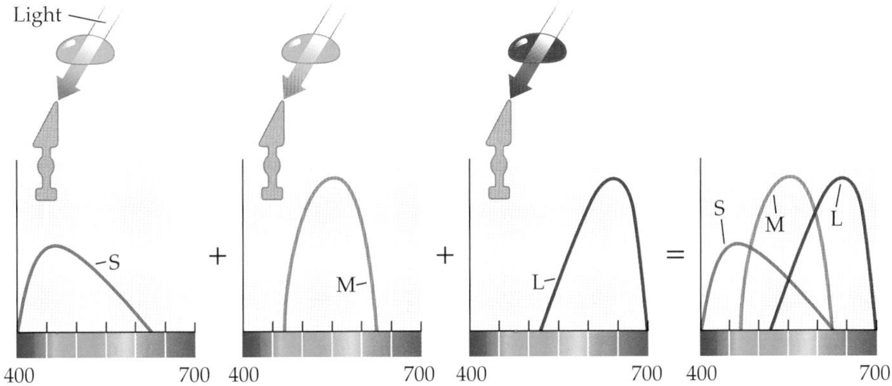

FIGURE 5.34 Two ways to make photoreceptors with different spectral sensitivities (A) Our S-, M-, and L-cones are different because they contain different photopigments. (B) Some animals have only one type of photopigment. These animals can have color vision because colored oil droplets sitting on top of photoreceptors create groups of photoreceptors with different sensitivities to wavelength.

Our S-, M-, and L-cones are different because they contain different photopigments (**FIGURE 5.34A**). It is also possible to use a single photopigment to create more than one functional type of cone. The trick is to put a different filter in front of each type of cone so that some wavelengths are subtracted before light reaches the photoreceptor (**FIGURE 5.34B**). A cone with a reddish oil droplet in front of it will respond more vigorously to long-wavelength light than will a cone covered by a greenish droplet. Chicks and other birds have these droplets, as do a variety of reptiles (Govardovskii, 1983).

Even fireflies get into this act in a limited way. Fireflies signal each other with bioluminescence: they make their own light. Different species have different lights, and each species' visual system appears to be tuned to its particular wavelength signature. A combination of a photopigment and a colored filter makes signals from conspecifics (members of the same species) appear brighter than the flashes of other fireflies in the vicinity (Cronin et al., 2000). With this sort of visual system, the firefly will never appreciate the palette of colors in a sunset. But it will be able to locate an appropriate mate, and that, after all, was the pressure shaping the development of this limited sensitivity to wavelength.

Scientists at Work

Filtering Colors

Question How well can you direct your attention to one color?

Hypothesis A "feature-based attention" mechanism should allow an observer to select all the items of one color and treat them as a group, effectively ignoring the other items.

Test The researchers showed their observers images like those in the first column of **FIGURE 5.35** (P. Sun, Chubb, et al., 2016). (The colors were much more carefully chosen than we can print here.) Observers were asked to mark the centroid of the three dots of a particular color. If you imagine the triangle formed by the three dots, the centroid is that triangle's center of mass. People can do this easily enough with three dots (as in the three dots in the upper right panel of Figure 5.35). If filtering by color worked, the dots of different colors would have no effect on ability to judge the centroid of one target color.

Results When the different dots varied in hue this task was quite easy. The researchers could calculate the impact of each color dot on the centroid, and in the hue condition, observers could create an attentional filter that effectively removed every dot except those of the correct hue (here, green). If the dots varied along a saturation axis, as they do in the second row, observers couldn't easily select just the dots of one saturation. (The actual experiment was a bit different from what is shown.)

Conclusion We can use our attention to select a group of items on the basis of hue. Other dimensions of color cannot be filtered as effectively. The authors speculate that "hue is a more reliable cue to material identity than either lightness or saturation" (P. Sun, Chubb, et al., 2016, p. E6717), so it might not be as useful to filter along those dimensions.

Future work Are there other features of the visual world for which it might be useful to have this kind of filtering ability? Suppose you were a product designer; might this result influence the way that you designed the bottles for a line of shampoo?

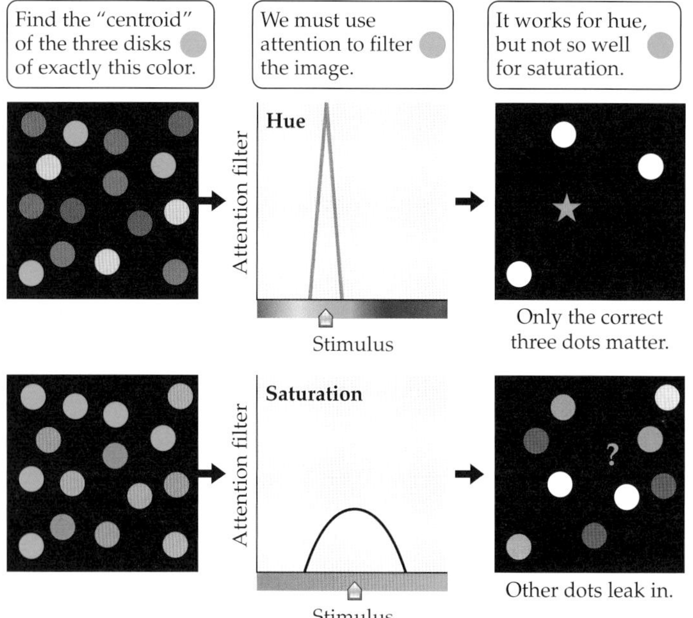

FIGURE 5.35 The Sun et al. (P. Sun, Chubb, et al., 2016) attention filter experiment Column 1 shows sample stimuli. Observers would be asked to pay attention to just three dots in each image, defined by their color. Column 2 shows the "attention filter" that can be inferred from the data. Column 3 shows the hypothetical strength of the dots in the mind of the observer when the filter has been applied. When the dots differ in hue (top row), the filter leaves only the target dots. When the dots vary in saturation (bottom row), nontarget dots get past the filter and influence behavior.

Summary

1. Probably the most important fact to know about color vision is that lights and surfaces look colored because a particular distribution of wavelengths of light is being analyzed by a particular visual system. Color is a mental phenomenon, not a physical phenomenon. Many animal species have some form of color vision. It seems to be important for identifying possible mates,

possible rivals, and good things to eat. Color vision has evolved several times in several different ways in the animal kingdom.

2. Rod photoreceptors are sensitive to low (scotopic) light levels. Humans have only one type of rod photoreceptor; it yields one "number" for each location in the visual field. Our rods can support only a one-dimensional representation of color, from dark to light. Thus, human scotopic vision is achromatic vision.
3. Humans have three types of cone photoreceptors, each having a different sensitivity to the wavelengths of light. Cones operate at brighter light levels than rods, producing three numbers at each location; the pattern of activity over the different cone types defines the color. Some animals have many more types of photoreceptors, but we know little about their color experience.
4. If two regions of an image produce the same response in the three cone types, they will look identical; that is, they will be metamers. And they will look identical even if the physical wavelengths coming from the two regions are different.
5. In additive color mixture, two or more lights are mixed. Adding a light that looks blue to a light that looks yellow will produce a light that looks white (if we pick the right blue and yellow). In subtractive color mixture, the filters, paints, or other pigments that absorb some wavelengths and reflect others are mixed. Mixing a typical blue paint and a typical yellow paint will subtract most long and short wavelengths from the light reflected by the mixture, and the result will look green.
6. Color-blindness is typically caused by the congenital absence or abnormality of one cone type—usually the L- or M-cone, usually in males. Most color-blind individuals are not completely blind to differences in wavelength. Rather, their color perception is based on the outputs of two cone types instead of the normal three.
7. A single type of cone cannot be used, by itself, to discriminate between wavelengths of light. To enable discrimination, information from the three cones is combined to form three cone-opponent processes. In the first, cones sensitive to long wavelengths (L-cones) are pitted against medium-wavelength (M) cones to create an $L - M$ process that is roughly sensitive to the redness or greenness of a region. In the second cone-opponent process, L- and M-cones are pitted against short-wavelength (S) cones to create an $(L + M) - S$ process roughly sensitive to the blueness or yellowness of a region. The third process is sensitive to the overall brightness of a region.
8. Color appearance is arranged around opponent colors: red versus green and blue versus yellow. This color opponency involves further reprocessing of the cone signals from *cone*-opponent processes into *color*-opponent processes.
9. The visual system tries to disentangle the properties of surfaces in the world (e.g., the "red" color of a strawberry) from the properties of the illuminants (e.g., the "golden" light of evening), even though surface and illuminant information are combined in the input to the eyes. Mechanisms of color constancy use implicit knowledge about the world to correct for the influence of different illuminants and to keep that strawberry looking red under a wide range of conditions.

Chapter 6

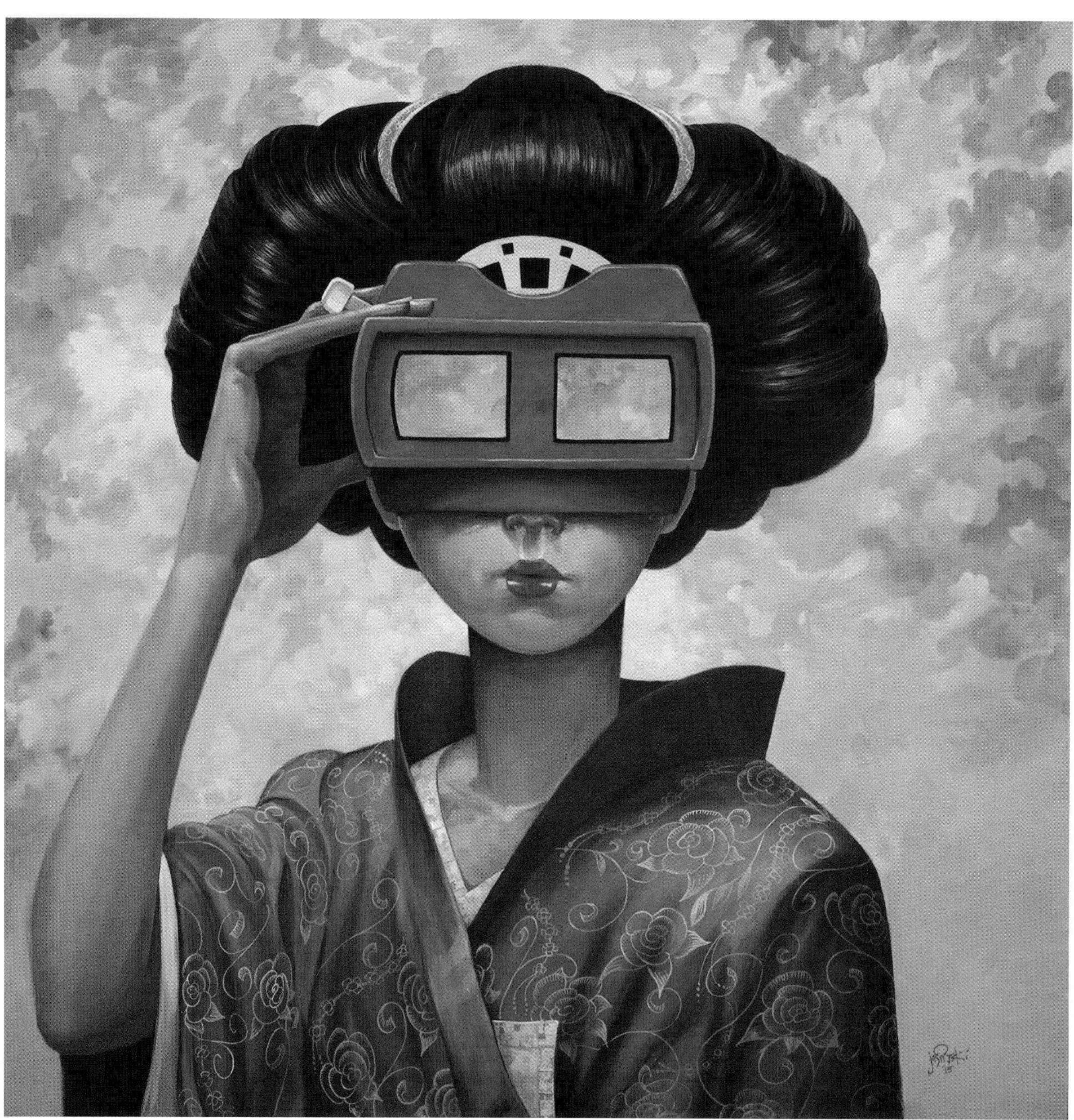

Aaron Jasinski, *Clarity II*, 2015

Space Perception and Binocular Vision

Questions to Contemplate

Think about the following questions as you read this chapter. By the chapter's end, you should be able to answer and discuss them.

- Given the curved, two-dimensional images on the retina of each eye, how does the brain reconstruct our rich three-dimensional world?
- What tricks do artists use to give the rich sense of depth in drawings and paintings?
- Why do we have two eyes?
- How does the brain combine different monocular cues to depth?
- How does the brain compute binocular cues to depth?
- How does three-dimensional vision develop?

Imagine that you're moving quietly through a meadow, trying to get close enough to a bear cub to get a good picture. Suddenly you discover that Mother Bear is not happy about your photo session (**FIGURE 6.1**). She charges, and you run—back across the field, through a thicket of trees. A quick leap across a stream brings you to a slope that leads down to the road where your partner is waiting in a Jeep. You dive into the passenger side and roar off down the track to safety. As the bear lumbers off and your heartbeat returns to normal, your thoughts naturally turn to the acts of visual space perception that you just performed: You picked a path through the three-dimensional world that brought you to safety. You behaved as though you knew where the trees were. You acted as though you understood how far it was across the stream. All in all, you demonstrated a sophisticated grasp of the layout of the physical world around you.

Humans share this sophistication with a large part of the animal kingdom. Faced with the same bear, a rabbit or deer would have shown a similar grasp of the relevant issues in space perception (without the Jeep). The ability to perceive and interact with the structure of space is one of the fundamental goals of the visual system. It is also quite a formidable accomplishment, and in this chapter we'll explore how we do it.

As a starting place, let's assume that the external world exists. This is a philosophical position known as **realism**. It is not the only possibility. The **positivists** note that all you really have to go on is the evidence of your senses, so the world could be nothing more than an elaborate hallucination. For less philosophical elaborations of this viewpoint, we watch *The Matrix* or *Inception*. In this book, however, we'll assume that there is a real world out there to perceive.

The problem that the visual system needs to solve is how to construct a three-dimensional world based on the inverted images on the retina of each eye. Parallel lines in the world do not necessarily remain parallel in the retinal image, as **FIGURE 6.2** illustrates. The angles of triangles don't always add up to 180 degrees. The retinal area occupied by an object gets smaller as the object moves farther away from the

realism A philosophical position arguing that there is a real world to sense.

positivism A philosophical position arguing that all we really have to go on is the evidence of the senses, so the world might be nothing more than an elaborate hallucination.

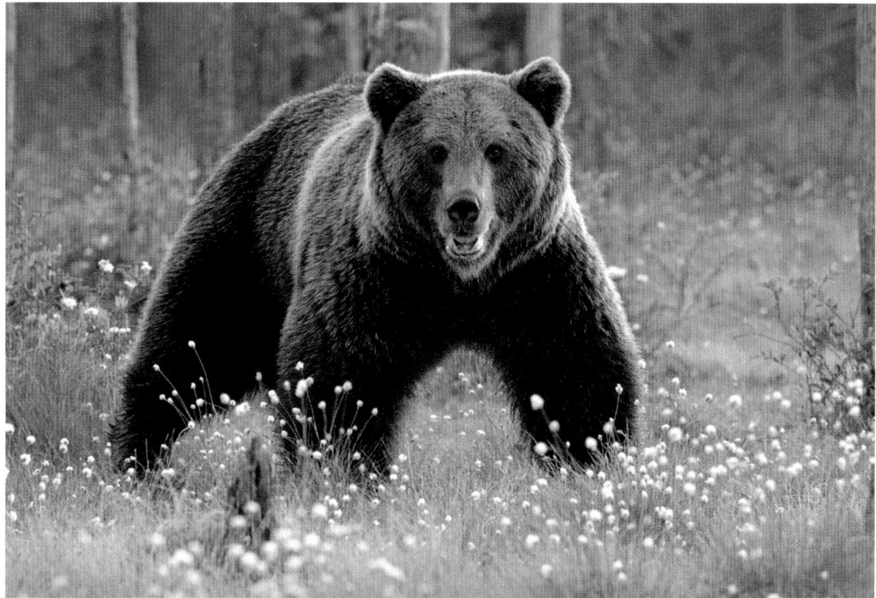

FIGURE 6.1 Bear necessities What do you do if the mother bear decides that you are in the wrong place?

eyeball. What all this means is that if we want to appreciate the three-dimensional world, we have to reconstruct it from the distorted retinal input.

To be more precise, as a general rule our visual experience is a reconstruction of the world based on two distorted inputs: the two distinct retinal images. Close your left eye, stretch your left arm out in front of you, and hold up your left index finger. Then hold up your right index finger about 6 inches in front of your face so that it appears to be positioned just to the left of the left index finger, as illustrated in **FIGURE 6.3**. Now quickly open your left eye and close your right eye. If you

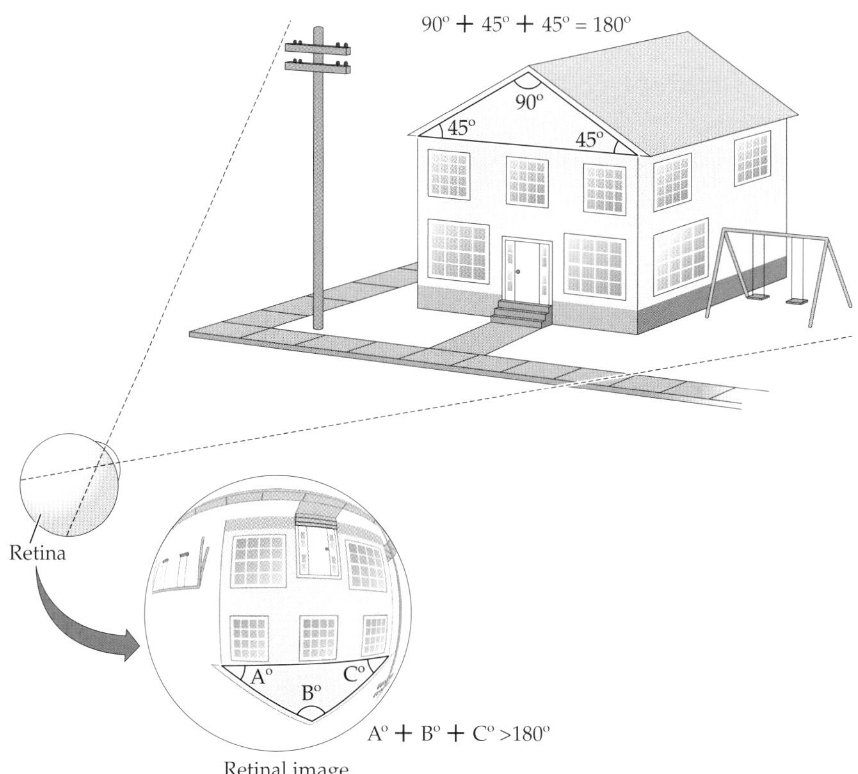

FIGURE 6.2 Geometries of visual space The Euclidean geometry of the three-dimensional world turns into something quite different on the curved, two-dimensional retina. In the Euclidean world, the angles of a triangle add up to 180 degrees. In the non-Euclidean world of the retinal image, this need not be so.

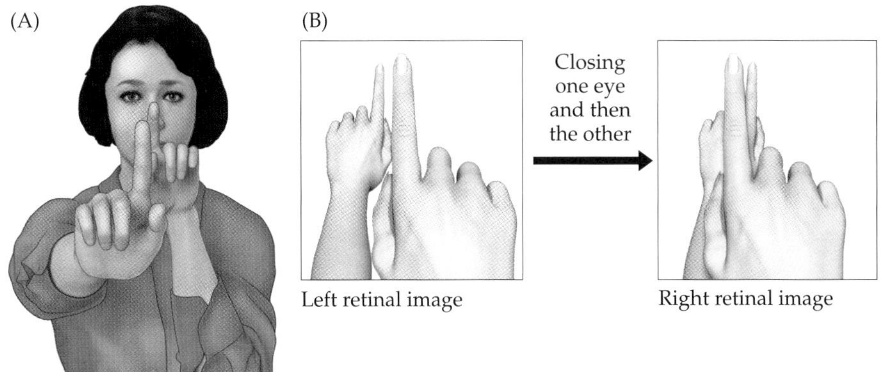

FIGURE 6.3 The two retinal images of a three-dimensional world are not the same You can demonstrate this by holding your fingers at different distances and closing first one eye and then the other, as described in the text.

positioned your fingers properly, your right finger will jump to the other side of your left finger. Although this demonstration is designed to exaggerate the different views of your two eyes, the point is a general one: the two retinal images always differ. They differ because your two eyeballs (and their two retinas) are in slightly different places in your head. Just as you and the person standing next to you see somewhat different views of the world, so do your two eyes. Much of this chapter will be devoted to explaining how the visual system goes to elaborate lengths both to exploit and to reconcile these differences.

Why have two eyes at all? Perhaps most fundamentally, having two eyes confers the same evolutionary advantage as having two lungs or two kidneys: you can lose one eye and still be able to see. A second advantage to doubling the number of eyes is that they enable you to see more of the world. This is especially true for animals like rabbits that have *lateral* eyes on the sides of their heads. A rabbit can actually see 360 degrees around its head (**FIGURE 6.4A**), which explains why it is so hard to sneak up on one. Moreover, the rabbit can also see straight up above its head

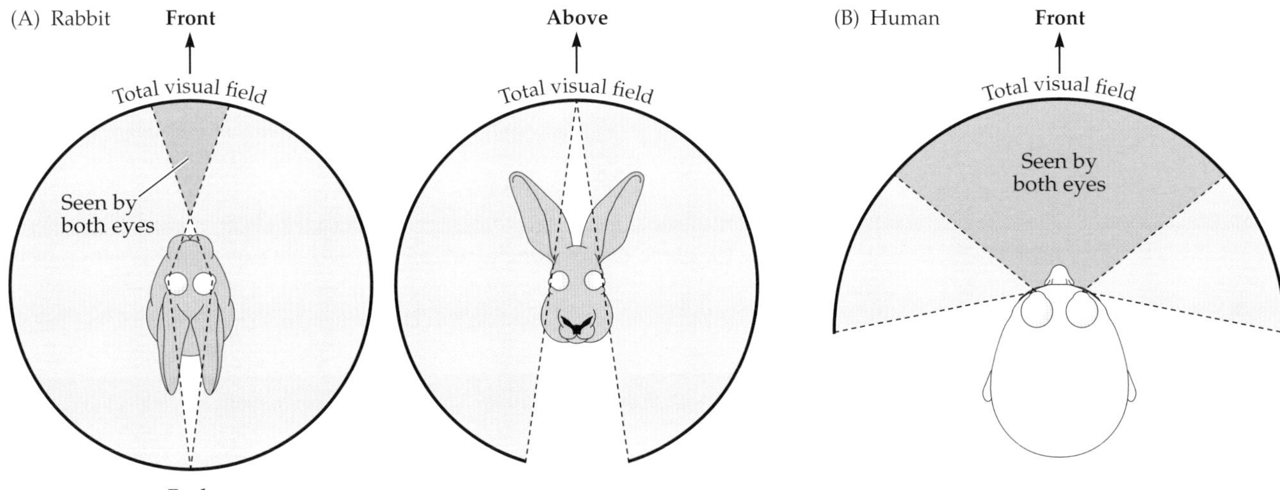

FIGURE 6.4 Comparing rabbit and human visual fields Light purple indicates the entire visual field and dark purple indicates the part of the visual field seen by both eyes. (A) A rabbit's lateral eyes can see all around its head. It can even see above its head, making its visual field something like a planetarium dome (with ears). (B) The human visual field is more like a windshield, covering a large region in front of the eyes.

binocular Referring to two eyes.

probability summation The increased detection probability based on the statistical advantage of having two (or more) detectors rather than one.

binocular summation The combination (or "summation") of signals from both eyes in ways that make performance on many tasks better than with either eye alone.

binocular disparity The differences between the two retinal images of the same scene. Disparity is the basis for stereopsis, a vivid perception of the three-dimensionality of the world that is not available with monocular vision.

monocular Referring to one eye.

stereopsis The ability to use binocular disparity as a cue to depth.

(Hughes, 1977)—a significant advantage for an animal that is hunted by birds of prey as well as by terrestrial predators.

Humans, with *frontal* eyes, still see more of the world with two eyes than with one. Our visual field is limited to about 190 degrees from left to right, 110 degrees of which is covered by both eyes (FIGURE 6.4B). The field is more restricted vertically: about 140 degrees, 60 degrees up to a limit defined by your eyebrows and 80 degrees down to your cheeks. The exact size of your visual field will be limited by the specific anatomy of your cheeks and eyebrows. Overlapping, frontal, **binocular** visual fields give predatory animals such as humans a better chance to spot small, fast-moving objects in front of them that might provide dinner. Prey animals like rabbits often have very wide visual fields, allowing them to monitor the whole scene for predators.

With frontal eyes and overlapping visual fields, you also get the advantage of two detectors looking at the same thing. For example, if two people each had a 50% chance of missing a target by themselves, the chance that both of them would miss it is 50% × 50% = 25%. So the chance that at least one of the two would *find* the target is 100% – 25%, or 75%. This is known as **probability summation**, and versions of it are used to improve the results in important tasks like breast cancer screening (Taylor-Phillips et al., 2018). Something similar happens if the two eyes both look for the same hard-to-see target. In vision, this would be called **binocular summation** (R. Blake, Sloane, and Fox, 1981). Binocular summation may have provided the evolutionary pressure that first moved eyes toward the front of some birds' and mammals' faces.

Under most circumstances, we do not get complete probability summation. The increase from a 50% chance to a 75% chance assumes two completely independent observers. Even two different people aren't completely independent, and the benefit you get from "double reading" will depend on a variety of factors, including how you combine the information from the two people (Corbett and Munneke, 2018). Certainly, our two eyes are not independent, because they are embedded in one person. Nevertheless, we can still do better at many tasks with two eyes than with just one (R. K. Jones and Lee, 1981).

Once the eyes had moved to the front, though, the overlapping visual fields provided another evolutionary advantage: the ability to use the slight differences between the eyes as a cue to three-dimensional depth. Try this: Take the top off a pen and hold the top in one hand and the pen in the other. Hold both about a foot in front of your face, with your elbows bent. Now, close one eye and try to quickly put the cap on the pen. Repeat the same task with both eyes open. For most (but not all) people, this task is easier with two eyes than with one. This is a quick demonstration of the usefulness of **binocular disparity**—the differences between the two retinal images of the same world. Disparity is the basis for a vivid perception of the three-dimensionality of the world that is not available with purely **monocular** (one-eyed) vision. The technical term for this binocular perception of a third dimension—depth—is **stereopsis**. The geometric and physiological bases for stereopsis are the topic of a large portion of this chapter (see also I. P. Howard and Rogers, 2001). Stereopsis is special in that it can provide very-high-resolution depth information in the absence of other cues (McKee, 1983).

When you decide you need a break from reading this chapter, take that break with one eye closed. You should be able to notice the loss of stereopsis (and of part of your visual field), but a period of one-eyed visual experience will also make it clear that stereopsis is not a necessary condition for depth or space perception. Rabbits do very well with very limited binocular vision, and painters and movie directors manage to convey realistic impressions of depth on flat canvases and movie screens.

However, stereopsis does add a richness to perception of the three-dimensional world, as vividly described by Oliver Sacks (2006) in his article about "Stereo Sue," a neuroscientist who regained stereopsis at the age of 48. We will talk about her later.

In this chapter, first we describe the set of **monocular depth cues** to three-dimensional space. After that, we turn to the more complicated topic of binocular stereopsis, a **binocular depth cue**. Finally, we consider how the various cues are combined to produce a unified perception of space.

monocular depth cue A depth cue that is available even when the world is viewed with one eye alone.

binocular depth cue A depth cue that relies on information from both eyes. Stereopsis is the primary example in humans, but convergence and the ability of two eyes to see more of an object than one eye sees are also binocular depth cues.

pictorial depth cue A cue to distance or depth used by artists to depict three-dimensional depth in two-dimensional pictures.

6.1 Monocular Cues to Three-Dimensional Space

The Dutch graphic artist M. C. Escher (1898–1972) was a master of the rules that govern our perception of space. In his 1953 work titled *Relativity*, shown in FIGURE 6.5, each bit of stairway, each landing, every person, is cleverly drawn using cues that enable us to infer three dimensions from two. But when we try to follow those stairs, we find that Escher's drawing fails to add up to a coherent representation of a place that could exist. Escher is playing tricks with us, but even when no one is trying to fool us, it is geometrically impossible for the visual system to create a perfectly faithful reconstruction of the true layout of space, given the distorted, two-dimensional input we receive through each eye. The best we can do is to use depth cues to infer aspects of the three-dimensional world from our two-dimensional retinal images. On the basis of the retinal images and an implicit understanding of physics and geometry, we collect cues that provide hints about the likely structure of the space in front of us and the disposition of objects in that space.

Unless we're stuck in an extremely impoverished perceptual environment (say, the Sahara during a sandstorm), every view of the world provides multiple depth cues. Usually the cues reinforce each other, combining to produce a convincing and reliable representation of the three-dimensional world. What cues does the visual system use to infer depth relations, and how do we use those cues to create a representation of the three-dimensional world?

Pictorial Depth Cues

Artists have long used clever tricks to depict depth in their paintings. These are known as **pictorial depth cues**. These cues work because they are the natural consequence of the projection of the three-dimensional world onto the two-dimensional surface of the retina. A realistic picture or photograph is the result of projecting the three-dimensional world onto the two-dimensional surface of film or canvas. When we look at the image from the correct position, the retinal image (in one eye, at least) formed by the two-dimensional picture will be the same as the retinal image that would have been formed by the three-dimensional world, and hence, we see depth in the picture. In theory, this means that a picture should look correct from only one, very precise viewing position. In fact, pictures look reasonable over quite a range of views. Were this not so, there would be only one good seat in the movie theater. As we will now discuss, pictorial depth cues include occlusion, size and position cues, and perspective cues.

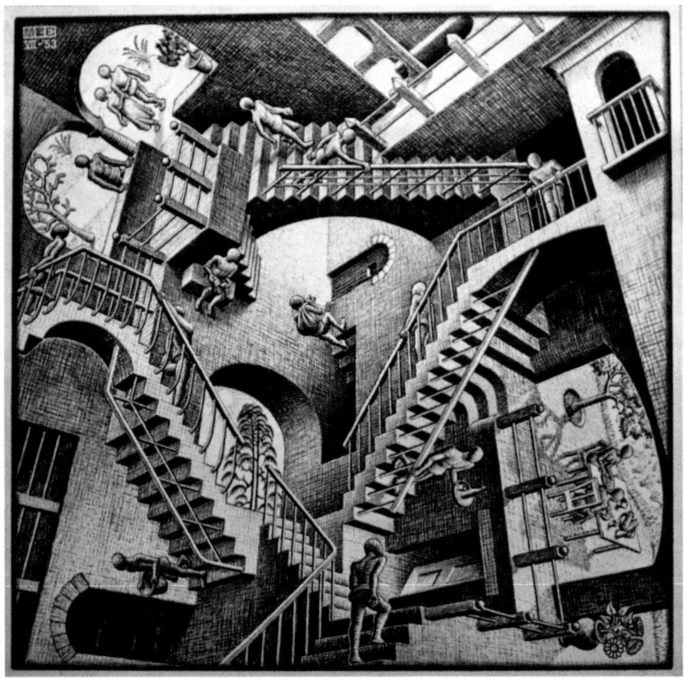

FIGURE 6.5 **M. C. Escher, *Relativity*, 1953** Escher deploys monocular cues to depth in a way that is essentially correct at each location, but these local cues add up to an impossible world.

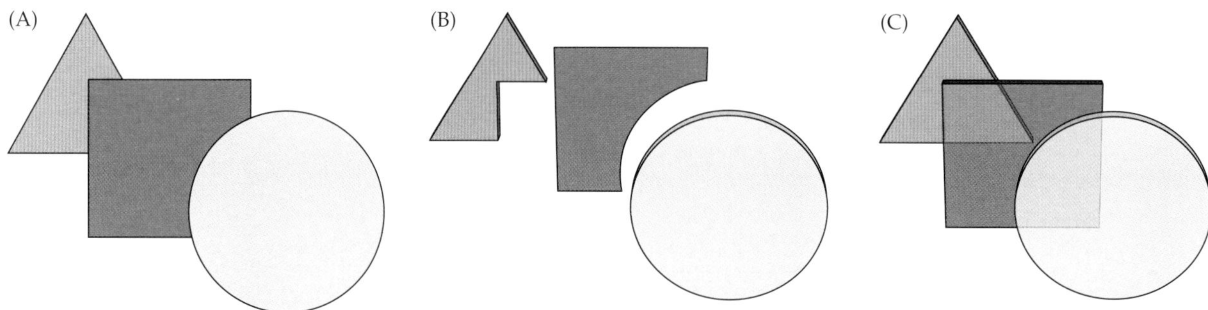

FIGURE 6.6 Accidental versus generic views Occlusion makes it easy to infer relative position in depth. (A) could be an "accidental" view of the pieces shown in (B). It is much more likely, however, that (A) is a generic view of circle, square, and triangle, as shown in (C).

occlusion A cue to relative depth order in which, for example, one object obstructs the view of part of another object.

nonmetrical depth cue A depth cue that provides information about the depth order (relative depth) but not depth magnitude (e.g., his nose is in front of his face).

metrical depth cue A depth cue that provides quantitative information about distance in the third dimension.

projective geometry For purposes of studying perception of the three-dimensional world, the geometry that describes the transformations that occur when the three-dimensional world is projected onto a two-dimensional surface. For example, parallel lines do not converge in the real world, but they do in the two-dimensional projection of that world.

Occlusion

Some of the cues to the layout of the three-dimensional world were introduced earlier in this book, because hints to the layout of space can also be hints about the structure of objects in that space. **Occlusion** is an example (see "Finding Edges" in Section 4.4). In Chapter 4, occlusion was a cue to the presence of an otherwise invisible edge. As a depth cue, occlusion gives information about the relative position of objects. Thus, in **FIGURE 6.6A**, we are happy to infer a circle in front of a square in front of a triangle. Occlusion is present in almost every visual scene (we challenge you to find a situation in normal life where nothing blocks your view of anything else), and many researchers argue that it is the most reliable of all the depth cues. It is misleading only in the case of "accidental viewpoints" (remember those from Section 4.4?). That is, the retinal image shown in Figure 6.6A could be produced by a circle and two oddly shaped puzzle pieces, as shown in **FIGURE 6.6B**. That scenario would require careful placement of the objects and the viewer. It is much more likely that Figure 6.6A would arise from a more generic view of a circle occluding a square occluding a triangle (**FIGURE 6.6C**).

We do not know from the occlusion cue alone whether the purple square in Figure 6.6A is in front of a small green triangle, a larger but more distant triangle (maybe a green tree), or an even larger, more distant green mountain. Occlusion is a **nonmetrical depth cue**; it just gives us the relative orderings of occluders and occludees. A **metrical depth cue** is one that does provide information about distance in the third dimension.

Size and Position Cues

The image on the retina formed by an object out in the world gets smaller as the object gets farther away. Moreover, your visual system knew this fact of **projective geometry** implicitly before you ever picked up this book and learned it explicitly. Projective geometry describes how the world is projected onto a surface. For example, a shadow is a projection of an object onto a surface. An implicit (nonconscious) understanding of the rules of projective geometry can be said to lie behind many of the depth cues described here. In this case, the visual system knows that, all else being equal, smaller things are farther away. To create **FIGURE 6.7A**, David McIntyre made a set of red balls of different sizes and placed them on a black surface. The depth cue of relative size makes them seem to form and arc in depth. We assume the little spheres are farther away. That assumption is added by the structure of Figure 6.7A. The effect is weaker in **FIGURE 6.7B**, where the balls are scattered more randomly.

FIGURE 6.7 **Depth from size** (A) This is a photograph of different-size red balls resting on the same flat surface at the same distance from the camera. Nevertheless, the small ones appear to be farther away. Some portion of the visual system assumes that all of these items are the same size. If one ball projects a smaller image on the retina, and if we assume that the balls really are the same size, then the smaller one must be farther away. This is the cue of relative size. (B) The effect is weaker if the balls are randomly scattered. The structure in (A) reinforces the appearance of depth.

(A)

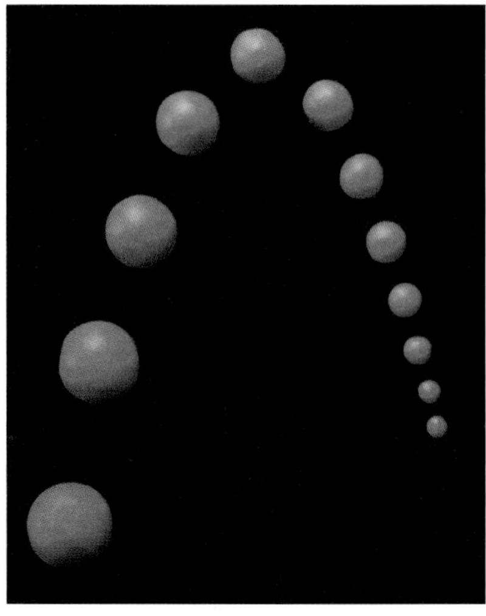

(B)

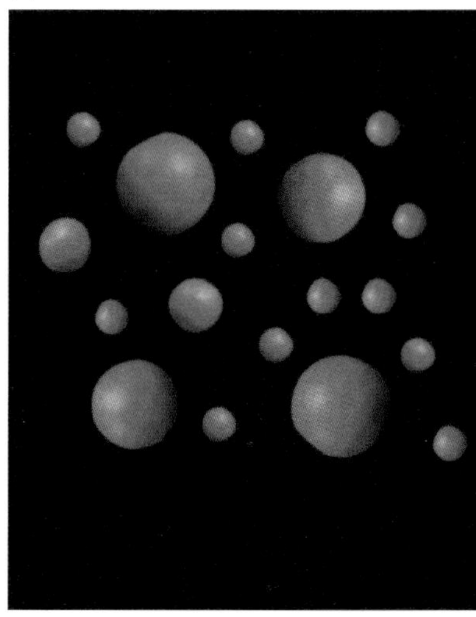

The impression of three-dimensionality returns in FIGURE 6.8 because we've added another cue. Here, the rabbits form an orderly **texture gradient**, with larger objects in one area and smaller objects in another. Because smaller is interpreted as farther away, this arrangement creates the perception of a ground plane receding into the distance.

In FIGURE 6.9, the rabbits are again arrayed in an orderly texture, but here we get less of a sense of depth. The difference between Figures 6.8 and 6.9 is that, while both form texture gradients, Figure 6.8 includes a depth cue that is not present in Figure 6.9: **relative height**. Imagine that you're actually standing in a field of rabbits. Consider the rabbit at your feet (FIGURE 6.10). It will project its image in your lower visual field. The smaller image of a more distant rabbit will be projected higher in your visual field. Here, then, is another geometric regularity, produced by projective geometry, that the visual system can exploit. If you have a set of objects lying on the ground plane, objects that are more distant in the world will be higher in the visual field. Indeed, Ooi, Wu, and He (2001) have shown that humans use the angle between the horizon and an object to judge that object's distance.

Texture fields that provide an impression of three-dimensionality are really combinations of **relative size** and relative height cues. Remember the metaphor of "perceptual committees" introduced in Section 4.4? Different modules in the visual system perform different tasks. The brain then combines the outputs to come up with a committee-like decision about the state of the world. In the case of a texture field, multiple cues interact to produce a final perception. FIGURE 6.11 shows how this interaction can give rise to a size illusion. The rabbit at the upper left of the figure is the same physical size on the page as the rabbit at the lower right, but the one at the bottom looks smaller to most of us than the one at the top. Why? We

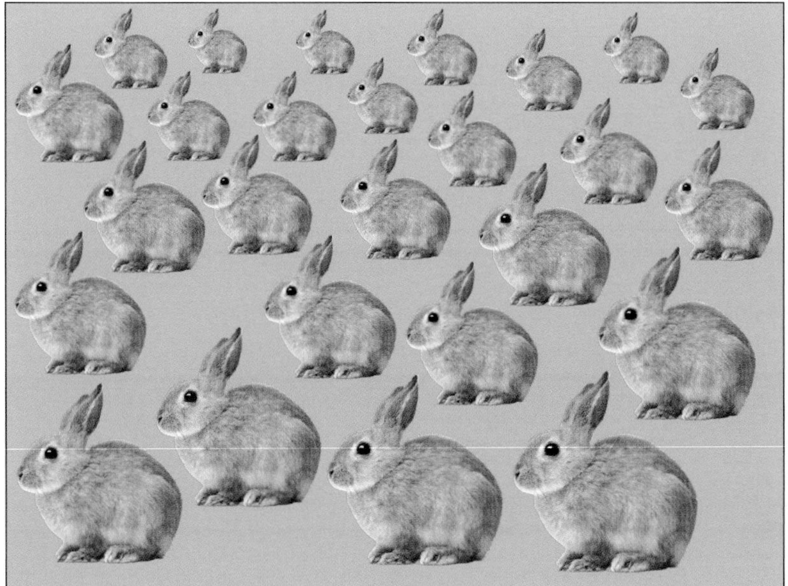

FIGURE 6.8 **Texture gradient** This rabbit texture gradient shows that the size cue is more effective when size changes systematically.

texture gradient A depth cue based on the geometric fact that items of the same size form smaller images when they are farther away. An array of items that change in size smoothly across the image will appear to form a surface tilted in depth.

relative height As a depth cue, the observation that objects at different distances from the viewer on the ground plane will form images at different heights in the retinal image. Objects farther away will be seen as higher in the image.

relative size A comparison of size between items without knowing the absolute size of either one.

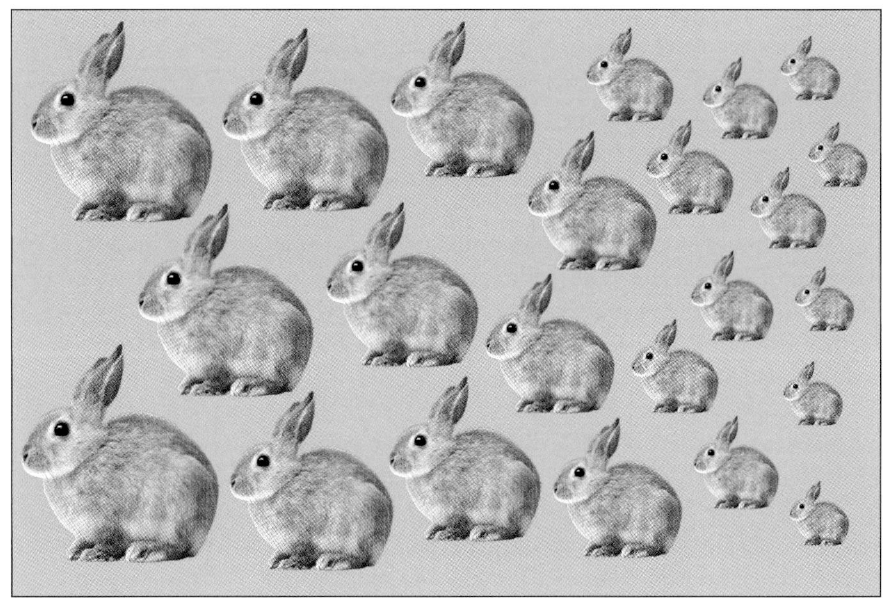

FIGURE 6.9 Texture gradients, continued Organized differently, the same rabbits as those shown in Figure 6.8 do not produce the same sense of depth. A size cue is most effective when it is consistent with objects arranged on the ground, not on a wall.

infer, on the basis of relative height, that the rabbit at the bottom must be closer. If it is closer and it forms an image of the same size as the little rabbit at the top, it follows that the little rabbit at the bottom must be really little.

If we know what size something *ought* to be, that knowledge can be a depth cue in its own right. We infer that the woman in **FIGURE 6.12A** is holding her hand out at the end of an outstretched arm. Why do we make this guess? One alternative is that she's holding her hand near her shoulder, as she is in **FIGURE 6.12B**. But if that were the case in Figure 6.12A, the hand would need to be a *very* big hand. Here, our knowledge of the normal relationship of hand size to head size makes all the difference. This is the depth cue of **familiar size**.

familiar size A depth cue based on knowledge of the typical sizes of objects, such as humans or pennies.

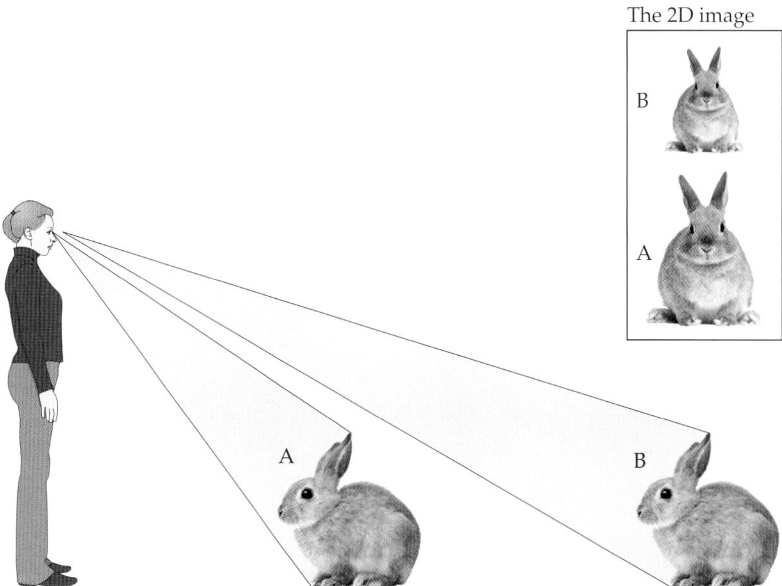

FIGURE 6.10 Relative height as a cue to depth If we're looking down at the ground plane, the image of a closer rabbit will lie above the image of a farther rabbit in the two-dimensional retinal image. Because the image is inverted, the closer rabbit lies lower in the visual field than the farther rabbit.

Recall that occlusion is a nonmetrical cue, providing only depth *order*. The relative size and relative height cues, especially taken together, provide some metrical information. This is illustrated in **FIGURE 6.13**, where the three balls appear to lie at measurable distances from each other. The blue ball seems closer to the red ball than to the green ball in depth, for example. Relative size and height do not tell us the *exact* distance to an object or between objects. These are **relative metrical depth cues**. Familiar size, however, could be an **absolute metrical depth cue**. If your visual system knew the actual size of an object and the visual angle of the object's projection on the retina, it could (at least in theory) calculate the exact distance from object to eye. In practice, however, even if you know that your friend is 5 feet 10 inches tall, the visual system does not seem to know that fact with a precision that would let you know he's standing exactly 12 feet away.

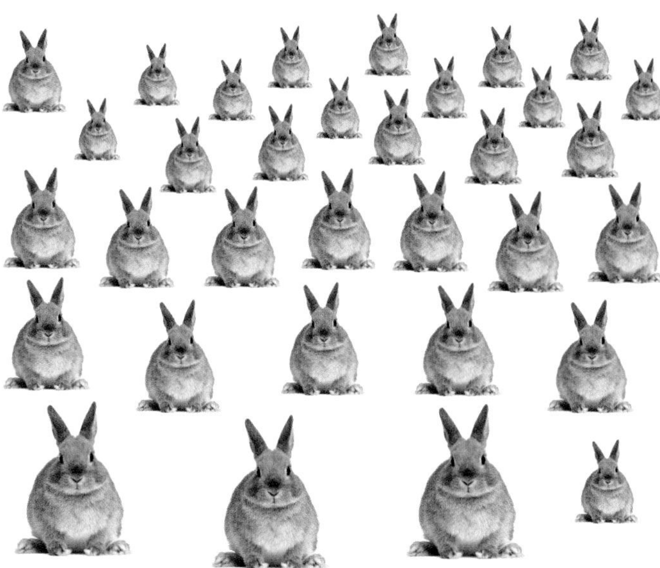

FIGURE 6.11 Apparent size is changed by apparent depth The rabbit image at the top far left is the same size as the one at the bottom far right. If they don't seem the same size, then you have been fooled by the depth cues.

Aerial Perspective

In addition to its implicit knowledge of geometry and its learned knowledge of familiar size, the visual system "knows" about properties of the atmosphere. Specifically, the depth cue known as **haze,** or **aerial perspective**, is based on an implicit understanding that light is scattered by the atmosphere and that more light is scattered when we look through more atmosphere. Thus, objects farther away are subject to more scatter and appear fainter and less distinct. Short wavelengths (blue) are scattered more than medium and long wavelengths (see Figure 2.1B). This is why the sky looks blue and why objects farther away look not only hazy but also bluish. **FIGURE 6.14** shows a real-world example. By now, it should be clear that the depth, seen in this image, is the product of multiple depth cues, such as occlusion and the known size of boats, in addition to bluish distant mountains that illustrate the aerial perspective cue.

Linear Perspective

It would not be difficult to imagine the six lines in **FIGURE 6.15** to be a sketch of the view out the windshield of a car moving down a road in a flat landscape. The depth cue in this case is **linear perspective**, which is based on the rules

relative metrical depth cue A depth cue that could specify, for example, that object A is twice as far away as object B without providing information about the absolute distance to either A or B.

absolute metrical depth cue A depth cue that provides quantifiable information about distance in the third dimension (e.g., his nose sticks out 4 centimeters in front of his face).

haze or aerial perspective A depth cue based on the implicit understanding that light is scattered by the atmosphere. More light is scattered when we look through more atmosphere. Thus, more distant objects are subject to more scatter and appear fainter, bluer, and less distinct.

linear perspective A depth cue based on the fact that lines that are parallel in the three-dimensional world will appear to converge in a two-dimensional image.

(A)

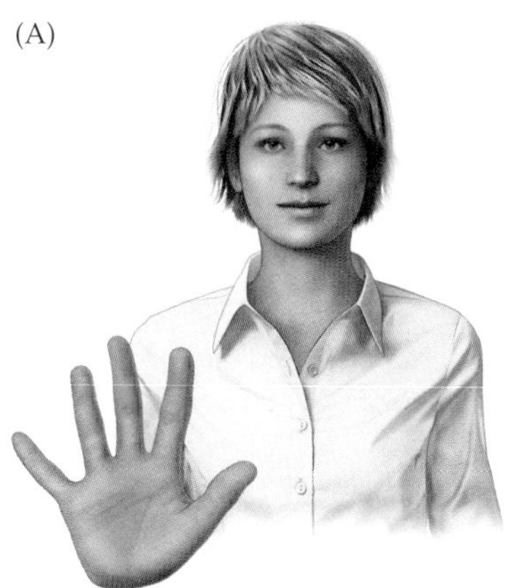

(B)

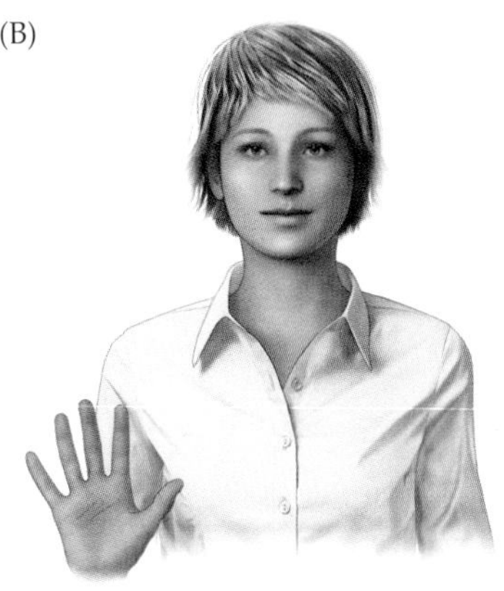

FIGURE 6.12 The cue of familiar size The hand in (A) looks closer than the one in (B) because we know how big hands should be relative to heads.

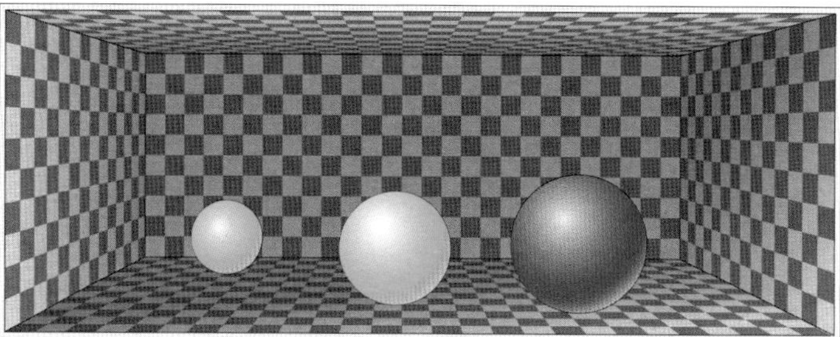

FIGURE 6.13 Metrical depth cues The metrical cues of relative size and height can give the visual system more information than a nonmetrical cue like occlusion can. Not only does the red sphere in this image appear to be closest and the green sphere farthest away, but the blue sphere is seen to be closer in depth to the red sphere than to the green sphere.

that determine how lines in three-dimensional space are projected onto a two-dimensional image. The core piece of projective geometry in this case is that lines that are parallel in the three-dimensional world will appear to converge in the two-dimensional image, except when the parallel lines lie in a plane that is parallel to the plane of the two-dimensional image. Artists of the Italian Renaissance are said to have "discovered" linear perspective. That is not quite right; your dog or cat knows about linear perspective. What Renaissance artists discovered was how to make the rules explicit, write them down, and turn linear perspective into a method for generating realistic depth in otherwise flat paintings.

Filippo di Ser Brunellesco (1377–1446) is typically given credit for bringing linear perspective into European art. Leon Battista Alberti (1404–1474) wrote the first book on the topic in 1435 (Alberti, 1970). **FIGURE 6.16** shows an example of what could be done. Painted around 1477, *Architectural View* by Francesco di Giorgio Martini (from the Italian city of Siena) is not the greatest work of Renaissance art, but it demonstrates the artist's use of the basic rules of linear perspective. Parallel lines in the image plane, like the two front center pillars, would be parallel in the

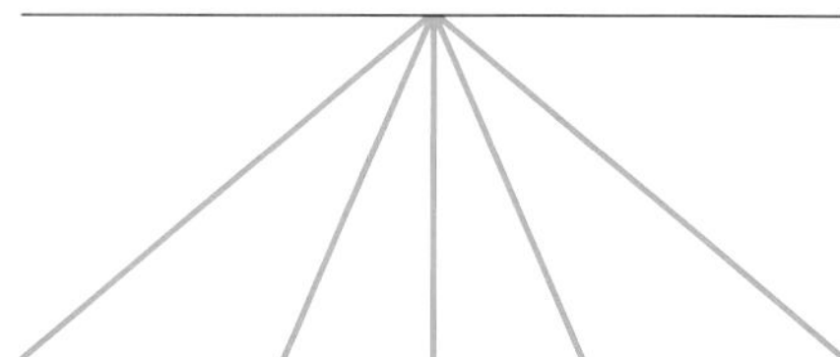

FIGURE 6.15 Linear perspective If we titled this image "Driving across Kansas," you would understand, because the converging lines give the impression of parallel lines receding toward the horizon.

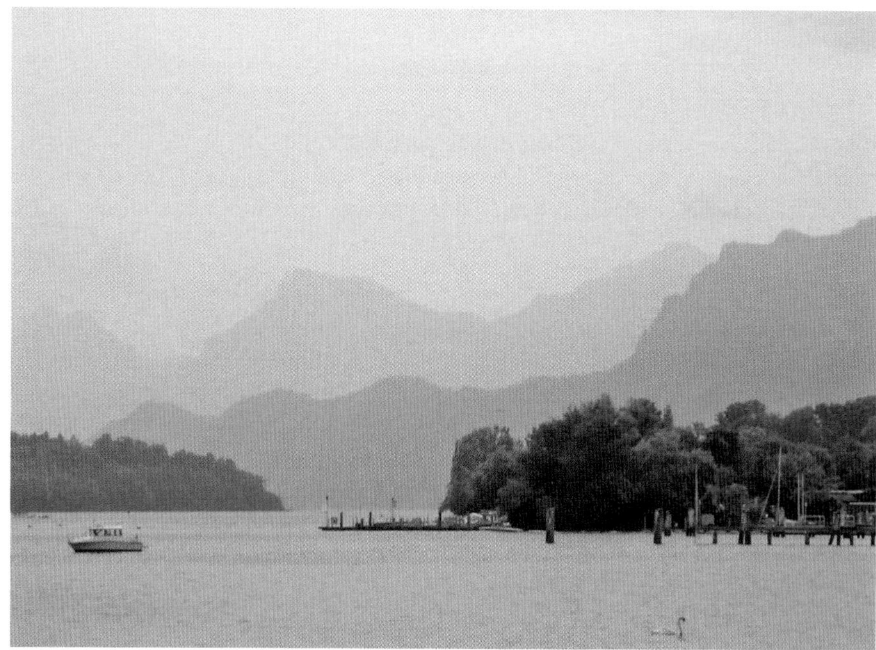

FIGURE 6.14 A real-world example of aerial perspective Scattering of light by the atmosphere makes more-distant features appear hazy and blue.

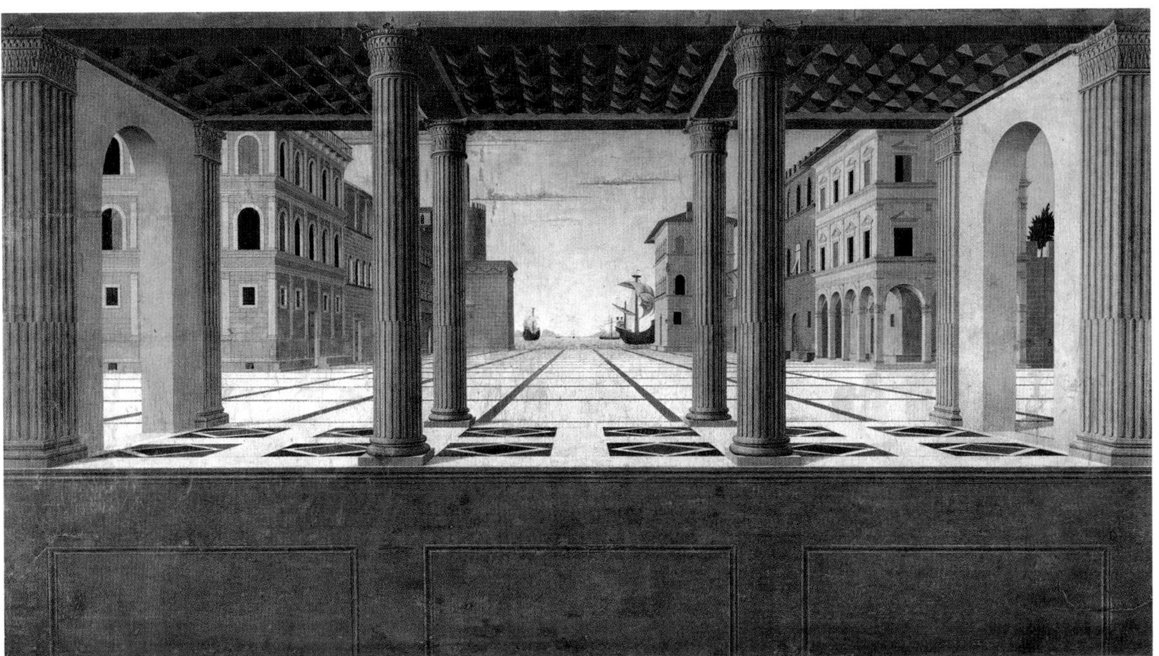

FIGURE 6.16 Linear perspective in art *Architectural View* by Francesco di Giorgio Martini (1477), a very clear example of linear perspective. Parallel lines in the image plane, such as the pillars at the front center, remain parallel in the image. Parallel lines that would recede in depth in the three-dimensional world converge to a single vanishing point in the two-dimensional image.

world. Look at all those other lines converging toward a **vanishing point**. Clearly, these are intended to show the parallel lines on the ground or on the sides of buildings running in depth. You can see occlusion, size, and texture cues at work, too.

vanishing point The apparent point at which parallel lines receding in depth converge.

In the real world, there isn't just one vanishing point (somewhere out in the harbor of Figure 6.16). The vanishing point will move as you move your eyes and head. This can be captured in a painting by having more than one vanishing point, as can be seen in **FIGURE 6.17** in a painting by Canaletto (1697–1768).

Seeing Depth in Pictures

To correctly interpret the shapes of three-dimensional objects from two-dimensional pictures, people take the orientation of the flat surface of the image into account. This allows them to understand that the picture is, in fact, a picture and not the real thing; at the same time, they can calculate an accurate impression of the thing that is portrayed (Vishwanath, Girshik, and Banks, 2005). To illustrate this point, **FIGURE 6.18A** is a photo of one of this book's authors standing alongside a picture of himself; here the "picture in the picture" appears reasonable. In **FIGURE 6.18B**, the same picture, stripped of its context, appears quite distorted. In Figure 6.18A, our visual system can compensate for

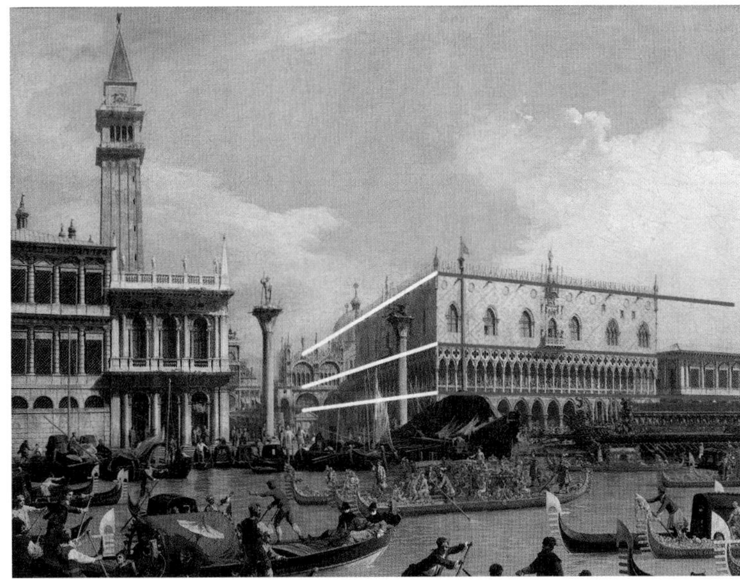

FIGURE 6.17 Two-point perspective *Bucentaur's Return to the Pier by the Palazzo Ducale* by Canaletto (1697–1768) is an example of two-point perspective. The pink and yellow lines are added to make the three vanishing points clear.

(A)

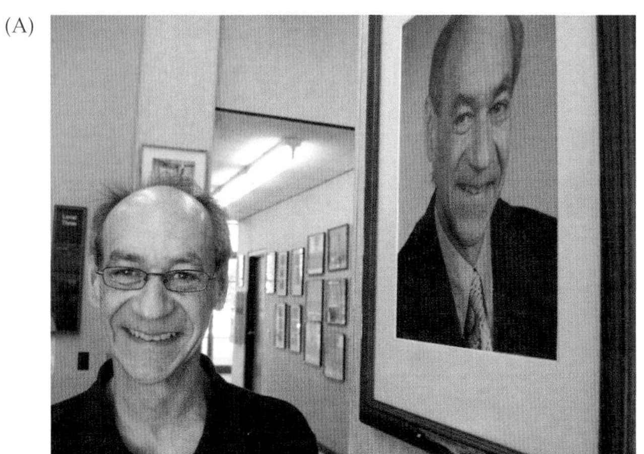

(B)

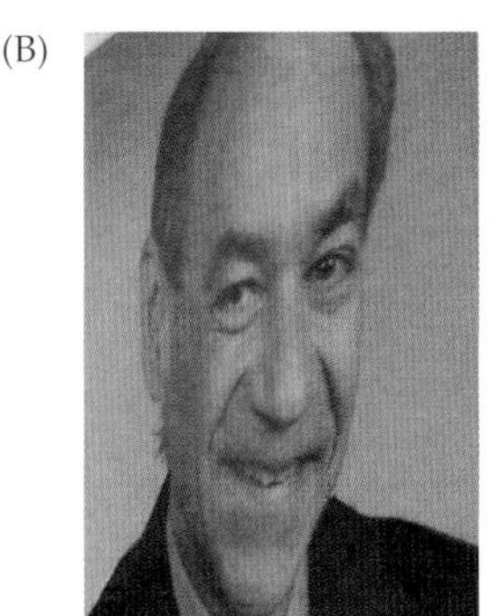

FIGURE 6.18 **Picture in a picture** (A) One of the authors, Dennis Levi, is seen standing next to a photograph of himself. In this panel, the "picture in the picture" appears reasonable. (B) The framed picture, isolated without the context. Does the picture appear distorted?

the perceptual distortion because there is enough context to enable the viewer to attribute the distortion to the slant of the picture surface.

The technique known as **anamorphosis**, or **anamorphic projection**, illustrates that our ability to cope with distortion is limited. In anamorphic projection, the rules of linear perspective are pushed to an extreme. Now the projection of three dimensions into two dimensions creates a two-dimensional image that is recognizable only from an unusual vantage point (or sometimes with a curved mirror). The results are known as anamorphic art. As an example, there is an odd diagonal smear in the lower center of Hans Holbein's sixteenth-century painting *The Ambassadors* (FIGURE 6.19A). If you could put your eye in exactly the right position to view the image, the smear would prove to be the skull shown in FIGURE 6.19B. Despite its successful recovery of the shapes in Figure 6.18A, the visual system cannot use knowledge about surface orientation to compensate for the distortion in Figure 6.19. In our own day, the sidewalk chalk artist Julian Beever creates amazing anamorphic images that look spectacularly real from the right vantage point and spectacularly distorted from elsewhere (FIGURE 6.20).

6.2 Triangulation Cues to Three-Dimensional Space

Beyond the pictorial depth cues, a number of additional sources of information are available to our visual system when we view real-world scenes—cues that cannot be reproduced in a static two-dimensional picture. We refer to these as **triangulation** cues because they arise from the viewing of the image from different vantage points. These cues can be either monocular (motion parallax and focus) or binocular (convergence and stereopsis).

(A)

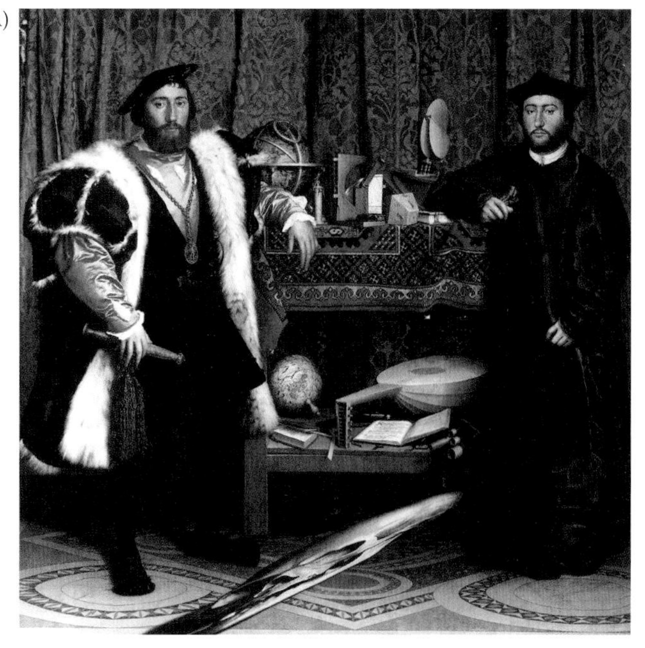

(B)

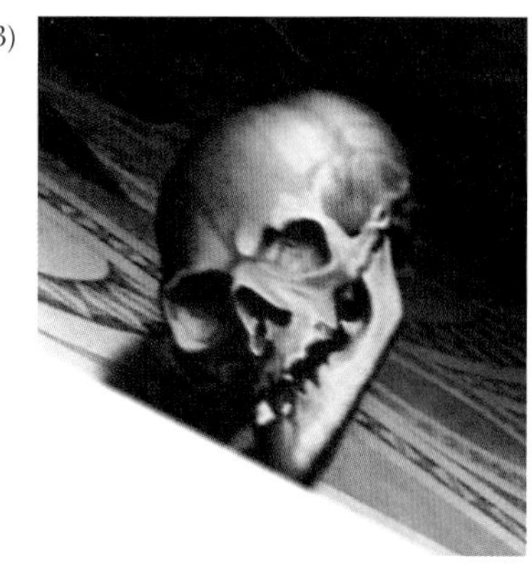

FIGURE 6.19 **Anamorphic art** In 1533, Hans Holbein painted the double portrait in (A) with an odd object (B) at the feet of the two men.

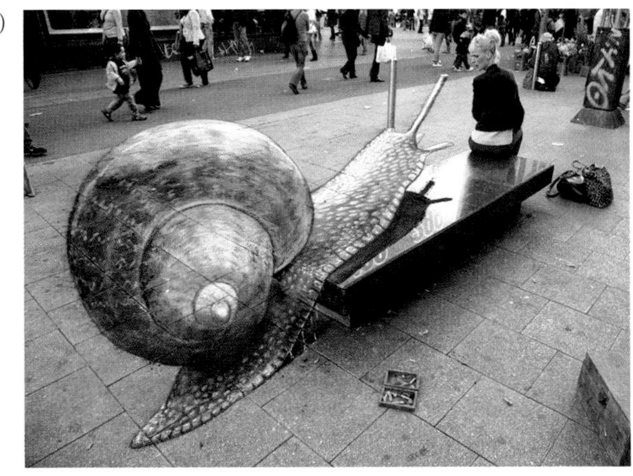

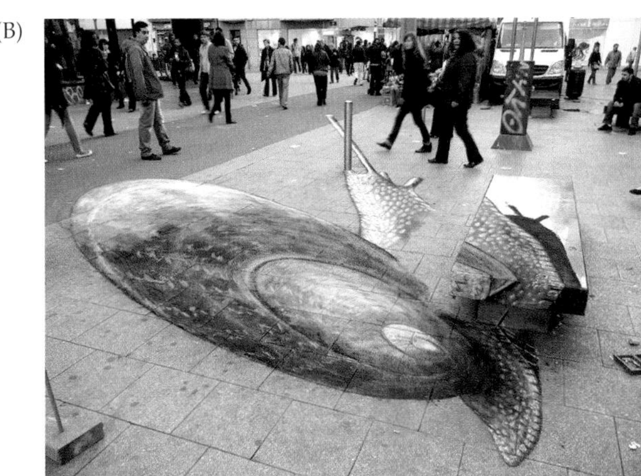

FIGURE 6.20 Modern-day anamorphic art (A) In this photograph, artist Julian Beever creates what appears to be a large three-dimensional version of a snail. (B) From this angle, we can see this is a clever bit of anamorphic art—a flat image that looks three-dimensional when viewed from the correct position.

Motion Cues

The first triangulation cue we will discuss is **motion parallax**. Motion parallax allows you to see the world from multiple viewpoints at different times by moving your head. To appreciate its power (and to understand why photographs of the forest often don't come out well), the best thing to do is to go outside and lie under a tree. Gaze up into the branches and leaves with one eye covered and your head stationary. You will notice that leaves and branches form a relatively flat texture. You can see all the details, but you may have trouble deciding whether one little branch lies in front of or behind another. If you open the other eye, stereopsis (introduced earlier and discussed in detail later in the chapter) will allow the branches and leaves to fill out a three-dimensional volume that was lacking before. Close the eye and the volume collapses again. Now move your head from side to side, and motion parallax will restore some of this sense of depth.

How does motion provide a cue for depth? Suppose you're sitting on a train, looking out the window at the countryside. At one instant you see the scene sketched in **FIGURE 6.21A**. A moment later, the scene has changed to the one in **FIGURE 6.21B**.

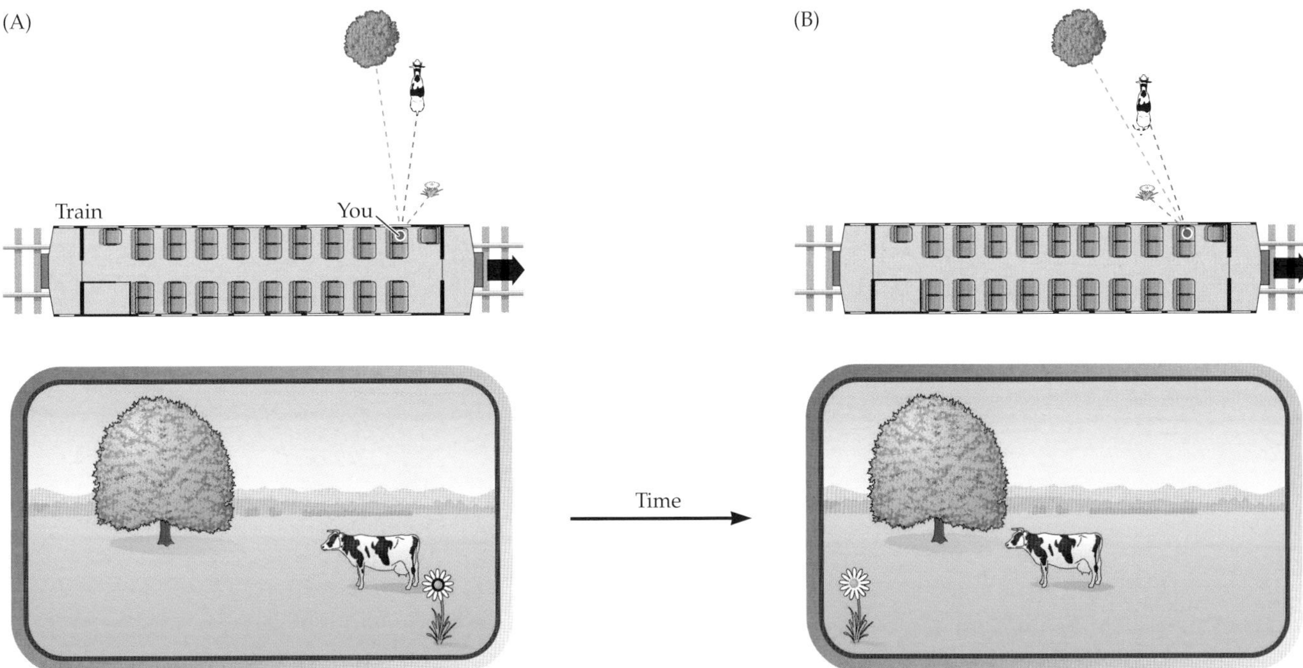

FIGURE 6.21 Motion parallax As you look out the window of a moving train, objects closer to you (like the flower in this illustration) shift position more quickly than do objects farther away (the tree) from one moment (A) to the next (B). This regularity can be exploited as a depth cue.

Notice that as your train moved from left to right in the figure, all the objects shifted from right to left. But note that some things shifted more than others. The flower moved almost all the way across your retinal image, the cow moved a much shorter distance, and the tree hardly changed position at all. The term *parallax* refers to the geometric relationship revealed here: when you change your viewpoint while rolling down the tracks, objects closer to you shift position more than objects farther away. Of course, you don't need to be on a train to experience motion parallax; just moving your head will do. The geometric information obtained from an eye in two different positions at two different times (motion parallax) is similar to the information from two eyes in different positions in the head at the same time (binocular stereopsis) (Durgin et al., 1995; Rogers and Collett, 1989).

Motion parallax provides relative metrical information about how far away objects are. As the experiment with the tree branches demonstrates, it can provide a compelling sense of depth in certain situations in which other cues are not very effective. The downside of motion parallax is that it works only if the head moves (just moving the eyes back and forth won't do, as you can easily prove to yourself). Now you know why a cat might bob its head back and forth as it plans a spectacular leap from the sofa to the table.

Other motion signals produce information about depth. For example, objects get bigger and smaller as they get closer and farther away, so an object that is simply getting bigger on a screen can appear to be looming toward you. If everything is looming at once in a large field, this **optic flow** may make you feel like you are moving toward the screen rather than like the objects on the screen are moving toward you. These topics are discussed in more detail in Chapter 8.

Accommodation and Convergence

Like a camera, the eyes need to be focused to see objects at different distances clearly. As we learned in Section 2.2, the human eye focuses via a process called **accommodation**, in which the lens gets fatter as we direct our gaze toward nearer objects (see Figure 2.3). We also need to point our eyes differently to focus on objects at different distances. As the schematic eyeballs in **FIGURE 6.22** move from the red dot to the blue dot, they rotate inward—a process called **convergence**

anamorphosis or anamorphic projection Use of the rules of linear perspective to create a two-dimensional image so distorted that it looks correct only when viewed from a special angle or with a mirror that counters the distortion.

triangulation In vision, this refers to the triangle formed by the two eyes and the point on which they fixate in the three-dimensional world. The angles of that triangle are related to the location of the fixated point in depth.

motion parallax An important depth cue that is based on head movement. The geometric information obtained from an eye in two different positions at two different times is similar to the information from two eyes in different positions in the head at the same time.

optic flow The pattern of apparent motion of objects in a visual scene produced by the relative motion between the observer and the scene.

accommodation The process by which the eye changes its focus (in which the lens gets fatter as gaze is directed toward nearer objects).

convergence The ability of the two eyes to turn inward, often used to place the two images of a feature in the world on corresponding locations in the two retinal images (typically on the fovea of each eye). Convergence reduces the disparity of that feature to zero (or nearly zero).

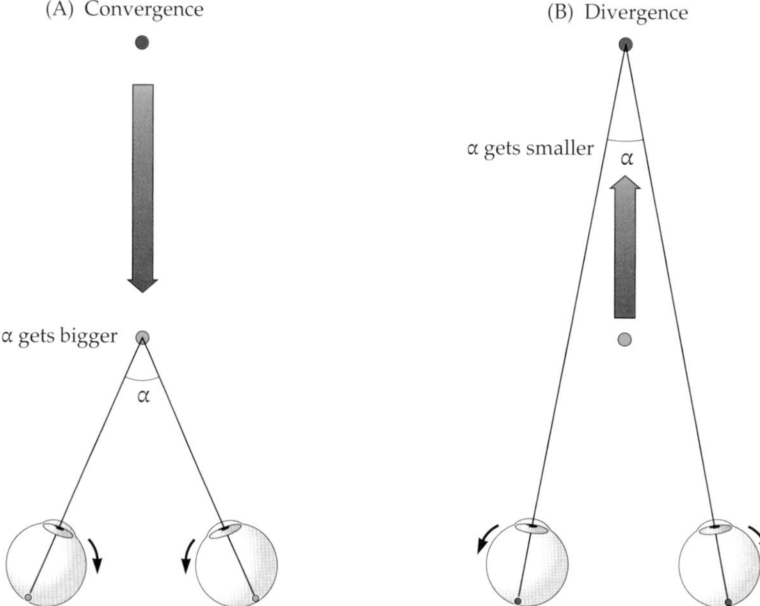

FIGURE 6.22 Vergence (A) As we shift focus from a far to a near point, our eyes converge. (B) As we go from near to far, the eyes diverge. The size of this vergence angle (labeled α) is a cue to depth.

(Figure 6.22A). Refocusing on the red dot would require rotation outward, which is known as **divergence** (Figure 6.22B). The angle, alpha, in Figure 6.22 is called the **vergence angle**.

In principle, focus cues can enable us to see depth because we see the image from various points across the pupil. If we could monitor our state of accommodation and/or the extent to which our eyes were converged, we could use this information as a cue to the depth of the object we were trying to bring into focus: the more we have to converge and the more the lens has to bulge in order to focus on the object, the closer it is. In fact, we do use this information. For example, D. M. Hoffman and Banks (2010) showed that depth discrimination improves when the focus is correct. However, when we focus on objects more than 2 or 3 meters away, the lens is as thin as it can get and the eyes are diverged about as much as possible, so neither cue provides much useful information. But studies have shown that the visual system takes advantage of both cues for objects closer than this limit. Convergence is used more than accommodation (Fisher and Ciuffreda, 1988; Owens, 1987). Moreover, in principle these cues can tell us the exact distance to an object. However, humans are not particularly precise about measuring the exact angles shown in Figure 6.22. Chameleons, however, do use the absolute metrical depth information from convergence to catch prey insects with their sticky tongues. Harkness (1977) showed this by fitting a chameleon with glasses that distorted the angle of convergence. The result was that the poor chameleon flicked out its tongue to the wrong distance and missed its intended dinner.

Interestingly, the pattern of blur can tell us something about the size of the space we are looking at. If you look at **FIGURE 6.23A**, you will see an aerial view of a train. At that distance, accommodation doesn't do much work. If one distant object is in focus, they will all be in focus. However, if we artificially blur the image (**FIGURE 6.23B**), something interesting happens. The visual system notices that the blue train car is in focus but things farther away and closer are not. Normally, that can only happen if the blue car is quite close to the viewer. If it is close, it must be small. Now, the scene looks like a toy train set. Blur is telling you about the size of the space (Held et al., 2010; Hafri, Wadhwa, and Bonner, 2022).

Artist Adrian Borda is playing with our estimation of space in **FIGURE 6.24**. Here, everything is in focus, so that pillar and that far wall must be quite far away,

divergence The ability of the two eyes to turn outward, often used to place the two images of a feature in the world on corresponding locations in the two retinal images (typically on the fovea of each eye). Divergence reduces the disparity of that feature to zero (or nearly zero).

vergence angle The angle formed by lines from each eye to the current object of fixation. A larger vergence angle implies a closer object.

(A)

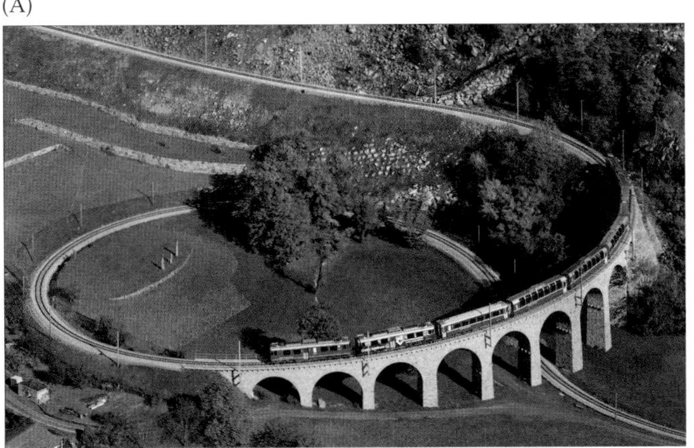

(B)

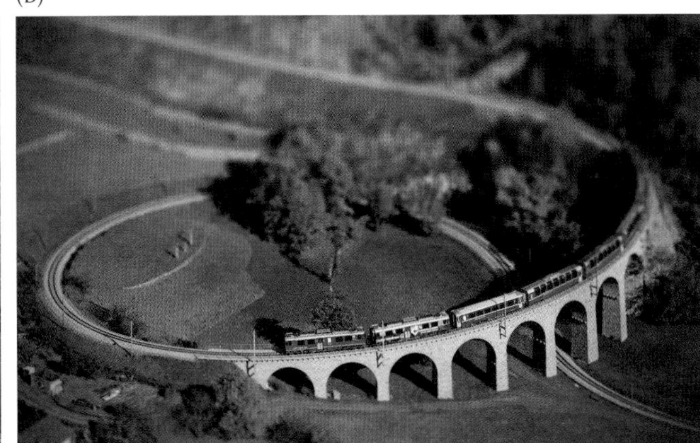

FIGURE 6.23 Inferring space from blur (A) A photo of a Swiss railroad. (B) When the same picture is strategically blurred at top and bottom, the scene looks more like a view of a vastly smaller, model railway.

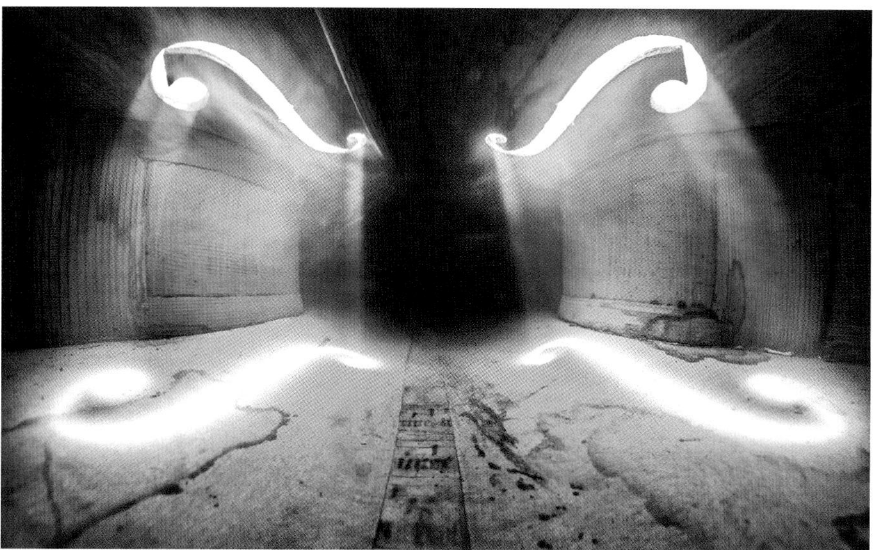

FIGURE 6.24 An interesting space What are you looking at?

right? Actually, no. You are looking at the inside of a cello. The absence of the right blur fools us into imaging a much larger space.

6.3 Binocular Vision and Stereopsis

As defined earlier, the term *binocular disparity* refers to differences between the images falling on our two retinas, and *stereopsis* refers to the impression of three-dimensionality—of objects "popping out in depth"—that most humans get when they view real-world objects with both eyes. Like the accounts of other depth cues, the story of the route from binocular disparity to stereopsis is a story of the visual system exploiting the regularities of projective geometry to recover the three-dimensional world from its projections—this time, onto a pair of two-dimensional surfaces. We will illustrate the translation from disparity to stereopsis using the situation shown in **FIGURE 6.25A**, in which the viewer (let's call him Bob) is facing a scene that includes four colored crayons at different depths. Suppose that Bob is

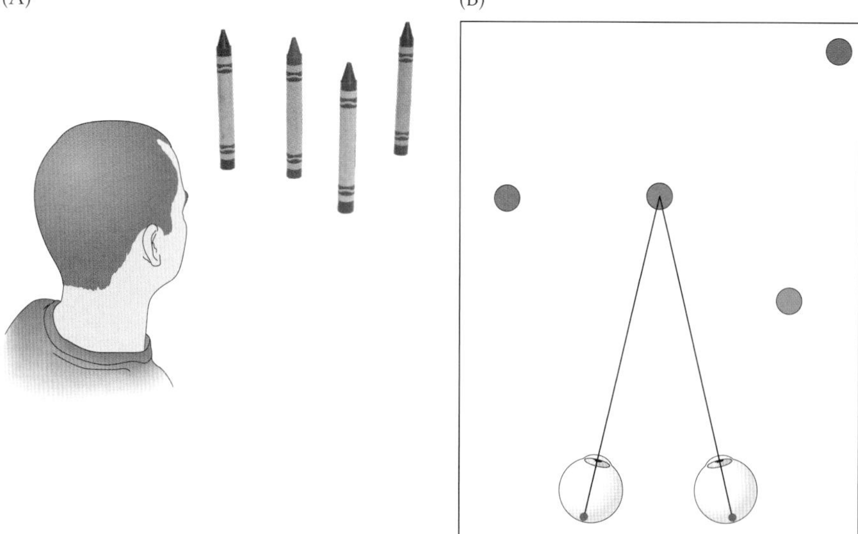

FIGURE 6.25 Binocular disparity This simple visual scene illustrates how geometric regularities are exploited by the visual system to achieve stereopsis from binocular disparity. (A) The viewer, Bob, is assumed to be fixing his gaze on the red crayon. (B) This "top looking down" view traces the rays of light bouncing off the red crayon onto Bob's retinas.

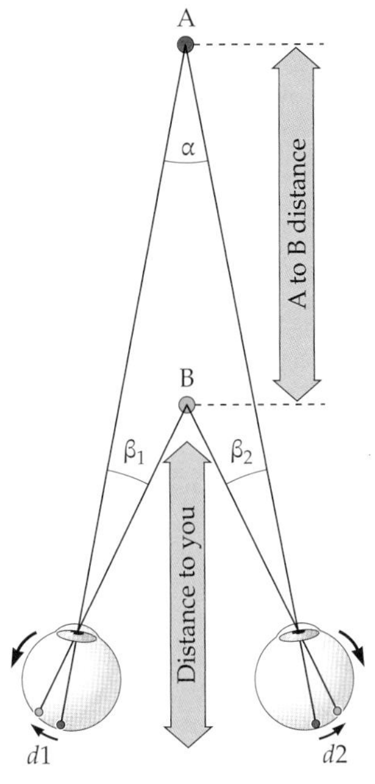

FIGURE 6.26 Absolute disparity If your eyes are converged on A with a convergence angle of α, point B, which is closer to you, will have an absolute disparity defined by the β angle (or by the distances *d*1 and *d*2 on the two retinas). If you know α, you know how far away point A is from you, based on the absolute disparity. If you know α *and* β (or *d*1 and *d*2), then you know how far point A is from point B and, as a result, you will know exactly how far point B is from point A—that is, the relative disparity.

focusing his gaze on the red crayon, as shown in **FIGURE 6.25B**. The two lines in this figure trace the paths of the light rays that reflect off the red crayon and onto Bob's two retinas.

We need to introduce one more concept: relative disparity versus absolute disparity. **Absolute disparity** is illustrated in **FIGURE 6.26**. Suppose you are fixating on point A. Your eyes will be converged on A with a vergence angle of α. Point B, which is closer to you, will have an absolute disparity defined by the β angles (or by the distances *d*1 and *d*2 on the two retinas). If you know the value of angle α, you know how far away point A is from you. If you know α and β (or *d*1/*d*2), then you know how far point A is from point B and, as a result, you know, absolutely, how far point B is from you. As you might expect, however, we are not very good at making perceptual judgments based on absolute disparity because we do not have a conscious readout of absolute disparities for judging depth. This has been termed the absolute disparity anomaly (Chopin et al., 2016).

It seems weird that our eyes would "know" where to converge based on absolute disparity, but that information would not be consciously available for making perceptual judgments. Why should we discard this information, especially since it is thought that relative disparities are calculated from absolute disparities? The likely explanation is that absolute disparities are corrupted by convergence noise, whereas relative disparities are not. Because the convergence noise is common to both point A and point B, it can be disregarded.

For **relative disparity**, let's get back to Bob and his crayons. Because the visual system is designed so that the object of our gaze always falls on the fovea, the rays from the red crayon fall on the fovea in each of Bob's eyes. **FIGURE 6.27** shows the retinal image for the crayons in each eye. The red crayon is in the center of both images. We've added a dashed vertical line in front of this crayon in each image to emphasize the fact that this is the location of the fovea.

Now consider the retinal images of the blue crayon. As you saw in Chapter 2, the optics of the eye reverse left-right and up-down (see Figure 2.2A). Thus, the blue crayon on the right side of the scene in Figure 6.25 falls on the left side in each of the two retinal images in Figure 6.27. In our imaginary scene, the blue crayon is placed so that the monocular retinal images of that crayon are formed at the same distance from the fovea in both eyes. We say that this crayon's images fall on **corresponding retinal points**. The same can be said of the images of the red

absolute disparity The difference in the angular distance of the images of an object from the foveas of the two eyes.

relative disparity The difference in the absolute disparities of two objects.

corresponding retinal points Two monocular images of an object in the world are said to fall on corresponding points if those points are the same distance from the fovea in both eyes. The two foveas are also corresponding points.

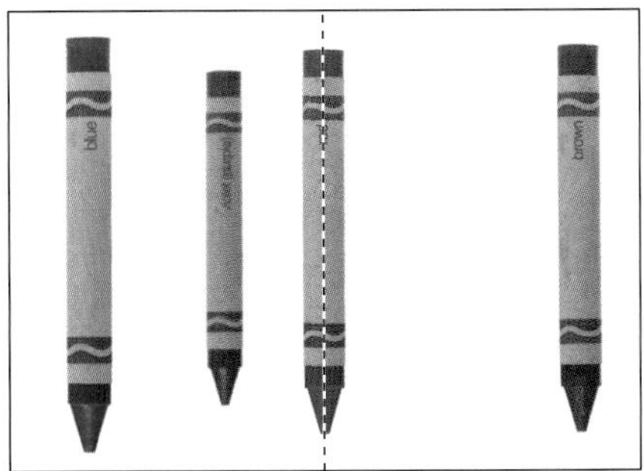

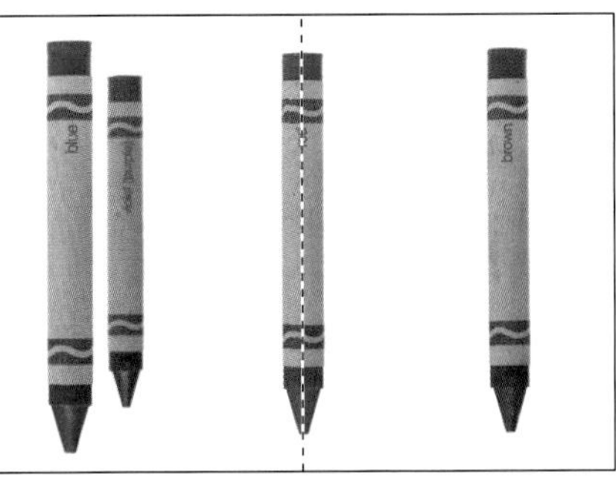

FIGURE 6.27 What's on Bob's retinas? The figure shows overlapping portions of the images falling on Bob's left and right retinas. Because the retinal image is reversed, the blue and purple crayons on the right side of the scene in Figure 6.25 project to the left side of each retina, whereas the brown crayon on the left projects to the right side of each retina. The size differences between the retinal images of the crayons are exaggerated in this figure compared with the differences we would observe if we saw this scene in the real world.

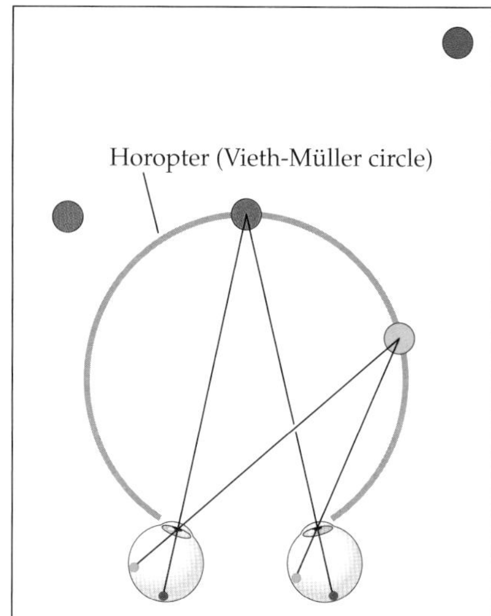

FIGURE 6.28 Vieth-Müller circle Bob is still gazing at the red crayon. This view from above traces the light rays reflecting from the red and blue crayons onto Bob's retinas. The blue crayon projects to corresponding retinal points—positions that are equidistant from and on the same side of the fovea. The same would be true of any object falling on the gray curve shown in the figure. (The horopter and Vieth-Müller circle are not exactly the same, but they would be very similar in this case.)

crayon, which fall on the two foveas. (Oh, and you do know why the crayons are upside down here, right? See Section 2.2.)

In fact, any object lying on the **Vieth-Müller circle**—the imaginary circle that runs through the two eyeballs and the object on which Bob is fixated—should project to corresponding retinal points. This imaginary circle is drawn in gray in **FIGURE 6.28**. Objects that fall on corresponding retinal points are said to have *zero binocular disparity*. If the two eyes are looking at one spot (such as the red crayon), then there will be a surface of zero disparity running through that spot. Any object placed on that imaginary surface will form images on corresponding retinal points. That surface is known as the **horopter**, and in Figure 6.28 it corresponds closely to the Vieth-Müller circle. As it happens, however, the horopter and the Vieth-Müller circle are not quite the same. If you are *extremely* fond of complicated geometry, you may want to pursue this topic in I. P. Howard and Rogers (1995 or 2001) or in Tyler (1991). Otherwise, the important point is that there is a surface of zero disparity whose position in the world depends on the current state of convergence of the eyes.

Objects that lie on the horopter are seen as single objects when viewed with both eyes. Objects significantly closer to or farther away from the surface of zero disparity form images on decidedly noncorresponding points in the two eyes, and we see two of each of those objects. This double vision is known as **diplopia**. Objects that are close to the horopter but not quite on it can still be seen as single objects. This region of space in front of and behind the horopter, within which binocular single vision is possible, is known as **Panum's fusional area** (Panum, 1940). You can check this ability quite simply by holding a red crayon (or pen) directly in front of you with your left hand, at a distance of about 20 centimeters (cm), and keeping both eyes on it. Now hold a blue crayon (or pen) about 5 cm to either side of the red one with your right hand and slowly move it nearer to your eyes and then farther away, while maintaining careful fixation on the red one. You should initially see the blue crayon/pen as single when it is about the same distance from you as the red one, because it is within Panum's fusional area. However, when it falls outside Panum's area, it will appear double. Panum's area provides a little room for small errors in eye alignment while still maintaining single vision.

Armed with this terminology, it's back to Bob and his crayons. Consider the retinal images of the brown crayon, lying just off the horopter. As **FIGURE 6.29A** shows, rays of light bouncing off this crayon do *not* fall on corresponding retinal points: the crayon's image is farther away from the fovea on the left retina than from the fovea on the right retina. Relative to the horopter, this crayon forms retinal images with a nonzero binocular disparity. The purple crayon is even farther off the horopter (**FIGURE 6.29B**) and forms retinal images that are even more disparate (**FIGURE 6.30**).

The geometric regularity that the visual system uses to extract metrical depth information from binocular disparity should now be growing clear. The larger the disparity, the greater the distance in depth of the object from the horopter.

The direction in depth is given by the *sign*—"crossed" or "uncrossed"—of the disparity, as illustrated in **FIGURE 6.31**. Suppose that Bob is looking at a red crayon with his eyes converged so that the red crayon falls on the fovea in each eye. The closer blue crayon will form images on noncorresponding, disparate points. On the

Vieth-Müller circle The location of objects whose images fall on geometrically corresponding points in the two retinas. If life were simple, this circle would be the horopter, but life is not simple.

horopter The location of objects whose images lie on corresponding points. The surface of zero disparity.

diplopia Double vision. If visible in both eyes, stimuli falling outside Panum's fusional area will appear diplopic.

Panum's fusional area The region of space, in front of and behind the horopter, within which binocular single vision is possible.

(A)

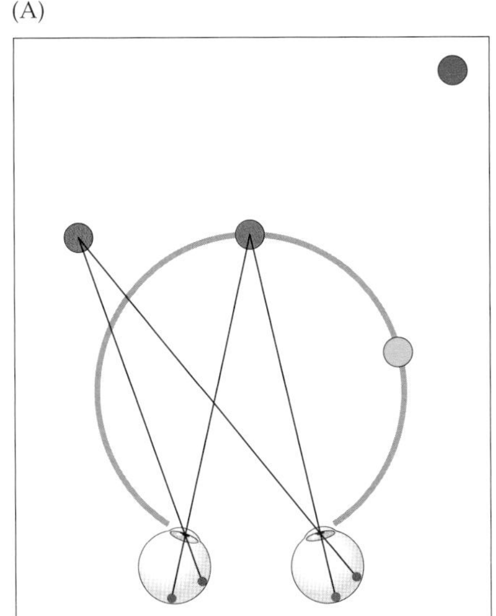

(B)

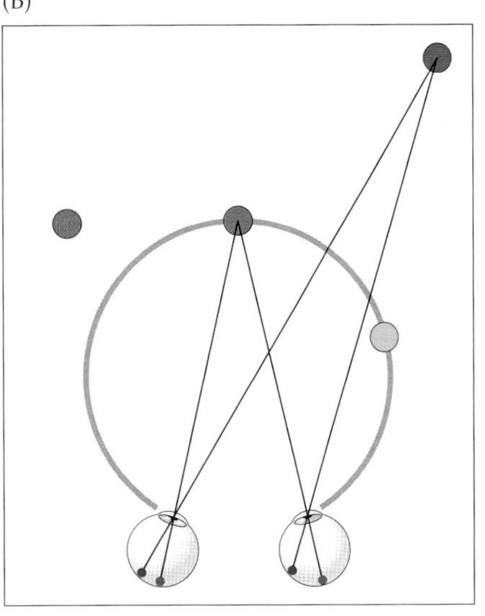

FIGURE 6.29 **Projecting objects to Bob's retinas** Light rays projecting from the brown (A) and purple (B) crayons onto Bob's retinas as he continues to gaze at the red crayon.

left retina, blue will lie to the left of red. Because the image is reversed, this means that, viewed from the left eye, blue is to the right of red. Viewed from the right eye, blue is to the left. Right in left and left in right is known as **crossed disparity** (Figure 6.31A); crossed disparity always means "in front of the horopter." In Figure 6.31B, Bob is looking at the blue crayon, and the red is seen to the left with the left eye and to the right with the right eye. That's **uncrossed disparity**, and uncrossed disparity always means "behind the horopter." Note that if we change our fixation, the horopter is now at a different location in space. Stereopsis is a relative depth cue that provides very-high-resolution depth information for objects that are close to the horopter.

crossed disparity The sign of disparity created by objects in front of the plane of fixation (the horopter). The term *crossed* is used because images of objects located in front of the horopter appear to be displaced to the left in the right eye and to the right in the left eye.

uncrossed disparity The sign of disparity created by objects behind the plane of fixation (the horopter). The term *uncrossed* is used because images of objects located behind the horopter will appear to be displaced to the right in the right eye and to the left in the left eye.

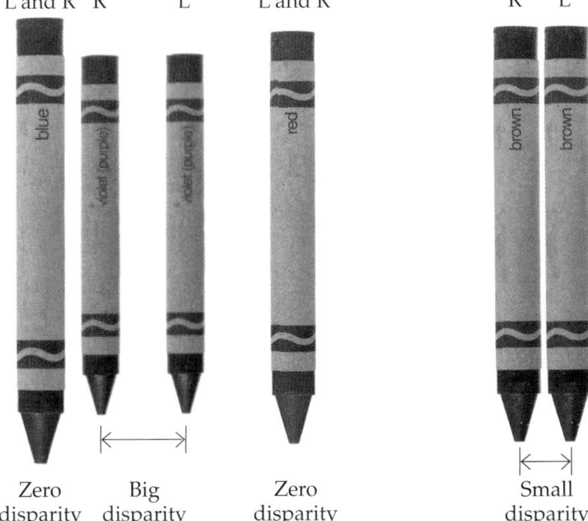

FIGURE 6.30 **Superposition of Bob's retinal images** Combining the left (L) and right (R) retinal images of the crayons in Figure 6.27 to show the relative disparity for each crayon. Size differences are ignored here. The red and blue crayons sit on the horopter and have zero disparity. They form retinal images in corresponding locations. The brown crayon forms images with a small binocular disparity. The purple crayon, farther from the horopter, has larger binocular disparity.

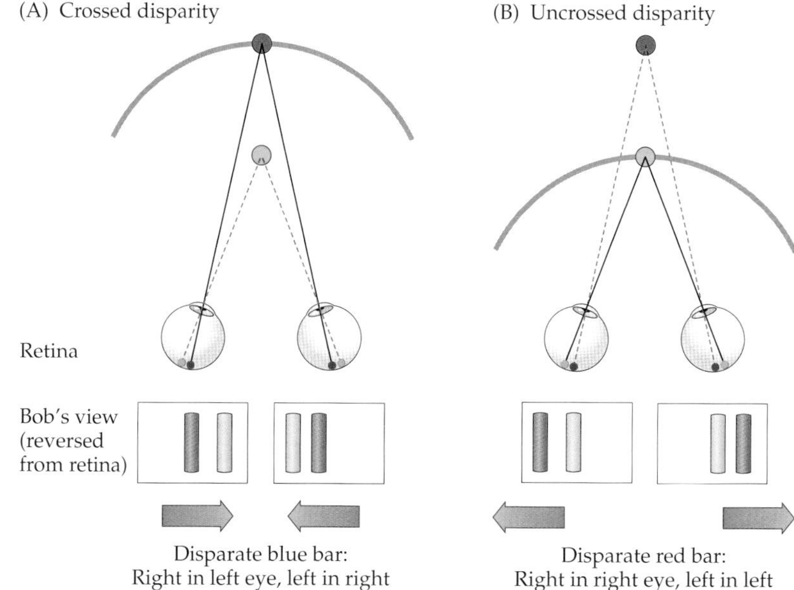

FIGURE 6.31 Crossed and uncrossed disparity (A) Here Bob is foveating the red crayon. In the Bob's-eye views, the closer, blue object is seen to the right in the left eye and to the left in the right eye. In this scenario the disparity is crossed. (B) Here Bob has shifted his gaze and his horopter to the blue crayon. In the Bob's-eye views, the farther, red object is seen to the left in the left eye and to the right in the right eye. In this scenario the disparity is uncrossed.

FIGURE 6.32 illustrates the relationship between binocular disparity and perceived relative depth. In the middle of the graph, just to either side of the horopter, are the lower limits of stereopsis—the smallest crossed and uncrossed disparities that can be detected (i.e., the stereo thresholds). Farther from the center in either direction, disparity increases. The limit of Panum's fusional area (the purple zone in Figure 6.32) marks the end of the zone of single vision. Beyond that, the images are diplopic. Items will look doubled but, interestingly, they are still seen in relative depth. When the disparity is not too large (the gray zones in Figure 6.32), the depth information from stereopsis is quantitative. Here, stereopsis still provides an accurate estimate of the relative depth. As disparity increases beyond this range into the blue zones, it still provides usable depth order information, but the information is now qualitative

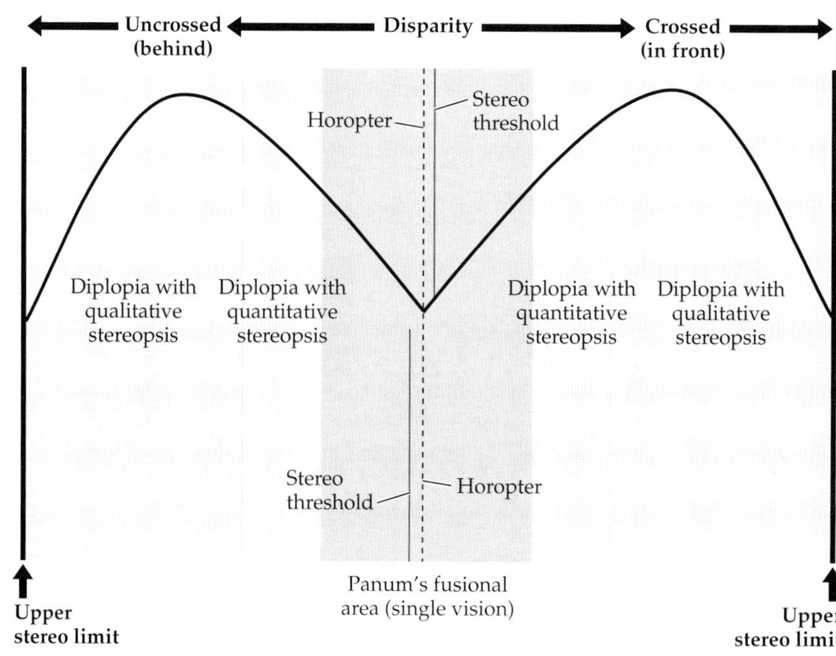

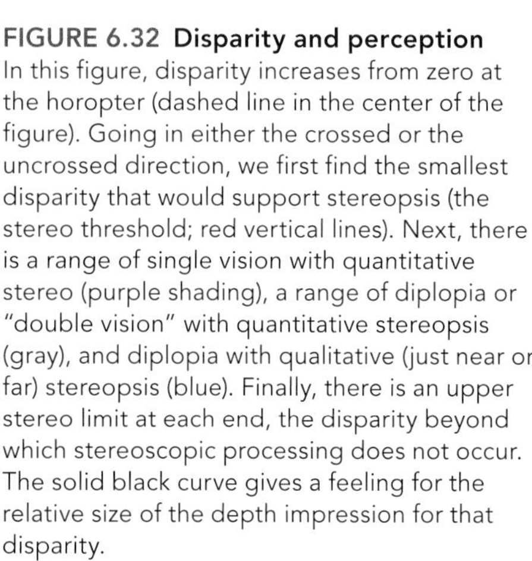

FIGURE 6.32 Disparity and perception In this figure, disparity increases from zero at the horopter (dashed line in the center of the figure). Going in either the crossed or the uncrossed direction, we first find the smallest disparity that would support stereopsis (the stereo threshold; red vertical lines). Next, there is a range of single vision with quantitative stereo (purple shading), a range of diplopia or "double vision" with quantitative stereopsis (gray), and diplopia with qualitative (just near or far) stereopsis (blue). Finally, there is an upper stereo limit at each end, the disparity beyond which stereoscopic processing does not occur. The solid black curve gives a feeling for the relative size of the depth impression for that disparity.

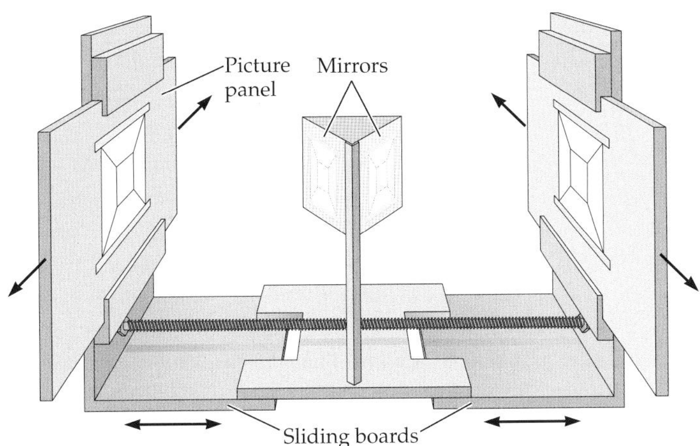

FIGURE 6.33 Wheatstone's stereoscope The viewer would bring her nose up to the vertical rod at the center of the apparatus so that each eye was looking at the image reflected in one of the two mirrors.

rather than quantitative. An item will appear to be in front or behind, but that is about all that stereopsis can provide in this range. Finally, once disparities are larger than the upper disparity limit, there is no longer any useful depth information.

Stereoscopes and Stereograms

Interestingly, although scientists had studied the geometry of binocular vision for millennia (the geometer Euclid was at it in the third century BCE), not until the nineteenth century was binocular disparity properly recognized as a depth cue. In the 1830s, Sir Charles Wheatstone invented a device called the **stereoscope** (FIGURE 6.33) that presented one image to one eye and a different image to the other eye. The stereoscope confirmed that the visual system treats binocular disparity as a depth cue, regardless of whether the disparity is produced by actual or simulated images of a scene.

For the average citizen at the time, the stereoscope was not science; it was home entertainment. The Wheatstone stereoscope held two different images in two different places. In the 1850s, however, David Brewster and Oliver Wendell Holmes invented viewers (FIGURE 6.34A) that held a card with a double image like that shown in FIGURE 6.34B. The double images were captured by cameras with two lenses separated by about 63 millimeters, which is the distance between the average human's eyes. This arrangement allows stereo cameras to take a pair of pictures that mimic the images produced by the projective geometry of human

stereoscope A device for simultaneously presenting one image to one eye and another image to the other eye. Stereoscopes can be used to present dichoptic stimuli for stereopsis and binocular rivalry.

(A)

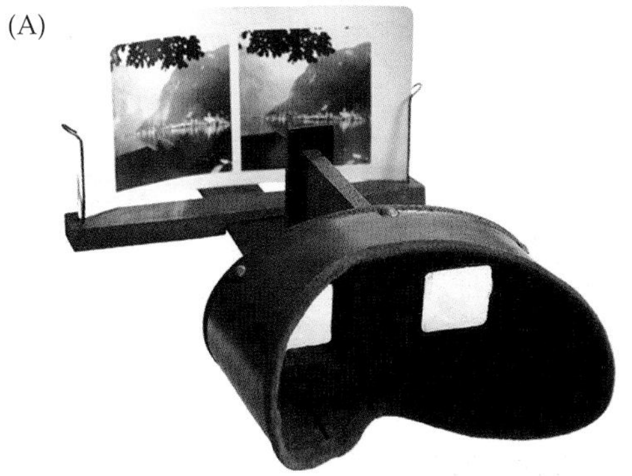

(B)

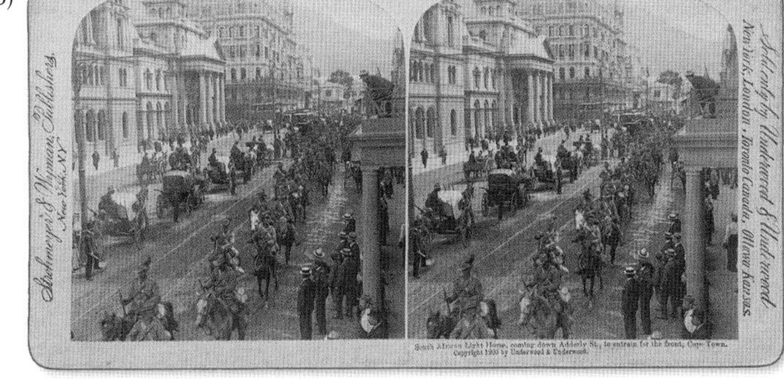

FIGURE 6.34 Stereopsis for the masses (A) This Holmes stereoscope—among others—brought stereo photos into many mid-nineteenth-century homes. (B) A stereo photo of South African Light Horse, a scouting regiment of the British Army, on Adderly Street in Cape Town, South Africa, in 1900. If you can free-fuse (see the text and Figure 6.35), you will be able to see this scene jump out in depth.

free fusion The technique of converging (crossing) or diverging the eyes in order to view a stereogram without a stereoscope.

stereoblindness An inability to make use of binocular disparity as a depth cue. This term is typically used to describe individuals with vision in both eyes. Someone who has lost one or both eyes is not typically described as "stereoblind."

binocular vision. Photographers traveled the world with these stereo cameras, capturing far-off scenes in a way that enabled a London schoolchild to see, for example, a vivid three-dimensional image of the British Army in Cape Town, South Africa.

A stereoscope is helpful, but you don't need one to experience stereopsis. You can teach yourself a technique known as **free fusion**, which John Frisby (1980) called "the poor man's stereoscope." **FIGURE 6.35** contains two almost identical sets of squares. If you cross your eyes hard, you should see four sets of squares. This is the phenomenon of double vision (diplopia), described in the previous section. Two sets of squares are seen with the left eye and two with the right. The trick is to relax just a bit until you see just three sets of squares. The far-left set is seen only in the left eye and the far-right set only in the right, but the middle set is the fusion of two sets, one seen by the left eye and another by the right eye. This fusion of the separate images seen by the two eyes makes stereopsis possible.

Achieving the perception of three, instead of four or two, sets of squares in Figure 6.35 is the first step toward free fusion. The second step is to bring the middle set into focus. Convergence and accommodation, discussed earlier, normally work in lockstep, so crossing your eyes automatically leads your ciliary muscles to make your lenses more spherical (unless you are presbyopic; see Section 2.2). Similar problems (in the opposite direction) will occur if you diverge your eyes. To see the middle set of squares clearly, you have to decouple accommodation and convergence. This can be a bit hard to do, but if you can manage it, the image will come into focus and the three white squares will appear to lie at different depths in the middle set of squares. When you view them normally, notice that the white squares in the left and right panels look misaligned in opposite directions. Those are the monocular views. When you free-fuse, the opposite misalignments become the binocular disparity, and your visual system converts that disparity into a perception of depth.

The depth that you see depends on whether you converged or diverged your eyes. We described crossing, or converging, the eyes. It is also possible to free-fuse the images in Figure 6.35 by *diverging* your eyes. Divergence requires focusing on a point beyond the plane of the page so that the image of the left-hand set of squares falls on the left fovea and the image of the right-hand set falls on the right fovea. Because the images falling on the two retinas in the divergence method are reversed compared with the convergence situation, the disparities are reversed and the perceived depth will be reversed. That is, if you converge, the top square will be the farthest back. If you diverge, it will appear closest to you. Either converging or diverging will produce a clear stereoscopic effect, so give it a try.

Before we go on, we should note that approximately 3–5% of the population lacks stereoscopic depth perception—a condition known as **stereoblindness**. Stereoblind

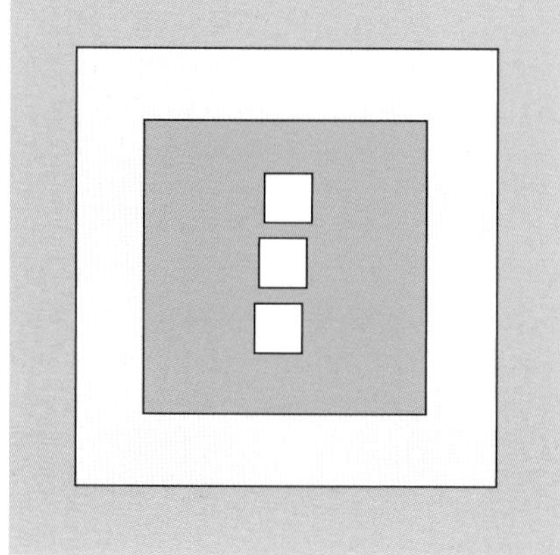

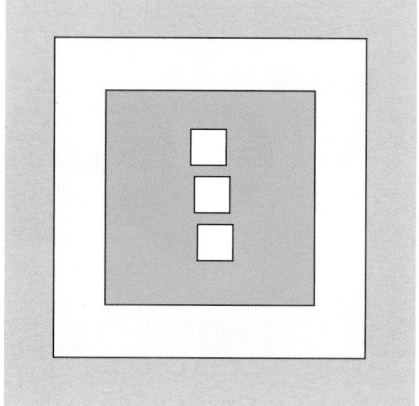

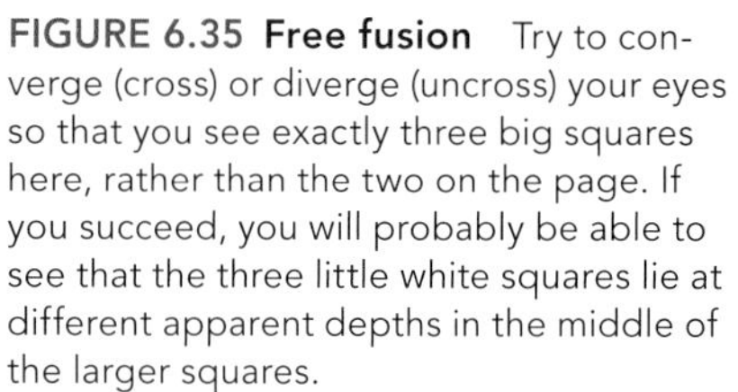

FIGURE 6.35 Free fusion Try to converge (cross) or diverge (uncross) your eyes so that you see exactly three big squares here, rather than the two on the page. If you succeed, you will probably be able to see that the three little white squares lie at different apparent depths in the middle of the larger squares.

Sensation & Perception in Everyday Life

Recovering Stereo Vision

About 3–5% of the population are stereoblind, meaning that they cannot use binocular disparity as a cue to depth. This is usually as a result of early childhood visual disorders. Can stereo vision be recovered later in life? Meet Stereo Sue and Binocular Bruce.

Susan Barry, a professor of neurobiology, had strabismus as an infant and had been stereoblind essentially all her life. Her book *Fixing My Gaze* (2009) provides a fascinating, informative, and beautifully written account of her acquisition of stereopsis following vision therapy. It describes her transformative journey from the many visual, social, and psychological challenges of a turned eye (a squint or strabismus) early in life, to the sudden enrichment of her perceptions of the world following successful unconventional visual therapy she began at the age of 48. (A 2006 article about her visual recovery, by the neurologist and noted author Oliver Sacks, was published in *The New Yorker* under the title "Stereo Sue.")

Barry vividly recounts how acquiring stereoscopic vision led to a dramatic improvement of her perception of depth, or the appreciation of the "space between objects." A particularly valuable insight is her argument for the inability of people with normal vision to appreciate the visual experience of being stereoblind. Naively, one might think that this experience could be duplicated simply by closing one eye so all information about depth was conveyed by monocular cues. Not so, Barry argues: The monocular experience of a typically reared person who closes one eye has been informed by a lifetime of experience with stereoscopic vision and so is far different from that of a person who is stereoblind. As a result, Barry's new stereoscopic vision brought much more to her life than just depth perception. Objects became clearer, motion perception became more veridical (that is, more true to the objects as they actually exist), and her movement around the world became more confident. Even more poignant is her vivid description of the enhanced sense of touch she had developed over the years and its key role in informing her newly acquired sense of stereo vision.

Barry did not simply "recover" stereopsis, but rather had to relearn to see with stereo vision. As blind or deaf individuals often describe, individuals deprived of a sense are not just "missing" a sense. Rather, they have developed an entirely different way of sensing the world. Upon sensory restitution, a fascinating but rather disturbing experience unfolds as the brain has to adapt to a new way of functioning.

Even more dramatic is the experience of Binocular Bruce (the late Bruce Bridgeman), a very perceptive vision scientist who had been stereo-deficient all his life. Remarkably, he spontaneously recovered stereopsis after watching the 3D movie *Hugo* (Bridgeman, 2014). Whether this sort of immersive experience, with very large disparities along with many other depth cues, will be a generally effective treatment for abnormal stereopsis remains to be tested. However, these case studies, along with lab studies of perceptual learning that have resulted in the recovery of stereopsis (Ding and Levi, 2011; Vedamurthy et al., 2016; reviewed in Levi, 2022), call into question the notion that recovery of stereopsis can only occur during early childhood. The idea, dating back to the early twentieth century, has been that there is a "critical period" of development when the visual system is still plastic and capable of change. After that, it was thought, our basic visual capabilities are fixed. This received wisdom led a number of practitioners to tell Susan Barry and her mother that "nothing could be done" about her vision (one even suggested she might need a psychiatrist). Since binocular neurons are present in the visual cortex of primates within the first week of life (see Section 6.5), Barry surmises that some of the innate wiring of her binocular connections remained intact and that vision therapy taught her to move her eyes into position for stereo vision, "finally giving these neurons the information they were wired to receive" (Barry, 2009).

individuals might be able to achieve the perception of three sets of squares in Figure 6.35, but the little white squares will not pop out in depth. Stereoblindness is usually a secondary effect of childhood visual disorders such as strabismus, in which the two eyes are misaligned (see Section 6.5). If you had such a visual disorder during childhood and/or you've been diagnosed with stereoblindness, we apologize, but you just won't perceive depth in the stereograms presented here and on the website. But being stereoblind does not preclude artistic achievement; indeed, some researchers have suggested that painters generally tend to have poor stereo vision, giving them an edge in working in two dimensions. No less distinguished an artist than the Dutch master, Rembrandt (1606–1669) is thought to have suffered from strabismus and stereoblindness. This hypothesis is based on his self-portraits that often show him with one eye wandering off the canvas.

That said, many people who try and fail to see depth in stereograms have "normal" vision (wearing glasses doesn't count as "abnormal" in this case). Those people just need practice, so don't give up.

Random Dot Stereograms

For 100 years or so after the invention of the stereoscope, it was generally supposed that stereopsis occurred relatively late in the processing of visual information. The idea was that the first step in free-fusing images such as those in **FIGURE 6.36** would be to analyze the input as a face. We would then use the slight disparities between the left-eye and right-eye images of the nose, eyes, chin, and other objects and body parts to enrich the sense that the nose sticks out in front of the face, that the eyes are slightly sunken, and so on.

Bela Julesz, a Hungarian radar engineer who spent most of his career at Bell Labs in New Jersey, thought the conventional wisdom might be backward. He theorized that stereopsis might be used to *discover* objects and surfaces in the world. Why would this be useful? Julesz thought that stereopsis might help reveal camouflaged objects. A mouse might be the same color as its background, but out in the open it would be in front of the background. A cat that could use stereopsis to break the mouse's camouflage would be a more successful hunter. (Cats do have stereopsis, by the way; see R. Blake, 1988; and R. Fox and Blake, 1971.) To prove his point, Julesz (1964, 1971) made use of **random dot stereograms (RDSs)**. An example is shown in **FIGURE 6.37**. If you can free-fuse these images, you will see a pair of squares, one sticking out like a bump and the other looking like a hole in the texture. Which one is the bump and which one is the hole depends, again, on whether you converge or diverge your eyes.

The important point about RDSs is that we cannot see the squares in either of the component images. We cannot see the squares using any monocular depth cues. These are shapes that are defined by binocular disparity alone. Julesz called such stimuli **Cyclopean**, after the one-eyed Cyclops of Homer's *Odyssey*. Wheatstone showed with his stereoscope that binocular disparity is a necessary condition for stereopsis. Julesz demonstrated with RDSs that disparity is *sufficient* for stereopsis.

random dot stereogram (RDS) A stereogram made of a large number (often in the thousands) of randomly placed dots. Random dot stereograms contain no monocular cues to depth. Stimuli visible stereoscopically in random dot stereograms are Cyclopean stimuli.

Cyclopean Referring to stimuli that are defined by binocular disparity alone. Named after the one-eyed Cyclops of Homer's *Odyssey*.

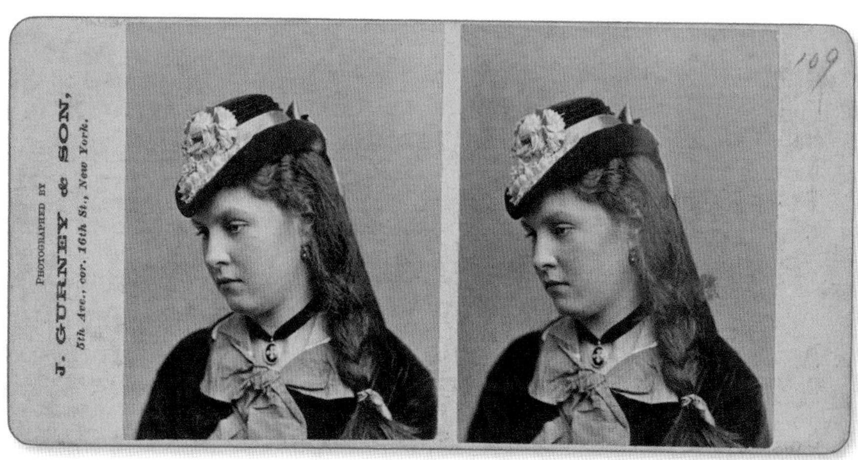

FIGURE 6.36 **Free-fusing images**
A stereo photograph of a woman's face.

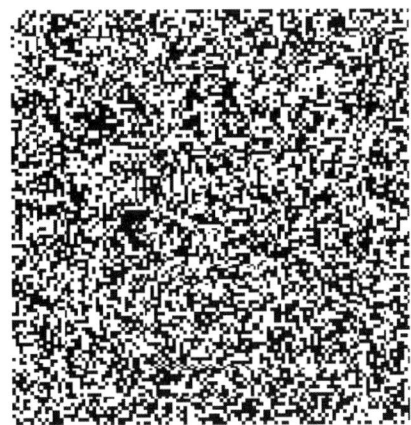

FIGURE 6.37 A random dot stereogram If you can free-fuse this random dot stereogram, you will see two rectangular regions: one in front of the plane of the page and the other behind the page. Which is which depends on whether you converge or diverge in order to fuse the two squares.

Using Stereopsis

Stereopsis has been put to work in a number of fields. The military has known for a long time that you can get more information out of aerial surveillance if your view of the ground is stereoscopic. However, if you've ever looked out the window from thousands of meters in the air, you may have noticed the ground looks rather flat. This is caused by yet more geometry. Stereopsis can provide useful information about metric depth only for distances up to 40 meters (Palmisano et al., 2010). With eyes a few centimeters apart, you don't get adequate disparity from more distant targets. What you need are eyes separated by hundreds of meters. This can be done if you have an airplane and a special camera. **FIGURE 6.38** reprints a figure from a 1951 issue of *Popular Mechanics* in which Colonel George W. Goddard showed the public how images taken from two vantage points produced stereo images during the Korean War.

A different use of the same trick has been tried as a way to improve airport baggage screening. Looking for threats in luggage is a difficult visual search task (see Section 7.2). As shown in **FIGURE 6.39**, the screeners search using two-dimensional X-ray images of the jumbled three-dimensional contents of your bag. One possible way to make the task a bit easier would be to create a three-dimensional image. This could be done by taking advantage of the fact that the bag is moving

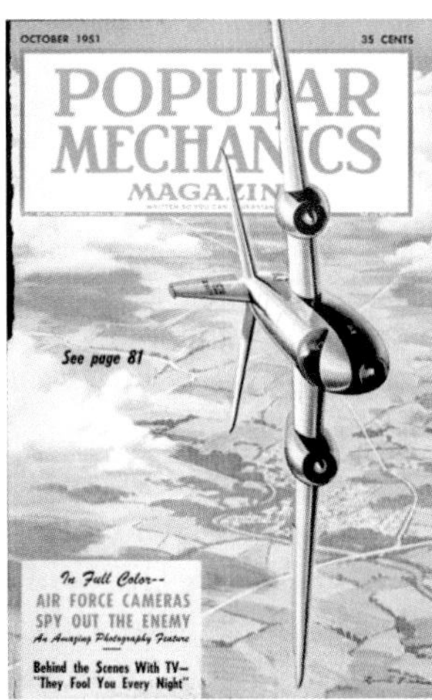

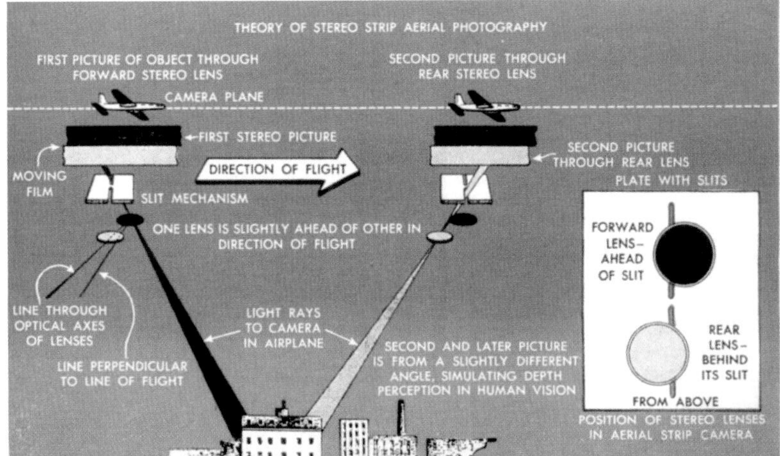

FIGURE 6.38 Stereoscopic depth from an airplane It is possible to make effective stereoscopic images of terrain by taking two aerial pictures from two, quite widely separated viewpoints.

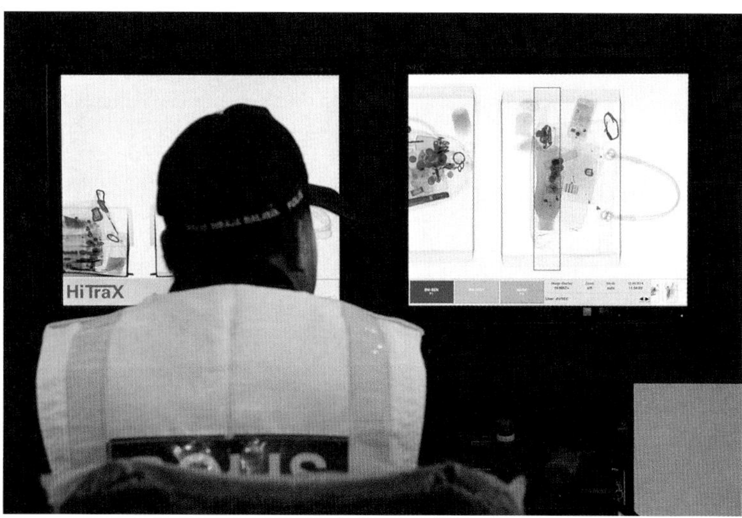

FIGURE 6.39 Baggage screening Could stereopsis help in the hunt for threats in baggage?

along a conveyor belt. If two X-rays are taken from different positions on the belt, a stereogram can be created and delivered to the inspector (Gittinger et al., 2017).

Is stereopsis useful in everyday life? In people with normal binocular vision, visually guided hand movements are significantly impaired when viewing is restricted to one eye (Fielder and Mosely, 1996; Niechweij-Szwedo, Colpa, and Wong, 2019), likely because binocular depth thresholds are about ten times better than monocular thresholds (McKee and Taylor, 2010). These results are mirrored in patients with amblyopia ("lazy eye"), for whom many observed visuomotor deficits are the result of impaired stereopsis, and in particular impaired visual feedback control of movements, rather than visual acuity loss (Grant and Moseley, 2011). Loss of stereopsis may also result in unstable gait, especially reduced accuracy when a change of terrain (e.g., steps) occurs, and difficulties for children in playing some sports. Indeed, how far ahead you look when walking in medium to rough terrain (like hiking in the woods) is highly correlated with stereoacuity. The worse your stereoacuity, the closer you look to find stable footholds (Bonnen et al., 2021).

Stereopsis is particularly important for reaching and grasping. In observers with normal binocular vision, studies of visual cue integration consistently demonstrate that stereoscopic disparities contribute strongly to depth and shape perception when presented in conjunction with other depth cues (Hillis et al., 2004; Johnston, Cumming, and Parker, 1993; Knill and Saunders, 2003; Lovell, Bloj, and Harris, 2012; Vuong, Domini, and Caudek, 2006). Despite these laboratory demonstrations, the functional importance of stereopsis is still much debated.●

FURTHER DISCUSSION of stereo sensation can be found in Section 10.1 (sound localization) and Section 14.3 (binaral rivalry).

Stereoscopic Correspondence

correspondence problem In reference to binocular vision, the problem of figuring out which bit of the image in the left eye should be matched with which bit in the right eye. The problem is particularly vexing when the images consist of thousands of similar features, like dots in random dot stereograms.

If you successfully free-fused the random dot patterns in Figure 6.37, you solved a truly daunting problem. Even if you didn't, if you have normal binocular vision, you are solving the **correspondence problem** all the time. The correspondence problem involves figuring out which bit of the image in the left eye should be matched with which bit in the right eye. **FIGURES 6.40** and **6.41** use an extremely simple situation to illustrate why correspondence is so tricky. There are just three dots in Figure 6.41—the same three dots presented by themselves in Figure 6.40. Figure 6.41A traces the paths of the rays of light from the printed circles on the page to the images on the viewer's retinas. The retinal images of the circles are labeled to make it clear which image on the left retina corresponds to which image on the right retina, but your visual system has no such labels. All it knows about is the retinal images, as shown in Figure 6.41B. Figure 6.41C shows another possible geometric interpretation of the situation: if the left retinal image of circle 2 is matched to the right retinal image of circle 1, and the left retinal image of circle 3 is matched to the right retinal image of circle 2, you will perceive four circles, with the inner pair of circles perceived as floating in front of the outer pair. In fact, you may be able to experience this for yourself, if you can cross your eyes correctly.

FIGURE 6.40 Three purple dots Is this a simple picture or a complicated computational problem?

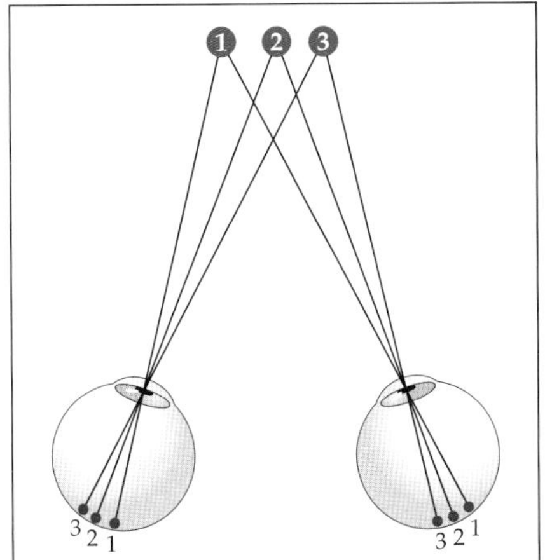

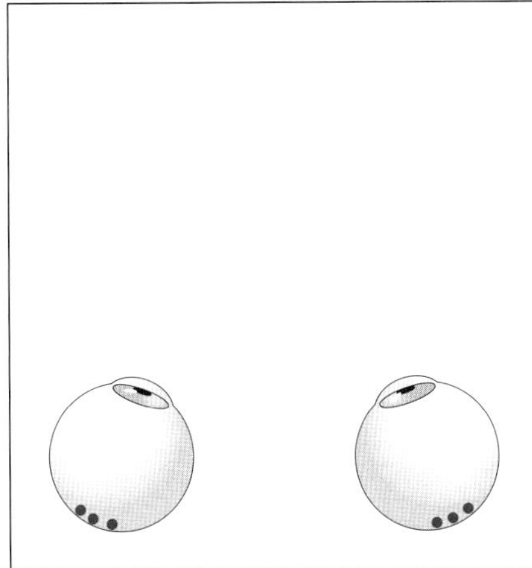

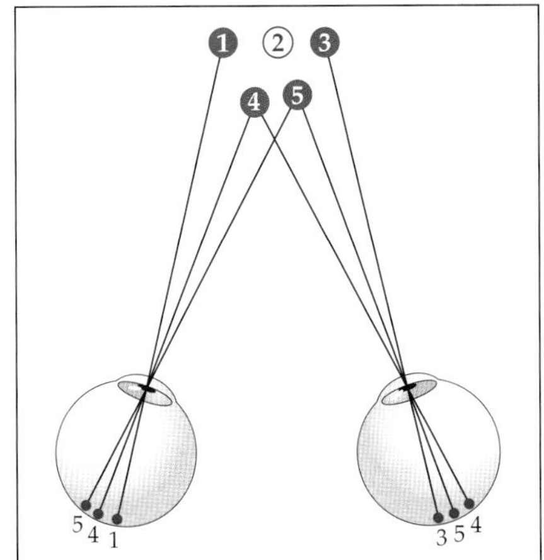

FIGURE 6.41 The problem with three dots Interpreting the visual information from the three circles in Figure 6.40. It would require careful placement, but four dots in the world, if lined up just right, could produce images of just three dots in each eye, as in (C).

With only three elements in the visual scene, it isn't hard to imagine how the visual system might achieve the proper correspondence: first match the two circles whose images fall on the foveas; then match the two images to the left of the foveas with each other; then match the two images to the right of the foveas. Before the introduction of random dot stereograms, a similar logic seemed reasonable for more complex scenes, too. Go back to the face in Figure 6.36. Our visual systems could solve the correspondence problem by first finding the parts of the two faces and then matching nose to nose, mouth to mouth, and so forth. The random dot stereogram in Figure 6.37, however, contains thousands of identical black and white dots falling on each retina. How can we be sure that the dot in the center of the fovea of one eye corresponds to the dot in the center of the other eye? Even if we could determine that, could we really match each dot in the right eye with just one dot in the left eye? If there were a little dirt on the page, would the whole process collapse? How in the world does our visual system succeed in making the proper matches?

Matching thousands of left-eye dots to thousands of right-eye dots in Figure 6.37 would require a lot of work for any computational system. However, the problem is simpler if we look at a blurred version of the stereogram, as shown in **FIGURE 6.42**. Blurring leaves only the low-spatial-frequency information. Now, rather than the thousands of dots of Figure 6.37, we have fewer and larger blobs. Now you could imagine a process that, for example, matched the black blob in the upper left corner of the left image with the very similar blob in the right image. Crude matches of this sort could act as anchors, allowing the visual system to fill in the finer (high-spatial-frequency) matches from there. The task still isn't trivial, but it could help.

FURTHER DISCUSSION of spatial frequency and retinal perception can be found in Sections 3.1 and 3.2.

In addition to starting with low-spatial-frequency information, David Marr and Tomaso Poggio (1979) suggested two more heuristics for solving the correspondence problem: the uniqueness and continuity constraints. The **uniqueness constraint** acknowledges that a feature in the world is represented exactly once in each retinal image. Working in the opposite direction, the visual system knows that each monocular image feature (e.g., a nose or a dot) should be paired with exactly one feature in the other monocular image. Notice that Figure 6.41C would not violate uniqueness.

uniqueness constraint In reference to stereopsis, the observation that a feature in the world is represented exactly once in each retinal image. This constraint simplifies the correspondence problem.

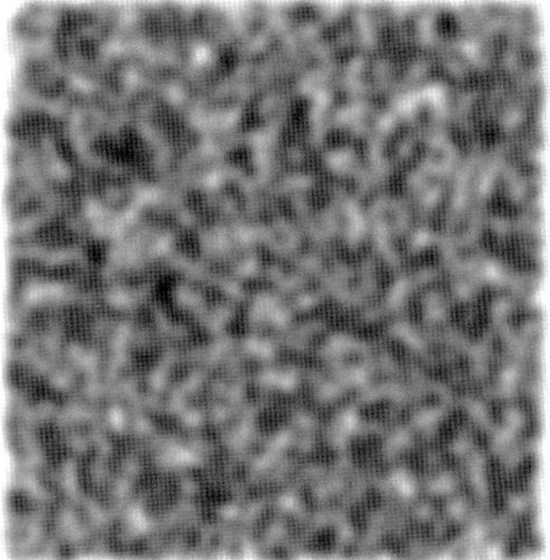
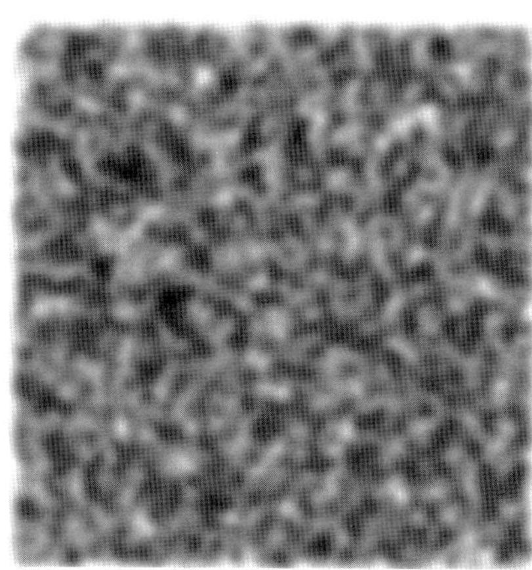

FIGURE 6.42 Matching blobs A low-spatial-frequency filtered version of the stereogram in Figure 6.37 contains bigger blobs that might be easier to match between the eyes.

continuity constraint In reference to stereopsis, the observation that, except at the edges of objects, neighboring points in the world lie at similar distances from the viewer. This is one of several constraints that have been proposed as helpful in solving the correspondence problem.

Each dot in the world would be represented exactly once in each retinal image. The odd thing is that two dots in the real world could be represented by the same dot in the retinal image. The **continuity constraint** holds that, except at the edges of objects, neighboring points in the world lie at similar distances from the viewer. Accordingly, disparity should change smoothly at most places in the image.

With the uniqueness and continuity constraints, the correspondence problem is not entirely solved, but it is made more tractable, because there are not so many possible solutions. However, recent work suggests that identifying correct matches may not be the optimal strategy (Goncalves and Welchman, 2017). Rather, they suggest that the brain uses "what *not*" detectors that sense dissimilar features in the two eyes. These perceptions suppress unlikely interpretations of a scene and facilitate stereopsis by providing evidence against interpretations that are incompatible with the true structure of the scene.

We've been illustrating stereopsis with static examples on a textbook page. Much of the time, however, we are moving in the three-dimensional world, and this motion gives us more cues to help us solve the problems of getting three dimensions out of two-dimensional retinal images. We already talked about *motion parallax*. Motion gives us dynamic disparity clues as the relative disparities change with movements of the observer. These will reduce the realm of possible solutions to the correspondence problem. Moreover, when you move, the velocities on each retina are slightly different; this *motion disparity* is another cue that can help (Cormack et al., 2017).

The Physiological Basis of Stereopsis and Depth Perception

Now that we know something about the theoretical basis of stereopsis, we can ask how it is implemented by the human brain. The most fundamental requirement is that input from the two eyes must converge onto the same neuron. As noted in Chapter 3, this convergence does not happen until the primary visual cortex (= V1, striate cortex), where most neurons can be influenced by input from both the left and the right eyes—that is, V1 neurons are binocular (Hubel and Wiesel, 1962). Usually, when we say a cell is binocular, we mean it can be excited by either eye, but the situation is more complicated than that. Some cells can only be stimulated by both eyes together. Other cells can only be excited by one eye, but they can be inhibited by stimulation of the other eye (Dougherty et al., 2019). Binocular neurons have two receptive fields, one in each eye. In binocular V1 neurons, the receptive fields in the two eyes are generally very similar, sharing nearly identical orientation and spatial-frequency tuning, as well as the same preferred speed and direction of motion (Hubel and Wiesel, 1973). Thus, these cells are well suited to the task of matching images in the two eyes.

Many binocular neurons respond best when the retinal images are on corresponding points in the two retinas, thereby providing a neural basis for the horopter. However, many other binocular neurons respond best when similar images occupy slightly *different* positions on the retinas of the two eyes (Barlow, Blakemore, and Pettigrew, 1967; Pettigrew, Nikara, and Bishop, 1968). In other words, these neurons are tuned to a particular binocular disparity (**FIGURE 6.43**).

Recall the distinction, described in Section 6.1, between metrical and nonmetrical depth cues. Stereopsis can be used both metrically and nonmetrically. Nonmetrical stereopsis might tell you only that a feature lies in front of or behind the plane of fixation. Poggio and Talbot (1981) found disparity-tuned neurons of this sort in visual area 2 (V2) and some higher cortical areas. Some neurons responded positively to disparities near zero—that is, to images falling on corresponding retinal points. Other neurons were broadly tuned to a range of crossed (near) or uncrossed (far) disparities. However, stereopsis can also be used in a very precise, metrical manner. Indeed, stereopsis is a "hyperacuity" like Vernier acuity with thresholds smaller than the diameter of a cone photoreceptor (see Section 3.1), with thresholds smaller than the size of a cone. Both metrical and nonmetrical forms of stereopsis have their uses, and functional magnetic resonance imaging data suggest that the dorsal *where* pathway is most interested in metrical stereopsis, while the ventral *what* pathway (see Section 4.2) makes do with more categorical, near-versus-far information (Preston et al., 2008).

Recall that we also made the distinction between absolute and relative disparity cues (see Section 6.3). Binocular neurons in V1 are generally responsive to absolute disparities, whereas neurons in V2 and many other higher cortical areas are sensitive to relative disparities. Relative disparities provide the basis for very fine stereoacuity (Parker, Smith, and Krug, 2016). The V1 signals, based on absolute disparity, feed into both the ventral and the dorsal streams. The absolute disparity information is sent to the dorsal stream and is thought to be used to control vergence eye move-

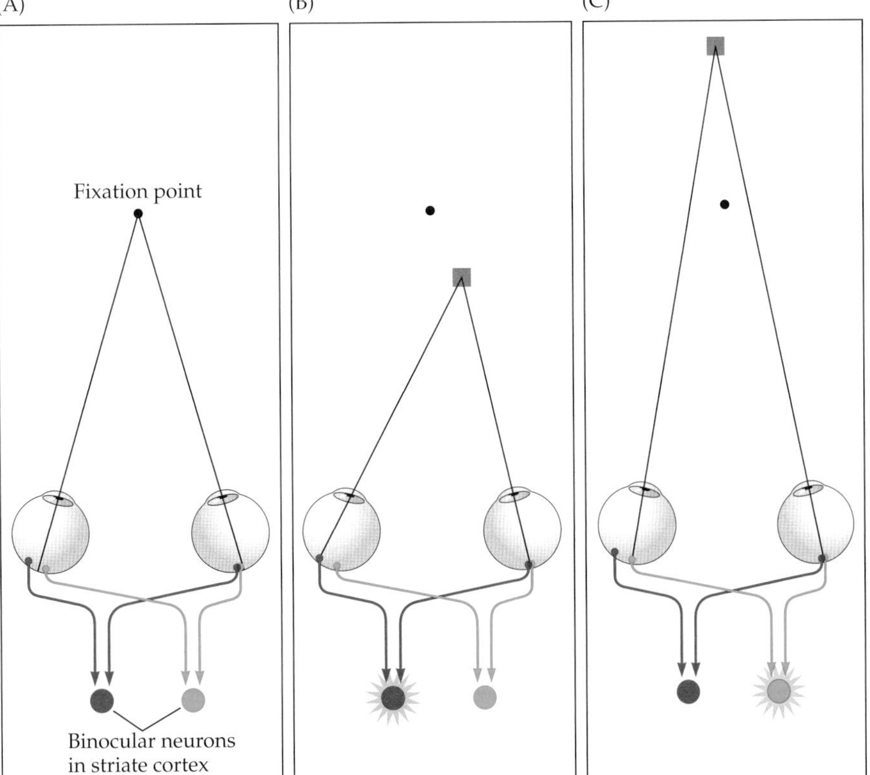

FIGURE 6.43 Receptive fields sensitive to disparity In these simplified diagrams of receptive fields for two binocular disparity–tuned neurons in primary visual cortex, the red neuron "sees" stimuli falling on the red receptive fields, and the blue neuron responds to stimuli falling on the blue receptive fields (these receptive fields overlap on the right retina). (A) The overall picture, showing the fixation point in relation to the two retinas. (B) The red neuron responds best to a stimulus closer to and slightly to the right of the fixation point. (C) The blue neuron responds best if its preferred stimulus is behind and slightly to the left of fixation.

ments (see Section 8.4) to get the images in the two eyes into registration. Relative disparity in V2 moves into the ventral pathways to form the neural basis for more complex, three-dimensional shape perception farther along in cortical processing in inferotemporal cortex (see Section 4.2) (Verhoef, Vogels, and Janssen, 2016). Indeed, areas in both dorsal and ventral pathways have been implicated in stereopsis in both monkeys and humans, and neuroimaging studies suggest that area V3/V3A may be especially important (Anzai, Chowdry, and DeAngelis, 2011; Henderson et al., 2019).

The neural bases of other depth cues have also been investigated. For example, when we discussed motion parallax earlier, we suggested moving your head back and forth while looking into the branches of a tree to create a more vivid impression of the depth relationships among the branches and twigs. To exploit that cue properly, you need to know both how your head is moving (see Chapter 12) and how items in the visual field are moving (see Chapter 8). Nadler, Angelaki, and DeAngelis (2008) looked for the neural substrate of parallax in the middle temporal area (area MT) of the brain of macaque monkeys. As we will see in Chapter 8, this area is very important in the perception of motion. Nadler and colleagues set up an apparatus where the monkey was moved from side to side while items on the screen also moved. If the monkey was integrating signals about its head movement with the motion signals, then the objects on the screen should have been seen in depth. Otherwise, they would have been seen as just moving in the plane of the screen. It turns out that cells in area MT can signal the sign of depth (near or far) based on this motion parallax signal alone.

Other visual areas also contribute to the complex business of inferring the three-dimensional world from two-dimensional retinal images. Anzai and DeAngelis (2010) suggest that early visual areas, particularly V2, are involved in computing depth order (who's in front?), based on the contour completion and border ownership process we discussed in Chapter 4 (see Figure 4.5). Intermediate visual areas such as V4 (visual area 4) encode depth intervals, based on relative disparities, and higher cortical areas such as inferotemporal cortex are involved in the representation of complex three-dimensional shapes. **FIGURE 6.44** shows the many cortical areas that are activated by stereoscopic depth in humans.

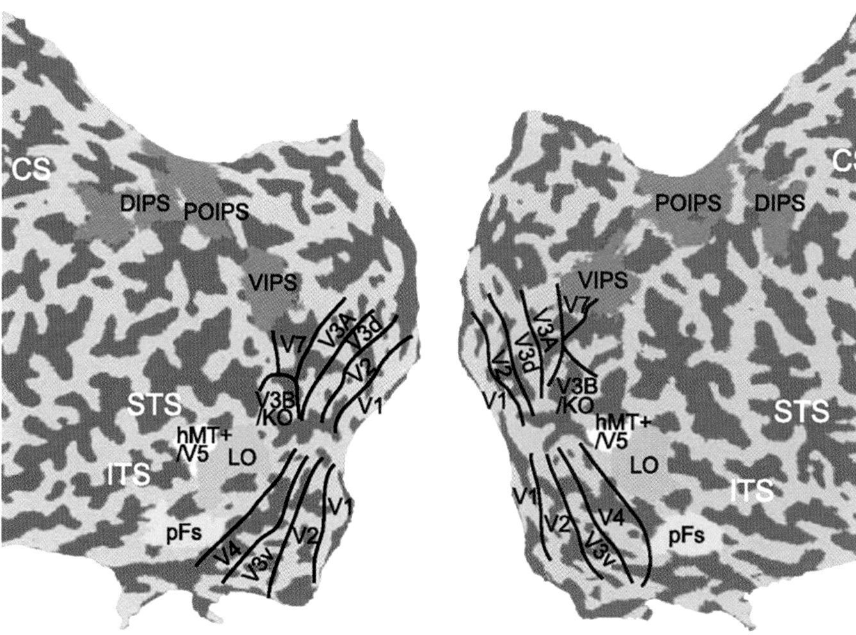

FIGURE 6.44 Brain regions sensitive to random dot stereograms Functional magnetic resonance imaging (fMRI) showing cortical brain regions in retinotopic areas and in V3B/KO, hMT /V5, and LO that respond to binocular disparity signals. Also shown are areas in the parietal cortex (VIPS, POIPS, and DIPS) that respond to three-dimensional shapes.

While many areas of our large brains are involved in stereopsis, it should be noted that many animals with much smaller brains (such as insects; see "Scientists at Work: Stereopsis in a Hunting Insect") can extract depth from disparity. One recent report (Feord et al., 2020) shows that the cuttlefish, a relative of the octopus, is a member of the stereoscopic club. As shown in **FIGURE 6.45A**, the Feord lab outfitted cuttlefish with a pair of stylish colored glasses ("anaglyphic glasses," used to restrict red stimuli to one eye and blue to the other). **FIGURE 6.45B** diagrams the method. Red and blue images of a shrimp were drawn with the disparity between the two images designed to place the fused, stereoscopic image of a shrimp in front of or behind the computer screen. Because the cuttlefish captures its prey by shooting out a pair of arms the right distance to grab the shrimp, the researchers could tell that the cuttlefish was using the depth cue by noting where in depth it attacked the shrimp image.

(A)

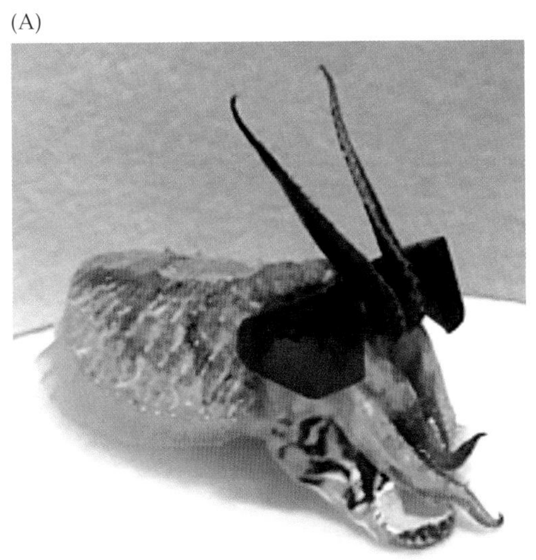

(B)

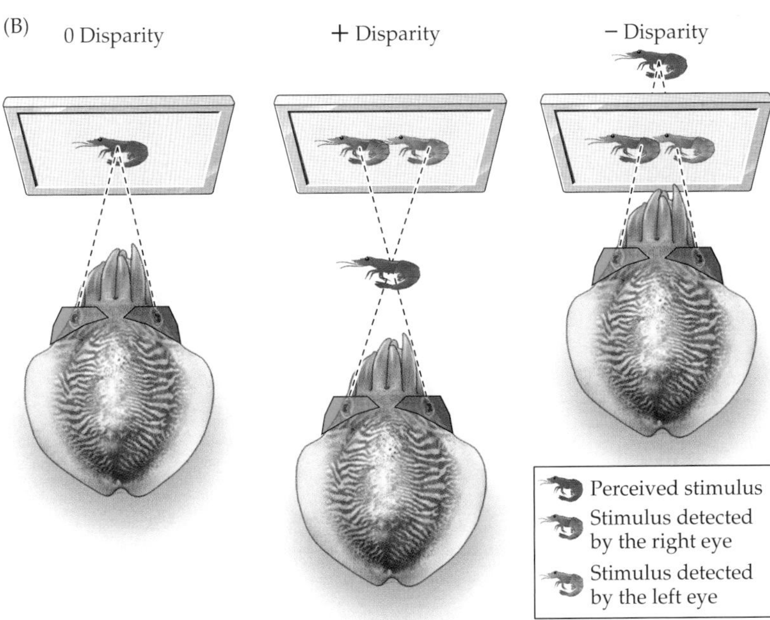

FIGURE 6.45 Stereopsis in the cuttlefish (A) A cuttlefish wearing stylish anaglyphic glasses. (B) The cuttlefish sees cartoon shrimp that should appear at different distances if the cuttlefish can use the disparity cue.

Scientists at Work

Stereopsis in a Hunting Insect

Question How can you tell if a praying mantis has stereopsis?

Hypothesis Praying mantises catch and eat bugs, leading to the hypothesis that the praying mantis should have stereoscopic depth perception. *At this point, you should be able to design this experiment yourself.*

Test Just as in the cuttlefish experiment, the researchers gave the mantises very, very small anaglyphic glasses (**FIGURE 6.46**)—in this case, with one lens blue and the other green (Nityananda et al., 2016). For each trial, they then placed a mantis in hunting position in front of a computer screen showing three-dimensional movies of simulated bugs. Binocular disparity was used to move the bugs to different virtual distances from the mantis. If the mantis had stereoscopic depth perception, it should attempt to strike its prey when it perceived that the bug was at exactly the right distance. That would be about 2 cm away, the grabbing distance of the mantis's extended front claws. (Notice how this a bit different from the cuttlefish. Cuttlefish were striking at fake shrimps at different distances. The mantis waited for a bug at the right distance. You need to really understand the normal behavior of your animal to do this kind of research.)

Results When the researchers played two-dimensional movies of simulated bugs, the mantises didn't react. However, when they played three-dimensional movies, they struck in attempts to nab their dinners when virtual bugs were at the apparently correct distance.

Conclusions This experiment provides clear and dramatic proof that the praying mantis has stereoscopic vision and will respond to depth defined by disparity.

Future work Mantises, cuttlefish, and humans are far apart on the evolutionary tree. Further research of this sort with other species will help us understand the forces that shape the number of eyes an organism has and how those eyes work together. Indeed, jewel wing damselflies have binocular neurons (although it is not known whether they actually have three-dimensional vision), while their close cousins, the dragonflies, do not (Supple et al., 2020).

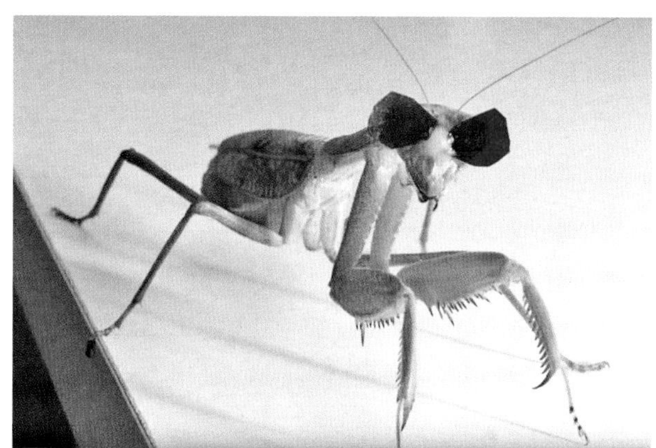

FIGURE 6.46 Stereopsis in praying mantis A praying mantis wearing stylish anaglyphic glasses (all the best invertebrates have them). Can an insect with a tiny brain still use disparity as a cue to depth?

6.4 Combining Depth Cues

If the chapters of this book were novels, this chapter could be said to have the same plot as the discussion of object recognition in Chapter 4, but with different characters. In Chapter 4 we talked about a set of cues that enable us to group local features together into possible objects and then recognize those objects. We described the process as a sort of committee effort, in which different sources of information all contribute their opinions and we see the committee's decision without necessarily knowing how that decision was reached. In this chapter, we've covered multiple sources of depth information and they, too, need to be combined. Any or all of these cues might be available to the visual system when we're viewing any visual scene. None of the cues is foolproof, and none works in every possible situation. For example, relative height produces inconsistent or misleading information if we can't see the point at which an object touches the ground. All we really have is a collection of guesses about possible depth relations between different objects in our visual field.

By carefully combining and weighting these guesses, the visual system generally arrives at a coherent, and more or less accurate, representation of three-dimensional space. Helmholtz, writing in the nineteenth century (and translated into English in the twentieth), called this automatic cue combination process "unconscious inference" (Helmholtz, 1924). In recent years, a number of vision researchers have been attempting to put this sort of argument on the more rigorous mathematical footing of the **Bayesian approach** that we mentioned in Section 4.4.

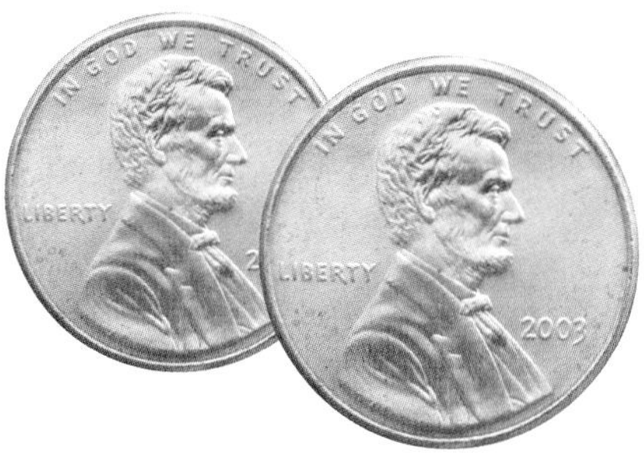

FIGURE 6.47 Two coins Retinal image of a simple visual scene.

Bayesian approach A way of formalizing the idea that our perception is a combination of the current stimulus and our knowledge about the conditions of the world—what is and is not likely to occur. The Bayesian approach is stated mathematically as Bayes' theorem—$P(A|O) = P(A) \times P(O|A)/P(O)$, which enables us to calculate the probability (P) that the world is in a particular state (A) given a particular observation (O).

The Bayesian Approach Revisited

Recall that the basic insight of Reverend Thomas Bayes was that prior knowledge can influence estimates of the probability of a current observation. Let's apply this idea to a concrete depth perception example. Suppose our visual system is confronted with the retinal image shown in **FIGURE 6.47**. There are infinite possible ways to produce this retinal image, and this is a bit of a problem for the use of Bayes' theorem. We don't *really* know the prior probabilities (M. Jones and Love, 2011). Still, we can acknowledge that limitation, and yet make good use of the basic insight that some hypotheses are more likely than others and that these prior probabilities can shape our interpretation of the world. Three hypotheses about our pennies are shown in **FIGURE 6.48**. Maybe the two pennies are the same size, but the one on the left is slightly farther away than the one on the right (Figure 6.48A). Maybe the penny on the right is much smaller, but also much closer, than the penny on the left (Figure 6.48B). Maybe the two pennies are equidistant, but the penny on the left is smaller and has had a bite taken out of it (Figure 6.48C). If you don't see how the set of possibilities could be infinite, remember that size and distance can vary continuously over a very large range. In Figure 6.48B, the big penny could be on the moon—but it would have to be a *really* big, *really* unlikely penny.

How does the visual system decide what we're actually seeing? Which interpretation seems most likely? That is the core of the Bayesian approach (except that it's all automatic; our conscious selves do not get to make the decision). In our experience, all pennies are the same size. This cue of familiar size is one source of prior knowledge in this case. This makes the prior probability of the hypotheses shown in Figure 6.48A higher than the prior probabilities of the other two hypotheses. Furthermore, for the scene in Figure 6.48C to produce the retinal image in Figure 6.47, we would have to be seeing the scene from one of those unusual and unlikely "accidental viewpoints" (see Section 4.4). It is much more likely that the points of contact between the images of the two pennies reflect occlusion. If we were to plug all these probabilities into Bayes' equation, we would find that, given the image in Figure 6.47, the most likely answer is the scene depicted in Figure 6.48A.

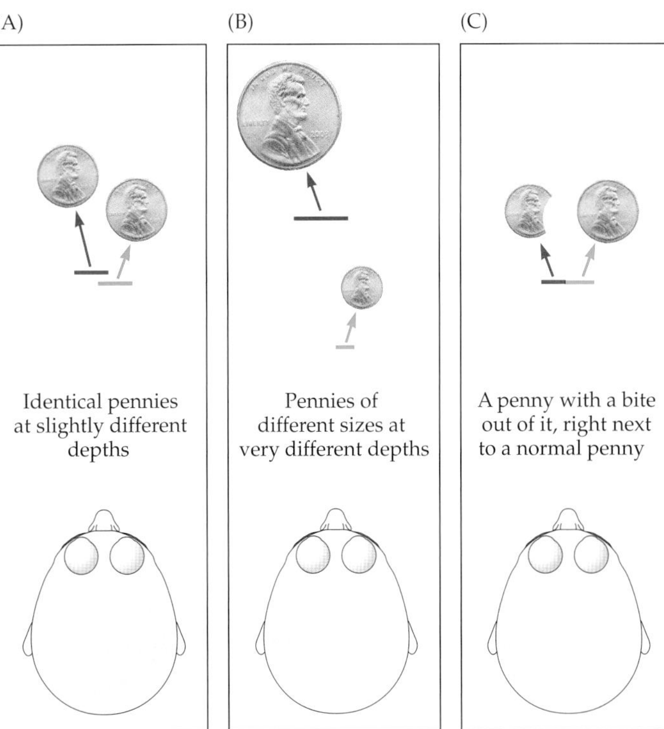

FIGURE 6.48 Bayesian prior probabilities Three of the infinite number of scenes that could generate the retinal image in Figure 6.47. Is (A), (B), or (C) the most probable?

In thinking about combining depth cues, our choice of the metaphor of a committee is not arbitrary. We could have talked about an election, but that would have implied something like "one cue, one vote." On a committee, you might have one member who is stronger than the others and wins all the arguments. You might give more weight to the committee member who comes prepared with the best information. The committee might defer to one member on one topic and another member on a different topic. Something like this last option is described by Held, Cooper, and Banks (2012). Binocular disparity information can be very precise, but that is only true near the plane of fixation (remember Panum's fusional area from Section 6.3?). Blur can be quite a good cue, too, but it is actually better away from the plane of fixation. When Held et al. (2012) made stimuli that had disparity cues, blur cues, or both, they found that disparity drove responses where disparity was more reliable and that blur drove responses in parts of the three-dimensional world where blur was more reliable. This is different from just letting every cue have its say, and it makes us realize that the visual system must be estimating how reliable each depth cue might be.

Sometimes the committee doesn't quite get things right. **FIGURE 6.49** shows a case where prior information about known size of cats seems to have been overruled by cues that seem to show the cat on the right, standing right next to the box containing the other cat. In fact, the cat on the right is some distance farther away, but we didn't get the correct cues and we don't arrive at the right answer.

Illusions and the Construction of Space

If our visual perception of the world is our best guess about the causes of visual input, then interesting things should happen when a guess is wrong. In some sense, as with the pennies we just discussed, a guess is wrong whenever we look at a two-dimensional picture and see it as three-dimensional. As noted,

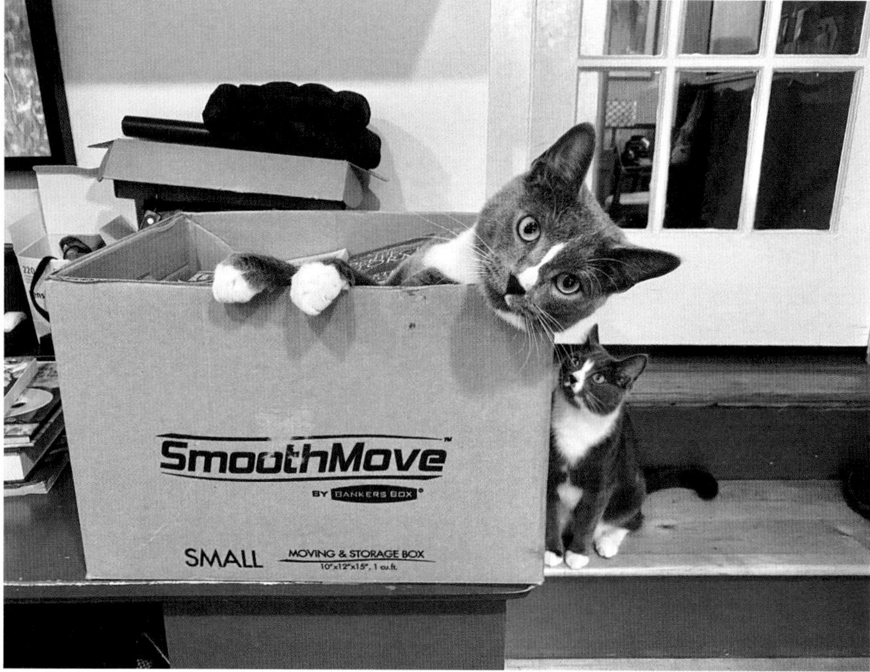

FIGURE 6.49 Big cat, little (?) cat The apparently smaller cat is actually substantially further away. We are misinterpreting the depth cues.

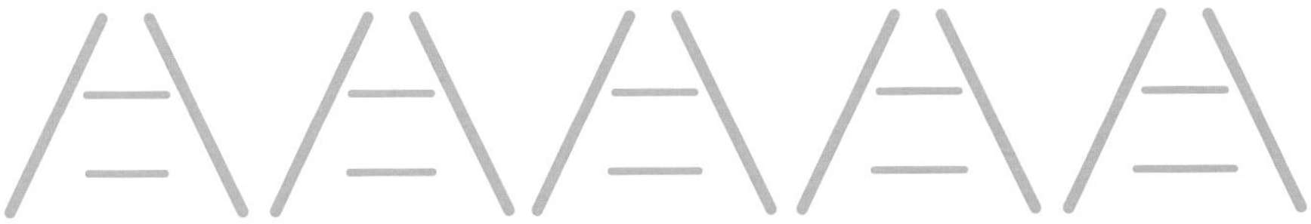

FIGURE 6.50 The Ponzo illusion In which image are the two horizontal lines the same length?

however, we are not really fooled into thinking that the picture is three-dimensional. It would be more accurate to say that we make a plausible guess about the three-dimensional world that is being represented in the two-dimensional picture.

What about a situation like that shown in FIGURE 6.50? One of the five pairs of horizontal lines (and only one) shows two lines of the same length. Can you pick the correct pair (without using a ruler)? In fact, it is the second from the left. Odds are you picked the third or fourth pair, even though the bottom line in both of those images is physically longer than the top line. This is known as the Ponzo illusion, named after Mario Ponzo, who described the effect in 1913. What causes this illusion? For many years, a popular family of theories held that the illusion is another case of a guess gone wrong—a situation in which we overinterpret the depth cues in a two-dimensional image. The basic idea is illustrated in FIGURE 6.51. Maybe the two tilted lines that induce the illusion in each image of Figure 6.50 are being interpreted by the visual system as linear-perspective cues like edges of the hall in Figure 6.51. If so, then objects that were the same size in the two-dimensional image would represent objects of different sizes in the three-dimensional world and the far red sphere would be much bigger (and more disturbing) than the closer one.

Such accounts are very compelling and exist for a wide range of visual illusions (Gillam, 1980). They are consistent with the idea that the job of the visual system is to use available cues to make an intelligent guess about the world (Gregory, 1966, 1970). Just because an answer is plausible, however, doesn't mean it's entirely correct. In FIGURE 6.52, line 2 looks longer than line 1 within the scene in Figure 6.52A, though we can see that they are the same length in Figure 6.52B. That makes sense if we're interpreting these lines as lines lying at different distances on the wall of the colonnade. As in the Ponzo illusion, if line 2 is farther away than 1, then the same image size implies a larger size in the real world. But what about lines 3 and 4? Surely 4 would be interpreted as farther away than 3, but it does not look convincingly larger.

Prinzmetal, Shimamura, and Mikolinski (2001) use a demonstration like this as part of their argument that the Ponzo illusion is not really a by-product of depth cues. They argued that it reflects a more general aspect of the visual system's response to tilted lines and is related to illusions like the Zollner and Hering illusions illustrated in FIGURE 6.53 (which we will *not* try to explain; see Prinzmetal and Beck, 2001). The point is debatable. After all, in Figure 6.52A, line 5 looks very big down there at the apparent end of the colonnade. Who is right? It could be that both arguments hold a piece of the truth. Perhaps the visual system's response to tilted lines is related to the role of those lines in creating an impression of depth. Going back to Figure 6.50, that would mean that the Ponzo illusion was not based on some version of the railroad track story, but that the processes that give rise to a three-dimensional interpretation of Figure 6.50 also give rise to illusions like those in Figures 6.51 to 6.53.

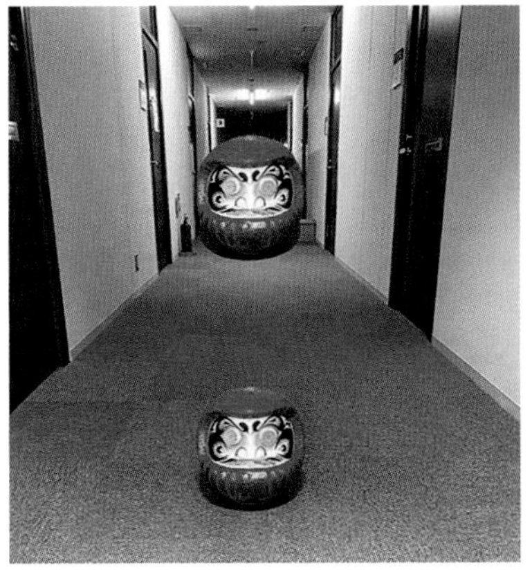

FIGURE 6.51 A real-world Ponzo illusion The two red objects are the same size in the image but your inferences about their distance in the world make them appear very different.

The Ames Room, shown in FIGURE 6.54A, is one of the most compelling illusions based on depth cues. The room is an unusual trapezoidal shape (FIGURE 6.54B), but when you look through a peephole with one eye to eliminate binocular depth information, your visual system makes the guess that this is a normal-size

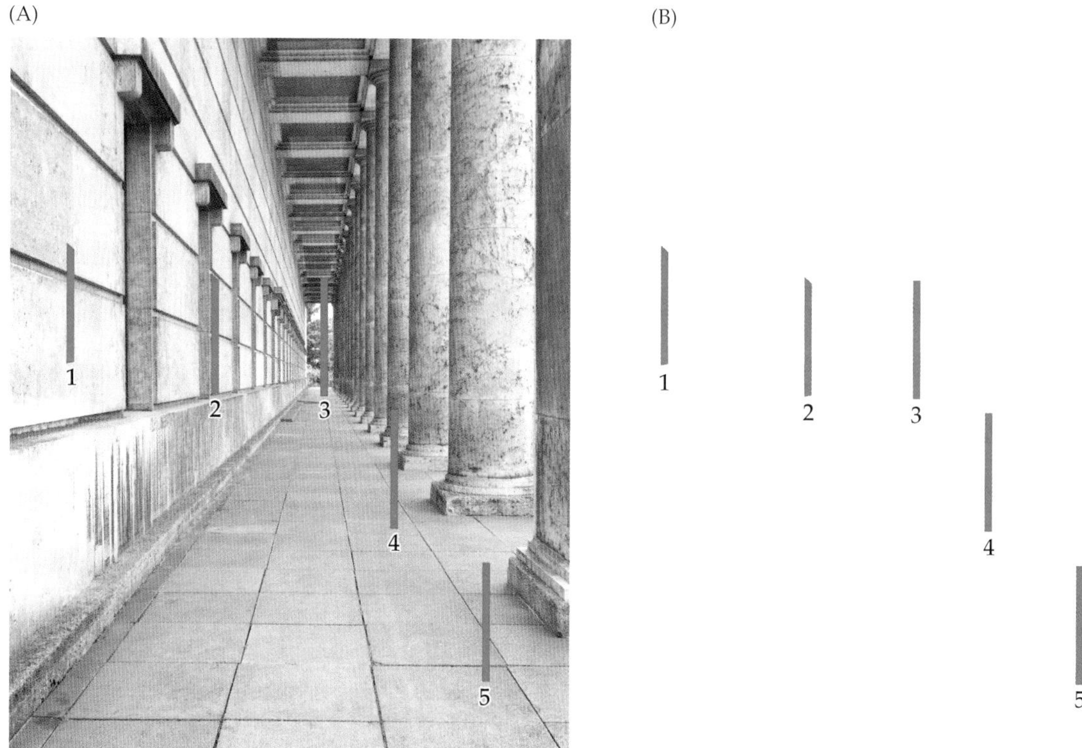

FIGURE 6.52 Explaining the Ponzo illusions All of the blue lines in this illustration (A) are the same length, as you can see in (B). Line 3 looks bigger than 2, which looks bigger than 1 (similar to the red object that is farther back in Figure 6.51). But line 4 does not look bigger than 5, revealing a limit to the perceived-distance account of the Ponzo illusion.

room. However, this "normal room" assumption causes you to make some decidedly abnormal inferences about these sizes of the people in the room.

Binocular Rivalry and Suppression

The preceding sections demonstrated that objects in the world often project images on our two retinas that do not overlap (that is, the images fall on noncorresponding retinal points) and that the visual system is physiologically prepared to deal with these discrepancies via disparity-tuned neurons in the primary visual cortex and beyond. But what happens when completely different stimuli are presented to the two eyes? You can answer this question for yourself by fixating on a small object across the room, such as a clock, and moving your hand up so that your fingers occlude the object in the right eye (making sure the left eye still has an unobstructed view). It would be a mistake for the visual system to fuse the images of your

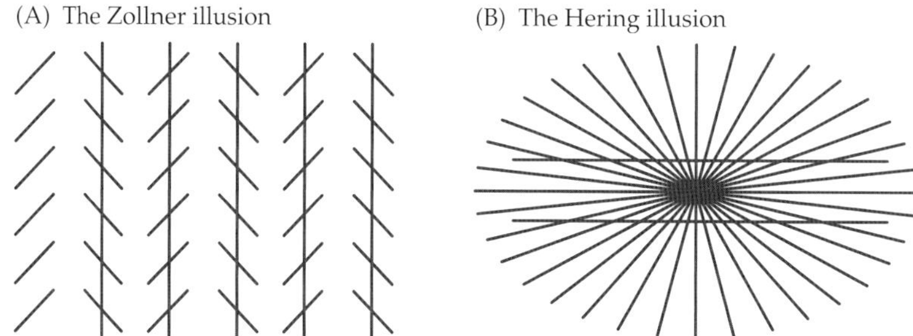

FIGURE 6.53 Zollner and Hering illusions Despite what you think you see, the five vertical lines are parallel in (A), as are the three horizontal lines in (B).

(A)

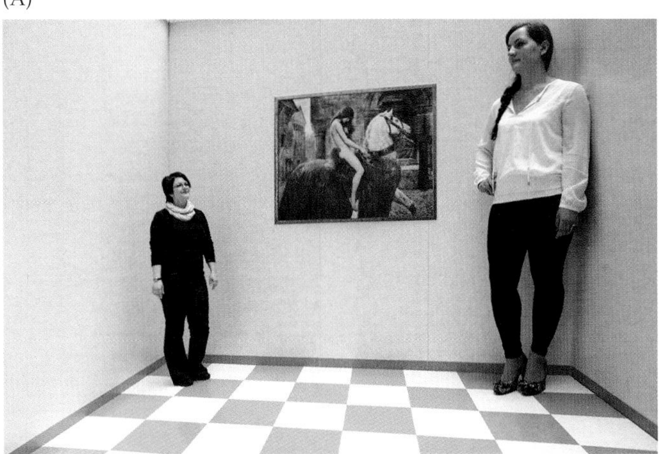

(B) (C)

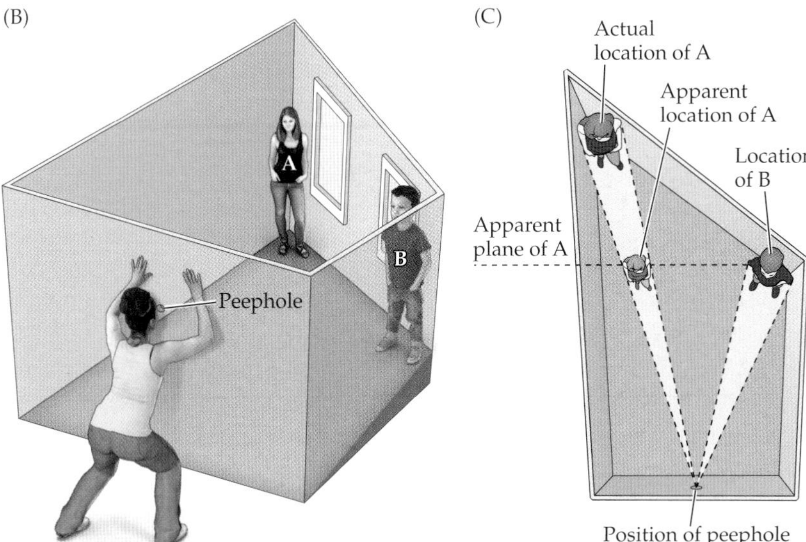

FIGURE 6.54 The Ames Room (A) The size of these people is distorted because you are looking at a very distorted room (B) but assuming that it is a normal room. (C) That makes the far-away person on the left appear closer and smaller than she is.

fingers and the clock into a single perception of something that does not exist in the world. Accordingly, the visual system chooses to *suppress* one image and perceive the other. In the present situation, you probably see the clock as though you were looking through a hole in your hand.

How does the visual system "decide" what to see? The more interesting of the two stimuli is likely to be dominant. *Interesting* in this case has several meanings. The most important factor is which stimulus is more salient to the early stages of cortical visual processing. High contrast is more salient than low contrast, bright is better than dim, moving objects are more interesting than stationary ones, and so forth (Fahle, 1982). The meaning of the stimulus also has an effect (Yu and Blake, 1992), as does what you're attending to (Ooi and He, 1999).

The competition between the two eyes for control of visual perception, known as **binocular rivalry**, is never completely won by either eye (Alais and Blake, 2005; Wheatstone, 1852) or either stimulus (R. Blake and Logothetis, 2002). If you stare at the combination of the clock and hand long enough, your fingers will eventually conquer the visual territory, only to surrender it back to the clock a moment later. The battle is easier to see if the two combatants are more closely matched. If you

binocular rivalry The competition between the two eyes for control of visual perception, which is evident when completely different stimuli are presented to the two eyes.

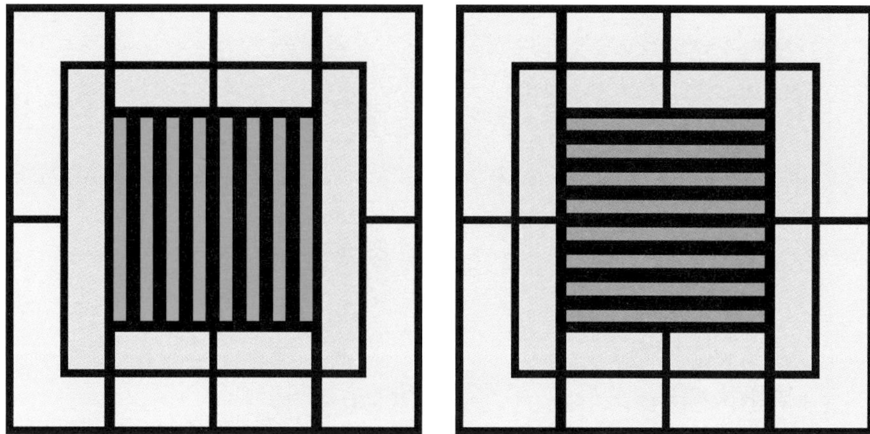

FIGURE 6.55 Binocular rivalry If you free-fuse these two images, you will be able to watch the blue vertical bars and orange horizontal bars engage in the perceptual battle known as binocular rivalry.

free-fuse the two panels of **FIGURE 6.55**, your visual system will not actually combine the perpendicular stripes in the two center squares. Instead, you will see a battle between the vertically and horizontally striped patches, with regions of dominance growing and shrinking over time, something like the cartoon in **FIGURE 6.56**.

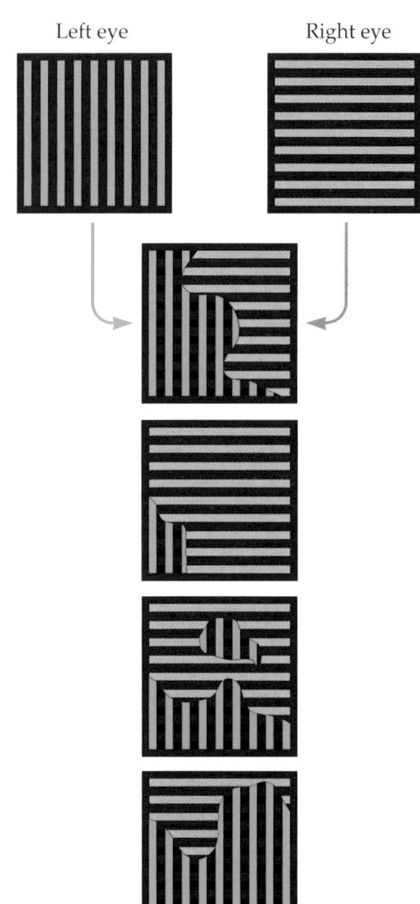

FIGURE 6.56 The dynamics of rivalry If the blue vertical bars are shown to one eye while the orange horizontal bars are shown to the other, the two stimuli will battle for dominance.

Binocular rivalry might seem an odd situation that would arise only in a vision lab or a perception course, but a moment's reflection should convince you that the stimuli for rivalry are actually very common. If you cover one eye and then the other while looking at the three-dimensional world, you should notice that there are various features visible to only one eye (for example, near the edges of nearby objects). If something is visible in only one eye, something else is present in the corresponding location in the other eye. When the stimuli presented to corresponding points in the two eyes are unrelated, rivalry occurs. The classic demonstrations of rivalry pit a stimulus in one eye against a stimulus in the other eye. More recently, it has become clear that rivalry is part of a larger effort by the visual system to come up with the most likely version of the world, given the current retinal images (sounds Bayesian again, doesn't it?) (Clifford, 2009). If you can free-fuse **FIGURE 6.57A**, you will see the chimp and the text battle each other. That is just standard binocular rivalry. Interestingly, you will see a similar chimp/text rivalry if you free-fuse **FIGURE 6.57B**. In that case, the chimp is being put together from bits in the two eyes. Your brain is not trying to pick a winner in a battle between the eyes. It is trying to figure out the world, and if that interesting chimp is seen with one eye in one spot and the other eye in another spot, the brain can put those different bits together into a coherent perception (Blake and Wilson, 2011).

In addition to the visual and cognitive factors that influence binocular rivalry, you might not be surprised to find out that input from other senses can bias the fight between the two eyes. Hense, Badde, and Röder (2019) had observers viewing bars going up in one eye and down in the other. The winner of the rivalry battle between these two motions could be influenced by the sensation of motion created by feeling a ridged wheel as it rotated under the fingers. ●

Rivalry is a very useful tool for probing one of the more vexing problems in the neuroscience of perception and consciousness: What parts of the visual system give rise to the conscious experience of seeing something? For these purposes, the great feature of rivalry is that it dissociates the stimulus on the retina from the stimulus that you see. Imagine that you record from single cells somewhere in the monkey visual system (Logothetis and Schall, 1989) or you use functional magnetic resonance imaging to look at the working human brain. If you train the monkeys or ask humans to monitor their perception ("Do you see vertical or

(A)

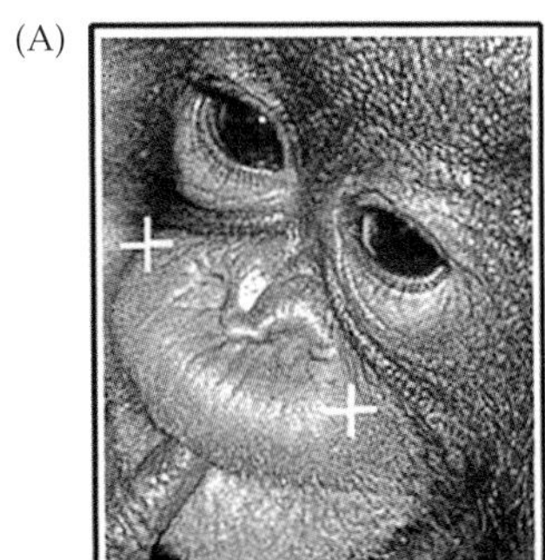

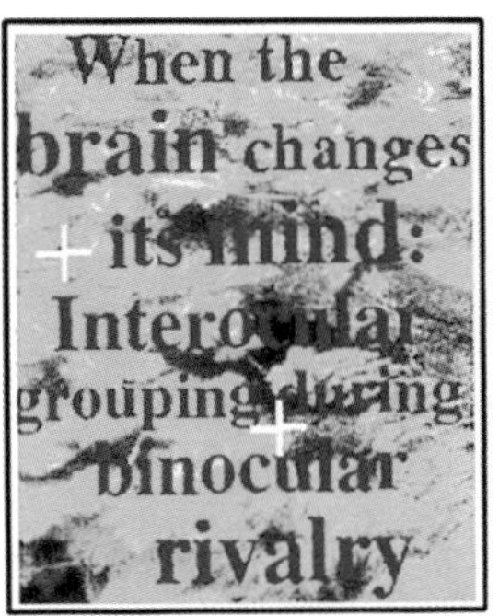

(B)

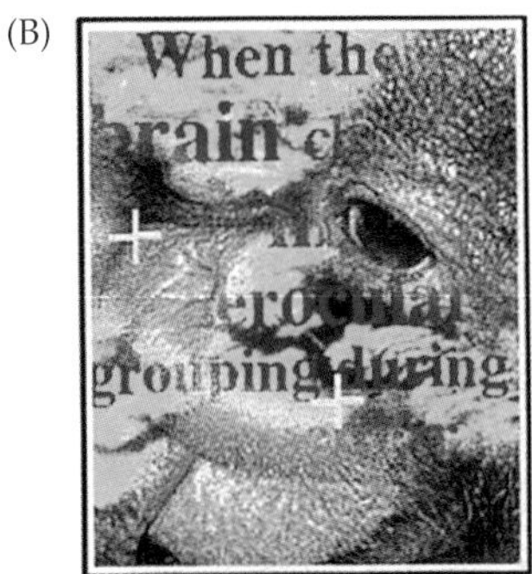

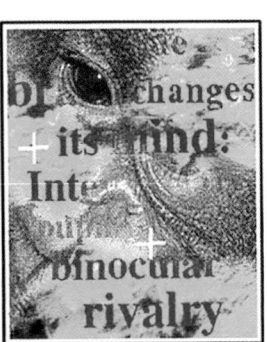

FIGURE 6.57 Binocular cooperation? Binocular rivalry is not just a fight between the two eyes. If you can free-fuse these pairs of images, you will see a typical example of rivalry. (A) Different images in each eye struggle for dominance. (B) The chimp and the text struggle for dominance in this panel also, but this is pattern rivalry: the two eyes are actually cooperating to put together coherent views of the chimp or the text.

horizontal?"), you can ask whether the neural signal in a specific part of the visual pathway follows the physical stimulus or the perceived stimulus. It is a complex and evolving story, but one that clearly shows that conscious visual awareness is not something that happens in one discrete step in a chain of visual processing (Tong, Meng, and Blake, 2006).

6.5 Development of Binocular Vision and Stereopsis

What is binocular vision like in infants? Babies are born with two eyes, but are they born with stereopsis? If not, how does binocular function develop? In a wonderful conversation about visual development, Davida Teller and Tony Movshon (1986) recalled a lecture by a disillusioned developmental psychologist, John McKee, who argued that the field could be summed up by three laws:

1. As children get older, they get better at things.
2. Whatever it is, girls do it before boys.
3. Everything develops along with everything else.

To these "laws," Teller added a summary statement: "Things start out badly, then they get better; then, after a long time, they get worse again" (Teller and Movshon, 1986).

As it turns out, research over the past 30 years or so has shown that visual development provides support for the first and second laws, but not for a strict form of the third. The development of binocular vision and stereopsis provides one of the strongest violations of that third law.

Most visual functions indeed start off badly (but not as badly as we used to think) and then improve steadily until they reach adult levels. However, the development of stereopsis is surprising, in that infants are essentially blind to disparity until about 3–4 months of age. At that point, stereopsis appears quite suddenly—almost out of the blue. Of course, measuring stereopsis (or anything else) in infants is no

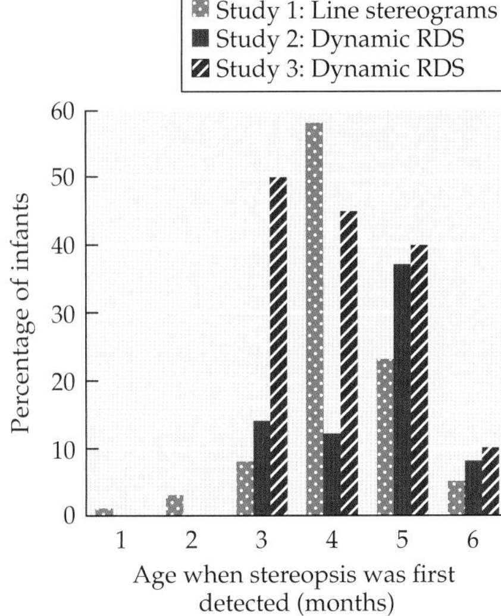

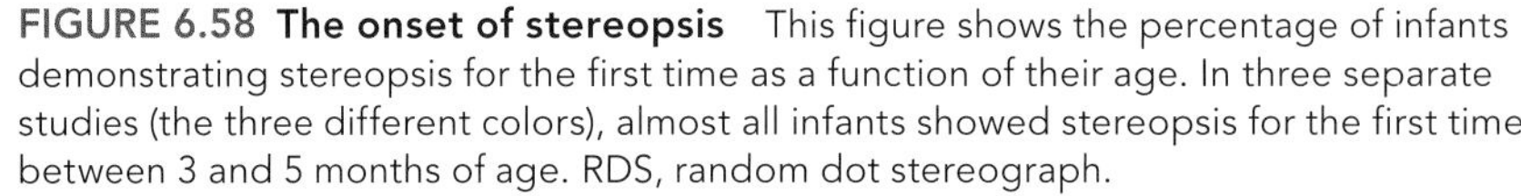
FIGURE 6.58 The onset of stereopsis This figure shows the percentage of infants demonstrating stereopsis for the first time as a function of their age. In three separate studies (the three different colors), almost all infants showed stereopsis for the first time between 3 and 5 months of age. RDS, random dot stereograph.

easy task, but developmental psychologists have been very inventive in designing methods for assessing development.

It is now quite well established that infants 6 months and older are sensitive to depth based on pictorial cues, and more recent studies show that infants as young as 4 months are sensitive to relative height (Tsuruhara et al., 2014). But how about stereoscopic depth, based on binocular disparity? Despite differences in techniques and procedures, most investigators agree about the onset of stereoscopic depth. **FIGURE 6.58** summarizes the results of several studies, showing the age at which stereopsis can first be detected. These studies (and others like them) looked for evidence indicating that infants could reliably detect a large binocular disparity (typically on the order of 30–60 arc minutes). The agreement among the studies is remarkable. Infants are essentially stereoblind before 3 months, with most infants showing a sudden onset of stereopsis between 3 and 5 months.

stereoacuity A measure of the smallest binocular disparity that can generate a sensation of depth.

Stereopsis is not an all-or-none phenomenon. Just as an individual's acuity is a measure of his ability to resolve spatial detail, **stereoacuity** is a measure of the smallest binocular disparity that can generate a sensation of depth. Once an infant develops stereopsis, stereoacuity increases rapidly to near adult levels (**FIGURE 6.59**). Birch and Petrig (1996) found that stereoacuity rose from essentially nothing before 4 months to near adult levels by 6 months. This time course is very different from the time course seen in the development of simple acuity. Though coarsely present at birth, basic acuity takes years to reach adult levels. The same difference between basic acuity and stereoacuity is seen in monkeys (O'Dell and Boothe, 1997), but the overall rate of development is faster in monkeys. Interestingly, not only stereoacuity but also several other visual functions develop at a rate approximately four times faster than in humans, as if one monkey week were the equivalent of one human month. In keeping with this rule of one human month being equal to one monkey week, stereopsis can be detected in monkeys within the first 3–5 weeks of life, compared with the 3- to 5-month window of onset observed in humans.

How, then, do we explain the sudden emergence of stereopsis in humans at about 4 months? Although a newborn infant makes convergence eye movements to track a target as it approaches her nose, accurate and consistent convergence probably does not occur until 3–4 months of age (Sreenivasan et al., 2016). But we can't conclude that inaccurate convergence prevents stereopsis from developing earlier than 4 months, because convergence does not need to be very accurate to detect large disparities. Moreover, several studies used repeating gratings, which would be fused at some disparity even

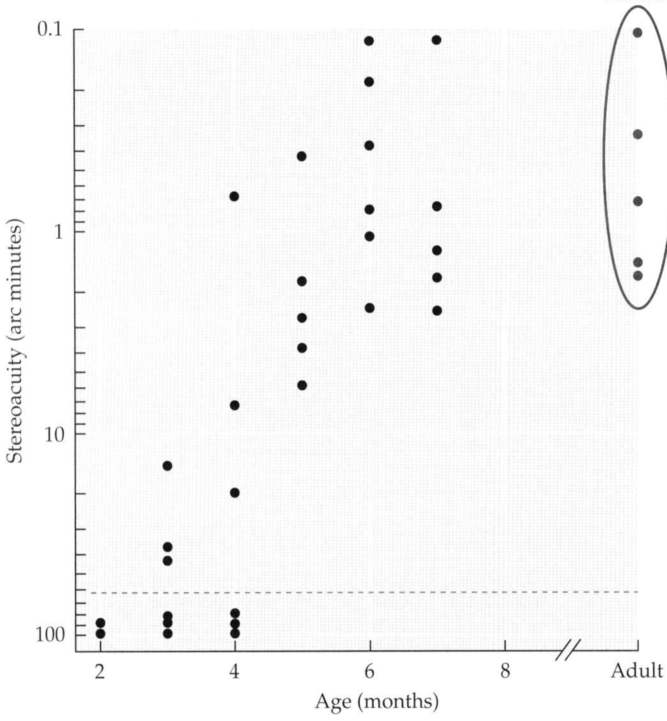

FIGURE 6.59 The development of stereoacuity Stereoacuity develops to adult levels within the first 6–7 months of life. Data points below the dashed line indicate unmeasurable stereoacuity.

if convergence were inaccurate. Before 4 months, babies don't respond to these stereoscopic stimuli either.

An alternative view is that the failure of stereopsis to develop prior to 4 months might mean that some part of the visual system is immature. Disparity-sensitive neurons in the primary visual cortex (V1) are one plausible candidate for that immature part, but recent anatomical and physiological data suggest that we need to look beyond V1 for an explanation of why infants don't exhibit stereopsis.

Yuzo Chino and his colleagues made the most detailed quantitative study of the binocular responses of V1 neurons of infant monkeys (Chino et al., 1997). They presented a pair of drifting sine wave gratings **dichoptically** (one to each eye). The sine waves were identical in spatial frequency, orientation, contrast, and velocity, and each of the values was chosen to maximize the cell's response. A phase difference between the two monocular gratings will also create binocular disparity. Some cells in the visual cortex are sensitive to this phase shift (Ohzawa and Freeman, 1986a, 1986b). When Chino et al. (1997) varied the relative spatial phase of the two drifting sine waves (**FIGURE 6.60A**), the response of a binocular neuron waxed and waned (**FIGURE 6.60B**). The dashed lines in Figure 6.60B show the levels of response for the two eyes, stimulated alone. Notice that for some

dichoptic Referring to the presentation of two different stimuli, one to each eye. Different from *binocular* presentation, which could involve both eyes looking at a single stimulus.

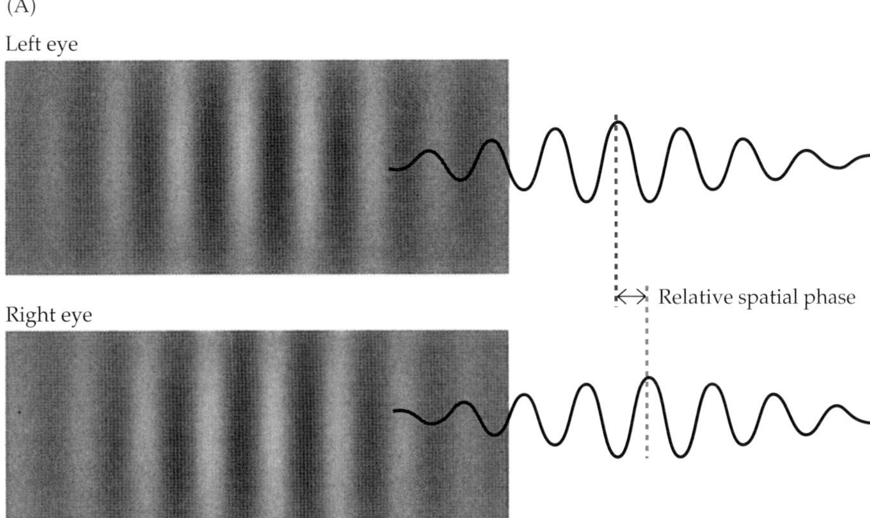

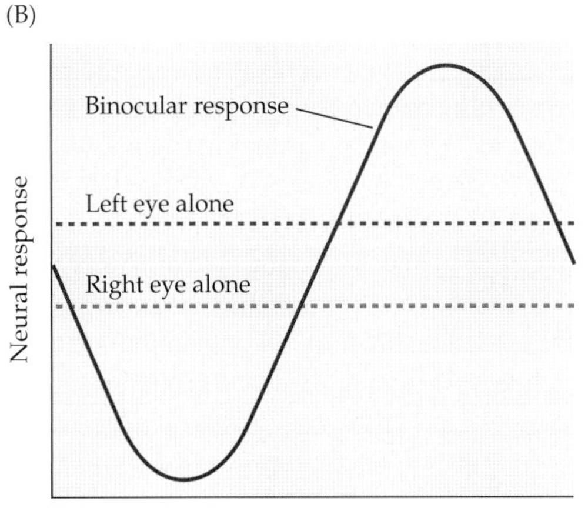

FIGURE 6.60 Interocular phase difference gratings These gratings can be used to study disparity tuning. (A) The sinusoidal grating drifts differently in one eye than in the other, producing a sinusoidal change in spatial phase disparity. (B) The response of a binocular neuron. Notice that the binocular response varies with phase, whereas the monocular responses do not.

interocular phase differences, the binocular response was considerably higher than the response through either eye alone. At other interocular phase differences, the binocular response was lower than the response through either eye alone. This sinusoidal binocular phase tuning is the hallmark of this type of binocular neuron in the visual cortex. Using this sensitive method, Chino et al. found that within the first week of life—well before the onset of stereopsis—infant monkeys had practically the same proportion of phase disparity–sensitive neurons that adults have in primary visual cortex.

In addition, the ocular dominance properties of these infant monkeys were essentially identical to those of adults. Other investigators have also found that ocular dominance columns in the input layers of V1 are essentially adult-like at birth (Horton and Hocking, 1996).

FURTHER DISCUSSION of ocular dominance can be found in Section 3.5.

What do these studies tell us about the development of stereopsis? The results suggest that the neural apparatus in a newborn's V1 is capable of combining signals from the two eyes and that it is sensitive to interocular disparities. So why are newborns blind to disparity? One possibility is that the extraction of relative disparity, which is needed for stereoacuity, takes place beyond V1, possibly in V2. At this time we do not know much about how V2 neurons in newborns respond to disparity, but emerging evidence suggests that other receptive-field properties mature later in V2 than in V1 (Zhang et al., 2005; Zheng et al., 2007).

Another possibility is that the problem is in V1. Although V1 cells of newborn monkeys are adult-like in their response to interocular phase disparity, these neurons remain immature in several important ways. They do not have adult sensitivity to monocular spatial frequency or direction of motion. Moreover, they are much less responsive overall than are adult neurons—that is, their peak firing rates are considerably lower. In addition, these neurons display more interocular suppression than adult neurons do. Thus, it is also possible that because of the immaturity in V1 neurons, the signals they send to the next stage of processing are too weak or confused to support stereopsis.

It is noteworthy that even at 4 to 6 months of age, infants show quantitative and qualitative response immaturities for relative disparity information, becoming adult-like by 4 to 7 years of age (Norcia et al., 2017). Moreover, integration of different cues to depth, such as disparity and texture cues, appears to develop later. For example, while 6-year-old children are sensitive to both disparity and slant information, they do not integrate them, and integration does not emerge until age 12 (Nardini, Bedford, and Mareschal, 2010), and children less than 10.5 years old show no evidence of integrating disparity and relative motion cues to depth, whereas older children showed evidence for integrating them in cortical area V3B (Dekker et al., 2015).

Abnormal Visual Experience Can Disrupt Binocular Vision

The presence of all this binocular hardware, even if it is immature, strongly suggests that extensive binocular visual experience is not necessary for binocular connections to form in V1. These connections are present at birth or very shortly thereafter, so we don't need to "learn" or develop binocular vision. However, the normal development of adult binocular vision and stereopsis does require visual experience. In Section 3.8, we learned about Hubel and Wiesel's work on the **critical period**, the period during early visual development when normal binocular visual stimulation is required for normal cortical development. During this period, the visual cortex is

critical period A period of time during development when the organism is particularly susceptible to developmental change. There are critical periods in the development of binocular vision, human language, and so on.

highly susceptible to any disorder that alters normal binocular visual experience. In cats and monkeys, this critical period is approximately the first 3–4 months of life.

We cannot study a child's visual cortex the way we might study a monkey's or a cat's. How, then, can we estimate the critical period in humans? Some humans are born with two eyes that do not point at the same spot in the world. This not-uncommon disorder (its incidence is about 3%) is known as **strabismus**, and we mentioned it in connection with stereoblindness in Section 6.3. In **esotropia**, one eye is pointed too far toward the nose ("cross-eyed"). In **exotropia**, the deviating eye is pointed too far to the side. There are various ways to treat strabismus. For example, it is possible to surgically correct the position of the eyes. For the present discussion, however, the important point is that it is possible to test adults who had misaligned eyes at different times and for different durations during childhood.

strabismus A misalignment of the two eyes such that a single object in space is imaged on the fovea of one eye and on a nonfoveal area of the other (turned) eye.

esotropia Strabismus in which one eye deviates inward.

exotropia Strabismus in which one eye deviates outward.

tilt aftereffect The perceptual illusion of tilt, produced by adaptation to a pattern of a given orientation.

FIGURE 6.61A shows a circa 1940s synoptophore (left panel), a Wheatstone stereoscope used in clinical settings for assessing and treating strabismus. The synoptophore allows separate images to be presented to the two eyes (an example is shown in Figure 6.61B, top) and alignment of the images on corresponding areas in the two eyes by adjusting the positions of the mirrors to enable fusion. In addition, the synoptophore is used to try to reduce suppression, encourage fusion and stereopsis, and increase the range of fusional vergence. These functions can (and have been) readily achieved using virtual reality display devices (an example is the Vive Pro Eye head-mounted display shown in Figure 6.61B, bottom).

FURTHER DISCUSSION of strabismus can be found in Section 3.8.

Recall from Section 3.7 that exposure to lines tilted to one side of vertical will make vertical lines appear tilted to the other side. This is known as the **tilt aftereffect**. One characteristic of the tilt aftereffect is that it shows interocular transfer (transfer of the effect from one eye to the other). If we show the adapting lines to one eye, we can measure an aftereffect through the other eye. This result is generally taken to show that the cells responsible for the effect are binocular: they receive input from both eyes (for some details, see Wolfe and Held, 1981). Individuals who exhibited strabismus during the first 18 months of life do not show normal interocular transfer (Banks, Aslin, and Letson, 1975; Hohmann and Creutzfeldt, 1975). This result provides an indirect estimate of the period during which binocular connections in humans are susceptible to abnormal input.

(A)

(B)

(C)

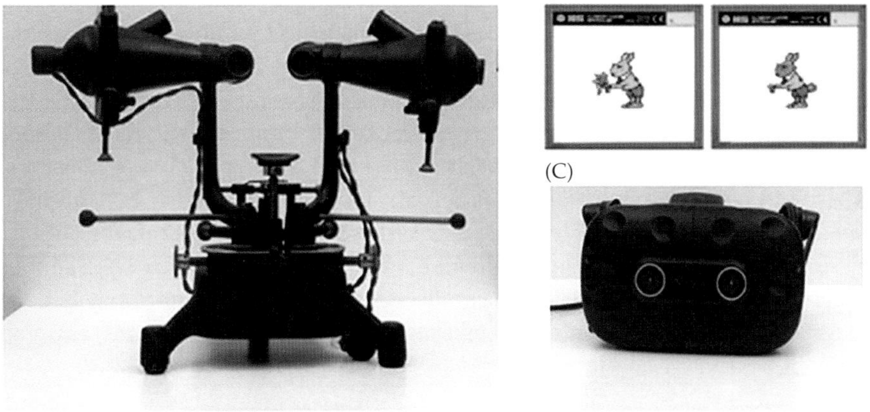

FIGURE 6.61 Stereoscopes for measuring and treating binocular anomalies (A) Vintage synoptophore (circa 1940s). (B) Fusion slides, one viewed by each eye in the synoptophore. (C) Vive Pro Eye virtual reality head-mounted display.

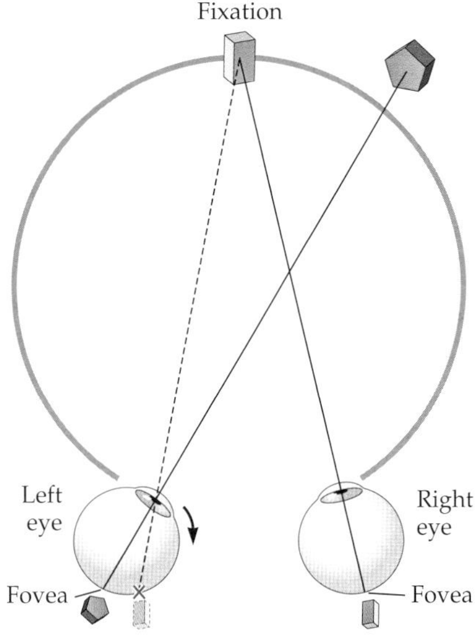

FIGURE 6.62 Left esotropia The person wants to fixate on the yellow brick, but the left eye is turned too far toward the nose; as a result, the left fovea is pointing at a different location (here, the purple pentagon), while the image of the yellow brick falls to the right of the left fovea.

Let's explore in a bit more detail why strabismus disrupts binocular vision. We will use left esotropia as an example. In left esotropia (**FIGURE 6.62**), the left eye is turned in. As a consequence, although the object of fixation (the yellow brick, in this case) lands on the fovea of the right eye, in the left eye it lands on a region in the "nasal" retina (i.e., the half of the retina closer to the nose). This means that the images of the yellow brick are in noncorresponding points in the two eyes. What will the person see? If an adult becomes esotropic (perhaps because of an injury), she will experience diplopia (double vision), seeing two bricks instead of one. However, people who exhibit strabismus early in life often experience no such problem. Why? Notice that something is present at the fovea of the left eye. In Figure 6.62, this "something" is a purple pentagon. Thus, in strabismus, normally corresponding points in the two eyes receive conflicting information (this situation is known—not unreasonably—as "confusion"). To eliminate diplopia and confusion, the brain suppresses one of the two images—it is simply not consciously perceived. Reasonably enough, this is known as **suppression**. In esotropia, the most common pattern is suppression of the input from the eye that is turned in. So, in the example in Figure 6.62, the person would most likely suppress visual input from the left eye.

suppression In reference to vision, the inhibition of an unwanted image. Suppression occurs frequently in people with strabismus.

Binocular rivalry is a form of suppression, so some suppression is an important part of normal visual experience. Unfortunately, early-onset strabismus can have other, more serious effects on the developing visual nervous system and on visual performance. For example, strabismus greatly reduces the number of binocular neurons in the visual cortex (Wiesel, 1982). Cells that would normally be driven by both eyes are dominated by only one. You would be correct if you suspected that this situation disrupts stereopsis. Birch and her colleagues (e.g., Stager and Birch, 1986) followed the development of stereopsis in normal and esotropic infants. **FIGURE 6.63** illustrates the percentage of infants who showed a measurable ability to perceive stereoscopic depth. The red line shows that by about 6 months of age, almost all normal infants demonstrate stereopsis. In contrast, infants with esotropia (all of whom were diagnosed by 6 months of age) initially demonstrated a normal pattern of stereopsis development. After 4 months, however, very few of the esotropic infants demonstrated stereopsis, although recent work suggests that "coarse" stereopsis—sensitivity to very large disparities—may be present in some children with strabismus and amblyopia (Giaschi et al., 2013).

This result has an interesting parallel in cortical physiology. Chino and his colleagues made otherwise normal monkeys strabismic (Kumagami et al., 2000). They found that a brief period of experimental strabismus shortly after the age of onset of stereopsis produced a greater loss of disparity sensitivity and more binocular suppression in V1 neurons than did an earlier episode of strabismus. These physiological and perceptual deficits appear to be permanent and have important implications for the surgical treatment of esotropia in infants. Almost all surgeons agree that treatment should happen early, but there has been a lot of debate about just how early. These results suggest that, to minimize the damage done by esotropia, treatment should take place before the age (~4 months) at which stereopsis normally develops.

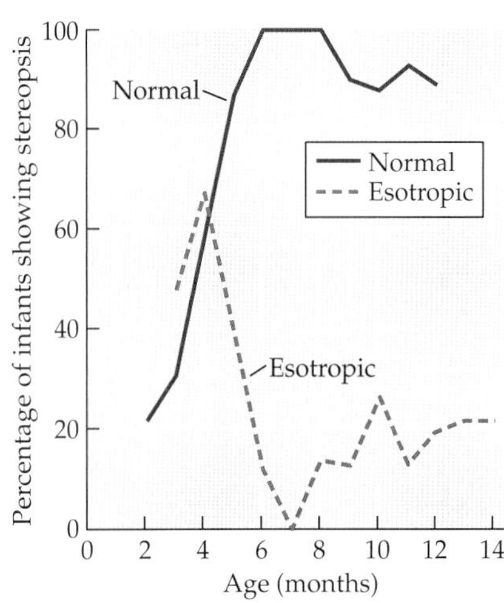

FIGURE 6.63 Development of stereopsis The solid red line shows normally developing infants. The dashed blue lines show infants with esotropia. Beyond 4 months, very few esotropic infants demonstrated stereopsis.

Summary

1. Reconstructing a three-dimensional world from two non-Euclidean, curved, two-dimensional retinal images is one basic problem faced by the brain.
2. A number of monocular cues provide information about three-dimensional space. These include occlusion, various size and position cues, aerial perspective, linear perspective, motion cues, accommodation, and convergence.
3. Having two eyes is an advantage for a number of reasons, some of which have to do with depth perception. It is important to remember, however, that it is possible to reconstruct the three-dimensional world from a single two-dimensional image. Two eyes have other advantages over just one: expanding the visual field, permitting binocular summation, and providing redundancy if one eye is damaged.
4. Having two laterally separated eyes connected to a single brain also provides us with important information about depth through the geometry of the small differences between the images in each eye. These differences, known as binocular disparities, give rise to stereoscopic depth perception.
5. Random dot stereograms show that we don't need to know what we're seeing before we see it in stereoscopic depth. Binocular disparity alone can support shape perception.
6. Stereopsis has been exploited to add, literally, depth to entertainment—from nineteenth-century photos to twenty-first-century movies. It has also served to enhance the perception of information in military and medical settings.
7. The difficulty of matching an image element in one eye with the correct element in the other eye is known as the correspondence problem. The brain uses several strategies to solve the problem. For example, it reduces the initial complexity of the problem by matching large "blobs" in the low-spatial-frequency information before trying to match every high-frequency detail.
8. Single neurons in the primary visual cortex and beyond have receptive fields that cover a region in three-dimensional space, not just the two-dimensional image plane. Some neurons seem to be concerned with a crude in-front/behind judgment. Other neurons are concerned with more precise, metrical depth perception.
9. When the stimuli on corresponding loci in the two eyes are different, we experience a continual perceptual competition between the two eyes, known as binocular rivalry. Rivalry is part of the effort to make the best guess about the current state of the world based on the current state of the input.
10. All of the various monocular and binocular depth cues are combined (unconsciously) according to what prior knowledge tells us about the probability of the current event. Making the wrong guess about the cause of visual input can lead to illusions. Bayes' theorem is the basis of one type of formal understanding of the rules of combination.
11. Stereopsis emerges suddenly at about 4 months of age in humans, and it can be disrupted through abnormal visual experience during a critical period early in life.

Chapter 7

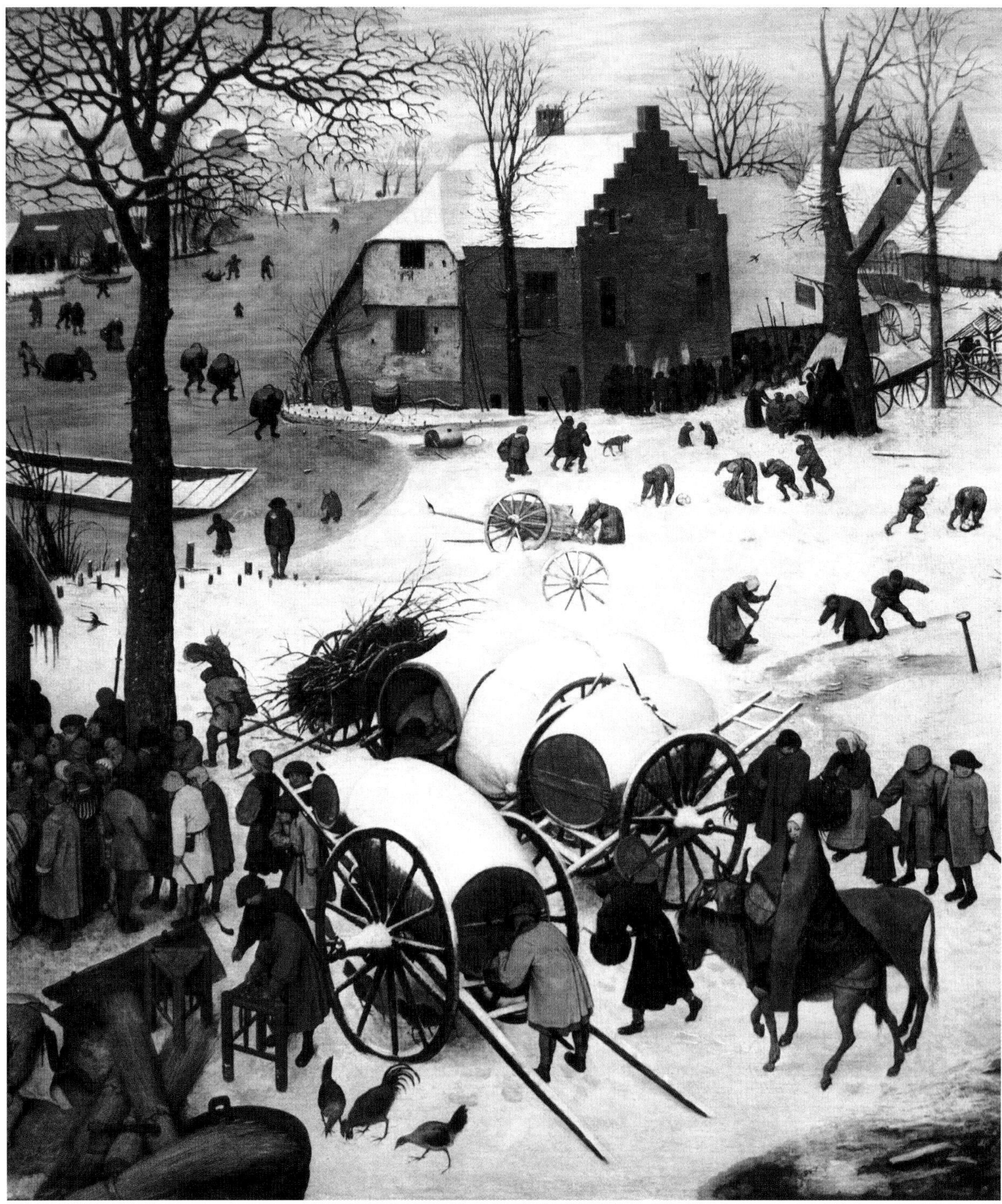

Painting "Census at Bethlehem", 1566 by Pieter Bruegel the Elder/ Sergi Reboredo/Alamy Stock Photo

Attention and Scene Perception

Questions to Contemplate

Think about the following questions as you read this chapter. By the chapter's end, you should be able to answer and discuss them.

- Why can't we process everything at once?
- Is attention really like a spotlight? What would that mean?
- How do we find what we are looking for?
- What changes in the brain when we "pay attention"?
- If we can attend to only one (or a very few) objects at once, why does the world seem to be filled with many, many clearly perceived objects?
- How much do we actually notice and/or remember of what we see?
- Are different kinds of scenes processed differently?

If you're reading this, you are probably a student. If you're a student, you are probably taking more than one course and are therefore very busy. Here's an idea: Why not read two books at the same time? Chapter 2 will have told you that the limit on peripheral acuity is one reason that this won't work. However, the acuity problem could be overcome if the size of the print were increased, as in **FIGURE 7.1**. Nevertheless, even with suitably large letters, it will be clear to you that you cannot look at the column of *X*s in the figure and read the two sentences *at the same time*. While looking at the *X*s, you can choose to read the words on one side or the other, but you can't read both sides simultaneously (White, Boynton, and Yeatman, 2019). This is a specific example of a more general problem—namely, that the retinal array contains far more information than we can process. **FIGURE 7.2** shows another example. We cannot possibly recognize all the objects in this picture at once, but if you are asked to find a horse, you can do that fairly easily. That's why "Where's Waldo?" and "I Spy" games are a challenge. This is not just a visual problem. All of the senses receive more input than we can handle (see Chapter 10 for a discussion of attention in hearing).

Why can't we process everything at once? Quite literally, we don't have the brains for it. Remember from Chapter 4 that recognizing a single object like an elephant requires a sizable chunk of the brain and its processing power, especially when that elephant could be seen in many different orientations, under different lighting conditions, at different retinal sizes, and so on. Moreover, to understand Figure 7.2, we also need to process the relationships between objects—like the fact that umbrellas are being held over people's heads. If we do the math for even a fairly small subset of all possible visual stimuli, it turns out that processing everything, everywhere, all at once requires a brain that will not fit in the human head (Tsotsos, 1990).

If it is not possible to process everything all at once, what *should* be processed? This matter can't be left to chance. If you are crossing a road, you need to determine that no car will hit you, so devoting your visual capacity to the vital tweet that just appeared on your phone is dangerous. (Many YouTube videos will demonstrate

These	X	Is
letters	X	it
are	X	time
big	X	for
and	X	a
easy	X	quick
to	X	snack
read.	X	yet?

FIGURE 7.1 Attentional limits Even though all the letters are big enough to resolve while looking at the Xs, we simply cannot read the left-hand and right-hand sentences at the same time.

this. Just remember to stop walking before you ask your browser to show you "texting while walking" videos.) To deal with this problem, we "pay attention" to some stimuli and not to others. As we will see in this chapter, **attention** is not a single *thing*, and it does not have a single locus in the nervous system (Chun, Golomb, and Turk-Browne, 2011). Rather, *attention* is the name we give to a family of mechanisms that restrict or bias processing in various ways.

Here are some of the distinctions we can make when considering varieties of attention:

- Attention can be internal or external. *External* attention refers to attention to stimuli in the world (our primary concern here), but we should not forget *internal* attention, our ability to attend to one line of thought as opposed to another or to select one response over another.
- Attention can be overt or covert. *Overt* attention usually refers to directing a sense organ at a stimulus—fixating the eyes on a single word, for example. However, you can direct your attention *covertly*, as, for example, when you pay attention to someone at a party while looking elsewhere.

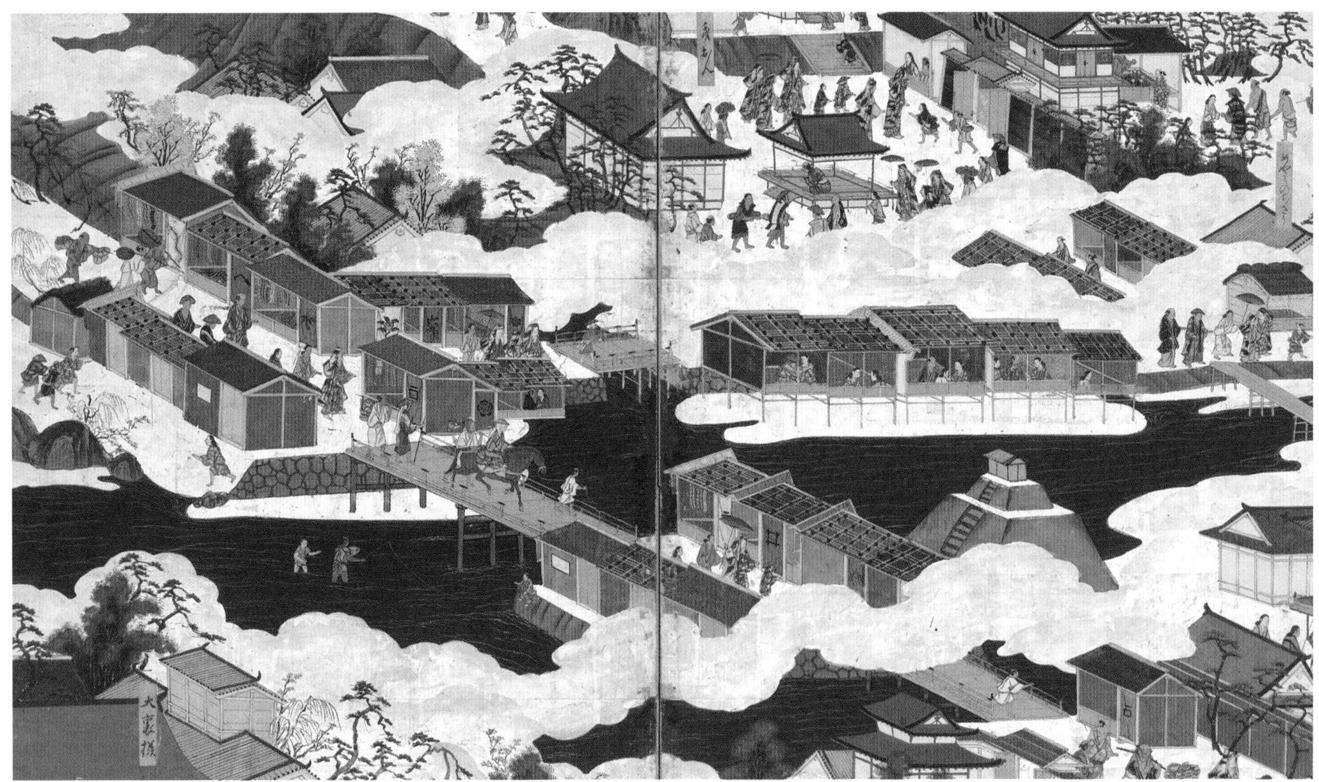

FIGURE 7.2 Where's the horse? We cannot possibly recognize all the objects in this picture at once, but if you are asked to find a horse, you can do that fairly easily.

- Reading this text while continuing to be aware of music playing in the room is an example of *divided* attention.
- Watching a pot on the stove, waiting for the water to boil, is a vigilance task requiring *sustained* attention.
- The ability to pick one (or a few) of many stimuli is a job for **selective attention**. This form of attention receives the most attention in this chapter.

attention Any of the very large set of selective processes in the brain. To deal with the impossibility of handling all inputs at once, the nervous system has evolved mechanisms that are able to bias processing to a subset of things, places, ideas, or moments in time.

selective attention The form of attention involved when processing is restricted to a subset of the possible stimuli.

These different forms of attention are not mutually exclusive. Choosing to stare straight ahead while choosing to attend only to an interesting person off to one side, to the exclusion of all else, might be described as an act of external, sustained, covert, selective attention.

Although we will focus on visual attention, it is important to remember that attentional mechanisms operate in all the senses. For example, the pain of getting a shot in the doctor's office may hurt more than a mild injury on the playing field because of the attention you focus on getting the shot. We can also use attentional mechanisms to give priority to one sense over others. Right now, you are probably selecting visual stimuli over auditory, even if you have music on in the background. And you didn't even notice the pressure of your posterior on the seat until we mentioned it (sorry for disrupting your attention). ●

In this chapter, first we discuss evidence that we attend to only one object (or perhaps a few) at any single moment. We consider attentional selection in space (I am attending to this object and not that object) and selection in time (I was attending to that object, but now I've selected this object). Next, we examine the changes that occur in the brain when we attend to one object rather than another, and we will see what happens when the neural substrate of attention is damaged. Finally, having argued that we can recognize only one object at a time, we will turn to scenes. If we're attending to one object, what does it mean to say that we *see* a whole scene?

7.1 Selection in Space

To begin, let's consider what it means to attend to a stimulus. A good place to start is with a cueing experiment of the sort pioneered by Michael Posner (1980). Start with the situation shown in **FIGURE 7.3A**. The participant in the experiment fixates on a central point (*). After a variable delay, a test probe (*X*) appears in one of the two boxes. All the participant needs to do is hit

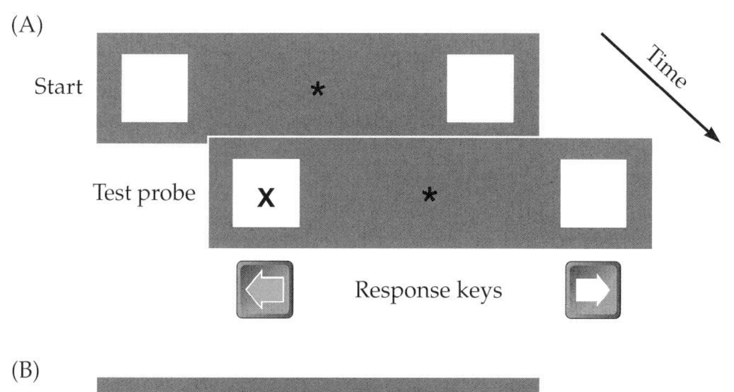

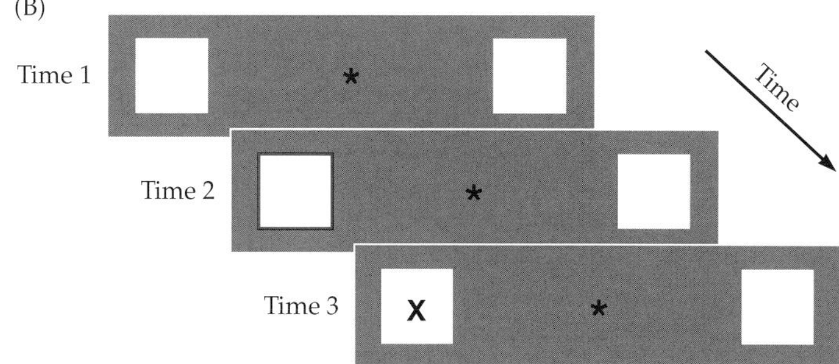

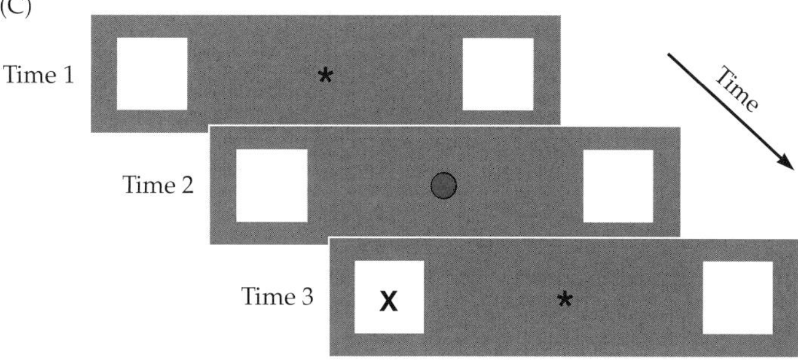

FIGURE 7.3 The Posner cueing paradigm (A) This simple probe detection experiment has two possible locations in which the test probe (X) can appear. All you have to do is hit one key if the probe appears on the left and another if it appears on the right. (B) A valid peripheral cue (red outline) indicates where the target will be. In this case the cue is valid; we are telling the truth. (C) An invalid cue points to the wrong side. Here the rule was this: If the cue (the central dot) is green, the probe is likely to be on the left; if the cue is red, the probe is likely to be on the right. This is also a different kind of cue—a symbolic cue—where color indicates the location. Symbolic cues direct attention more slowly (see Figure 7.4).

a response key as fast as possible when the probe appears. The measure of interest is the average **reaction time (RT)**—the amount of time that elapses between the point when the probe appears and the point when the participant hits the response key.

Suppose now that the situation is slightly changed: During the waiting period, the participant is given a **cue**, a stimulus that provides a hint about where the target might appear. In **FIGURE 7.3B**, the cue is a change in the outline color of one of the two boxes (a "peripheral cue"). Because the test probe appears in the cued location, this peripheral cue is said to be a "valid cue." Not surprisingly, Posner found that RT decreases with a valid cue. Compared with the no-cue control situation, the participant generally responds faster to the probe because she is "paying attention" to the correct location. In **FIGURE 7.3C**, we have a different kind of cue. The red dot is a "symbolic cue," but it can also direct attention. In Figure 7.3C, however, the cue is misleading, or "invalid," because the cued location is on the right but the probe appears on the left. RTs are slower here than in the control condition, because the participant has been fooled into attending to the wrong location.

The peripheral cue (the outlined box) is an example of an **exogenous cue**. Exogenous cues seem to summon attention automatically by virtue of their physical salience. The symbolic cue (the red dot) is an example of an **endogenous cue**. Endogenous cues can be considered something like instructions that can be voluntarily obeyed. The endogenous cue says "go right," so you go right, while the exogenous cue could drag you to the right, whether you wanted to go there or not. *Endo* and *exo* refer to "inside" and "outside," respectively, as in the vertebrate *endo*skeleton and the *exo*skeleton on the outside of an insect (Posner, 1980).

Peripheral/exogenous and symbolic/endogenous cues can be valid or invalid. As in Figure 7.3C, an invalid cue might tell you to go right, when the target actually appears on the left. In a typical experiment, the cue might be valid on 80% of the trials and invalid on the remaining 20%. Since the observer doesn't know if the cue is valid, it would be in the observer's interest to deploy attention on the assumption that the cue is valid. This means that the experimenter can compare RTs from trials that had valid cues, where attention was cued left and the stimulus appeared on the left, and trials that had invalid cues, where the cue moved attention to the left but the stimulus appeared on the right.

reaction time (RT) A measure of the time from the onset of a stimulus to a response.

cue A stimulus that might indicate where (or what) a subsequent stimulus will be. Cues can be valid (giving correct information), invalid (incorrect), or neutral (uninformative).

exogenous cue In directing attention, a cue that is located out (*exo*) at the desired final location of attention.

endogenous cue In directing attention, a cue that is located in (*endo*) or near the current location of attention.

stimulus onset asynchrony (SOA) The time between the onset of one stimulus and the onset of another.

How long does it take for a cue to redirect our attention? It depends on the nature of the cue. At the beginning of a trial in a Posner cueing experiment, the participant is attending to the fixation point (time 1 in Figures 7.3B and 7.3C). The cue appears at time 2, and the probe appears at time 3. We can measure the timing of the attentional shift by varying the interval between time 2 and time 3. This is called the **stimulus onset asynchrony**, a psychophysical variable that typically goes by its acronym, **SOA**. If the SOA is 0 milliseconds (ms), the cue and probe appear simultaneously. There is no time for the cue to be used to direct attention, and there is no difference between the effects of valid or invalid cues. As the SOA increases to about 150 ms, the magnitude of the cueing effect from a valid peripheral cue increases, as shown by the red line in **FIGURE 7.4**. After that, the effect of the cue levels off or declines a bit.

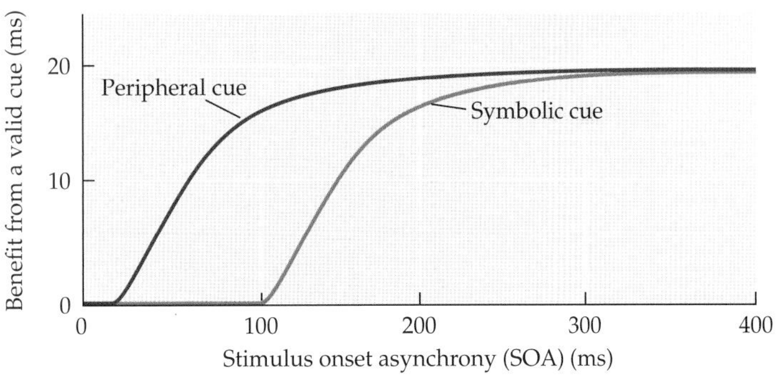

FIGURE 7.4 The time course of attentional cueing A peripheral cue (like that in Figure 7.3B) becomes fully effective 100–150 milliseconds after it appears. A symbolic cue (see Figure 7.3C) takes longer to get started and to rise to full effect.

Symbolic/endogenous cues, such as the colored dot, take longer to work (the blue line in Figure 7.4), presumably because we need to do some work to interpret them. Interestingly, some rather symbolic cues behave like fast peripheral cues. For example, we are very quick to deploy our attention to arrow cues and even faster to respond to a pair of eyes looking in one direction or another (**FIGURE 7.5**), as if we were built to get information from the gaze of others (Kuhn and Kingstone, 2009).

Interestingly, if you move your attention or your eyes to a location and then look away from that location, it is harder to look back at it again for a little while. This is known as **inhibition of return** (Klein, 2000). Inhibition of return helps to keep you from getting stuck continually revisiting one spot. For instance, suppose you were looking for those umbrellas, mentioned above, in Figure 7.2. If your attention was continually grabbed by the very salient, black river, that would be rather useless. Inhibition of return helps your search to move forward (Klein and MacInness, 1999).

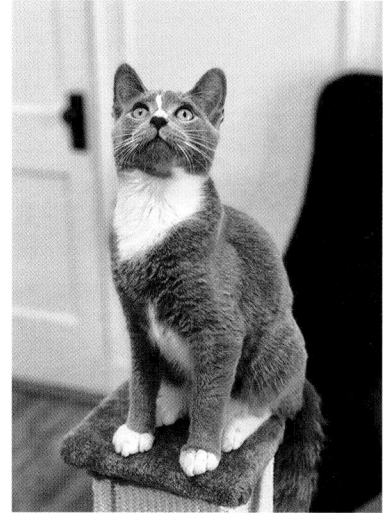

FIGURE 7.5 Gaze cueing Which way does your attention shift when you look at this photo?

The "Spotlight" of Attention

In a cueing experiment, attention starts at the fixation point and somehow ends up at the cued location. But does attention actually *move* from one point to the next? Attention could be deployed from spot to spot in a number of ways. It might move in a manner analogous to the movements of our eyes. When we shift our gaze, our point of fixation sweeps across the intervening space (although, as we will see in Section 8.4, "saccadic suppression" keeps us from noticing, and being disturbed by, this movement). Attention might sweep across space in a similar manner, like a spotlight beam (Posner, 1980).

The spotlight metaphor makes good sense and has become, perhaps, the most common way for cognitive psychologists to talk about attention. But there are other possibilities. For example, attention might expand from fixation, growing to fill the whole region from the fixation spot to the cued location, and then it might shrink to include just the cued location. This would be a version of a zoom lens model of attention (Eriksen and Yeh, 1985). Or, when attention is withdrawn from the fixation spot, it might not move at all. It might simply melt away at that location and then reappear at the cued location (Sperling and Weichselgartner, 1995). It is hard to say for sure which metaphor is "correct," because we have no direct way to measure the location and extent of attention. However, the best evidence suggests that attention is not *moving* from point to point in the brain in the way a physical spotlight would move across the world (Cave and Bichot, 1999). Moreover, there is no guarantee that there is just one "spotlight." It might be split (look ahead to Figure 7.18) (McMains and Somers, 2004), though most of the time, visual selective attention is probably directed to one thing in one location.

One last point to make about the spotlight metaphor is that you can see *something* even in the locations where the spotlight is not shining. The Nobel Prize winner Francis Crick put it nicely: "In this metaphor, the searchlight is not supposed to light up part of a completely dark landscape but, like a searchlight at dusk, it intensifies part of a scene that is already visible to some extent" (Crick, 1984). It seems that there are two pathways to your visual awareness: a selective pathway that constitutes the spotlight and a nonselective pathway that fills in the rest of your visual experience (Wolfe et al., 2011).

7.2 Visual Search

Cueing experiments provide important insight into the deployment of attention. But the situation is rather artificial, in that all of the experiments involve telling the observer exactly when and where to attend. **Visual search** experiments provide

inhibition of return The relative difficulty in getting attention (or the eyes) to move back to a recently attended (or fixated) location.

visual search A search for a target in a display containing distracting elements.

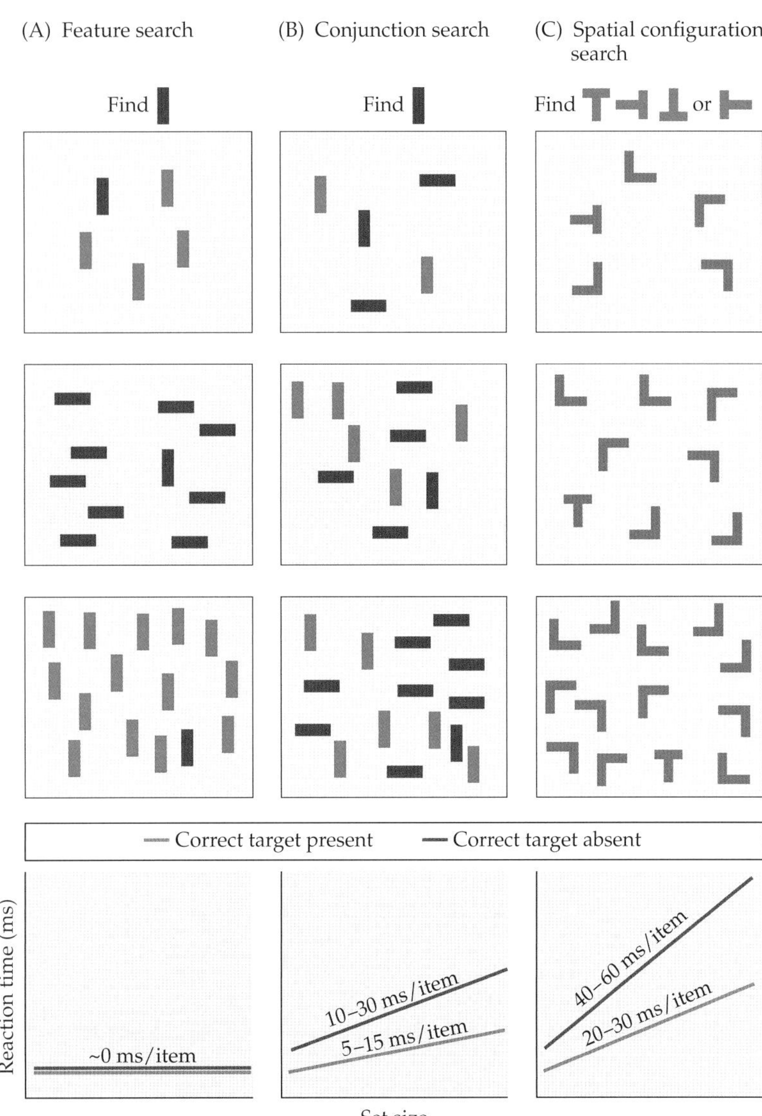

FIGURE 7.6 Laboratory visual search tasks Each part of the figure shows a different search task, with difficulty increasing from (A) to (C). Each row shows a different number of items (the set size), with difficulty increasing as set size increases. Here, we show only examples with the target present. In a typical experiment, a target might be absent in half of the trials. The graphs at the bottom depict typical patterns of results for each type of task. The purple line in each graph represents average reaction times for different set sizes on target-absent trials; the green line shows results for target-present trials.

a closer approximation of some of the actions of attention in the real world. In a typical visual search experiment, the observer looks for a **target** item among **distractor** items. Visual searches are ubiquitous in the real world; we look for faces in a crowd, mugs in a cupboard, books on a shelf, and so forth. Some searches are so easy that we hardly think of them as searches (e.g., finding the cold-water tap on a sink). Others, like finding the horse in Figure 7.2, are more demanding. Some are, quite literally, matters of life and death, as when radiologists look for tumors in X-rays or airport security officers look for threats in luggage.

The quest to understand what makes some search tasks easy and others hard has proven to be one of the most productive and interesting lines of cognitive psychology research in the past half century. **FIGURE 7.6** shows examples of the simplified visual search tasks often used in the lab. In Figures 7.6A and 7.6B, the target is a red vertical bar. In Figure 7.6C, the target is the letter *T* (in any of four possible rotations). Two factors are being varied in this figure: First, moving across the figure, the tasks increase in difficulty from left to right. Second, the **set size**—the number of items—increases as we move down each column. As a general (and unsurprising) rule, it is harder to find a target as the set size increases.

To measure the efficiency of a visual search, often we ask how much time is added (on average) for each item added to the display. To find out, the experimenter measures the RT required for the observer to say "yes" if the target is present or "no" if there is no target in the display, and observers perform the same type of search over and over. The functions relating RT to set size are graphed at the bottom of Figure 7.6. The efficiency of the search is described by the slope of the function relating RT to set size (higher slopes mean lower efficiency). *Efficiency* describes the ease with which we can work our way through a display. It is a way to compare search tasks. If we can direct attention to the target as soon as the display appears, regardless of the set size, then we have an efficient search, like the feature searches in Figure 7.6A. Here, the slope is near zero because adding more blue distractors or more horizontal distractors does not seem to make it any harder to find a red or a vertical target. If we must examine each item in turn until we find the target,

target The goal of a visual search.

distractor In a visual search, any stimulus other than the target.

set size The number of items in a visual display.

then we have an inefficient search. Figure 7.6C shows an inefficient search where each *L* needs to be examined until the observer stumbles upon a *T*. Notice that being able to say "Yes, the target is present" is typically faster and more efficient than saying "No, it is not." This is because even in the hardest task, a lucky observer might stumble on the presence of the target with her first deployment of attention, but it is not possible to stumble on the *absence* of the target in the same way.

Although all the displays in Figure 7.6 include a target, in a typical experiment the target might be present in 50% of the trials and absent in the other 50%.

feature search Visual search for a target defined by a single attribute, such as a salient color or orientation.

salience The vividness of a stimulus relative to its neighbors.

parallel search Visual search in which multiple stimuli are processed at the same time.

Feature Searches Are Efficient

The task in Figure 7.6A is a simple **feature search**. Here, the target is defined by the presence of a single feature. Each example contains an item with a unique color or orientation. If the unique item is sufficiently **salient** (if it stands out visually from its neighbors), it almost doesn't matter how many distractors there are. The target seems to "pop out" of the display. Actually, it does get a little harder in ways that are theoretically important, but not really noticeable by the average searcher (Buetti et al., 2016). Apparently, we can process the color or orientation of all the items at once (often called a **parallel search**). When we measure the RT, it barely changes with the set size. The results will approximate the flat lines plotted at the bottom of Figure 7.6A; more technically, the slope of the function relating RT to set size is near 0 ms per item.

Between one dozen and two dozen basic attributes seem able to support parallel visual search (Wolfe and Horowitz, 2017). These include obvious stimulus properties such as color, size, orientation, and motion (A. Treisman, 1986a, 1986b) and some less obvious attributes, like lighting direction (Enns and Rensink, 1990). In **FIGURE 7.7A**, the bar that is lit from below pops out of the display. In **FIGURE 7.7B**, a similar set of shapes shows no depth and no pop-out of the odd item (did you find it?).

Many Searches Are Inefficient

When the target and distractors in a visual search task contain the same basic features, as in Figure 7.6C, search is inefficient. Here, we are looking for *T*s among *L*s where both targets and distractors are composed of a vertical and a horizontal bar. It is not hard to distinguish a *T* from an *L*, but we need to attend to each item until we stumble on the target. Even if, as in Figure 7.1, the letters are big enough that we don't have to move our eyes to distinguish *T* from *L*, each additional distractor adds about 20–30 ms to a successful search for a target and about twice that amount of time (40–60 ms) to a search that ends without finding a target. We call this an inefficient search.

(A)

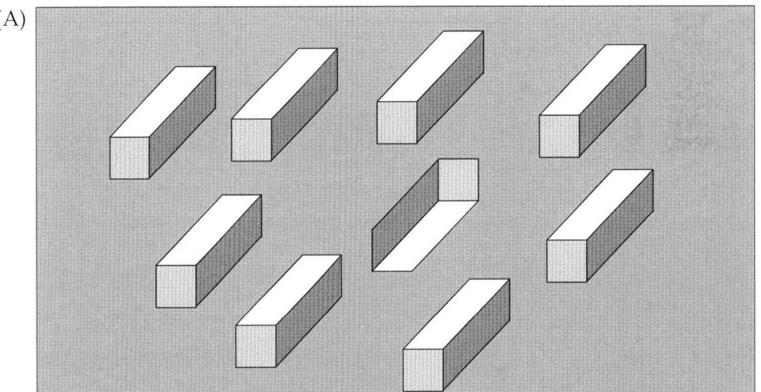

(B)

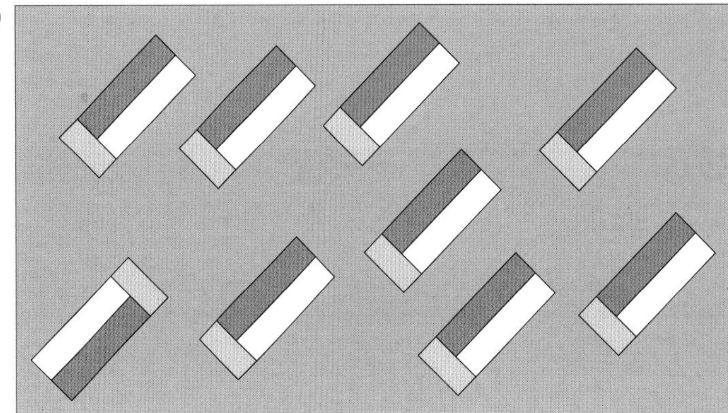

FIGURE 7.7 Three-dimensional orientation
(A) The oddly oriented bar in this image is easy to find, even though all the bars have the same orientation in the two-dimensional image plane. (B) To show that the ease of the task in (A) had to do with the three-dimensional effects and not just with the relative positions of different regions, the experiment was repeated with apparently two-dimensional items composed of similar parts in similar positions. This made it harder to find the odd item.

serial self-terminating search A search from item to item, ending when a target is found.

Why do we get the particular pattern of results seen in Figure 7.6C? One straightforward proposal is that these tasks involve a **serial self-terminating search**, in which items are examined one after another (serially) either until the target is found or until all items have been checked. Consider the case in which a target is present. Sometimes the observer will get lucky and find the target on the first deployment of attention. Sometimes she will be unlucky and have to search all the items before stumbling on the target. On average, she will have to search through about half the items on each trial before the search can be terminated. When no target is present, our observer will always need to search through all the items. There are other models of this behavior that would not propose an exhaustive examination of each item (J. Palmer, 1995). The important point is that some searches are inefficient, meaning that each additional item in the display imposes a measurable cost on the searcher.

The inefficient search for a *T* among *L*s is nothing like the hardest search we could devise. For starters, if we need to spend a lot of time with each item, search will be much slower, as it is in the search for a particular Chinese character in **FIGURE 7.8** (unless, of course, you happen to read Chinese). Other search tasks, like spotting missile sites in satellite images, could take days, even if, once you found one, the missile site was readily identifiable. The *T*-among-*L*s search is interesting because it is a simpler case where a target can "hide in plain sight." The items are easy to see and very familiar, but search is still inefficient.

Guided Searches in the Real World

In the real world, it would be rare to have a true feature search for the only red item among homogeneous distractors that are not red. How often do you have to find the strawberry among the limes? What elements guide our visual searches in the complex environment outside the laboratory?

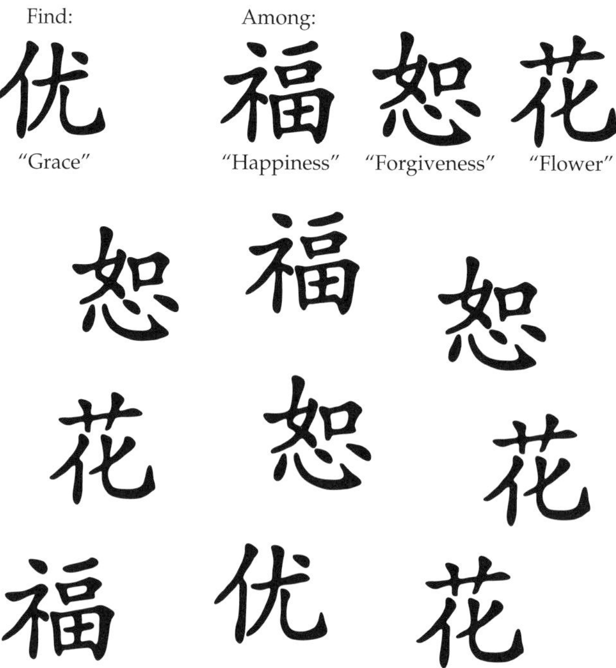

FIGURE 7.8 Chinese characters Search can be much more laborious if you're not familiar with what you're searching for. Here, the search for the target—the Chinese character for "grace"—will be much easier if you can read Chinese.

Scientists at Work

How Would You Study Visual Search by a Fish?

Question Humans are not the only animals that perform visual searches. When other animals search for visual stimuli, are the rules of visual search the same as the rules used by humans?

Hypothesis Visual search by the archerfish will be at least broadly similar to visual search by humans.

Test First, why test archerfish (genus *Toxotes*)? Archerfish cruise around streams, rivers, and mangrove swamps in South Asia. The fish feed on insects and have evolved the amazing hunting strategy of spitting a stream of water at a bug on a branch above the water's surface, knocking the prey into the water, where the fish can gobble it up. Researchers were able train individuals of one species (*Toxotes chatareus*) to spit at a computer screen (**FIGURE 7.9**). The behavior is accurate enough that stimuli like those you saw in Figure 7.6 can be put on the monitor and, in return for snacks, the fish will perform classic search tasks and spit at the target image that provides the reward. Adam Reichenthal and his colleagues in Israel asked if basic features pop out for these fish (Reichenthal et al., 2019). Specifically, they tested color, size, orientation, and motion—all features that pop out for humans. They also tested conjunctions as in Figure 7.6B, though they used color and size (e.g., find the big blue circle among big black and small blue circles). As you might guess, there are challenges to testing even a well-trained fish. After approximately 40 trials, the fish get full and stop playing the game, so it takes many days to collect the amount of data that you could get from a human in a few minutes. Moreover, with a human, you don't need to keep wiping down the screen. Nevertheless, the experiment can be done.

Results To a first approximation, the fish data show similar patterns to the human data (**FIGURE 7.10**). If you look at *y*-axes, you will notice that fish responses are slower than those of humans (not a big surprise). Still, the fish are best at what humans are best at and least efficient where humans are least efficient. The fish were fastest at identifying color targets and slowest for detecting motion. For conjunctions, the fish were much better at finding the big blue target than they were at finding a small black target among the same small blue and big black distractors. This "search asymmetry" is also similar to results from human studies. For shapes, archerfish seem particularly poor at identifying the difference between a disk and a "Pac-Man" dingbat (Reichenthal et al., 2019).

Conclusion Even though the brain of a fish is very different from that of a human, it is interesting that this study indicates that the rules of visual search seem to be fairly similar. This similarity leads to the hypothesis that there may be "universal search rules" among visual animals. There are data from other species—from

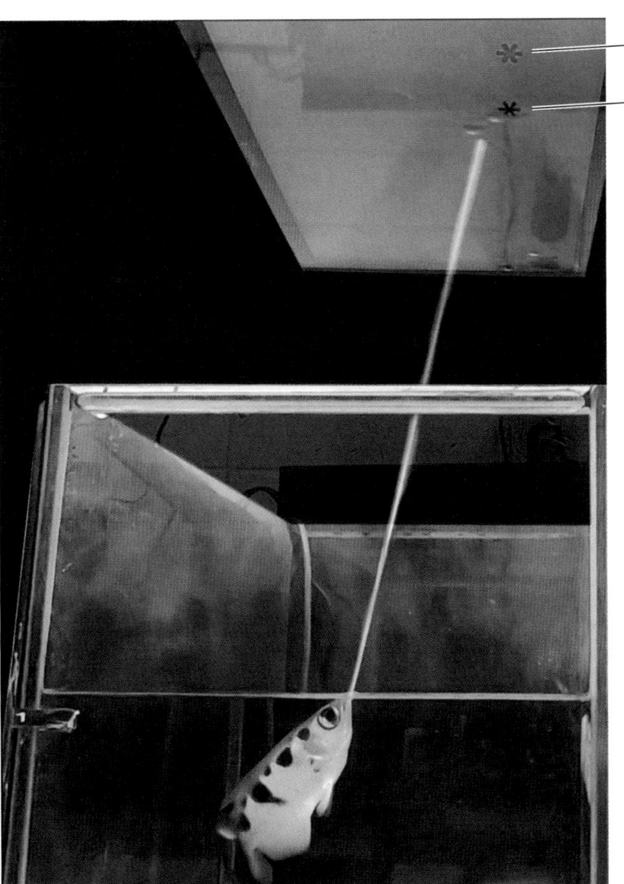

FIGURE 7.9 Archerfish search for targets Archerfish spit a jet of water to knock prey off plants hanging over the water. Researchers trained individuals to shoot at targets on a computer screen. The fish had to search for and hit a specific target (among several) to trigger a reward.

(*Continued*)

Scientists at Work (continued)

owls to monkeys to bees—that support this idea (Reichenthal, Segev, and Ben-Shahar, 2020).

Future work There are many fine-grained properties of human search that could be tested in fish. For example, faces seem to be special stimuli for humans. Would fish shapes be special stimuli for archerfish?

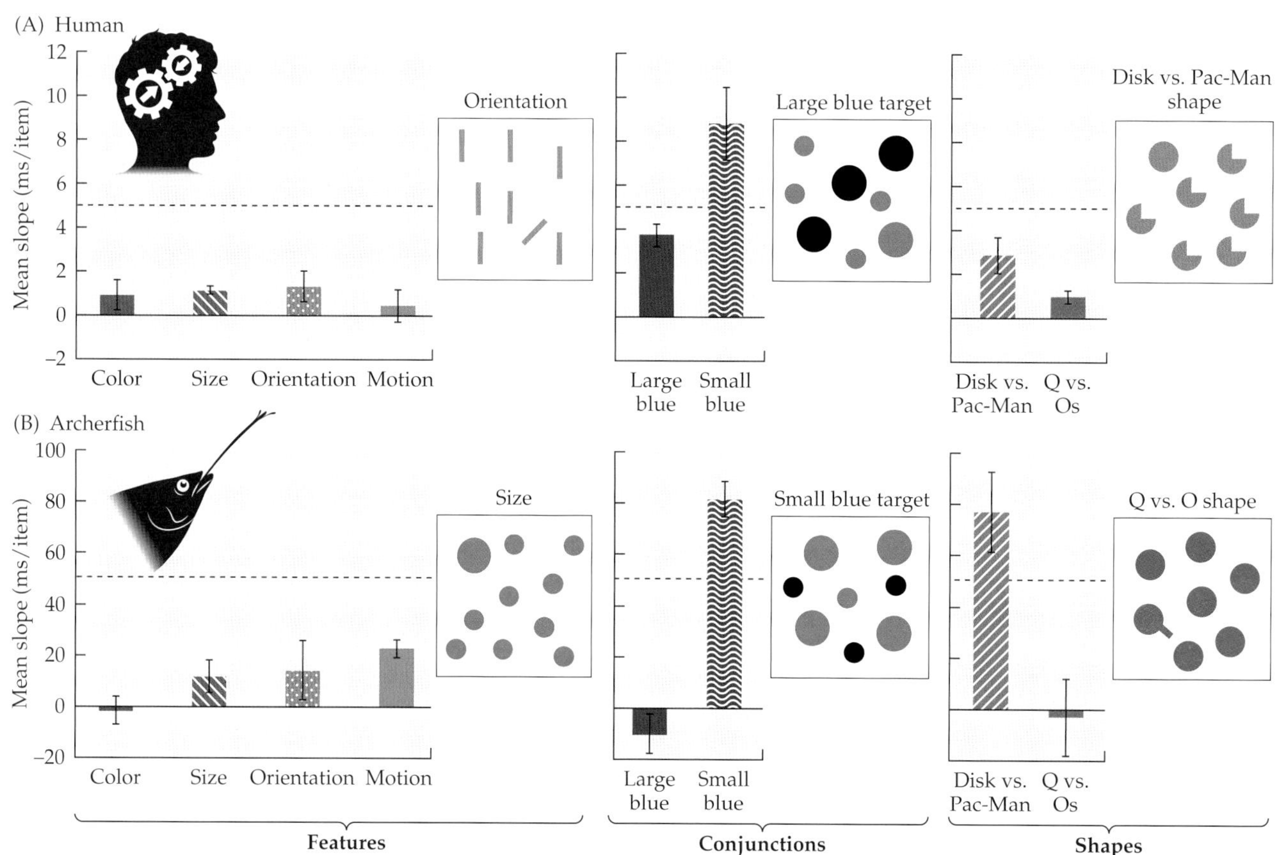

FIGURE 7.10 Human and archerfish visual search data Although archerfish are slower and less efficient than humans in search tasks, you can see that the pattern of results is similar between the two species. Error bars represent the standard deviation from the mean.

guided search Search in which attention can be restricted to a subset of possible items on the basis of information about the target item's basic features (e.g., its color).

conjunction search Search for a target defined by the presence of two or more attributes (e.g., a *red*, *vertical* target among *red* horizontal and blue *vertical* distractors).

BASIC FEATURES GUIDE VISUAL SEARCH Very seldom do we have to search through a scene containing objects that all share the same basic features (the proverbial needle in a haystack). Usually, an object's basic features can be used to narrow down the search, even if they cannot eliminate all distractions. This is known as **guided search** (Wolfe, 2021; Wolfe, Cave, and Franzel, 1989). If you're looking for a tomato in **FIGURE 7.11**, you will be able to find it quite quickly, even though it is not defined by any one feature—it is not the only red thing or round thing or big thing in this scene. Tomatoes are distinguished from most of the distractors by a *conjunction* of several features. If you guide your attention to things that are red *and* round *and* large, you will have eliminated most of the competition and performed a **conjunction search**, like those in the lab experiment cartooned in Figure 7.6B. In a conjunction search, no single feature defines the target. Instead, the target is defined by the conjunction—the co-occurrence—of two or more features (such as

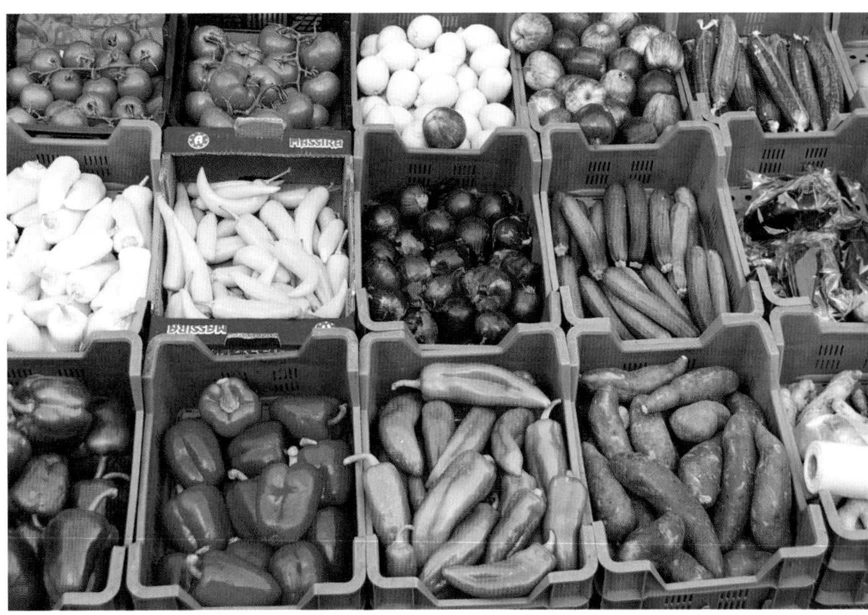

FIGURE 7.11 **A real-world conjunction search** Find the big, round, red tomatoes among things that might be big or round or red but do not have all three basic features.

red, vertical items in Figure 7.6B). In terms of efficiency, conjunction searches tend to lie between the very efficient feature searches and the inefficient serial searches.

HISTORY GUIDES VISUAL SEARCH

Now take a look at FIGURE 7.12 and find the monkey puppets. It may take you a moment to find the first one, but after that, the other two may seem immediately obvious. Finding something once **primes** you to find it again. This is one example of the way that the history of what you have looked for guides your search for the next target (Awh, Belopolsky, and Theeuwes, 2012). It is not just that those monkeys were salient. If you now look for salt and pepper shakers, the second and third instances will seem to jump off the page.

prime A stimulus that might make it easier or faster to respond to a subsequent stimulus. If you are primed by the word "cat," you will respond more quickly to the word "mouse" than to "broom" or some other unrelated word.

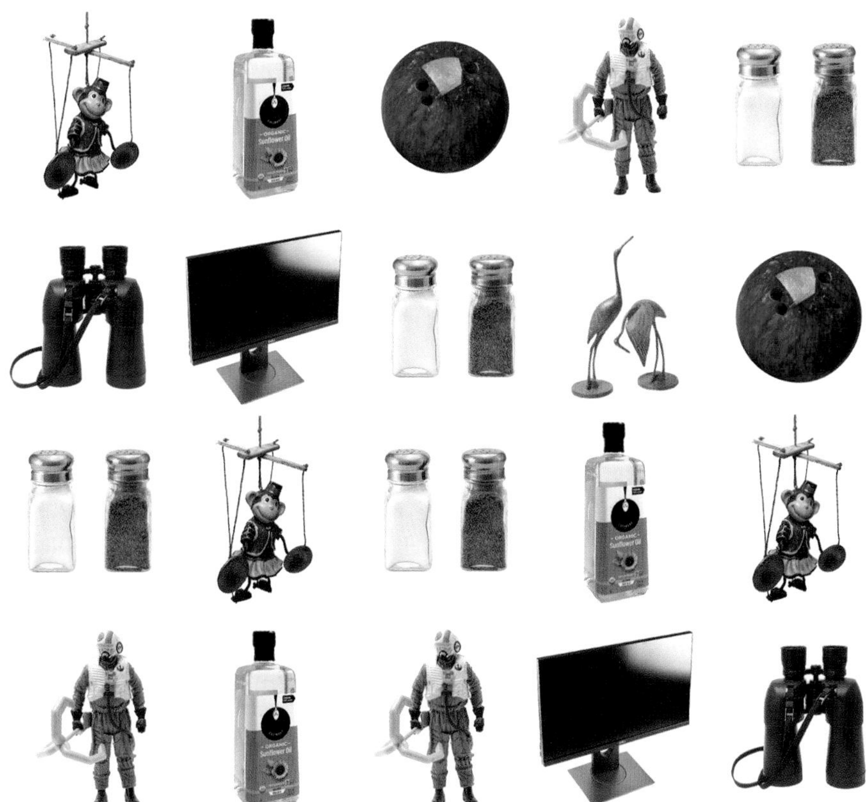

FIGURE 7.12 **History guides search** Finding one monkey puppet primes you to find more monkey puppets.

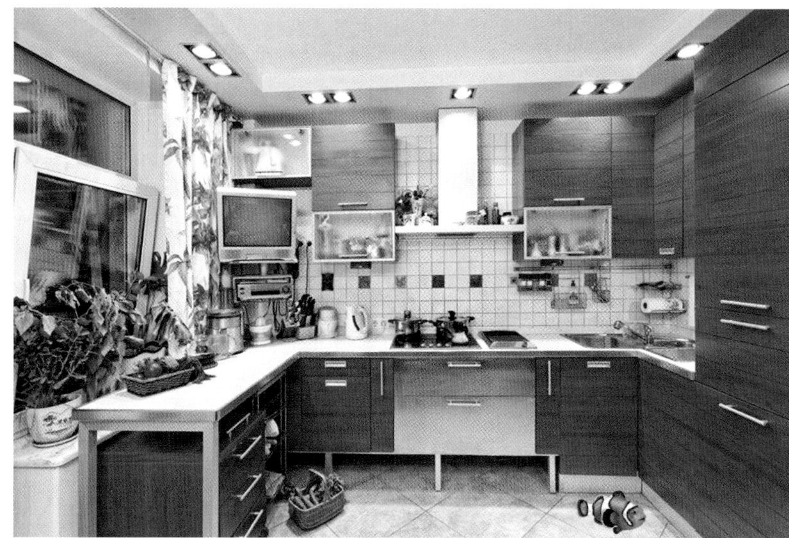

FIGURE 7.13 **Scene-based guidance** Understanding kitchens makes it fairly easy to find the faucet in this scene. You should also look for carrots, a white kettle, and bowls.

REWARD GUIDES VISUAL SEARCH Looking back at Figure 7.12, if we rewarded you every time you found a shiny, round blue ball, you would be motivated to find them, of course. More interestingly, if you were now asked to find those monkey puppets, your attention would still be guided to shiny, round, and blue, even though those features would be irrelevant or even detrimental to the monkey puppet task (D. S. Lee, Kim, and Anderson, 2022). Of course, you can still find the monkey puppets. There would just be a bit of a pull to the previously rewarded stimuli.

PROPERTIES OF SCENES GUIDE VISUAL SEARCH In the real world, we are not usually confronted by random collections of objects like those in Figure 7.12. You search in scenes, and you are helped by various forms of **scene-based guidance** (Castelhano and Krzyś, 2020). For example, find the faucet in **FIGURE 7.13**. It is small and inconspicuous, but easy enough to spot. Why? Even though you've never seen this particular kitchen before, you know about kitchens. They have sinks in typical places. Sinks are **anchor objects** (Vo, Boettcher, and Draschkow, 2019): relatively big objects in predictable locations that tell you about the location of other objects. You also know that sinks have faucets in typical places. Melissa Vo (2021) and her colleagues talk about a **scene grammar**. Just like the rules of grammar in language help you to understand a sentence, the structural rules of scenes help you to understand and to find what you are looking for in a novel scene. If you search for the white kettle in Figure 7.13, you would be guided by the color feature, white, and by the scene grammatical knowledge that a kettle must rest on a surface; they do not float. A floating bowl would be a syntactic violation of scene grammar, a violation of the normal structure ("**syntax**") of the world.

The fish in the lower right of the image would be semantic violation. The fish could physically be in that location, but it violates the meaning (the "**semantics**") of the scene. If you were asked to search for carrots, the feature "orange" would help, but your search might be a bit harder because those vegetables on the floor are not in a typical location. That is a mild version of a semantic violation.

When you first encounter a scene, you rapidly understand the three-dimensional layout of the surfaces (Castelhano and Krzyś, 2020) and you have

scene-based guidance Information in our understanding of scenes that helps us find specific objects in scenes (e.g., objects do not float in air, faucets are found near sinks).

anchor objects Typically, a relatively big object that provides information about the location of other objects. For instance, the toilet provides information about the location of the toilet paper.

scene grammar A set of implicit rules about what can be where that allow you to understand a scene, just as linguistic grammar allows you to understand language.

scene syntax In language, syntax refers to the structure of sentences. In scenes, it refers to what is normal in the structure of the world.

scene semantics In language, semantics refers to the meaning of an utterance. In scenes, it refers to the meaning of the scene.

a rapid understanding about what parts of the image are likely to be meaningful, in the sense of giving you information about what is going on in the scene (Henderson and Hayes, 2018). So, now suppose you were asked to search for bowls. You know that bowls need the support of a surface. You know about the average size of bowls and you know about the three-dimensional shape of the space. This knowledge would allow you to figure out that only a few objects in Figure 7.13 are plausibly bowl-sized. These various sources of guidance would speed your conclusion that there are no bowls.

We can think of all of these various forms of scene guidance as constituting a Bayesian "prior probability" that tells you how likely it is that any given object in the scene is the target (Ehinger et al., 2009).

FURTHER DISCUSSION of the Bayesian approach can be found in Sections 4.4 and 6.4.

The Binding Problem in Visual Search

We will return to complicated stimuli like kitchen scenes later in this chapter. First, we need to step back and consider what selective attention does for us. One answer, championed by Anne Treisman (1996), is that selective attention allows us to solve the **binding problem**. This problem is illustrated in FIGURE 7.14. A quick glance tells us that we're looking at *pluses* whose components are purple and green, and vertical and horizontal. It is also easy to spot the one slightly tilted plus sign. However, if we need to find green/vertical, purple/horizontal items, we will need to search, directing attention to the individual items (Wolfe and Bennett, 1997). In the language of Treisman's **feature integration theory** (A. Treisman and Gelade, 1980), the basic features of color and orientation are available in a **preattentive stage** of processing. Notice that it is easy to find the one slightly tilted item because of its distinctive orientation. With those upright pluses, we don't recognize how their features are bound together until we attend to a specific plus. To recognize almost any object, you must "bind" its features, and that requires attention.

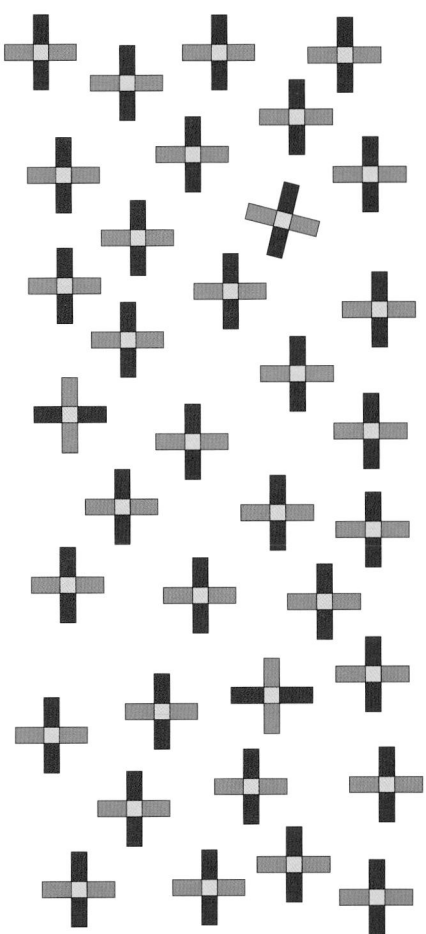

FIGURE 7.14 **A conjunction search with a binding problem** In this image, it is hard to find the plus that contains green verticals and purple horizontals (there are two of them), because all of the items have the features purple and green and vertical and horizontal. Notice that the tilted object is easy to find.

By the way, did you find *both* of the pluses with the green vertical bar? If you missed one, you fell victim to what is called a **satisfaction of search** error (Berbaum et al., 2019). Finding one item can actually make it less likely that you will find a second target in the same display. This can be a serious problem in real-world search tasks, like those in radiology. It is not good if finding signs of pneumonia in a lung X-ray makes you less likely to report a broken rib in the same image.

The idea of guided search described in the preceding section fits into this framework. We can use some preattentive feature information to guide the choice of what should be attended and bound next. If we're searching for a *little, brown* mouse, we should guide our attention to little stuff and brown stuff and not devote attention to shiny, red things or large, square things. Even before attention can enable binding, the mere presence of the right collection of unbound features might, in some cases, very quickly give us a pretty good idea that there is a mouse (or at least an animal) present (F. F. Li et al., 2002), but full object recognition is going to require attention.

If attention is needed to bind features correctly, what happens if we don't have enough time to complete the job? We'll see something, but what? DON'T look at FIGURE 7.15 yet. It is a demonstration of part of the answer. *After you have read these instructions,* look *quickly* at the figure. Then look away and write down as many of the letters and their colors as you can. Try that now.

binding problem The challenge of tying different attributes of visual stimuli (e.g., color, orientation, motion), which are handled by different brain circuits, to the appropriate object so that we perceive a unified object (e.g., red, vertical, moving right).

feature integration theory Anne Treisman's theory of visual attention, which holds that a limited set of basic features can be processed in parallel preattentively, but other properties, including the correct binding of features to objects, require attention.

preattentive stage The processing of a stimulus that occurs before selective attention is deployed to that stimulus.

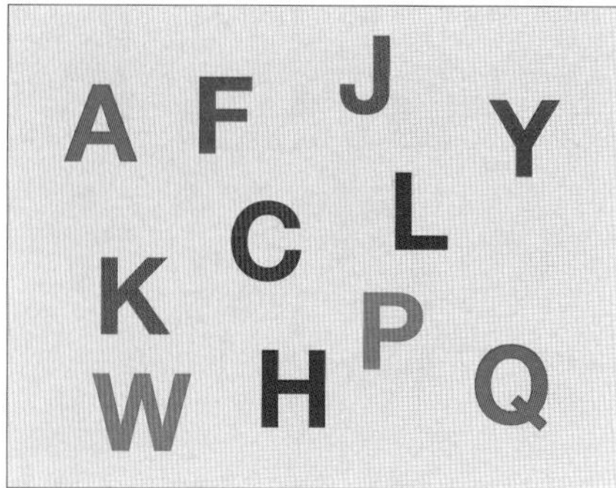

FIGURE 7.15 Illusory conjunctions Look at this figure quickly. Then, without looking, try to recall what you saw. You may remember what colors were there, and you also may remember the letters, but you are quite likely to pair a color and a letter incorrectly. This is an example of a binding error.

If you compare your list to the actual figure, you may find that you matched the wrong color to a letter. For example, you might be quite sure that you saw a green *H*. If so, you have experienced an **illusory conjunction**, a false combination of the features from two or more different objects (A. M. Treisman and Schmidt, 1982). You are unlikely to think that you have seen a yellow *H* or a green *T*, because neither the color yellow nor the letter *T* is present in the figure. We conjoin only those features that are actually in the display. When we can't complete the task of binding, we do the best we can with the information we have.

Binding between the Senses

Out in the world, there are many objects that are experienced as multisensory objects. Think about squeezing a rubber duck toy. Its color, sound, and feel are somehow part of a unified experience. Speech is a more critical example. Certainly, you can usually understand speech if you only hear the speaker. However, your comprehension improves if you can see the movements of the speaker's face and/or the gestures they make with their hands. There is a lot to be said about this (for instance, in Chapter 11). For present purposes, it is interesting to think about speech comprehension as a binding problem. You have mechanisms in vision and audition that extract many visual and auditory features. Then these features must be bound into comprehensible speech (Holler and Levinson, 2019). This binding differs from the binding of color and orientation we experienced in Figure 7.14. Here, the stimuli occur over time, and, among other things, the system must figure out how to bind features that do not occur at the same time. This leads us to our next topic, attending in time. ●

7.3 Attending in Time: Rapid Serial Visual Presentation and the Attentional Blink

Imagine the following situation: You're looking at a stream of letters that all appear at the same location in space. Showing the stimuli in this way is known as **rapid serial visual presentation (RSVP)**. Your task is to decide whether there's an *X* in the stream of letters. How fast can the characters be presented and still permit you to do the task with high accuracy? With fairly large, clearly visible stimuli, we can reliably pick an *X* out of letters when the characters are appearing at a rate of eight to ten items per second. The task does not need to be limited to simple characters. If we're watching a stream of photographs flash by at this rate, we can monitor that stream for the appearance of a picnic photograph. We don't even need to know which particular picnic we're looking for. The general idea of "picnic" is adequate for the task (Potter, 1976).

Returning to simple letters, let's change the task a bit. Instead of looking for one target in a stream of letters, now we're looking for two. We can call the first "T1" (for "target 1") and call the second "T2." In this example, T1 is a white letter in a stream of black letters, and T2 is the letter *X* (**FIGURE 7.16A**). The *X* will be present in 50% of the trials. The critical variable is the interval between T1 and T2, and the somewhat surprising result of the experiment is shown in **FIGURE 7.16B**. If T2 appears 200–500 ms after T1 and if T1 is correctly reported, we are very likely to miss T2. (Note that each frame in Figure 7.16A and each position on the *x*-axis in Figure 7.16B represents 100 ms of time, since letters appear every 100 ms.) This phenomenon is known as the **attentional blink (AB)** (Shapiro, 1994); it is as if our ability to visually attend to the characters in the RSVP sequence is temporarily knocked out, even though our eyes remain wide open.

satisfaction of search A type of error that occurs when detection of one target makes an observer less likely to find a second target in the same display or scene.

illusory conjunction An erroneous combination of two features in a visual scene—for example, seeing a red *X* when the display contains red letters and *X*s but no red *X*s.

rapid serial visual presentation (RSVP) An experimental procedure in which stimuli appear in a stream at one location (typically the point of fixation) at a rapid rate (typically about 8 per second).

attentional blink (AB) The tendency not to perceive or respond to the second of two different target stimuli amid a rapid stream of distracting stimuli if the observer has responded to the first target stimulus 200–500 milliseconds before the second stimulus is presented.

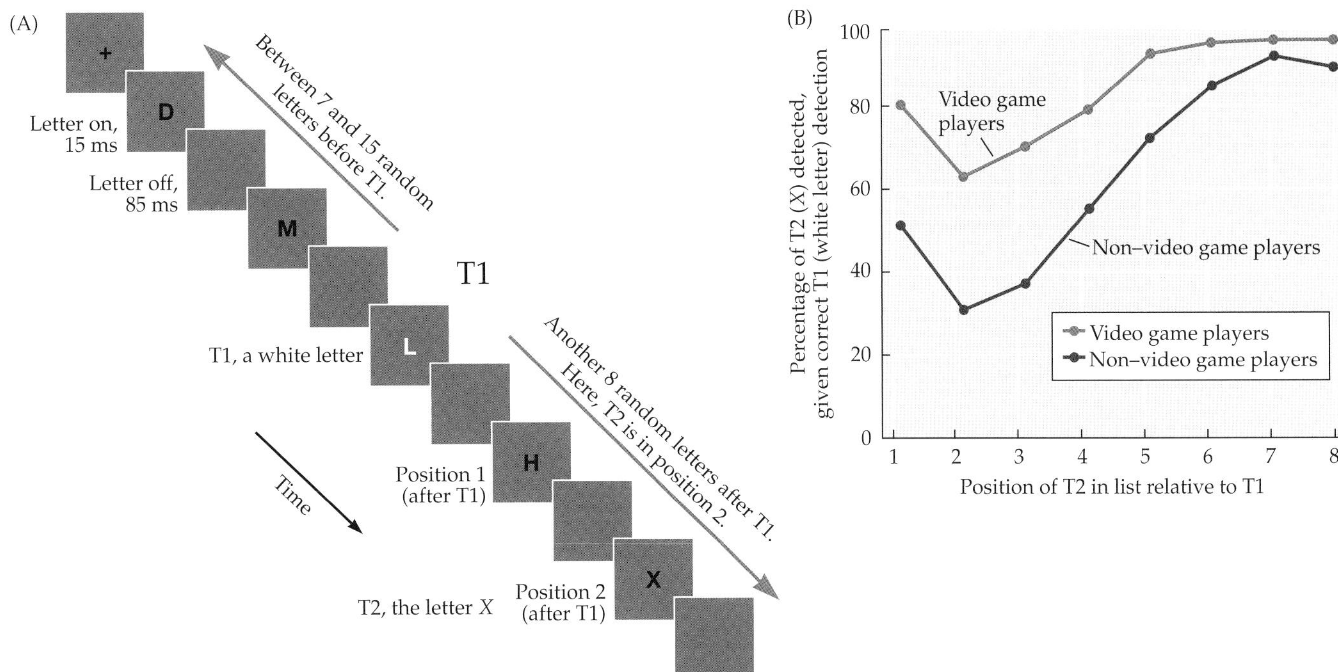

FIGURE 7.16 The attentional blink (AB) in video game and non–video game players (A) In this AB task, observers try to report two targets: a white letter (T1) and an *X* (T2) coming in the stream after that white letter. Letters appear every 100 ms. T2 can appear in various positions in the list after T1. Here, T2 is in position 2. (B) If the *X* appears within 500 ms (positions 1–5 after T1), detection is impaired. That impairment is known as the attentional blink. Video game players (blue) show less of a blink.

To show that missing T2 in this scenario is an attentional problem, we can do a control experiment in which participants report only T2. If participants are asked to monitor the RSVP stream for the T2 letter *X*, they pay no particular attention to the (now irrelevant) white letter, and T2 performance is uniformly good at all delays between T1 and T2.

Somehow, the act of attending to T1 makes it very hard to attend to T2 if T2 appears 200–500 ms later in the stream. What is happening? Marvin Chun suggests the following metaphor (Chun and Potter, 1995): Imagine you're fishing with a net in a less-than-pristine stream, with boots and tires and the occasional fish floating or swimming by. You can monitor the stream and identify each item as it passes—boot, tire, boot, fish, boot, and so on. You can also dip your net in and catch a fish (**FIGURE 7.17A**). Once you have a fish in the net, however, it takes some time before you can get the net back into the water to catch fish number 2. As a result, you might miss fish 2 if it swims by too soon after you've caught fish 1 (**FIGURES 7.17B** and **7.17C**).

Looking back at Figure 7.16B, notice that performance is quite good if T2 appears immediately after T1. In Chun's metaphorical account, this would be a case in which one scoop nets two fish. This metaphor illustrates the idea that two processes are at work. Notice the interesting difference between the role attention plays here and the role it plays in the spatial example of visual search. In search, there is a capacity limit: you just don't seem to be able to recognize more than one object at a time. In AB, though, the problem is probably not the size of the metaphorical net. The problem is that, once attention has dipped that net into the river, there is a temporary inhibition (Olivers and Meeter, 2008) or a temporary loss of control (Di Lollo et al., 2005) that makes it impossible to

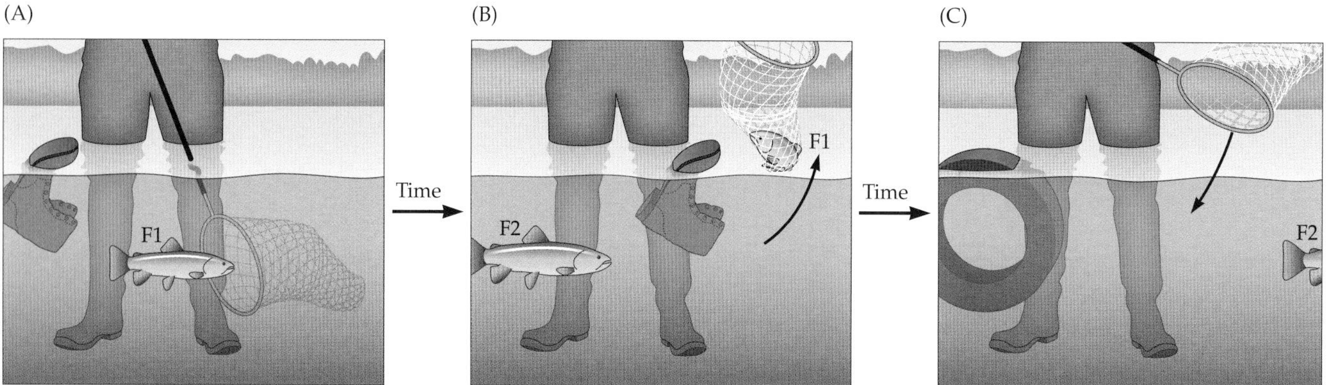

FIGURE 7.17 Marvin Chun's fishing metaphor for the attentional blink (A) You can see all the stuff in the river as it drifts by (e.g., the boot and the fish). (B) You commit to netting fish number 1 (F1). The boot drifts by, and fish 2 (F2) appears. (C) Because you're tied up with F1, you will not be able to capture F2, and that second fish swims away—detected perhaps, but uncollected.

coordinate a second dip for several hundred milliseconds. The blink might reflect a disruption of the ability to attend to the item or it might be a disruption of the ability to move the T2 item into memory. That is, you might "see" the item, but you might have no memory of it. In fact, both sorts of disruption probably occur (Zivony and Lamy, 2022).

Figure 7.16B shows data from two groups of participants who performed differently on the AB task. Interestingly, the group that shows a smaller AB consists of players of "first-person shooter" video games. Indeed, those gamers seem to do better on a range of attentional tasks (C. S. Green and Bavelier, 2003). Why? A variety of factors make some people less subject to the blink (Willems and Martens, 2016). It could be that people who choose to play these video games have better attentional resources. It could also be that the games themselves enhance attention. To test this idea, C. S. Green and Bavelier (2003) conducted a study with two groups of non–video game players. One group got experience with a first-person shooter game, and the other group played the game *Tetris*. The first-person shooter group improved on attentional tasks; the *Tetris* group did not. Of course, this is not an endorsement of violent video games, but it does suggest that attentional abilities can be changed by training and that those first-person shooter video games produced change for reasons that remain to be worked out.

Effects like the AB are important because they tell us something about the time required for acts of attention and/or selection. From these RSVP experiments alone, we can see that there are several "speed limits" in our mental life. The single-target RSVP experiments tell us that if we are just watching a stream of stimuli over time, we can speed along at a rate of many images per second (perhaps as many as 75 per second; Potter et al., 2014). A much slower rate describes the speed with which we can act on items, even if we are just grabbing them to report about their presence. Here, the RSVP data suggest a speed limit of 2–5 items per second.

7.4 The Physiological Basis of Attention

In an oft-quoted passage, William James declared, "Everyone knows what attention is." This great nineteenth-century psychologist went on to say, "It is the taking possession by the mind, in clear and vivid form, of one out of what seem several simultaneously possible objects or trains of thought" (James, 1890, vol. 1, pp. 403–404). That seems fair enough, but what does it mean for the mind to "take possession" of a possible object? If we try to get specific, we discover that this attention that everyone "knows" can be rather difficult to pin down. In part, it is difficult to know what attention does because, as already discussed, attention performs a variety of tasks. But we also need to deal with the physiological question of what the brain is actually doing when it selects one location in space, or one object, or one moment in time, for further processing (Nobre and Kastner, 2014). Let's consider some of the neural possibilities.

Attention Could Enhance Neural Activity

If we are asked to attend to one location in the visual field, as in a Posner cueing task (see Figure 7.3), the neurons that respond to stimuli in that part of the field will become more active. This will be true even in the first stages of visual cortical processing, since those stages are influenced by attention (**FIGURE 7.18**) (Brefczynski and DeYoe, 1999; Gandhi, Heeger, and Boynton, 1998; Haenny and Schiller, 1988; McMains and Somers, 2004). As we progress farther into the visual areas of the cortex, even larger attentional effects are seen (Reynolds and Chelazzi, 2004). In fact, the effects seen at the early stages in the cortex are quite possibly the results of feedback from these later stages of processing (Martinez-Trujillo, 2022). Such feedback may be a very important part of visual processing (Ahissar and Hochstein, 2004; Di Lollo, Enns, and Rensink, 2000).

Attention Could Enhance the Processing of a Specific Type of Stimulus

The mechanisms of attention described in Section 7.3 might suffice if we want to keep watch "out of the corner of the eye" by enhancing activity in a specific region of visual cortex. But let's go back to looking for tomatoes in Figure 7.11 (reprinted in **FIGURE 7.19A**). For a tomato search, you would want to highlight all the red *color* information (**FIGURE 7.19B**) and all the round *shape* information (**FIGURE 7.19C**) (and maybe shininess and some size information, not shown

Subject A

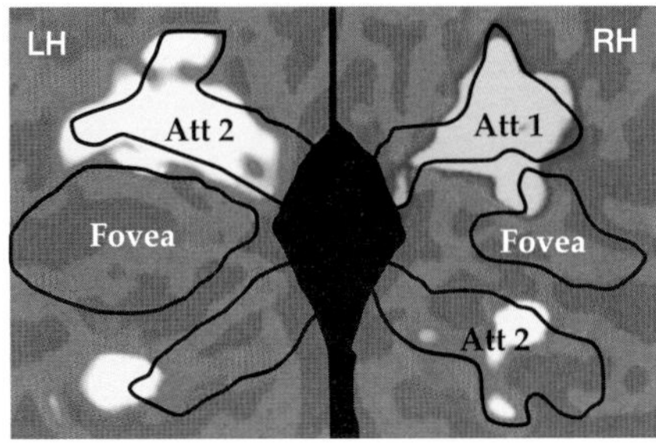

Subject B

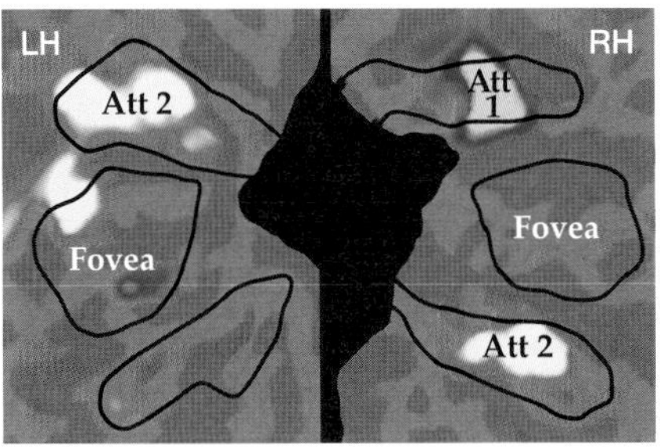

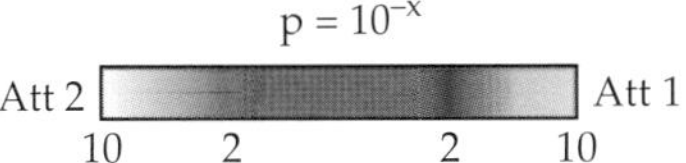

FIGURE 7.18 Spotlights of attention in the human brain These functional magnetic resonance images of human visual cortex (V1, or striate, and some extrastriate) show activity in the brain while participants paid attention to one stimulus (Att 1) or two stimuli (Att 2). The stimuli were outside the fovea, so the regions of activity don't include the fovea.

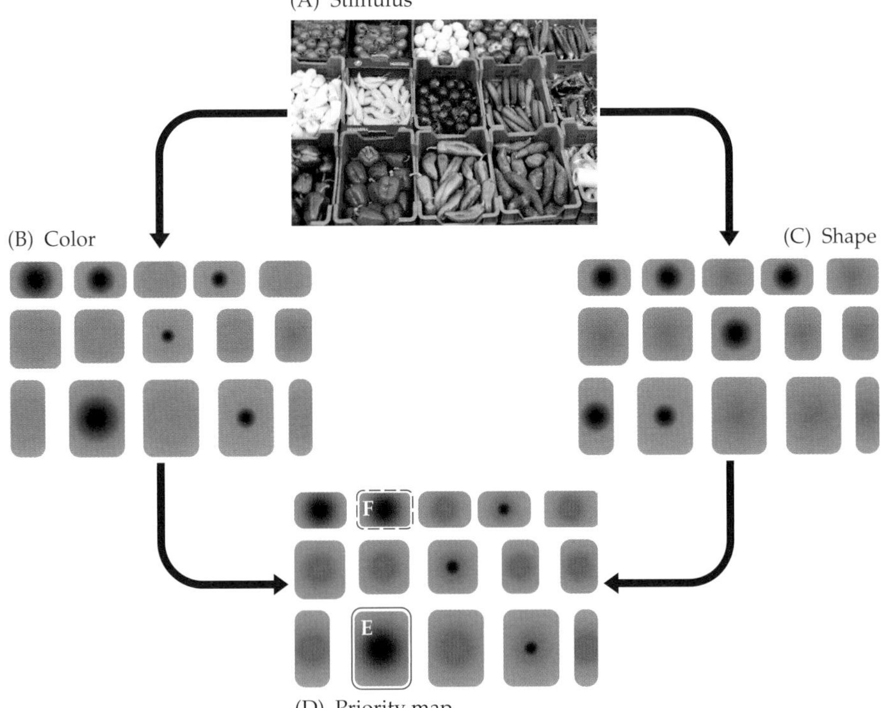

FIGURE 7.19 Building a priority map (A) Early in the visual system, basic feature information is gathered from the stimulus. Here we show only color (B) and shape (C) information. Those sources are combined to produce a priority map (D). Attention is attracted to the most active spot in the map (E, red outline) and then to the next most active (F, dashed red outline) and so on.

priority map A hypothetical neural representation of visual space in which the activity at each point reflects how much that location (or object) will attract attention.

lateral interparietal area A brain region, present in both parietal lobes, that serves an important role in the control of visual attention.

frontal eye fields Brain regions in both frontal lobes that help to coordinate visual selective attention with the movements of the eyes.

superior colliculus A structure in the midbrain that is important in initiating and guiding eye movements.

fusiform face area A region of extrastriate visual cortex in humans that is specifically and reliably activated by human faces.

parahippocampal place area A region of extrastriate visual cortex in humans that is specifically and reliably activated more by images of places than by other stimuli.

response enhancement An effect of attention on the response of a neuron in which the neuron responding to an attended stimulus gives a bigger response.

here). Then you might combine all that information into a **priority map** (**FIGURE 7.19D**) (Serences and Yantis, 2006). Your attention would then be directed to the most active spot in that map (marked E in Figure 7.19D). When that spot turned out to hold red peppers, you might inhibit that location in the map (Klein, 2000) and move on to the next most active spot, where you would find some tomatoes (marked F).

Many neurophysiologically inspired models of this kind of guided search have an architecture like that shown in Figure 7.19 (albeit more complicated; see Itti, Koch, and Niebur, 1998; Miconi, Groomes, and Kreiman, 2016) and candidate priority maps have been found in many parts of the visual system. Important candidates include the **lateral interparietal area** in the parietal lobe of the brain, the **frontal eye fields** in the frontal lobe, and the **superior colliculus** in the midbrain (Bisley and Mirpour, 2019). The frontal eye fields and superior colliculus are also important in the control of eye movements (see Section 8.4).

Attentional selection can also differentially activate parts of the brain that are specialized for the processing of more complex stimuli. Recall from Chapter 4 that functional magnetic resonance imaging has shown that the **fusiform face area** is especially important in the processing of faces (Kanwisher, McDermott, and Chun, 1997), while the **parahippocampal place area** is especially important in the processing of places (**FIGURE 7.20**) (Epstein et al., 1999). If participants view an image of a face superimposed on an image of a house (**FIGURE 7.21**), the fusiform face area becomes more active when the participant is attending to the face, and the parahippocampal place area becomes more active when the participant is attending to the house (O'Craven and Kanwisher, 2000). Beyond these specific areas, it is quite startling how many parts of the brain are involved in the control of attention. Attention "is implemented by a large-scale network that consists of areas spanning across all major lobes . . . of the cerebral cortex as well as subcortical regions" (Boshra and Kastner, 2022).

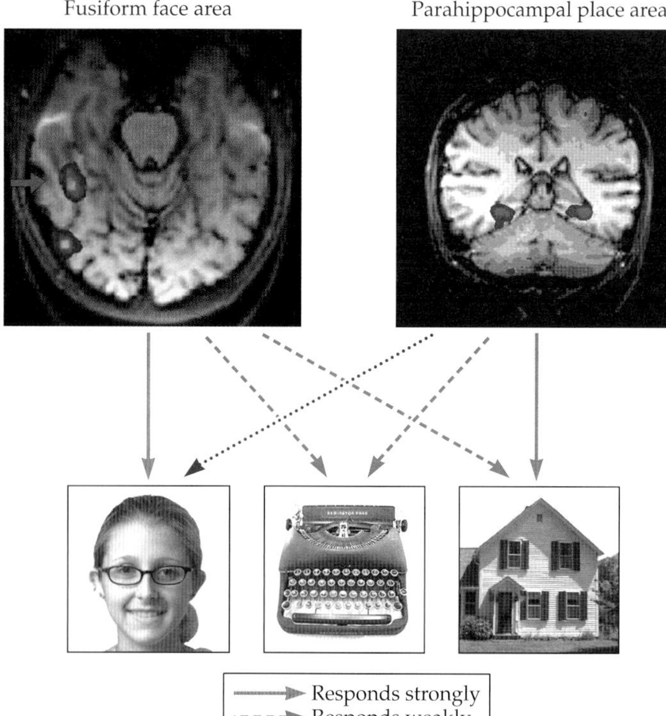

FIGURE 7.20 **Attending to faces or places** Functional magnetic resonance imaging reveals that different locations within the cortex are activated by faces and by places. This is true even when both stimuli are present at the same time (as in Figure 7.21) and the observer merely alters his mental set from faces to places.

FURTHER DISCUSSION of fusiform face area and parahippocampal place area can be found in Section 4.5.

Attention and Single Cells

We have been talking about areas of the brain. On a finer scale, we can ask how attention might change the responses of a single neuron. **FIGURE 7.22** shows one set of possibilities. Suppose a cell responded to a range of different orientations but was maximally responsive to vertical lines (see Section 3.5). Attention might make the cell more responsive across the board (Figure 7.22A). This sort of **response enhancement** has been seen in visual cortex cells, but simple response enhancement seems like a rather indiscriminate change. Alternatively, a cell might become more precisely (more sharply) tuned. In the example in Figure 7.22B, **sharper tuning**

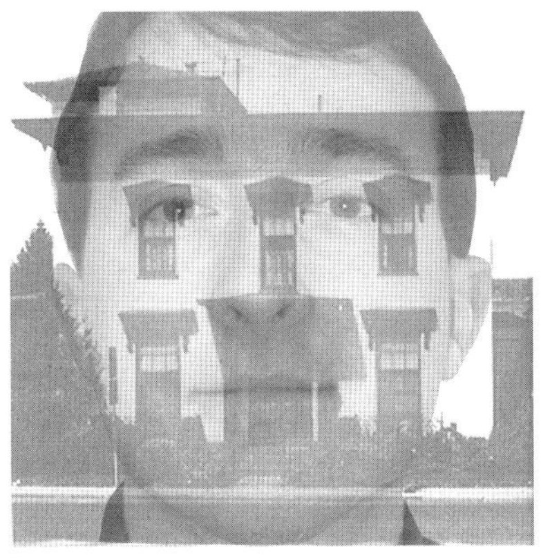

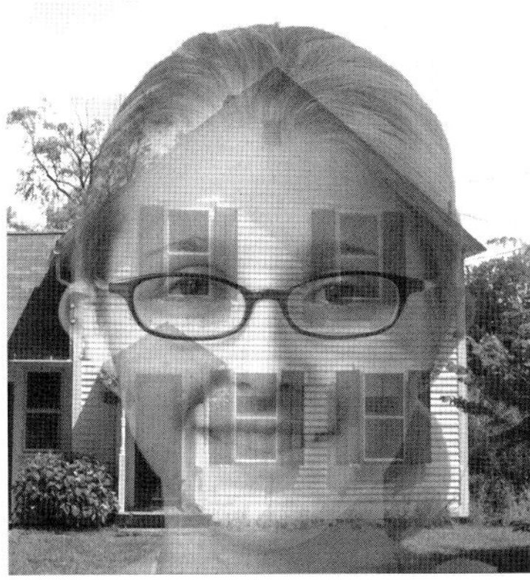

FIGURE 7.21 Attending to faces or places These images combine faces and houses. In both cases you can use attention to enhance the perception of one or the other. As you switch your attention from one type of object to the other, you also change the activation of different parts of the brain, as shown in Figure 7.20.

would mean that attention could make it easier for the neuron to find a weak vertical signal amid the noise of other orientations. Lu and Dosher (1998) carried out elegant psychophysical experiments showing that attention does make it possible to exclude noise in this way, though some efforts to find physiological evidence for sharper tuning have found only response enhancement (Treue and Trujillo, 1999).

A more radical possibility is **altered tuning**: that attention changes the preferences of a neuron. As illustrated in Figure 7.22C, under the influence of attention, a cell that was initially tuned to vertical lines might come to respond better to a different orientation. The best evidence for a change in the fundamental preferences

sharper tuning An effect of attention on the response of a neuron in which the neuron responding to an attended stimulus responds more precisely. For example, a neuron that responds to lines with orientations from −20 degrees to +20 degrees might come to respond to ±10-degree lines.

altered tuning An effect of attention on the response of a neuron in which the neuron responds differently to the features of an attended versus an unattended stimulus. For example, a neuron that responds strongly to lines with orientations from −20 degrees to +20 degrees might shift to respond strongly to −10- to +30-degree lines.

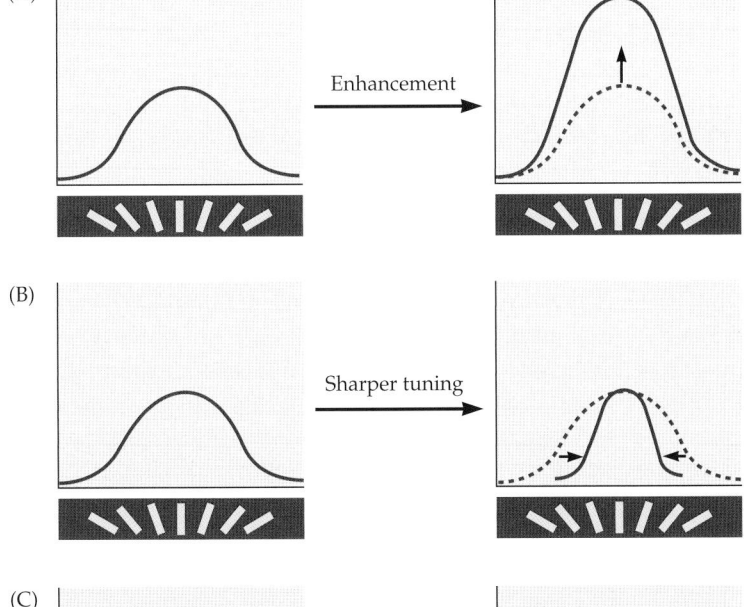

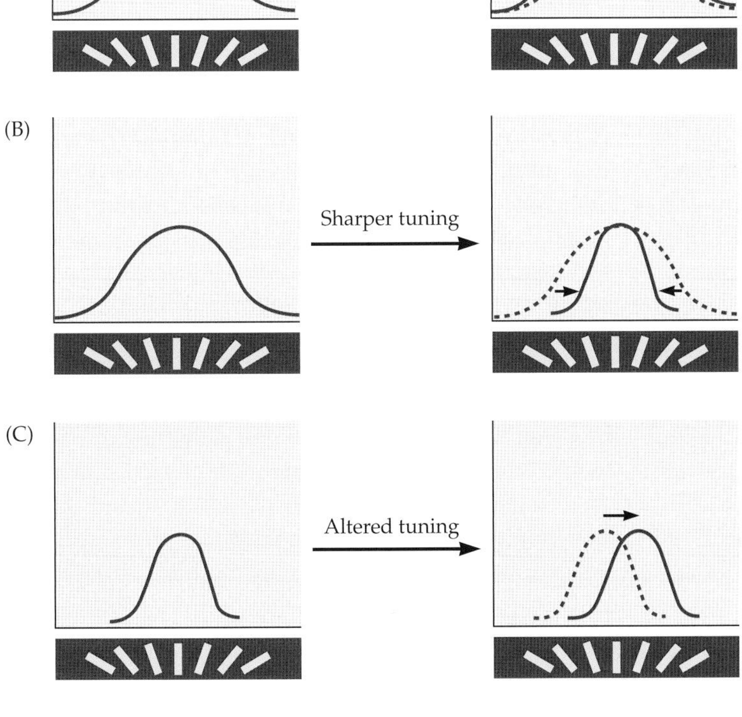

FIGURE 7.22 Three ways a cell's response could be changed as a result of attention (A) Enhancement. (B) Sharper tuning. (C) Altered tuning. In each row, the red line shows the response of a single cell to lines of different orientations. The left column shows the cell's response without attention, and the right column is with attention.

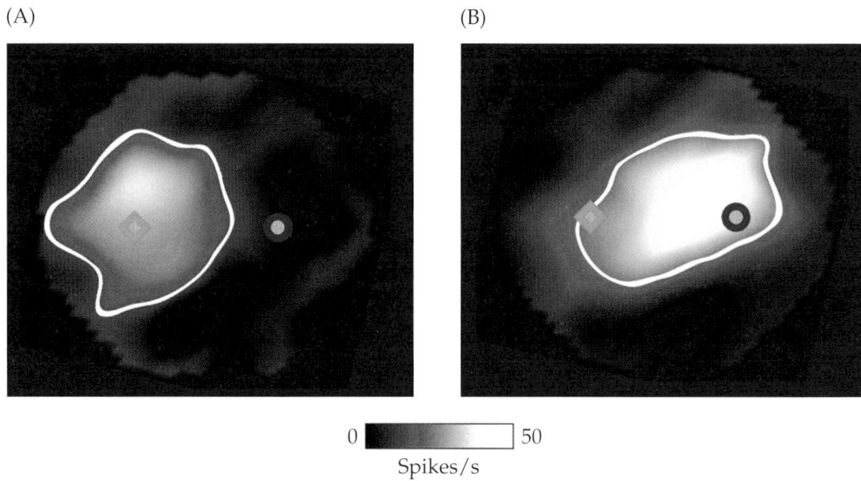

FIGURE 7.23 Attention can move receptive fields Each of these images is a receptive-field map of the responses of one cell in a monkey. In this experiment, the investigators flashed little spots of light at different locations and measured the responses of the cells. Brighter, whiter locations are areas of greater response. The only difference between (A) and (B) is that in (A) the monkey was attending to the location marked by the diamond, while in (B) it attended to the location of the circle. This change in attention caused the receptive field of the cell to "shrink-wrap" itself around the attended stimulus location.

of a neuron comes from studies of its preferences in space—that is, the size and shape of a neuron's receptive field (Moran and Desimone, 1985). FIGURE 7.23 shows just such a change in a specific area of monkey cortex. When the monkey attends to one stimulus, the cell's sensitivity is enhanced around that location. When attention is shifted to another location, the receptive field shifts too (Womelsdorf et al., 2006). If cells are restricting their processing to the object of attention, then sensitivity to neighboring items might be reduced as resources are withdrawn from them. This prediction is borne out: mapping the effects of attention reveals inhibition surrounding the object of attention (Mounts, 2000).

The three hypotheses about the microcircuitry of attention discussed here are not mutually exclusive. Different neurons perform different parts of the task of attending, and each subtask may require a different type of change in neuronal responses. As a hypothetical example, simple response enhancement from one neuron might be the "command" that causes another neuron to sharpen its tuning and/or to change the shape of its receptive field. In fact, these may not even be different functions, say John Reynolds and David Heeger (2009). Reynolds and Heeger's "normalization" theory says that the current response of a neuron is the product of that neuron's built-in receptive field and the effects of attention. This product must then be "normalized" by neural suppression. Otherwise, the numbers (or the level of excitation of the cell) can get too big. The results of this single process of multiplying and dividing can look like response enhancement, like sharper tuning, or like changes in receptive-field size and shape—all depending on the specific stimuli that are used in the experiment. For present purposes, the main message is that *attention can change the activity of single cells.*

Attention May Change the Way Neurons Talk to Each Other

We have discussed how attention can modulate the activity of a neuron and of an area of the brain. Now, let's think about how attention might modify the interactions between neurons and/or between brain areas. For example, how might the brain implement a solution to the binding problem? More specifically, if different brain areas perform different tasks, such as processing faces or places or color or orientation, how might those areas be coordinated if, for instance, we want to think about how the windows and door of a certain red house look like two eyes and a mouth? One possibility is that this binding and coordination of areas involves synchronizing the temporal patterns of activity in those areas (Singer, 1999).

One role of attention appears to be to control what is synchronized with what. For instance, Baldauf and Desimone (2014) showed that attention to faces or places could change whether the fusiform face area or parahippocampal place area were synchronized with a third brain area. More locally, within a brain area, attention may serve to desynchronize neurons. If neurons are synchronized, it is as if they are all doing more or less the same thing. A group of properly desynchronized neurons can more accurately represent a stimulus if different neurons contribute different bits of information (M. R. Cohen and Maunsell, 2009). We can imagine a set of synchronized neurons saying, in effect, "That is a face" while other neurons, roused into desynchronized action by attention, might be working on different aspects of recognition: "Hey, that is Mom's face. Her expression looks angry. We better check with memory and find out if we forgot to take out the trash."

7.5 Disorders of Visual Attention

What would happen if you could no longer pay attention? A complete inability to attend would be devastating. Because we cannot recognize objects or find what we're looking for without attention, complete inattention would be something near to functional blindness. Brain damage that produces a deficit this severe is very rare. More common is the attentional equivalent of a **visual-field defect**. As you may recall, a person who is unfortunate enough to lose primary visual cortex (= V1, striate cortex) in the right hemisphere will be blind on the opposite (left) side of visual space. Suppose, however, that the lesion is in the right **parietal lobe**. People with this sort of lesion (FIGURE 7.24) are not blind on their left side, but they have problems directing attention to objects and places in that field. These problems manifest themselves in a curious set of clinical symptoms, including *neglect* and *extinction.*

visual-field defect A portion of the visual field with no vision or with abnormal vision, typically resulting from damage to the visual nervous system.

parietal lobe In each cerebral hemisphere, a lobe that lies toward the top of the brain between the frontal and occipital lobes.

neglect In reference to a neurological symptom, in visual attention: 1. The inability to attend or respond to stimuli in the contralesional visual field (typically, the left field after right parietal damage). 2. Ignoring half of the body or half of an object.

Neglect

Patients with **neglect** behave as if part of the world were not there. Asked to describe what he is seeing, a patient experiencing neglect of the left visual field will tend to name objects to the right of fixation and ignore objects on the left. A "line cancelation test" is a more systematic way to assess this problem. The patient is given a piece of paper full of lines and asked to draw an intersecting line through each one. He might produce something like the drawing in FIGURE 7.25, in which the lines on one side (the right, in this case) are crossed out, but those

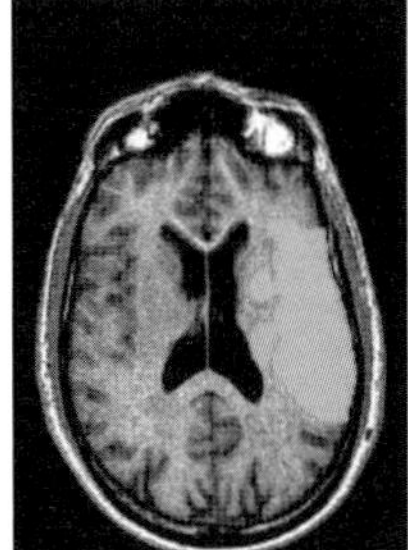
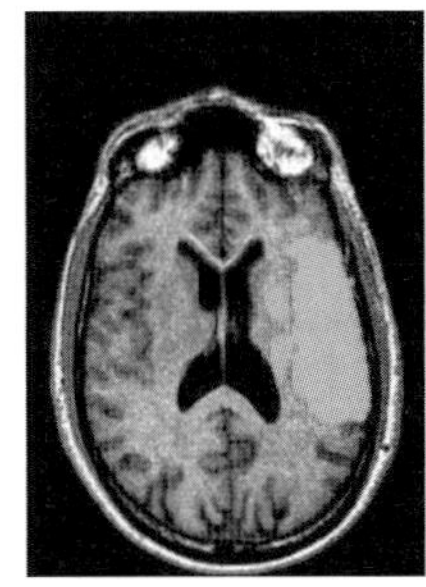
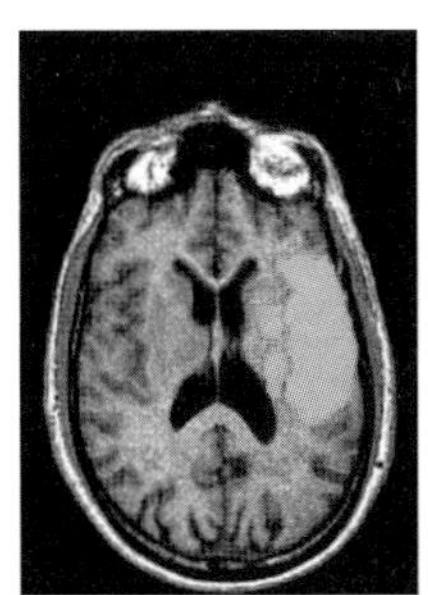
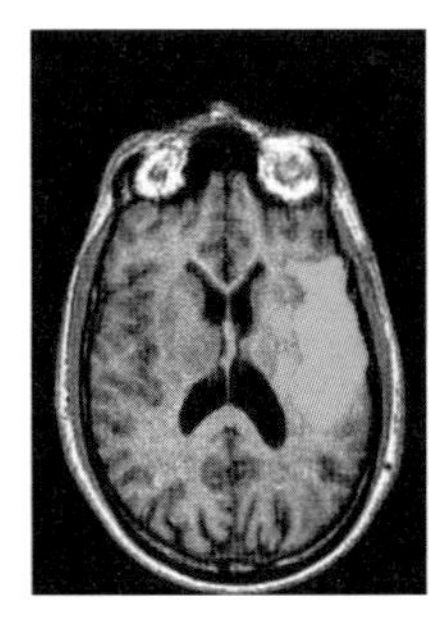
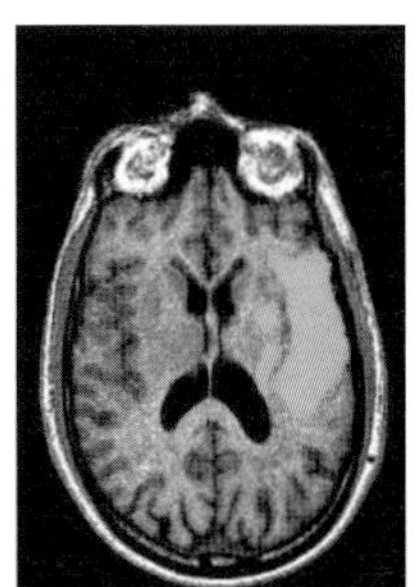

FIGURE 7.24 A parietal lobe lesion Five "slices" through the brain of a patient with neglect (magnetic resonance imaging viewed as though from above). The damage, shown here in yellow, includes the right parietal and frontal lobes. The patient neglects the left side of space.

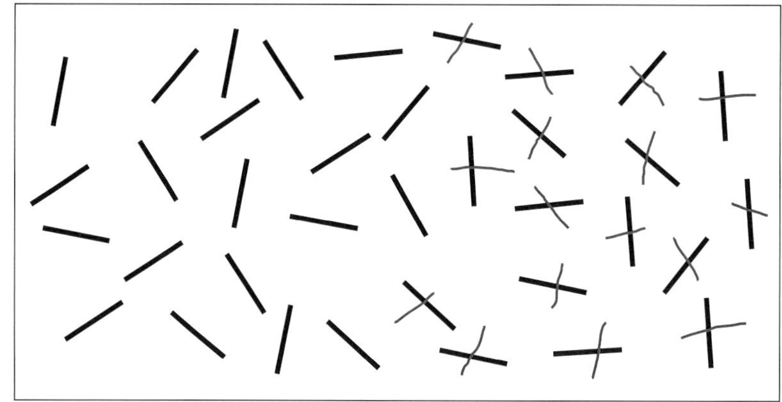

FIGURE 7.25 The cancelation task A patient with neglect would probably produce this sort of result if asked to cross out all the lines. The patient might neglect the lines in the left side of the image following damage to the right parietal lobe.

on the other side (here, the left) are overlooked. **FIGURE 7.26** shows what might result if a patient experiencing neglect of the left visual field were asked to copy a simple line drawing. Again, the right side is reproduced fairly faithfully, but the left side is missing. Such a patient might also eat only what's on the right side of her dinner plate or shave only the right side of his face. These are all forms of neglect, though they may be the result of different damage to the brain (M. J. Moore et al., 2023).

It is not always clear whether neglect affects one side of the visual world or one side of objects. Most likely, neglect can be either or both. In one elegant illustration of this point, Steve Tipper and Marlene Behrmann (1996) asked patients with neglect to detect changes on one or the other side of a barbell. When the barbell had one ball in the left field and one in the right, patients with neglect paid better attention to the right. Tipper and Behrmann's clever trick was to rotate the barbell, while the patients were watching, so that the left ball moved into the right field and the right ball moved into the left (**FIGURE 7.27**). Now, the patients paid better attention than they should have to the piece of the object in the normally neglected, **contralesional field** (the field on the side opposite the lesion). Apparently, they were neglecting half of the object, and the neglect somehow moved with the object.

contralesional field The visual field on the side opposite a brain lesion. For example, points to the left of fixation are contralesional to damage in the right hemisphere of the brain.

extinction In reference to visual attention, the inability to perceive a stimulus to one side of the point of fixation (e.g., to the right) in the presence of another stimulus, typically in a comparable position in the other visual field (e.g., on the left side).

Extinction

The phenomenon of **extinction** is related to neglect; it might even be neglect in a milder form (Driver, 1998). A neurologist might test for neglect by having a patient fixate on her (the neurologist's) nose. She might then hold up a fork in the patient's good (in this case, right) visual field and ask, "What do you see?" "A fork," would

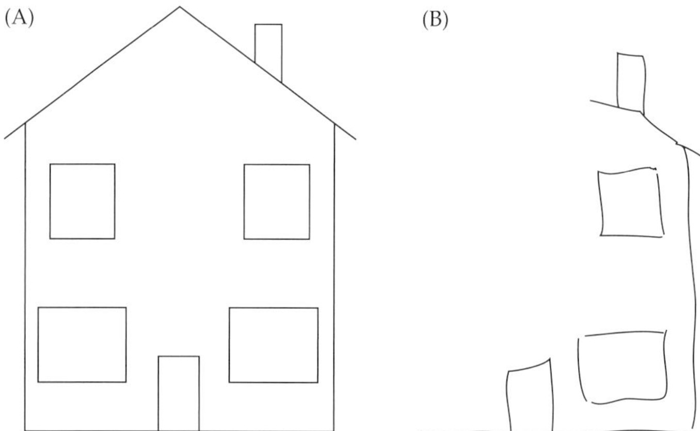

FIGURE 7.26 The object copying task In copying a drawing like the one in (A), a patient with neglect often omits one side of the object, as in (B).

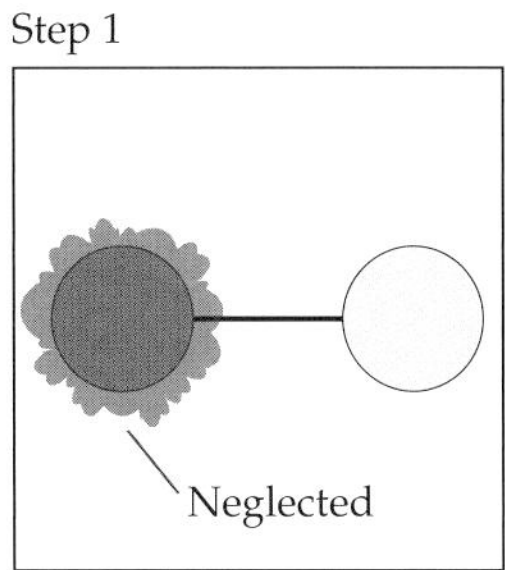

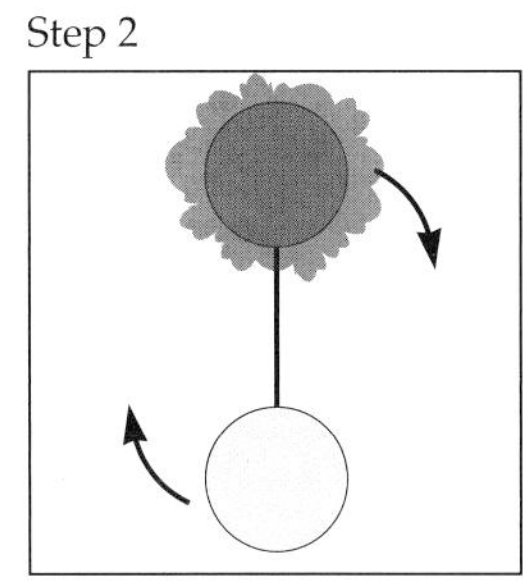

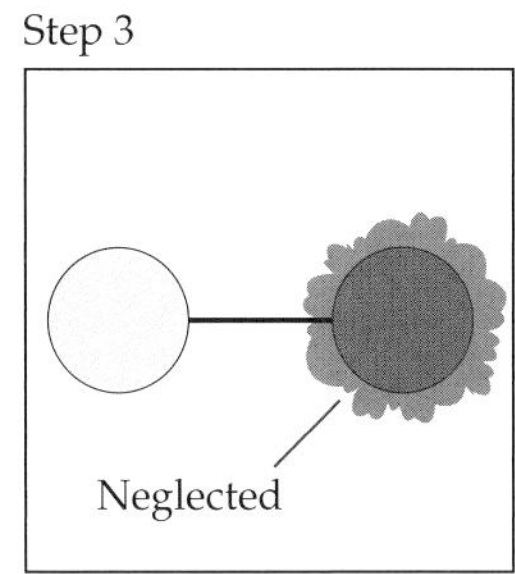

FIGURE 7.27 Tipper and Behrmann's (1996) experiment Step 1: The patient neglected the left side of the barbell. Step 2: The barbell was rotated through 180 degrees. Step 3: The neglect rotated with the object, indicating that, in this case, the neglect was relative to the object, not to the whole scene.

be the reply. Next the neurologist might present a spoon in the bad (left) field. A patient with left-visual-field extinction would be able to report "spoon," while a patient with neglect would not. However, if the neurologist were to hold up a fork in one hand and a spoon in the other, the extinction patient would report only the object in the good field. The object in the left field would be perceptually "extinguished" by the presence of the object in the right field.

In neglect, the patient may be entirely unable to deploy attention to the contralesional side of the world or the object. In extinction, the patient may be able to deploy attention to an object in the contralesional field if it is the only salient object. However, if there is competition from a similar object in the **ipsilesional field** (the same side as the lesion), then the two objects compete for attention and the ipsilesional object wins. Objects are always competing for our attention, but as a general rule it is no great matter for us to redeploy attention from one object

ipsilesional field The visual field on the same side as a brain lesion.

attention deficit hyperactivity disorder (ADHD) A quite common childhood disorder that can continue into adulthood, symptoms of which include difficulty focusing attention and problems controlling behavior.

Sensation & Perception in Everyday Life

Selective Attention and Attention Deficit Hyperactivity Disorder

Neglect and extinction are relatively rare consequences of damage to the nervous system. There are much more common disorders of attention; the best known of these is **attention deficit hyperactivity disorder**, or **ADHD**. Recall that, early in this chapter, we said that attention was not a single thing, but a name for a family of processes that restrict or bias our mental activities. That is demonstrably true, but at the same time, we have the intuition that there is some general attentional resource that is being summoned when our mother or our teacher or our significant other says, "Pay attention!" Some people seem to have more difficulty paying attention in this sense than others. If that difficulty is severe enough, they may be diagnosed with ADHD, which is diagnosed in North American children more than any other behavioral disorder. It is characterized by three kinds of symptoms: impulsivity (an inability to control behavior), hyperactivity, and, of most interest to us, inattentiveness. An inattentive child or adult might fail to carry out a set of instructions or tasks (like homework). They might have problems organizing activities, be easily distracted or forgetful, and may seem not to listen (i.e., they are inattentive) when spoken to (Feldman and Reiff, 2014; Volkow and Swanson, 2013).

How does the sort of attention that is disrupted in ADHD relate to the attentional processes that we have been discussing here? For instance, if you have trouble organizing a task, might you have trouble organizing a visual search? Mullane and Klein (2008) analyzed the results of a number of different studies of this question. These researchers found that there were differences between observers with and without a diagnosis of ADHD, but that these differences were fairly subtle. Doing search tasks like those shown in Figure 7.6, ADHD observers produced a pattern of results that was qualitatively similar to the pattern shown at the bottom of Figure 7.6. Feature searches were basically the same, and highly efficient, in both ADHD and non-ADHD observers. Inefficient searches were a little more inefficient in ADHD observers, but the difference was not dramatic. ADHD and non-ADHD observers seem to search in pretty much the same manner. So it appears that although it is a disorder with significant attentional components, the major components of ADHD seem to lie outside the realm of visual spatial attention.

Balint syndrome A disorder where everything except the current object of attention seems to be blocked from conscious perception.

to the next. In extinction, the object that loses the competition is far less likely to attract attention than is normally the case. When the parietal lobe is damaged on both sides of the brain, patients can develop **Balint syndrome**, a disorder where everything except the current object of attention seems to be blocked from conscious perception.

7.6 Perceiving and Understanding Scenes

We said at the beginning of this chapter that we need attention to deal with the vast amount of information in the visual scene in front of our eyes. The rest of this chapter is devoted to the problem of scenes—how we understand them and what it is that we are actually *seeing* at any moment in time.

It would be convenient if we could divide visual perception into the object-based processes described in Chapter 4 and the scene-based processes we've discussed in this chapter. However, just as with defining "objects" in Chapter 4, we have a problem defining the term "scene." The flower in **FIGURE 7.28A** is an *object*; the Japanese Temple Courtyard in **FIGURE 7.28B** is a *scene*, if we define a scene as a space that could contain objects. **FIGURE 7.28C** represents an intermediate case. We could think of this picture of an airline meal as space containing objects. However, it is a special kind of space that Emilie Josephs and Talia Konkle call a "reachspace"

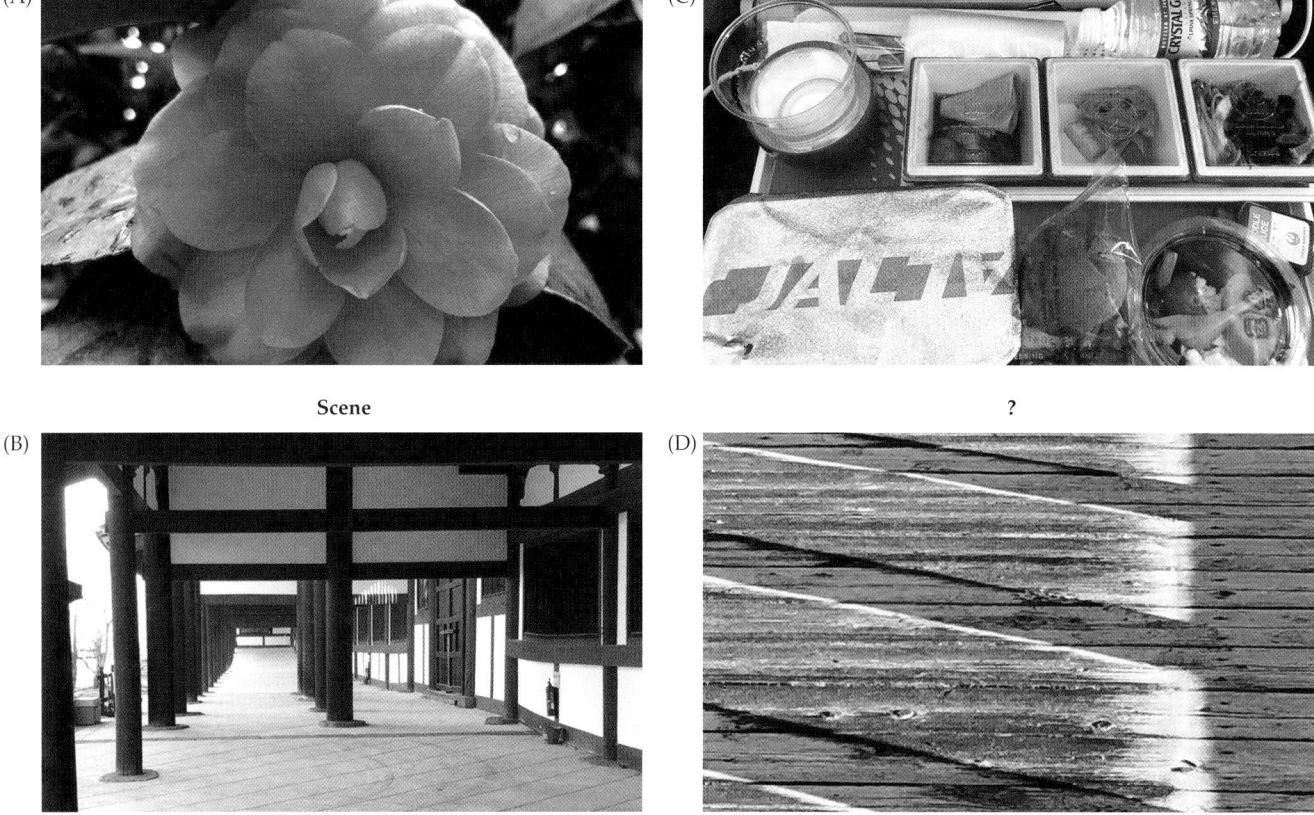

FIGURE 7.28 What defines a scene? (A) The single flower is clearly an "object." (B) This is pretty clearly a "scene." (C) A "reachspace" is a scene within a space that allows objects to be touched and, perhaps, manipulated. (D) Is this patch of wooden decking an object, a scene, or something else?

(Josephs and Konkle, 2019). **Reachspaces** are relatively small and, importantly, we can interact with them in ways that you cannot interact with a bigger scene. Reachspaces are treated differently by our visual system than either objects or scenes and shouldn't be thought of as a purely visual concept. As is obvious in the name, you can *reach* for things in a reachspace, which typically would mean you could *touch* those things. We know there are multimodal neurons that can be stimulated both by touch and by visual input, but only when the stimuli are in **peripersonal space**—that part of the world that is near your body, especially your hands (Graziano and Gross, 1994). The effects of brain damage, discussed in Section 7.5, interact with the multimodal nature of the space around your body. Thus, some parietal damage might produce visual neglect, but other lesions might cause the patient to neglect one side of the body or a combination of space and the body (Grusser, 1983). ●

reachspace A region of visual space that is within arm's reach: bigger than most objects, smaller than a typical scene, and critically positioned where the arms can reach.

peripersonal space That part of the world that is near your body—especially your hands.

Finally, it is worth pointing out that the categories of "object," "scene," and "reachspace" still don't capture the full range of what we see. For example, what should we call the view of a wooden deck with frost in **FIGURE 7.28D**? It doesn't seem to be object, scene, or reachspace. Moreover, the "scenes" in Figure 7.28 are also objects: they are all photographs, embedded in a figure that is in a book (or on the screen) that is part of the real-world scene in which you find yourself right now.

Two Pathways to Scene Perception

To come at this problem in a different way, let's go back to the two-pathway idea introduced at the very end of Section 7.1, where we stated that visual experience can be thought of as a combination of the work of a selective and a nonselective pathway (Wolfe et al., 2011). The initial stages of vision (as described in the preceding chapters) are shared by both pathways (**FIGURE 7.29A**). The spotlight of attention is associated with the selective pathway (**FIGURE 7.29B**): specific locations or objects are selected for the processing that allows for binding and object recognition. The visual scene outside the current spotlight is brought to you via the nonselective pathway (**FIGURE 7.29C**): What do you see away from the current focus of attention?

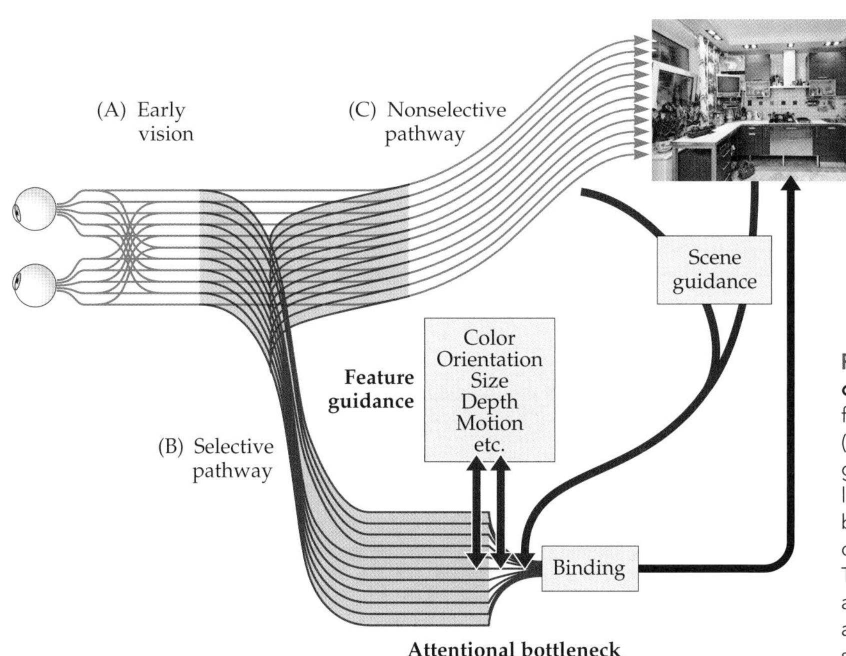

FIGURE 7.29 Two pathways to our perception of the world Early stages of the visual system feed our retinal images (A) into two pathways. (B) The selective pathway has a bottleneck that is governed by selective attention. (C) The nonselective pathway is not subject to this attentional bottleneck. The selective pathway permits the recognition of one or a very few objects at one time. The nonselective pathway contributes information about the distribution of features across the scene, as well as information about the rough gist of the scene.

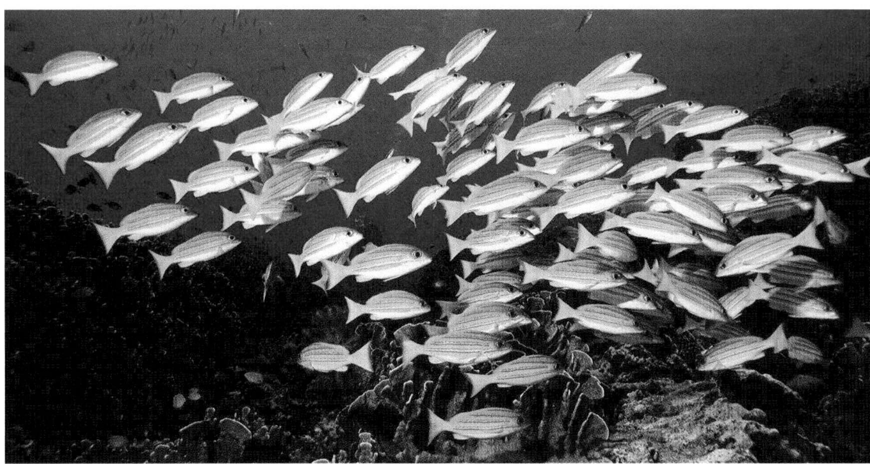

FIGURE 7.30 **Some "fishy" ensemble statistics** In a glance you can tell that, as a group, these fish are oriented roughly horizontally, even though you cannot tell, in that glance, which specific fish are oriented *exactly* horizontally. Similarly, you know in a glance that some fish are more tilted, and some are small. Selective attention is required to determine whether any one fish is both strongly tilted and small.

ensemble statistics The average and distribution of properties like orientation or color over a set of objects or over a region in a scene.

proto-object A term used to refer to object-like stimuli before they are attended and recognized.

The Nonselective Pathway Computes Ensemble Statistics

Look at FIGURE 7.30. You very rapidly know several things about this school of fish. You know that the school is oriented to the right, perhaps slightly up from horizontal. You know the average size and color of the fish. You also know something about the distribution of orientations, sizes, and colors. That is, you know that a range of fish orientations is present—they are not all pointed in exactly the same direction. To know these things, you are computing **ensemble statistics** (Whitney and Yamanashi Leib, 2018). Ensemble statistics represent knowledge about the properties of a group (ensemble) of objects or, perhaps we should say, an ensemble of **proto-objects**. Our estimates of these statistics are surprisingly accurate (Chong and Treisman, 2003; Chubb and Landy, 1994).

These are *ensemble* statistics because we know them without knowing the properties of the individual fish. For example, you would have to search to find a fish that was pointed exactly horizontally, even though that fish's orientation contributes to the estimate of the ensemble orientation. Features are not bound in ensemble statistics. You would have no idea, without attentional scrutiny, if the most strongly tilted fish is also the smallest fish. You know there are smaller fish and more tilted fish, but appreciating conjunctions of those features requires the *selective* pathway. Your analysis of the ensemble statistics in front of you helps you to deploy the limited capacity of your selective pathway (Corbett, Utochkin, and Hochstein, 2023).

FURTHER DISCUSSION of our ability to perceive the characteristics of a group of objects can be found in Section 4.4.

The Nonselective Pathway Computes Scene Gist and Layout—Very Quickly

As was mentioned earlier in our discussion of attending in time (Section 7.3), people can monitor a stream of images for one particular image or type of image at rates of one image every 100 ms (see Figure 7.16). In fact, in some cases you don't need as much as 100 ms. Holle Kirchner and Simon Thorpe (2006) presented observers with two side-by-side scenes and found that the observers could reliably move their eyes to fixate on whichever scene included an animal (any animal) in as little as 120 ms. The fact that most of that 120 ms was taken up in generating the eye movement implies that the processing of the scene was extremely rapid. Michelle Greene and Aude Oliva (2009) presented single scenes very briefly, followed by masking stimuli. They found that people could differentiate between natural and urban scenes with just 19

(A)

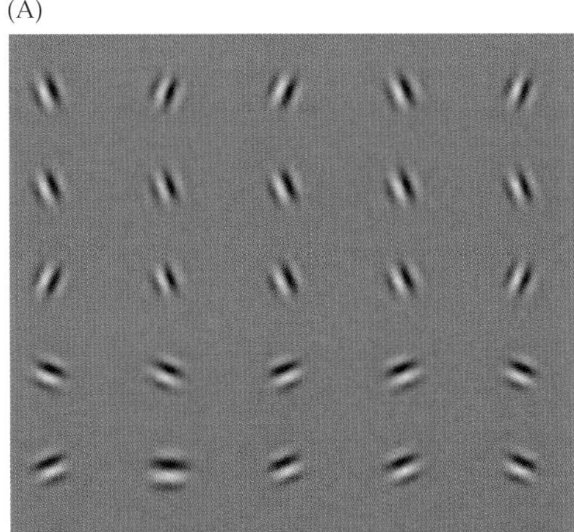

(B)

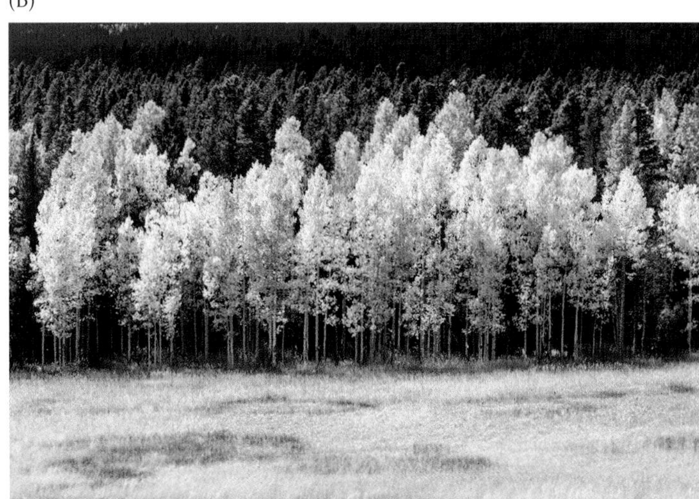

FIGURE 7.31 **Ensemble statistics and scene perception** (A) It is quite clear that the little patches of spatial frequency (Gabor patches) are roughly vertical on the top half of the image and horizontal on the bottom. You rapidly extract these ensemble statistics, though it would take you longer to determine whether any one Gabor patch was actually vertical or horizontal. (B) Similarly, you rapidly see the vertical trees and horizontal line of the field, but analysis of any one tree would require attention.

ms of exposure to a scene (<1/50th of a second). Global properties that described the **spatial layout** of the scene (e.g., was it a navigable or non-navigable space?) could be extracted a bit more quickly than could basic categories like "desert" or "lake," but all of these could be appreciated within about 50 ms. It probably takes 20–50 ms to recognize just one object, so observers are certainly not recognizing scenes by recognizing a string of objects and putting them together. What are they doing?

An interesting potential answer comes from the work of Aude Oliva and Antonio Torralba (2001). Look quickly at FIGURE 7.31A. In a glimpse, it is clear that the field is divided in two, with a roughly vertical top and a roughly horizontal bottom. You get that from the ensemble statistics as in Figure 7.30; it will take you longer to use your selective pathway to determine whether any one item is actually vertical or horizontal. Now look at FIGURE 7.31B. Again, it is clear from a glimpse that the upper part of the image contains a lot of vertical stuff and a horizontal line divides the image. Oliva and Torralba (2001) argued that the same processes that allowed you to process all the local spatial frequency components could also allow you to distinguish beaches from city streets from bedrooms, and so forth. There was a straight line from ensemble statistics to the **gist**, or essential character, of what a scene contains. (The concept of visual "gist" is complex, and we'll return to it in the final paragraphs of this chapter.) Thus, wide-open scenes like beaches, fields, parking lots, and so on tend to have a lot of strong horizontal components corresponding to the horizon. Oliva and Torralba (2001) called this dimension "openness" and defined a number of other dimensions, including "naturalness" (versus "man-made") and "roughness." They could measure the amount of each of these dimensions by examining the local spatial frequency components that made up the stimulus.

When Oliva and Torralba (2001) measured the properties of thousands of scenes, they observed something very useful: scenes with the same meaning tended to be neighbors in the space defined by their scene dimensions. Suppose we define a simple two-dimensional space using the dimensions of openness and expansion. FIGURE 7.32 graphs a set of man-made scenes using these two dimensions. Look at how the scenes organize themselves. The frontal views of buildings fall in the

spatial layout The description of the structure of a scene (e.g., enclosed, open, rough, smooth) without reference to the identity of specific objects in the scene.

gist The essential or primary character of a scene. In vision, gist typically refers to information that can be gleaned in a very brief glimpse, without voluntary eye movements.

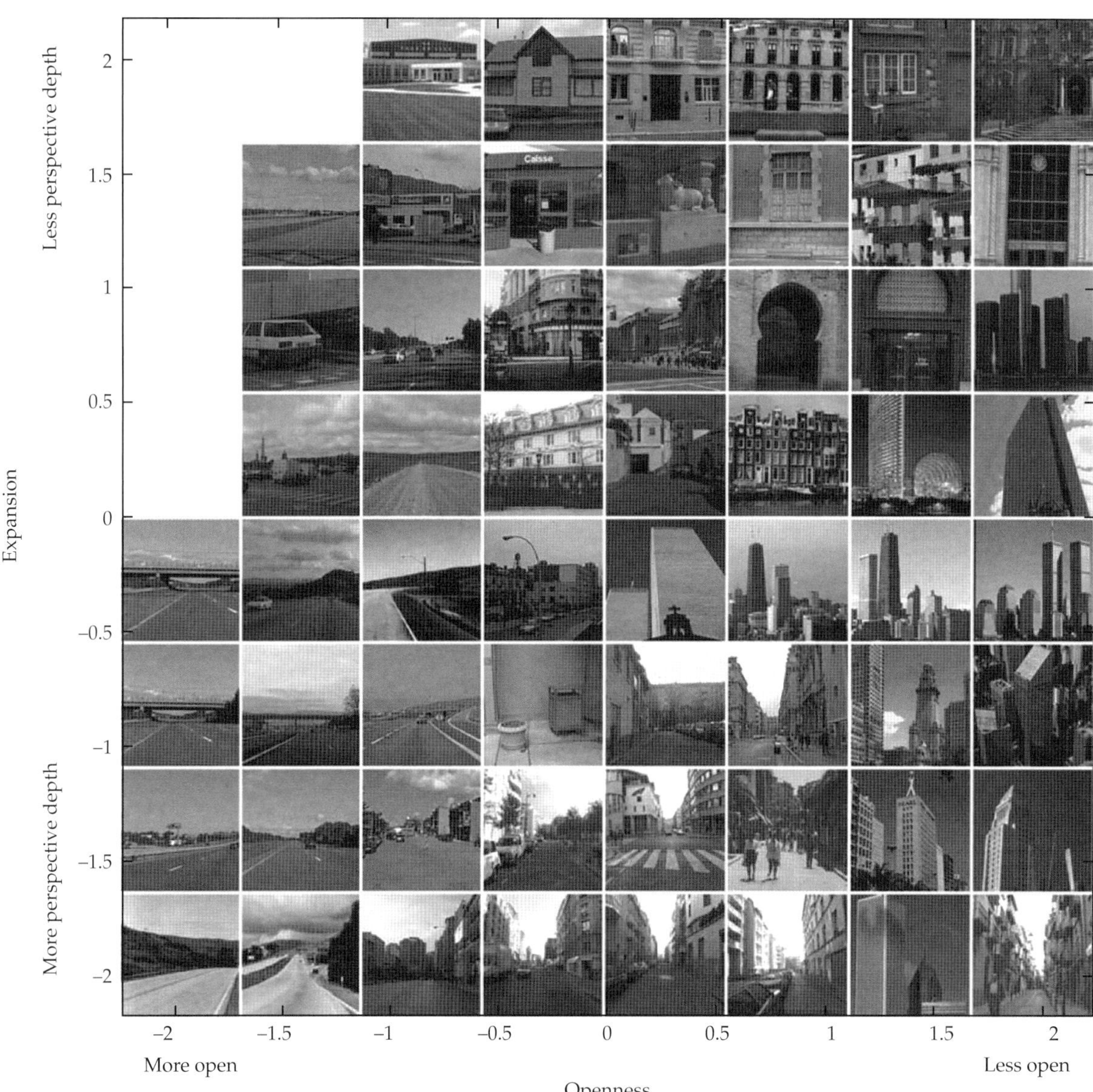

FIGURE 7.32 Spatial layout from global information In this collection of urban scenes, the *x*-axis represents a measure of "openness," from panoramic scenes to vertically structured scenes, derived from spatial-frequency information. The *y*-axis represents "expansion" (capturing a sense of depth from perspective). Scenes with the same meaning cluster together in this space.

upper right (low openness, low expansion). Highways fall in the lower left (high openness, high expansion). The rules that make this arrangement don't include anything about buildings or highways, just sine waves. Nevertheless, scenes with the same gist tend to cluster together.

Memory for Objects and Scenes Is Amazingly Good

The representation of scenes generated by information from the selective and non-selective pathways is very powerful. First, it gives rise to our perception of a world full of coherent objects in a coherent scene, even before we have a chance to attend to most of those objects. Second, it is easily stored in memory. Have a look at **FIGURE 7.33**. It contains photographs of 16 scenes. Spend about one second on

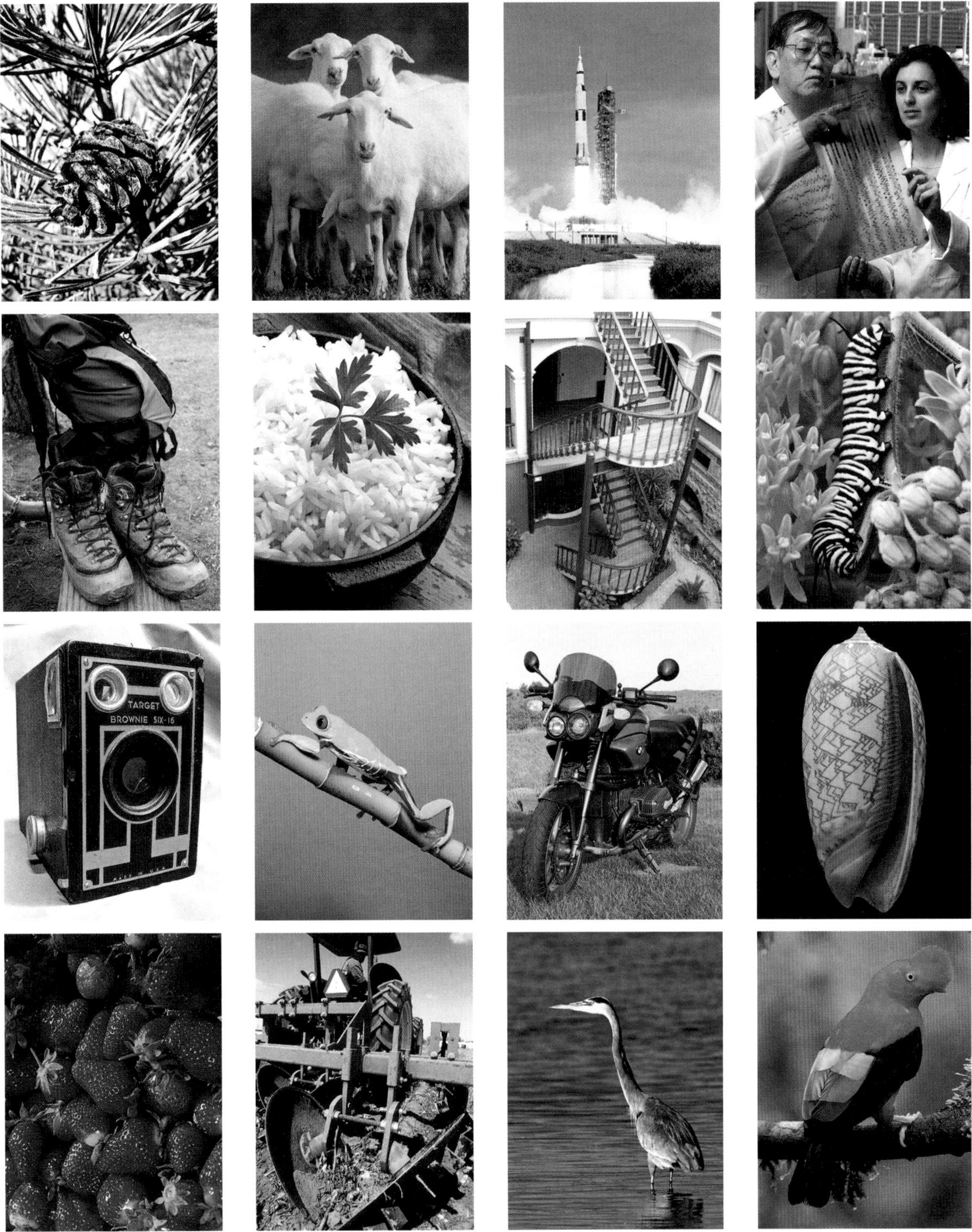

FIGURE 7.33 Picture memory Spend a second or two looking at each of these pictures. Then move on to Figure 7.34.

each scene, and then go to **FIGURE 7.34**, where you will find another set of 16 scenes. Your job is to determine which 8 of the 16 in Figure 7.34 you saw in Figure 7.33. You probably won't need the answer key (it's in Figure 7.34). It is likely that you will correctly classify 14 or more of the images as "old" or "new." That's pretty quick learning of fairly complicated stimuli. Yet it is a mere fraction of what you could do if

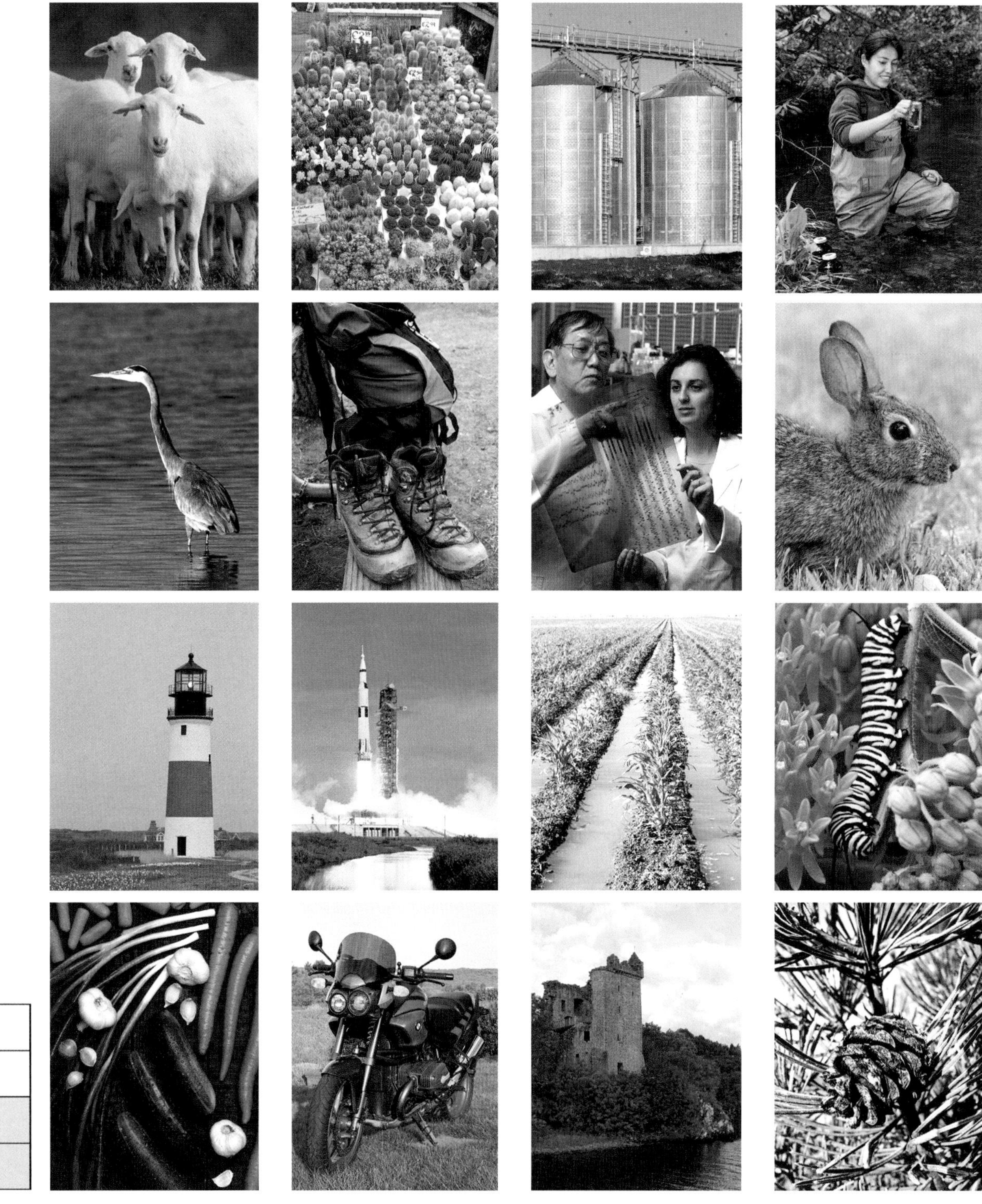

FIGURE 7.34 **Picture memory test** Without referring back to Figure 7.33, try to identify which of these pictures you already saw. Decide whether each picture is "old" or "new." You can check your answers on the grid to the left. The shaded squares show the locations of old pictures.

you had the time and we had the pictures. Roger Shepard (1967) conducted the original version of the test with 612 pictures and found that his observers were 98% correct. They were 90% correct when quizzed a week later. Standing, Conezio, and Haber (1970) got 85% accuracy after showing their observers 2500 pictures for 2 seconds apiece, and Standing (1973) later obtained similar results with 10,000(!) images.

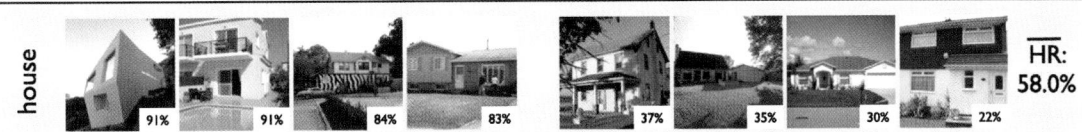

FIGURE 7.35 Memorable houses The percentage values give the probability that this house would be remembered in a picture memory experiment. Is it obvious, for example, why house 4 is much more memorable than house 7?

In his studies, Standing used a diverse collection of scenes clipped from magazines of the time. Consider what might happen if we restricted the "scenes" to single objects (an apple, a backpack) or if we included other examples of these objects in the test set (Did I see *that* apple?) or, worse yet, if we used the same objects in different poses (Was that backpack lying down before?). Aude Oliva and her students (Brady et al., 2008) tried this with 2500 objects. When asked to pick between an old item and a new one, their observers got 92% correct if the new item was an object of a type that had not been seen before in the experiment. Amazingly, observers were still 88% correct at remembering which example of a category they had seen and 87% correct at remembering which state of a specific object they had seen.

Interestingly, some scenes are much more memorable than others. Some aspects of memorability are pretty intuitive. On average, scenes with people in them are more memorable, as are scenes where a lot is going on. Objects and buildings are somewhat less memorable and wide-open spaces still less. This matches our intuition of what objects might make an image memorable (Khosla et al., 2015). Within categories of scenes, things can be a lot less intuitively clear. For instance, it is not obvious what makes one face more memorable than another, even though some faces are more memorable than others (Bainbridge, 2017). Or take a look at **FIGURE 7.35**. That first house does look pretty memorable, but it is not immediately obvious why house 4 should stick in memory so much better than house 7 (Bylinskii et al., 2015).

But . . . Memory for Objects and Scenes Can Be Amazingly Bad: Change Blindness

From the findings just described, we could conclude that pictures can be understood very rapidly and that, given enough time—perhaps a few seconds—we can code them into memory in sufficient detail to be able to recognize them days later. That is true, but it is not the whole story. In the 1990s, Ron Rensink and his colleagues introduced a different sort of picture memory experiment (Rensink, O'Regan, and Clark, 1997). They showed observers just one picture at a time. The observers would look at the picture for a while, and then it would vanish for 80 ms and be replaced by a similar image. The observer's task was to determine what had changed. The two versions of the same image would flip back and forth, separated by a brief interval in which a blank screen was presented, until the observer spotted the change or time ran out. A static version of the task is illustrated in **FIGURE 7.36**. Try to find the differences between the two pictures in this figure. The answers are in **FIGURE 7.37**.

(A)

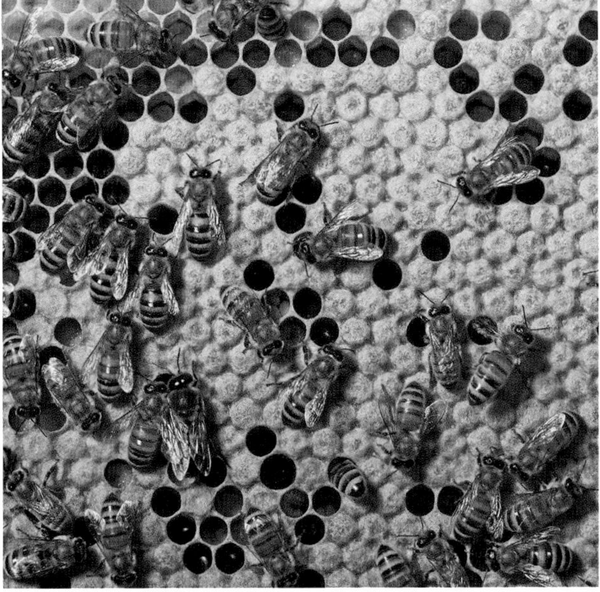

(B)

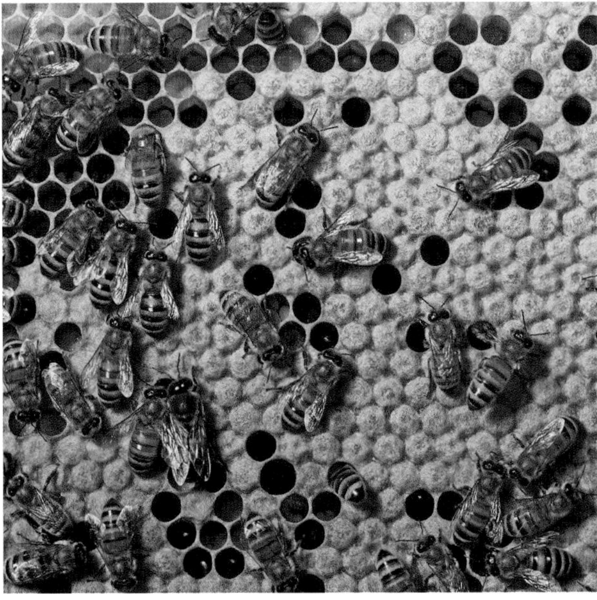

FIGURE 7.36 Change detection There are four differences between these two images. Can you find them?

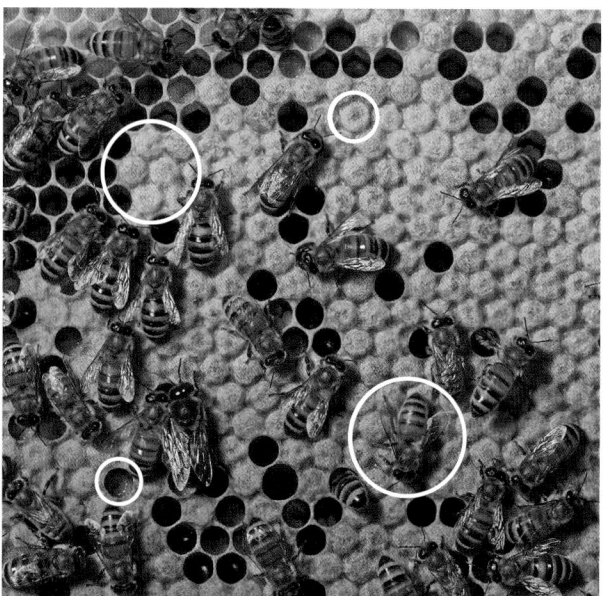

FIGURE 7.37 **Change detection answers** Here are the locations of the differences between the two images in Figure 7.36. When you go back to Figure 7.37 with this information, you will have no trouble seeing what was altered.

It may have taken you a while to discover all four changes circled in in Figure 7.37. That's what happened in Rensink's experiment: participants took several seconds on average to find the changes, and some never managed the task at all in the time they were given. This phenomenon is known as **change blindness.** If the blank screen between the two images is removed, the changes are more obvious because observers experience a kind of apparent-motion effect (see Chapter 8) when an object changes position, disappears, or changes color. But once we've taken care of that low-level factor by inserting the blank screen, viewers can be oblivious to jet engines that vanish from airplanes, branches that jump from tree to tree, and boats that change color.

Actually, we can eliminate the need for a blank screen if the change is made while the eyes are moving. We are virtually blind during an abrupt (saccadic) eye movement. McConkie and Currie (1996) took advantage of this fact to make dramatic changes in a scene while an observer was just looking around. If they made the changes while the eye was in motion, observers often failed to notice.

FURTHER DISCUSSION of eye movements can be found in Section 8.4.

What Do We Actually See?

It is not immediately obvious how these various facts can all be true of the same visual system. This is a topic of current controversy in the field. We can remember thousands of objects after a mere second or two of viewing, but we can't tell if a clearly visible bee or a black hole is changing from Figure 7.36A to 7.36B.

change blindness When one scene is replaced by another version of the same scene, observers may be unable to report what changed between the two versions.

Maybe we don't see changes when they don't change the gist of the scene. For this idea to be part of a convincing theory, it would help if we really understood what the gist of a scene might be. Gist is something different from the brief verbal description we might give if asked to "describe the gist" of an image. Describe the gist of **FIGURE 7.38**. Now look at **FIGURE 7.39** and decide which one of these two photographs is the same as Figure 7.38. You can probably do this quite easily, even though the gist descriptions of Figures 7.38A and 7.38B would be very similar: both are scenes of rowers in a boat on a sunny day. There is something about gist that we cannot trivially put into words.

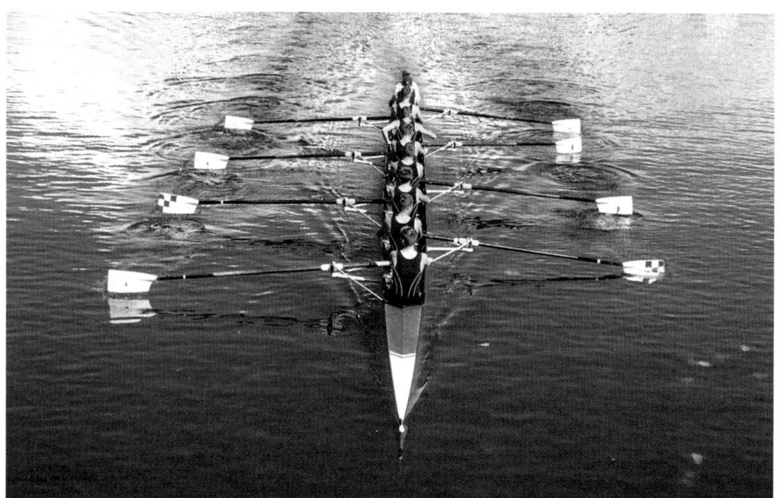

FIGURE 7.38 **Gist** Look at this picture for a couple of seconds. Describe it to yourself in a sentence. Then look at Figure 7.39.

We have already suggested what that "something" might be. The nonselective pathway (see Figure 7.29) gives us some sort of texture of *ensemble statistics* across the entire visual field. Combining that rough representation with a stream of objects recognized by way of the selective pathway, we *infer* a coherent world, filled with recognized objects (M. A. Cohen, Dennett, and Kanwisher, 2016). This act of inference gives us the experience a full-color, in-focus, three-dimensional scene filled with clearly identifiable

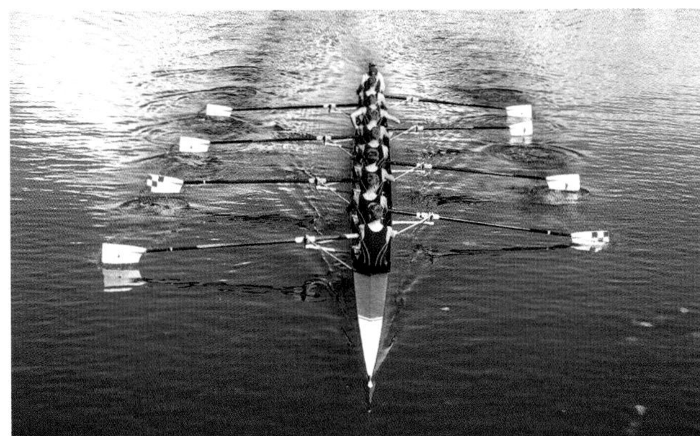

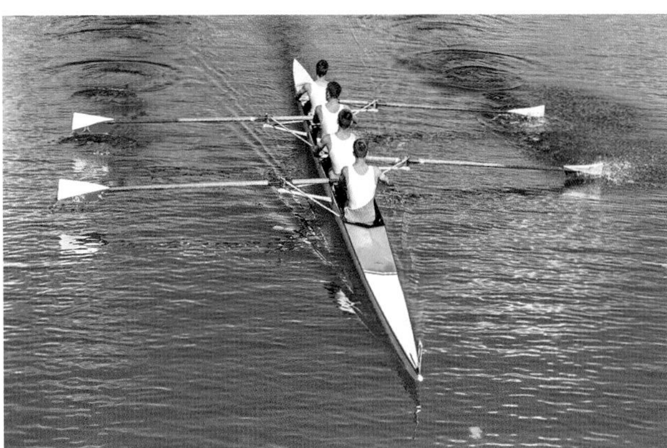

FIGURE 7.39 **Two pictures, one gist?** Which of these two images is the one you saw in Figure 7.38? You probably know, even though your verbal description of the new image would be very similar to the description you gave for Figure 7.38. Apparently, the gist of a scene contains more than is captured by our usual verbal descriptions.

objects. We do not have a perceptual experience of a few objects, floating in a sea of ensemble statistics. We know, from the research described in other chapters, that this experience must be a construction of the mind, not an exact copy of the stimulus. We know from Chapter 2 that the world is decently focused only at the fovea and that high-resolution processing occurs only in the central 1 degree or so of the visual field. We will see in Chapter 8 that the scene before us is smeared across the retina three or four times each second as we move our eyes. We know from Chapter 6 that we're getting two slightly different copies of the scene from our two retinas and that both copies are really two-dimensional.

Over and over in this book, we say that a particular aspect of perception is an inference, a guess about the world. Our conscious experience of the world is the mother of all inferences. This realization is hard for us to accept, because perception doesn't *feel* like an inference; it feels like it must be showing us what's really out there. It feels like Truth. Phenomena like change blindness are important because they show us the gap between perception and reality. Experiments investigating change blindness show us that we don't see all of what *is* there. Rather, in some spots, we see what *was* there when we last paid attention, and even then, we may not remember it perfectly (Irwin, Zacks, and Brown, 1990). In other spots, we perceive what we think should be there.

Moreover, we can fail to perceive what we do not expect to see—what does not fit with the current inference. This failure to notice the unexpected is an example of **inattentional blindness**. The great example of inattentional blindness comes from another experiment of Dan Simons, this time in collaboration with Christopher Chabris. They had observers keeping track of ball movements in a basketball passing game. Many of these participants failed to notice an actor in a gorilla suit who wandered into the middle of the scene, waved, and wandered off (Simons and Chabris, 1999).

Outside the lab, the bottleneck between the world and our perception is not usually much of a problem, because the world is a pretty stable and predictable place—at least on a moment-to-moment basis. If you put your coffee mug down on the desk and turn your attention to the computer screen, the mug will still be there when you choose to attend to it again. Only in the lab does the coffee mug vanish during an eye movement. This means that the physical world can serve as an "external memory" that backs up the perceptual world we create in our minds (O'Regan, 1992).

When the world does change, it tends to change in very predictable ways. If we've just driven past Second Avenue and then Third Avenue, we don't need to look at the next street sign to know that it probably says "Fourth Avenue." At a rate of about 20 objects per second, we can monitor the relevant items in this relatively stable

inattentional blindness A failure to notice—or at least to report—a stimulus that would be easily reportable if it were attended.

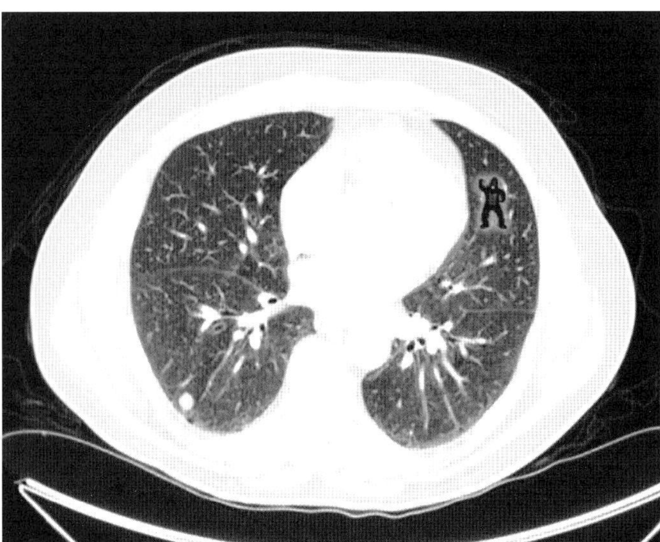

FIGURE 7.40 Gorillas in the lung? Radiologists tended to miss the silhouette of a gorilla in the lung, not because they were poor radiologists, but because even experts must perform their expert acts of attention and perception within the capacity limits of the human visual system.

world and be reasonably sure that we are up to date. And if something surprising does occur (like a gorilla leaping into the middle of Fourth Avenue), the event will probably be marked by a visual transient that grabs our attention so that we can update our internal representation pretty quickly and maintain our grasp on reality (Yantis, 1993).

A certain amount of work needs to be done to induce us to miss gorillas. Still, we should not feel too complacent about our inference of the perceptual world. Let's end with two examples. In an odd version of the gorilla experiment, Drew, Vo, and Wolfe (2013) put the image of a gorilla in a computed tomography image of a lung (**FIGURE 7.40**). Most radiologists, looking for small, white, round signs of lung cancer, missed the big, black, shaggy gorilla. That such an oversight is possible shows, among other things, that experts are faced with the same attentional limits on perception as the rest of us. They have learned to do remarkable things with their visual systems, but experts do their expert tasks using the same visual and cognitive systems as the rest of us.

Finally, let's consider eyewitness testimony. The basic assumption of eyewitness testimony is that you can report what *was* there, not what you inferred, guessed, hoped, or feared was there. Sadly, if unsurprisingly, we know that eyewitness testimony is subject to the same sorts of effects discussed here and that these factors are probably the cause of errors with real consequences (Wixted and Wells, 2017). In an effort to illustrate this point, Chabris and Simons (2011) gave people the task of following a jogger down a track and found that those observers could easily fail to notice a very visible apparent beating that was occurring along their route. The researchers picked this particular scenario because of a real case in which a policeman reported that, as he chased a suspect, he never saw his colleagues beating another man. At the time, people didn't believe that he could have been so blind. Now you know that such a scenario is, at least, possible.

Summary

1. Attention is a vital aspect of perception because we cannot process all of the input from our senses. The term *attention* refers to a large set of selective mechanisms that enable us to focus on some stimuli at the expense of others. Though this chapter talked almost exclusively about visual attention, attentional mechanisms exist in all sensory domains.
2. In vision, it is possible to direct attention to one location or one object. If something happens at an attended location, we will be faster to respond to it. It can be useful to refer to the "spotlight" of attention, though deployments of attention differ in important ways from movements of a physical spotlight, and the shape and size of that spotlight is not easy to define.
3. In visual search tasks, observers typically look for a target item among a number of distractor items. If the target is defined by a salient basic feature, such as its color or orientation, search is very efficient and the number of distractors has little influence on the reaction time (the time required to find the target). If no basic feature information can guide the deployment of attention, then search is inefficient, as if each item needed to be examined

one after the other. Search can be of intermediate efficiency if some feature information is available to guide your attention (e.g., if we're looking for a red car, we don't need to examine the blue objects in the parking lot).

4. Search for objects in real scenes is guided by the known features of the objects, by the salient features in the scenes, by your history of searching and your history of reward, and by a variety of scene-based forms of guidance. For example, if you're looking for your coffee mug, you will guide your attention to objects with the right color, shape, and size, and located in physically plausible locations (horizontal surfaces) and in logically sensible places (the desk or counter, but probably not the floor).
5. Attention varies over time as well as over space. In the attentional blink paradigm, observers search for two items in a rapid stream of stimuli that appear at the point of fixation. Attention to the first target makes it hard to find the second if the second appears within 200–500 ms of the first. When two identical items appear in the stream of stimuli, a different phenomenon makes it hard to detect the second instance.
6. The effects of attention manifest themselves in several different ways in many different parts of the brain. In some cases, attention is marked by a general increase in neural activity or by a greater correlation between activity in different brain areas. In other cases, attention to a particular attribute tunes cells more sharply for that attribute. And in still other cases, attention to a stimulus or location causes receptive fields to shrink so as to exclude unattended stimuli.
7. Damage to the parietal lobe of the brain produces deficits in visual attention. Damage to the right parietal lobe can lead to neglect, a disorder in which it is hard to direct attention into the contralesional (in this case, the left) visual field. People with neglect may ignore half of an object or half of their own body.
8. Scene perception involves both selective and nonselective processing. Tasks like visual search make extensive use of selective processing to recognize specific objects. Nonselective processing allows observers to appreciate the mean and variance of features across many objects (or proto-objects). Thus, you know the average orientation of trees in the woods (vertical) before knowing whether any particular tree is oriented perfectly vertically. Using these ensemble statistics, even without segmenting the scene into regions and objects, the nonselective pathway can provide information about the gist of a scene (e.g., whether it's natural or man-made).
9. Picture memory experiments show that people can remember thousands of images after only a second or two of exposure to each. In contrast, change blindness experiments show that people can miss large changes in scenes if those changes do not markedly alter the meaning of the scene.
10. Our perceptual experience of scenes consists of nonselective processing of the layout and ensemble statistics of the scene, combined with selective processing of a very few objects at each moment. Our experience can be thought of as an inference based on all of the preceding processing. Usually this inference is adequate because we can rapidly check the world to determine whether the chair, the book, and the desk are still there. In the lab, however, we can use phenomena like inattentional blindness and change blindness to reveal the limits of our perception, and it is becoming increasingly clear that those limits can have real-world consequences.

Chapter 8

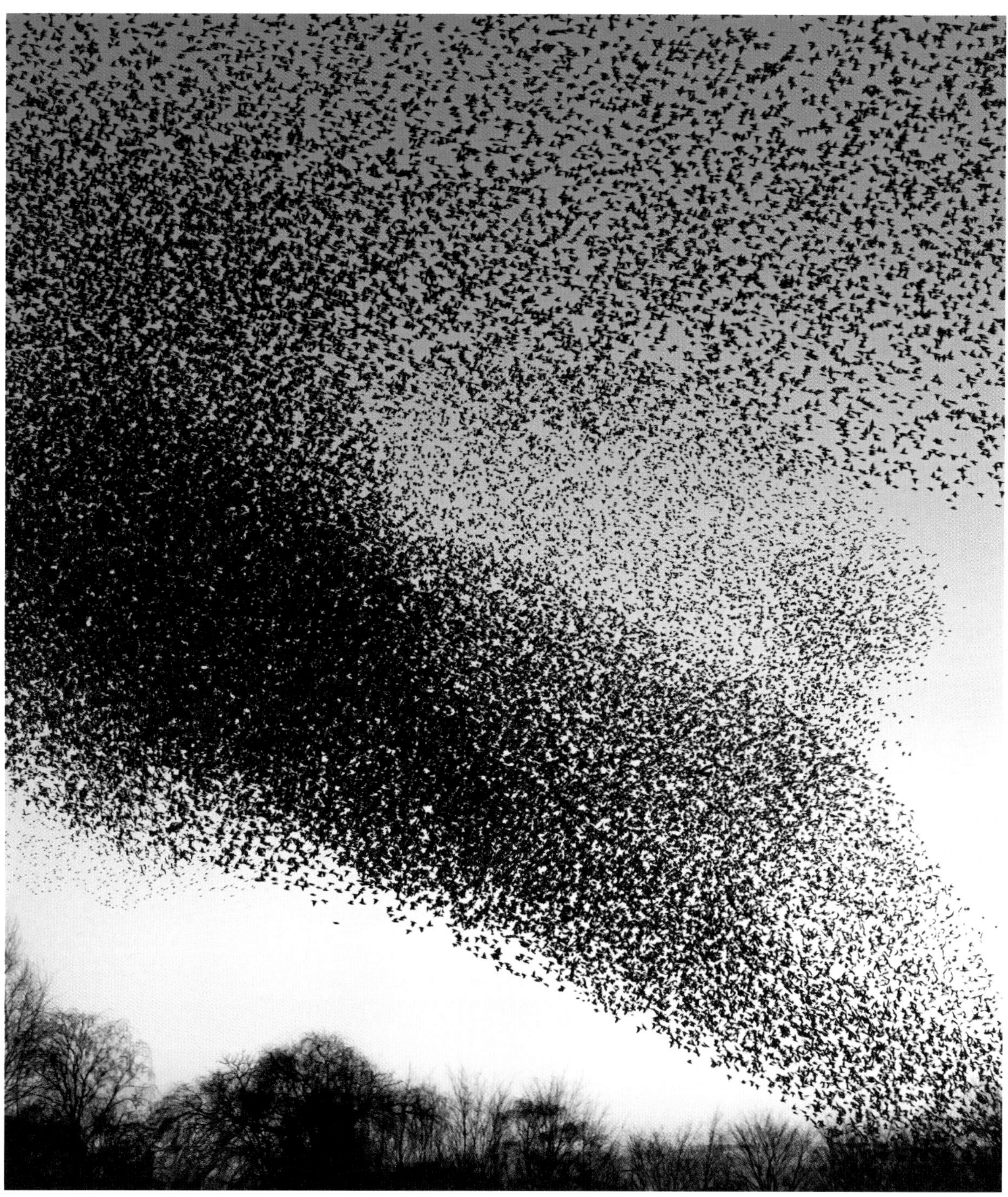

Albert Beukhof, *Starling Murmuration*, 2022

Visual Motion Perception

Questions to Contemplate

Think about the following questions as you read this chapter.
By the chapter's end, you should be able to answer and discuss them.

- Is motion a fundamental perceptual dimension?
- How is it that the world stands still when we move our eyes?
- What do beetles, flies, and humans have in common?
- How do the movies create the perception of objects in motion?

Like any self-respecting ladybug, the one in **FIGURE 8.1** flits around from leaf to leaf. At time 1 it is on the lowermost leaf; at time 2 it has moved to the middle leaf. Our visual system distinguishes the bug by a number of features, such as its shape, its location in space, and its color. Previous chapters have established these features as fundamental perceptual dimensions: characteristics of visual stimuli that are directly encoded by neurons fairly early in the visual system.

Is the ladybug's motion also a fundamental perceptual dimension? At first glance, we might think not. After all, motion is really just a change in an object's location over time. If we already have neural mechanisms set up to determine position, why go to the extra expense of adding more low-level machinery to process motion?

Though the added investment might seem unnecessary, consider this question from the position of the primordial vertebrates whose visual system we eventually inherited. Many bugs move pretty quickly, so if we depend on catching them for our supper, fast detection of their direction of motion will be important to our survival. Similarly, if other animals are trying to catch us for their supper, we also need to be adept at detecting the motion of these predators. In Section 6.2 we saw that motion parallax is an important cue for depth perception. And from a different perspective, it would be hard to believe that hockey goalies, baseball batters facing knuckleball pitchers, and boxers trying to avoid being pummeled by their opponents could do their jobs without having a mechanism for very quickly determining and predicting the movements of pucks, balls, and fists, respectively.

8.1 Motion Aftereffects

In fact, we've already seen some indications that motion is a low-level perceptual phenomenon; we mentioned in Chapter 3 that many cells in the primary visual cortex (= V1; striate cortex) selectively respond to motion in one particular direction. A phenomenon called the waterfall illusion provides another piece of evidence

Time 1

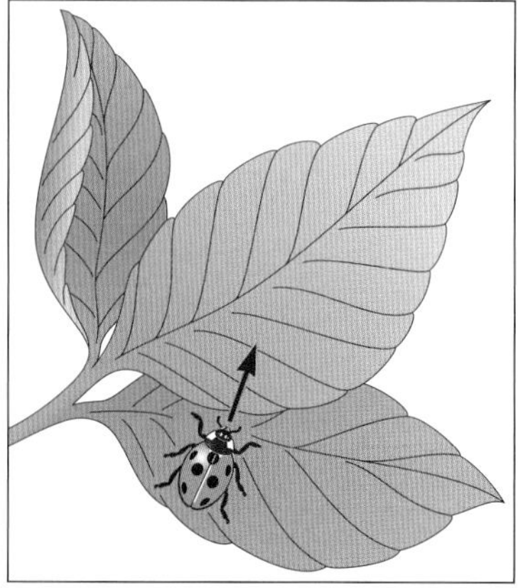

Time 2

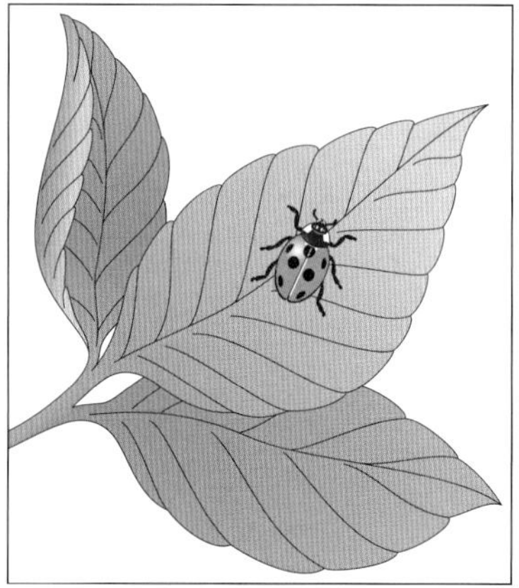

FIGURE 8.1 Motion As the movements of this ladybug demonstrate, motion is a change in position over time.

that there is something special about motion. Here's how Robert Addams (1834) described this illusion after a visit to the waterfall of Foyers (**FIGURE 8.2**):

> Having steadfastly looked for a few seconds at a particular part of the cascade, admiring the confluence and decussation of the currents forming the liquid drapery of waters, and then suddenly directed my eyes to the left, to observe the face of the sombre age-worn rocks immediately contiguous to the water-fall, I saw the rocky surface as if in motion upwards, and with an apparent velocity equal to that of the descending water, which the moment before had prepared my eyes to behold that singular deception.

The "deception" that Addams described—which had also been noted by Aristotle (384–322 BCE)—was later dubbed the **motion aftereffect (MAE)**. After viewing motion in a constant direction for a sustained period of time (at least 15 seconds), we see any stationary objects that we view subsequently (like the rocks around the waterfall) as moving in the opposite direction. This phenomenon may seem a lot like the color aftereffects we studied in Section 5.6, and that's no coincidence. Just as color aftereffects are caused by opponent processes for color vision, MAEs are caused by opponent processes for motion detection.

We know that the monkey brain is very similar to the human brain, but it is always nice to establish converging evidence suggesting that results from monkey labs apply to human vision as well. In the case of motion perception, researchers have looked for this evidence using the MAE. As noted earlier, the existence of the MAE implies an opponent-process system much like the one that plays a role in color vision. Neurons tuned to different directions of motion generally do not respond to a stationary object, so they simply continue to fire at their spontaneous rate, and the spontaneous rates for upward- and downward-sensitive cells are normally balanced. That is, neurons sensitive to upward motion fire at about the same rate as neurons sensitive to downward motion, so the signals cancel out and no motion is perceived. But when we look at a waterfall for a prolonged period, the detectors sensitive to downward motion become adapted. When we then switch our gaze to a stationary object, such as the rocks next to the waterfall, the neurons sensitive to upward motion fire faster than the adapted downward-sensitive neurons, and we therefore perceive the rocks as drifting up.

motion aftereffect (MAE) The illusion of motion of a stationary object that occurs after prolonged exposure to a moving object.

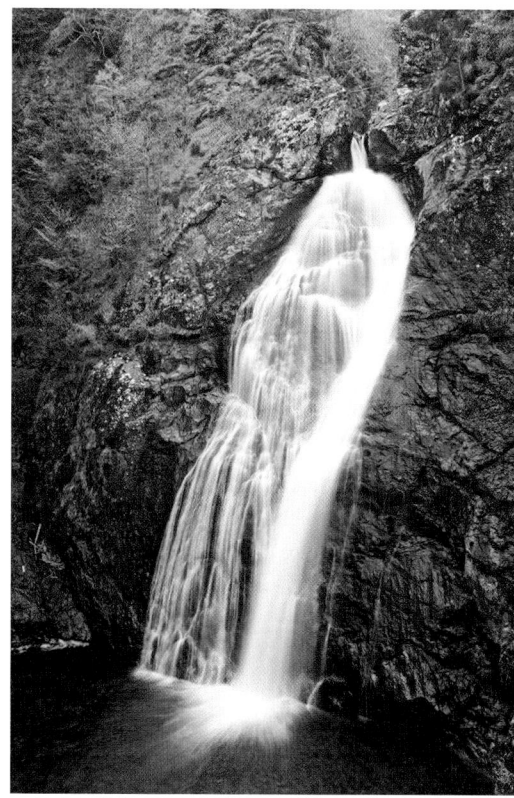

FIGURE 8.2 The waterfall illusion The lower falls of Foyers, where Addams discovered (or rediscovered) the motion aftereffect.

interocular transfer The transfer of an effect (such as adaptation) from one eye to the other.

middle temporal area (MT) (V5) An area of the brain thought to be important in the perception of motion. Also called V5 in humans.

You might wonder why *any* motion detectors would fire in response to a stationary rock, but as we will see in a bit, our eyes are constantly drifting around, so there is always a small amount of retinal motion to stimulate motion detectors, at least slightly. You might also wonder what happens when we adapt to downward motion and then see something moving horizontally. Make a prediction, and then test your hypothesis.

Here's another experiment to try. Adapt for 15 seconds or so to rightward motion with your right eye open but your left eye closed, and then quickly switch eyes, closing your right eye and opening your left. You should experience an aftereffect that is only slightly reduced in magnitude compared with the aftereffect you get with both eyes open the whole time. What does this **interocular transfer** tell us about the locus of the MAE in the visual system? Could MAEs subserved by neurons in the retinas? What about neurons in the lateral geniculate nucleus?

The fact that a strong MAE is obtained when one eye is adapted and the other is tested means that the effect must be reflecting the activities of neurons in a part of the visual system where information collected from the two eyes is combined (Raymond, 1993). As we learned in Chapter 3, input from both eyes is not combined until the primary visual cortex, where neurons show a preference for input from one eye or the other, but respond to some extent to stimuli in both eyes. Advances in functional imaging techniques may make it possible to locate the site of MAEs even more precisely. The emerging evidence suggests that the MAE in humans is caused by the same brain region shown to be responsible for global-motion detection in monkeys: the **middle temporal area** of the cortex, an area commonly referred to as **MT** or **V5** (Culham et al., 1999). For example, David Heeger and colleagues, after controlling for the important effects of attention, demonstrated that the direction-selective adaptation produced a selective imbalance in the functional magnetic resonance imaging signal in human MT, providing evidence that MAEs are the result of a population imbalance in area MT (Huk, Ress, and Heeger, 2001). Remarkably, more recent work shows that MAEs can occur even after very brief exposures—as little as 25 milliseconds—and that these can be explained by direction-selective responses of neurons in MT to subsequently presented stationary stimuli (Glasser et al., 2011).

FURTHER DISCUSSION of the role of the primary visual cortex in combining input from both eyes can be found in Section 3.5.

The waterfall illusion is just one of many motion illusions. *Induced motion* is another, and you've probably experienced it. For example, you're sitting in your stationary car when an SUV in the adjacent parking place backs out. Although your car is not moving, you get the strong illusion that it is going forward and is about to smash into the wall. This motion illusion can give you quite a scare.

Akiyoshi Kitaoka's art shows powerful illusions of motion (see https://www.ritsumei.ac.jp/~akitaoka/index-e.html). Kitaoka's pictures are stationary on the page, but they can produce a strong illusion of motion if you allow your eyes to drift across them. How does this work? We don't yet have a consensus, but studies suggest that patterns like Kitaoka's Rotating Snakes elicit directional responses from neurons in monkey cortex that correspond closely to the directions perceived by humans (Conway et al., 2005).

8.2 Computation of Visual Motion

What are the minimum requirements for an effective motion detector? Because motion involves a change in position over time, a logical place to start is with two adjacent receptors (call them neurons 1 and 2), separated by a fixed distance.

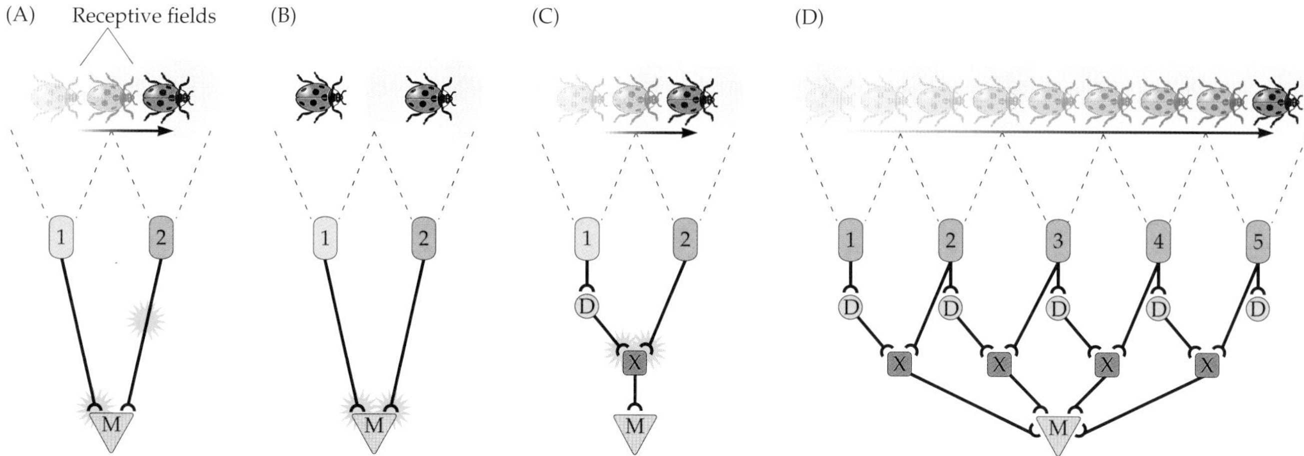

FIGURE 8.3 A neural circuit for the detection of rightward motion
(A) When an object such as a ladybug moves, it is logical to suppose that the object is perceived by the receptive fields of separate but adjacent neurons 1 and 2. (B) Motion-detection neuron M responds identically to a single moving ladybug and to two separate stationary ladybugs. (C) To distinguish motion, the circuit needs additional neurons. The first (D) delays neuron 1's input to M, while the second (X) fires only when both neurons (1 and 2) are stimulated. This combination of inputs allows M to detect motion. (D) In detecting longer-range motion, a single M cell fires continually as the bug moves across the receptive fields of five distinct neurons.

Getting back to ladybugs, a bug (or a spot of light) moving from left to right would first pass through neuron 1's receptive field, and then a short time later it would enter neuron 2's receptive field (**FIGURE 8.3A**). In theory, a third cell that "listens" to both neurons should be able to detect this movement.

However, our motion detection cell (call it M) cannot simply add up excitatory inputs from cells 1 and 2. Given such a neural circuit, M would indeed fire in response to the moving bug—but it would also respond to two stationary bugs, one in each receptive field (**FIGURE 8.3B**). To solve this problem, we need two additional components in our neural circuit, as shown in **FIGURE 8.3C**. The first new cell, labeled D in Figure 8.3, receives input from neuron 1 and delays transmission of this input for a short period of time. Cell D also has a fast adaptation rate. That is, it fires when cell 1 initially detects light, but it quickly stops firing if the light remains shining on 1's receptive field. Neuron 2 and cell D are then connected to cell X, which is a multiplication cell. This multiplication cell will fire only when both cells 2 and D are active. Multiplication seems to be a common feature of neural networks. Precisely how multiplication neurons work physiologically is not altogether clear; however, Christof Koch considers this to be one of the most important and challenging questions in neurobiology (Koch, 1999).

By cell D delaying receptor 1's response and then cell X multiplying 1's input by receptor 2's input, we create a mechanism that is sensitive to motion. This mechanism is direction-selective: it would respond only to motion from left to right, not from right to left. A bug moving from cell 2's receptive field into cell 1's receptive field would cause cells 2 and D to fire in the wrong order, so X would not receive the two inputs simultaneously, and M would not fire. The mechanism would also be tuned to speed, because when the bug moved at just the right speed, the delayed response from receptor 1 and the direct response from receptor 2 would occur at the same time and thus reinforce each other. If the bug moved too fast or too slow, the outputs from cells 2 and D would be out of sync.

A more realistic circuit would include additional receptors to detect longer-range motion, as shown in **FIGURE 8.3D**. Here, the M cell fires continually as the bug moves across the fields of the five receptors at the top of the circuit. If you were the "circuit designer," how would you change the speed tuning of this circuit?

This simple "bug" motion detector is based on a model initially developed by Werner Reichardt in the 1950s to explain how beetles and flies detect motion (Reichardt, 1986). Almost all models of human motion detection are, at their core, elaborations of Reichardt's model adapted to the spatial-frequency filtering properties of the human visual system (see Chapter 3). Indeed, much of our current understanding about motion processing derives from studies of insects.

One elaboration, developed by Barlow and Levick (1965), uses what electrical engineers would call an "AND gate." Cell X fires if and only if both its inputs (cells 2 *and* D) are firing simultaneously, and it passes this message on to the motion detection cell M. The AND concept is almost certainly not correct, and a more elaborate version—developed by Adelson and Bergen (1985) and based on linear filters that delay, sum, and then are followed by nonlinearities—seems closer to the "truth."

Origins of Direction Selectivity

A critical feature of motion detectors is their ability to detect the direction of motion. In nonhuman primates, direction selectivity starburst amacrine cells in the retina selectively inhibit direction-selective retinal ganglion cells, giving rise to direction selectivity. Recent work (Patterson et al., 2022) suggests that a similar circuit is present in the primate retina. This circuit then projects to the accessory optic tract.

Apparent Motion

One possible objection to the Reichardt model is that it does not, in fact, require continuous motion in order to fire. An image of a bug that appears in A's receptive field, then disappears, and then reappears in B's receptive field a short time later will drive M to respond just as strongly as if the image had moved smoothly across the two receptive fields. Although it raises a valid concern, this observation turns out to be a virtue rather than a liability for the Reichardt model, because it provides an excellent explanation for a visual illusion, called apparent motion, that modern humans experience on a daily basis.

Apparent motion was first demonstrated by Sigmund Exner in 1875. Exner set up a contraption that would generate electrical sparks separated from each other by a very short distance in space and a very short period of time. Even though there were two separate sparks—that is, two different perceptual objects—observers swore that they saw a single spark moving from one position to another.

We in the twenty-first century experience apparent motion every time we watch television, go to a movie, or use a computer. You are probably aware that an animated cartoon is really a series of still drawings (**FIGURE 8.4**). Objects such as Daffy Duck change positions each frame, and when the frames are shown to us at a sufficiently fast speed (e.g., 30 frames per second), we perceive these position changes over time as motion. Live-action movies and television programs work the same way, except that the frames are still photographs rather than drawings.

Interestingly, visual apparent motion signals can be integrated with signals from audition to change the perceived direction of auditory apparent motion (Soto-Faraco et al., 2002), and conversely, auditory signals can alter the perceived direction of illusory motion. For example, a sound that is perceived to move from left to right induces the illusion that a stationary bar moves in the direction of the sound and shifts the landing positions of saccadic eye movements (Fracasso et al., 2013). (We will discuss saccadic eye movements in detail in Section 8.4.) ●

The Correspondence Problem: Viewing through an Aperture

Although apparent motion turns out to be a win for our motion detection circuit, one of the classic perceptual "problems" that we've discussed over and over in this book remains an issue for the Reichardt model. We can illustrate this problem with

apparent motion The illusory impression of smooth motion resulting from the rapid alternation of objects that appear in different locations in rapid succession.

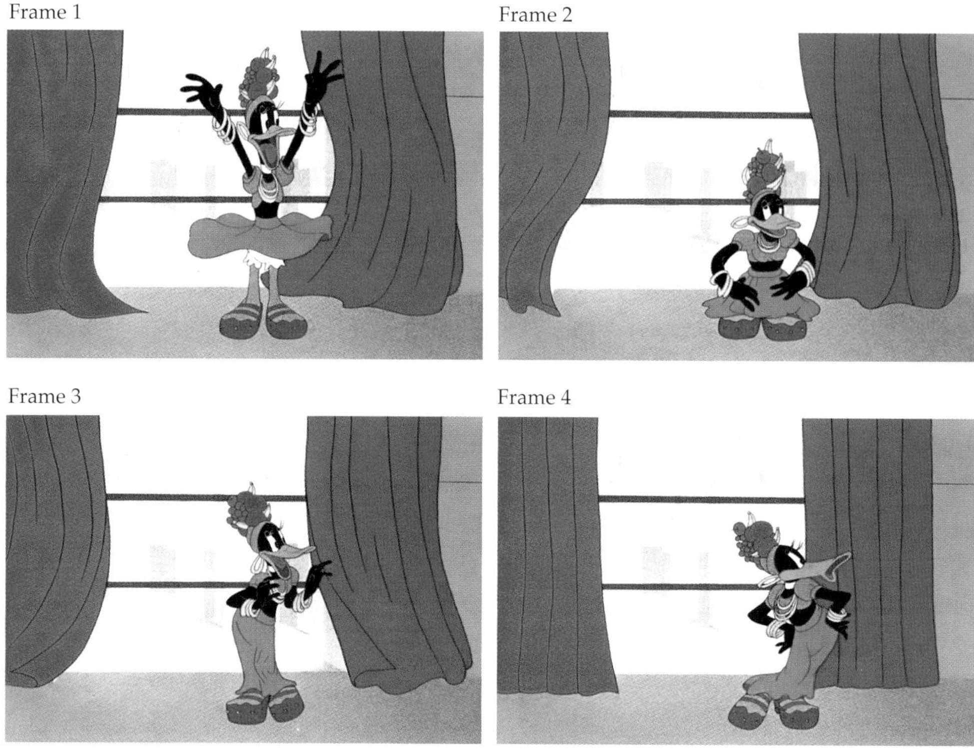

FIGURE 8.4 Apparent motion A series of still images played one after the other at a fast rate produces the apparent motion of cartoons, like these four stills from the Looney Tunes animation *Yankee Doodle Daffy*, showing Daffy Duck impersonating Carmen Miranda.

the movies diagramed in **FIGURE 8.5**. Each movie has two frames that alternate back and forth. The only difference between the two frames is that the only object in the movie—the red square studded with small circles—has been shifted diagonally by a short distance.

If you view the first version of the movie (Figure 8.5A), you will clearly detect diagonal motion. This scenario appears to present no problem to our motion detector: the square moves down and to the right, and then back up and to the left, and detectors sensitive to these directions pick up and signal this movement. Now consider movie 2 (Figure 8.5B), where we cover most of the square with a black "mask," leaving three of the circles viewable through a small window, or **aperture**

aperture A windowlike opening that allows only a partial view of an object.

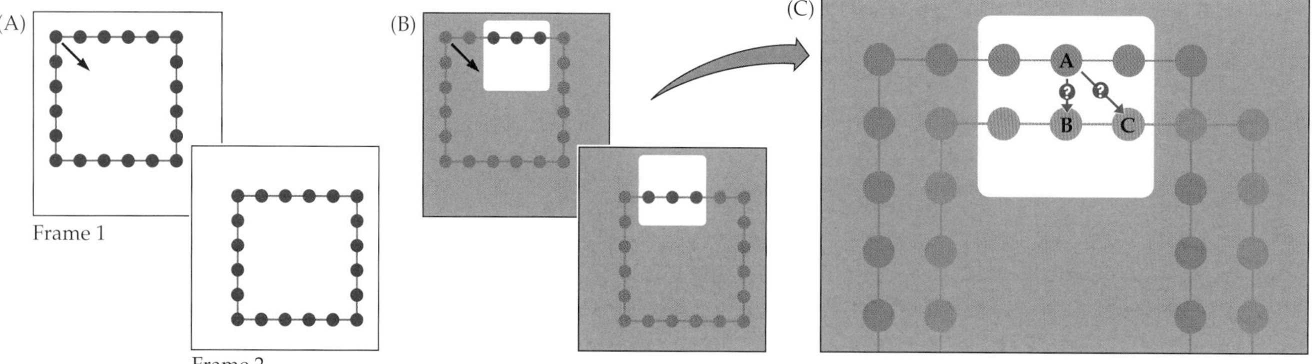

FIGURE 8.5 The correspondence problem (A) The square moves down and to the right. (B) For a detector that "sees" only the contents of the white square, the motion is ambiguous. (C) What the detector sees is consistent with both motion straight down and motion down and to the right.

(in Figure 8.5, the mask is illustrated as transparent so that you can see what's behind it, but in the movie the mask is opaque). Beneath the mask, the square moves exactly as before, but if you view the movie, you will quite clearly perceive up-and-down, *not* diagonal, motion.

The larger issue that these movies bring up is called the **correspondence problem** for motion detection. Consider Figure 8.5C, which is a close-up view of the situation in Figure 8.5B. Here we superimposed the two frames, coloring the circles blue in their frame 1 positions and green in their frame 2 positions. The difficulty for our motion detection system is this: How does it know which circles in frame 2 correspond to which circles in frame 1? Because we have motion detectors for all directions, one detector will sense the diagonal motion implied by matching the circle labeled A in Figure 8.5C with the circle labeled C. But another detector will sense the vertical motion implied by matching circle A with circle B. These detectors compete to determine our overall perception.

correspondence problem In reference to motion detection, the problem faced by the motion detection system of knowing which feature in frame 2 corresponds to a particular feature in frame 1.

aperture problem The fact that when a moving object is viewed through an aperture (or a single receptive field), the direction of motion of a local feature or part of the object may be ambiguous.

FURTHER DISCUSSION of correspondence as it relates to stereoscopic depth perception can be found in Section 6.3.

An important example of the correspondence problem is known as the **aperture problem**. It gets its name from the fact that a different detector may win this competition when an object is viewed through an aperture than would win if we could see the whole object. Consider the demonstration illustrated in **FIGURE 8.6**. Here the object is a grating moving behind an aperture. The motion direction of the grating is ambiguous—the grating could be moving up and to the left (perpendicular to the stripes, but diagonally overall; Figure 8.6A), but it could also be moving just up (Figure 8.6B) or just to the left (Figure 8.6C). The motion component parallel to the grating cannot be inferred from the visual input, because there are no perpendicular contours or features on the grating. This means that a variety of contours of different orientations moving at different speeds can cause identical responses in a motion-sensitive neuron in the visual system. Without the aperture, there's no ambiguity and no problem. But when we view the grating through the aperture, the system appears to impose some kind of shortest-distance constraint, and the vertical-motion detector wins.

At this point you may be thinking it's rather silly to claim that an artificial situation such as the one we've set up here poses a broad challenge to the visual system. After all, how often is our view of a moving object limited to a small window, as in the examples presented here? To understand the broader implications of the correspondence and aperture problems, consider the fact that every neuron in V1

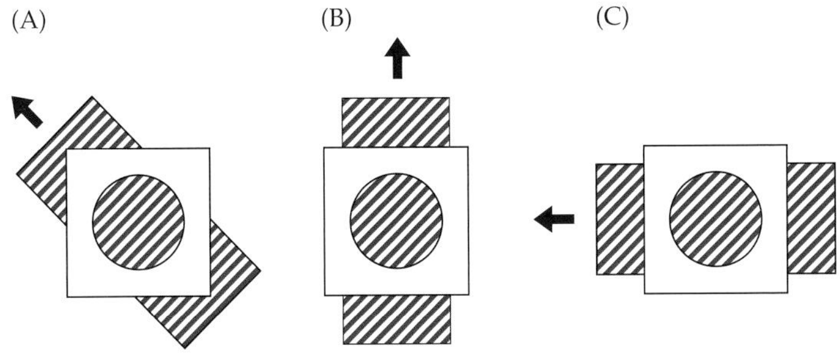

FIGURE 8.6 The aperture problem The contents of the aperture (circle) are the same in (A), (B), and (C), even though the physical motion of the patterned rectangle is quite different.

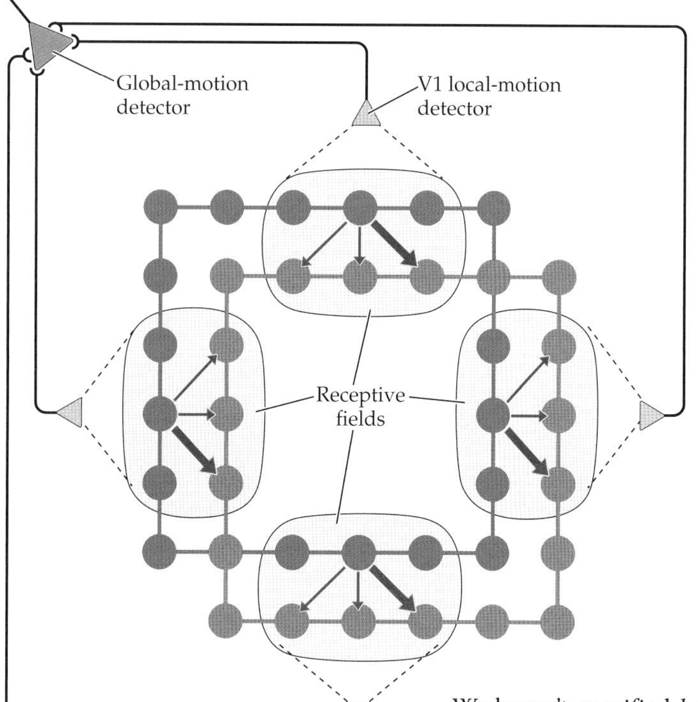

FIGURE 8.7 A global-motion detector As the thicker red arrows show, only one direction—movement down and to the right—is consistent with the receptive fields (shaded rectangles) of all four V1 cells, and this is the motion we perceive when we see the object as a whole. If a single neuron—the "global-motion detector," represented by the orange triangle—has access to all the V1 cells detecting local-motion directions, it will be in a position to compare their outputs and find this common denominator.

has a limited receptive field. In other words, *every V1 cell sees the world through a small aperture*. Therefore, as **FIGURE 8.7** illustrates, none of the V1 cells (represented in the figure as gray triangles) can tell with certainty which visual elements correspond to one another when an object moves, even when no mask is present.

The solution to this problem is to have another set of neurons, each of which "listens" to several V1 neurons and integrates their potentially conflicting signals. Such an integrative neuron is known as a global-motion detector, represented by the orange triangle in Figure 8.7. We haven't specified *how* this global-motion detector performs this comparison, but that question would lead us beyond the scope of this book.

The aperture problem is like the Indian parable about the blind men and the elephant, which we introduced in Chapter 4 (see Figure 4.10A). In one version of this parable, the king asks six blind men to determine what an elephant looks like by feeling different parts of the elephant's body. The first blind man feels a leg and says the elephant is like a tree trunk; the second feels the tail and says the elephant is like a rope; the third feels the trunk and says the elephant is like a snake; the fourth feels the ear and likens the elephant to a fan; the fifth climbs the body and says the elephant is like a wall; and the sixth feels the tusk and says the elephant is like a solid pipe. The king explains to them, "You are all correct. Each of you describes it differently because each one of you touched a different part of the animal. But, in fact the elephant has all the features you mentioned." In the aperture problem, each of the V1 cells is a blind man, and the correct answer comes only from combining their responses.

Detection of Global Motion in Area MT

Though a discussion of how global-motion detectors work would be too broad for this text, we can say something about *where* the global-motion detectors are. We saw in Chapter 3 that lesions to the magnocellular layers of the lateral geniculate nucleus impair the perception of large, rapidly moving objects. Information from magnocellular neurons feeds into V1 and is then passed on to (among other places) the middle temporal area of the cortex, an area commonly referred to as MT in nonhuman primates, and then to the medial superior temporal area, MST. MT and MST are considered the hub for motion processing (Ilg, 2008). The human equivalent of MT has been localized using functional magnetic resonance imaging and variously labeled as hMT+ or V5 (**FIGURE 8.8**). Recent work suggests that this motion-sensitive area may have at least two separate maps located on the lateral surface at the temporal–occipital boundary. The vast majority of neurons in the MT are selective for motion in one particular direction, but they show little selectivity for form or color. But do these MT cells correspond to the orange neuron in

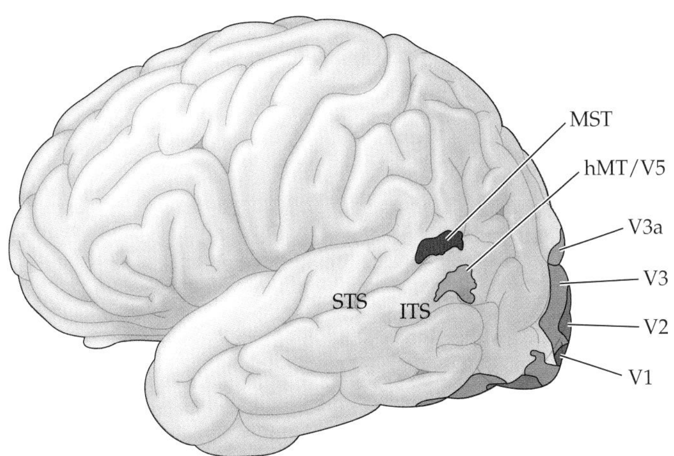

FIGURE 8.8 Motion-sensitive areas in the human brain The middle temporal area (hMT/V5, green) and medial superior temporal area (MST, red) are shown in relation to other visual areas (V1, V2, V3, and V3a). STS (superior temporal sulcus), ITS (inferior temporal sulcus).

Figure 8.7, which responds to large-scale motion of whole objects? Or are they more like the low-level motion detectors represented by the gray triangles in Figure 8.7?

To find out, Newsome and Paré (1988) trained a group of monkeys to respond to correlated-dot-motion displays (**FIGURE 8.9**). In Figure 8.9A, all the dots (100%) are moving to the right. In Figure 8.9B, 50% of the dots have correlated motion (they are moving in the same direction), while the motion of the rest of the dots is uncorrelated (they are moving in random directions). In Figure 8.9C, only 20% of the dots have correlated motion. Just as in the aperture problem demonstration, no single dot in these displays is sufficient to determine the overall direction of correlated motion. To detect the correlated direction, a neuron must integrate information from many local motion detectors.

Once they were fully trained, the monkeys in Newsome and Paré's study could recognize the correlated-motion direction when only 2–3% of the dots were moving in this direction. The researchers then lesioned the monkeys' MT areas. Following the surgery, the monkeys needed about ten times as many correlated dots to correctly identify the direction of motion. However, the monkeys' ability to discriminate the orientation of stationary patterns was generally unimpaired. Interestingly, the monkeys' performance in the correlated-dot-motion task improved markedly during the weeks following the lesion, presumably because they learned to use other brain areas to discriminate motion.

Lesion studies have been central to our understanding of the specificity of brain areas. However, such studies are often less than completely compelling, because lesions (even "clean" chemical lesions like those used by Newsome and Paré) may be incomplete or may influence other structures. To test the involvement of MT neurons in global-motion perception more directly, Newsome and colleagues trained

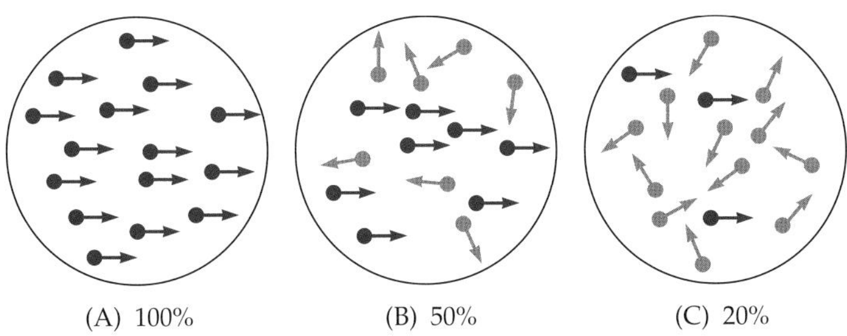

FIGURE 8.9 The Newsome and Paré paradigm Initially described by Williams and Sekuler (1984), the monkey's task was to identify the direction of motion of the correlated dots (i.e., those moving in the same direction). Correlated dots are shown in purple here, but in the actual study stimuli, all the dots were the same color and there were no arrows. The monkeys' ability to determine correlated direction was impaired after researchers lesioned areas in the middle temporal cortex.

Sensation & Perception in Everyday Life

The Man Who Couldn't See Motion

Recall what it's like to experience a motion aftereffect. You stare at a waterfall and then shift your gaze to the cliff next to the falls. You know that the rocks are not moving, and you can see that they aren't going anywhere, yet you still experience an otherworldly sense of "disembodied" motion.

Now imagine the opposite experience: objects change position, and you are fully aware of these location shifts, but you experience *no* perception of motion. As bizarre as it seems, this is exactly what happens in a rare neuropsychological disorder known as **akinetopsia**, described in the following case report (Horton and Trobe, 1999):

> A 47-year-old man reported seeing streams of multiple, frozen images trailing in the wake of moving objects. As soon as motion ceased, the images collapsed into each other. He compared his vision to a scene lit by a flashing strobe, except that stationary elements were perceived normally. In fact, if nothing was in motion and he held perfectly still, his vision was entirely normal. The moment anything moved, however, it left a stream of static copies in its path. For example, while out for an evening stroll, he saw a pack of identical dogs lined up behind his West Highland terrier. Driving was impossible because he was confused by multiple snapshots of cars, streets, and signs. Moving lights were followed by a long comet trail.

Another patient reported that when she watched her own arm moving, "passage of the limb would be reduplicated by multiple, fuzzy images, the way a cartoonist might draw motion."

Not surprisingly, akinetopsia appears to be caused by disruptions to V5, the area corresponding to visual area MT in monkeys. For the two patients described here, the disruptions were side effects of a prescription antidepressant drug, and their motion perception problems disappeared once they stopped taking the drug. In other cases, akinetopsia is brought on by direct trauma to V5 as a result of stroke or elective brain surgery (e.g., surgery to alleviate epileptic seizures). Patients in the latter category sometimes regain normal motion perception abilities several weeks after surgery, indicating that, as in Newsome's monkeys, the human brain can sometimes rearrange its connections so that different areas take over the MT's motion-processing functions.

a new group of monkeys to discriminate correlated-motion directions and then poked around in the monkeys' MT areas to find groups of neurons that responded to one particular direction (Salzman, Britten, and Newsome, 1990). Once they had found a group of neurons that responded, for example, to rightward motion, they showed the monkey a new set of stimuli and electrically stimulated the identified MT neurons. Remarkably, the monkeys showed a strong tendency to report motion in the stimulated neurons' preferred direction, even when the dots they were seeing were moving in the opposite direction. These results make a very strong case that the MT is critically involved in the processing of global motion.

Up to this point, our discussion has focused on **first-order motion**—the change in position of **luminance-defined objects** over time. In the next section, we describe another interesting motion phenomenon: **second-order motion**, in which **texture-defined objects**, also called **contrast-defined objects**, change position over time.

akinetopsia A rare neuropsychological disorder in which the affected individual cannot perceive motion.

first-order motion The motion of an object that is defined by changes in luminance (reflected light).

luminance-defined object An object that is delineated by differences in reflected light.

second-order motion The motion of an object that is defined by changes in contrast or texture, but not by luminance.

texture-defined object or **contrast-defined object** An object that is defined by differences in contrast or texture, but not by luminance.

Second-Order Motion

The three frames in FIGURE 8.10 look like collections of random black and white dots, which is what they are. The movie is constructed from a combination of two patterns: a random collection of small white and black dots and a series of wide white and black stripes. The patterns are overlaid and combined in such a way that

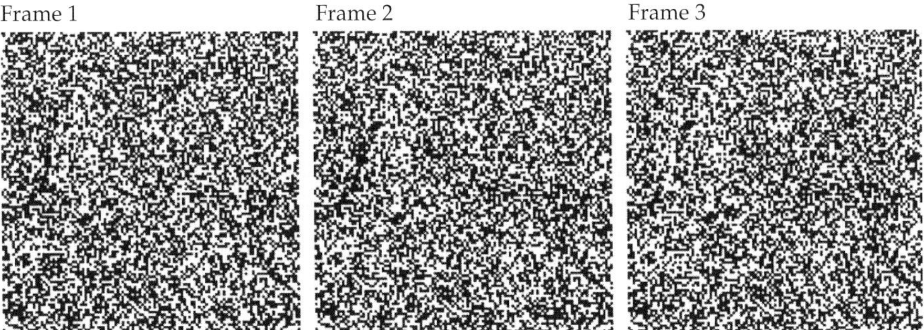

FIGURE 8.10 Second-order motion Three frames of a movie made by shifting the bars to the left while the dots remain stationary. The resulting perception is of a set of leftward-moving stripes. This perceived movement is called second-order motion.

dots covered by white bars are inverted (black dots turn white and vice versa), and dots covered by black bars are left alone. The frames of the movie are made by the process of shifting the bars to the left while the dots remain stationary. The resulting perception is of a set of leftward-moving stripes. This perceived movement is called second-order motion.

As in first-order apparent-motion displays, nothing actually moves in second-order motion. Even more incredibly, there is nothing *to* move in second-order motion. As FIGURE 8.11 shows, the only thing that changes in our second-order motion movie is that strips of dots are inverted from one frame to another: from frame 1 to frame 2, the dots in the red strip are inverted; then from frame 2 to frame 3, the dots in the blue strip are inverted. Just as random dot stereograms prove that matching discrete objects across the two eyes is not necessary for stereoscopic depth perception (see Section 6.3), second-order motion proves that matching discrete objects across movie frames is not necessary for motion perception.

Several lines of evidence suggest that the visual system includes specialized mechanisms for second-order motion. For example, Lucia Vaina and colleagues described a neurological patient who displayed brain damage that impaired the perception of first-order motion but not second-order motion (Vaina et al., 1998; Vaina and Cowey, 1996). A second patient showed the opposite pattern—that is, impaired second-order but spared first-order motion perception. These two patients had lesions in different brain areas, and together they demonstrate a **double dissociation** of function, which would not be possible if there were a single motion mechanism. Tim Ledgeway demonstrated an MAE for second-order motion and found that the second-order MAE transfers even more completely between eyes than does the first-order MAE (Ledgeway, 1994; Ledgeway and Smith, 1994).

double dissociation The phenomenon in which one of two functions, such as first- and second-order motion, can be damaged without harm to the other, and vice versa.

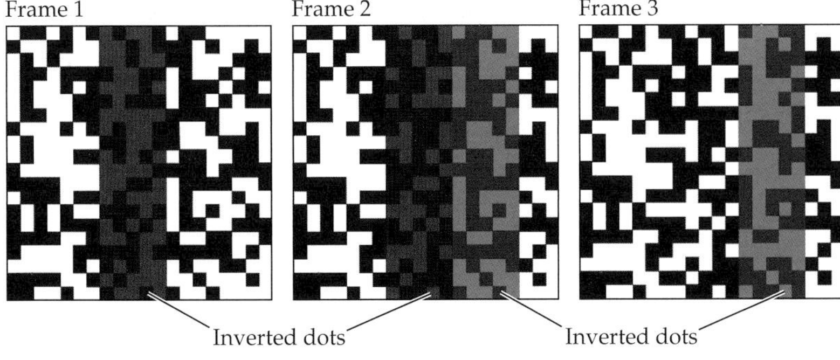

FIGURE 8.11 Movie frames Close-ups of one section of the frames in Figure 8.10, illustrating the changes from frame to frame.

optic array The collection of light rays that interact with objects in the world that are in front of a viewer. The term was coined by J. J. Gibson.

optic flow The changing angular positions of points in a perspective image that we experience as we move through the world.

focus of expansion The point in the center of the horizon from which, when we're in motion (e.g., driving on the highway), all points in the perspective image seem to emanate. The focus of expansion is one aspect of optic flow.

What might explain the evolution of a motion detection system for something as esoteric as second-order motion? It turns out that second-order-like motion does occur in the real world, especially when an object is effectively camouflaged.

8.3 Using Motion Information

Now that we know something about how the motion perception system works "under the hood," let's consider some ways we might use motion information to interpret the world around us.

Going with the Flow: Using Motion Information to Navigate

For sighted people, getting around is easy. Our vision effortlessly guides our motion through space, whether we're walking or driving, so that we usually reach a destination safely. Indeed, safe navigation is one of the primary functions of the visual system. What information does the visual system use to help us navigate our way across a busy intersection? Or consider the challenge that confronts a pilot landing an airplane at high speed. In an attempt to improve World War II pilots' performance in such situations, J. J. Gibson (1957), who was working for the US Army at the time, developed an influential theory about the **optic array**, the collection of light rays that interact with objects in the world in front of a viewer. Some of these rays strike our retinas, enabling us to see. Gibson argued that when we move through our environment, we experience patterns of **optic flow** that our visual systems use to determine where we're going.

Consider a pilot coming in to land a plane. As the plane approaches the ground, the optic array expands outward, in a pattern known as radial expansion (FIGURE 8.12). The heading—the specific point at which the pilot is aiming the plane—will always be the center, or **focus of expansion**, of the optic array. As indicated in Figure 8.12, the focus of expansion is the one place in the visual field that will be stationary, and if the pilot's visual system can locate this stationary point, that point can determine the heading.

Gibson (1957) was able to derive a number of optic flow heuristics that the visual system might use to navigate. At the most basic level, the mere presence of optic flow indicates locomotion, and a lack of flow is a signal that you are stationary. If you have ever been sitting in a stationary train at a busy railroad station when the train beside you moves, you may have experienced a situation in which optic flow alone gives you the illusion that you (rather than the neighboring train) are in motion. Outflow (flow toward the periphery, as depicted in Figure 8.12) indicates that you are approaching a particular destination; inflow indicates retreat (assuming that your head is facing forward). And the focus of expansion, mentioned already, or focus of constriction if you're looking forward while driving in reverse, tells you where you're going to or coming from.

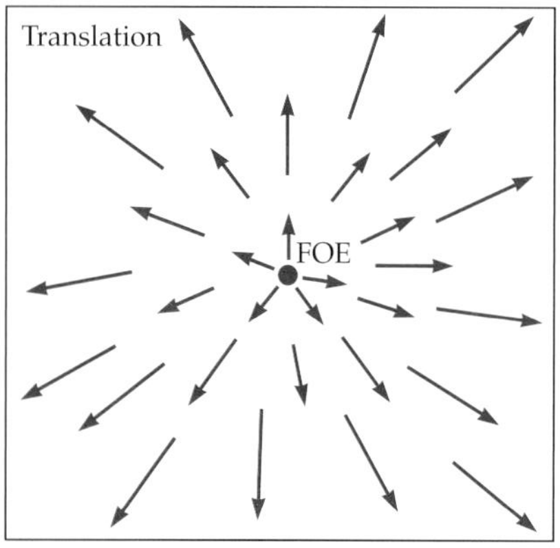

Are humans able to make use of optic flow information? Using elaborate computer-generated displays of moving dots and lines to simulate optic flow information, laboratories like that of W. H. Warren have made a good deal of progress in understanding both the utility and the complexity of optic flow information. For example, W. H. Warren, Morris, and Kalish (1988) demonstrated that humans could estimate their direction of heading to within about 1 or 2 degrees, using as their sole guide the pattern of optic flow simulated by the moving dots, even when the display contained only a very small number of dots.

Of course, the nice, clean optic flow pattern diagrammed in Figure 8.12 occurs only if the head and eyes remain fixed and pointed straight ahead. As soon as gaze shifts to one side, a new radial component is introduced to the optic flow.

Translation

FOE

FIGURE 8.12 The optic flow field The flow patterns produced by movement forward in space. FOE = focus of expansion.

However, W. H. Warren showed that observers were able to discount these radial components, both when the observers moved their own eyes and when the computer-generated display mimicked the radial flow caused by an eye movement (W. H. Warren and Hannon, 1990). If the radial shift is relatively slow, observers can compensate for simulated eye movements just as readily as they do for real eye movements, but with faster simulated eye movement speeds, performance breaks down (Royden, Banks, and Crowell, 1992). This result implies that the visual system can make use of the copies of eye muscle signals when it is processing optic flow information. (We'll discuss this notion later in the chapter, in the section titled "Saccadic Suppression and the Comparator.")

Interestingly, in humans, early visual cortical areas are not sensitive to optic flow; however, the MST gyrus visual area appears to be sensitive to both rotation and expansion (Wall et al., 2008).

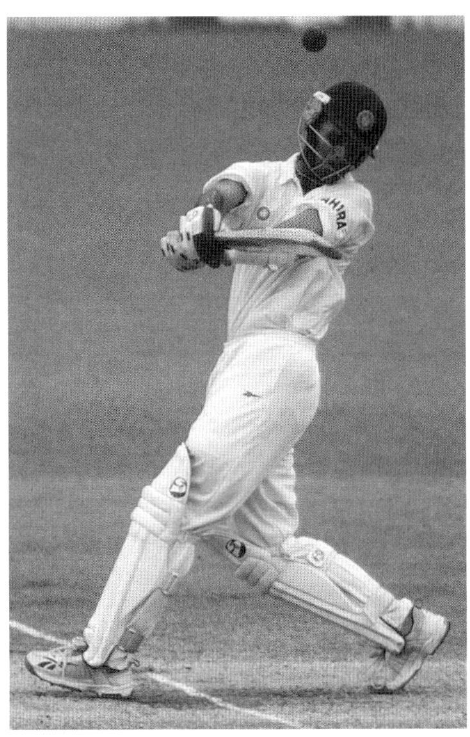

FIGURE 8.13 Ouch! This batsman has just been hit by a very hard cricket ball.

Avoiding Imminent Collision: The Tao of Tau

In cricket, as in so much of life, the object is to keep your eye on the ball and to stay out of trouble. Indeed, much of our visual apparatus may be designed to do just that. Accidents like the one shown in FIGURE 8.13 are not common, because cricketers are extremely good at judging precisely when a tiny ball, hurtling toward them at speeds approaching 100 miles per hour, is about to collide with their head (D. Regan, 1991). What visual information do we use to avoid imminent collisions, or to achieve collision when catching or batting a ball? To rephrase somewhat more precisely, how do we estimate the **time to collision (TTC)** of an approaching object?

Consider a small, red cricket ball, thrown by a large, rather angry-looking man on the other team, that bounces off the ground about 10 feet away from you. At this distance, if the ball hurtles toward the bridge of your nose at a constant rate of 50 feet per second, it will collide with your face in 0.20 second (TTC = distance/rate = 10/50). The most direct way to estimate TTC would therefore be to estimate the distance and speed of the ball. However, determining absolute distances in depth is a tricky proposition, as we saw in Chapter 6, and humans are far better at judging TTC than would be predicted on the basis of their ability to judge distance.

In an attempt to reconcile this apparent discrepancy, D. N. Lee (1976) and others have pointed out that there is an alternative source of information in the optic flow that could signal TTC without the need for absolute distances or rates to be estimated. Lee called this information source **tau** (**τ**), and here's how it works. As the ball approaches your nose, the image of the ball on your retina grows larger (if you don't believe this, have someone throw a ball—preferably a soft one—at your face and see for yourself). The ratio of the retinal image size at any moment to the rate at which the image is expanding is tau, and TTC is proportional to tau. The great advantage of using tau to estimate TTC is that it relies solely on information available directly from the retinal image; all you need to do is track the visual angle subtended by the cricket ball as it approaches your eye.

Do we make use of tau? The jury is still out. It is clear that estimating the time to imminent collision is critically important to animals and humans, and almost every species tested will attempt to avoid a simulated collision. There is also evidence that certain neurons in the visual systems of pigeons and locusts respond to objects on a collision course with them and can signal a particular time to collision (Rind and Simmons, 1999; Y. Wang and Frost, 1992). Interestingly, a looming object on a collision path with an observer captures his attention, whereas a looming object on

time to collision (TTC) The time required for a moving object (such as a cricket ball) to hit a stationary object (such as a batsman's head). TTC = distance/rate.

tau (τ) Information in the optic flow that could signal time to collision (TTC) without the necessity of estimating either absolute distances or rates. The ratio of the retinal image size at any moment to the rate at which the image is expanding is tau, and TTC is proportional to tau.

a near-miss path does not, even when the observer is not aware of any difference between collision and near-miss objects (Lin, Murray, and Boynton, 2009).

However, J. R. Tresilian (1999) has noted that tau is just one of a number of different sources of visual information that can be used to judge the TTC. For example, consider depth perception. Imagine that a bee is flying toward you, aimed directly at your nose at high speed. There are two distinct ways that you can detect how it is moving in depth: through changing binocular disparity over time (the closer the bee, the larger the disparity) and the difference in velocity between the images of the two eyes (also known as the interocular velocity difference) (Cormack et al., 2017; J. M. Fernandez and Farell, 2005).

FURTHER DISCUSSION about how motion cues contribute to depth perception can be found in Section 6.2.

Something in the Way You Move: Using Motion Information to Identify Objects

The fact that we use motion information to guide us as we move through our environment is not all that surprising. What may be less obvious is that motion can also provide information about the nature of objects. Almost 50 years ago, Gunnar Johansson (1975) recognized that there might be something special about the motion of animals and people—**biological motion**—that helps us identify both the moving object and its actions.

Consider the tennis player in **FIGURE 8.14A**. It's clear from the contours of her body that she's just smashed an innocent little tennis ball in the direction of her opponent. **FIGURE 8.14B** shows the same tennis player in the dark. All we can see are the little lights attached to her ankles, knees, hips, elbows, wrists, and shoulders. There's not very much in the static pattern of the lights to inform us that the contour is a human (let alone a woman), or that she/it is engaged in athletic activity. What Johansson discovered, however, is that when the lights move, their motion gives the viewer an immediate and very compelling impression of a live human in action.

biological motion The pattern of movement of living beings (humans and animals).

(A)

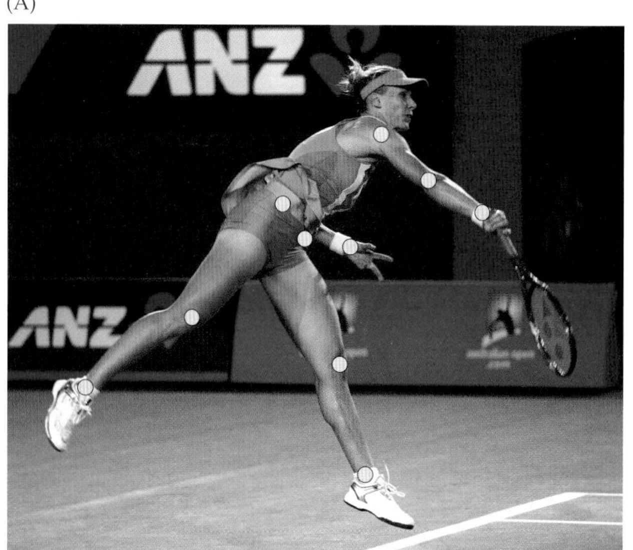

(B)

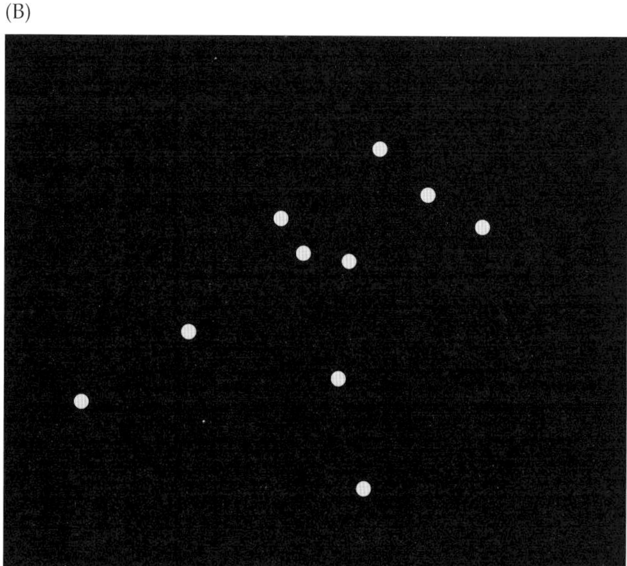

FIGURE 8.14 Biological motion For a compelling demonstration of biological motion, first attach lights to a moving human (A). When the moving lights are viewed in total darkness (B), the image of a moving human becomes evident.

Biological motion activates a number of brain areas, including the MT/V5 and other visual cortical areas. Moreover, in humans, biological motion also evokes signals in "action observation" networks in frontal regions of the brain considered to be premotor cortex (Saygin et al., 2004), leading to the suggestion that the observer's motor system may "fill in" the point light displays.

Importantly, the perceptual mechanisms that analyze biological motion obey different rules for integrating motion over space and time than do mechanisms for other forms of complex motion (Neri, Morrone, and Burr, 1998). There is even evidence that observers can use biological motion to identify whether a set of moving lights is attached to a male or female walker. How do they do that? As we walk, when the right leg is in front of the left leg, the right shoulder is behind, and vice versa. If we draw one line connecting the left shoulder with the right hip and another connecting the right shoulder with the left hip, the intersection of the two lines is the center of the walker's motion. Because males typically have broader shoulders and narrower hips than females, the average male's center of motion is higher than that of females. James Cutting and his colleagues suggested that observers use estimates of the center of motion as a cue to the walker's gender (Barclay, Cutting, and Kozlowski, 1978). Other studies (e.g., Mather and Murdoch, 1994) suggest that, in certain views, the amount of body sway might provide an even more salient gender cue.

Biological motion appears to play an important role in how we interpret human actions. For example, studies of biological motion with two "actors" either dancing or fighting show that we are much more efficient in discriminating biological motion of a human when two humans are acting in synchrony (e.g., fighting or dancing) than when they are out of sync. We can think of this phenomenon as proof of the old adage that "it takes two to tango" (Neri, Luu, and Levi, 2006). There are many other ways in which motion signals provide useful information, including camouflage breaking, figure-ground segregation, and shape from motion, to name a few.

Motion-Induced Blindness

Although it may seem hard to believe, motion can make you temporarily blind! Bonneh, Cooperman, and Sagi (2001) discovered that if you carefully fixate on a central target, stationary targets in the periphery will simply disappear, as if erased, when a global moving pattern is superimposed. You can check out this remarkably compelling illusion at https://michaelbach.de/ot/mot-mib/index.html.

While there is no clear explanation, motion-induced blindness seems to be somewhat related to the well-known Troxler effect, in which an unchanging target in peripheral vision will fade and disappear if you steadily fixate on a central target. This effect can be observed under conditions in which the retinal image is stabilized (or relatively stabilized when the target is in the periphery) so that the involuntary eye movements that occur during fixation (discussed in Section 8.4) do not move the target onto new receptive fields. The result is that the target is effectively not changing, and the underlying neurons become adapted.

8.4 Eye Movements

A key function of vision is to tell us when to move and where to move to, and a critical aspect of this involves *controlling where we are looking*. Because high-acuity vision falls off rapidly with eccentricity (the distance between the retinal image and the fovea; see Section 3.1), we must constantly move our eyes to fixate on the object of interest with our fovea and to follow that object as it moves from place to place. We make very fast (ballistic) eye movements known as **saccades** to change fixation

saccade A type of eye movement, made both voluntarily and involuntarily, in which the eyes rapidly change fixation from one object or location to another.

smooth pursuit A type of voluntary eye movement in which the eyes move smoothly to follow a moving object.

from one place to another. Saccades are one of several types of eye movements, as we will describe in this section.

When our eyes move, the image on the retina moves too. So how does our brain figure out which motions on the retina belong to real moving objects and which are caused by our own eye and head movements? Let's try a simple experiment: Place a blank piece of paper on the desk in front of you and draw a small black dot right in the center of the paper. Close your left eye and focus your right eye's gaze on the dot; then position a pencil so that it is near the bottom right corner of the paper. Keeping your eye trained on the dot, move the pencil slowly across the sheet to the left side, as shown in **FIGURE 8.15A**. What did you perceive? The image of the pencil just swept across your retina from right to left, so assuming that your rightward-motion detectors are functioning correctly, you should have perceived movement in this direction. (You may have thought that the word *rightward* in the previous sentence was a typo, but technically the image sweeps across the retina in the opposite direction from the actual movement, since the right side of the world projects to the left side of the retina and vice versa. To avoid confusion, we'll ignore this inconvenient bit of physics for now and pretend that images move on the retina in the same direction that the objects in the world are moving.)

Now try a slightly different demonstration. Start with the pencil near the bottom left corner of the paper, fixate on the eraser, and track the fixation point with your eye as you move the pencil back across the sheet of paper to the right corner (**FIGURE 8.15B**). Congratulations! You have just executed a type of eye movement called **smooth pursuit**, which kept the pencil's image stationary on the retina while the pencil was in motion. But think about what happened to the image of the dot just above your pencil. When the pencil was on the left side of the page, the dot was to the right of your fixation point. As you tracked the pencil, the dot shifted to the center of your retina, and then it slid to the left of your fixation point once the pencil reached the right side of the paper. However, you should *not* have perceived the dot to be moving in this case, even though the image of the dot made essentially the same journey across your retina that the image of the pencil did in Figure 8.15A.

We hope you've convinced yourself that the retinal image movement of the pencil when you keep your gaze centered on the dot (see Figure 8.15A) is essentially the same as the retinal image movement of the dot when you keep your gaze centered

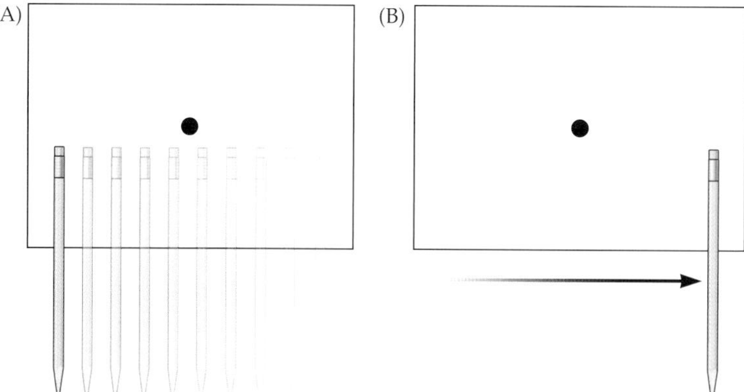

FIGURE 8.15 Eye movements (A) Fixing our gaze on the dot while the pencil moves to the left causes the pencil to generate motion across the retina, and we perceive movement of the pencil in this direction. (B) Fixating our gaze on the pencil while it moves to the right causes the dot to generate motion in the same direction across the retina, but we do not perceive movement of the dot.

on the pencil (see Figure 8.15B). The question is, Why do we perceive motion of the pencil in the first case but perceive that the dot is stationary in the second case? The reason is that in one case there's an eye movement. Think about how the visual system might accomplish this balancing act while we back up and describe eye movements in a bit more detail. (By the way, you may want to save the piece of paper with the dot for another exercise later in this chapter.)

superior colliculus A structure in the midbrain that is important in initiating and guiding eye movements.

Physiology and Types of Eye Movements

As **FIGURE 8.16A** shows, six muscles are attached to each eye, arranged in three pairs. These muscles are controlled by an extensive network of structures in the brain. One way to get some inkling of the role of these brain structures is to stimulate them with small electrical signals and observe the movements of the eyes. For example, if a cell in the **superior colliculus** (**FIGURE 8.16B**) of a monkey is stimulated, the monkey's eyes will move by a specific amount in a specific direction. Every time that cell is stimulated, the same eye movement will result. Stimulating a neighboring cell will produce a different eye movement (Stryker and Schiller, 1975). (The superior colliculus also gets some input directly from retinal ganglion cells; this input presumably helps with the planning of eye movements.) By contrast, in response to stimulation of some of the cells in the frontal eye fields (Figure 8.16B)—and in certain superior colliculus cells as well—the monkey will move its eyes to fixate on a specific spot in space. Depending on where the eyes

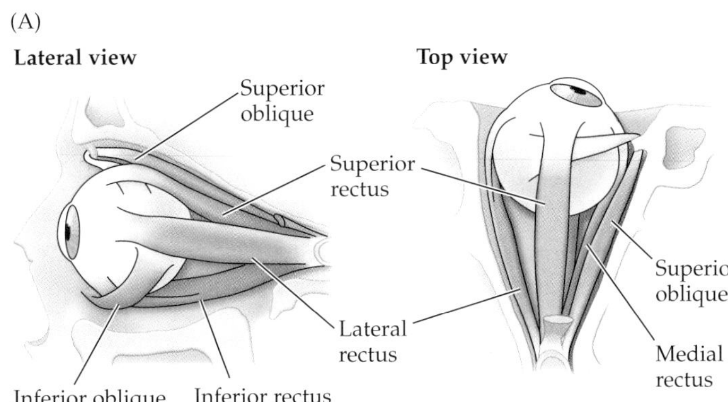

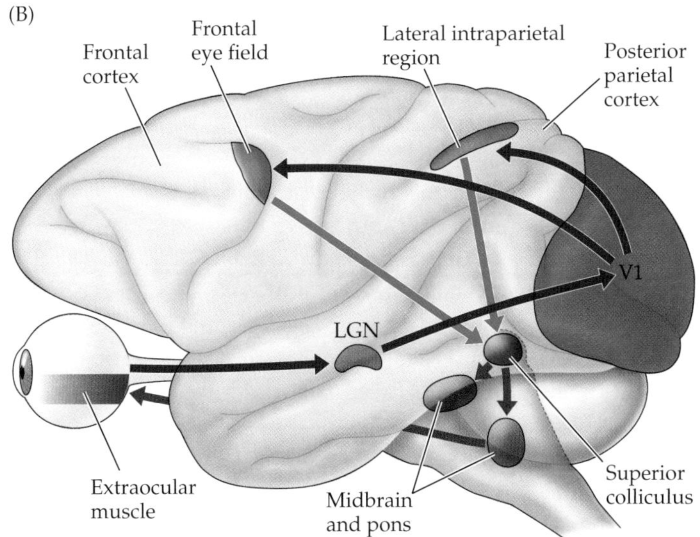

FIGURE 8.16 Muscles of the eye (A) Six muscles—arranged in three pairs (superior and inferior oblique, superior and inferior rectus, and medial and lateral rectus)—are attached to each eye. (B) Brain circuits for visually guided saccades.

microsaccade An involuntary, small, jerky eye movement.

reflexive eye movement A movement of the eye that is automatic and involuntary.

optokinetic nystagmus A reflexive eye movement in which the eyes will involuntarily track a continually moving object.

vergence A type of eye movement in which the two eyes move in opposite directions; for example, both eyes turn toward the nose (convergence) or away from the nose (divergence).

start, this adjustment may require an eye movement up, down, left, or right. In this case, it is the destination and not the movement that is coded (Mays and Sparks, 1980; Schiller and Sandell, 1983).

This description merely scratches the surface of a motor system that is not only very complex, but also very active. For example, even when we try to hold our eyes completely stationary, they continue to execute small but important movements. Specifically, there are involuntary eye drifts and small jerks called **microsaccades**. If the eye muscles are temporarily paralyzed—say, as a result of taking curare (it's amazing what some people will subject themselves to in the name of science!)—the entire visual world gradually fades from view (Matin et al., 1982). As noted in the discussion of motion-induced blindness (see Section 8.3), small peripheral targets may fade and disappear during steady fixation—an illusion known as the Troxler effect. In normal viewing, image velocities are often fast enough to prevent fading without the need for microsaccades (Kowler and Collewijn, 2010). So what are microsaccades good for? Recent work suggests that they may be important for very fine spatial judgments, such as threading a needle, because they precisely move the eye to nearby regions of interest (Ko, Poletti, and Rucci, 2010); for compensating for the very rapid falloff of acuity even a few minutes outside the fovea (Poletti, Listorti, and Rucci, 2013); and for changing the spatiotemporal pattern of information that arrives at the retina, in order to redistribute spatial information across temporal frequencies (Rucci and Victor, 2015). Other recent work suggests that microsaccades are directed toward objects we are attending (Engbert and Kliegl, 2003; Hafed and Clark, 2002), thus playing an important role in attention.

There are also **reflexive eye movements**—for example, when the eyes move to compensate for head and body movement while maintaining fixation on a particular target. These are known as vestibular eye movements and operate via the vestibulo-ocular reflex (see Section 12.8). **Optokinetic nystagmus** is another reflexive eye movement in which the eyes will involuntarily track a continually moving object, moving smoothly in one direction (e.g., to the right) in pursuit of the object moving in that same direction, and then snap back. The presence of optokinetic nystagmus in response to moving stripes has often been used as a measure of visual acuity in infants.

In addition to involuntary and reflexive eye movements, there are three types of eye movements over which we have at least some level of voluntary control. Most obvious, perhaps, are the previously discussed smooth-pursuit movements that we make when tracking a moving object. Observing these smooth-pursuit eye movements in patients is often used by doctors as a simple screening for neurological impairments, and they can even help identify individuals with schizophrenia (Benson et al., 2012). **Vergence** eye movements occur when we rotate our eyes inward (converging the eyes) or outward (diverging the eyes) to focus on a near or far object. The third type of voluntary movement is the saccade mentioned at the start of this section. A saccade is an explosively fast (ballistic) jump (up to 1000 degrees per second; Bahill and Stark, 1979) of the eye that shifts our gaze from one spot to another. We can decide to make a saccade deliberately, but whether we're thinking about it or not, we will make three or four saccades every second of every minute of every waking hour of the day. That's something like 3 saccades × 60 seconds × 60 minutes × 16 hours = 172,800 saccades per day—and that doesn't include the saccades we make during our dreams in rapid-eye-movement sleep (Maquet et al., 1996).

When we view a scene, our saccades are not random. We tend to fixate on the "interesting" places in the image. Thus, the eyes are more likely to make saccades in response to contours than to broad, featureless areas of an image (**FIGURE 8.17**).

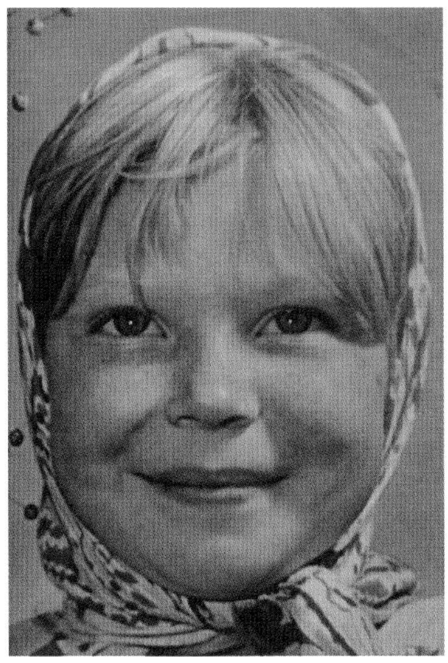

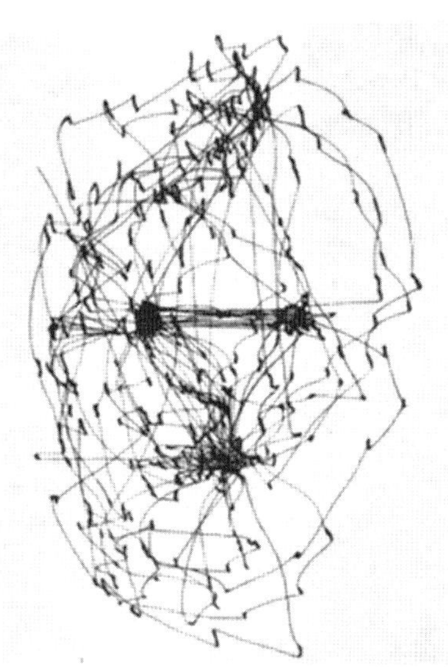

FIGURE 8.17 Where do we look? A classic scan path (right) showing the pattern of eye movements during inspection of the picture of the girl on the left.

Interesting also has a richer semantic meaning: we make eye movements that are based on the content of a scene and on our specific interests in that scene (Yarbus, 1967). Our pattern of eye movements as we enter the cafeteria will be different if we're looking for lunch than if we're looking for love.

Eye Movements and Reading

If you are reading this chapter, your eyes are doing a lot of moving. Reading English involves fixating for roughly a quarter of a second, then making a saccade of about 7–9 letter spaces—and then doing it over and over again. We make saccades to bring the text onto our fovea, because print that's too far from our fixation cannot be read, in part because of visual crowding (see Section 3.4) (Levi, 2008). Interestingly, readers of English are able to gain information from up to 15 characters to the right of fixation, but only 3–4 characters to the left. Thus, the perceptual span is asymmetrical. Readers of Hebrew (which is read from right to left) have the reverse asymmetry. Readers of both Hebrew and English can switch asymmetry depending on which language they're reading (Rayner, 1978), so this asymmetry is attentional, not a product of limitations imposed by the visual system.

As we discuss next, there is no information processing during saccades, so while we're reading, all of the information processing must take place during the fixations. Interestingly, such processing occurs during only a small fraction of each fixation. "Disappearing text" experiments (in which the words actually disappear from the computer screen while participants are reading) reveal that if a word remains on the screen for only 50 milliseconds after it is first fixated, reading proceeds normally (Rayner et al., 2003). There are many other interesting aspects of eye movements in scene perception and in visual search and attention (see Chapter 7).

Saccadic Suppression and the Comparator

Now let's return to the tricky problem of discriminating motion across the retina that is caused by eye movements versus object movements. Let's do one more demonstration using that white piece of paper with the dot in the middle from Figure 8.15. Close your left eye and gaze just to the left of the dot; then execute some saccades, shifting your eye back and forth to the right and then to the left of the dot. The dot will be moving across your retina, but you should not experience any perception of movement. Now, with your left eye still closed, fixate on the dot,

saccadic suppression The reduction of visual sensitivity that occurs when we make saccadic eye movements. Saccadic suppression eliminates the smear from retinal image motion during an eye movement.

efference copy or corollary discharge signal The phenomenon in which outgoing (efferent) signals from the motor cortex are copied as they exit the brain and are rerouted to other areas in the sensory cortices.

comparator An area of the visual system that receives one copy of the command issued by the motor system when the eyes move (the other copy goes to the eye muscles). The comparator compares the image motion signal with the eye motion signal and can compensate for the image changes caused by the eye movement.

place your right index finger on the right side of your right eye socket, and gently "jiggle" your eyeball. *Now* the dot (as well as the paper and the desk the paper is sitting on) should appear to move back and forth! What's going on here?

Part of the answer is thought to be **saccadic suppression**. When we make a saccade, the visual system essentially shuts down for the duration of the eye movement (visual activity is suspended in a similar way when we blink). To be a bit more precise, the visual system does not shut down altogether; saccadic suppression acts mainly to suppress information carried by the magnocellular pathway (see Section 3.3).

To observe saccadic suppression, you need to find a mirror. As you look at yourself in the mirror, fixate on first one eye and then the other. You will notice that you do not see the saccadic eye movements that you must be making. If you're concerned that the saccades might be too small to see, find a friend to help you. Have this person stand in front of you and move his or her fixation from one of your eyes to the other. You will have no trouble seeing your friend's saccades, even though you are quite blind to your own.

Although saccadic suppression eliminates the "smear" of the moving world during a saccade, it seems as if we should still be disturbed by the sudden displacement of the objects in front of us. In any case, no suppression takes place when we execute smooth-pursuit eye movements, as in the earlier exercise with the pencil. Although many scientists believe suppression to be an active process, others argue that saccadic suppression is little more than masking and that the magnocellular pathway is not suppressed during saccades (Castet, Jeanjean, and Masson, 2001).

By sending out two copies of each order to move the eyes, the motor system is thought to solve the "problem" of why an object moving across the retina may appear stationary. One copy goes to the eye muscles; another (often referred to as the **efference copy** or the **corollary discharge signal**) goes to an area of the visual system that has been dubbed the **comparator** (**FIGURE 8.18**). The comparator can then compensate for the image changes caused by the eye movement, inhibiting any attempts by other parts of the visual system to interpret the changes as object motion. When we jiggle the eyeball with a finger, no signal is sent from the eye

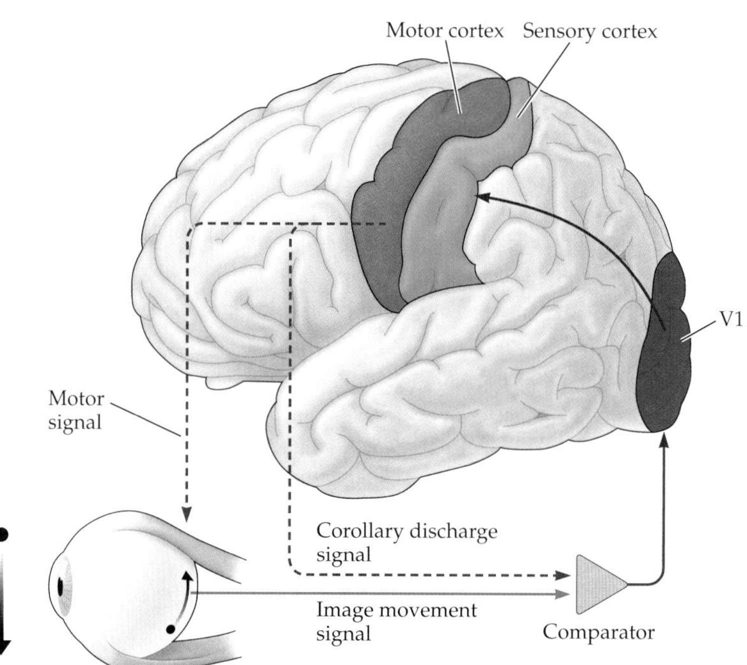

FIGURE 8.18 The comparator The brain sends two copies (dashed red lines) of each command to move the eyes. One copy (the motor signal) goes directly to the extraocular muscles; the other (known as the efference copy or the corollary discharge signal) goes to the comparator, which compares the image motion signal with the eye motion signal and can compensate for image changes produced by the eye movement.

muscles to the comparator (the eye muscles are not what move the eye in this case), so the visual input is interpreted as our world being rocked. Although a lot of work has been dedicated to the analysis of extraretinal signals during smooth pursuit, visual stability during saccades remains a matter of active research, and attention (as described in Chapter 7) seems to play an important role (Cavanagh et al., 2010; Gegenfurtner, 2016; Poletti, Listorti, and Rucci, 2010; Schütz, Braun, and Gegenfurtner, 2011).

Updating the Neural Mechanisms for Eye Movement Compensation

How does the brain compensate for eye movements in order to preserve the stability of our visual world? Over a century ago, Hermann von Helmholtz (1863) suggested that since the brain generates the neural signals for saccadic eye movements, it can perceptually compensate for them (by using the efference copy described in the paragraph above). One way this compensation could occur is through the "remapping" of visual receptive fields. We've discussed the receptive field—the region in space in which a visual stimulus causes a neuron to change its firing rate—throughout Chapters 2–7 of this book. Receptive fields are generally considered to be fixed in space relative to a fixation point (stars in **FIGURE 8.19**), so if the eyes move to a new fixation point, the receptive fields (ovals in Figure 8.19) should shift in lockstep so that they maintain the same positions relative to the fovea. Thus, shifting fixation from the sculpture on the bow (Figure 8.19A) to the roof of the boat (Figure 8.19B) results in a lockstep shift of the receptive fields. However, the receptive fields of some neurons in the parietal cortex actually shift to the new locations before the saccade. Duhamel, Colby, and Goldberg (1992) referred to this anticipatory shift as predictive remapping or updating. A key assumption about this spatial-updating hypothesis is that the neural representation of the visual field is rigidly translated just prior to the eye movement. However, a recent study suggests a different view, illustrated in Figure 8.19C. Zirnsak et al. (2014) found that the receptive fields of neurons in the frontal eye fields shift transiently toward the target location. In this view, the receptive-field shifts do not predict the retinal displacements produced by saccades, but rather reflect the fact that space is perceived to be compressed just before a saccade (J. Ross et al., 2001).

Updating has generally been thought to be accomplished in higher visual areas, such as parietal and temporal areas, because receptive fields in early visual areas such as V1 are fixed on the retina. However, a recent study showed that V1 neurons are sensitive to eye position, even when stimulation of their receptive fields does not change. Morris and Krekelberg (2019) showed that V1 eye position signal could be used as an eye tracker, to take into account the sensory consequences of eye movements and remap the transient positions of images on the retina onto their stable position in the world. (For more on eye movements and perception, see Schütz, Braun, and Gegenfurtner [2011].)

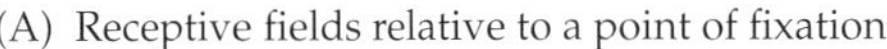
(A) Receptive fields relative to a point of fixation

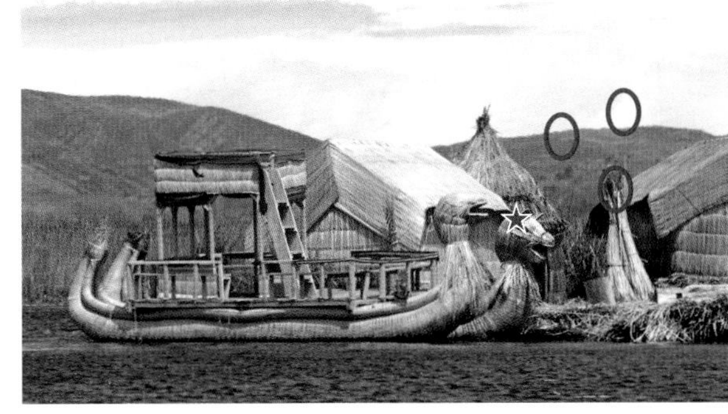

(B) Receptive fields shift with the point of fixation

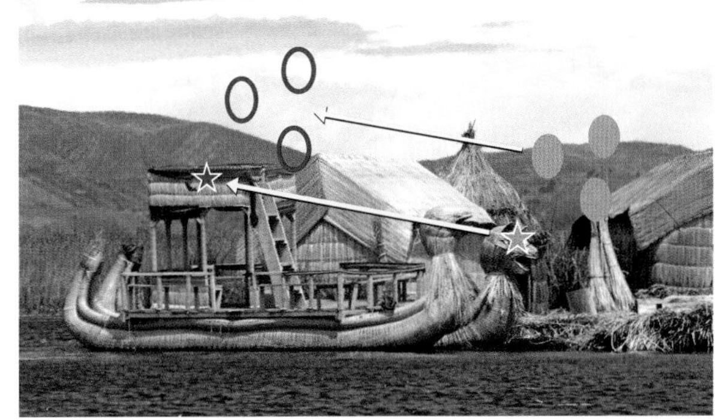

(C) Receptive fields transiently remap toward the new point of fixation

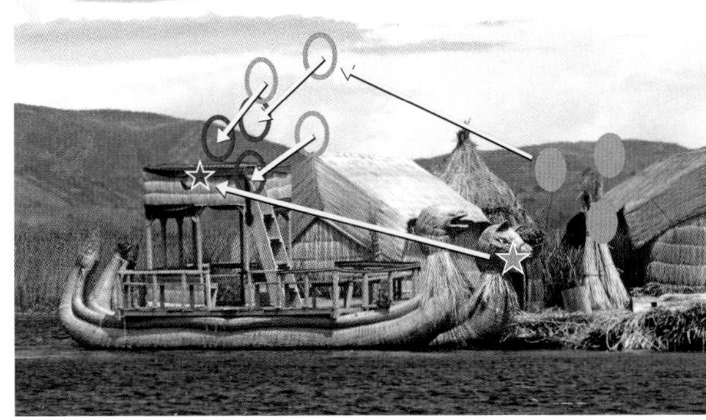

FIGURE 8.19 Receptive-field updating Receptive fields (ovals) are generally considered to be fixed in space, relative to the fixation point (stars) (A), so if the eyes move to a new fixation point, the receptive fields should shift in lockstep so that they maintain the same positions relative to the fovea (B). Shifting fixation from the sculpture on the bow of the boat (A) to the roof of the boat (B) results in a lockstep shift of the receptive fields. Recent work suggests that receptive fields of neurons in the frontal eye fields shift toward the target location (C).

8.5 Development of Motion Perception

Sensitivity to visual motion does not develop all at once. Some aspects of motion perception are already evident at birth. For example, reflexive eye movements to moving targets (optokinetic nystagmus; see the previous section) are present in newborns (as long as the targets are sufficiently large), and physiological studies show that neurons in V1 have adultlike sensitivity to motion direction. However, sensitivity to global motion, which is thought to reflect processing in the MT area (V5), appears to develop more slowly, reaching maturity at about 3–4 years of age, and sensitivity to motion-defined form and biological motion takes even longer

Scientists at Work

Guess Who's Coming to Dinner

Question How does a stationary praying mantis spot its moving dinner?

Hypothesis The African praying mantis *Sphodromantis lineola* is a predator that stays stationary for long periods of time while waiting to ambush its fast-moving prey (bugs). This behavior is different from that of predatory insects that are constantly in motion, leading to the hypothesis that the mantis's motion detection system might be different from that of other insects.

Test The researchers evaluated *S. lineola*'s optomotor response to drifting gratings with different spatial and temporal frequencies and contrasts (Nityananda et al., 2015). On each trial, a researcher (who was unaware of the stimulus direction) coded whether the mantis turned its body to the left or to the right. After the session, these responses were compared with the actual direction the drifting grating was moving on each trial. This enabled the researchers to generate psychometric functions showing the probability of eliciting an optomotor response as a function of stimulus contrast and to estimate the mantis threshold for each spatial and temporal frequency.

Results The contrast sensitivity of the mantis depended on both the spatial and the temporal frequencies present in the stimulus rather than on the object's speed (**FIGURE 8.20**).

Conclusions Mantis sensitivity to motion differs from that of humans and bees, but is similar to that of hoverflies and hawkmoths in that it allows them to respond to stimuli at low and high velocities. This may be especially useful in enabling a stationary mantis to spot a fast-moving bug and catch it for dinner!

Future work It would be interesting to compare the properties of the early neuronal mechanisms of the praying mantis to their behavior, as measured here, to determine the specific mechanisms that underlie their sensitivity.

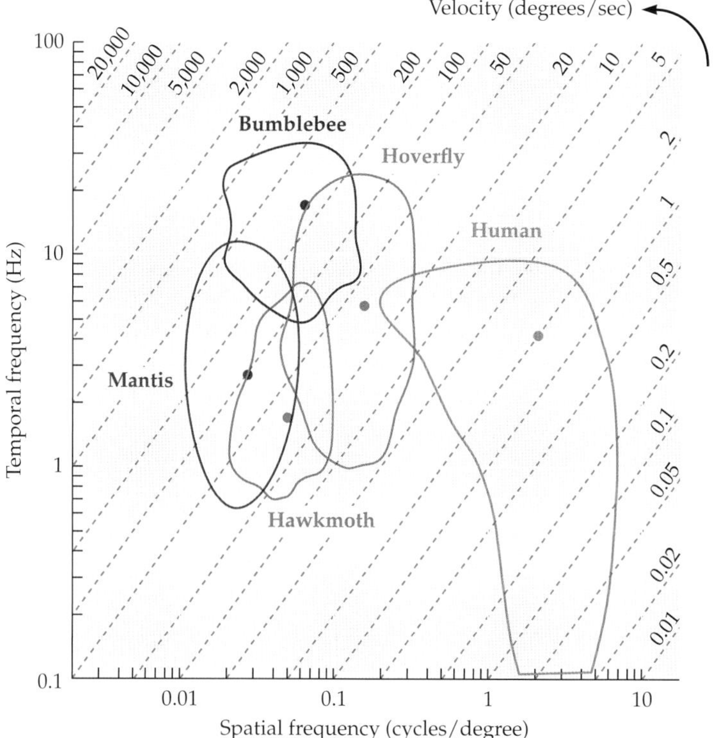

FIGURE 8.20 Praying mantis spatiotemporal sensitivity Contour isolines bounding the spatiotemporal frequencies where mantis sensitivity is half of its maximum value, along with similar isolines for other species. Colored dots indicate the maximum sensitivity for each species.

(Freire et al., 2006; Parrish et al., 2005). Differences in the rate of development of different forms of motion may be related to speed, with sensitivity to slow speeds developing more slowly, and may be more susceptible to altered visual input (for example, because of congenital cataracts) than faster speeds (Hadad et al., 2015).

Summary

1. Like color or orientation, motion is a primary perceptual dimension that is coded at various levels in the brain. Motion information is used to determine where objects are going and when they're likely to get there.
2. We can build a simple motion-detecting circuit by using linear filters that delay and sum information (and are followed by nonlinearities).
3. V1 neurons view the world through a small window, leading to the well-known aperture problem (that is, a V1 neuron is unable to tell which elements correspond with one another when an object moves through its receptive field).
4. Strong physiological and behavioral evidence suggests that the middle temporal area (MT/V5) is involved in the perception of global motion.
5. Aftereffects for motion, like those for orientation or color, can provide important insights into the underlying mechanisms of perception in humans.
6. Luminance-defined (first-order) motion and contrast- or texture-defined (second-order) motion appear to be analyzed by separate systems.
7. The brain has to figure out which retinal motion arises in the world and which arises because of eye movements. Moreover, the brain must suppress the motion signals generated by our eye movements, or the world will be pretty "smeared."
8. Motion information is critically important to us for navigating around our world, avoiding imminent collision, and recognizing the movement of animals and people.
9. Eye movements that provide motion information include reflexive movements such as optokinetic nystagmus, involuntary microsaccades, and movements over which we have varying levels of control, including vergence movements, smooth-pursuit movements, and saccades.
10. Saccades are rapid-fire eye shifts that occur constantly throughout our waking hours and during rapid-eye-movement sleep. Saccadic suppression masks saccadic images being processed in the brain so that we do not perceive the world as a blur.

Chapter 9

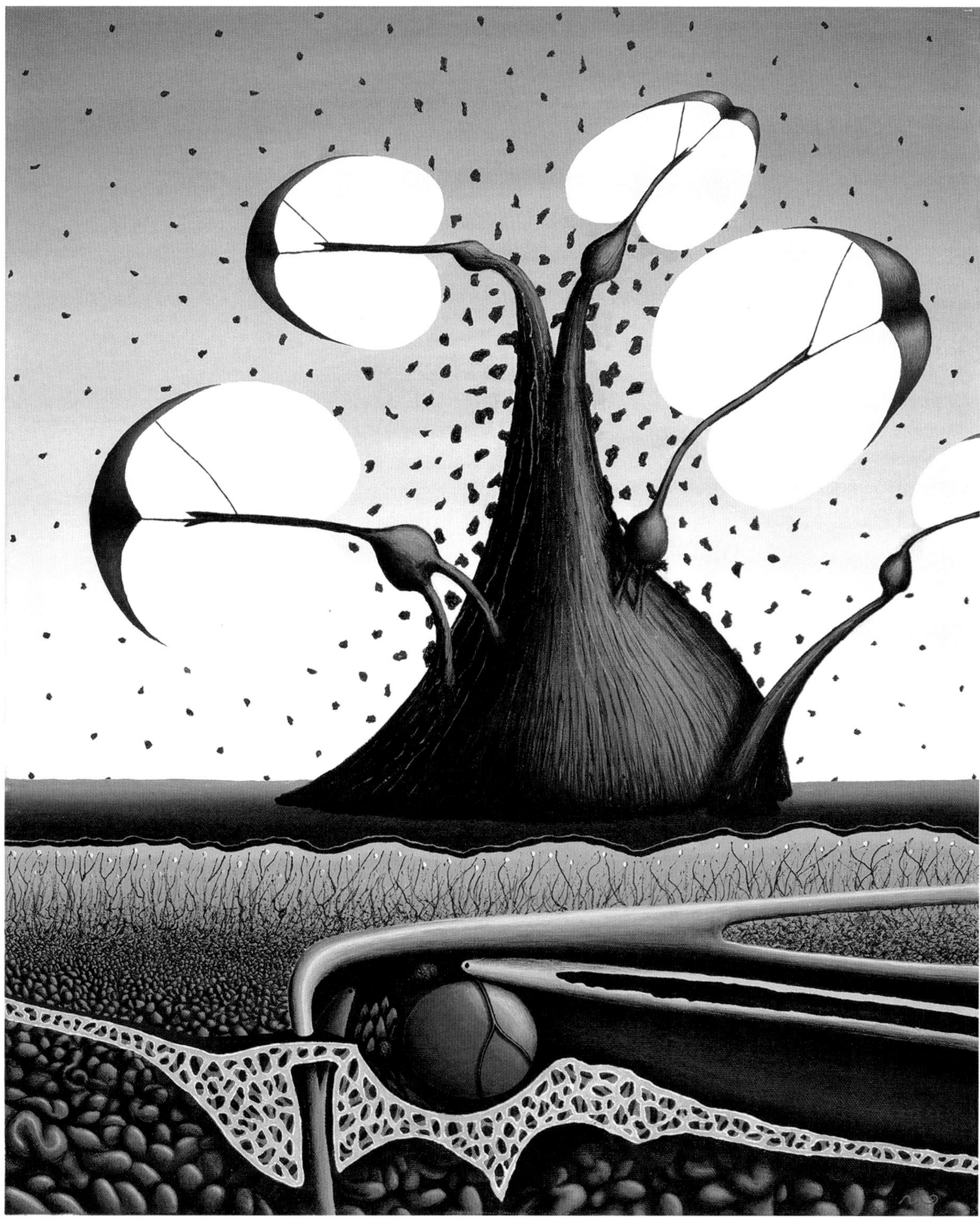

Micah Ofstedahl, *Sounds Like Infinity*, 2011

Hearing: Physiology and Psychoacoustics

Questions to Contemplate

Think about the following questions as you read this chapter.
By the chapter's end, you should be able to answer and discuss them.

- What are the physical and psychological qualities of sound?
- How is sound energy turned into neural firing for the brain to interpret?
- How does the brain encode pitch and loudness?
- How is hearing loss caused, and what can be done about it?

We are reminded of the importance of vision whenever we close our eyes or awaken in the night, because so much of what we know about our environment is suddenly gone. In contrast, those who hear have fewer reminders of the importance of hearing. We hear perfectly well in the dark, and our ears are always "open." Sounds can rouse us even from sleep. Awakening in the night, we can detect soft sounds that alert us that we are not alone. We can hear around obstacles and corners and through barriers that light cannot penetrate (like the thin walls of an apartment).

Though it is easy to take hearing for granted, sound delivers important information. It carries speech and music, and it alerts us to danger with honking horns and screeching brakes. For the deaf community that lives without the sense of hearing and for those with hearing impairments, disrupted access to information coming from sound can introduce challenges that the hearing population takes for granted.

The next three chapters are all about hearing. In this chapter we cover the basics: the nature of sound, the anatomy and physiology of the auditory system, and how we perceive the two fundamental sound qualities: loudness and pitch. We conclude this chapter by looking at some of the ways hearing can be impaired. In Chapter 10, we will discuss how sounds help us to learn about our surroundings. Then, in Chapter 11, we will cover the higher-level auditory functions that we use when we're listening to speech and music.

9.1 The Function of Hearing

Many fundamental principles in hearing apply to all senses. However, each sense developed at different periods in our evolutionary history and in response to different environmental challenges. So, although you should find that much of what you've learned thus far will help you to understand hearing, you also will be impressed by how biology has provided some very different (and very clever) solutions to the challenges of sensing and interpreting sound.

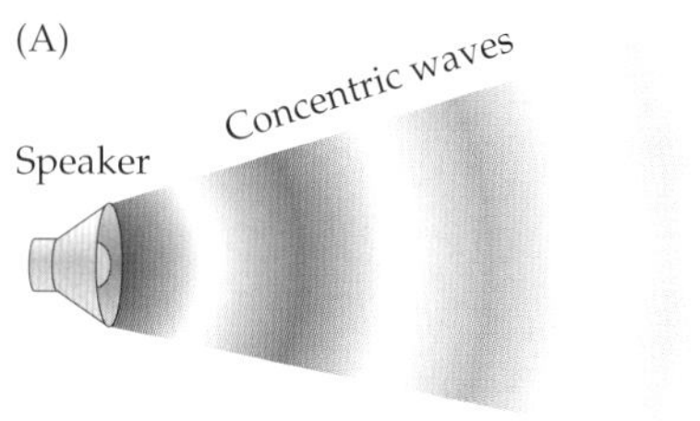

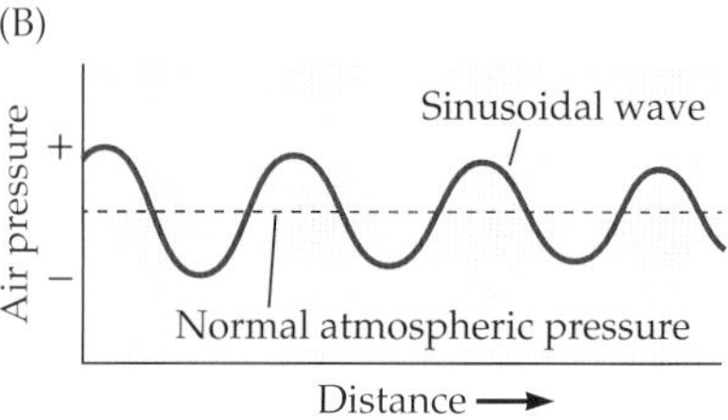

FIGURE 9.1 Sounds moving away from sources The pattern of pressure fluctuations of a sound, distances peak to peak, stays the same as the sound wave moves away from the source (A), but the amount of pressure change, the height of peaks relative to the depth of valleys, decreases with increasing distance (B).

9.2 What Is Sound?

When an object vibrates, it creates sound. Even tiny, invisible vibrations cause molecules surrounding the object to vibrate as well. For humans, these molecules are usually the Earth's atmosphere, the "air." This vibration causes pressure fluctuations in the medium (**FIGURE 9.1**). These pressure changes are best described as waves, and they are like the waves on a pond caused by dropping a rock into the water. Water molecules displaced by the rock do not themselves travel very far, but the *pattern* of displacement moves outward from the source until something (the shore, a boat, a swimming duck, or anything else) gets in the way. Although the patterns of pond and sound waves do not change as they spread out, the initial amount of pressure change is dispersed over a larger and larger area as the wave moves away, so the wave becomes less prominent as it moves farther from its source.

Sound waves travel through different media at different speeds, moving faster through denser substances. For example, the speed of sound through air is about 340 meters per second, depending on the humidity level (sounds travel a bit faster on muggy days), but the speed of sound through water is about 1500 meters per second. Light waves move through air almost a million times faster than sound waves do. This is why you see lightning before hearing thunder—the difference is almost 5 seconds per mile.

Basic Qualities of Sound Waves: Frequency and Amplitude

Sound waves are simply fluctuations in air pressure across time. The magnitude of the pressure change in a sound wave—the difference between the highest pressure and the lowest pressure of the wave—is called the **amplitude** or **intensity** (**FIGURE 9.2**). Pressure fluctuations may be very close together or spread apart over longer periods. For light, the sensation of color relates to the distance between peaks in the waves—that is, the "wavelength." Sound waves also have wavelengths, but we describe their patterns by noting how quickly the pressure fluctuates; this rate of fluctuation is known as the **frequency** of the wave (see Figure 9.2). To see an example of frequency, dangle a thread in front of a stereo speaker. As the speaker creates fluctuations in air pressure, the thread waves back and forth. The tempo of this waving is the thread's frequency. Sound wave frequencies are measured by these back-and-forth cycles, and the unit of measure is called a **hertz** (**Hz**), where 1 cycle per second equals 1 Hz. For example, the pressure in a 500 Hz wave goes from its highest point down to its lowest point and back up to its highest point 500 times every second.

amplitude or **intensity** In reference to sound, the magnitude of displacement (increase or decrease) of a pressure wave. Amplitude is perceived as *loudness*.

frequency In reference to sound, the number of times per second that a pattern of pressure change repeats. Frequency is perceived as *pitch*.

hertz (Hz) A unit of measure for frequency; 1 hertz equals 1 cycle per second.

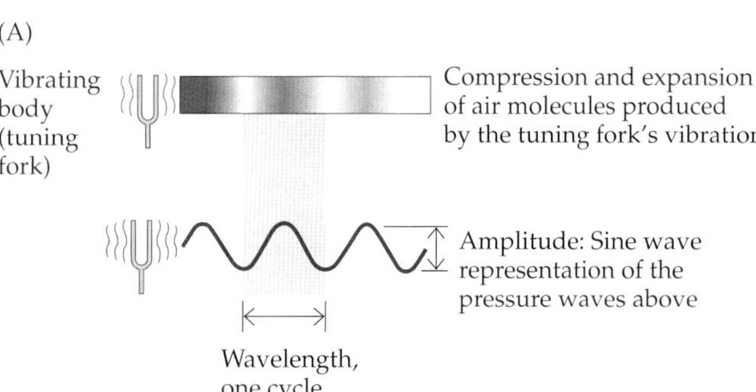

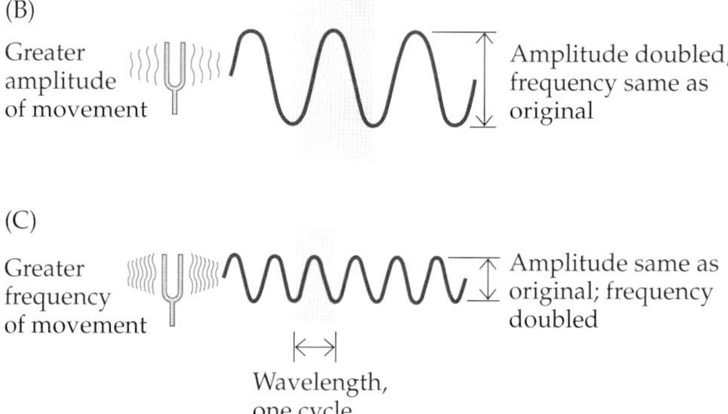

FIGURE 9.2 Amplitude and frequency (A) Sound waves are described by the frequency and amplitude of pressure fluctuations. Changes in amplitude (B) and frequency (C) are shown for sine waves, the simplest kind of sound wave.

FIGURE 9.3 **Range of human hearing** Humans can hear frequencies that range from about 20 to 20,000 Hz across a very wide range of intensities, or sound pressure levels (dB SPL, where dB = decibels).

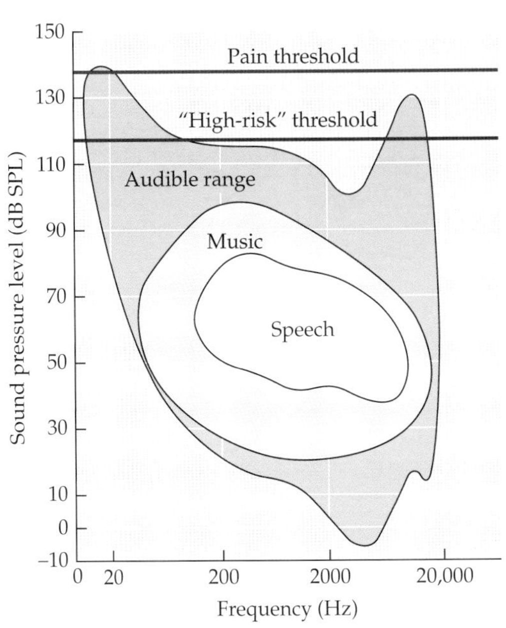

Just as the amplitude and wavelength of light waves correspond to perceptual qualities in vision (brightness and color, respectively), the amplitude and frequency of sound waves are closely related to auditory characteristics. Amplitude is associated with the perceptual quality of **loudness**: the more intense a sound wave is, the louder it will sound. Frequency is associated with **pitch**: low-frequency sounds correspond to low pitches (e.g., low notes played by a tuba), and high-frequency sounds correspond to high pitches (e.g., the high notes from a piccolo). We will have much more to say about the relationships between amplitude and loudness and between frequency and pitch later in this chapter.

In Chapter 2, you learned how visible light makes up only a small portion of the much broader range of electromagnetic energy. Similarly, human hearing uses a limited range of the frequencies present in environmental sounds. If you are relatively young and you've been careful about your exposure to loud sounds, you may be able to detect sounds that vary from about 20 to 20,000 Hz (**FIGURE 9.3**). Some animals hear sounds that have lower and higher frequencies than those heard by humans. In general, larger animals are better at hearing low frequencies, and smaller animals are better at hearing high frequencies. Elephants hear vibrations at very low frequencies that help them detect the presence of large animals, such as other elephants. Dogs can be called with whistles that emit sounds at frequencies too high for humans to hear, and the sonar systems used by some bats use sound frequencies above 60,000 Hz.

Humans hear across a very wide range of sound intensities. The intensity ratio between the faintest sound humans can detect and the loudest sounds that do not quickly do damage is more than 1:1,000,000. To describe differences in amplitude across such a broad range, sound levels are measured on a logarithmic scale using units called **decibels** (**dB**). Using a logarithmic scale allows us to describe such a large range of intensities compactly because it is nonlinear (that is, it is compressed). Compressing the scale helps to measure things that increase very rapidly, like sound intensity. Decibels define the *difference* between two sounds in terms of the ratio between sound pressures. Each 10:1 sound pressure ratio is equal to 20 dB, so a 100:1 ratio is equal to 40 dB. The range of human hearing extends from 0 dB (very quiet sounds like breathing) to more than 120 dB (like a jet engine).

An important thing to remember about logarithmic scales such as decibels is that relatively small decibel changes can correspond to large physical changes. For example, there is a roughly 44 dB difference between a heavy truck and a jet at takeoff, but the sound pressure level of the jet is 158 times as great as that of the truck (**FIGURE 9.4**).

Sine Waves and Complex Sounds

In Chapter 3 you were introduced to Fourier analysis and sine waves. Sine waves are crucial for understanding human hearing. A single **sine wave** is often called a **pure tone**, and all sounds, even those as complex as the sounds produced by musical instruments, human speech, and city traffic, can be described as combinations of sine waves with different frequencies and intensities. A complex sound is best described in a **spectrum** (plural *spectra*) that displays how much energy, or amplitude, is present at multiple frequencies, as shown in **FIGURE 9.5**.

loudness The psychological aspect of sound related to perceived intensity (amplitude).

pitch The psychological aspect of sound related mainly to the perceived frequency.

decibel (dB) A unit of measure for the physical intensity of sound. Decibels define the difference between two sounds as the ratio between two sound pressures. Each 10:1 sound pressure ratio equals 20 dB, and a 100:1 ratio equals 40 dB.

sine wave or **pure tone** The single waveform for which variation as a function of time is a sine function. In hearing research, this is sometimes referred to as a pure tone.

spectrum A representation of the relative energy (intensity) present at each frequency.

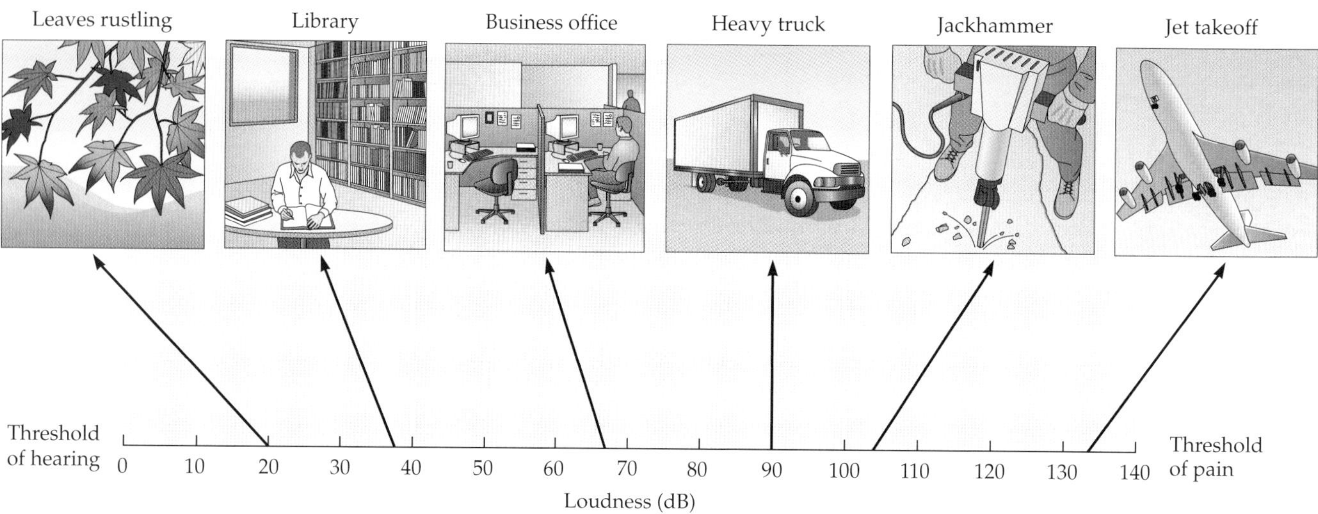

FIGURE 9.4 Sounds around us Sounds that we hear in our daily environments vary greatly in intensity.

harmonic spectrum The spectrum of a complex sound in which energy is at integer multiples of the fundamental frequency.

fundamental frequency The lowest-frequency component of a complex periodic sound.

timbre The psychological sensation by which a listener can judge that two sounds with the same loudness and pitch are dissimilar. Timbre quality is conveyed by harmonics and other high frequencies.

Many common sounds have **harmonic spectra** (FIGURE 9.6). These are typically caused by a simple vibrating source, such as the string of a guitar, the reed of a saxophone, or the vocal cords of a voice. Each frequency component in such a sound is called a harmonic. The first harmonic, called the **fundamental frequency**, is the lowest-frequency component of the sound. All the other harmonics have frequencies that are integer multiples of the fundamental. The shape of the spectrum is one of the most important qualities that distinguish different sounds.

Properties of sound sources determine the spectral shapes of sounds, and these shapes help us identify sound sources. For example, Figure 9.6 illustrates harmonic spectra from three musical instruments. Each instrument is producing a note with the same fundamental frequency (262 Hz, which corresponds to the note C_4, or middle C) and the same harmonics (524 Hz, 786 Hz, 1048 Hz, and so on). However,

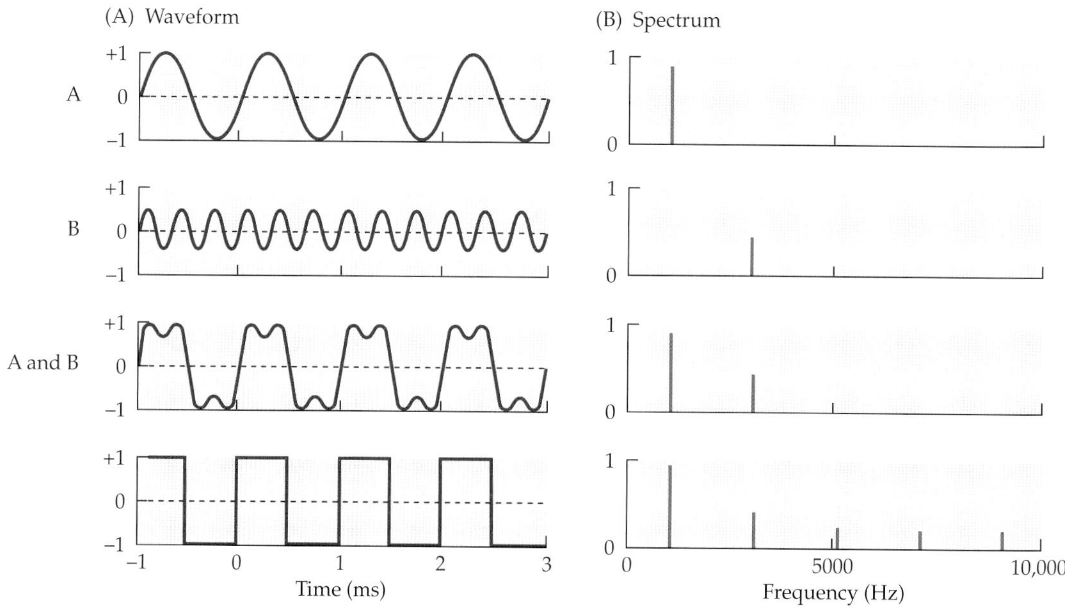

FIGURE 9.5 Waveforms and spectra A spectrum displays the amplitude for each frequency present in a sound wave. Each signal is shown as a waveform (A) and as a spectrum (B).

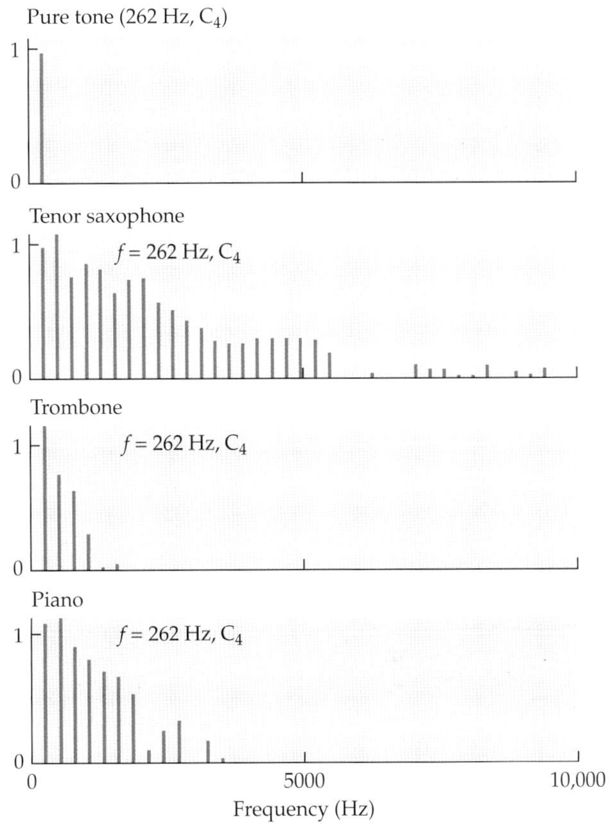

FIGURE 9.6 Spectral shapes and timbre Harmonic sounds with the same fundamental frequency can sound different because amplitudes of individual frequency components are different, resulting in different spectral shapes. For example, different musical instruments playing the same note (the same fundamental frequency, abbreviated *f*) sound different. C_4 = middle C.

the shapes of the spectra (the patterns of amplitudes for each harmonic) vary. **Timbre** (pronounced "tamber," like "amber") is a term used to describe the quality of a sound that depends, in part, on the shape of the spectrum.

We will return to harmonics, timbre, and other aspects of complex sounds in Chapter 10. In this chapter we'll stick mainly to the story of how the auditory system processes simple sounds such as sine wave tones.

9.3 Basic Structure of the Mammalian Auditory System

Our sense of hearing has evolved over millions of years to be able to do some amazing things. We are about to describe quite a few anatomical structures that are essential to understanding how sequences of tiny air pressure changes are turned into meaningful sound perception. The discussion may occasionally be a bit confusing if you are new to the ear, but if you consult the figures often, you will soon know the parts and how they fit together.

Outer Ear

Sounds are first collected from the environment by the **pinna** (plural *pinnae*), the curly structure on the side of the head that we typically call an ear. Only mammals have pinnae, and they vary widely in shape and size across species; they also vary (although less dramatically) across individuals within species (**FIGURE 9.7**). As we will see in Chapter 10, the shapes of pinnae play an important role in our ability to localize sound sources.

The pinna funnels sound waves into and through the external **ear canal**, which extends about 25 millimeters (mm) into the head (**FIGURE 9.8**). Together, the pinna and ear canal make up the **outer ear**. The length and shape of the ear canal enhance sound frequencies between about 2000 and 6000 Hz, but the main purpose of the canal is to protect the structure at its end, the **tympanic membrane** (eardrum), from damage. The tympanic membrane is a thin membrane that moves in and out in response to the pressure changes of sound waves. Remember that sounds are vibrations. When they reach the tympanic membrane, these vibrations set the tympanic membrane in motion with vibration.

Middle Ear

The tympanic membrane is the border between the outer ear and the **middle ear**, which consists of three tiny bones, the **ossicles**, that amplify sound waves (see Figure 9.8). The first ossicle, the **malleus**, is connected to the tympanic membrane on one side and to the second ossicle, the **incus**, on the other. The incus is connected in turn to the third ossicle, the **stapes**, which transmits the vibrations of sound waves to the **oval window**, another membrane, which forms the border between the middle ear and the **inner ear**.

pinna The outer, funnel-like part of the ear.

ear canal The canal that conducts sound vibrations from the pinna to the tympanic membrane and prevents damage to the tympanic membrane.

outer ear The external sound-gathering portion of the ear, consisting of the pinna and the ear canal.

tympanic membrane The eardrum; a thin sheet of skin at the end of the outer ear canal. The tympanic membrane vibrates in response to sound.

middle ear An air-filled chamber containing the middle bones, or ossicles. The middle ear conveys and amplifies vibration from the tympanic membrane to the oval window.

ossicle Any of three tiny bones of the middle ear: malleus, incus, and stapes.

malleus The most exterior of the three ossicles. The malleus receives vibration from the tympanic membrane and is attached to the incus.

incus The middle of the three ossicles, connecting the malleus and the stapes.

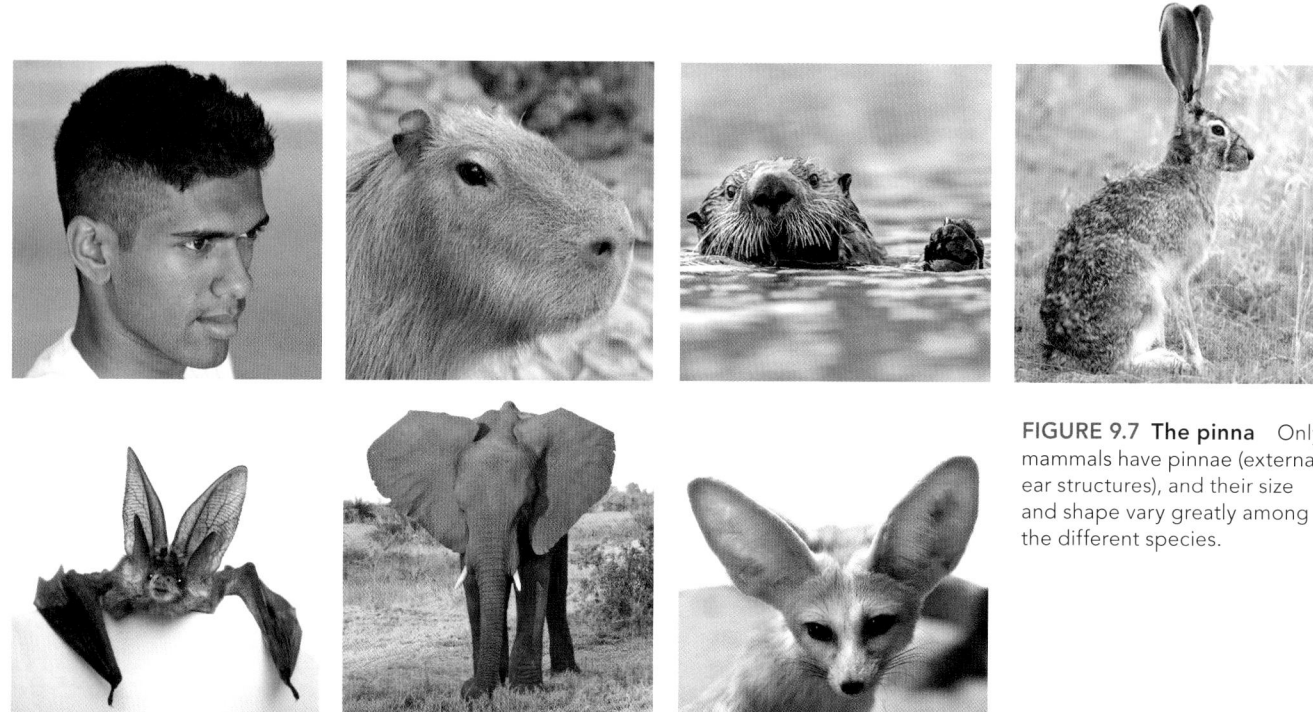

FIGURE 9.7 The pinna Only mammals have pinnae (external ear structures), and their size and shape vary greatly among the different species.

FIGURE 9.8 Structures of the human ear The three parts of the outer ear are the pinna, external ear canal, and tympanic membrane. The middle ear is composed of the oval window and three tiny bones (the ossicles) that connect it to the tympanic membrane (eardrum). Note that the tympanic membrane has about 18 times as much surface area as the oval window beneath the stapes. The cochlea is the major structure of the inner ear, where sound waves (vibrations) are transduced into neural signals that are then sent to the auditory cortex of the brain.

The ossicles are the smallest bones in the human body, and they amplify sound vibrations in two ways. First, the joints between the bones are hinged in ways that make them work like levers: a modest amount of energy on one side of the fulcrum (joint) becomes greater energy on the other side. This lever action increases the amount of pressure change by about a third. The second way the ossicles increase the energy transmitted to the inner ear is by concentrating energy from a larger to a smaller surface area. The tympanic membrane, which moves the malleus, is about 18 times as large as the oval window, which is moved by the stapes (see Figure 9.8). Therefore, pressure on the oval window is magnified 18 times relative to the pressure on the tympanic membrane. This is the same principle that makes stiletto heels a danger to wood floors (think of the tympanic membrane as the heel of the foot and the oval window as the tip of the stiletto heel), in contrast to the way snowshoes keep feet on top of the snow.

Amplification provided by these physical properties (leverage and different surface areas) is essential to our ability to hear faint sounds, because the inner ear—as we will see in a moment—is made up of a collection of fluid-filled chambers. Because it takes more energy to move liquid than it does to move air, this fluid creates a mismatch. If sound waves were transmitted to the oval window directly, many would simply bounce back, hardly moving the oval window and the liquid behind it.

Ossicles play an important role for loud sounds, too. The middle ear has two muscles: the **tensor tympani** (attached to the malleus) and the **stapedius** (attached to the stapes) (see Figure 9.8). As might be expected because they are attached to the smallest bones in the body, the tensor tympani and the stapedius are the smallest muscles in the body. Their main purpose is to tense when sounds are very loud. They restrict movement of the ossicles and thus muffle pressure changes that might be large enough to damage the delicate structures in the inner ear. Unfortunately, this **acoustic reflex** follows the onset of loud sounds by about one-fifth of a second. So, muscles help in environments like a concert that are loud for sustained periods, but the acoustic reflex cannot protect against abrupt loud sounds, such as the firing of a gun. Muscles of the middle ear are also tensed during swallowing, talking, and general body movement, helping to keep the auditory system from being overwhelmed by sounds generated by our own bodies.

Inner Ear

The inner ear is where minute changes in sound pressure are translated into neural signals that inform the listener about the world. The function of the inner ear with respect to sound waves is roughly analogous to that of the retina with respect to light waves in vision: both structures translate the information carried by waves into neural signals.

COCHLEAR CANALS AND MEMBRANES The major structure of the inner ear is the **cochlea** (from the Greek *kochlos*, "snail"), a tiny, coiled structure embedded in the temporal bone of the skull (see Figure 9.8). Rolled up, the cochlea is the size of a baby pea, about 4 mm in diameter in humans. Uncoiled, it would be a tube almost ten times as long—about 35 mm, running from its base (at the oval window) to its apex (at the top of the coil). The cochlea is filled with watery fluids in three parallel canals (FIGURE 9.9): the **tympanic canal** (or scala tympani), the **vestibular canal** (scala vestibuli), and the **middle canal** (scala media). The tympanic and vestibular canals are both filled with a fluid called perilymph and are connected by a small opening, the **helicotrema**. These two canals are effectively wrapped around the middle canal. Think of the tympanic and vestibular canals as one long, skinny balloon (the kind clowns use to make hats and animals), blown up and folded back

stapes The most interior of the three ossicles. Connected to the incus on one end, the stapes presses against the oval window of the cochlea on the other end.

oval window The flexible opening to the cochlea through which the stapes transmits vibration to the fluid inside.

inner ear A hollow cavity in the temporal bone of the skull and the structures within this cavity: the cochlea and the semicircular canals of the vestibular system.

tensor tympani The muscle attached to the malleus. Tensing the tensor tympani decreases vibration.

stapedius The muscle attached to the stapes. Tensing the stapedius decreases vibration.

acoustic reflex A reflex that protects the ear from intense sounds via contraction of the stapedius and tensor tympani muscles.

cochlea A spiral structure of the inner ear containing the organ of Corti.

tympanic canal One of three fluid-filled passages in the cochlea. The tympanic canal extends from the round window at the base of the cochlea to the helicotrema at the apex. Also called *scala tympani*.

vestibular canal One of three fluid-filled passages in the cochlea. The vestibular canal extends from the oval window at the base of the cochlea to the helicotrema at the apex. Also called *scala vestibuli*.

middle canal One of three fluid-filled passages in the cochlea. The middle canal is sandwiched between the tympanic and vestibular canals and contains the cochlear partition. Also called *scala media*.

helicotrema The opening that connects the tympanic and vestibular canals at the apex of the cochlea.

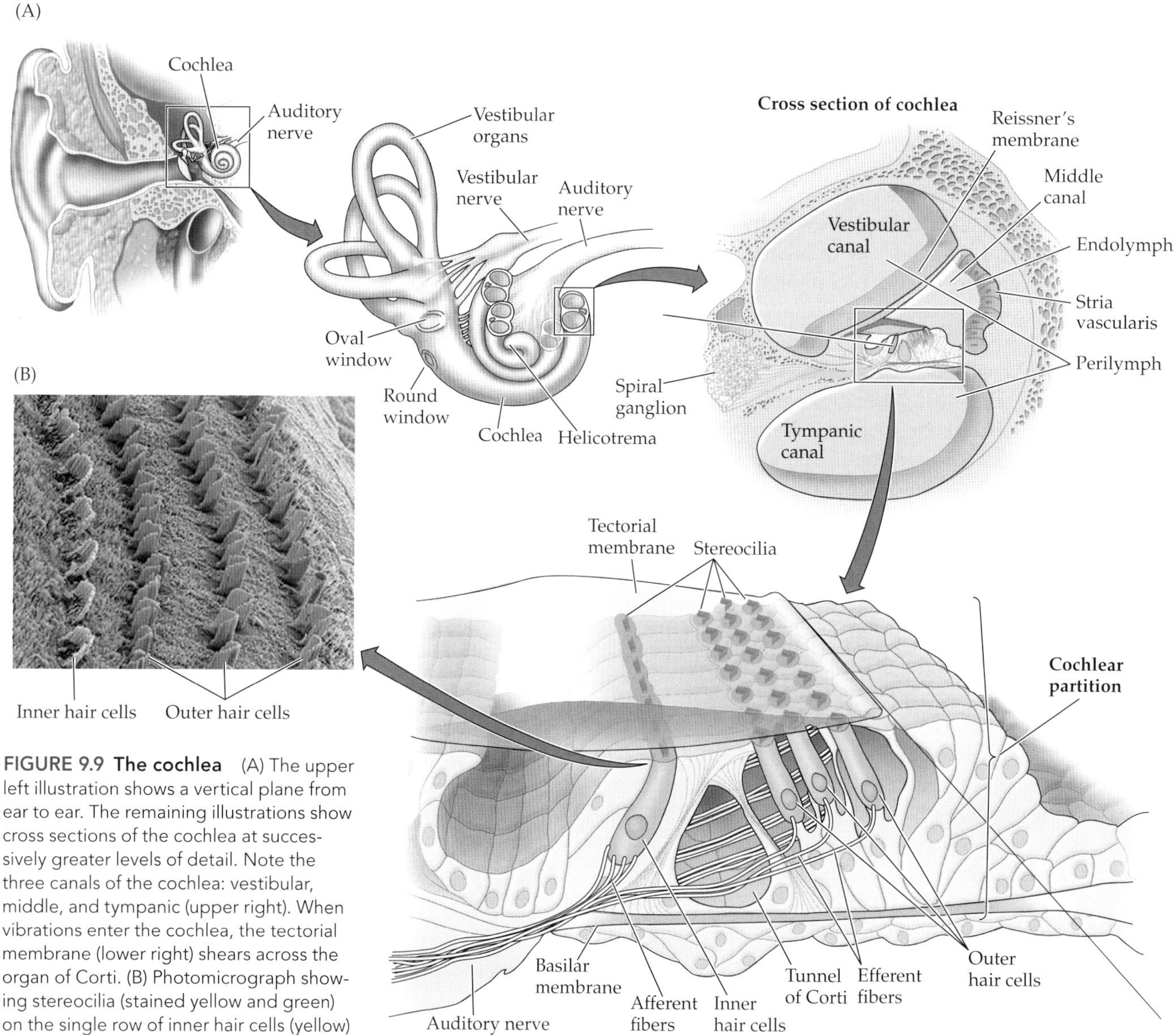

FIGURE 9.9 The cochlea (A) The upper left illustration shows a vertical plane from ear to ear. The remaining illustrations show cross sections of the cochlea at successively greater levels of detail. Note the three canals of the cochlea: vestibular, middle, and tympanic (upper right). When vibrations enter the cochlea, the tectorial membrane (lower right) shears across the organ of Corti. (B) Photomicrograph showing stereocilia (stained yellow and green) on the single row of inner hair cells (yellow) and three rows of outer hair cells (green).

on itself. The middle canal is another long balloon that is sandwiched, lengthwise, between the two halves of the first balloon. The middle canal is filled with a different fluid called endolymph, which bathes the most important parts of the inner ear. Specialized tissue called **stria vascularis** lines one side of the middle canal. It keeps the cells that translate sound to a neural signal working at their best by maintaining the right balance of charged ions.

The three canals of the cochlea are separated by two membranes (see Figure 9.9): **Reissner's membrane** between the vestibular canal and the middle canal, and the **basilar membrane** between the middle canal and the tympanic canal. The basilar membrane is not really a membrane like the tympanic membrane, oval window, and Reissner's membrane. Instead, it is a plate made up of stiff fibers. The basilar membrane forms the base of the **cochlear partition**, a complex structure through which sound waves are transduced into neural signals.

stria vascularis Specialized tissue lines one side of the middle canal and maintains the right balance of charged ions in the endolymph to keep hair cells working at their best.

Reissner's membrane A thin sheath of tissue separating the vestibular and middle canals in the cochlea.

basilar membrane A plate of fibers that forms the base of the cochlear partition and separates the middle and tympanic canals in the cochlea.

Vibrations transmitted through the tympanic membrane and middle-ear bones cause the stapes to push and pull the flexible oval window in and out of the vestibular canal at the base of the cochlea. This movement of the oval window causes waves of pressure changes, called traveling waves, to flow through the fluid in the vestibular canal, in much the same way that the membrane of a loudspeaker moves air to create sound waves. Because the cochlea is a closed tube, changes in pressure cannot spread out in all directions. Instead, a displacement, or "bulge," forms in the vestibular canal and extends from the base of the cochlea down to the apex (look ahead to Figure 9.12). If sounds are extremely intense, any pressure that remains at the apex passes through the helicotrema and back to the cochlear base through the tympanic canal, where it is relieved by stretching yet another membrane, the **round window** (see Figure 9.9).

Because the vestibular and tympanic canals are wrapped tightly around the middle canal, when the vestibular canal bulges out, it puts pressure on the middle canal. This pressure has the effect of displacing the basilar membrane (which, recall, lies at the bottom of the middle canal), pushing down when the vestibular-canal bulge is created.

THE ORGAN OF CORTI Movements of the basilar membrane are translated into neural signals by structures in the **organ of Corti**, which extends along the top of the basilar membrane (see Figure 9.9). The organ of Corti is made up of a scaffold of cells that support specialized neurons called **hair cells**. Axons and dendrites of **auditory nerve (AN)** fibers terminate at the bases of hair cells (more about these fibers as the chapter progresses). Hair cells in each human ear are arranged in four rows that run down the length of the basilar membrane: one row of about 3500 inner hair cells and three rows with a total of about 10,500 outer hair cells.

Inner and outer hair cells provide the foundations for minuscule hairlike bristles called **stereocilia** (singular *stereocilium*). On an inner hair cell, stereocilia are arranged as if posing for a group photo, in several nearly straight rows, with the shorter stereocilia in front and the taller ones peering over their shoulders in the back. On an outer hair cell, stereocilia stand in rows that form the shape of a *V* or *W* (see Figure 9.9B).

The **tectorial membrane** extends atop the organ of Corti. Like the basilar membrane, it isn't really a membrane. Rather, it is a gelatinous flap that is attached on one end and rests atop the outer hair cells on the other end. Taller stereocilia of outer hair cells are embedded in the tectorial membrane, and the stereocilia of inner hair cells are nestled just below it. Because the tectorial membrane is attached on only one end, it sweeps sideways across the width of the cochlear partition whenever the partition moves up and down. This shearing motion causes the stereocilia of both inner and outer hair cells to bend back and forth (**FIGURE 9.10**).

HAIR CELLS Like photoreceptors in the retina, hair cells are specialized receptor cells that transduce one kind of energy (in this case, sound pressure) into another form of energy (neural firing). Hair cells in the vestibular organs also report head movements to the brain, as you will learn in Chapter 12. Deflection of a hair cell's stereocilia causes a change in voltage potential that initiates the release of neurotransmitters, which in turn encourages firing by AN fibers that have dendritic synapses on hair cells (Eggermont, 2017). However, it is the *differences* between photoreceptors and hair cells, not their similarities, that are the most interesting.

cochlear partition The combined basilar membrane, tectorial membrane, and organ of Corti, which are together responsible for the transduction of sound waves into neural signals.

round window A soft area of tissue at the base of the tympanic canal that releases excess pressure remaining from extremely intense sounds.

organ of Corti A structure on the basilar membrane of the cochlea that is composed of hair cells and dendrites of auditory nerve fibers.

hair cell Any cell that has stereocilia for transducing mechanical movement in the inner ear into neural activity sent to the brain. Some hair cells also receive inputs from the brain.

auditory nerve (AN) A collection of neurons that convey information from hair cells in the cochlea to the brainstem (afferent neurons) and from the brainstem to the hair cells (efferent neurons).

stereocilium Any of the hairlike extensions on the tips of hair cells in the cochlea that, when flexed, initiate the release of neurotransmitters.

tectorial membrane A gelatinous structure, attached on one end, that extends into the middle canal of the cochlea, floating above inner hair cells and touching outer hair cells.

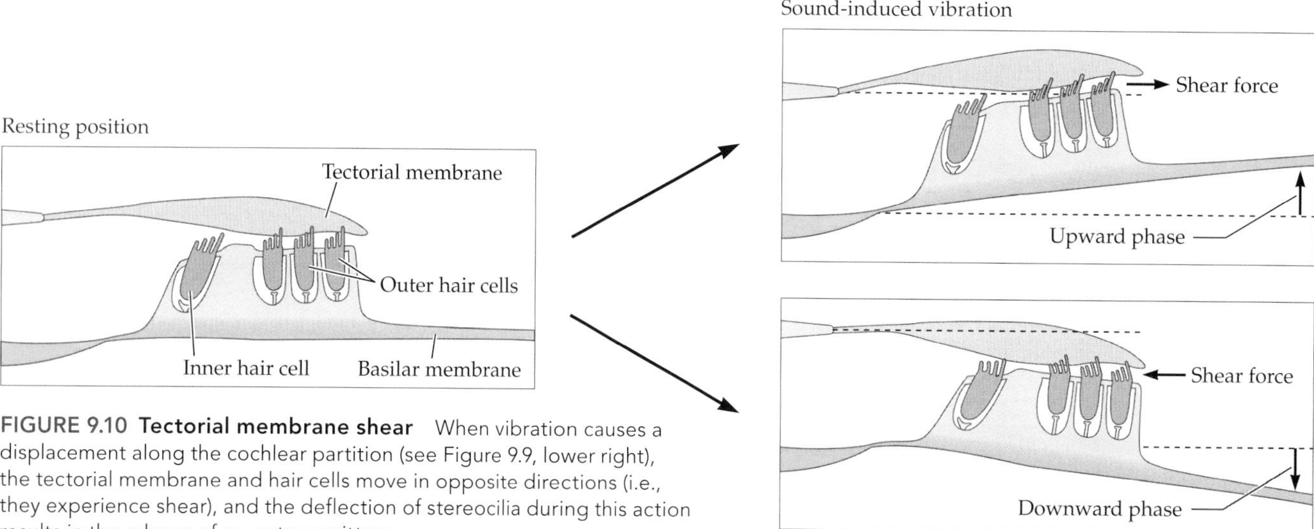

FIGURE 9.10 Tectorial membrane shear When vibration causes a displacement along the cochlear partition (see Figure 9.9, lower right), the tectorial membrane and hair cells move in opposite directions (i.e., they experience shear), and the deflection of stereocilia during this action results in the release of neurotransmitters.

While the retina has almost 100 million photoreceptors, each cochlea has only about 14,000 hair cells. Although outnumbered, stereocilia of hair cells blow away the photoreceptor competition when it comes to speed and sensitivity. Listeners can detect differences between onsets of two sounds as small as 1 millisecond (ms) (Zera and Green, 1993), and they can detect gaps between sounds as brief as 2–3 ms (Schneider and Hamstra, 1999). In contrast, when we watch a movie, pictures shown at 24 frames per second (over 40 ms apart) appear continuous to the visual system. Hair cells are not only extremely fast, but also extremely sensitive. It may take 30 minutes for our eyes to fully adjust to a dark theater, but our ears are always ready for the slightest sound.

Recall that the shortest stereocilia are in front of slightly taller stereocilia that are in front of still taller stereocilia (**FIGURE 9.11**). Each stereocilium is connected to its neighbor by a tiny filament called a **tip link**, so the stereocilia connected by tip links bend together as a set when deflected by the shearing motion of the tectorial membrane. Because what happens next is very difficult to observe—tiny parts of tiny structures atop single tiny hair cells—what follows is only a current hypothesis. When a stereocilium deflects, the tip link pulls on the taller stereocilium in a way that opens an ion pore, somewhat like opening a gate for just a tiny fraction of a second. This action permits potassium ions (K^+) to flow rapidly into the hair cell, causing rapid depolarization because potassium carries a positive charge (see Figures 9.11B and 9.11C). In turn, depolarization leads to a rapid influx of calcium ions (Ca^{2+}) and initiation of the release of neurotransmitters from the base of the hair cell to stimulate dendrites of the AN (Fettiplace and Hackney, 2006; Hudspeth, 1997). The firing of the AN fibers completes the process of translating sound waves into patterns of neural activity.

The opening of ion pores that results from the direct connection between stereocilia via tip links is known as mechanoelectrical transduction, which is responsible for both the extreme speed and the sensitivity of hair cells. Unlike the case in vision, depolarization in hearing does not await a cascade of biochemical processes such as those in photoactivation. Mechanoelectrical transduction is extremely sensitive: ion pores open when deflection is as little as 1 nanometer (nm). For comparison, a sheet of paper is about 100,000 nm thick.

tip link A tiny filament that stretches from the tip of a stereocilium to the side of its neighbor.

Here's a summary of the process of sound transmission. An air pressure wave is funneled by the pinna through the ear canal to the tympanic membrane, which

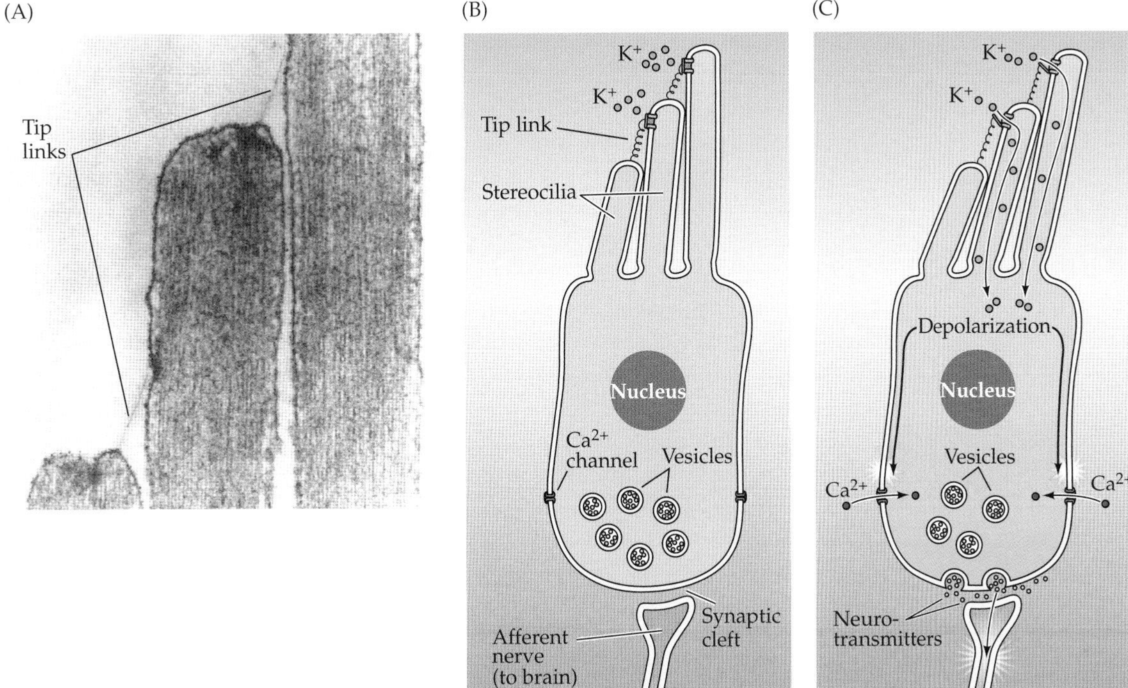

FIGURE 9.11 Mechanoelectrical transduction in hair cells Stereocilia regulate the flow of ions into and out of hair cells. (A) This photomicrograph shows the threadlike tip links that connect the tip of each shorter stereocilium to its taller neighbor. (B, C) Bending the stereocilia atop a hair cell opens the ion pores, permitting a rapid influx of potassium ions (K^+) into the hair cell. This depolarization opens channels that allow calcium ions (Ca^{2+}) to enter the base of the hair cell, causing the release of neurotransmitters into the synaptic cleft between the hair cell and an afferent auditory nerve (AN) fiber, resulting in the nerve fiber firing, sending a signal to the brain. Between 5 and 30 AN fibers synapse with each inner hair cell; only one is shown here.

vibrates back and forth in time with the sound wave. The tympanic membrane vibrates the malleus, which vibrates the incus, which vibrates the stapes, which pushes and pulls on the oval window. The movement of the oval window causes pressure bulges to move down the length of the fluid-filled vestibular canal, and these bulges in the vestibular canal move the middle canal up and down. This up-and-down motion forces the tectorial membrane to shear across the organ of Corti, moving the stereocilia atop hair cells back and forth. The pivoting of the stereocilia opens ion pores that allow entry of positively charged potassium ions. This rapidly depolarizes the hair cell and results in spurts of neurotransmitter released into synaptic clefts between the hair cells and dendrites of AN fibers. These neurotransmitters initiate action potentials in the AN fibers, and these signals are carried to the brain. This completes the chain of translating sound pressure to a neural code.

CODING OF AMPLITUDE AND FREQUENCY IN THE COCHLEA Now that we know more about how ears work, we can return to the two fundamental characteristics of sound waves—amplitude and frequency—and learn how they are encoded by the cochlea.

Sounds with greater amplitude have greater pressure changes. If the amplitude of a sound wave is increased, the tympanic membrane and oval window move farther in and out with each pressure fluctuation. The result is that the bulge in the vestibular canal becomes bigger, which causes the cochlear partition (with the basilar membrane) to move farther up and down, which causes the tectorial membrane to shear across the organ of Corti more forcefully, which causes the hair cells to pivot farther back and forth, which causes more neurotransmitters to be released, which causes AN fibers to initiate action potentials more quickly. (We will discuss some complications of this simple explanation in the next section, where we discuss the AN in more detail.)

Coding for frequency is a bit more interesting. Depending on the frequencies of a sound, the basilar membrane is displaced up and down in different places along the length of the cochlea. High frequencies cause the largest displacements closer to the oval window, near the base of the cochlea by the oval window. Lower frequencies cause displacements farther away and nearer the apex, at the top of the snail shell–like cochlear twist. In other words, different places on the cochlea are "tuned" to different frequencies. This tuning is known as the **place code** for sound frequency.

Cochlear tuning to frequency is caused, in large part, by differences in the structure of the basilar membrane along the length of the cochlea. If we were to unroll the snail shell–like cochlea, it would be apparent that the all-important basilar membrane widens toward the apex (FIGURE 9.12). In addition, the basilar membrane is stiff at the base and becomes floppier as it widens toward the apex. These physical qualities of the basilar membrane cause the cochlea to separate frequencies like an acoustic prism. Higher frequencies have the most effect on displacing the narrower, stiffer regions of the basilar membrane near the base, and lower frequencies cause greater displacements in the wider, more flexible regions near the apex.

When you look at displacements from sounds of different frequencies along the basilar membrane in Figure 9.12B, they are labeled as traveling waves. This is because the displacement really does travel from base to apex—faster near the base where the basilar membrane is narrower and slower toward the wider apex. Because it takes time for the traveling wave to travel down the basilar membrane, high-frequency regions (base) are stimulated earlier than lower-frequency regions. This fact will become important when, in Chapter 10, you learn about how you know from what direction sounds are coming.

In addition to this passive, structural way of being tuned to frequency, the cochlea has processes that actively sharpen tuning. Remember that there are two different types of hair cells: inner and outer. Over 90% of the **afferent fibers** in the AN—fibers that take information *to* the brain—synapse on the 3500 inner hair cells (5–30 AN fibers "listen" to each inner hair cell; see Figure 9.11). If the inner hair cells are conveying almost all the information about sound waves to the brain, then what do the 10,500 outer hair cells do?

To a large extent, outer hair cells do what they are told by the next stages in the auditory pathway. Most of the nerve fibers that synapse with the outer hair cells are **efferent fibers**, conveying information *from* the brain. These efferent fibers play a special role in determining what kind of information is sent on to the brain by the afferent fibers (Fettiplace and Hackney, 2006); this will become easier to understand in just a few paragraphs.

place code Tuning of different parts of the cochlea to different frequencies, in which information about the particular frequency of an incoming sound wave is coded by the place along the cochlear partition that has the greatest mechanical displacement.

afferent fiber A neuron that carries sensory information to the central nervous system.

efferent fiber A neuron that carries information from the central nervous system to the periphery.

The Auditory Nerve

Now that we've covered the mechanics of how the auditory system translates air pressure changes into AN firing, let's discuss what we know about AN fibers. More specifically, we'll consider the type of information conveyed by afferent AN fibers from the cochlea to the brain.

Remember that sounds with different frequencies displace different places along the basilar membrane. Inner hair cells, which provide most of the information

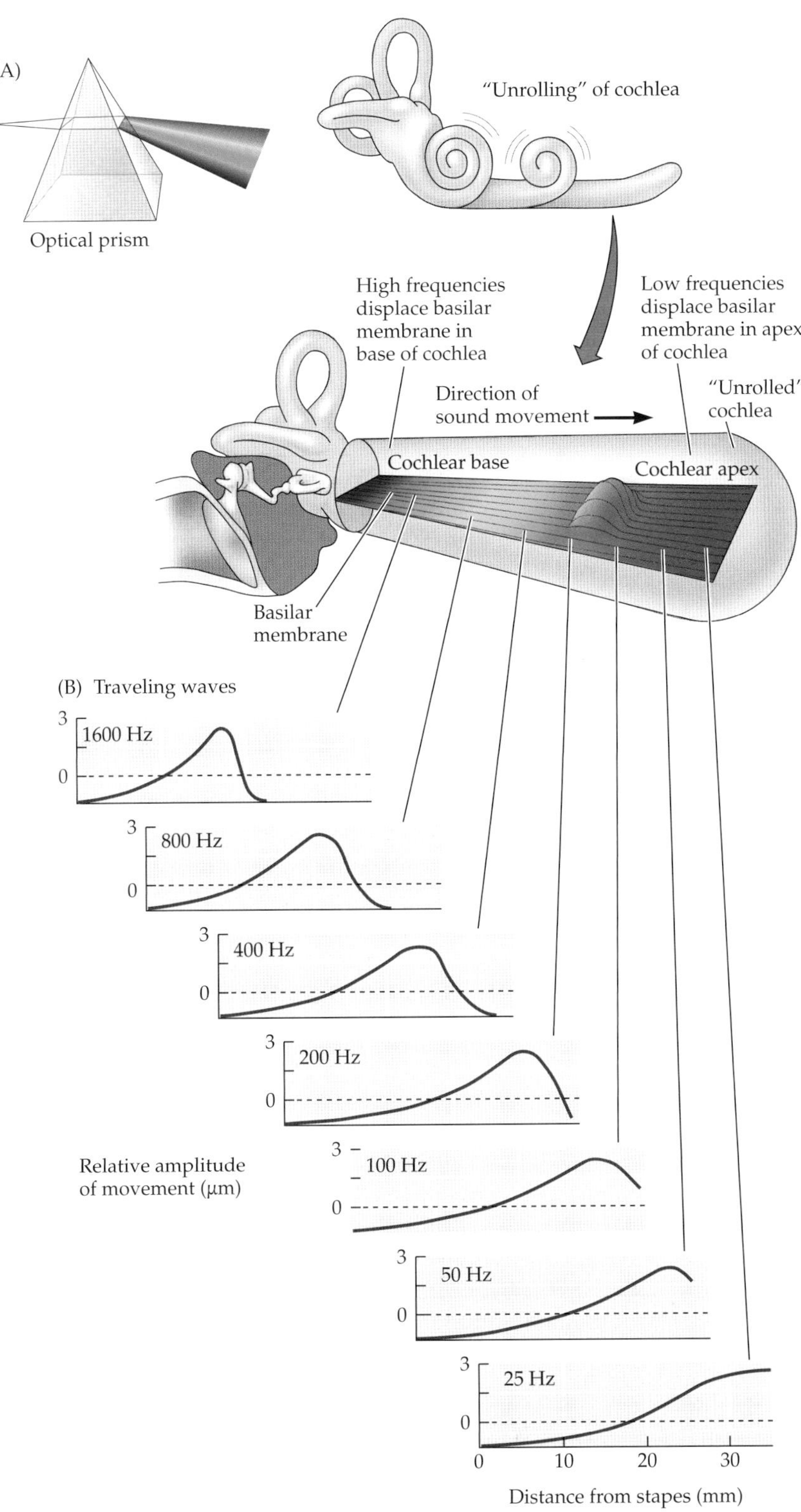

FIGURE 9.12 Frequencies along the cochlea The cochlea is like an acoustic prism in that its sensitivity spreads across different sound frequencies along its length. (A) The cochlea is illustrated as if it were uncoiled. The narrower end of the basilar membrane toward the base is stiffer and most sensitive to higher frequencies. The wider, more flexible end toward the apex is most sensitive to lower frequencies. (B) The shapes of the traveling waves for different frequencies of vibration are shown.

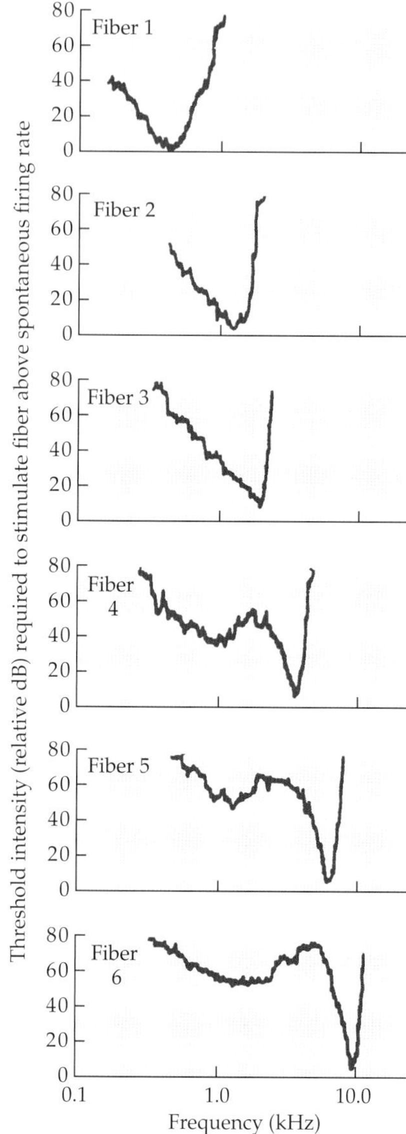

FIGURE 9.13 Threshold tuning curves Tuning curves for six auditory nerve fibers on inner hair cells are shown, each tuned to a different frequency. Curves define the lowest intensity necessary for the neuron to fire above its spontaneous rate at each frequency. The characteristic frequency for each of these six nerve fibers is at the lowest point of the tuning curve.

to the brain via AN fibers, are lined up single file along the length of the basilar membrane, and responses of individual AN fibers to different frequencies should be related to their place along the cochlea. Indeed, when scientists record from individual AN fibers in animals, they find that different fibers selectively respond to different sound frequencies.

This frequency selectivity is clearest when sounds are very faint: at very low intensity levels, an AN fiber will increase firing to only a very restricted range of frequencies. **FIGURE 9.13** shows **threshold tuning curves** for six AN fibers. To graph one of these curves, a researcher inserts an electrode very close to a single AN fiber and then measures how intense sine waves of different frequencies must be for the neuron to fire action potentials faster than its normal, spontaneous firing rate. The frequency that increases the neuron's firing rate at the lowest intensity (the lowest *y*-axis point on the threshold tuning curve) is called the neuron's **characteristic frequency (CF)**.

Let's go back to those outer hair cells that receive their instructions from the brain. The sharp tuning measured from outputs of inner hair cells in Figure 9.13 greatly depends on the outer hair cells. In **FIGURE 9.14**, the shallow dashed line illustrates tuning when outer hair cells are absent. You can see how outer hair cells are required for threshold tuning curves to be focused on a narrow range of frequencies. The way that they do this is with a remarkable ability to lengthen and contract in response to changes in electric potential, an ability called **electromotility** (Brownell, 2017). When outer hair cells are stimulated, they actually lengthen, extending farther into the tectorial membrane. Through lengthening and contracting, outer hair cells cause parts of the cochlear partition to stiffen in ways that make the responses of inner hair cells more sensitive (Dong and Olson, 2013) and more sharply tuned to specific frequencies (Eggermont, 2017).

But what "stimulates" the outer hair cells to change their shape and influence how the cochlea responds to sound? Remarkably, the brain sends efferent electrical potentials to the cochlea. That means that the brain is playing an active role in shaping its own input! We do not yet understand all the circumstances that lead the brain to communicate with the cochlea in this way, but it is an essential aspect of healthy hearing. The movement of outer hair cells even *creates* sounds, called otoacoustic emissions, that *exit* the ears. Audiologists can use these emissions to diagnose impaired versus healthy hearing.

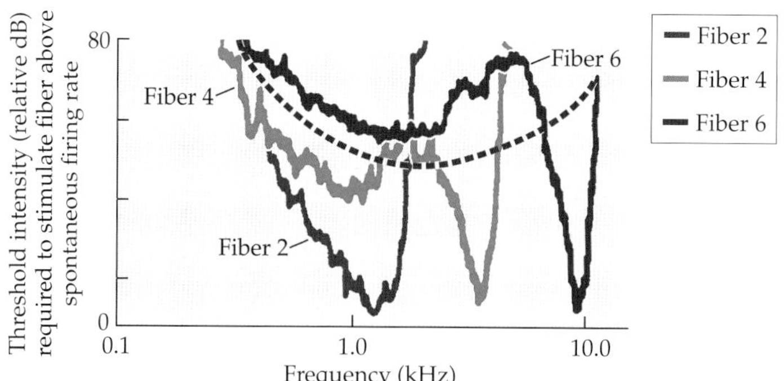

FIGURE 9.14 Function of outer hair cells Outer hair cells improve both sensitivity and frequency selectivity. Threshold tuning curves for three of the nerve fibers in Figure 9.13 show responses when outer hair cells are active. The dashed line shows what the rightmost tuning curve (for fiber 6) would look like if outer hair cells were not active. Higher-intensity tones would be required to excite the auditory nerve fiber, and the fiber would be less selective in frequencies to which it would fire.

threshold tuning curve A graph plotting the thresholds of a neuron in response to sine waves with varying frequencies at the lowest intensity that will give rise to a response.

characteristic frequency (CF) The frequency to which a particular auditory nerve fiber is most sensitive.

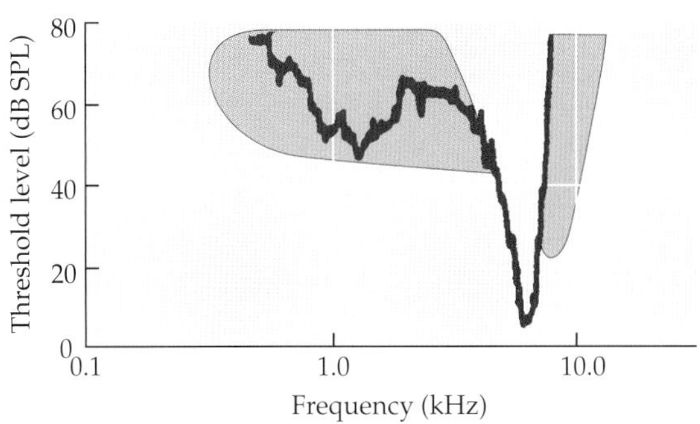

FIGURE 9.15 Two-tone suppression The threshold tuning curve (dark red) plots the responses of one auditory nerve fiber with a characteristic frequency of 8000 Hz. Whenever a second tone is played at the frequencies and levels within the light-red areas to each side, the response of this AN fiber to an 8000 Hz tone is reduced (suppressed). SPL, sound pressure level.

BEYOND SIMPLE SOUNDS AT LOW INTENSITY Up to this point, the way the ear transduces acoustic energy at different frequencies into a pattern of neural responses seems straightforward. A low-intensity sine wave tone with a certain frequency will cause certain AN fibers to increase their firing rates, while other AN fibers continue to fire at their spontaneous rates. As long as the brain knows which AN fibers have which characteristic frequencies, it can interpret the pattern of firing rates across all the AN fibers to determine the frequency of any tone (as long as it is within the range of frequencies picked up by the human cochlea).

Unfortunately, it's not quite this simple. Almost all sounds in the environment are more complex than single sine waves, and most sounds we hear are also much louder than the very quiet sound waves used to measure threshold tuning curves. So, although the previous paragraph captures the gist of how AN fibers code for sound frequencies, we must do a bit more work to understand how higher-intensity, complex sounds are encoded in the AN. Let's consider two of the specific complications. Then, we'll look at one additional mechanism, related to timing rather than place along the cochlea, that the auditory system uses to convey low-frequency components of sound waves.

electromotility The ability of outer hair cells to extend and contract, which changes the stiffness and sensitivity of the cochlear partition.

two-tone suppression A decrease in the response (firing rate) of one auditory nerve fiber to one tone when a second tone is presented at the same time.

TWO-TONE SUPPRESSION The rate at which an AN fiber responds changes when energy is introduced at nearby frequencies. When a second tone of a slightly different frequency is added, the rate of neural firing for the first tone decreases—a phenomenon called **two-tone suppression** (FIGURE 9.15). Suppression effects are particularly pronounced when the second (suppressor) tone has a lower frequency than the first tone. In other words, if we're recording from an AN fiber whose characteristic frequency is 8000 Hz and we use an 8000 Hz test tone, adding a 1000 Hz suppressor tone decreases the neuron's firing rate more than adding a 15,000 Hz suppressor tone. You can see how understanding the response of the whole AN to complex sounds that involve frequency combinations is more complicated than simply adding up the responses of individual AN fibers to individual pure tones.

RATE SATURATION Sounds that matter most to listeners—most conversational speech, for example—are usually heard at intensities (say, 60–70 dB) that are over 1000 times greater than the threshold for just detecting sounds. At higher intensities, AN fibers become much less selective about the frequencies to which they will respond. FIGURE 9.16 shows

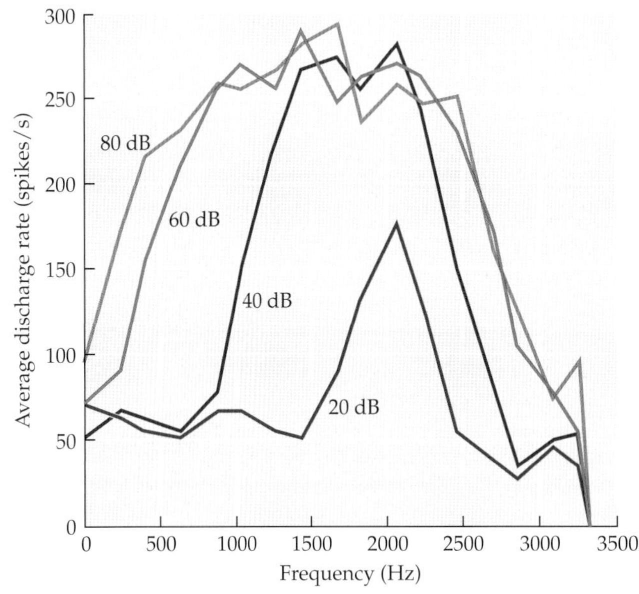

FIGURE 9.16 Isointensity functions Neurons become less sharply tuned with increasing sound level. For one auditory nerve fiber with a characteristic frequency of 2000 Hz, tones of varying frequencies are presented at 20, 40, 60, and 80 dB. The neuron fires vigorously to a wider range of frequencies (mostly lower) when intensity is increased. Note that the 20 dB curve resembles an upside-down threshold tuning curve (compare with Figure 9.13) because 20 dB is almost as low as the intensities at which thresholds are measured.

isointensity curve A map plotting the firing rate of an auditory nerve fiber against varying frequencies at varying intensities.

rate saturation The point at which a nerve fiber is firing as rapidly as possible and further stimulation is incapable of increasing the firing rate.

rate-intensity function A graph plotting the firing rate of an auditory nerve fiber in response to a sound of constant frequency at increasing intensities.

low-spontaneous fiber An auditory nerve fiber that has a low rate (less than 10 spikes per second) of spontaneous firing. Low-spontaneous fibers require relatively intense sound before they will fire at higher rates.

high-spontaneous fiber An auditory nerve fiber that has a high rate (more than 30 spikes per second) of spontaneous firing. High-spontaneous fibers increase their firing rate in response to relatively low levels of sound.

mid-spontaneous fiber An auditory nerve fiber that has a medium rate (10–30 spikes per second) of spontaneous firing. The characteristics of mid-spontaneous fibers are intermediate between those of low- and high-spontaneous fibers.

a family of **isointensity curves** for one AN fiber with a CF of 2000 Hz. The bottom curve shows the average firing rate (number of action potentials per second) of the neuron in response to 20 dB tones with frequencies between 50 and 3300 Hz. The other curves track firing rates for 40, 60, and 80 dB tones over the same frequency range.

We learn from these curves that for relatively quiet, 20 dB sounds (this is below the sound level of leaves rustling in the wind), the neuron is still quite narrowly tuned, firing much faster in response to its CF (2000 Hz) than to neighboring frequencies. At 80 dB, however, the neuron appears to fire at about the same rate for any frequency in the range of 800–2500 Hz. In other words, frequencies such as 1000 Hz, to which the AN fiber had almost no response at low intensity levels, evoke quite substantial—and less frequency-selective—responses when intensity is increased.

The phenomenon behind this broadening of frequency selectivity is called **rate saturation**. Remember that AN fibers fire in response to the displacement of stereocilia on hair cells. The farther stereocilia pivot, the faster AN fibers linked to that hair cell fire. For a 20 dB tone at 1000 Hz, the stereocilia on the hair cell feeding the AN fiber featured in Figure 9.16 will not bend at all, so the fiber's firing rate remains at its resting level. The firing rate rises above this resting level when the frequency of the 20 dB tone is increased to 1700 Hz, and it reaches its highest level at the AN fiber's characteristic frequency, 2000 Hz.

When the intensity is increased to 40 dB, however, the bulge in the vestibular canal is so large that stereocilia start displacing even to a 1000 Hz tone (see Figure 9.16). If we increase the frequency to 1250 Hz, the firing rate increases, and it increases even more at 1500 Hz. The problem is that at about 1500 Hz, the fiber's firing rate maxes out, or *saturates*. At this point, stereocilia are pivoting as much as they can, so increasing the frequency of the tone has no additional effect on the AN fiber's firing rate until we increase the frequency above the fiber's CF and the firing rate starts dropping again. For 80 dB tones, the fiber is maxed out at a range between even lower and higher frequencies relative to the CF of 2000 Hz.

This means that for moderately intense sounds, such as speech, the brain cannot rely on a single AN fiber to determine whether there is energy at a particular frequency. For example, we can't use the rule "if an AN fiber with a characteristic frequency of 2000 Hz is firing very fast, the sound must be 2000 Hz" because, as Figure 9.16 illustrates, this neuron will also fire at its maximum rate to a 1000 Hz tone if the sound wave has a large enough amplitude.

One way the auditory system gets around this problem is to use AN fibers with different spontaneous firing rates. FIGURE 9.17 shows **rate-intensity functions** for six fibers, all of which listen to the same hair cell (remember that dendrites from 5–30 auditory neurons are synapsing with each inner hair cell). To plot these curves, the intensity level of a tone at the AN fiber's CF is slowly raised from 0 dB up to 90 dB. As you can see, the resting rates of some fibers (those plotted in red) are less than 10 spikes per second. These are **low-spontaneous fibers**. The blue lines plot firing rates for **high-spontaneous fibers**, which fire 30 or more times per second, even in silence. **Mid-spontaneous fibers** have resting rates between these levels.

High-spontaneous AN fibers are somewhat analogous to rods in the retina: they are especially sensitive to low levels of sound, responding at rates above resting level even when decibel levels are quite low. The trade-off is that the firing rates of these fibers quickly reach saturation, so their frequency selectivity is relatively poor when intensity is relatively high. Low-spontaneous fibers are more like cones, requiring more energy (higher-intensity sound waves) to start responding, but retaining their frequency selectivity over a broader range of intensity.

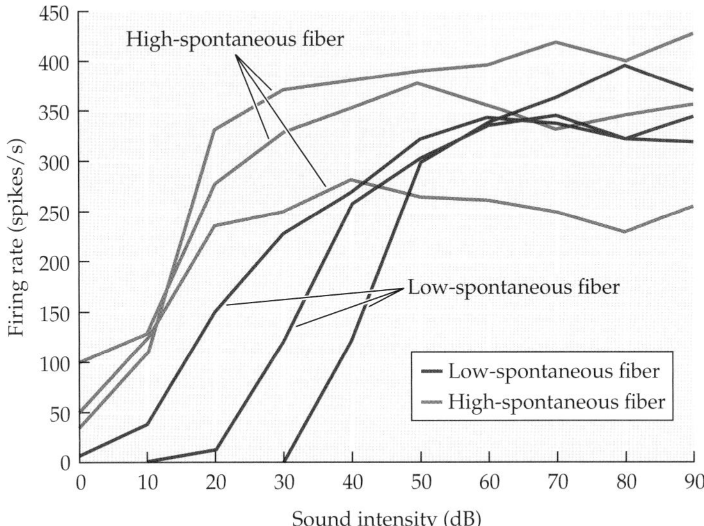

FIGURE 9.17 Firing rate across intensities Neural firing rate is shown at increasing sound intensities for six auditory nerve fibers (three low-spontaneous fibers and three high-spontaneous fibers). Firing rates for all six neurons increase with increasing sound level. Low-spontaneous neurons require higher-intensity sounds before they begin to fire, and they continue to increase firing rate to higher sound levels.

In addition to having different AN fibers with different spontaneous rates, the auditory system can accurately determine the frequency of incoming sound waves by integrating information across many AN fibers and using the *pattern* of firing rates across all these fibers. Remember that in the visual system, we use the pattern of firing across only three types of cones to calculate the wavelength of light. The auditory system uses the same principle, but it has some 14,000 AN fibers in each ear to discern acoustic frequency. Consequently, the human auditory system has exquisite frequency sensitivity across a wide range of intensity levels despite the coarse selectivity of individual AN fibers.

TEMPORAL CODE FOR SOUND FREQUENCY In addition to the cochlear place code, the auditory system has another way to encode frequency. As **FIGURE 9.18** illustrates, many AN fibers tend to fire action potentials at one particular point in the amplitude fluctuation of a sound wave (also called *phase*). This is called **phase locking**. Phase locking may occur because AN fibers fire when the stereocilia of hair cells move in one direction (e.g., as the basilar membrane moves up toward the tectorial membrane), but do not fire when the stereocilia move in the other direction. Recall from our discussion above that the encoding of time is extremely accurate.

The existence of phase locking means that the firing pattern of an AN fiber carries a **temporal code** for the sound wave frequency. For example, if the AN fiber fires an action potential 100 times per second, then downstream neurons listening to the AN fiber can infer that the sound wave includes a frequency component of 100 Hz (which cycles in pressure fluctuations 100 times per second).

phase locking Firing of a single neuron at one distinct point in the period (cycle) of a sound wave at a given frequency. (The neuron need not fire on every cycle, but each firing will occur at the same point in the cycle.)

temporal code Tuning of different parts of the cochlea to different frequencies, in which information about the particular frequency of an incoming sound wave is coded by the timing of neural firing as it relates to the period of the sound.

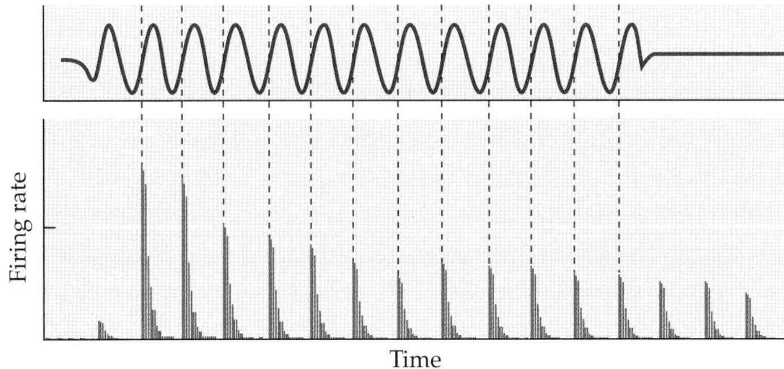

FIGURE 9.18 Phase locking The histogram (bottom) shows neural spikes for an auditory nerve fiber in response to the same low-frequency sine wave (top) being played many times. Note that the neuron is most likely to fire at one particular phase of each cycle of the sine wave. This phase locking provides a temporal code to sound frequency.

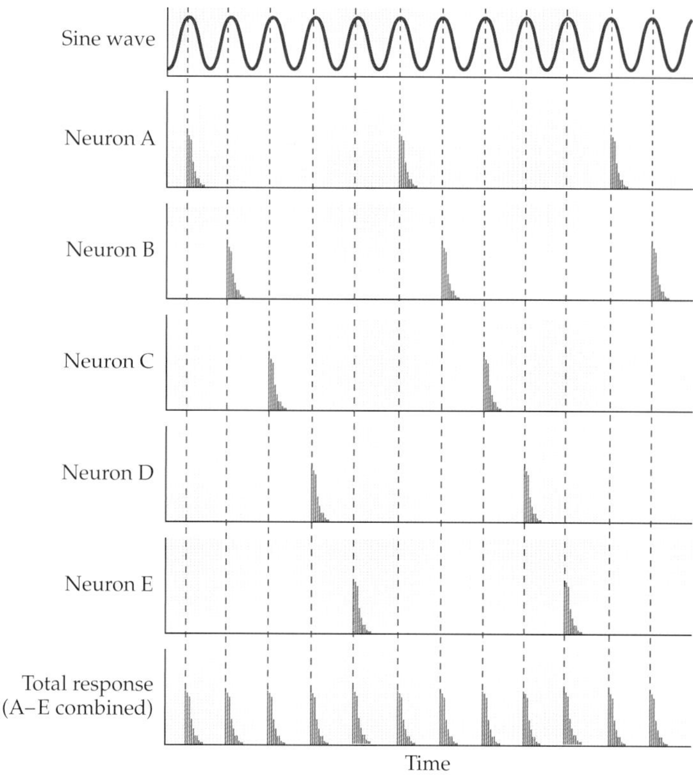

FIGURE 9.19 The volley principle Even if one neuron cannot fire in response to every cycle of a higher-frequency tone, multiple auditory nerve fibers together can provide a temporal code for frequency if different neurons (A, B, C, D, E) fire at different periods of the sine wave.

While reliable for lower frequencies, temporal coding becomes inconsistent for frequencies higher than 1000 Hz and is virtually absent above 4000 or 5000 Hz. In large part, this inconsistency is a result of the refractory period of the AN fiber, the brief period after an action potential during which the AN cannot fire again. For high frequencies, fibers simply cannot produce action potentials quickly enough to fire on every cycle of the sound. However, multiple neurons could, in principle, encode higher frequencies as a group. For example, four neurons could each fire only once every fourth cycle of a 2000 Hz sound. If the four neurons "took turns," each would have to fire only 500 times per second to fully encode the 2000 Hz sound in their combined temporal pattern. This idea has a long history (Wever, 1949), and it is referred to as the **volley principle** (**FIGURE 9.19**). According to this hypothesis, neurons sustain a temporal pattern of firing much like the pattern of Revolutionary War–era soldiers firing guns from the front line of a formation while the second and third lines took time to reload.

When it comes to temporal coding, neurons along the full length of the cochlea can participate. Even AN fibers with relatively high-frequency CFs encode lower-frequency energy in the temporal pattern of their responses. For example, if you are listening to a fairly loud sound that is a combination of 200 and 8000 Hz sine wave tones, a neuron near the base of the cochlea that becomes wildly excited by the 8000 Hz component of the sound will also tend to be phase-locked to the 200 Hz component. This neuron thus carries information about both the high-frequency component (via place coding, because the brain knows the AN fiber's CF) and the low-frequency component (via temporal coding).

Auditory Brain Structures

The nerve fibers that make up the auditory nerve share cranial nerve VIII, the vestibulocochlear nerve, with nerve fibers for the vestibular system (discussed in Chapter 12). All AN fibers initially synapse in the **cochlear nucleus** (**FIGURE 9.20**). The cochlear nuclei (we have two, right and left) contain several different types of specialized neurons. Some of these neurons are especially sensitive to onsets of sound at particular frequencies. Some are sensitive to the coincidence of sound onsets across many frequencies (they fire when multiple frequencies initially begin, but stop firing if the sound continues playing). Some cochlear nucleus neurons sharpen the tuning to one frequency by suppressing nearby frequencies—a mechanism reminiscent of that used by retinal ganglion cells to respond to spots of light instead of broad fields of light. Others respond in exactly the same way as the AN fibers that relay action potentials to the cochlear nuclei.

Some neurons appear to serve as little more than quick relays from the cochlea to the **superior olives**, another pair of brainstem nuclei important for interpreting the locations of sounds in the world. As Figure 9.20 shows, some of the neurons that project from the cochlear nuclei to the superior olives cross over to the opposite

volley principle The idea that multiple neurons can provide a temporal code for frequency if each neuron fires at a distinct point in the period of a sound wave but does not fire on every period.

cochlear nucleus The first brainstem nucleus at which afferent auditory nerve fibers synapse.

superior olive An early brainstem region in the auditory pathway where inputs from both ears converge.

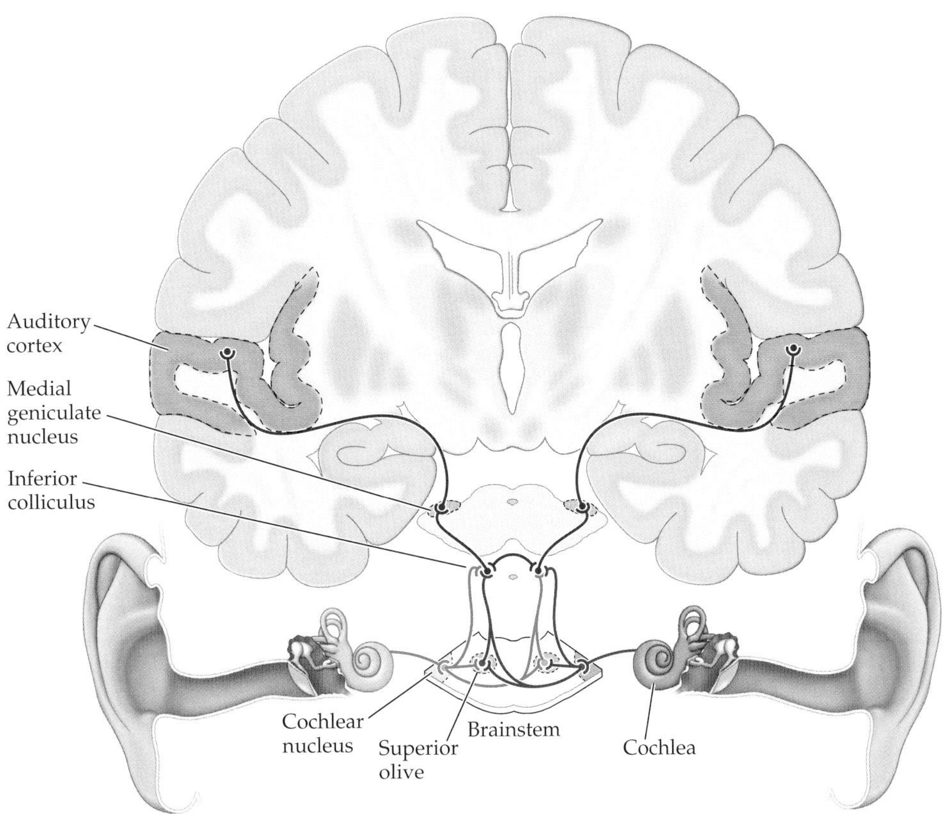

FIGURE 9.20 Pathways in the auditory system Only a few auditory pathways are shown here. Red and blue pathways indicate input from the left and right ears, respectively, and purple indicates integration of input from both ears. Although there are two parallel pathways, information from both ears comes together very early in the auditory system, at the superior olives. Cerebral processing of auditory information begins in the primary auditory cortex, or A1 (see Figure 9.21).

side of the brain. Thus, unlike the visual system, where inputs from each visual field remain separate until they have extended a fair distance in the visual cortex, signals from both cochleas reach both sides of the brain after only a single synapse. As we will see in Chapter 10, this direct relay of information across both ears is essential to using tiny differences between the two ears to detect the location of a sound.

Neurons from the cochlear nucleus and superior olive travel up the brainstem to the **inferior colliculus**. Most (but not all) of the input to each inferior colliculus comes from the opposite (contralateral) ear; that is, the *left* inferior colliculus listens mostly to the *right* ear, and vice versa.

The **medial geniculate nucleus** of the thalamus is the last stop in the auditory pathway before the cerebral cortex. Like the lateral geniculate of the visual system, there are many more neurons that project from the cortex to the medial geniculate (efferent neurons) than project from the medial geniculate to the cortex (afferent neurons). These efferent connections, some of which convey information back to lower stages of the auditory system, provide further anatomical evidence that sensory systems are two-way streets, in which feedback from the brain is tightly integrated with sensory information flowing up to the brain.

All structures of the auditory system, beginning with the basilar membrane and continuing through the cochlear nucleus, superior olive, inferior colliculus, and medial geniculate nucleus, show a consistent organizational pattern in which neurons are aligned based on the frequencies to which they are most sensitive. That is, neurons most responsive to low-frequency energy lie on one edge of each structure, neurons responding to high frequencies lie on the other edge, and

inferior colliculus A midbrain nucleus in the auditory pathway.

medial geniculate nucleus The part of the thalamus that relays auditory signals to the temporal cortex and receives input from the auditory cortex.

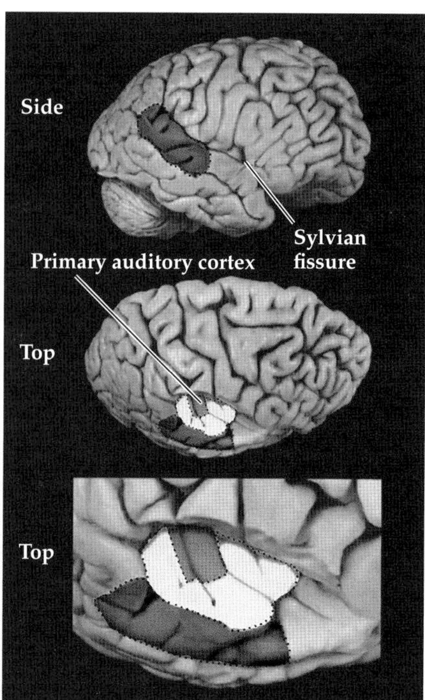

FIGURE 9.21 **Primary auditory cortex** The first stages of auditory processing begin in the temporal lobe of the cerebral cortex within the Sylvian fissure. The top picture is a side view of the brain's right hemisphere (the front of the brain faces right). The lower two pictures are looking down at the interior of the right hemisphere, with the parietal cortex cut away. Primary auditory cortex (A1) is surrounded by belt regions, and parabelt regions extend past the belt to the front and side. These belt regions are sometimes called secondary or associational auditory areas.

neurons responding to other frequencies are spread out in an orderly fashion in between. The pervasiveness of this **tonotopic organization** reflects both the early mechanical properties of the basilar membrane (with its narrow, thick base and wide, floppy apex coding frequency) and the importance of the frequency composition of sounds for auditory perception.

Primary auditory cortex is often referred to as **A1**, just as primary visual cortex is called V1. Tonotopic organization is maintained in A1, but its organization is a bit more complicated, with interdigitated "fingers" of high and low frequencies (Dick et al., 2017). Neurons from A1 project to the surrounding **belt area** of cortex, and neurons from this belt synapse with neurons in the adjacent **parabelt area** (FIGURE 9.21). Tonotopic organization is maintained in these higher auditory cortical regions, too. Just about any sound will cause activation in some part of A1. In the belt and parabelt areas, referred to as *secondary* or *associational auditory areas*, simple sounds such as sine waves elicit less activity, particularly if the stimuli don't change much over time. Thus, we see that, as in other sensory systems, processing proceeds from simpler to more complex stimuli as we move farther along the auditory pathway. We also find greater evidence of cross-modal processing (e.g., combining sound and light information), particularly in parabelt areas. ●

Comparing the overall structure of the auditory and visual systems shows that a relatively large proportion of auditory processing is done before A1. By contrast, as you learned in Chapter 3, the most important visual processing occurs in cortical areas V1 and beyond. We will return to the role of the cortex in auditory processing when we discuss speech and music perception in Chapter 11.

9.4 Psychoacoustics

Up to this point, we have discussed the anatomy of the auditory system and the physiology of how the system encodes the two basic physical attributes of sound waves: amplitude (intensity) and frequency. We've learned this through direct observation of anatomical structures. We turn now to the findings of researchers who have approached the auditory system from a different perspective. Instead of playing a sound and trying to determine how neurons respond, we can instead play the sound and ask human listeners—each of whom is the sum total of a great many neurons—what they hear. When humans are asked to report their auditory sensations, their answers are partly a result of the acoustic properties of the sound signal and partly a result of the sounds' psychological characteristics. This method of investigation is thus called **psychoacoustics**.

Psychoacousticians, scientists who study psychoacoustics, are always careful to distinguish between the physical characteristics of sounds and the impressions of these sounds for listeners. As we noted earlier, whereas frequency, measured in hertz, is a physical description of the spectral composition of a sound, the subjective attribute of frequency for listeners is *pitch*. Sounds are measured with respect to frequency, but listeners hear pitch. Similarly, the intensity of sound is measured as sound pressure in decibels, but listeners hear *loudness*. If the auditory system operated like an electronic measuring device, we could use the terms *frequency* and *pitch* and the terms *intensity* and *loudness* interchangeably. But biological auditory systems do not work exactly like electronic measuring devices. Two sounds with identical amplitude may be heard as having different loudness. Careful study of the differences between the responses of electronic devices that measure sound acoustics and human responses that measure psychological properties of sound provides insight into how the human auditory system works.

tonotopic organization An arrangement in which neurons that respond to different frequencies are organized anatomically in order of frequency.

primary auditory cortex (A1) The first area within the temporal lobes of the brain responsible for processing acoustic information.

belt area A region of cortex, directly adjacent to the primary auditory cortex (A1), with inputs from A1, where neurons respond to more complex characteristics of sounds.

parabelt area A region of cortex, lateral and adjacent to the belt area, where neurons respond to more complex characteristics of sounds, as well as to input from other senses.

Intensity and Loudness

The bottom curve in FIGURE 9.22 shows the human **audibility threshold**, which graphs the lowest sound pressure level that can be reliably detected across the frequency range of human hearing (20–20,000 Hz). Note that the best (lowest) absolute thresholds for human hearing are between 2000 and 6000 Hz (2–6 kilohertz). Remember that these frequencies are enhanced by the physical properties of the ear canal. Thresholds rise on both sides of this range, meaning that higher- and lower-frequency sound waves must have larger amplitudes to be heard.

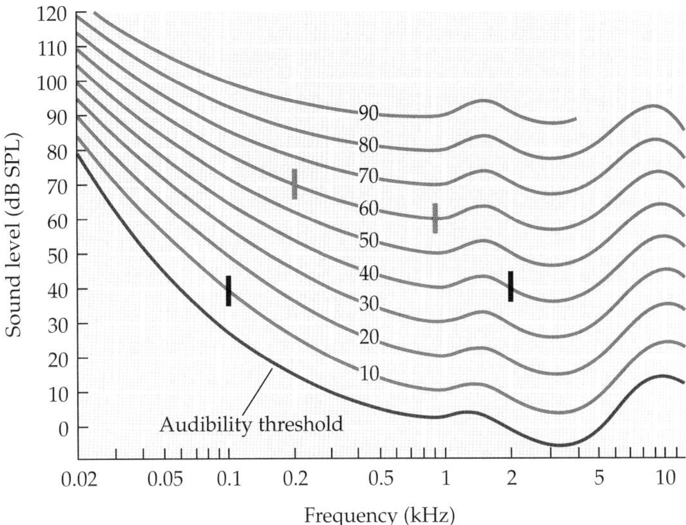

FIGURE 9.22 Equal-loudness curves The lowest curve (red) illustrates the threshold for hearing sounds at varying frequencies. The curves labeled 10, 20, 30, and so on are equal-loudness curves. For a single contour, tones of different frequencies have different physical intensities, but they sound equally loud. Thus, the two orange tick marks indicate that a 200 Hz tone presented at 70 dB sounds about as loud as a 900 Hz tone presented at 60 dB (that is, both points fall on the equal-loudness curve marked 60), whereas a 2000 Hz tone presented at 40 dB sounds much louder than a 100 Hz tone presented at the same level (black tick marks). SPL, sound pressure level.

The other lines in Figure 9.22 are **equal-loudness curves** (Suzuki and Takeshima, 2004). We obtain these curves by asking listeners to equate the loudness of sounds with different frequencies. The starting point for each curve is always 1000 Hz, so the curve marked 40 shows the amplitude necessary to make tones at other frequencies sound exactly as loud as a 1000 Hz, 40 dB tone; the curve marked 60 represents the decibel levels necessary to match a 1000 Hz, 60 dB tone, and so on. As Figure 9.22 shows, the same pattern of frequency-dependent sensitivity that we see in the audibility threshold curve extends to sounds above threshold. These observations demonstrate that physical sound pressure level is not one and the same as loudness: equal-amplitude sounds can be perceived as softer or louder than each other, depending on the frequencies of the sound waves. Doubling the perceived loudness of a sound requires more than a doubling in the amount of acoustic energy present in a sound wave, especially above 40 dB. The same kind of relationship holds in vision: the number of photons must be more than doubled to double the perceived brightness of a light.

The loudness of a sound also depends on its duration. Within limits, longer sounds are heard as being louder. Again, the same thing happens in vision: flashes of light appear brighter when they last longer. The reason for this general phenomenon is that the perception of loudness or brightness depends on the summation of energy over a brief, but noticeable, period of time—a process called **temporal integration.** For hearing, temporal integration occurs over an interval of 100 to 200 ms. So, if a sound is presented for less than 100 ms, it will be perceived as softer than a sound with the same amplitude and frequency presented for 200 ms. However, there will be little difference in loudness perception if the duration of the sound is increased from 300 to 1000 ms or longer.

In addition to studying absolute loudness judgments, psychoacousticians are interested in how well humans discriminate between loudness levels of two sounds. There are several ways to measure the smallest differences in intensity that can be detected, and many measures show sensitivity to changes of less than 1 dB. This ability is quite impressive, given the wide range of sound intensities (from 0 to over 100 dB) that humans can perceive and the fact that, unlike the visual system, the auditory system is always sensitive to this entire range. (We will see in Chapter 10 how the auditory system uses differences between the intensity levels of sounds reaching the left and right ears to determine *where* sound sources are located.)

psychoacoustics The branch of psychophysics that studies the psychological correlates of the physical dimensions of acoustics in order to understand how the auditory system operates.

audibility threshold The lowest sound pressure level that can be reliably detected at a given frequency.

equal-loudness curve A graph plotting sound pressure level against the frequency for which a listener perceives constant loudness.

temporal integration The process by which a sound at a constant level is perceived as being louder when it is of greater duration. The term also applies to perceived brightness, which depends on the duration of light.

Scientists at Work

Why Don't Manatees Get out of the Way When a Boat Is Coming?

Question Manatees, also known as sea cows (**FIGURE 9.23A**), are loved by children and adults alike. Sadly, about 100 manatees are killed each year when they are struck by motorboats. Why is it that manatees cannot seem to hear boat motors and get out of the way?

Hypothesis Manatees either do not hear very well or cannot hear the particular sounds made by boat motors.

Test Train manatees to listen for sounds at different frequencies and respond when they hear (or do not hear) a sound (Gerstein, 2002) (**FIGURE 9.23B**).

Results Manatees have quite good hearing, generally better than that of humans underwater. Manatees, however, are not very good at hearing low frequencies (**FIGURE 9.23C**).

Conclusion Laws that require boaters to slow down in manatee zones result in motors running slower and producing softer sounds with lower frequencies. This may not have the desired effect of saving manatees. To the contrary, creating lower-frequency sounds is a good way to sneak up on a manatee without being heard.

Future work Driving boats faster is not a solution, because even if the manatees can hear faster boats better, they still need time to get out of the way. Instead, boats should have manatee alerting devices that project a band of sound in front of the boats as they move, and this sound should comprise one or more of the higher frequencies that manatees hear very well (Florida Atlantic University, 2017).

(A)

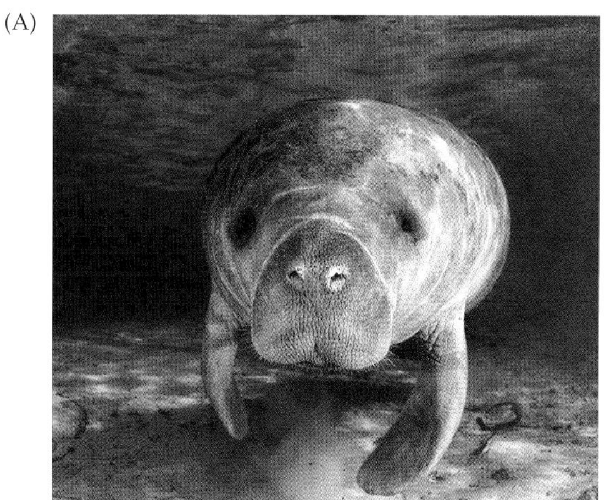

(B)

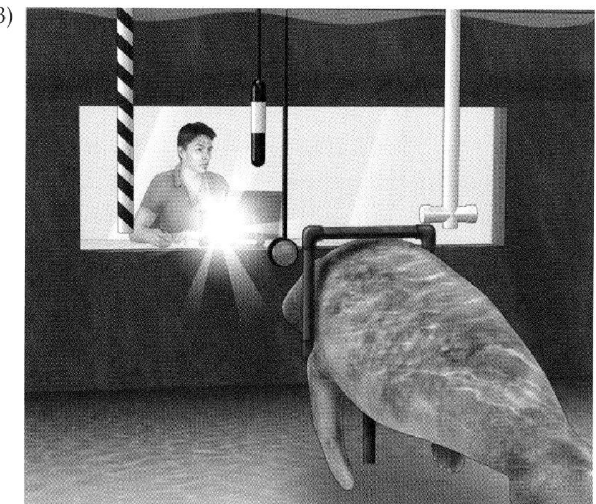

(C)

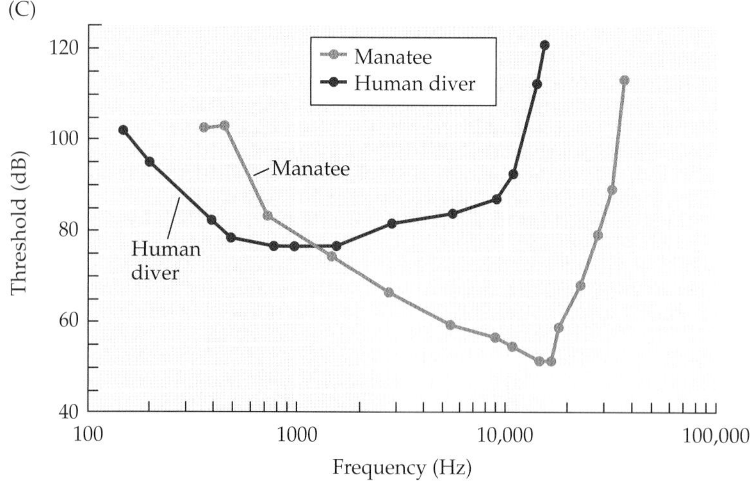

FIGURE 9.23 Manatee hearing The hearing of a manatee (A) can be tested in a special underwater setup (B) and compared with human hearing (C).

For a time, it was difficult to understand how listeners could be sensitive to such small differences in loudness over such a large range. Sound wave intensity is generally signaled by the firing rate of AN fibers: larger intensities (loud sounds) correspond to higher firing rates, and smaller intensities (quiet sounds) correspond to lower firing rates. You should recall that the intensities required to fire (the thresholds) vary from one AN fiber to the next. For example, one fiber might selectively respond to the range of amplitudes between 0 and 25 dB, another might span the range of 15–40 dB, a third might cover 38–65 dB, and so on (see Figure 9.17). A full population of fibers with different thresholds can encode a much broader range of intensities than is possible with any single fiber. In addition, remember that fibers become responsive to a broader range of frequencies when intensity is higher (see Figure 9.16). One result is that, as sounds become more intense, more AN fibers respond.

Frequency and Pitch

The tonotopic organization of the auditory system, from basilar membrane to primary auditory cortex and beyond, is a very big hint that frequency composition is a fundamental determinant of how we hear sounds. More than anything else, psychoacousticians have studied how listeners perceive pitch, the psychological counterpart to frequency. As is the case with intensity and loudness, the frequency of a sound is related to, but not perfectly associated with, the perceived pitch of the sound. For any given frequency increase, say 50 Hz, listeners will perceive a greater rise in pitch for lower frequencies than they do for higher frequencies. Consequently, listeners perceive a greater pitch difference when a tone shifts from 500 to 1000 Hz than when a tone shifts from 4000 to 4500 Hz.

Research done using pure tones (each composed of a single sine wave) indicates that humans are remarkably good at detecting very small differences in frequency. For example, listeners can discriminate between tones of 1000 and 1001 Hz—a difference of only one-tenth of 1%! Frequency discrimination at the lower and higher ends of the auditory system's frequency range is not quite as good, but it is still impressive.

Psychoacousticians also use **masking** experiments to investigate frequency selectivity. In the research described in the previous paragraph, listeners always hear only one sound frequency at a time. In a masking experiment, multiple frequencies are combined, and we see how well listeners can pick out certain frequencies. We look at how effective one sound—the masker—is at hiding another sound.

In the classic approach to measuring frequency selectivity using masking, a single sine wave tone is placed in the middle of a band of acoustic noise (Fletcher, 1940). **White noise** is a signal that includes equal energy of every frequency in the human auditory range (20–20,000 Hz), just as white light includes light rays of all frequencies in the visible spectrum. A more limited band of noise might include all frequencies in the range of 1200–2800 Hz; an even smaller band could span 1900–2100 Hz.

In a typical experiment, we might start with a 2000 Hz sine wave test tone presented along with a very narrow 50 Hz band of noise—say, 1975–2025 Hz. We would then adjust the intensity of the test tone until listeners could just hear it over the noise. Next, we would increase the width of the noise, perhaps from 50 to 100 Hz, so that now the noise would include frequencies between 1950 and 2050 Hz. As we might expect, the intensity of the test tone must be increased for listeners to be able to hear it over this broader range of noise frequencies.

If we keep widening the width of the noise, however, we will eventually reach a point at which adding more frequencies to the noise stops affecting the detectability of the test tone. The size of the noise band at this point is called the

masking Using a second sound, frequently noise, to make the detection of another sound more difficult.

white noise Noise consisting of all audible frequencies in equal amounts. White noise in hearing is analogous to white light in vision, for which all wavelengths are present.

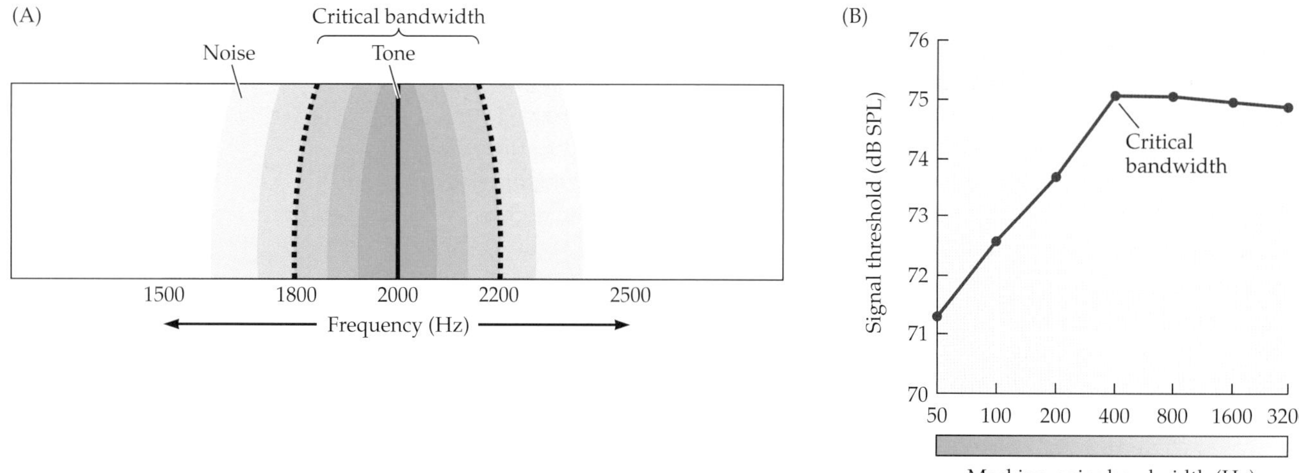

FIGURE 9.24 Critical bandwidth and masking (A) To measure the width of a critical band, participants listen for a tone in the center of a band of noise of constant intensity. It is harder to detect the tone as the band of noise widens up to a point, after which further widening has no effect on detecting the tone. This point defines the critical bandwidth. (B) For this plot of bandwidth data, a 2000 Hz tone was used. The bandwidth of the noise had no effect on detection of the tone when it exceeded 400 Hz, so 400 Hz is the width of the critical band at 2000 Hz. SPL, sound pressure level.

critical bandwidth (**FIGURE 9.24A**). For the experimental data plotted in **FIGURE 9.24B**, the critical bandwidth is 400 Hz. In this case, to pick out a 2000 Hz tone from the background noise, listeners must increase the intensity of the tone when the bandwidth is widened from 50 to 100 Hz and from 200 to 400 Hz. But going from a 400 Hz noise band to an 800 Hz band does *not* require the listener to make the test tone any louder. In fact, the 400 Hz noise band is just as effective a masker as white noise covering the entire spectrum of human hearing.

Results from the masking paradigm have helped cement the role of place coding in pitch perception by revealing similarities between perceptual effects and biological findings. First, the width of the critical bandwidth changes depending on the frequency of the test tone, and these widths correspond to the physical spacing of frequencies along the basilar membrane. For example, we know that a greater proportion of the basilar membrane vibrates in response to low frequencies, and higher frequencies vibrate smaller portions of the membrane. Correspondingly, masking studies show that the critical bandwidths for low frequencies are smaller than the critical bandwidths for high frequencies because the spacing between low frequencies is larger on the basilar membrane.

Another important finding is that masking effects are asymmetrical. Masking sounds at frequencies lower than the test tone are more effective—a phenomenon called the *upward spread of masking*. This phenomenon may seem counterintuitive, but a look back at Figure 9.12 shows how displacement of the basilar membrane (the traveling wave) extends from the high-frequency base to the low-frequency apex. Displacement for low-frequency sounds toward the apex leaves a trail of displacement across high-frequency regions toward the base.

9.5 Hearing Loss

critical bandwidth The range of frequencies conveyed within a channel in the auditory system.

Roughly 30 million Americans, 1 in every 8 people, experience hearing impairment. When we talk about hearing loss, we typically do not mean the total loss of hearing (deafness), but rather the elevation of sound thresholds. For example, frequencies that once were audible at 20 dB may become inaudible unless they are presented at 40 or 60 dB. Of course, in the end, we do not just need to detect sounds; the term *hearing* really refers to using spectral and temporal differences between sounds to learn about and react to events going on in the environment.

Hearing can be impaired by damage to any of the structures along the chain of auditory processing, from the outer ear all the way up to the auditory cortex. As we describe the most common forms of hearing loss, you will have the opportunity to review much of what you have learned in this chapter.

conductive hearing loss Hearing loss caused by problems with the bones of the middle ear.

otitis media Inflammation of the middle ear, common in children as a result of infection.

otosclerosis Abnormal growth of the middle-ear bones that causes hearing loss.

sensorineural hearing loss Hearing loss caused by defects in the cochlea or auditory nerve.

metabolic hearing loss Hearing loss caused by degraded ability of the stria vascularis to provide sufficient nutrients and ions to the cochlear partition.

Types of Hearing Loss

The simplest way to introduce hearing loss is to obstruct the ear canal, thus inhibiting the ability of sound waves to exert pressure on the tympanic membrane. Many people do this on purpose by wearing earplugs. A less intentional hearing loss can be created by the excessive buildup of earwax (cerumen) in the ear canal. This problem is easy for clinicians to remedy, so long as the effort to clear out the ear canal does not damage the tympanic membrane.

Another type of hearing impairment, called **conductive hearing loss**, occurs when the middle-ear bones lose (or are impaired in) their ability to freely convey (conduct) vibrations from the tympanic membrane to the oval window. Because you now know how the bones in the middle ear work, you understand why this is sometimes to referred to as *mechanical loss*. Such impairment occurs most often when the middle ear fills with mucus during ear infections—a condition known as **otitis media**. The oval window usually still vibrates under these conditions, but without the amplifying power of the ossicles, hearing thresholds can be elevated such that sounds need to be 50 dB louder to be heard. Thankfully for the millions of young children who suffer ear infections, normal hearing returns after mucus is absorbed back into surrounding tissues; however, this reabsorption can take up to several months. A more serious type of conductive loss, **otosclerosis**, is caused by abnormal growth of the middle-ear bones, most typically around the oval window next to the stapes. Surgery can free the stapes from these bone growths and improve hearing.

By far the most common, and most serious, form of auditory impairment is **sensorineural hearing loss**, which most commonly occurs inside the cochlea and sometimes is the result of damage to the AN. We can begin by dividing sensorineural loss into the first and second halves of *sensorineural*. "Sensory loss" refers to the injury and loss of hair cells, mostly outer hair cells. (Refer back to Figure 9.14 to see the effects of losing outer hair cells.) As a result, AN responses are decreased and less selective for frequency. Damage to inner hair cells also occurs. With fewer inner hair cells, the neuronal firing pattern described by the volley principle for temporal coding of frequency would become more difficult to maintain, because there would be fewer neurons available to take turns firing (Sayles and Heinz, 2017).

"Neural loss" is the actual loss of AN fibers. This is a significant part of hearing loss resulting from aging, because a little more than 2000 auditory nerve cells are lost every decade. Thank goodness that we begin with around 35,000.

In recent years, we have learned much more about a third major component to sensorineural loss; this **metabolic hearing loss** is caused by the stria vascularis (see Figure 9.9) losing its ability to perform its job of bathing the cochlear partition with sufficient nutrients and ions (Dubno et al., 2013; Vaden et al., 2017). Hair cell activity decreases as a result of their surrounding fluid being compromised.

Causes of Hearing Loss

A major cause of sensorineural hearing loss is damage to the hair cells by excessive noise exposure (Eggermont, 2017). Those exquisitely fast and sensitive hair cells are very vulnerable to damage from excessive sound levels. It is no coincidence that so many aging rock stars (including Dave Grohl of Nirvana and the Foo Fighters) and race car drivers (including Richard Petty) suffer hearing loss. It is a wise and important trend that more people who work with loud sounds or enjoy loud music at concerts are wearing ear protection. Unfortunately, it is not yet possible to state exactly how much exposure to sounds is safe. Readers of this textbook are especially likely to become the listeners from whom we learn what levels are unsafe. This is because of the increasing use of earbuds delivering sounds directly to eardrums. Right now, there is extensive debate concerning the contribution of these devices to hearing loss, in part because consequences may be years down the road. At present, we know that use of earbuds and hearing loss are related (Ivory, Kane, and Diaz, 2014). It is always wise to listen at a safe level, with the volume low.

Disorders such as diabetes as well as bacterial and viral infections can also cause sensorineural hearing loss (Eggermont, 2017). For some people, hearing loss can be present at birth, or it can appear during adolescence or early adulthood and progressively worsen over one or more decades. Over 150 different genes have been linked to hereditary hearing loss in humans.

Hearing loss is a natural consequence of aging for many people, and it is difficult to separate a person's age from the amount of exposure to noise. Age-related hearing loss is called **presbycusis** (also spelled presbyacusis, from Greek *presbys* "old" + *akousis* "hearing"), and on average, it is more severe in men than in women. Typically, age-related hearing loss first affects the perception of high frequencies (**FIGURE 9.25**). The 20–20,000 Hz frequency range for human hearing really applies only to young people; by the time most of us reach college age, we may have already

presbycusis Age-related hearing loss.

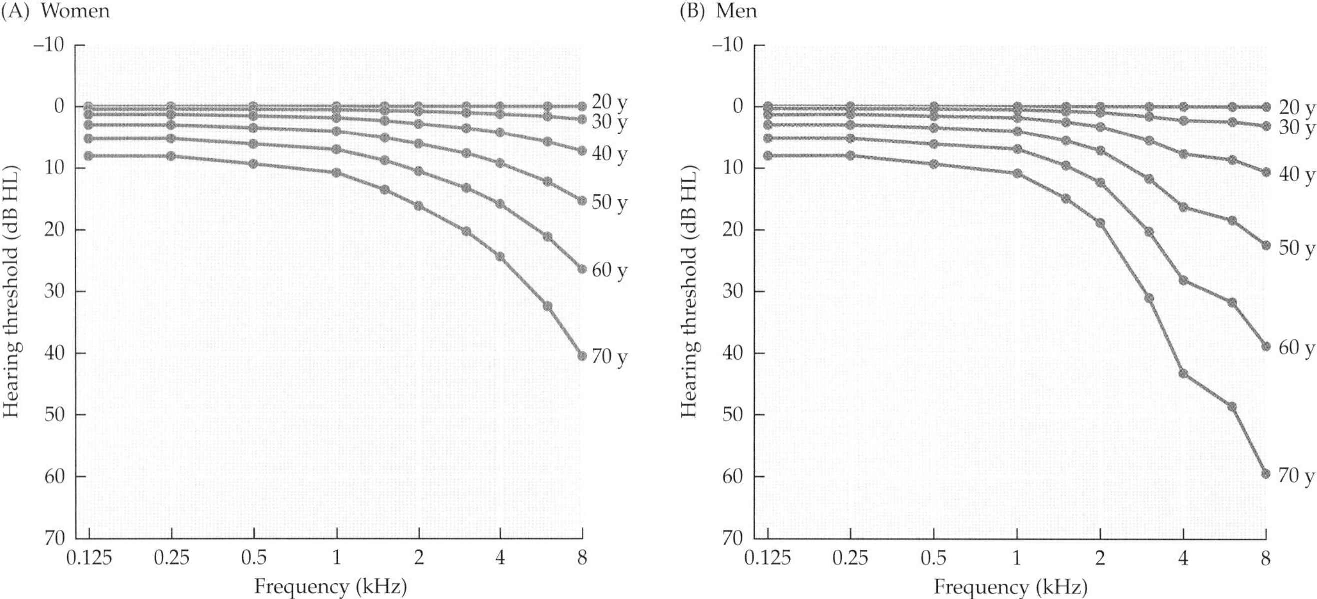

FIGURE 9.25 Presbycusis In general, hearing sensitivity decreases as people age. This decrease begins with higher frequencies and affects men more severely than women.

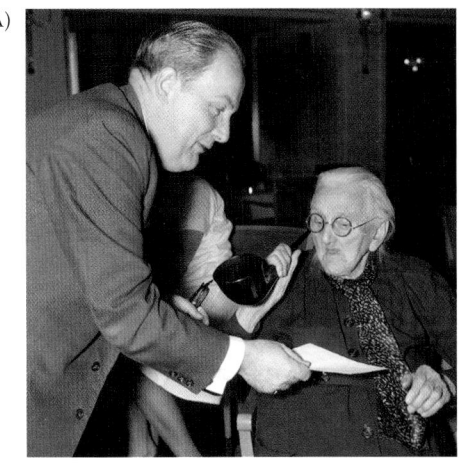

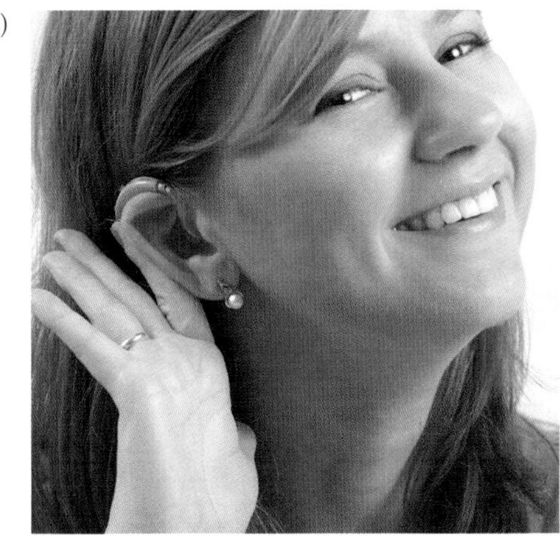

FIGURE 9.26 Hearing aids (A) The first hearing aids were "ear trumpets" or "ear horns" that funnelled more sound into the ear than a normal pinna and permitted listeners to direct the device to the source that they wished to hear. (B) Modern hearing aids are much less conspicuous and can be tuned to an individual's specific hearing loss.

lost some ability to hear frequencies above 15,000 Hz. The decrease in the ability to hear higher-frequency sounds continues throughout life, with the highest audible frequency becoming lower and lower as we grow older. Fortunately, many of the sounds that people care most about, including speech and music, are composed predominantly of lower frequencies.

Treating Hearing Loss

The earliest devices for helping people with hearing loss were simple horns. The small end of the horn would be held at the entry to the ear canal, and the wide end would be used to funnel more acoustic energy toward the listener's ear (**FIGURE 9.26A**). Although effective, these horns were obviously cumbersome. Electronic hearing aids are much more convenient (**FIGURE 9.26B**), but they must be designed to do more than simply amplify all sounds, because extremely loud sounds (above 100 dB) are just as annoying (or painful) for impaired listeners as they are for listeners with normal hearing. For a person who cannot hear sounds until their intensity is at least 70 dB, compared with about 0 dB for healthy hearing, sounds that could normally vary between 0 and 100 dB must be squeezed between 70 and 100 dB (**FIGURE 9.27**). All quality hearing aids use some means to amplify the signal while also compressing intensity differences to keep the highest intensities within a comfortable listening level.

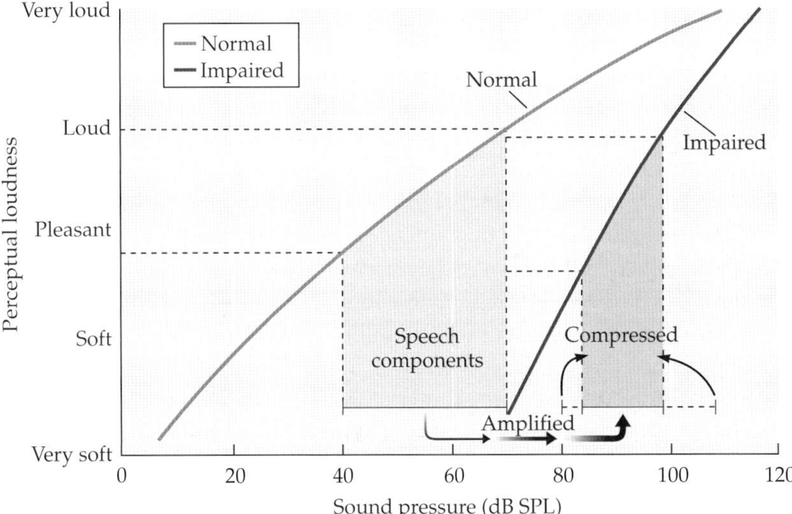

FIGURE 9.27 Modern hearing aids compress sound levels When hearing thresholds are increased by impairment, a sound must have more energy to be heard, but loudness increases faster than it does with healthy ears. When a hearing aid is used to increase the intensity of sounds, all variation in sound levels must be compressed into a smaller range of intensity because very loud sounds can be just as painful for listeners with hearing impairment as they are for listeners with healthy hearing.

Hearing aids are typically tuned to provide the greatest amplification only for frequencies in the region of greatest loss (for most people, higher frequencies will need greater amplification). An additional method is to move energy from frequency regions in which hearing is poor (usually high frequencies) into regions where hearing is normal (Alexander, 2016). Because the lower-frequency region is already being used for lower-frequency sounds, this strategy requires squeezing together some lower-frequency sounds to make room for the high-frequency sound that is being moved down.

One advantage of the old horns over electronic hearing aids was that they permitted listeners to direct their hearing toward the sound source they were most interested in. We may think about hearing aids as amplifying the voice to which one is listening, but they also amplify all the other sounds in the environment. The background noise in a car, or even the sound of a refrigerator, can become loud enough to compete with the sound of a person's voice. When the entire range of hearing is compressed from a range of 100 dB to only 30 dB, a 10 dB difference between the rumbling of the car's engine and the voice of the person in the passenger seat becomes compressed into only a 3 dB difference.

Hearing aids are always improving, and they have provided relief to millions of Americans. However, despite researchers' many clever innovations for improving the signal that arrives at the tympanic membrane, damage to the mechanisms that transduce sound waves into neural signals is proving difficult or impossible to overcome completely. By analogy to vision, the best eyeglasses, contact lenses, or even laser surgery cannot change an image enough to overcome retinal degeneration. The best advice is to protect your ears by avoiding exposure to loud sounds and using hearing protection such as earplugs or earmuffs when necessary. If someone else can sing along to the song you're listening to on over your earbuds, turn it down!

Using versus Detecting Sound

Even the best hearing aids serve mostly to amplify sounds for frequencies where thresholds are elevated by the hearing loss. However, the ability to detect sounds is not the same as the ability to listen to and use sounds. The audiogram, our measure of the softest detectable tones at different frequencies, is not a perfect predictor of listeners' abilities to *use* sounds. Understanding speech or enjoying music, especially when there is background noise, can be good with poor audiograms and weak with normal audiograms.

A great deal of recent research activity concerns what is called **hidden hearing loss**. Research from nonhuman animal models, like mice, is demonstrating that even brief periods of exposure to loud noise can result in a loss of synapses between AN fibers and hair cells (**FIGURE 9.28**). Unlike damage to hair cells, which results in decreased sensitivity, loss of synapses with AN fibers results in a loss of connectivity to the brain. It has been hypothesized that this hidden hearing loss might explain some of the difficulties that human listeners have in noisy situations even when their audiograms are normal (Bharadwaj et al., 2014). Unfortunately, improving a person's ability to *detect* sounds is unlikely to improve the ability of people with hidden hearing loss to *process* and *use* sounds effectively.

hidden hearing loss A recently described auditory disorder associated with loss of synapses between hair cells and AN fibers, disrupting connectivity to the brain

Before noise exposure

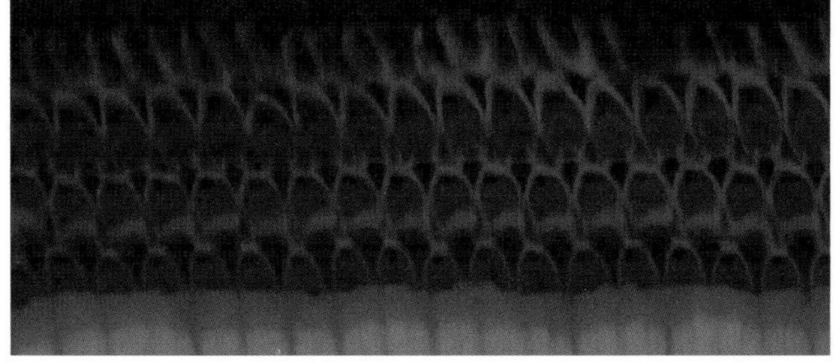

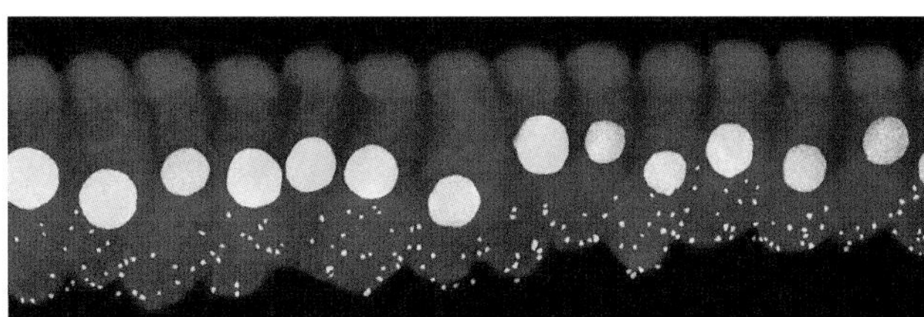

After noise exposure

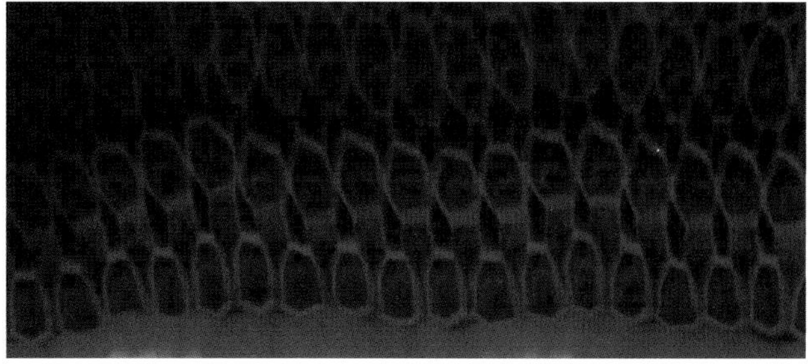

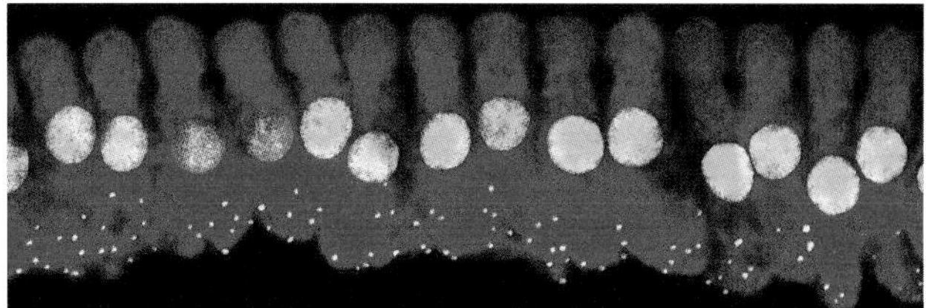

FIGURE 9.28 **Hidden hearing loss** Following exposure to loud sounds, listeners can have difficulty using sounds even when hair cells appear to be undamaged. This is because some of the synapses between hair cells and neurons in the auditory nerve are lost, resulting in a breakdown of connectivity between the signal and its processing by the brain's auditory cortex. The top (purple) photos are of healthy hair cells before and after exposure to noise. The bottom photos show synapses highlighted as small yellow dots, with more yellow dots indicating greater numbers of synapses. There are fewer synapses following noise exposure (right) compared to before noise exposure.

Sensation & Perception in Everyday Life

Electronic Ears

Modern medical science and engineering are providing some degree of hearing to many people who are deaf. Cochlear prosthetics, more commonly known as cochlear implants (**FIGURE 9.29A**), are tiny flexible coils with about two dozen miniature electrode contacts along their length. Surgeons delicately thread these electrode arrays through the round window as far toward the apex of the cochlea as possible. The electrode array is connected to a tiny radio receiver under the scalp, and signals are transmitted from a small microphone device on the outside of the head behind the ear (**FIGURE 9.29B**). Signals coming in from the microphone activate the miniature electrodes at appropriate positions along the cochlear implant, which in turn stimulates associated AN fibers.

Although cochlear implants are a modern medical miracle, the quality of hearing they provide cannot approach what nature provides. We should not be surprised, however, that a handful of electrodes cannot replace the function of 14,000 hair cells. Some people benefit more than others from implants, and many adults with electrical hearing converse flawlessly over the phone. Children receiving implants as young as 1 or 2 years of age do best of all, because young brains are particularly plastic. Children's brain circuitry develops to get the most information possible from their electronic ears.

(Continued)

Sensation & Perception in Everyday Life *(continued)*

(A)

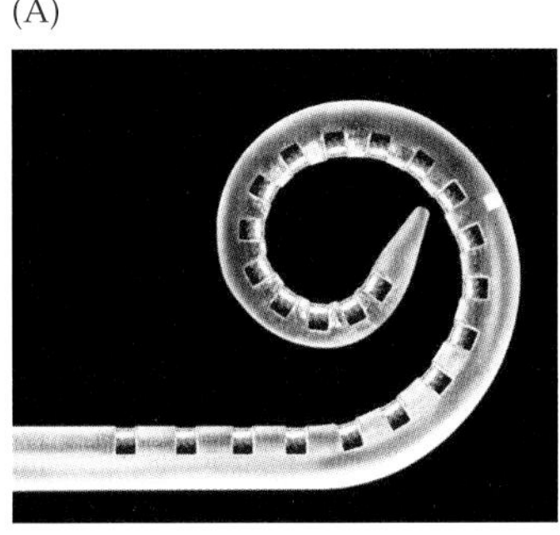

(B)

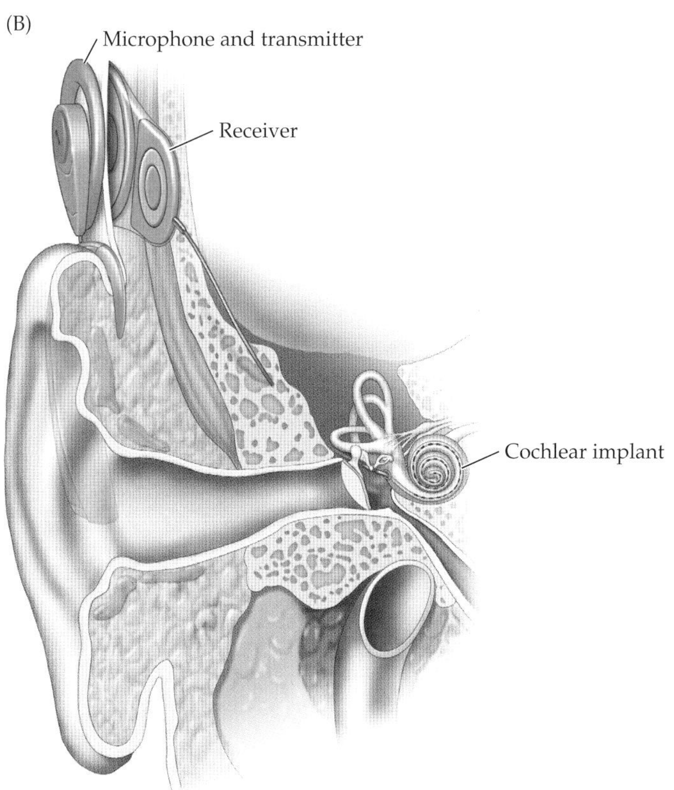

FIGURE 9.29 Cochlear prosthetics (A) A cochlear implant's flexible array of electrodes is inserted through the round window as far as possible toward the apex of the cochlea. (B) The electrode array is connected to a small receiver beneath the scalp, and a small microphone and transmitter are placed over the receiver on the outside of the head.

Summary

1. Sounds are fluctuations of pressure. Sound waves are defined by the frequency, intensity (amplitude), and phase of fluctuations. Sound frequency and intensity correspond to our perceptions of pitch and loudness, respectively.
2. Sound is funneled into the ear by the outer ear, made more intense by the middle ear, and transformed into neural signals by the inner ear.
3. In the inner ear, cilia on the tops of inner hair cells pivot in response to pressure fluctuations in ways that provide information about frequency and intensity to the auditory nerve and the brain. Auditory nerve fibers convey information through both the rate and the timing patterns with which they fire.

4. Different characteristics of sounds are processed at multiple places in the brainstem before information reaches the cortex. Information from both ears is brought together very early in the chain of processing. At each stage of auditory processing, including primary auditory cortex, neurons are organized in relation to the frequencies of sounds (tonotopically).
5. Humans and other mammals can hear sounds across an enormous range of intensities. Not all sound frequencies are heard as being equally loud, however. Hearing across such a wide range of intensities is accomplished by the use of many auditory neurons. Different neurons respond to different levels of intensity. In addition, more neurons overall respond when sounds are more intense.
6. Series of channels (or filters) process sounds within bands of frequency. Depending on frequency, these channels vary in how wide (many frequencies) or narrow they are. Consequently, it is easier to detect differences between some frequencies than between others. When energy from multiple frequencies is present, lower-frequency energy makes it relatively more difficult to hear higher frequencies.
7. Hearing loss is caused by damage to the bones of the middle ear, to hair cells in the cochlea, to neurons in the auditory nerve, or to the stria vascularis that provides nourishment and ions to the hair cells. Although hearing aids are helpful to listeners with hearing impairment, there is only so much that can be done to help when damage to hair cells cannot be repaired.

Chapter 10

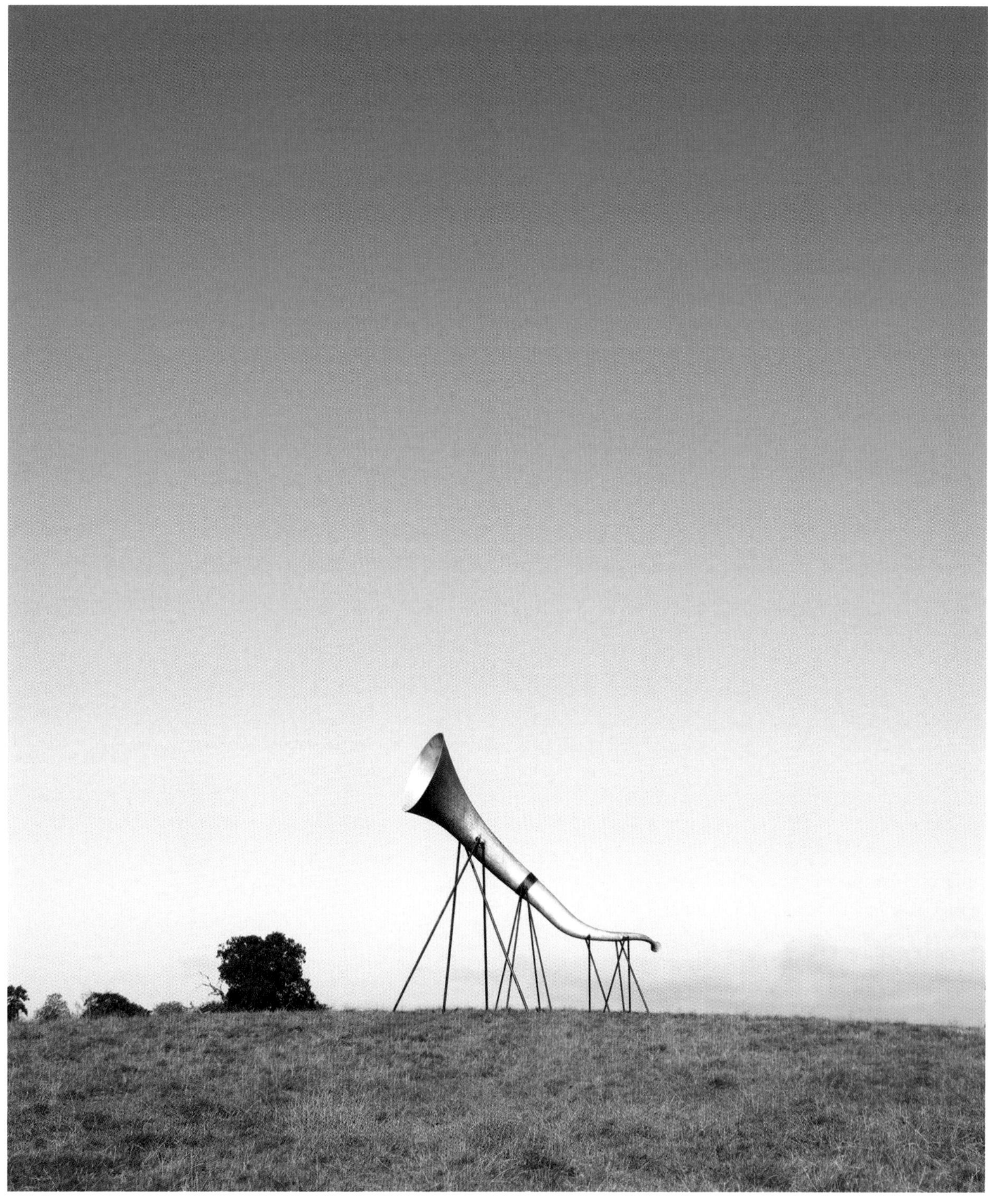

Studio Weave, Listening to the Sounds of the Sky, 2013

Hearing in the Environment

Questions to Contemplate

Think about the following questions as you read this chapter.
By the chapter's end, you should be able to answer and discuss them.

- How does your auditory system use tiny differences in time, amplitude, and frequency to make you aware of your world?
- How do we define the characteristics of complex natural sounds on which you depend the most?
- How can you separate the many sounds in your environment when they all overlap one another when entering your ears?

The auditory system's ability to transform tiny air pressure changes into a rich perceptual world is a wonder of evolution. From the funneling of sound waves by the pinnae, to the mechanics of middle-ear bones, to the traveling wave creating tiny perturbations of the basilar partition and hair cells, to the sophisticated neural encoding in the brainstem and cerebral cortex, some remarkable mechanisms have evolved to interpret acoustic information about the world around us.

Much of what we know about these inner workings of the auditory system comes from studying simple sounds in constrained listening contexts. Although these methods are valuable for understanding how the auditory system functions, this is obviously not the way we experience sounds in our daily lives. In this chapter, we investigate how hearing helps us learn about the real world.

We start by looking at how it is possible to determine the location of a sound. In many respects, sound localization parallels visual depth perception, which you learned about in Chapter 6. We next turn from *where* to *what*: how perceptual aspects of complex sounds are composed of simpler sounds in much the same way that visual representations of objects are built up from simple features (see Chapter 4). The third part of the chapter deals with auditory scene analysis, where we will see why some sounds group together while separating from others, in ways that resemble the Gestalt principles introduced in Chapter 4. We will see how the auditory system seamlessly fills in gaps to form a complete and coherent "picture" of our auditory environment in an auditory analog of how the visual system deals with occlusion (see Section 6.1). Finally, we explore how auditory attention has much in common with the visual attention that you learned about in Chapter 7, while also serving a special role in keeping us vigilant for surprises in the world.

10.1 Sound Localization

Suppose you were camping in your local state park one mild summer night, enjoying the last embers of a campfire, when an owl hoots. You might be startled, or you may turn your head toward the owl without even thinking about it. You would instantly know whether the owl was perched to the left, to the right, or directly behind the

interaural time difference (ITD) The difference in time between arrivals of sound at one ear versus the other.

fire pit. Moreover, if you were willing to leave the comfort of the fire, and if the owl were cooperative enough to sit still and keep hooting, you could easily walk to the exact location of the sound even though you wouldn't be able to see the owl until you were very close to it (and maybe not even then).

When you think about it, you will realize that our ability to locate a sound source is quite different from locating a visual object. If you could see the owl in front of you, you would know that it was to the left or the right of your fovea because its image would appear on the right or left side of your retina (**FIGURE 10.1**). But the owl's hoots enter your ears in exactly the same place (funneled through the pinnae into the middle and inner ear), regardless of where the owl is.

You may recall that we face a similar dilemma in determining the distance of a visual object. As we learned in Chapter 6, visual depth perception involves processing and integrating a set of cues that provide indirect evidence about how far away an object is. The auditory system uses a similar approach to determine a sound's location in space.

Having two eyes turns out to be important for determining visual depth perception. And having two ears is critical to determining auditory location. For most positions in space, a sound source will be closer to one ear than to the other. A sound coming from your left will be closer to your left ear than your right ear. Thus, there are two types of information (**FIGURE 10.2**). First, even though sound travels fast, the sound pressure waves do not arrive at both ears at the same time. Sounds arrive *very slightly* sooner at the ear closer to the source. Second, the intensity of a sound is greater at the ear closer to the source. These are our first two auditory localization cues.

Interaural Time Difference

Let's first consider what we can learn from the **interaural** (between ear) **time difference** (**ITD**). If the source is to the left, the sound will reach the left ear first. If it's to the right, it will reach the right ear first. Thus, we can tell whether a

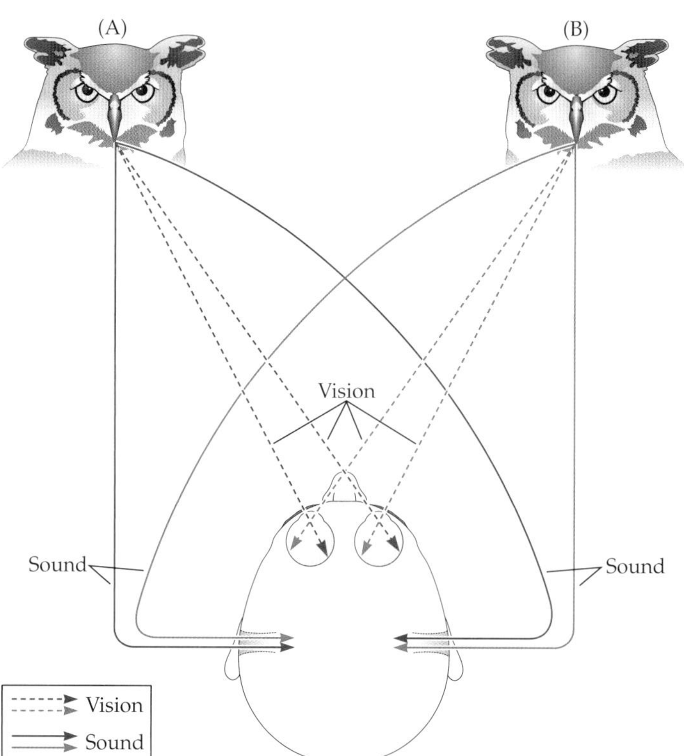

FIGURE 10.1 Eyes and ears The position of the owl is easily encoded by the visual system because the owl's image falls on different parts of the retina (and thus activates different receptors) depending on whether it is to the left (A) or to the right (B) of the observer. In the auditory system, however, the same receptors are activated regardless of the owl's position.

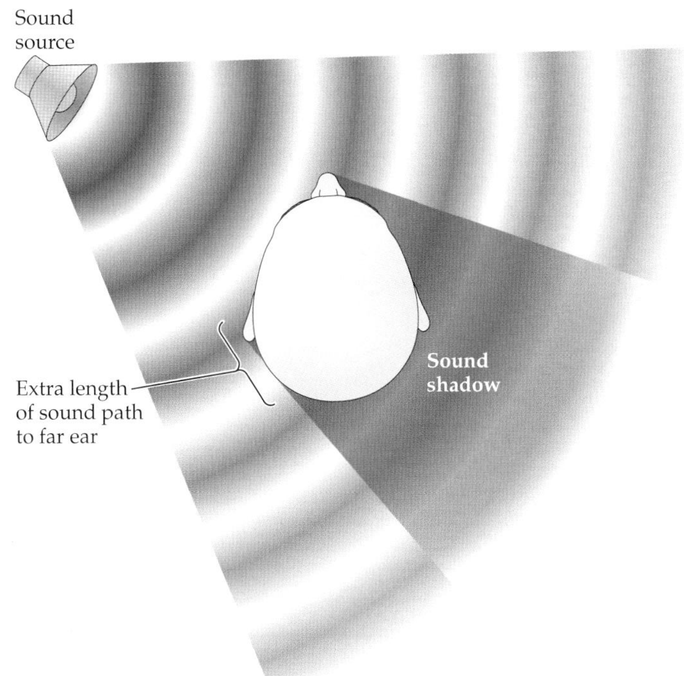

FIGURE 10.2 Two different inputs The two ears receive slightly different inputs when the sound source is located to one side or the other. For frequencies greater than 1000 Hz, the head blocks some of the energy from reaching the opposite ear, creating a sound shadow.

sound is coming from our right or left by determining which ear receives the sound first.

The term that is used to describe locations on an imaginary circle extending around us in a horizontal plane—front, back, left, and right—is **azimuth** (**FIGURE 10.3**). Which azimuth locations produce no ITD? Which would produce the maximum ITDs? Figure 10.3 illustrates the answers to these questions. The ITDs for sounds coming from various angles are represented by colored circles. Red circles indicate positions from which a sound will reach the right ear before the left ear; blue circles show positions from which a sound will reach the left ear first. The size and brightness of each circle represent the magnitude of the ITD.

azimuth The angle of a sound source on the horizontal plane relative to a point in the center of the head between the ears. Azimuth is measured in degrees, with 0 degrees being straight ahead. The angle increases clockwise toward the right, with 180 degrees being directly behind.

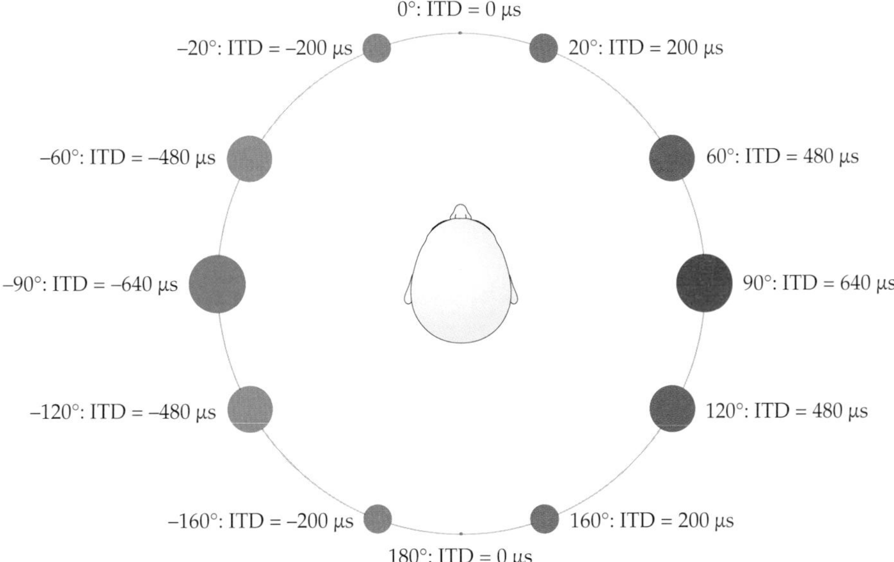

FIGURE 10.3 Interaural time differences (ITDs) along the azimuth ITDs are shown for different azimuth positions encircling the head. Blue indicates locations from which sound reaches the left ear first; red indicates locations from which sound reaches the right ear first. The size and brightness of each circle represent the magnitude of the ITD. (Data from W. E. Fedderson et al. 1957. *J Acoust Soc Am* 29: 988–991.)

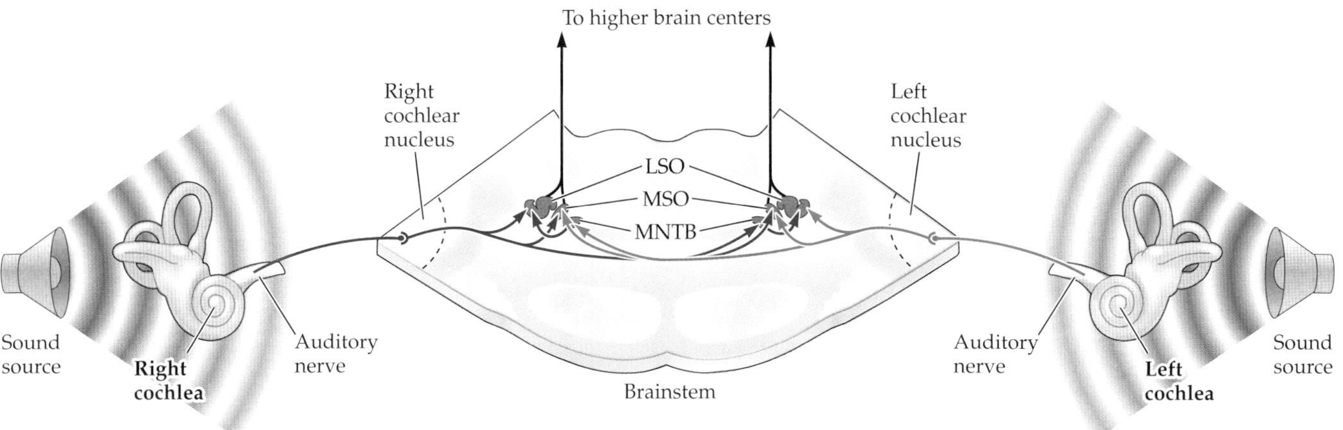

FIGURE 10.4 Brain circuits for localization After only a single synapse in the cochlear nucleus, information from each ear travels to both the medial superior olive (MSO) and the lateral superior olive (LSO) on each side of the brainstem. The medial nucleus of the trapezoid body (MNTB) generates inhibitory inputs from the ear on the opposite side of the head (the contralateral ear).

As Figure 10.3 shows, ITDs are largest—about 640 microseconds (millionths of a second, abbreviated μs)—when sounds come directly from the left or directly from the right, although this value varies depending on the size of your head. A sound coming from directly in front of or directly behind the head produces an ITD of 0; that is, the sound reaches both ears simultaneously. For intermediate locations, the ITD will be somewhere between these two values. Thus, a sound source located at an angle of 60 degrees will produce an ITD of 480 μs, and a sound coming from –20 degrees will produce an ITD of –200 μs. That might not seem like much of a time difference, but listeners can detect ITDs of as little as 10 μs for tones around 1000 hertz (Hz) (Brughera, Dunai, and Hartman, 2013), which is good enough to detect the angle of a sound source to within 1 degree, a very slight change in sound location.

THE PHYSIOLOGY OF ITD The portion of the auditory system responsible for calculating ITDs obviously needs to receive input from both ears. As we saw in Chapter 9, input from both ears enters almost every stage of the auditory nervous system after the auditory nerve (see Figure 9.20). However, as information moves upward through the system, with every additional synapse the timing between the two ears is likely to become less precise. The **medial superior olives** (**MSOs**) in the brainstem are the first places in the auditory system where inputs from both ears converge (**FIGURE 10.4**), and sure enough, firing rates of neurons in the MSOs increase in response to very brief time differences between inputs from the two ears (T. C. Yin and Chan, 1990).

How do these MSO neurons discover such tiny delays across the two ears? After all, a single action potential lasts about 1 millisecond (ms), and 10 μs is a mere 1/100 of 1 ms. Many years ago, Jeffress (1948) hypothesized an ingenious way this could be possible. If an array of inputs from both ears formed a "ladder," then small differences between the lengths of axons could provide a way to delay input from one ear compared with the other; inputs would arrive at the MSO at the same time only when input to one ear was delayed relative to the other (**FIGURE 10.5A**). Unfortunately, anatomical and physiological evidence for this clever idea has been elusive (Joris, Smith, and Yin, 1998), so most researchers have

medial superior olive (MSO) A relay station in the brainstem where inputs from both ears contribute to detection of the interaural time difference.

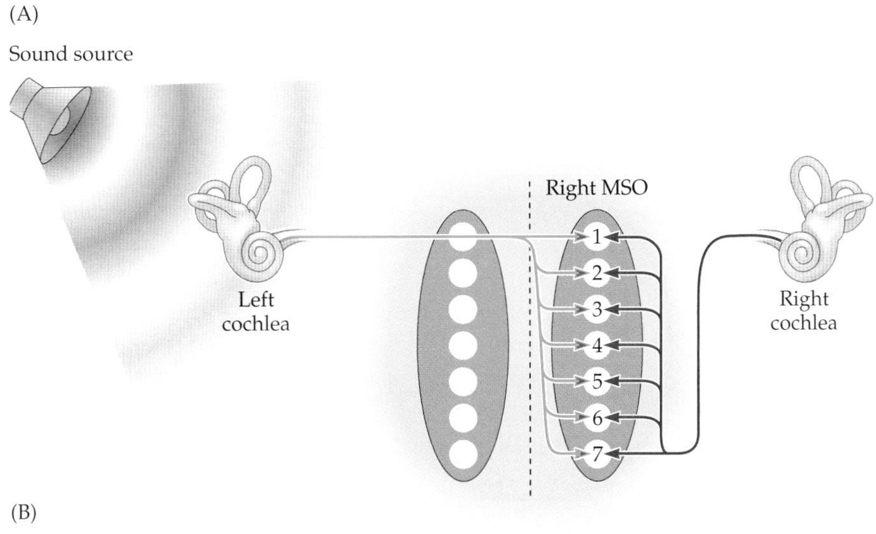

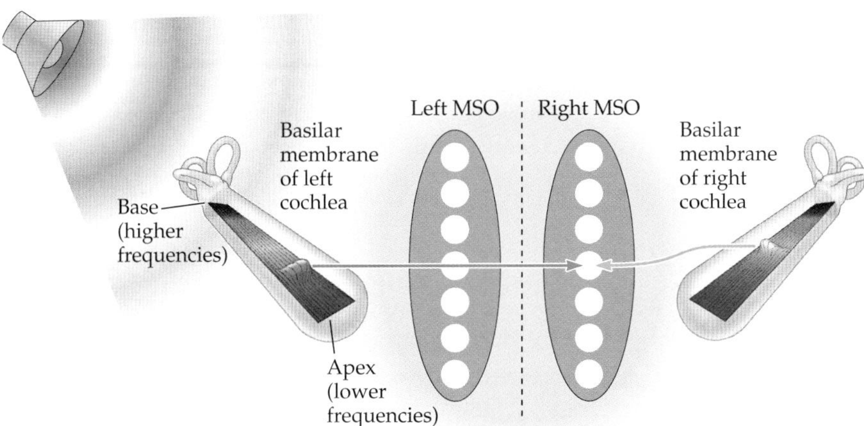

FIGURE 10.5 Two models for detecting timing differences The models describe two different ways neurons in the medial superior olive (MSO) may detect time difference between two ears. (A) It was long thought that differences between the lengths of neural axons (red and blue lines) coming from the two ears might provide a time delay to detect tiny time differences used to localize sounds. (B) The most recent evidence suggests that, instead, the brain takes advantage of the time it takes for the sound wave to travel from high to low frequencies along the basilar membrane of the cochlea. Then, the brain uses small differences in frequencies across the two ears to measure time.

become quite skeptical. Current research is investigating the possibility that the MSO may be tuned to capture slight frequency differences across the ears that arise from differences in the basilar membrane traveling wave (Joris and van der Heijden, 2019; Sayles et al., 2017) (**FIGURE 10.5B**).

Interaural Level Difference

The second cue to sound localization is the **interaural level difference** (**ILD**) in sound intensity. Sounds are more intense at the ear closer to the sound source because the head partially blocks the sound pressure wave from reaching the opposite ear. The properties of the ILD relevant for auditory localization are like those of the ITD:

- Sounds are more intense at the ear that is closer to the sound source and less intense at the ear farther away from the source.
- The ILD is largest at 90 and −90 degrees. It is nonexistent at 0 degrees (directly in front) and 180 degrees (directly behind).
- Between these two extremes, the ILD correlates with the angle of the sound source, but because of the irregular shape of the head, the correlation is less precise than it is with ITDs.

interaural level difference (ILD) The difference between levels (intensities) of sound at one ear versus the other.

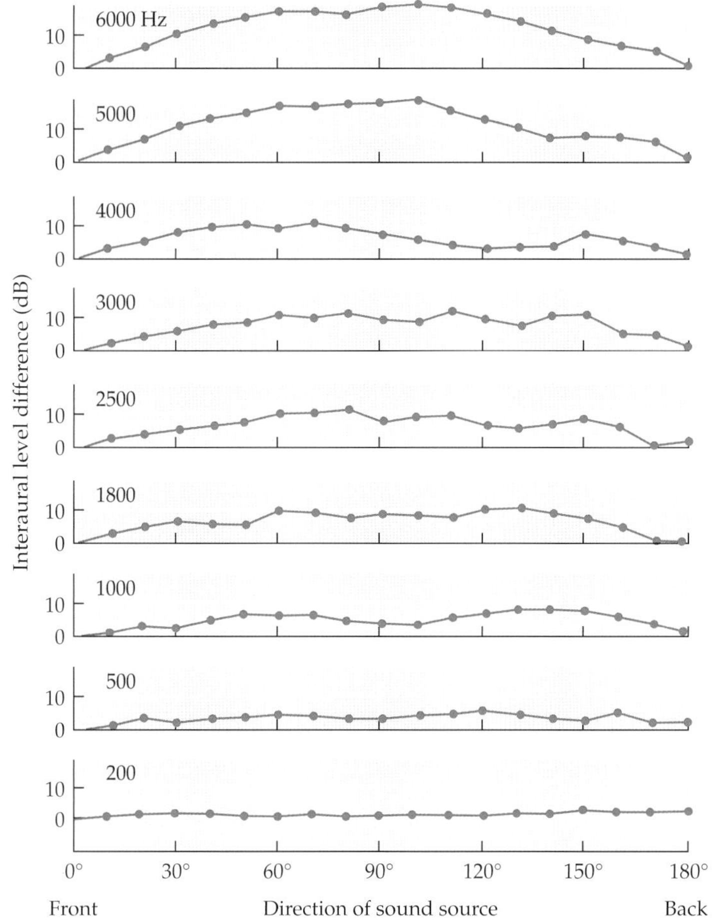

FIGURE 10.6 Intensity differences Interaural level (intensity) differences for tones of different frequencies presented at different positions around the head. Note that the biggest differences are for frequencies greater than 1000 Hz, at which point the head creates a sound shadow. The curves are not symmetrical toward the front and back, because of filtering characteristics of the pinnae.

Although the general relationship between ILD and sound source angle is a lot like the relationship between ITD and angle, there is an important difference between the two cues: the head blocks high-frequency sounds much more effectively than it blocks low-frequency sounds. This is because the long wavelengths of low-frequency sounds "wrap around" the head in much the same way that a large ocean wave rolls over a piling near the shore. Thus, as shown in **FIGURE 10.6**, ILDs are greatest for high-frequency tones, and ILD cues work well to determine location as long as the sounds have higher-frequency energy. ILDs are greatly reduced for low frequencies, becoming almost nonexistent below 1000 Hz. Our inability to localize low frequencies is the reason it does not matter where in a room you place the low-frequency subwoofer of your audio system.

THE PHYSIOLOGY OF ILD Neurons that are sensitive to intensity differences between the two ears can be found in the **lateral superior olives** (**LSOs**; see Figure 10.4), which receive both excitatory and inhibitory inputs. Excitatory connections to each LSO come from the ipsilateral ear—that is, excitatory connections to the left LSO originate in the left cochlea, and excitatory connections to the right LSO come from the right cochlea. Inhibitory inputs come from the contralateral ear (the ear on the opposite side of the head) via the medial nucleus of the trapezoid body.

Neurons in the LSOs are very sensitive to differences in intensity across the two ears because excitatory inputs from one ear (ipsilateral) and inhibitory inputs from the other ear (contralateral) are wired to compete. When the sound is more intense at one ear, connections from that ear are better both at exciting LSO neurons on that side and at inhibiting LSO neurons on the other side.

Cones of Confusion

If you examine Figures 10.3 and 10.6, you should see a potential problem with using ITDs and ILDs for sound localization: An ITD of −480 μs arises from a sound source that is located at either an angle of −60 degrees from the line of sight (10 o'clock in Figure 10.3) or an angle of −120 degrees (8 o'clock). Adding information from intensity differences does not help us here, because the ILDs for these two angles are also identical. If we also consider the elevation of a sound source (how far above or below our head the sound source is—a factor we've been ignoring up to now), we find that a given ITD or ILD could arise from any point on the surface of a **cone of confusion** that extends perpendicularly from the left or right

lateral superior olive (LSO) A relay station in the brainstem where inputs from both ears contribute to detection of the interaural level difference.

cone of confusion A region of positions in space where all sounds produce the same time and level (intensity) differences.

(A)

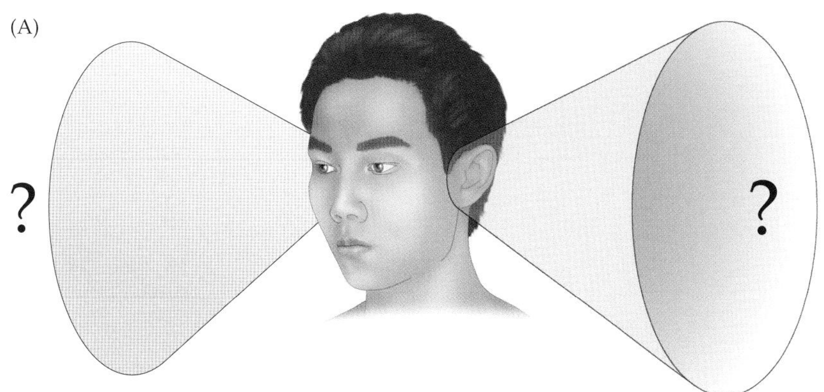

(B)

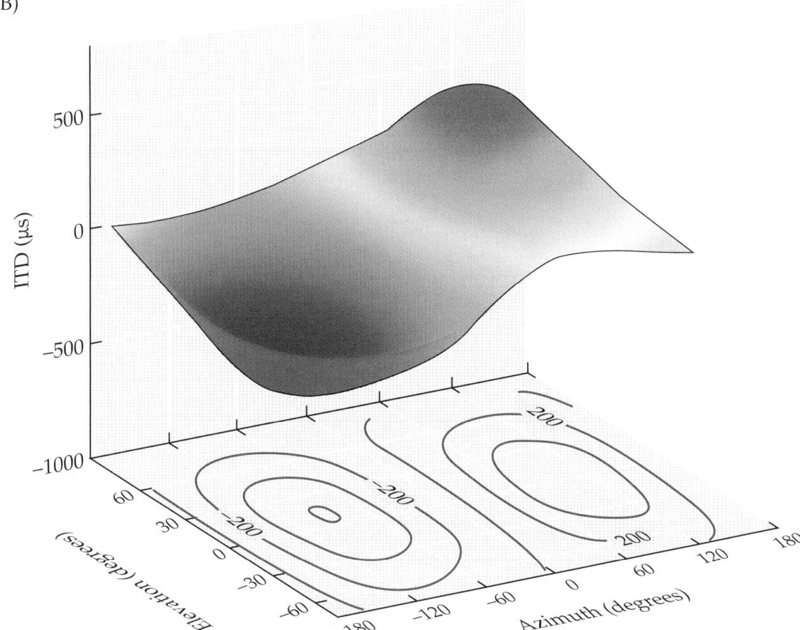

FIGURE 10.7 Cones of confusion Elevation adds another dimension to sound localization. (A) Cones of confusion exist because, for a sound at any point in space, there is a different point in space for which the interaural time differences (ITD) and the interaural level difference are the same. (B) ITDs are plotted here across azimuth and elevation. A sound with zero azimuth and elevation is directly in front of a listener's head. All of the locations in space that share the same color provide the exact same ITDs. Red contours plotted beneath the colored surface illustrate how all the locations on the red line give rise to the same ITD.

ear (**FIGURE 10.7**). This means that it is possible to confuse whether sounds are coming from in front of you or behind you because they carry the same ITD and ILD information. Thankfully, as soon as you move your head, the ITD and ILD of a sound source shift, and only one spatial location will be consistent with the ITDs and ILDs perceived before and after you move your head (**FIGURE 10.8**).

Pinnae and Head Cues

Another reason cones of confusion are not a major practical problem for the auditory system is that time and intensity differences are not the only cues for pinpointing the location of sound sources. Take a look at one of your pinnae (or, more realistically, take a look at a friend's pinna). You'll see that the shape of the pinna is quite complex, with lots of personalized nooks and crannies (**FIGURE 10.9**). Remember that the pinnae funnel sound energy into the ear canal (see Section 9.3). Because of their complex shapes, the pinnae funnel certain sound frequencies more efficiently than others. In addition to pinnae, the size and shape of the rest of the body, especially the upper torso, affect which frequencies reach the ear

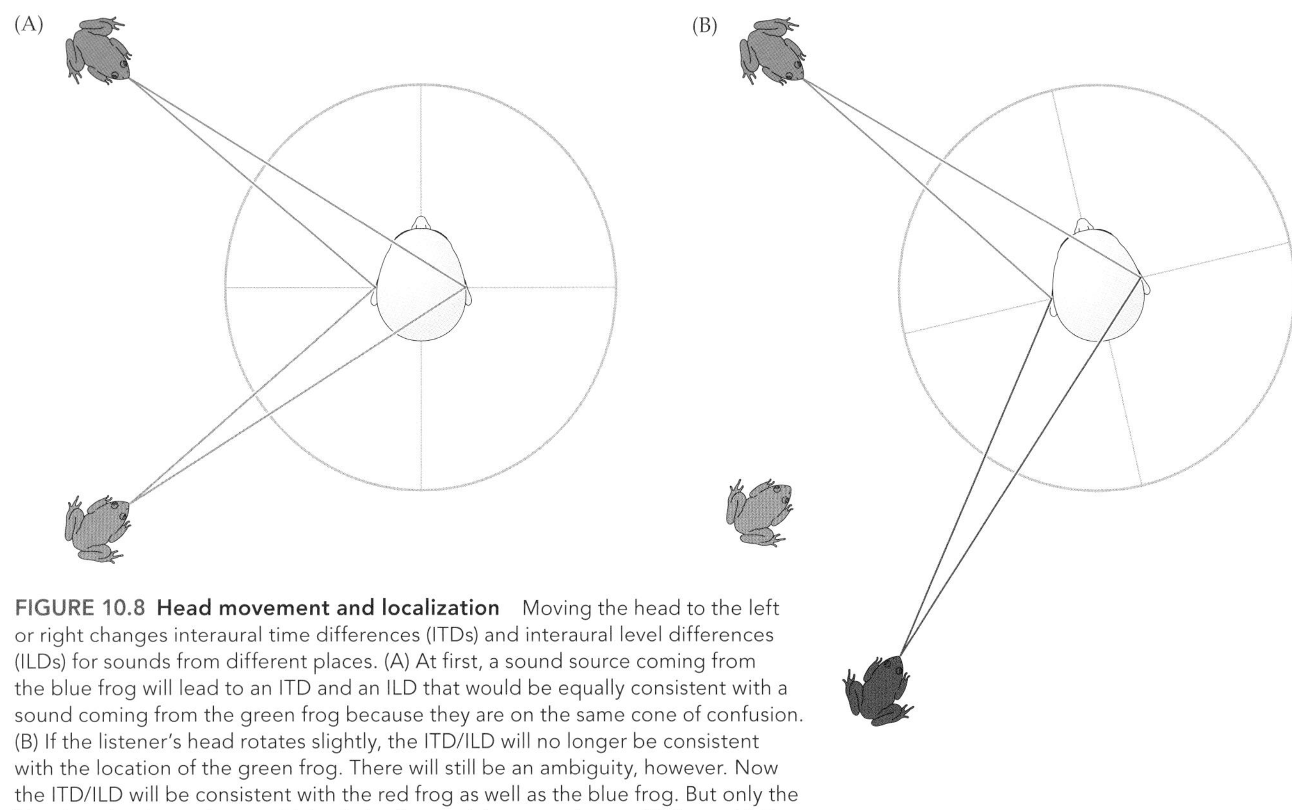

FIGURE 10.8 Head movement and localization Moving the head to the left or right changes interaural time differences (ITDs) and interaural level differences (ILDs) for sounds from different places. (A) At first, a sound source coming from the blue frog will lead to an ITD and an ILD that would be equally consistent with a sound coming from the green frog because they are on the same cone of confusion. (B) If the listener's head rotates slightly, the ITD/ILD will no longer be consistent with the location of the green frog. There will still be an ambiguity, however. Now the ITD/ILD will be consistent with the red frog as well as the blue frog. But only the blue location is consistent with both the first and the second sets of ITDs and ILDs.

most easily. Because of these effects, the intensity of each frequency varies slightly according to the direction of the sound. This variation provides us with another auditory localization cue.

To measure how the pinnae and upper body shape sounds from different locations, listeners sit in an anechoic room—a room in which the walls and even

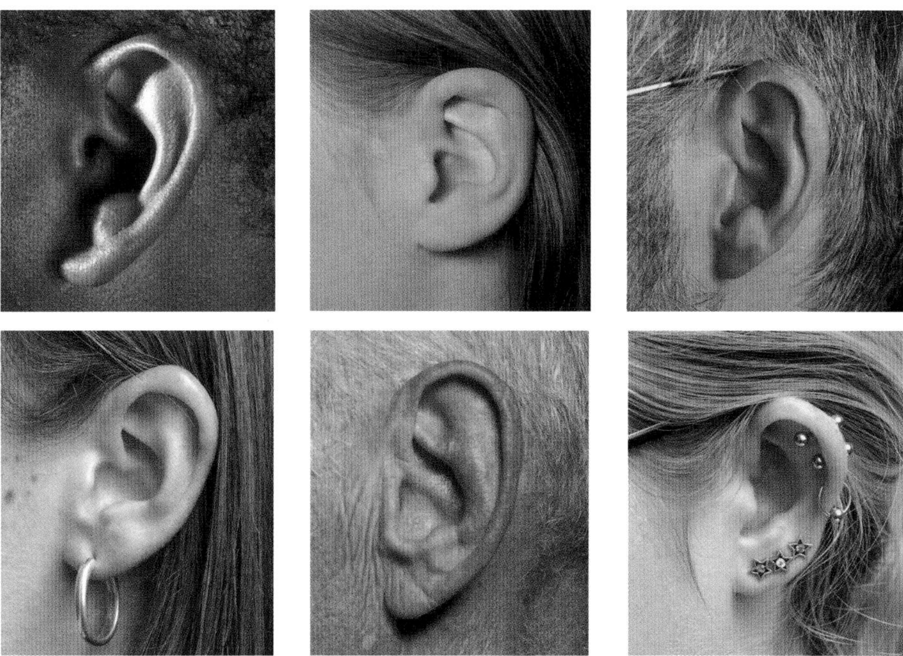

FIGURE 10.9 Pinna shapes Listeners learn how their personal pinnae affect how they hear sounds from different places in the environment.

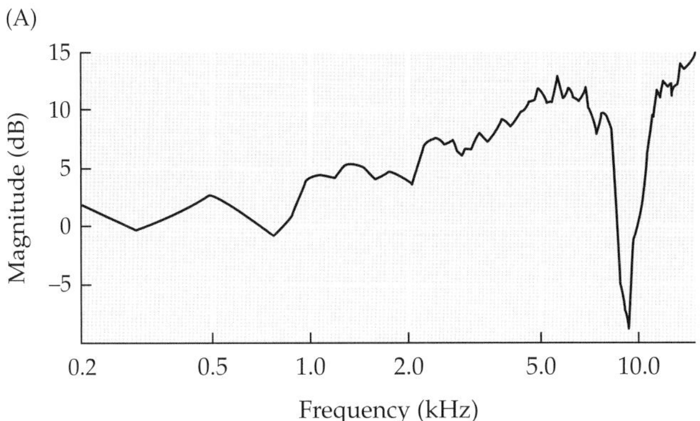

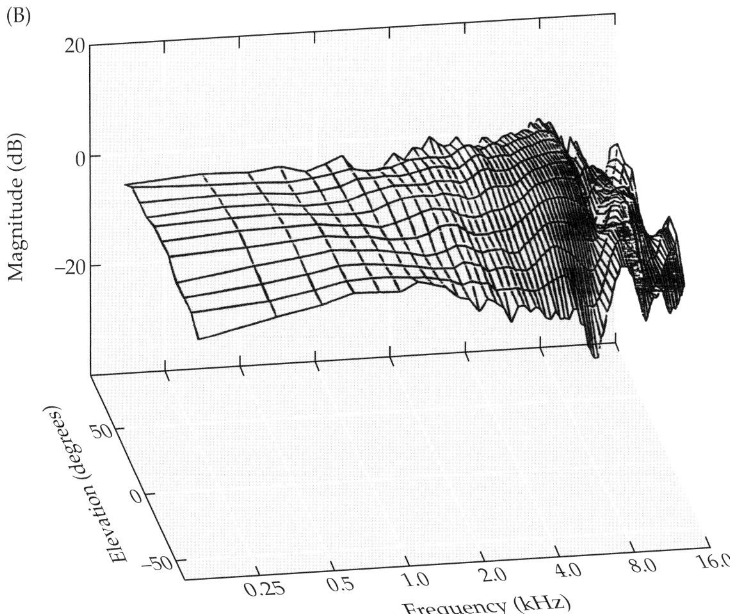

FIGURE 10.10 Directional transfer functions (DTFs) (A) Differences in intensity at the eardrum for sounds of varying frequency are plotted in this DTF for a single point along the azimuth. Acoustic energy is exaggerated at some frequencies and diminished at others. (B) The series of DTFs plotted here is for the same azimuth point, but at different elevations.

the floor are padded so that sounds do not bounce (reverberate) off the walls. The room is filled with speakers at locations up, down, and all around the listener. If we insert tiny microphones next to the listener's tympanic membrane (eardrum) and play sounds from different points in space, we can measure just how much energy from different frequencies actually reaches the eardrum from different locations. **FIGURE 10.10A** shows the measurements at the eardrum in a similar experimental setup—in this case, for sounds played over a speaker 30 degrees to the left of a listener and 12 degrees up from the listener's head. Although the amounts of energy at all frequencies were equally intense coming from the speaker, you can see that the amounts of energy were *not* equally intense at the eardrum. Some frequencies (e.g., 5 kilohertz [kHz]) had higher intensity when they arrived at the eardrum; others (e.g., 8 kHz) had less intensity.

These changing spectral shapes provide information about where a sound comes from on the elevation (up-down) plane. Figure 10.7 showed how relative intensities of different frequencies change depending on azimuth and illustrated that those curves are not symmetrical toward the front and back, the result of the filtering characteristics of the pinnae. For the final piece of the puzzle, look at **FIGURE 10.10B**, which shows the sound recorded by in-ear microphones as the speaker was moved up and down in elevation. As you can see, the relative intensities

directional transfer function (DTF) A measure that describes how the pinna, ear canal, head, and torso change the intensity of sounds with different frequencies that arrive at each ear from different locations in space (azimuth and elevation).

of different frequencies continuously change with changes in elevation, as well as in azimuth. These intensity shifts can be measured and combined to determine what we call an individual's **directional transfer function** (**DTF**). The DTF describes how the shape of your pinna and ear canal amplifies some frequencies and diminishes others before sounds reach the eardrum. Since each of us has a unique pinna shape (Figure 10.9), individual DTFs vary substantially.

The importance of the DTF in sound localization is easily understood if we consider the difference between hearing a live concert and listening to music through headphones. In person, we perceive the sound of the French horn as coming from one side of the orchestra and the sound of the cello as coming from the other side. But when we wear headphones (especially the type inserted directly inside the auditory canals), sounds are delivered directly to the eardrums, bypassing the pinnae. Auditory engineers can use multiple microphones to simulate the ITDs and ILDs that result from the musicians' different locations (the Beatles were early users of this type of technology), but DTFs are not simulated. As a result, you may be able to get some sense of direction when listening to a concert through headphones, but the sounds will seem to come from inside your skull rather than from out in the world. The situation is akin to that of visual depth perception. Pictorial cues can give a limited sense of depth, but to get a true perception of three-dimensionality, we need the binocular-disparity information (see Section 6.3) that we normally get only when we're seeing real objects.

Just as stereoscopes can be designed to simulate binocular disparity, it is possible to simulate DTFs. Instead of using two camera lenses in place of two eyes, two microphones are placed near the eardrums, as described earlier. Then the sound source, such as a concert, is recorded from these two microphones. When this special stereo recording, called a binaural recording, is played over headphones, the listener experiences the sounds as if they were back out in the world. This works best when the simulation is tailored to your unique DTF, but even approximations based on an average of many DTFs can produce a strong experience of auditory space over headphones. Developers are using this knowledge of the auditory system to deliver realistic three-dimensional sound experiences in contemporary video games.

Just as heads (and their corresponding ITDs and ILDs) grow to be larger, ears grow and change during development. It is hypothesized that listeners learn about the way DTFs relate to places in the environment through their experience listening to sounds, while other sources of information, such as vision, provide feedback about location (Wightman and Kistler, 1998). This learning through experience suggests that, as they grow, children may update the way they use DTF information. ●

Auditory Distance Perception

How do listeners know how far away a sound is? Although it is important to know what direction a sound is coming from, none of the cues we've discussed so far (ITD, ILD, and DTF) provides much information concerning the distance between a listener and a sound source that is much more than an arm's length away. At the risk of ruining a good story, begin by knowing that listeners are not nearly as good at judging auditory distance as they are at judging auditory direction. Listeners are best at judging the distance to a sound source when it is about 1 meter away. Closer than that, listeners overestimate distance. At distances greater than 1 meter, they underestimate distance (Kolarik et al., 2016). Auditory perception of distance also is relatively sloppy compared with visual perception

Scientists at Work

Vulcan Ears

Questions After their heads stop growing, can adults adjust to changing pinnae? Do people with radical piercings or large holes caused by stretching have a difficult time localizing sounds (**FIGURE 10.11A**)? What about damage to the ear (**FIGURE 10.11B**) or prosthetics (**FIGURE 10.11C**)?

Hypothesis Even after becoming full-grown adults, people can still adjust to changing ears when localizing sound.

Test Artificially change the shape of adult ears by inserting plastic ear molds and test whether listeners can still localize sounds as well as they could before the molds were inserted (Hofman, Van Riswick, and Van Opsal, 1998).

Results Listeners immediately became much poorer at localizing sounds. However, by 6 weeks of living with these molds in their ears, the listeners' localization abilities had greatly improved. Somewhat surprisingly, these listeners also remained quite good at localizing with their "old" ears when the molds were removed.

Future work Unfortunately, there are some limits to the ability to adjust to growing or remolded pinnae. Larger ears help older adults use lower-frequency cues; however, this improved ability to use low frequencies is insufficient to offset the effects of age-related hearing loss, and older individuals are poorer at localizing elevation (Otte et al., 2013). How can older adults with poorer hearing retain more of their ability to localize (and attend to) sounds?

(A)

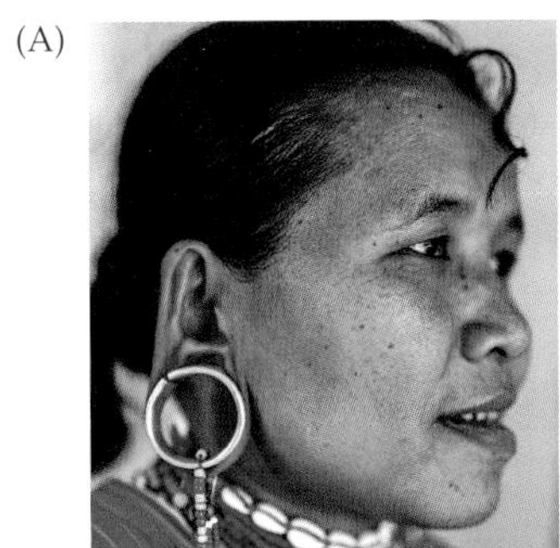

(B)

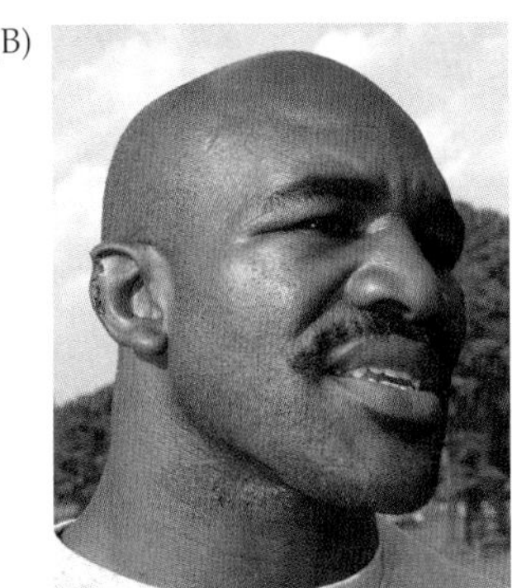

(C)

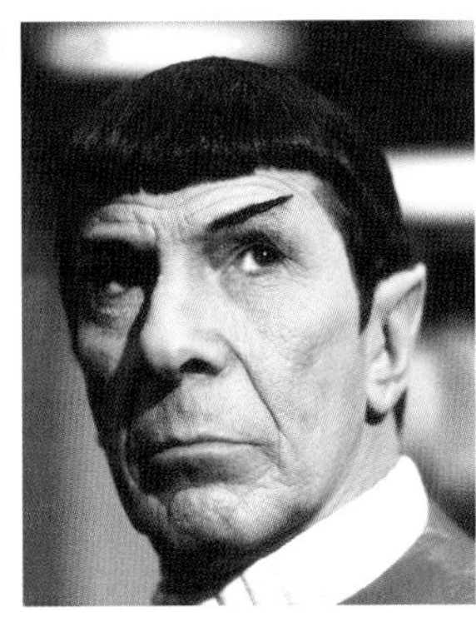

FIGURE 10.11 When pinnae are changed Listeners with altered pinnae initially experience difficulty localizing sounds but soon adjust to the new shape of their pinnae. (A) Stretching and piercing can radically alter pinna shape. (B) If you are a boxing fan, you might ask if Evander Holyfield could localize sounds as well following his fight with Mike Tyson. (C) It would be interesting to know how well the actor Leonard Nimoy (Spock in the original *Star Trek* series) could localize sounds while equipped with Vulcan ear molds. The experience of participants in the study by Hofman, Van Riswick, and Van Opsal (1998) suggests that switching between human and Vulcan pinnae may have become just a normal part of Nimoy's auditory life.

of distance—about twice as variable for hearing as for vision (P. W. Anderson and Zahorik, 2014).

The simplest cue for judging the distance of a sound source is *relative intensity*. Because sounds become less intense with greater distance, listeners have little difficulty perceiving the relative distances of two identical sound sources. For example, if you hear a pair of croaking bullfrogs, the louder croaks should be coming from the closer frog. Unfortunately, this cue suffers from the same problem as relative size in depth perception: interpreting the cue requires one to make assumptions about the sound sources that may turn out to be false (e.g., the softer-sounding frog might be very close, with its croaks muffled by surrounding vegetation).

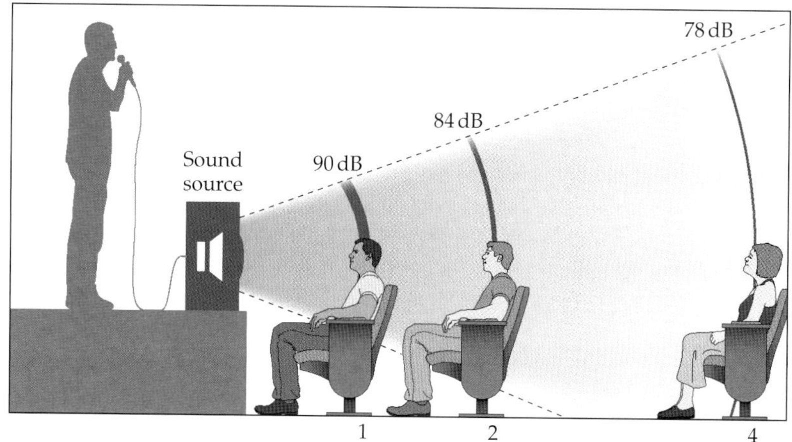

FIGURE 10.12 Sound and distance The intensity of a sound drops very quickly with greater distance from the sound source. Level decreases by half every time distance is doubled. (Recall that a 6 dB difference is a factor of 2 in sound pressure.) This relationship, which also holds for light energy, is called the inverse-square law.

In Figures 6.8 and 6.9, you saw lots of rabbits when learning about the use of relative size in visual depth perception, and the problem in hearing is much the same. At the end of this section, we will return to the challenge of figuring out just how loud (big) a sound is perceived to be when distance changes. But first, we will continue to consider distance perception.

The effectiveness of relative intensity decreases quickly as distance increases because sound intensity decreases according to the **inverse-square law** (**FIGURE 10.12**). When sound sources are close to the listener, a small difference in distance can produce a relatively large intensity difference. For example, a sound that is 1 meter away is more intense by 6 decibels (dB) than a sound that is 2 meters away. But the same 1-meter difference between sound sources 39 and 40 meters away produces an intensity change of only a fraction of 1 dB. The inverse-square law helps you to understand why listeners are good at using intensity differences to determine distance when sounds are presented within 1 meter of the head (Brungart, Durlach, and Rabinowitz, 1999) but tend to consistently underestimate the distance to sound sources farther away. And, not surprisingly, the amount of underestimation grows as distance becomes longer (Zahorik, 2002).

Intensity works best as a distance cue when either the sound source or the listener is moving. If a croaking frog starts hopping toward you, its croaks will become louder and louder. Listeners also get some information about how far away a source is when they move through the environment. This is because, in a manner akin to motion parallax in the perception of visual depth (see Section 6.2), sounds that are farther away do not seem to change direction in relation to the listener as much as nearer sounds do.

Another possible cue for auditory distance is the *spectral composition* of sounds. The sound-absorbing qualities of air dampen high frequencies more than low frequencies, so when sound sources are far away, higher frequencies decrease in energy more than lower frequencies as the sound waves travel from the source to the ear. Thus, the farther away a sound source is, the "muddier" it sounds. This change in spectral composition is noticeable only for large distances greater than 1000 meters. You experience the change in spectral composition when you hear thunder from near your window or from far away: you hear thunder as a loud "crack" nearby, but thunder from farther away sounds more like a "boom." Note that this auditory cue is analogous to the visual depth cue of aerial perspective, which involves the fact that more-distant objects look blurrier (see Section 6.1).

inverse-square law A principle stating that as distance from a source increases, intensity decreases faster, such that decrease in intensity is equal to the distance squared. This general law also applies to optics and other forms of energy.

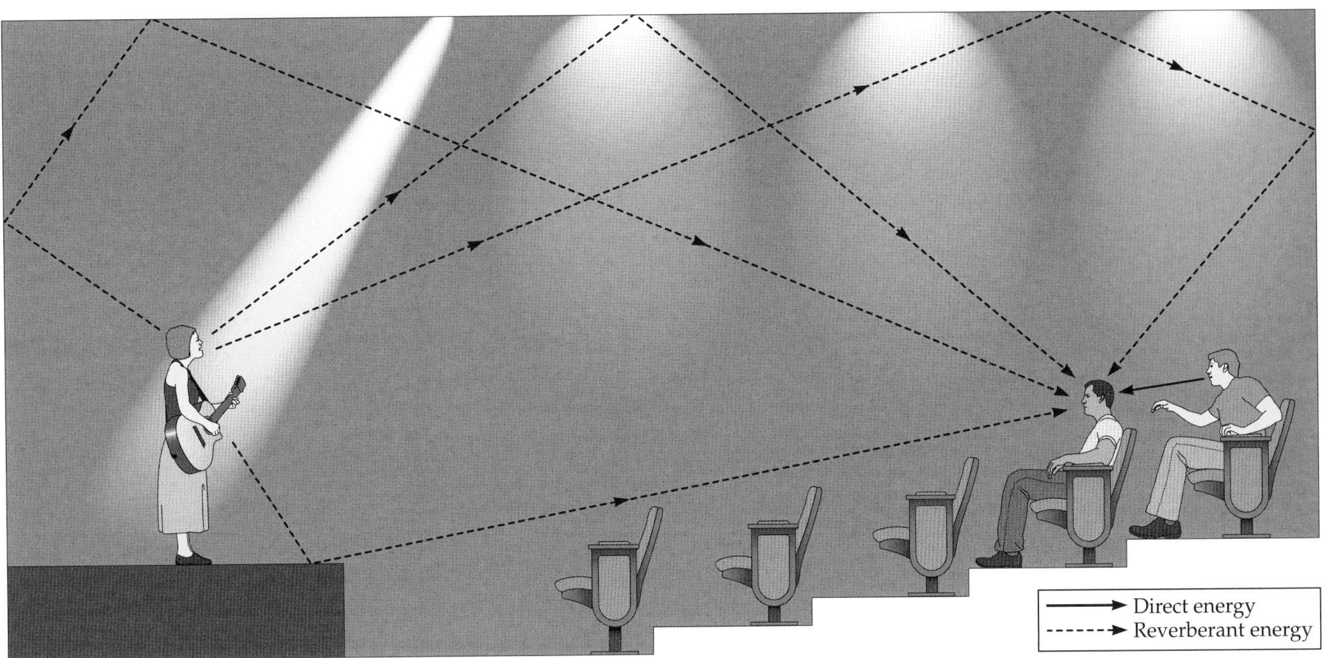

FIGURE 10.13 Sounds bounce The relative amounts of direct and reverberant energy coming from the listener's neighbor and the singer will inform the listener about the relative distances of the two sound sources.

A final distance cue stems from the fact that, in most environments, the sound that arrives at the ear is some combination of direct energy (which arrives directly from the source) and reverberant energy (which has bounced off surfaces in the environment). The *relative amounts of direct versus reverberant energy* inform the listener about distance, because when a sound source is close to a listener, most of the energy reaching the ear is direct, whereas reverberant energy provides a greater proportion of the total when the sound source is farther away. Suppose you're attending a concert. The intensities of the musician's song and your neighbor's whispered comments might be identical, but the singer's voice will take time to bounce off the concert hall's walls before reaching your ear, whereas you will hear only the direct energy from your neighbor's whispers (FIGURE 10.13).

Spatial Hearing and Blindness

Many studies have shown that severe loss of vision can result in improved auditory perception of localization of sounds in space (Kolarik et al., 2016). There is even evidence that regions of occipital (visual) cortex are recruited to process auditory input when visual inputs are no longer available (Voss and Zatorre, 2012). The most impressive demonstration of enhanced auditory perception of the spatial environment by visually impaired listeners is echolocation. You likely know about echolocation by bats and dolphins; they produce sounds in air or water and use the sounds that bounce back at them to gain information about their environments. Did you know that humans can do it, too? Some blind people learn to make clicks with their mouths and to use returning echoes to sense obstacles and even particular objects in their environment. Expert human echolocators can distinguish sizes and shapes of objects, as well as differences between the materials that comprise those objects (Thaler and Goodale, 2016). Measurement of human brain activity using functional magnetic resonance imaging has shown that visual regions of the brain are especially recruited to the task engaged by echolocation experts (FIGURE 10.14) (Thaler, Arnott, and Goodale, 2011).

Echolocation expert

Visual brain areas

Auditory brain areas

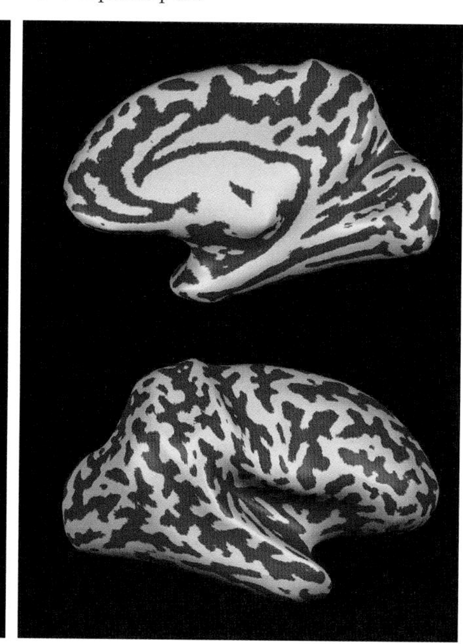

FIGURE 10.14 Echolocation and sightlessness Functional magnetic resonance imaging scans. The brain on the left is that of an echolocation expert who lost vision very early in life. The brain on the right belongs to a nonexpert who lost vision much later in life. When listening to sounds such as clicks and echoes, brain regions typically associated with vision became very active only in the brain of the echolocation expert.

Sensation & Perception in Everyday Life

Sounds from Wind Farms

Increasingly, clean renewable energy sources are replacing fossil fuels, especially coal. The amount of electricity generated by wind farms is expected to double in the next decade. That means that more and more people will live near wind farms. But do they *want* to live near wind farms? This gets personal, and in the United States more than 3000 counties are separately responsible for wind turbine zoning regulations.

Luckily, you've now learned about sound and hearing and should be able to help your neighbors decide what's best for your community. Today's wind turbines create a lot of sound (**FIGURE 10.15**). If you are perched right at the top of one, the sound is over 100 dB, about the same as a gas lawnmower. But what if you get farther away? Once you are about 300 m away (about three American football fields, including end zones), the level drops to about 43 dB. Move another 300 m away, and the level is down to 37 dB. Because sound level decreases by the inverse-square law, you know that you have to move another 600 m away (six football fields) before the sound is cut in half again to 31 dB.

How far is far enough? The answer depends on two things. First, how quiet do you think quiet should be? The level of background sound in a quiet library is about 37 dB—about the same as standing 600 m from a wind turbine. Second—and this is the important part—what really matters is whether the sound of the wind turbine is more intense than the sounds that are already around you. This is because we only detect sounds that are not masked by sounds that are more intense. A window air conditioner is about 50 dB. Although you rarely notice it because other sounds are around you, your refrigerator is about 40 dB. So you probably wouldn't hear the 37 dB wind turbine sound when either of these appliances is operating.

So much for sounds you can hear. Wind turbines also create infrasound. Infrasound is sound with frequencies lower than 20 Hz, the lowest frequencies humans can hear. You now know that very low frequency sounds have long wavelengths that wrap

Sensation & Perception in Everyday Life *(continued)*

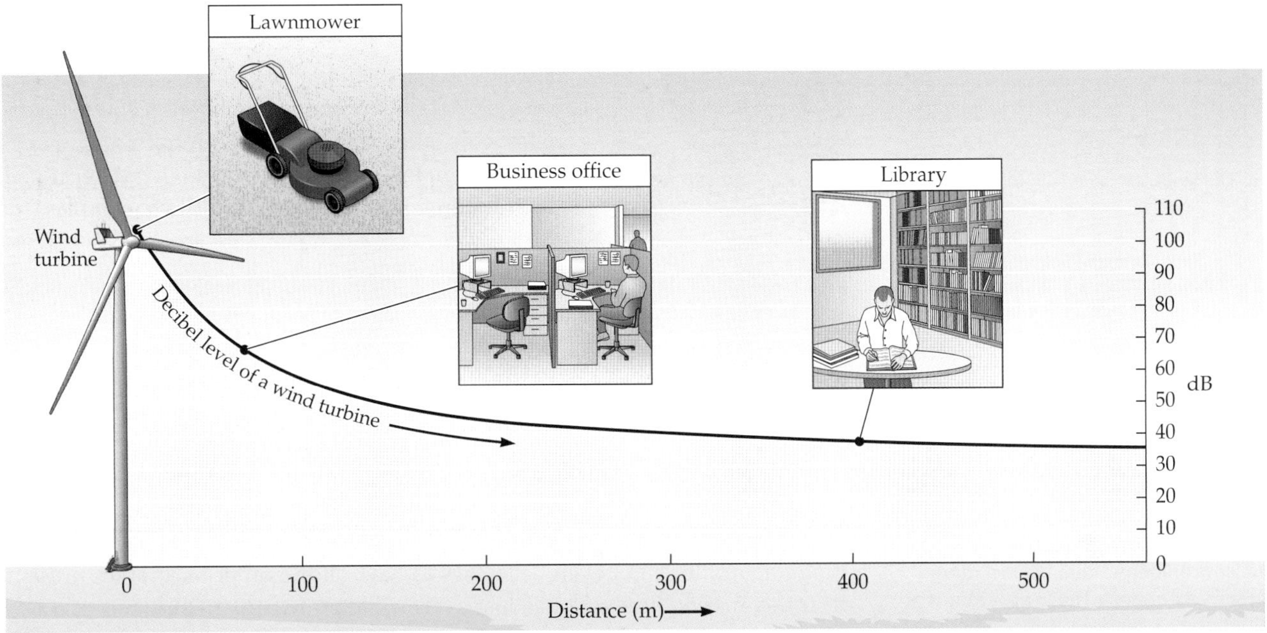

FIGURE 10.15 Wind farms Wind turbines are quite loud when you are close to them. Because the intensity of sound drops by half with every doubling of distance following the inverse-square law, sound levels become lower than those from household appliances such as window air conditioners and refrigerators as distance from the turbine increases.

around objects, so they are not easily stopped. And just because you cannot hear them does not mean they are safe; after all, you wear sunscreen even though you cannot see UV light. We do know that infrasound occurs naturally from storms, waterfalls, and ocean waves and less naturally from ceiling fans and washing machines. While it is impossible to say that anything is completely safe, there are no known health consequences from infrasound. We cannot say that about air pollution from burning fossil fuels.

10.2 Complex Sounds

Simple sounds like sine waves and bands of noise are very useful for exploring the fundamental operating characteristics of auditory systems (see Section 9.2), just as sine wave gratings and single-wavelength light sources are essential tools for vision researchers. But pure sine wave tones, like pure single-wavelength light sources, are rare in the real world, where objects and events that matter to listeners are more complex, more interesting, and more challenging for researchers to study.

Harmonics

Many environmental sounds, including the human voice and the sounds of musical instruments, have a **harmonic spectrum** (FIGURE 10.16). In fact, harmonic sounds are among the most common types of sounds in the environment. The lowest frequency of a harmonic spectrum is the **fundamental frequency.** With natural vibratory sources (as opposed to pure tones created in the laboratory), there

harmonic spectrum The spectrum of a complex sound in which energy is at integer multiples of the fundamental frequency.

fundamental frequency The lowest-frequency component of a complex periodic sound.

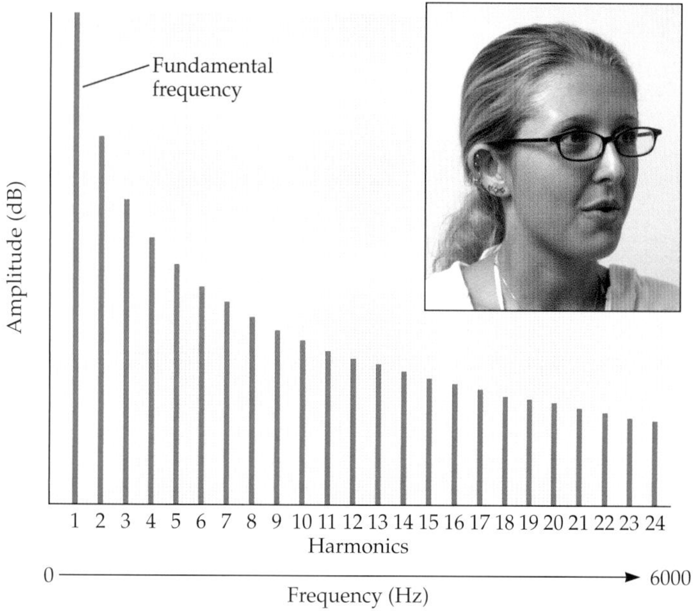

FIGURE 10.16 Harmonic spectra Many environmental sounds, including voices, are harmonic. The lowest frequency of a harmonic sound is the fundamental frequency, and there are peaks of energy at integer multiples of the fundamental.

is also energy at frequencies that are integer multiples of the fundamental frequency. For example, a female speaker may produce a vowel sound with a fundamental frequency of 250 Hz. Her vocal cords will produce the greatest energy at 250 Hz, less energy at 500 Hz, less still at 750 Hz, even less at 1000 Hz, and so on. In this case, 500 Hz is the second harmonic, 750 is the third harmonic, and 1000 is the fourth harmonic. For harmonic complexes, the perceived pitch is determined by the fundamental frequency, and the harmonics (often called *overtones* by musicians) add to the perceived richness, or timbre, of the sound.

The auditory system is acutely sensitive to the natural relationships between harmonics. In fact, if the first harmonic (fundamental frequency) is removed from a series of harmonics, as shown in **FIGURE 10.17**, and only the others (second, third, fourth, and so on) are presented, the pitch that listeners hear corresponds to the fundamental frequency—even though it is not part of the sound, listeners hear a phantom *missing fundamental*. It is not even necessary to have all the other harmonics present to hear the missing fundamental; just a few will do (**FIGURE 10.18A**).

The most straightforward explanations of the missing-fundamental effect involve the temporal code for sound frequency (pitch) discussed in Section 9.3. One thing that all harmonics of a fundamental have in common is fluctuations in sound pressure at regular intervals corresponding to the fundamental frequency. For example, the waveform for a 500 Hz tone has a peak every 2.0 ms (**FIGURE 10.18B**). The waveforms for 750 and 1000 Hz tones have peaks every 1.3 and 1.0 ms, respectively (**FIGURES 10.18C** and **10.18D**). As shown in **FIGURE 10.18E**, these three waveforms come into alignment every 4 ms, which, conveniently, happens to be the period of the fundamental frequency for these three harmonics: 250 Hz. Indeed, *every* harmonic of 250 Hz will have an energy peak every 4 ms. Some neurons in the auditory nerve and cochlear nucleus will fire action potentials every 4 ms to the collection of waves shown in Figure 10.18E, providing an elegant mechanism to explain why listeners perceive the pitch of this complex tone to be 250 Hz, even though the tone has no 250 Hz component.

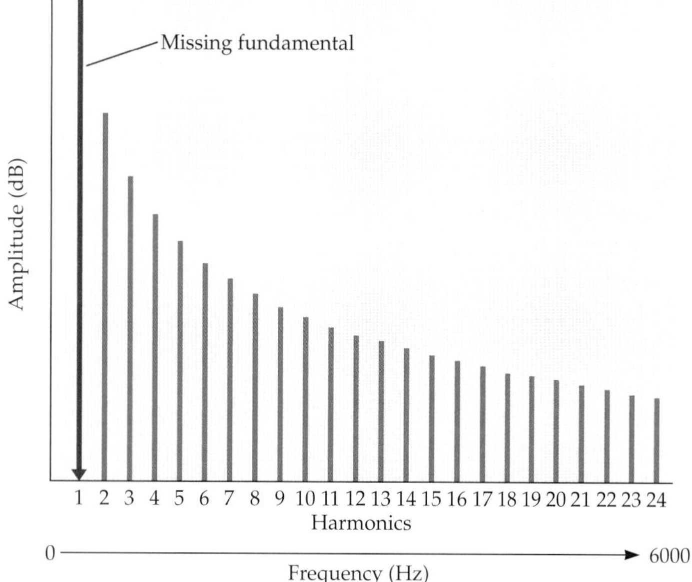

FIGURE 10.17 The missing fundamental If the fundamental (lowest frequency) of a harmonic sound is removed, listeners still hear the pitch of this "missing fundamental."

Timbre

Loudness and pitch are relatively easy to describe because, as you learned in Chapter 9, they correspond fairly well—although not perfectly—to simple acoustic dimensions (amplitude and frequency, respectively). But the richness of complex sounds like those in our world depends on more than simple sensations of loudness and pitch. For example, if a trombone and a tenor saxophone play the same note (that is, their two notes

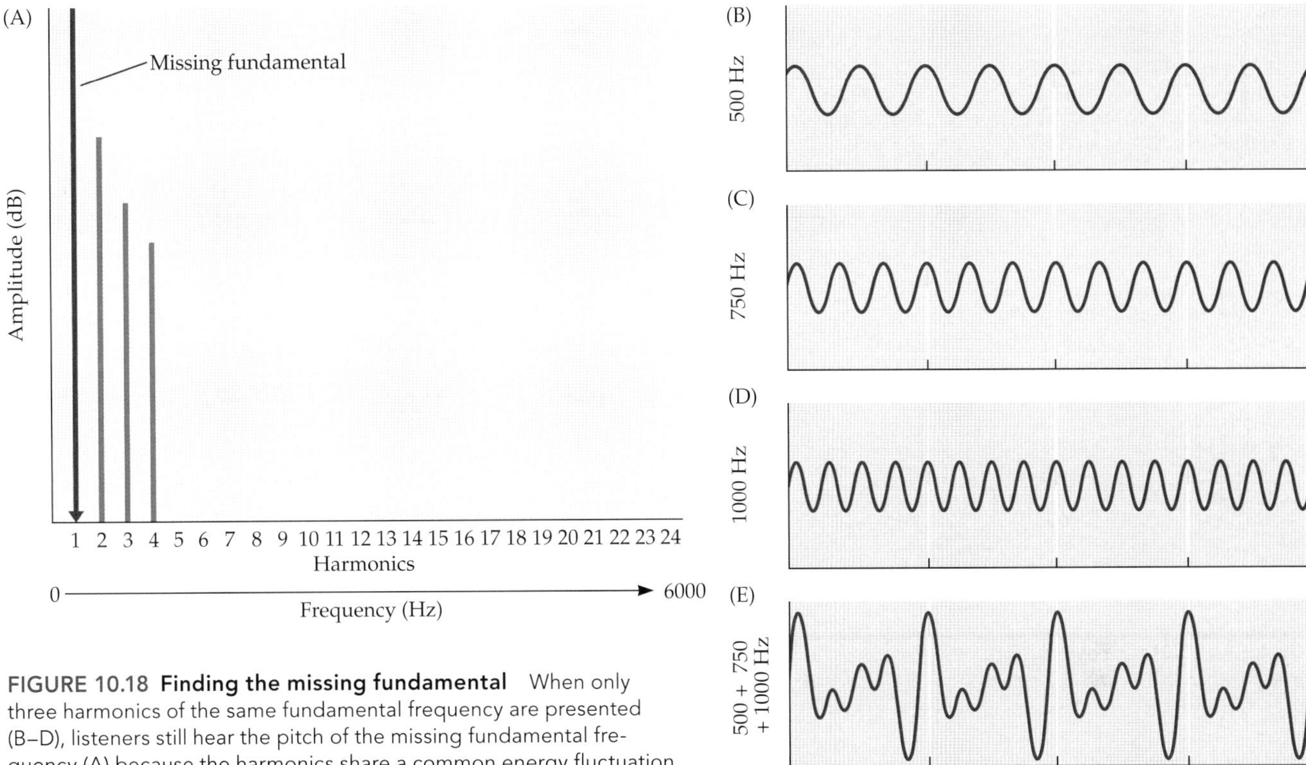

FIGURE 10.18 Finding the missing fundamental When only three harmonics of the same fundamental frequency are presented (B–D), listeners still hear the pitch of the missing fundamental frequency (A) because the harmonics share a common energy fluctuation every 4 ms, the period of a 250 Hz signal (E).

will have the exact same fundamental frequency) at exactly the same intensity, we have no trouble discerning that two different instruments are being played. The perceptual quality that differs between these two musical instruments, as well as between vowel sounds such as those in the words *hot*, *heat*, and *hoot*, is known as **timbre**.

What exactly is timbre? You won't find a good answer to this question in the dictionary, because the official definition of *timbre* is "the quality that makes listeners hear two different sounds even though both sounds have the same pitch and loudness" (American Standards Association, 1960). However, differences in timbre between musical instruments or vowel sounds can be estimated closely by comparison of the extent to which the overall spectra of two sounds overlap (Plomp, 1976). Perception of visual color depends on the relative levels of energy at different wavelengths (see Chapter 5), and very similarly, perception of timbre is related to the relative energies of different acoustic frequency components (**FIGURE 10.19**). For example, the trombone and tenor saxophone notes plotted in Figure 10.19A share the same fundamental frequency (middle C, 262 Hz). However, notice that the trombone's third (786 Hz) component is more intense than its fourth (1048 Hz) component, whereas for the saxophone, the relationship between the energies of these two components is reversed.

timbre The psychological sensation by which a listener can judge that two sounds with the same loudness and pitch are dissimilar. Timbre quality is conveyed by harmonics and other high frequencies.

attack The part of a sound during which amplitude increases (onset).

decay The part of a sound during which amplitude decreases (offset).

Attack and Decay

Another important quality of a complex sound is the way it begins (the **attack** of the sound) and ends (the sound's **decay**) (**FIGURE 10.20**). For example, important contrasts between speech sounds in the words *bill* and *will* or the words *chip* and

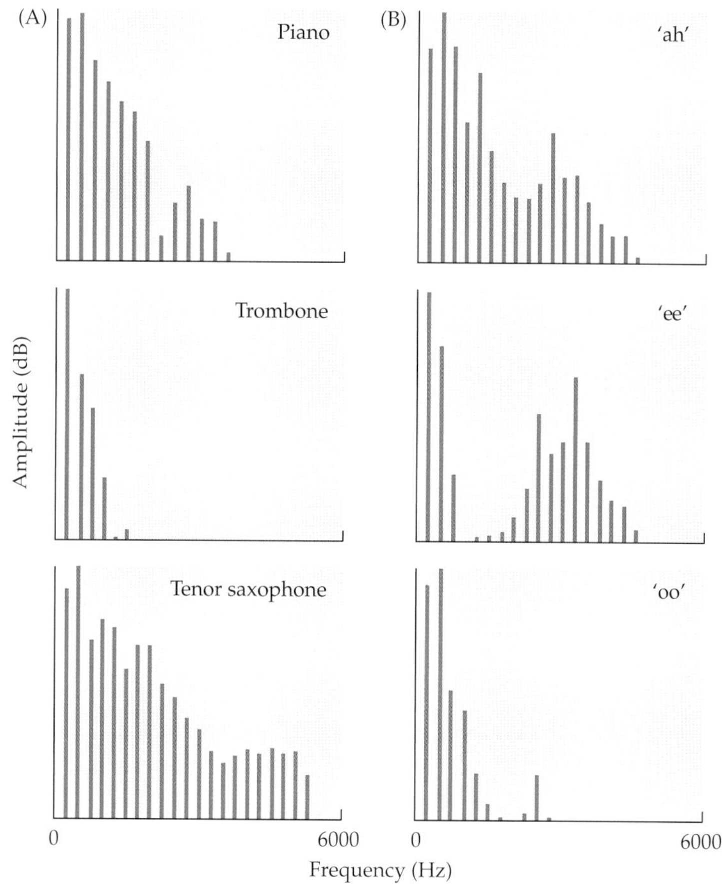

FIGURE 10.19 Timbre (A) Three different musical instruments playing the same note (middle C, 262 Hz) sound different because they have different spectral shapes. (B) Three vowels produced by the same female talker, also with a fundamental frequency of 262 Hz, sound very different to listeners.

ship relate to differences in how quickly sound energy increases at the onset—that is, the rate of attack.

The same musical instrument can have quite different attacks, from the rapid onset of a plucked violin string to the gradual onset of a bowed string (Figures 10.20A and 10.20B). How quickly a sound decays depends on how long it takes for the vibrating object creating the sound (the violin string, for example) to dissipate energy and stop moving. One of the more challenging aspects of designing music synthesizers that mimic real musical instruments was learning how to mimic the attacks and decays of the different instruments.

The sound of a piano note is caused by a small hammer hitting a string. The amplitude of the resulting sound increases very quickly before more gradually dissipating. If a recording of a piano note is played backward, the sound no longer even remotely resembles a piano. Instead, it sounds more like the same note played on an accordion.

10.3 Auditory Scene Analysis

The acoustic environment can be a busy place. In most natural situations, the sound source that one is listening to is not the only sound present. Consider chatting with a friend at a party where many other people are talking, music is playing, chips are being munched, the door is being opened and closed, and so on. Now consider simpler environments, such as those you choose for studying. You probably chose the spot where you are reading this chapter because it was relatively quiet. But stop

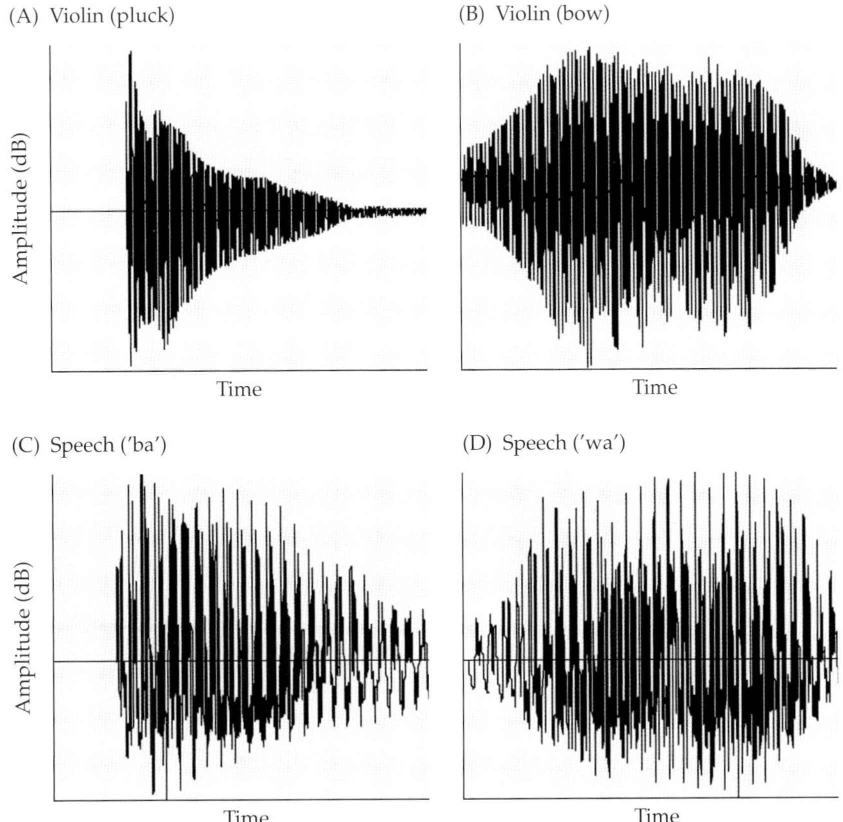

FIGURE 10.20 Sound onsets We use the onsets of sounds (attacks) to identify them. The attack is quite different when a violin string is plucked (A) versus bowed (B). Similarly, different speech sounds, such as 'ba' (C) and 'wa' (D), have different attacks.

and listen carefully. Is a heater, air conditioner, computer, or refrigerator humming in the background? Can you hear people talking somewhere in the vicinity? Are chair legs sliding across floors? Places with only a single sound source are very uncommon. Indeed, there are few truly quiet places outside the laboratories of hearing scientists and the testing chambers of audiologists. Environments with multiple sound sources are the rule, not the exception.

How does the auditory system sort out sources? The visual system contends with a busy world, but eyes can be directed to any part of the scene of interest. Moreover, the rods and cones on the right side of the retina always see the objects on the left, politely leaving the receptors on the other side of the retina to collect data about objects on the right. For an auditory scene, the situation is greatly complicated by the fact that all the sound waves from all the sound sources in the environment are summed together in a single complex sound wave (**FIGURE 10.21**). You can move your ears around all you want, but everyone's voice at the party must be picked up by the same two sets of cochlear hair cells. Separating different sounds from one another is like living in a world in which everything is made of glass: it is difficult to distinguish separate objects, because they all merge into a single combination of shapes, as Figure 10.21E illustrates.

Somehow, the auditory system contends quite well with the situation: Our perception is typically of a world with easily separable sounds. We can understand the conversation of a dance partner at a party, and we can pick out a favorite instrument in the band. This distinction of auditory events or objects in the broader auditory environment is commonly referred to as **auditory scene analysis**.

auditory scene analysis Processing an auditory scene consisting of multiple sound sources into separate sound images.

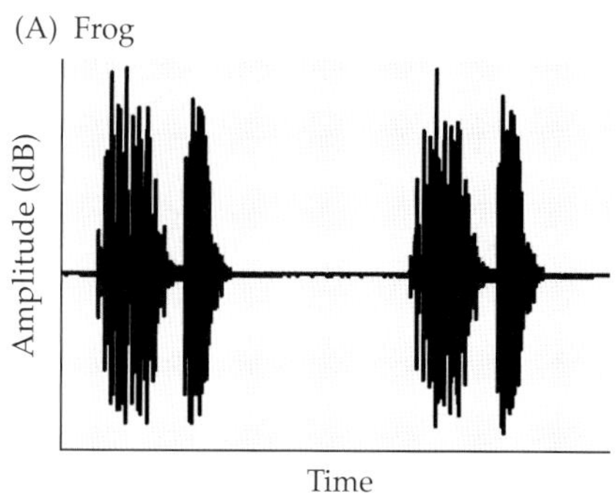

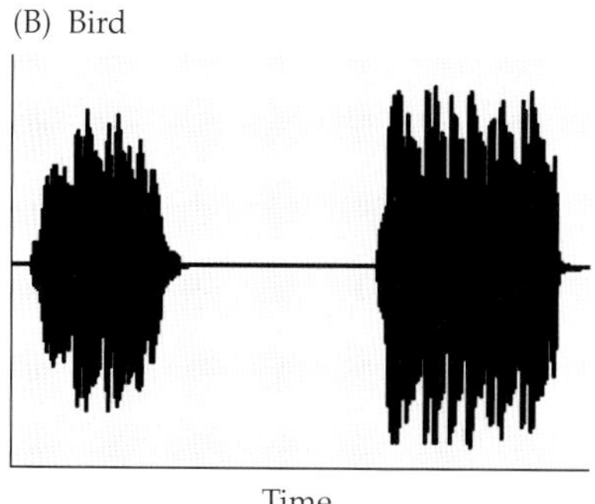

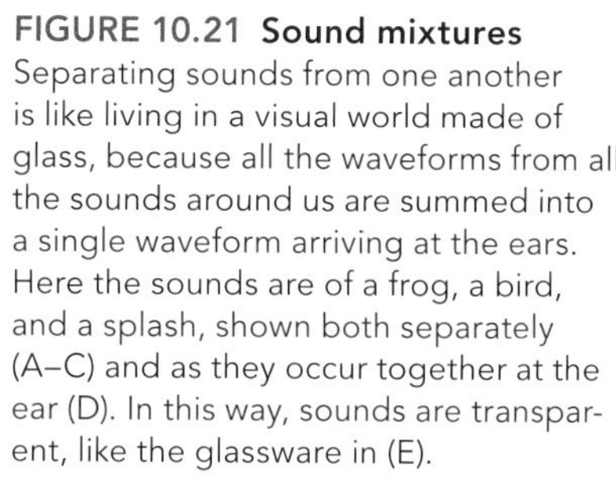

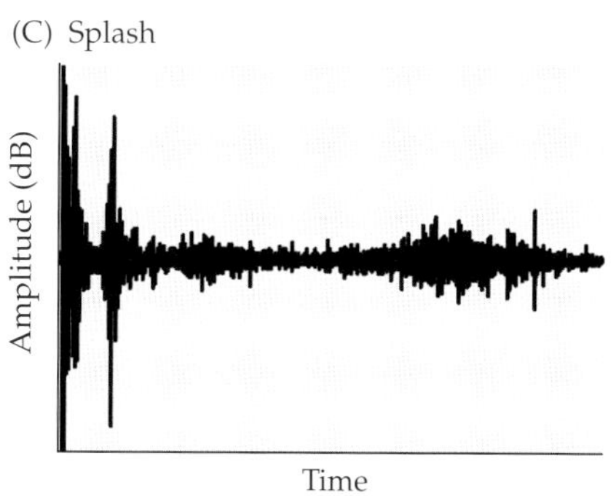

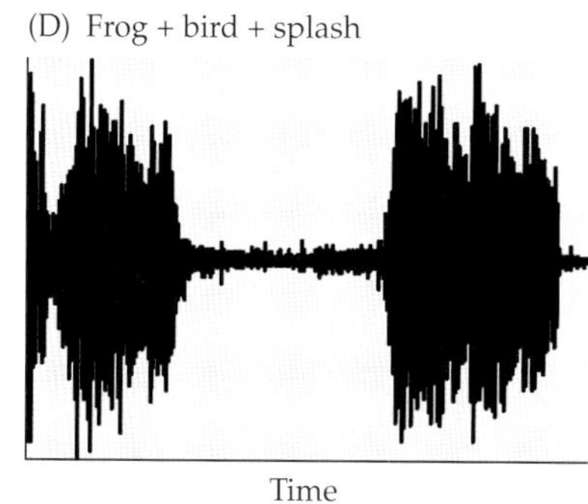

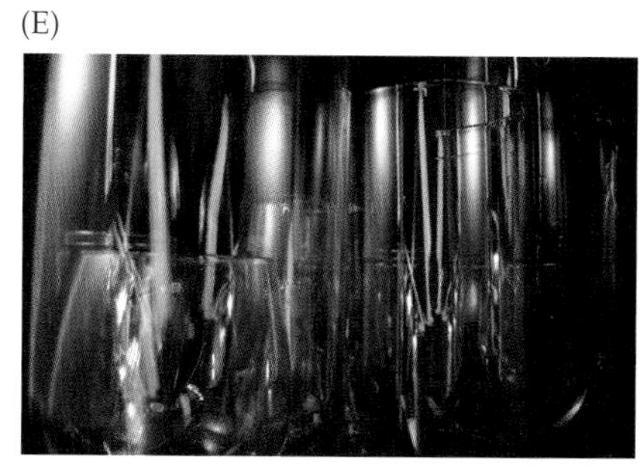

FIGURE 10.21 Sound mixtures Separating sounds from one another is like living in a visual world made of glass, because all the waveforms from all the sounds around us are summed into a single waveform arriving at the ears. Here the sounds are of a frog, a bird, and a splash, shown both separately (A–C) and as they occur together at the ear (D). In this way, sounds are transparent, like the glassware in (E).

auditory stream segregation The perceptual organization of a complex acoustic signal into separate auditory events for which each stream is heard as a separate event.

Spatial, Spectral, and Temporal Segregation

The auditory system uses several strategies to segregate sound sources. One of the most obvious strategies is spatial separation between sounds. Sounds that emanate from the same location in space can typically be treated as if they arose from the same source. Moreover, in a natural environment in which sound sources move, a sound that is perceived to move in space can more easily be separated from background sounds that are relatively stationary. Listeners move too, so if a sound stays in the same place relative to the path of a listener, it will be easier for that sound to be sorted out from other sounds.

In addition to being sorted by location, sounds can be segregated based on their spectral or temporal qualities. For example, sounds with the same pitch or similar pitches are more likely to be grouped as coming from the same source and to be segregated from other sounds. Familiarity is also helpful (everyone has the experience of being distracted by someone saying their name, even in a crowded room full of voices). As you learn about the ways listeners make sense of the cascade of sounds surrounding them, you will see that both the physical properties of sounds and the experiences learned by the brain work together (Kondo et al., 2017).

Sounds that are perceived to emanate from the same source are often described as being part of the same "auditory stream," and dividing the auditory world into separate auditory objects is known as **auditory stream segregation**. The challenge of sorting out the sound to which one is listening from all the competing sounds in the environment is common across all animals that hear, and variants of the examples that follow have been demonstrated to exist not only for humans, but also for birds, fishes, frogs, and nonhuman mammals (Itatani and Klump, 2017).

Perhaps the simplest example of auditory stream segregation involves two tones with similar frequencies that are alternated (**FIGURE 10.22A**). This sequence sounds like a single coherent stream of tones that warble up and down

FIGURE 10.22 **Auditory stream segregation** (A) When tones that are close in frequency occur in rapid succession, they are heard as a single warbling stream. (B) When successive, rapidly alternating tones have very different frequencies, they are heard as two separate streams.

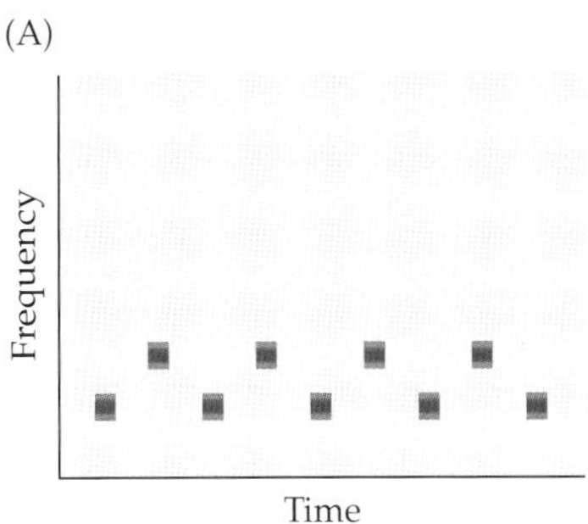

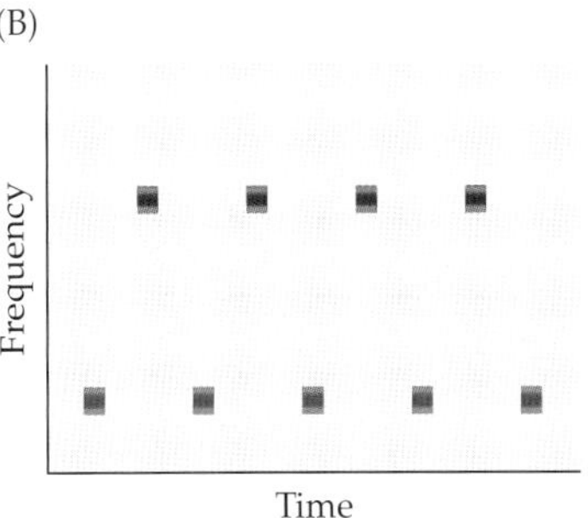

in frequency. But if the alternating tones are markedly different in frequency (**FIGURE 10.22B**), two simultaneous streams of tones are heard—one higher in pitch than the other (G. A. Miller and Heise, 1950). It is as if one "auditory object" becomes two objects.

Auditory stream segregation is a powerful perceptual phenomenon that is not limited to simple tones in the laboratory. Before stream segregation was "discovered" by auditory scientists, the composer Johann Sebastian Bach (1685–1750) exploited these auditory effects in his compositions (**FIGURE 10.23**). The same instrument, such as a pipe organ, would rapidly play interleaved sequences of low and high notes. Even though the musician played a sequence in the order H1-L1-H2-L2-H3-L3, listeners heard two melodies—one high (H1-H2-H3) and one low (L1-L2-L3). This bit of knowledge about auditory perception was understood not only by Bach, but also by other baroque composers of the seventeenth and early eighteenth centuries.

When thinking about auditory scene analysis, you may find it useful to describe effects using Gestalt principles such as those elucidated for vision in Section 4.4. The examples of auditory stream segregation presented in this section can be described as applications of the Gestalt principle of **similarity** (see Figure 4.22A): similar sounds tend to be grouped together into streams. While we use examples from vision to help you to better understand how the auditory system groups sounds together, these principles can be predicted based on regularities discovered by statistically analyzing a wide array of natural sounds such as speech and music (Młynarski and McDermott, 2019).

similarity Gestalt grouping rule stating that the tendency of two sounds to group together will increase as the acoustic similarity between them increases.

For example, auditory stream segregation based on groups of notes with similar timbres can be seen as another example of the Gestalt principle of similarity at work. As Figure 10.19 illustrated, timbres are very different for pianos, trombones, and saxophones. Grouping by timbre is particularly robust because sounds with

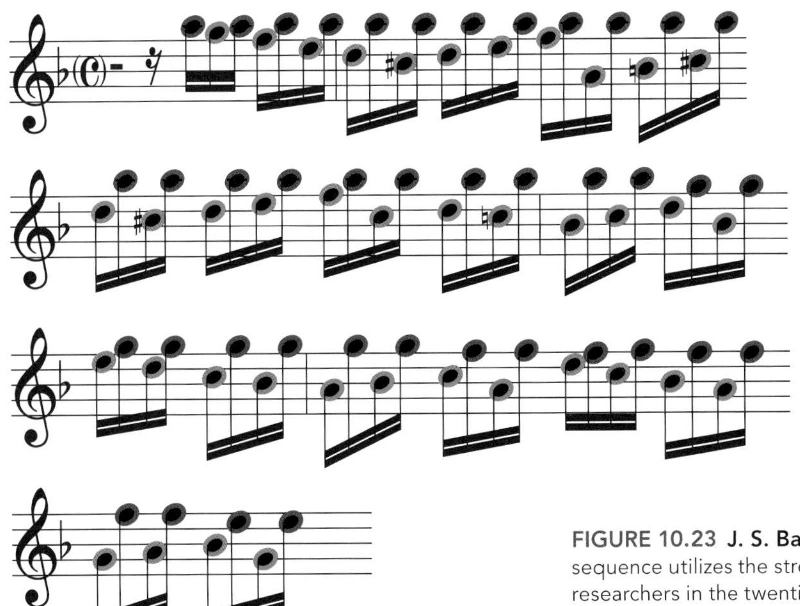

FIGURE 10.23 **J. S. Bach's Toccata and Fugue in D Minor** This musical sequence utilizes the stream segregation principles "discovered" by auditory researchers in the twentieth century. When played in rapid succession, the higher notes (red) are heard as one melody, separate from the lower notes (blue).

similar timbres usually arise from the same sound source. This principle explains why listeners can pick out the melody played on a single instrument—a trombone, for example—even when another instrument, such as a saxophone, plays a different or even opposite sequence of notes (Wessel, 1979).

Neural processes that give rise to stream segregation can be found throughout the auditory system—from the first stages of auditory processing to the primary auditory cortex (A1), to secondary areas of the auditory cortex such as the belt and parabelt areas (see Figure 9.21) (J. S. Snyder and Alain, 2007). The brainstem shows neural evidence of stream segregation based on simple cues such as the frequencies of different tones, but segregation based on more sophisticated perceptual properties of sounds, and based on familiarity, is more likely to take place in the cortex.

Grouping by Onset

Sound components that begin at the same time (or nearly the same time), such as the harmonics of a music or speech sound, will tend to be heard as coming from the same sound source. One way this phenomenon helps us is by grouping different harmonics into a single complex sound. Frequency components with different onsets are less likely to be grouped.

R. A. Rasch (1978) showed that it is much easier to distinguish two notes from one another when the onset of one precedes the onset of the other by at least 30 ms. He noted that musicians playing together in an ensemble such as a string quartet do not begin playing notes at exactly the same time, even when the musical score instructs them to do so. Instead, they begin notes slightly before or after one another, and this staggered start probably helps listeners pick out the individual instruments. Part of the signature style of the Rolling Stones has been to carry this practice to an extreme; members of the group sometimes begin the same beat with such widely varying onsets that it is unclear whether they are playing together or not.

Grouping of sounds with common onsets is consistent with the Gestalt principle of **common fate**. Consider the consequences of dropping a bottle on a hard surface and listening for whether the bottle breaks. When any object bounces, each bounce results in a set of overtones that relate to the size, shape, and material of the object. If the dropped bottle does not break (**FIGURE 10.24A**), this pattern of overtones repeats as a group, and the intensity of the sounds decreases with every additional bounce. But if the bottle breaks on landing (**FIGURE 10.24B**), individual shards of the bottle will have different spectral compositions, each shard being its own sound source. Onsets of the overtones for different shards will differ because the pieces bounce independently until they bounce no more. Thus, even when the initial burst of noise is removed from the sound of the bouncing and breaking bottles, listeners can use patterns of onsets to accurately determine whether the bottle broke (W. H. Warren and Verbrugge, 1984).

common fate Gestalt grouping rule stating that the tendency of sounds to group together will increase if they begin and/or end at the same time.

When Hearing Dominates Vision

Hearing is fast. In Chapter 9, you learned how sensitively and quickly hair cells respond to sounds. In this chapter, you learned how we use tiny differences between the times sounds arrive at the two ears to localize from where the sound was created. Hearing is our best sense when it comes to timing, and when we perceive events that involve timing, we appear to rely more heavily on sound than on light. For example, when observers are asked to judge the length of time that a visual pattern (such as that in Figure 3.7) is presented, they report seeing the visual pattern longer when a sound of longer duration is played (de Haas et al., 2013). When participants see a light flickering while hearing a fluttering sound, they "see" the light flickering faster or slower as the sound

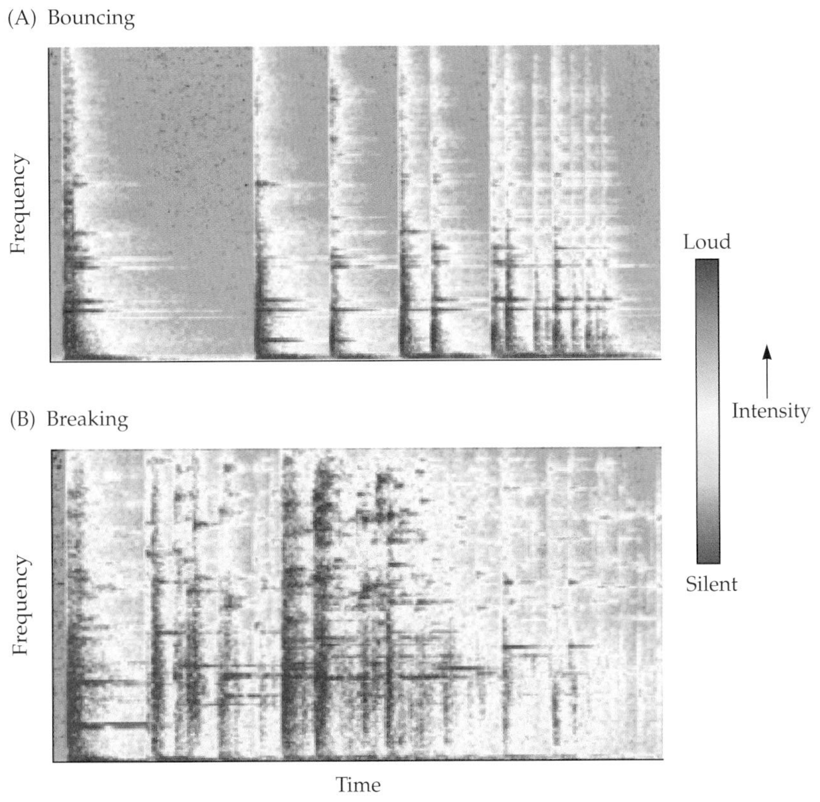

FIGURE 10.24 Bounce or break? Spectrograms of a bottle bouncing (A) and breaking (B). When the bottle breaks, there are multiple patterns of onset for multiple pieces of glass. Listeners can use patterns of onset to accurately determine whether the bottle broke.

flutters faster or slower (Welch, DuttonHurt, and Warren, 1986). Sounds can even make people see flashes of light that did not occur and see only one flash when more than one occurred. If a single flash of light is presented to the visual periphery while multiple beeps are played, participants will report seeing multiple flashes (Shams, Katimani, and Shimojo, 2000, 2002). When two brief flashes are presented in rapid succession (less than 1/10 of a second apart) and at the same time as a single sound, observers often perceive only a single flash (Andersen, Tiippana, and Sams, 2004).

Perhaps the most compelling example of hearing changing the way we see the world is the "bouncing balls" illusion. When viewing two disks approaching one another along the same direct trajectory (for example, one left to right and one right to left), what happens when they keep going past one another is visually ambiguous. The disks can be viewed as simply passing through one another, or they can be perceived as bouncing off one another, instantly repelling in the opposite direction. If a sound is played at the moment the disks meet, observers are far more likely to report that the disks bounced off one another (F. Zhou, Wong, and Sekuler, 2007). This effect is even greater if observers hear the sound of one pool ball striking another (Grassi and Casco, 2010). ●

When Sounds Become Familiar

In addition to the simple Gestalt principles we've already discussed, listeners make use of experience and familiarity to separate different sound sources. When you know what you're listening for, it's easier to pick out sounds from a background of other sounds. An obvious example is how quickly you recognize someone saying your name even when there are many other sounds, including other voices, in the room.

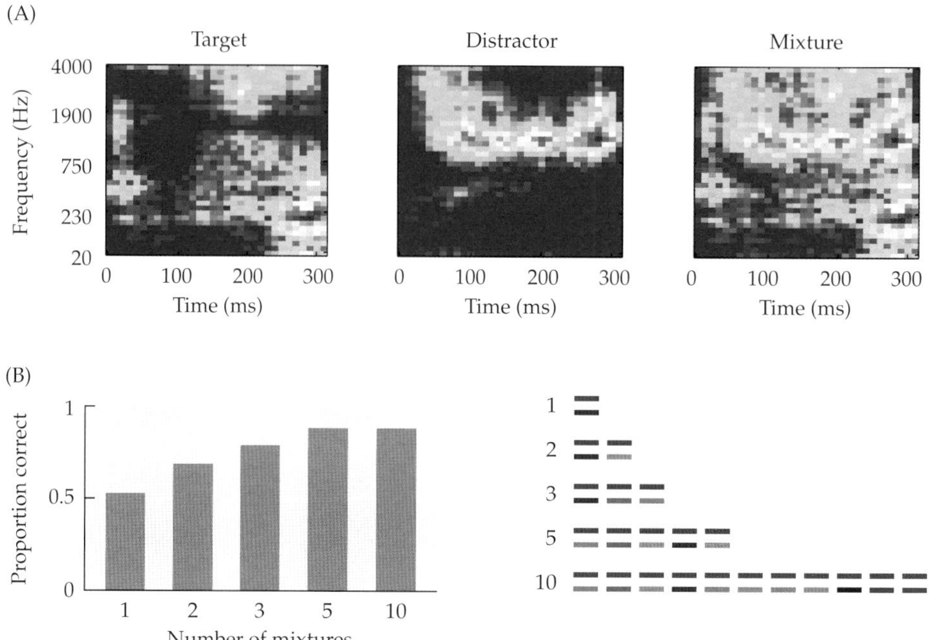

FIGURE 10.25 **Learning new sounds** (A) The listeners' task is to identify a novel complex sound (the target) when that target and a distractor overlap in one combined sound (the mixture). (B) When a new complex sound (red bars) is repeatedly played at the same time as different sounds (not-red bars) just a few times, listeners quickly become familiar enough with the target sound that they can pick it out from other sounds in the background.

You might be surprised to learn how quickly you can come to recognize a completely new sound once you've heard it a few times. Sounds in the environment, such as bird calls, often occur more than once. To test how much experience listeners need to benefit from familiarity, McDermott, Wroblewski, and Oxenham (2011) created complex novel sounds by combining natural sound characteristics in ways that listeners had never heard before. They repeatedly played these sounds at the same time and intensity as a background of other novel sounds that did not repeat, as shown in FIGURE 10.25. Although listeners could not segregate a sound from its background when they listened to a single instance, they could nonetheless segregate and identify the sound when it repeated. Listeners needed only a few repetitions to perform well above chance, even though they had never heard the complex sounds before they came to the laboratory.

10.4 Continuity and Restoration Effects

As already discussed, the sound we're trying to listen to at any given time is usually not the only sound in the environment. In addition to dealing with overlapping auditory streams, we also often must deal with cases when one sound completely obscures, or masks, another sound for brief periods. Suppose you're listening on your cell phone as a friend gives you directions to the restaurant where you're to meet for lunch. A car may honk, a baby may cry, or your cell phone may produce a short burst of static, but if you're paying attention and the interruption is not too long, you will probably be able to "hear through" the interruption. This effect is consistent with the Gestalt principle of **good continuation** (illustrated for vision in

good continuation Gestalt grouping rule stating that sounds will tend to group together as continuous if they seem to share a common path, similar to a shared contour for vision.

Figure 4.16): the continuous auditory stream is heard to continue behind the masking sound. Auditory researchers have labeled these phenomena "continuity effects" or "perceptual restoration effects"—the latter label arising because the auditory system appears to restore the portion of the continuous stream that was blocked out by the interrupting sound (R. M. Warren, 1984). In this sense, auditory restoration is analogous to the visual system's filling in the portions of a background object that is sitting behind an occluding object.

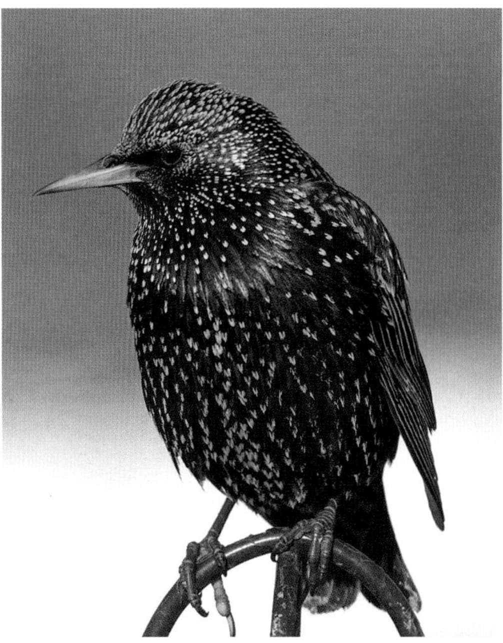

FIGURE 10.26 **Starlings can restore missing pieces of song** European starlings perceptually restore bits of starling songs and are more likely to restore song parts when familiar with the starling that produced them.

FURTHER DISCUSSION of Gestalt grouping rules as they pertain to vision can be found in Section 4.4.

Listeners maintain perceptual continuity for quite a long time (through longer than 2 seconds of noise) when listening to sounds that would sensibly continue for a while, such as applause, music, and sawing wood (McWalter and McDermott, 2019). The compelling nature of perceptual restoration suggests that at some point the restored missing sounds are encoded in the brain as if they were really present in the signal (Riecke et al., 2009). Macaque monkeys also hear tones being restored even when interrupted by noise (Petkov, O'Connor, and Sutter, 2003), and A1 neurons in monkeys show the same responses to real and restored tones (Petkov, O'Connor, and Sutter, 2007). These data from the auditory cortex cannot tell us whether the sounds were restored in the cortex or at a point earlier in auditory processing. However, they make it easier to understand why perceptually restored sounds really sound like they are present.

Restoration of Complex Sounds

Complex sounds such as music and speech can be perceptually restored, as well. When DeWitt and Samuel (1990) played familiar melodies with notes excised and replaced by noise, listeners perceived the missing notes as if they were present. Restoration was so complete that listeners could not report which notes had been removed and replaced with noise. The researchers also tested whether familiarity of the melodies mattered. As you might expect, listeners were much less likely to "hear" a missing note in an unfamiliar melody.

Just in case you think only human listeners care about melodies, listen up. Seeba and Klump (2009) trained European starlings (**FIGURE 10.26**) to peck when they heard a difference between two sections of starling song, called motifs. Then the starlings heard intact motifs and, for comparison, interrupted motifs with short snippets filled with either noise or silence. They were more likely to peck, indicating a difference between an intact and an interrupted motif, when silence filled the gap. This observation suggests that the starlings restored the missing bits of motifs when noise was inserted into the gap. Not all starling songs are equal, however. In the same set of experiments, the researchers used bits of song that were either familiar to the starling in the experiment (the bird's own song or the song of a cage mate) or unfamiliar (from starlings the subject had never heard). Just like humans listening to familiar and unfamiliar melodies, starlings are more likely to restore missing bits of a familiar song.

Listening to familiar melodies and to real speech sentences, as opposed to simple sounds such as sine waves and tonal glides, permits listeners to use more than just auditory processing to fill in missing information. Clearly, these "higher-order"

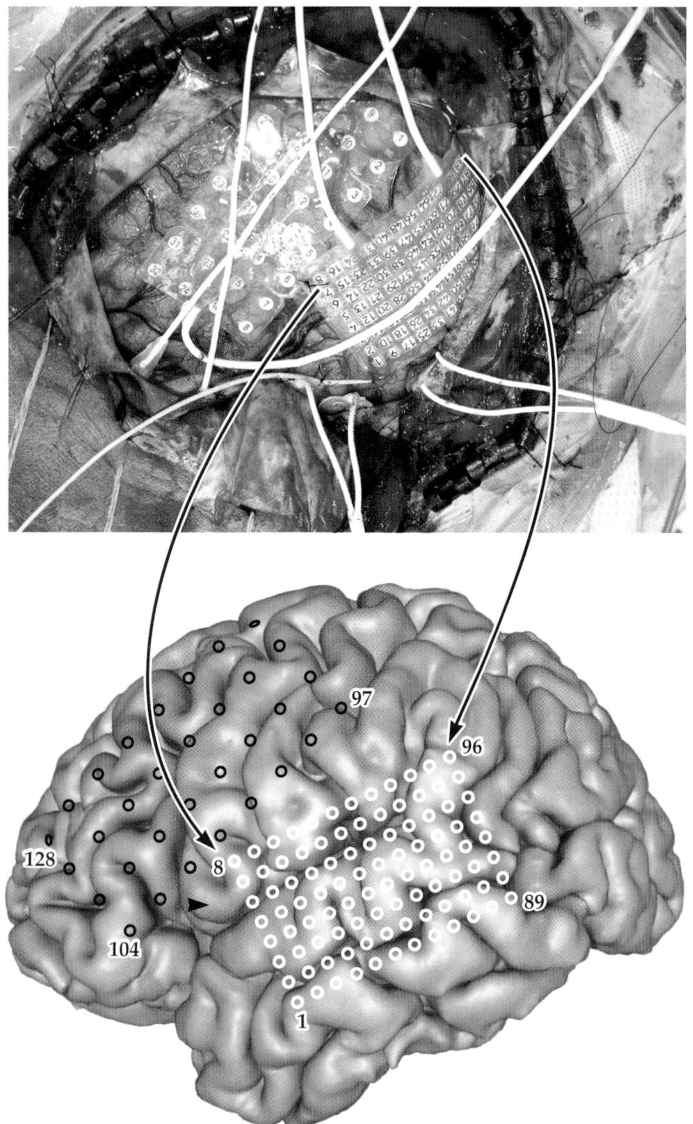

FIGURE 10.27 **Brain surface recording** Prior to performing brain surgery to remove a tumor or to reduce the effects of very severe epilepsy, neurosurgeons often place electrodes directly on the surface of the brain to localize regions of neural activity. Researchers can take advantage of these presurgical electrodes (which are medically needed) to record responses to experimental materials. The electrode grid shown here is similar to that used in the Leonard et al. (2016) study.

sources of information are used for listening to a sound in acoustically cluttered environments. Consider words that vary by only a single sound, such as *novel* versus *nozzle*. When the single sound that changes the word ('v' versus 'z' in this example) is replaced by noise (as in 'no#el'), listeners can report which of the two alternatives they "heard." What is happening in the brain? Matthew Leonard and colleagues (Leonard et al., 2016) found answers when they measured the activity of thousands of neurons recorded by electrodes placed on the surface of the brains of patients who were awaiting brain surgery (FIGURE 10.27). First, they recorded brain responses to the intact-word sounds 'novel' and 'nozzle.' Then they played the sounds of the words with noise replacing 'v' and 'z,' that is, 'no#el.' Listeners would report which word they heard when they listened to 'no#el,' and the researchers could predict which word the listeners would report by looking at whether brain activity in response to 'no#el' was more like activity in response to 'novel' or to 'nozzle.' The brain had filled in the missing sound so well that the response to a word missing a sound looked like the response to an intact word.

10.5 Auditory Attention

Have you ever been so engrossed by a task, such as reading this book, that you didn't even hear someone calling your name? At other times, maybe also while reading this book, have you ever noticed that it took only the barest distraction to draw your attention away? We said a lot about visual attention in Chapter 7. We will not delve so deeply into auditory attention, but there are some parallels to the visual case. Auditory attention can also differ from visual attention in ways that reflect the differences between senses. You just learned about how the auditory system is exquisitely fast and sensitive. In Chapter 9, we pointed out that hearing works great at a distance, in the dark, and around obstacles. These facts make hearing our primary sense for being vigilant in our surroundings—your first line of defense in a sensory world.

We see the auditory system playing the role of sentinel in the **acoustic startle reflex**. Just like its name implies, this is the very rapid bodily movement that arises following a loud, abrupt sound. The startle reflex is very fast: muscle twitches may follow the sound by as little as 10 ms (Musiek, 2003). Because the transmission time between ear (sound) and spinal cord (movement) is so brief, there can be no more than a few brainstem neurons between them. Being afraid increases the acoustic startle (M. Davis, 2006). Directors of horror movies know this, as they gradually ramp up your anxiety before the big event, and then the surprise is usually loud.

acoustic startle reflex The very rapid motor response to a sudden sound. Very few neurons are involved in the basic startle reflex, which can also be affected by emotional state.

The acoustic startle reflex is unselective—almost any loud sound will do. Auditory attention, however, is selective, picking one sound source out of several.

Many sounds occur at the same time in natural environments, with all sounds becoming merged at the ears. This makes listening to only one sound among many a serious challenge that is not solely solved by simple Gestalt grouping principles. This problem has much in common with the selective visual attention that you learned about in Chapter 7.

Effects of attending to a particular sound source can be so strong that we completely miss out on hearing other sounds in a kind of inattentional deafness. Skilled musicians were no better than untrained listeners at noticing an electronic guitar improvisation that was mixed in with Richard Strauss's "Thus Spoke Zarathustra" (the theme music from the sci-fi classic *2001: A Space Odyssey*) when both groups were asked to count (and, thus, to attend to) the number of timpani beats (Koreimann, Gula, and Vitouch, 2014). From this example, you see that task-specific "goals" can affect auditory attention in ways that may not be explained by only physical characteristics of sounds (Kaya and Elhilali, 2017). This **inattentional deafness** has its limits, because listeners had less trouble noticing the guitar when it was made sufficiently loud.

inattentional deafness The failure to notice a fully audible, but unexpected sound because attention was engaged on auditory stream.

While inattentional deafness might seem to be a bad thing, it really represents an extreme example of auditory processes that help us to listen in our acoustically crowded world. Imagine yourself in a room full of people who are speed dating in their search for true love (**FIGURE 10.28**). You earnestly focus on the person you are sizing up, but many other voices compete with the one voice you are trying to understand. Listeners can use the acoustic characteristics of a talker to track what that voice is saying despite the clutter of other voices. While we might think that this relies on being familiar with a talker or actively concentrating on that voice, this may not be necessary (Bressler et al., 2014). It appears that the brain does this automatically, following principles like those for auditory stream segregation described in Section 10.3.

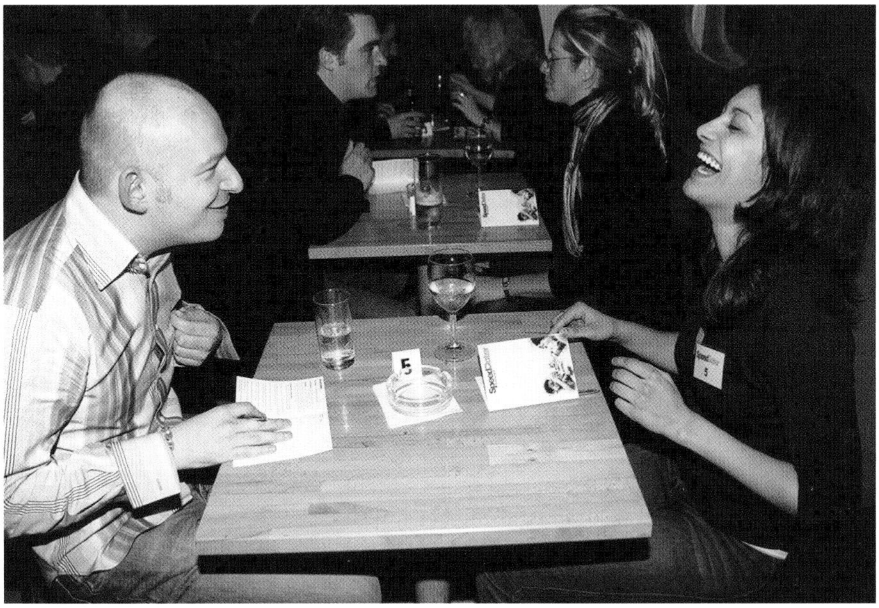

FIGURE 10.28 Auditory attention The organizers of this speed-dating event couldn't seat potential couples so close together if we didn't have the ability to attend to one voice among many. Note that although each of these individuals appears to be attending to the person across the table, any of them could be attending to one of the other conversations.

Suppose that, after sharing a brief exchange, you require no more time with the person to whom you've been listening. You begin to tune in to a neighboring conversation without moving away just yet from your currently assigned dating candidate. This requires shifting attention. There are several points to be made about this situation. First, there is a cost to moving to the next sound source: listeners become less accurate in understanding what they hear when they switch between talkers (Lawo and Koch, 2014). Second, your ability to look at one person while attending to a different conversation illustrates the flexibility of your attentional apparatus. Finally, if you are attending to another conversation, really embarrassing things can happen when you realize that your partner has stopped speaking and is waiting for a response to a question to which you have not attended. You can switch attention back and forth between streams, but you cannot fully process two streams of speech any more than you can read two sentences at the same time (see Figure 7.1).

Learning also affects attention. If the speed dating proceeds successfully and you enjoy years of conversations with your partner, the characteristics of their voice will affect your auditory attention. Compared to strangers' voices, the familiar voice of a spouse is better understood in noisy environments with competing sounds. On the flip side, it is also easier to *ignore* a spouse's voice than a stranger's voice when you are trying to focus on another sound. These effects of familiarity seem to grow greater with age, suggesting that the auditory system may rely on knowledge about patterns of voices to compensate for age-related auditory changes, like hearing loss (Johnsrude et al., 2013).

Summary

1. Listeners use small differences, in time and intensity, across the two ears to learn the direction in the horizontal plane (azimuth) from which a sound comes.
2. Time and intensity differences across the two ears are not sufficient to fully indicate the location from which a sound comes. In particular, they are not enough to indicate whether sounds come from the front or the back, or from higher or lower (elevation).
3. The pinna, ear canal, head, and torso alter the intensities of different frequencies for sounds coming from different places in space, and listeners use these changes in intensity across frequency to identify the location from which a sound comes.
4. Perception of auditory distance is similar to perception of visual depth because no single characteristic of the signal can inform a listener about how distant a sound source is. Listeners must combine intensity, spectral composition, and relative amounts of direct and reflected energy of sounds to estimate distance to a sound source.
5. Many natural sounds, including music and human speech, have rich harmonic structure with energy at integer multiples of the fundamental frequency, and listeners are especially good at perceiving the pitch of harmonic sounds.
6. Important perceptual qualities of complex sounds are timbre (conveyed by the relative amounts of energy at different frequencies) and the onset and offset properties of attack and decay, respectively.

7. Because all the sounds in the environment are summed into a single waveform that reaches each ear, a major challenge for hearing is to separate sound sources in the combined signal. This general process is known as auditory scene analysis. Auditory stream segregation succeeds by using multiple characteristics of sounds, including spatial location, similarity in frequency and timbre, onset properties, and familiarity.
8. In everyday environments, sounds to which a person is listening often are interrupted by other, louder sounds. Perceptual restoration is a process by which missing or degraded acoustic signals are perceptually replaced.
9. Auditory attention has many aspects in common with visual attention. It is a balance between being able to make use of sounds one needs to hear in the midst of competing sounds and being on alert for new auditory information.

Chapter 11

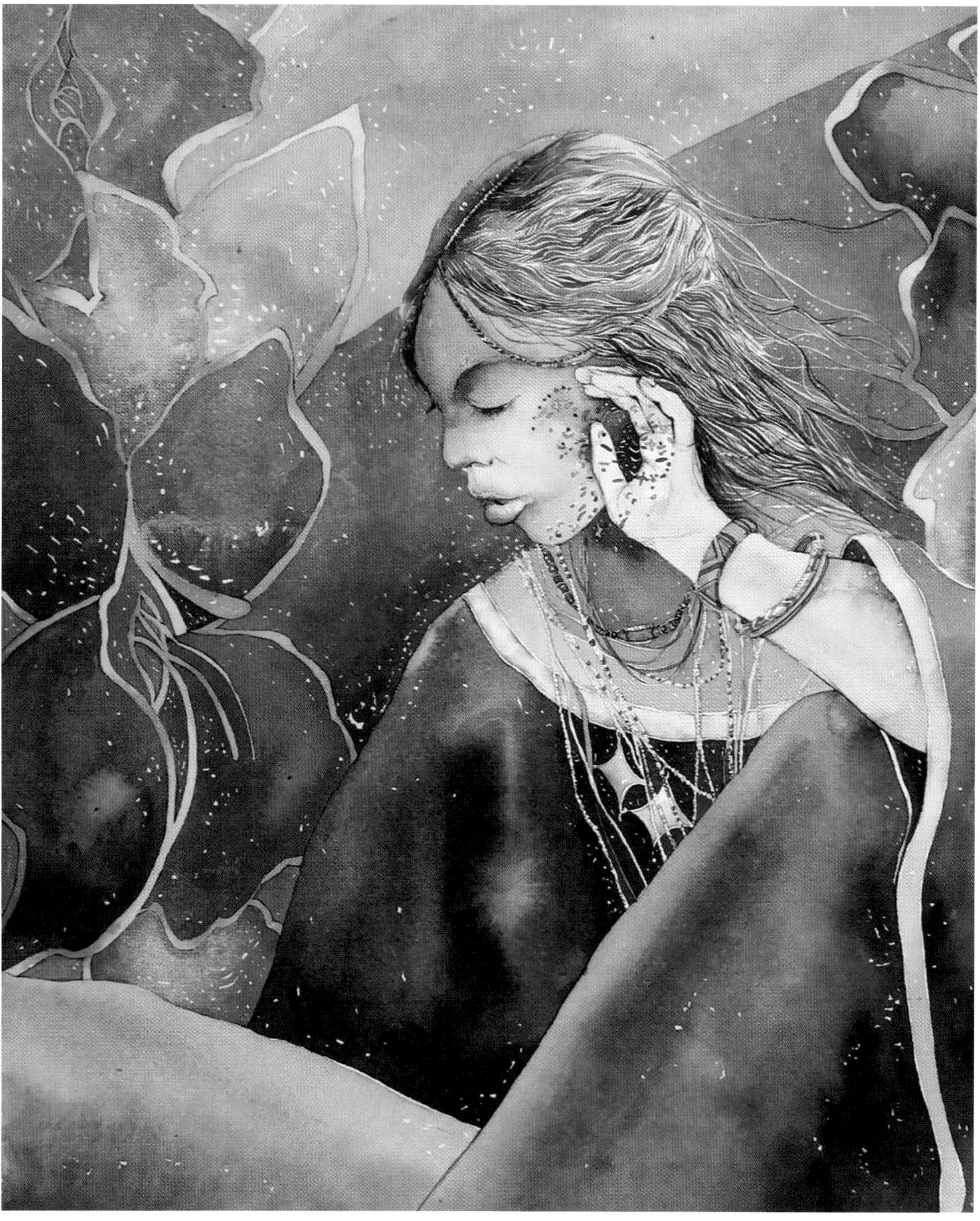

Meganne Forbes, Listening, 2001

Music and Speech Perception

Questions to Contemplate

Think about the following questions as you read this chapter.
By the chapter's end, you should be able to answer and discuss them.

- How is perception of music and speech different from perception of other sounds?
- What are the psychological dimensions of musical sounds?
- How are the psychological dimensions of music similar to and different from psychological dimensions of hearing for other sounds?
- What is the role of culture in determining how we hear music?
- In what ways are human speech sounds different from vocalizations by other creatures, and why?
- How are speech sounds described and in what ways do they vary?
- What are some differences and similarities between the way speech sounds are perceived compared to ways other acoustic stimuli are heard?
- Why and how is experience with speech important to how it is perceived?

Sounds from musical instruments and human voices obey the same laws of physical acoustics as all other sounds. Guitar strings and human vocal folds vibrate, with similarities to rubber bands and suspension bridges. Trombones and vocal tracts act as resonators following the same laws as empty bottles and hollow logs. In this sense, spoken words and musical notes are nothing more than very familiar, very complex sounds.

Music and speech also can be distinguished from most other environmental sounds. Just as visual art like paintings and sculpture is created to attract the eye, music and speech are created with listeners in mind. Both music and speech serve to communicate, and both can convey emotion and deeper meanings. In song, music and speech conspire to move the listener. Although dogs, birds, and whales share acoustic messages and even sing to one another, there is no question that the depth and breadth of human communication by music and speech has no rival in the acoustic world. In this chapter, we explore these communicative aspects of hearing.

11.1 Music

People have been using music to express themselves and influence the thoughts and emotions of others for a very long time. The oldest discovered musical instrument—a flute carved from the thighbone of a young cave bear—is perhaps 60,000 years old and created by Neanderthals (Turk, Dirjec, and Kavur, 1995). You probably know of the ancient Greek scholar Pythagoras (ca. 580–ca. 500 BCE) from the Pythagorean theorem in high school geometry. To say that Pythagoras was obsessed with numbers would be an understatement. And the numbers that he

Sensation & Perception in Everyday Life

Music and Emotion

What we hear has a powerful effect on how we feel. Emily Dickinson (1830–1886) (**FIGURE 11.1**), one of America's greatest poets, required only four lines to portray the bond between hearing and emotion.

An ear can break a human heart
As quickly as a spear
We wish the ear had not a heart
So dangerously near

—Excerpt from "The saddest noise, the sweetest noise"

We know listening to music affects people's moods (Eich, 1995; Pignatiello, Camp, and Rasar, 1986) and emotions (Sloboda, 1999). When listeners hear pleasant-sounding chords preceding a word, they are faster to respond that a word such as *charm* is positive and slower to respond that a word such as *evil* is negative (Sollberger, Reber, and Eckstein, 2003). Given the powerful effects of music on mood and emotion, some clinical psychologists practice music therapy, during which people sing, listen, play, and move to music in efforts to improve mental and physical health.

Music has deep physiological effects. Music can promote positive emotions, reduce pain, and alleviate stress, and it may even improve resistance to disease (Gangrade, 2011; Roy, Peretz, and Rainville, 2007). Evidence across many studies suggests that music can reduce pain (Lunde et al., 2019) and that it improves anxiety, mood, and overall quality of life for patients with cancer (Archie, Bruera, and Cohen, 2013). When people listen to highly pleasurable music, they experience changes in heart rate, muscle electrical activity, and respiration, as well as increases in blood flow to brain regions involved in reward and motivation (Blood and Zatorre, 2001). The strength of connections between auditory cortex and brain regions associated with reward and pleasure predicts how rewarding music is for an individual (Martínez-Molina et al., 2019).

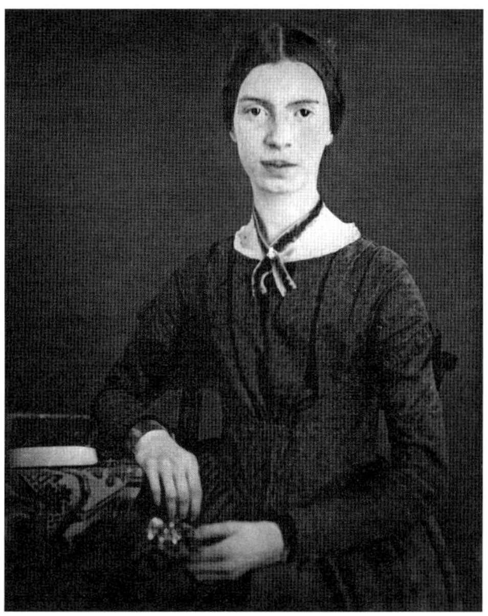

FIGURE 11.1 Emily Dickinson Although the people around her knew that she was often writing, only 11 of Emily Dickinson's 1775 poems were published during her lifetime. "The saddest noise, the sweetest noise" was her 1764th poem.

and his followers cared about most were those found in musical scales. They were convinced that the musical intervals they found most pleasing should provide the greatest insights not only into mathematics, but also into the universe. Although music may not explain the known universe, we all appreciate how important music is to culture and, perhaps, to one's personal cultural identity.

Musical Notes

From Chapter 9, you know that one of the most important characteristics of any sound is frequency. You also know that brain structures for processing sounds are tonotopically organized to correspond to frequency. The psychological quality of perceived frequency is **pitch**. When you imagined pitch while reading Section 9.2, you probably imagined musical pitch. **FIGURE 11.2** illustrates the extent of the frequency range of musical sounds in relation to human hearing.

pitch The psychological aspect of sound related mainly to perceived frequency.

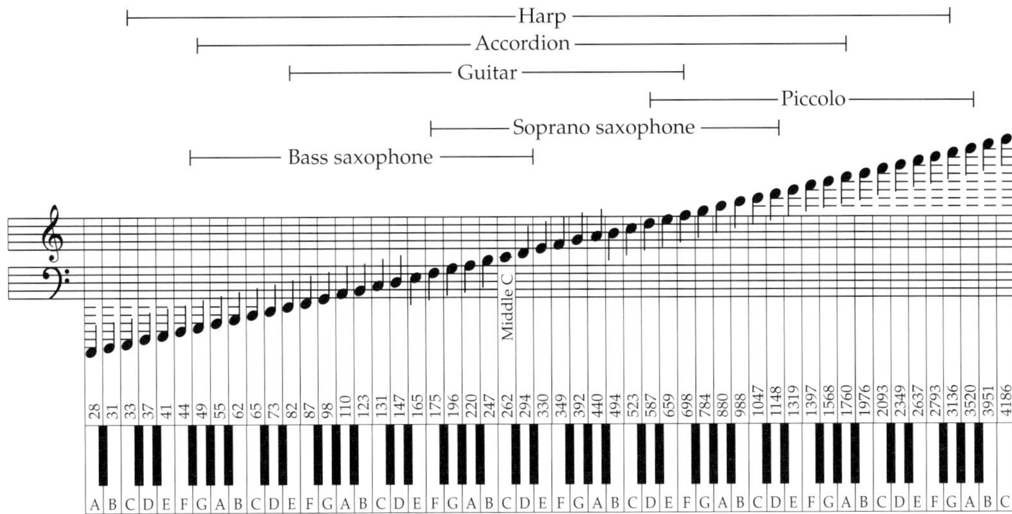

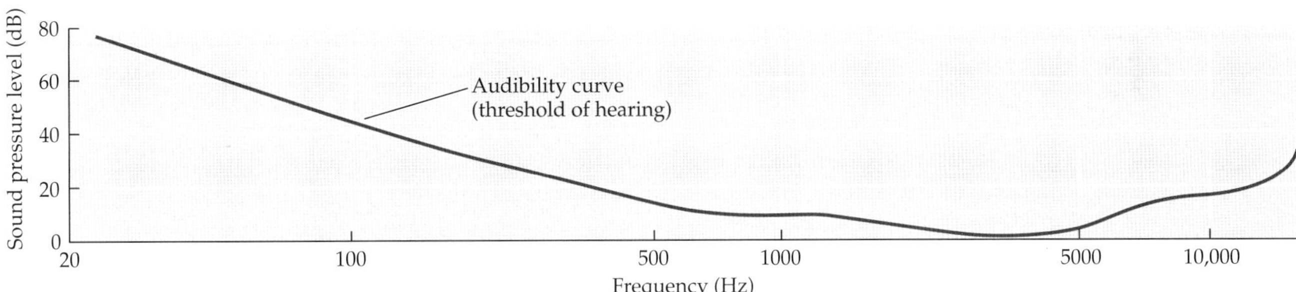

FIGURE 11.2 Frequency range of music The sounds of music extend across a frequency range from about 25 to about 4200 Hz. Although human hearing extends to much higher frequencies (bottom), sounds above 4000–5000 Hz are not perceived as musical.

TONE HEIGHT AND TONE CHROMA Musical pitch is one of the characteristics of musical notes, the sounds that make up a melody. A very important concept in understanding musical pitch is the **octave**. When we described pitch in Section 9.2, it seemed clear that the nearer any two sounds were in frequency, the nearer they were in pitch. Here's where octaves come in. When one of two periodic sounds is double the frequency of the other, those two sounds are one octave apart. For example, middle C (C_4) has a fundamental frequency of 261.6 hertz (Hz). Notes that are one octave below and above middle C are 130.8 Hz (C_3) and 523.2 Hz (C_5), respectively. Not only do these three sounds have the same name on the musical scale (C), but also they sound similar. In fact, C_3 (130.8 Hz) sounds more similar to C_4 (261.6 Hz) than to a sound with a closer frequency—for example, E_3 (164.8 Hz). Clearly there is more to musical pitch than just frequency.

The preceding example illustrates the concept of *just intonation*, in which frequencies of sounds are in simple whole-number ratios with one another (e.g., 2:1 for an octave). But in typical Western music, the frequencies of notes are adjusted slightly from simple ratios so that combinations of notes will sound equally good when played in higher- or lower-frequency ranges (i.e., a higher or lower key). The set of notes (the scale) commonly used in Western music is called *equal temperament*.

octave The interval between two sound frequencies having a ratio of 2:1.

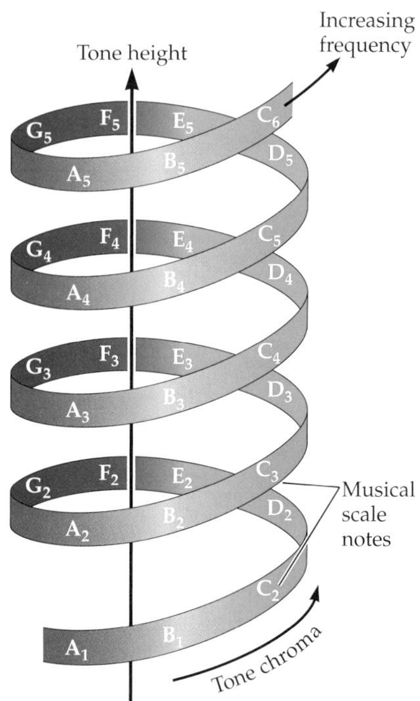

FIGURE 11.3 Musical helix This helix illustrates the two dimensions of musical pitch: tone height (related to frequency) and tone chroma (related to the octave).

Because of octave relations, musical pitch is typically described as having two dimensions. The first is **tone height**, which relates to frequency in a fairly straightforward way. The second dimension, related to the octave, is **tone chroma** (*chroma* is the Greek word for "color"). We can visualize musical pitch as a helix. Frequency and tone height increase with increasing height on the helix, as shown in FIGURE 11.3. The circular laps around the helix correspond to changes in tone chroma. At the same point along each lap around the helix, a specific sound lies on a vertical line, and all sounds along that line share the same tone chroma and are separated by octaves.

You may have learned to sing the notes of the musical scale: "do," "re," "mi," "fa," "sol," "la," "ti," "do." Perhaps you even tested how many times you could sing the scale at increasingly higher pitches. In that case, you were singing your way up the musical helix. Your pitch traveled a full turn upward with each repetition of a particular note—for example, "do" or "re." There is an upper limit on how high a note can be before it no longer sounds musical. Most musical instruments generally produce notes that are below 4000 Hz, and a sequence of pure tones with frequencies greater than 5000 Hz does not convey a melody very well (Attneave and Olson, 1971). It is also true that listeners have great difficulty perceiving octave relationships between tones when one or both tones have a frequency greater than 5000 Hz (W. D. Ward, 1954).

CHORDS Music is further defined by richer, complex sounds called **chords**, which are created when three or more notes are played simultaneously. (The simultaneous playing of two notes is called a dyad.) The major distinction between chords is whether they are consonant or dissonant. Perceived to be most pleasing, *consonant* chords are combinations of notes in which the ratios between the note frequencies are simple. This is why Pythagoras was so taken by the relationship between pleasantness and mathematics. You already know one of the consonant relationships, the octave, in which the frequencies of the two notes are in the simple ratio of 2:1. Other major consonant intervals are the perfect fifth (3:2) and the perfect fourth (4:3). *Dissonant* intervals are defined by less elegant ratios. For example, the minor second (16:15) and the augmented fourth (45:32) do not sound very pleasing. Indeed, during the Middle Ages the augmented fourth was called the "devil in music" (Seay, 1975).

Because chords are defined by the ratios of the note frequencies combined to produce them, they are named the same no matter what octave they're played in. For example, the G-major chord consists of the notes G, B, and D, and it can be played as $G_2 + B_2 + D_3$, $G_4 + B_4 + D_5$, $G_6 + B_6 + D_7$, or in any other octave, provided the ratios remain the same. Note that in the musical helix in FIGURE 11.4, the relationships between the notes of the chord on the helix stay the same, as in Figure 11.3; only the pattern's height changes.

CULTURAL DIFFERENCES Musical scales and intervals vary widely across cultures. Although potent relationships between notes such as octaves are relatively universal, different musical traditions use different numbers of notes and spaces between notes within an octave. Our discussion so far has concerned the heptatonic (seven-note) scale. Another common scale, pentatonic, has five notes per octave, and you've heard this scale in gospel, jazz, rock, and blues music, among other North American genres. The pentatonic scale is traditional in many other parts of the world, especially Asia.

In scales for which fewer notes comprise an octave, notes may be more loosely tuned than are notes in the heptatonic Western scale. When there are fewer notes

tone height A sound quality corresponding to the level of pitch. Tone height is monotonically related to frequency.

tone chroma A sound quality shared by tones that have the same octave interval.

chord A combination of three or more musical notes with different pitches played simultaneously.

to distinguish, a wider range of pitches can qualify for a given note. For example, the Javanese *sléndro* and *pélog* scales have fewer than seven notes within an octave, and there is greater variation in a note's acceptable frequencies.

Because people around the world have very different listening experiences, you might expect them to hear musical notes in different ways. Indeed, when Javanese and Western musicians hear intervals between notes, their estimates of the intervals vary according to how well those notes correspond to Javanese and Western scales, respectively (Perlman and Krumhansl, 1996). Furthermore, infants seem equipped to learn whatever scale is used in their environment. Lynch and Eilers (1990) tested the degree to which 6-month-old infants in Florida noticed inappropriate notes within both the traditional Western scale and the Javanese *pélog* scale. The infants appeared to be equally good at detecting "mistakes" within both Western and Javanese scales, but adults were reliably better at detecting deviations from the Western scale.

Even basic mathematical principles about musical intervals are not as fixed in stone as Pythagoras thought. Remember the "devil in music," the augmented fourth, that is so dissonant that it sounds unpleasant? Deep in the Amazon rain forest of Bolivia live the Tsimane′ forager-horticulturalist group. As shown in **FIGURE 11.5**, researchers made their way through the rain forest to test what Tsimane′ people like in their music (McDermott et al., 2016). Perception of pitch grows roughly logarithmically with frequency for Tsimane′ people, and they also hear sounds as being musical up to only about 4000 Hz (Jacoby et al., 2019). So far, this is nothing unusual. However, when Tsimane′ people sing, they seem not to recognize chroma, the characteristic that two notes sound similar when they are one octave apart. Further, Tsimane′ have no difficulty hearing the difference between consonant and dissonant chords, but they have no preference for consonant, dissonant, or even vocal harmonies. City dwellers in La Paz, however, have the same preferences as most other Westerners. While we cannot know whether this is a cause or an effect, you may find it interesting that Tsimane′ people do not tend to sing in groups.

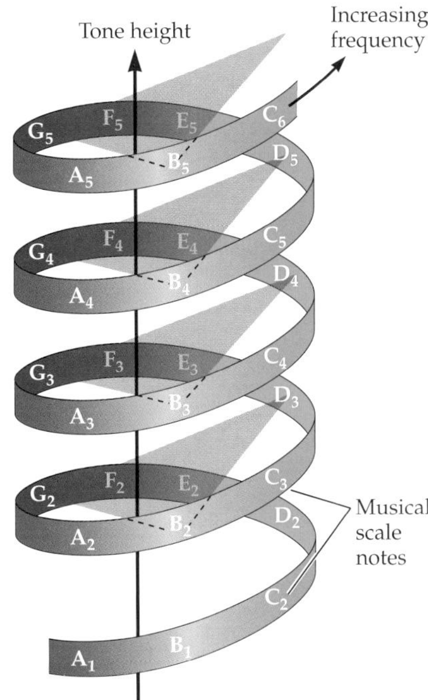

FIGURE 11.4 Chords Chords are made up of three or more notes and can be played with different tone heights while their chromatic relationships are maintained. Here, the G-major chord (purple shading) is shown being played at different tone heights.

ABSOLUTE PITCH You may have heard that some people are "gifted" with **absolute pitch (AP)**, often referred to as "perfect pitch." AP is an ability of some listeners to accurately name or recreate notes in isolation. In this way, *absolute* is used to distinguish AP from *relative pitch*, which is the way most people identify notes. AP relates specifically to musical notes, because people with AP share the same

absolute pitch (AP) A rare ability whereby some people are able to accurately name or produce notes without comparison to other notes.

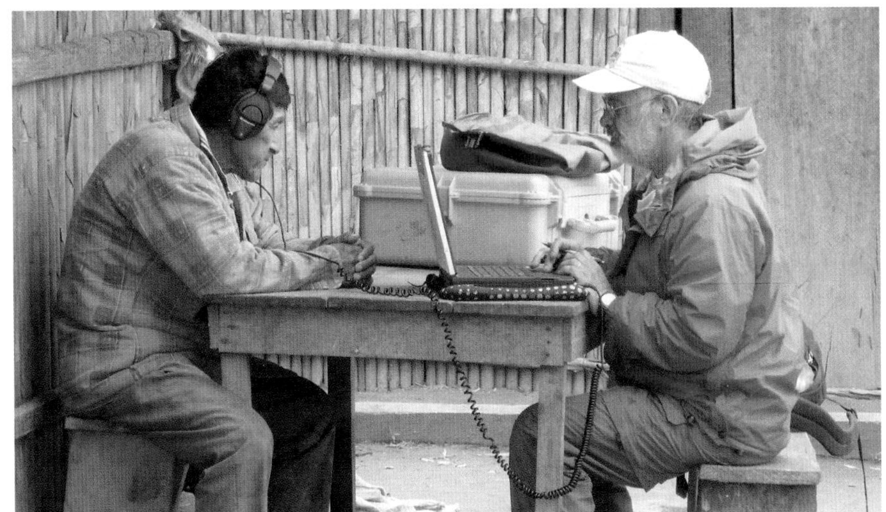

FIGURE 11.5 Are musical preferences influenced by culture? In Bolivia, a researcher (right) plays a variety of musical chords for a man of the Tsimane′ people of the Amazon rain forest. The Tsimane′ man is then asked about which chords, if any, he prefers over others.

basic sense of hearing as other people: their auditory systems are no more sensitive than normal, and they are no better than anyone else at detecting differences between sounds.

Absolute pitch is rare, occurring in less than one in 10,000 people (Takeuchi and Hulse, 1993). Among musicians, this rare skill is often considered highly desirable. Many believe that Beethoven had AP, and it appears that Mozart demonstrated AP by the time he was only 7 years old (Deutsch, 2013).

Researchers disagree on how some people come to have AP. One idea is that people might acquire AP following a great deal of practice. However, only some adults can be trained to have AP, even *with* practice (Van Hedger, Heald, and Nusbaum, 2019). Others have suggested that, in contrast to learning AP, some people are born with it (Athos et al., 2007), and this is consistent with the fact that AP appears to run in families (Theusch and Gitschier, 2011). However, children in the same family share more than genetics. In a home in which one child receives music lessons, it is likely that siblings also receive music lessons. There is variation in AP, and this variation presents a challenge for identifying possible genetic components. Most traits that are influenced by genes, such as height, show variation—they are not "all or none"—and variation in expertise also occurs for skills that are learned. The best explanation for AP might be that it is acquired through experience and (as we will soon learn is true about development of speech perception) the age at which experience occurs matters a great deal. In studies measuring abilities across many people, the age at which musical training begins is well correlated with future possession of AP (Deutsch et al., 2011; Lee and Lee, 2010).

Absolute pitch might not be so absolute, and adults with AP might be more flexible in their listening than typically thought. After first testing the identification of notes by listeners with AP, Van Hedger, Heald, and Nusbaum (2013) had their participants listen to Johannes Brahms's Symphony no. 1 in C minor and asked them to pay close attention to individual melodies. What the researchers did not tell their listeners was that, during the first part of the piece, they very gradually "de-tuned" the music by making all the notes a bit flat by playing the music at these lower frequencies for a while longer. After the musical passage was complete, AP listeners were more likely to judge flat notes as being in tune and to judge in-tune notes as being mistuned. While it may be very difficult to train adults to become AP listeners, perception of musical notes by adults with AP can be shifted by musical experience. Absolute pitch is apparently not as absolute as once was thought.

Making Music

Notes or chords can form a **melody**, a sequence of sounds perceived as a single coherent structure. The notes of "Twinkle, Twinkle, Little Star" (also known as "Now I Know My ABCs," "Baa Baa Black Sheep," and Variation K 265 by Wolfgang Amadeus Mozart) "belong together" perceptually because they form this familiar melody. Note that a melody is defined by its contour—the pattern of rises and declines in pitch—rather than by an exact sequence of sound frequencies (Handel, 1989).

You've already learned one simple way in which melody is not a sequence of specific sounds: shift every note of a melody by one octave, and the resulting melody is the same. When you sing with other people who have higher or lower voices, you all sing the same melody at very different pitches. Even within a single octave, the same melody can be perceived from different notes if the steps between notes stay the same.

In addition to varying in pitch, notes and chords vary in duration. The average duration of a set of notes in a melody defines the music's **tempo**. Any melody can be played at either a fast or a slow tempo. But the relative durations within

melody A sequence of notes or chords perceived as a single coherent structure.

tempo The perceived speed of the presentation of sounds.

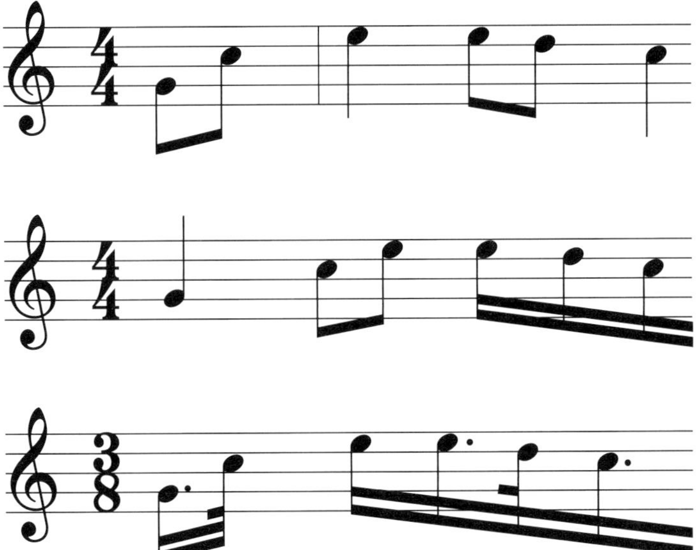

FIGURE 11.6 **Melody** The pattern of increasing and decreasing pitches can remain the same, but the melody will change if notes have different durations. Here, three series of notes with the same melody contour are shown with notes that differ only in duration.

a sequence of notes are a critical part of the melodies themselves. If the notes of a given sequence are played with different relative durations, we will often hear completely different melodies (FIGURE 11.6).

RHYTHM In addition to varying in speed, music varies in **rhythm**. The fact that music has rhythm should go without saying. After all, how else would we dance to it? Less obvious, perhaps, is that many—or even most—activities have rhythm. Walking and galloping have rhythm. So do finger tapping, waving, clapping, and swimming. Perhaps it is the very commonness of rhythm that causes us to hear nearly all sounds as rhythmic, even when they're not.

Over a century ago, Thaddeus Bolton (1894) conducted experiments in which he played a sequence of identical sounds perfectly spaced in time; they had no rhythm. Nevertheless, his listeners readily reported that the sounds occurred in groups of two, three, or four. Moreover, they reported hearing the first sound of a group as accented, or stressed, while the remaining sounds were unaccented, or unstressed. You've probably had a similar experience while riding in a train or car. Even though a train travels over junctions in the rails at nearly equal intervals, you hear the sound as "CLICK click CLICK click." When you ride in a car at a steady speed, you hear "THUMP thump THUMP thump" as your tires roll over cracks in a concrete road.

As Bolton's studies show, listeners are predisposed to grouping sounds into rhythmic patterns. Several qualities contribute to whether sounds will be heard as accented (stressed) or unaccented (unstressed). Sounds that are longer, louder, and higher in pitch all are more likely to be heard as leading their groups (Woodrow, 1909). The timing relationship between one sound and the others in a sequence also helps determine accent. For example, we are more likely to hear a series of three sounds as "Aaa Aaa Aaa" than as "aAa aAa aAa."

Listeners prefer, or at least expect, sequences of notes to be fairly regular, and this tendency provides opportunities for composers to get creative with beat. One way to be creative in deviating from a bland succession of regular beats is to introduce **syncopation**. Syncopation is any deviation from a regular rhythm, for example, by accenting a note that is expected to be unaccented or not playing a note (replacing it with a rest) when a note is expected. Syncopation has been used for

rhythm A repeated pattern of sounds composed of strong and weak elements.

syncopation Any deviation from a regular rhythm.

AaaAaaAaaAaaAaaAaaAaaAaaAaa

BbbbBbbbBbbbBbbbBbbbBbbbBbbb

← → ← →

FIGURE 11.7 Syncopated polyrhythms When two rhythms are played together and one rhythm (in this case Aaa) is dominant, listeners tend to perceive the timing of beats in the nondominant rhythm (Bbbb) adjusted to conform with the dominant rhythm. Arrows illustrate how accented B beats perceptually move backward or forward in time to align with the accented A in the dominant rhythm.

centuries and can be found in compositions by all the great composers, including Bach, Beethoven, and Mozart. You may be familiar with syncopation from jazz, reggae, and ska.

One particularly illustrative example of syncopation is syncopated auditory polyrhythms. When two different rhythms are overlapped, they can collide in interesting ways. For example, if one rhythm is based on 3 beats (AaaAaaAaaAaa) and the other on 4 (BbbbBbbbBbbb), the first accented sound for both rhythms will coincide only once every 12 beats. Across the 11 intervening beats, the two rhythms will be out of sync. When we listen to syncopated polyrhythms, one of the two rhythms becomes the dominant or controlling rhythm, and the other rhythm tends to be perceptually adjusted to accommodate the first (**FIGURE 11.7**). In particular, the accented beat of the subordinate rhythm shifts in time (Handel and Oshinsky, 1981). Thus, syncopation is the perception that beats in the subordinate rhythm have traveled backward or forward in time.

These findings reveal that rhythm is, in large part, psychological. We can produce sequences of sounds that are rhythmic and are perceived as such. But we also hear rhythm when it does not exist and notes effectively travel in time to maintain the perception of consistent rhythm.

Given the psychological nature of rhythm, at least with respect to syncopation, you might be wondering if the classic intervals of musical notes themselves are predestined or the result of experience. The durations of notes in Western musical notation are at very tidy intervals. A sixteenth note (𝅘𝅥𝅯) is half as long as an eighth note (♪), which is half as long as a quarter note (♩), which is half as long as a half note (𝅗𝅥), which is half as long as a whole note (𝅝). Just as octaves are defined by doubling frequency, musical notes represent doubling of duration. This relative change in duration illustrates Weber's law (see Section 1.2) in action.

Let's return to the Tsimane′ of Bolivia. We do not have Tsimane′ notes to look at, but we can ask whether they prefer certain rhythms more than others. Tsimane′ listeners do gravitate toward the simple rhythms that follow simple doubling of intervals (such as 1:1:1, 1:1:2, 1:2:1, 2:1:1, 1:2:2, 2:1:2, and 2:2:1). However, Tsimane′ listeners are much less inclined toward other simple rhythms (for example, 1:1:3, 1:2:3, or 2:2:3) that do not involve doubling when compared to listeners from the United States (Jacoby and McDermott, 2017). This is true even when the US listeners have no musical training.

MELODY DEVELOPMENT Like rhythm, melody is essentially a psychological entity (Handel, 1989). There is nothing about the sequence of notes in "Twinkle, Twinkle, Little Star" that makes them a melody. Rather, it is our experience with a particular sequence of notes or with similar sequences that helps us perceive coherence.

Studies of 8-month-old listeners reveal that learning of melodies begins quite early in life. Saffran et al. (1999) created six simple and deliberately novel "melodies" composed of sequences of three tones. Infants sat on their parents' laps while hearing only 3 minutes of continuous repetitions of the six melodies. Next, infants heard both the original melodies and a series of new three-tone sequences. These new sequences contained the same notes as the originals, but one part of the sequence

Sensation & Perception in Everyday Life

 Sonic Seasoning

Everyone believes they have good taste in music, but did you know that music literally affects your taste? People instinctively match basic tastes such as sweet, sour, bitter, and salty (see Section 15.3) with certain kinds of musical notes, chords, and melodies (Spence, 2020). This multisensory experience has been referred to as *sonic seasoning*, and much of what we've learned about it involves wine tasting. You can find descriptors such as "bright," "intense," "complex," "dense," and "structured" on a wine label—but these terms could also be used to describe music. And this is before claiming the wine has "notes" of almond.

Wine tasters are more likely to match Mozart's Flute Quartet in D Major, compared to Tchaikovsky's String Quartet no. 1, to a crisp white wine. However, they found the Tchaikovsky piece to be a better match to a rich red wine (Spence et al., 2013). Participants tasting red wines while hearing a 100 Hz bass note (around G_2) or a 1000 Hz high note (around B_5) felt that a pinot noir tasted fuller-bodied and a Spanish garnacha tasted more aromatically intense when either was paired with the bass note as compared to the high note (Burzynska et al., 2019). Remarkably, Q. Wang and Spence (2018) found no relation between degree of wine expertise (experts versus novices) and the amount of influence music has over taste.

Not a wine drinker? Sonic seasoning has also been documented for participants tasting chocolate ice cream (Italian gelato). Trained chocolate tasters rated milk chocolate, dark chocolate, and bittersweet chocolate gelati while listening to three different music samples. When tasters liked or were neutral about the music sample, they rated the chocolate's level of sweetness more highly; when they gave the music a low rating, the chocolate tasted more bitter (Kantono et al., 2016). ●

was taken from one melody and another part from another melody. Because the infants responded differently to the new melodies, we can deduce that they had learned something about the original melodies.

This ability to learn new melodies is not limited to simple sequences of tones. In a study with 7-month-old infants, parents played a recording of two Mozart sonata movements to their infants every day for 2 weeks (Saffran, Loman, and Robertson, 2000). After another 2 weeks had passed, the infants were tested in a laboratory to see whether they remembered the movements. Infant listeners responded differently to the original sonata movements than to similar Mozart movements introduced to them for the first time in the laboratory.

This learning is important because although music appears to be universal, it takes different forms across cultures. Even those of us who are nonmusicians progressively learn patterns and regularities of our culture's music through exposure. These patterns are different in Western music than, for example, in traditional Indian ragas. The knowledge of a culture's music patterns leads listeners to implicitly predict the probability of different possible continuations of the music (Pearce, 2018). When a melody or rhythm departs from expectations, it is surprising. Many human composers, and even computer algorithms that write music, capitalize on this "surprisal" to engage listeners' attention.

11.2 Speech

Among hearing people, speech is the principle basis of language. Language connects us to other people and forms a basis for culture. Whether catching up on a favorite television series, chatting with a friend at a cafeteria, or listening to a professor lecture, we consume a great deal of speech each day. A classic and oft-cited analysis attributes 70–80% of the workday to communication, with about 55% of this time devoted to speech listening (Klemmer and Synder, 1972). Even our own voice provides us with rich input; systematic recordings of natural conversations indicate that we utter an average of about 16,000 words each day (Mehl et al., 2007).

Most people who listen to speech also produce speech. Talkers speak so that they can be understood, and the relationship between the production and perception of speech is an especially intimate one. Therefore, it is important to know some things about speech production before trying to understand speech perception.

Humans can produce an incredible range of distinct speech sounds (the 5000 or so languages across the world use over 850 different speech sounds) (Maddieson, 1984). If you've ever heard Kenny Muhammad, the "Human Orchestra," you've experienced the unrivaled versatility of human sound production. This flexibility arises from the unique structure of the human larynx ("voice box") and the vocal tract that lies above it (Lieberman, 1984). Compared with that of other animals, the human larynx is positioned quite low in the throat. One notorious disadvantage of such a low larynx is that humans choke on food more easily than any other animal does. The fact that these life-threatening anatomical liabilities were evolutionarily trumped by the survival advantage of oral communication is a testament to the importance of language to human life.

Speech Production

The production of speech has three basic components: respiration (lungs), phonation (vocal folds), and articulation (vocal tract) (**FIGURE 11.8**). Speaking fluently requires an impressive degree of coordination among these components.

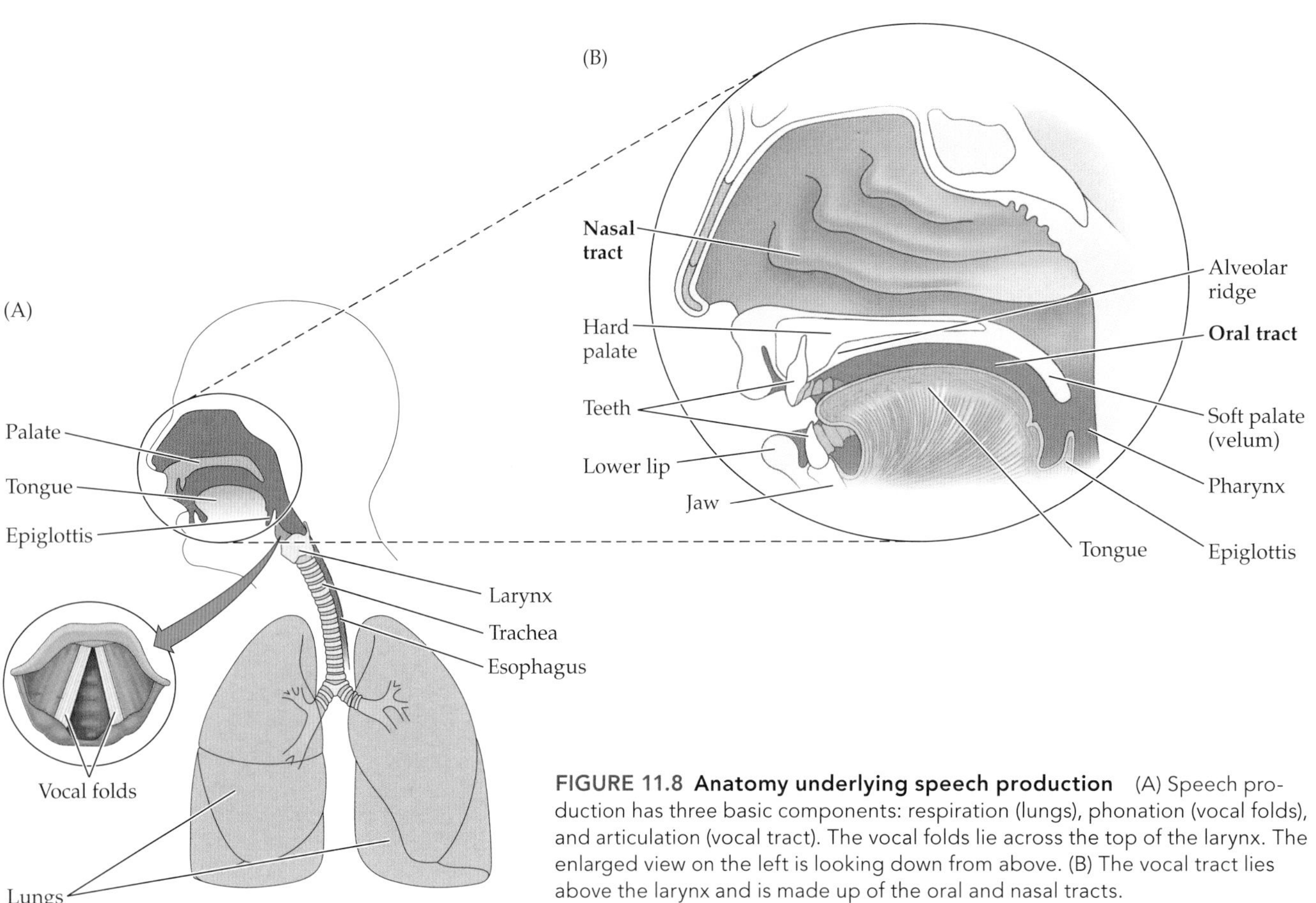

FIGURE 11.8 Anatomy underlying speech production (A) Speech production has three basic components: respiration (lungs), phonation (vocal folds), and articulation (vocal tract). The vocal folds lie across the top of the larynx. The enlarged view on the left is looking down from above. (B) The vocal tract lies above the larynx and is made up of the oral and nasal tracts.

RESPIRATION AND PHONATION To initiate a speech sound, air must be pushed out of the lungs, through the trachea, and up to the larynx. The diaphragm flexes to draw air into the lungs, and elastic recoil forces air back out. At the larynx, air must pass through the two **vocal folds**, which are made up of muscle tissue that can be adjusted to vary how freely air passes through the opening between them. These adjustments are described as types of **phonation**.

The rate at which vocal folds vibrate depends on their stiffness and mass. Consider guitar strings as an analogy. Just like guitar strings, vocal folds become stiffer and vibrate faster as their tension increases, creating sounds with higher pitch. The pitch of a guitar string also depends on its thickness, or mass. Thinner guitar strings vibrate more quickly and create higher-pitched sounds. Similarly, children, who have relatively small vocal folds, have higher-pitched voices than adults do. Adult men generally have lower-pitched voices than adult women, because one of the effects of testosterone during puberty is to increase the mass of the vocal folds. By varying the tension of vocal folds (stiffness) and the pressure of airflow from the lungs, individual talkers can vary the fundamental frequency of voiced sounds, like vowels.

If we were to measure the sound right after the larynx, we would see that vibration of the vocal folds creates a harmonic spectrum, described in Section 10.2 and illustrated in **FIGURE 11.9A**. If we could listen to just this part of speech, it would sound like a buzz. The first harmonic corresponds to the actual rate of physical vibration of the vocal folds—the fundamental frequency. Talkers can make interesting modifications in the way their vocal folds vibrate—creating breathy or creaky voices, for example—and singers can vary vocal-fold tension and air pressure to sing notes with widely varying frequencies. However, the extraordinary part of producing speech sounds occurs above the larynx and vocal folds.

ARTICULATION The area above the larynx—the oral tract and nasal tract combined—is referred to as the **vocal tract** (see Figure 11.8B). Humans have an unrivaled ability to change the shape of the vocal tract by manipulating articulators: the jaw, lips, tongue body, tongue tip, velum (soft palate), and other vocal-tract structures. These manipulations are referred to as **articulation**. Changing the size and shape of the space through which sound passes increases and decreases energy at different frequencies. We call these effects "resonance characteristics," and the spectra of speech sounds are shaped by the way people configure their vocal tracts as **resonators**. **FIGURE 11.9B** illustrates the filtering effects of the vocal tract for the vowel sound 'eh,' as in *wet*. **FIGURE 11.9C** portrays the net result of passing the periodic energy from the larynx through the vocal tract.

Peaks in the speech spectrum are referred to as **formants**. Formants are labeled by number, from lowest

vocal folds The pair of elastic tissues that vibrate as a result of airflow generated by lungs, depending on how close or apart and how tense or lax they are.

phonation The process through which vocal folds are made to vibrate when air pushes out of the lungs.

vocal tract The airway above the larynx used for the production of speech. The vocal tract includes the oral tract and nasal tract.

articulation The act or manner of producing a speech sound using the articulators—vocal tract structures including the mouth, tongue, soft palate, and jaw.

(A) Harmonic spectrum

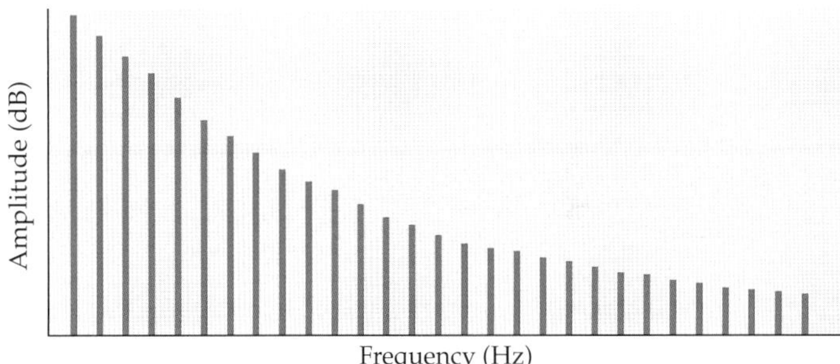

(B) Filter function

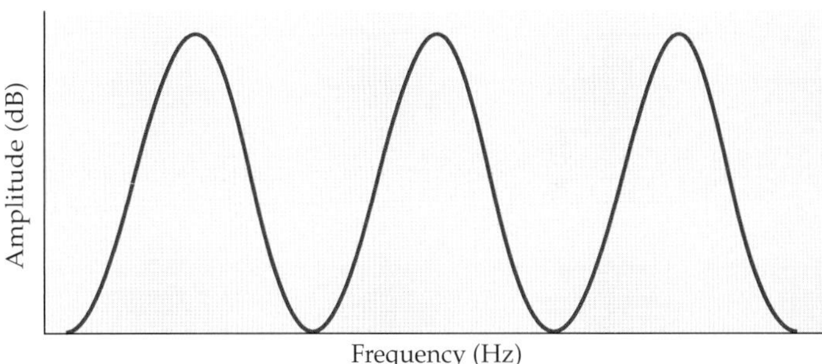

(C) Vowel output

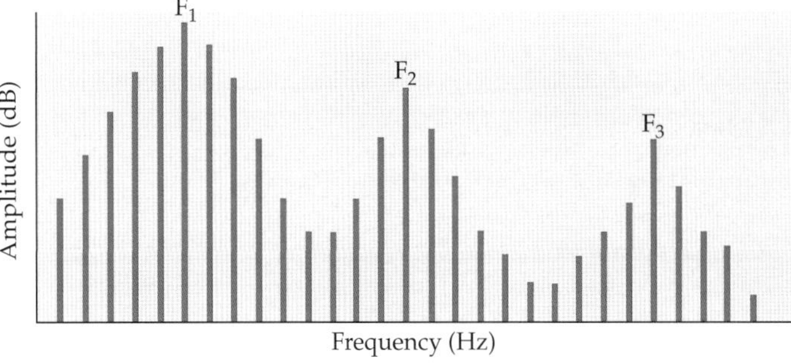

FIGURE 11.9 Source-filter model The spectrum of sound coming from the vocal folds is a harmonic spectrum (A). After passing through the vocal tract, which has resonances based on the vocal tract's shape at the time (B), there are peaks (formants; here F_1, F_2, and F_3) and troughs of energy at different frequencies in the sounds that come out of the mouth (C).

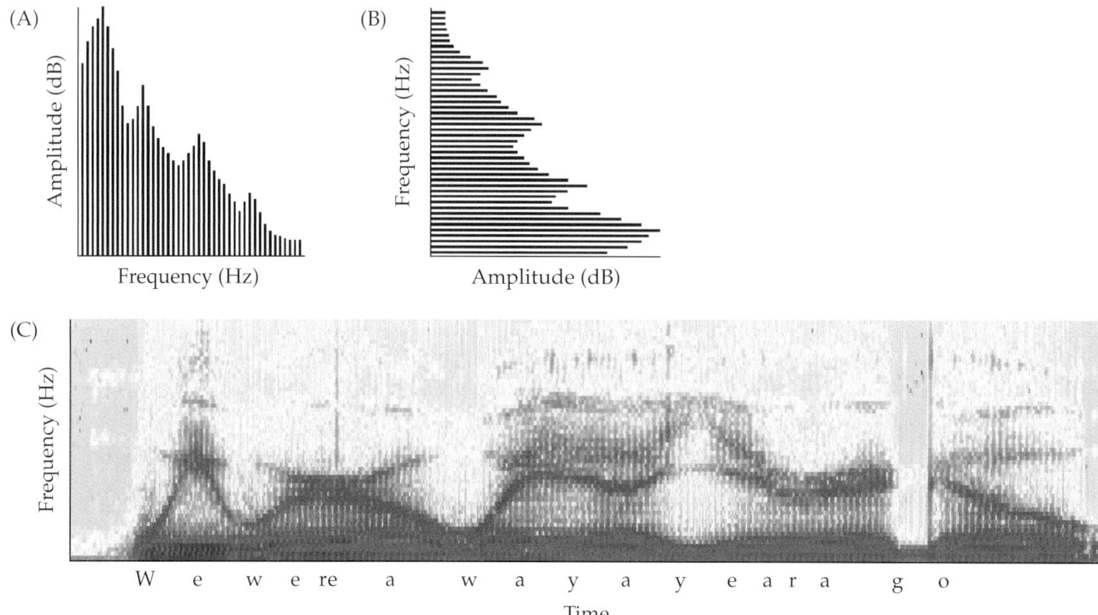

FIGURE 11.10 Spectrogram (A) For sounds that do not vary over time, frequency spectra can be represented by graphs that plot amplitude on the *y*-axis and frequency on the *x*-axis. (B) To graphically show sounds whose spectra change over time, first we rotate the graph so that frequency is plotted on the *y*-axis. (C) We can then plot time on the *x*-axis, with the amplitude of each frequency during each time slice now represented by color (darker red indicates greater intensity). The spectrogram in (C) shows the acoustic signal produced by a male uttering the sentence "We were away a year ago."

frequency to highest (F_1, F_2, F_3, and so on). These concentrations in energy occur at different frequencies, depending on the length of the vocal tract. For shorter vocal tracts (in children and smaller adults), formants are at higher frequencies than they are for longer vocal tracts. Because frequencies for each peak change depending on who's talking, listeners must use the relationships between formant peaks to perceive speech sounds. Only the first three formants are depicted in Figure 11.9C. For the most part, we can distinguish almost all speech sounds on the basis of patterns of energy in the region of these lowest three formants. However, additional formants do exist, at higher frequencies with lower amplitudes.

Many of the sounds we discussed in Chapters 9 and 10 had constant frequency spectra. That is, if a sound started with a 50 decibel (dB), 100 Hz component and a 60 dB, 200 Hz component, the two frequencies continued at these amplitudes for the duration of the sound. One of the most distinctive characteristics of speech sounds is that their spectra change over time. To represent this third dimension—time—in addition to the dimensions of frequency and amplitude represented in frequency spectra of static sounds, auditory researchers use a type of display called a **spectrogram**. In a sound spectrogram, frequency is represented on the *y*-axis, time is tracked on the *x*-axis, and amplitude is indicated by the color of any point on the graph (**FIGURE 11.10**). Formants show up clearly in spectrograms as intense bands of acoustic energy that undulate up and down, depending on the speech sounds being produced.

resonator Most objects such as musical instruments and vocal tracts are resonators because, as a result of their shape, they increase amplitude at some frequencies, called resonant frequencies, compared to other frequencies.

formant A resonance of the vocal tract. Formants are specified by their center frequency and are denoted by integers that increase with relative frequency.

spectrogram In reference to sound analysis, a three-dimensional display that plots time on the horizontal axis, frequency on the vertical axis, and amplitude (intensity) on a color or gray scale.

CLASSIFYING SPEECH SOUNDS Speech sounds are most often described in terms of articulation. This is because in the early days of studying speech, people

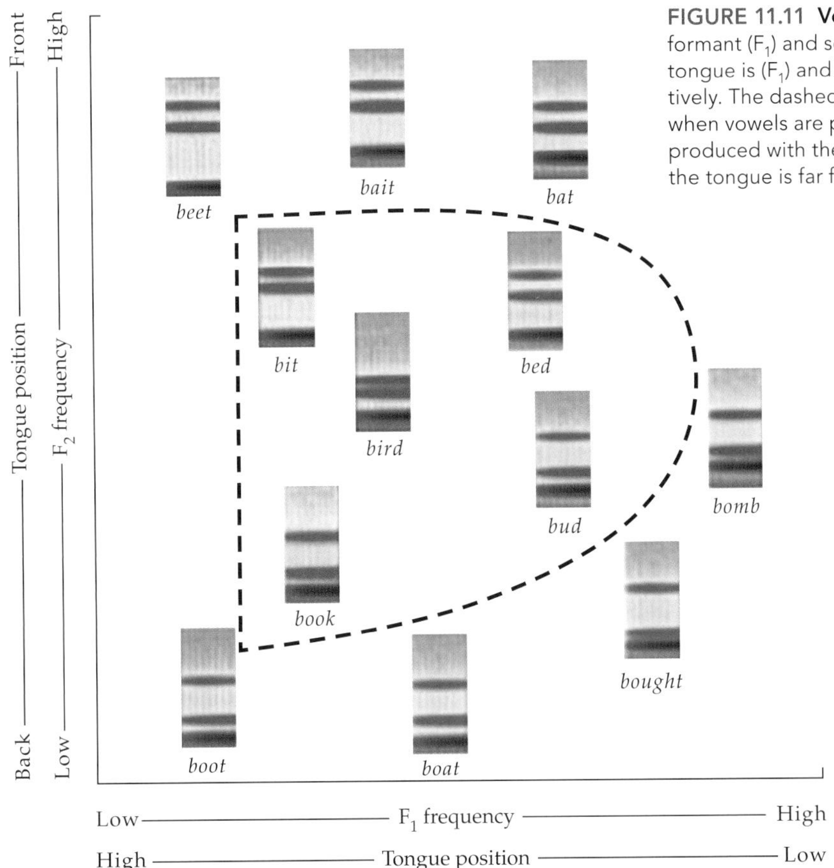

FIGURE 11.11 Vowel sounds of English Frequencies of the first formant (F_1) and second formant (F_2) relate to how high or low the tongue is (F_1) and how far forward or back the tongue is (F_2), respectively. The dashed line illustrates limits on how far the tongue moves when vowels are produced. For example, the vowels 'ee' and 'oo' are produced with the tongue very high in the mouth. In the case of 'ee,' the tongue is far forward, but for 'oo,' the tongue is far back.

did not have electronic recording or the ability to analyze sounds. Instead, they paid close attention to their own vocal tracts and described speech sounds in terms of the articulations necessary to produce them. You will get the most out of the following discussion if you "sing along" just as these early speech researchers did, producing the speech sounds yourself and feeling the various articulatory maneuvers necessary to speak them.

Vowel sounds are all made with a relatively open vocal tract, and they vary mostly in how high or low and how far forward or back the tongue is placed in the oral tract, along with whether or not the lips are rounded. We produce the 'ee' sound in the word *beet* by placing the tongue up and forward, the 'aw' in *bought* by moving the tongue down and back, and the 'oo' in *boot* by moving the tongue up and back while rounding the lips (**FIGURE 11.11**).

We produce consonants by obstructing the vocal tract in some way, and each consonant sound can be classified according to three articulatory dimensions. In English, for example:

1. *Place of articulation* (see Figure 11.9B). Airflow can be obstructed . . .
   - At the lips (bilabial speech sounds: 'b,' 'p,' 'm')
   - At the alveolar ridge just behind the teeth (alveolar speech sounds: 'd,' 't,' 'n')
   - At the soft palate (velar speech sounds: 'g,' 'k,' 'ng')
2. *Manner of articulation*. Airflow can be . . .
   - Totally obstructed (stops: 'b,' 'd,' 'g,' 'p,' 't,' 'k') (**FIGURE 11.12**)

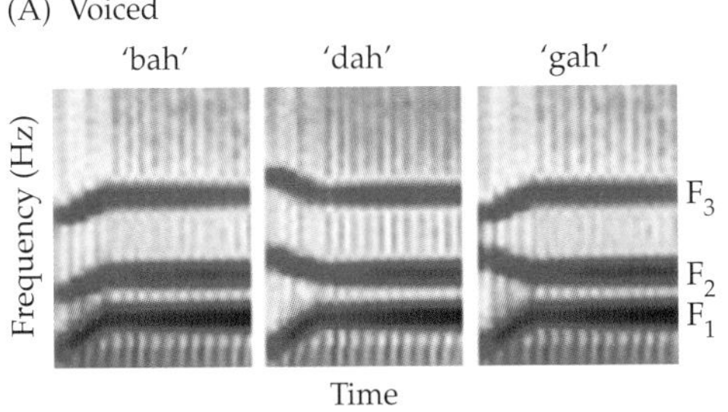

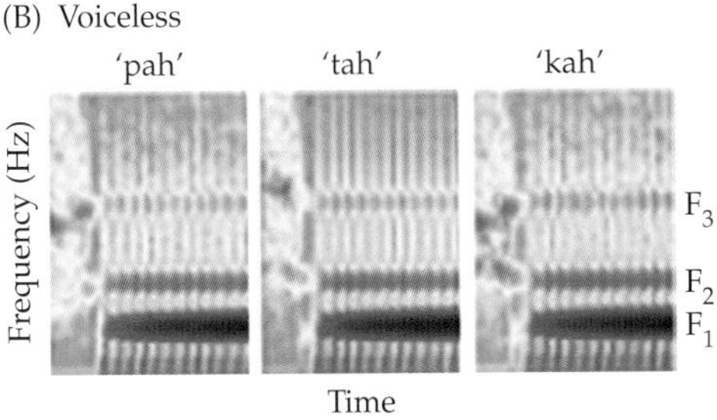

FIGURE 11.12 English stop consonants Stop consonants may be (A) voiced, as in 'bah,' 'dah,' and 'gah,' or (B) voiceless, as in 'pah,' 'tah,' and 'kah.' The main articulatory difference between voiced and voiceless stop consonants is that, for the latter, talkers delay vibration of the vocal folds by about 1/20 of a second after opening the vocal tract to begin the sound.

- Partially obstructed (fricatives: 's,' 'z,' 'f,' 'v,' 'th,' 'sh')
- Only slightly obstructed (laterals: 'l,' 'r'; and glides: 'w,' 'y')
- First blocked, and then allowed to sneak through (affricates: 'ch,' 'j')
- Blocked at first from going through the mouth, but allowed to go through the nasal passage (nasals: 'n,' 'm,' 'ng')

3. *Voicing* (see Figure 11.13). The vocal folds may be . . .
    - Vibrating (voiced consonants, which can be felt by a finger on the throat: 'b,' 'm,' 'z,' 'l,' 'r')
    - Not vibrating (voiceless consonants: 'p,' 's,' 'ch')

These speech sounds from English are only a tiny sample of the over 850 sounds used by languages around the world. Most languages use fewer consonants and vowels than are used in English. Some sounds are quite common across languages, and others, such as English 'th' as in *thin* and 'r' as in *run*, are uncommon around the world. When many or most languages include a particular set of speech sounds, the reason is often that they are particularly easy to perceive. Humans must sometimes communicate in difficult environments where the listener is far away or there are many competing sounds. To be effective, speech sound repertoires of languages have developed over generations of individuals to include mostly sounds that are relatively easy to tell apart.

In addition to using relatively easily distinguishable sounds, another way speech provides effective communication is by signaling all distinctions between vowels and consonants with multiple differences across sounds. Because more than one acoustic property can be used to tell two sounds apart, distinctions are signaled redundantly, and this redundancy helps listeners. The speech signal is so redundant that if we remove all energy below 1800 Hz, listeners will still perceive speech nearly perfectly, and the same is true if we remove all energy above 1800 Hz (**FIGURE 11.13**). You may already know this all too well if you have lived in an apartment with thin walls. Even though walls stop energy at higher frequencies, you may learn far more about your neighbors than you wish from their conversations on the other side.

Speech Perception

Speech production is very fast. In casual conversation, we produce about 10–15 consonants and vowels per second, and if we're in a hurry, we can double this rate. To achieve this acoustic feat, our articulators (tongue, lips, jaw, and so on) must

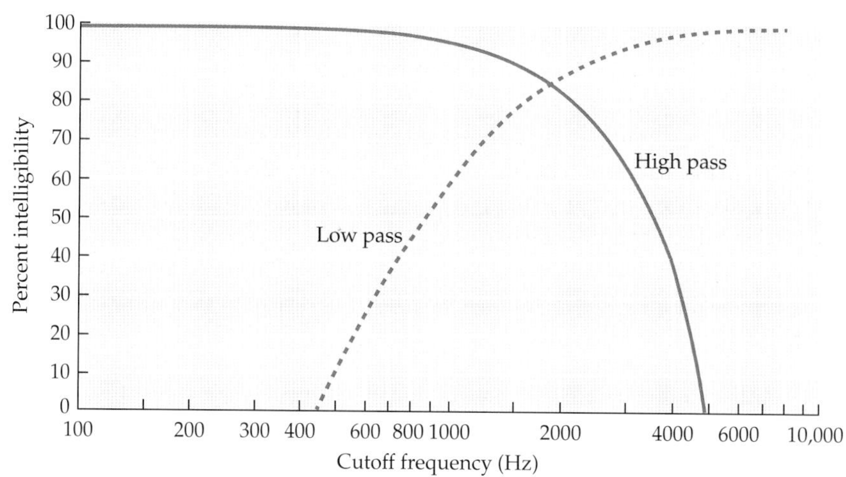

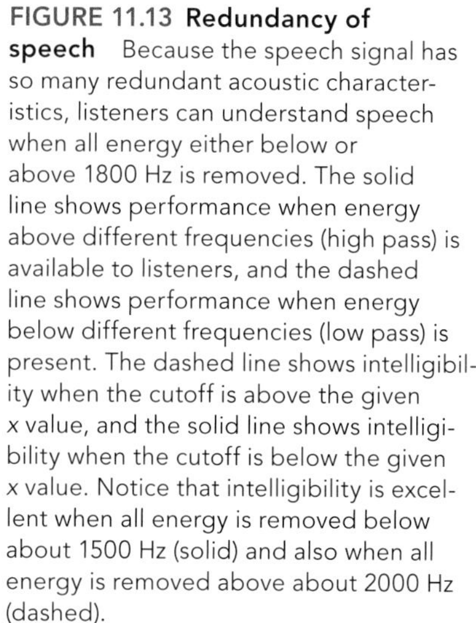
FIGURE 11.13 Redundancy of speech Because the speech signal has so many redundant acoustic characteristics, listeners can understand speech when all energy either below or above 1800 Hz is removed. The solid line shows performance when energy above different frequencies (high pass) is available to listeners, and the dashed line shows performance when energy below different frequencies (low pass) is present. The dashed line shows intelligibility when the cutoff is above the given x value, and the solid line shows intelligibility when the cutoff is below the given x value. Notice that intelligibility is excellent when all energy is removed below about 1500 Hz (solid) and also when all energy is removed above about 2000 Hz (dashed).

FIGURE 11.14 **Lack of invariance** Spectrograms of 'd' sounds (center column), along with stop-consonant cousins 'b' (left) and 'g' (right). Changes in formants across time (formant transitions) for these sounds differ dramatically depending on the following vowels: 'ah' (top row), 'oo' (middle), and 'ee' (bottom).

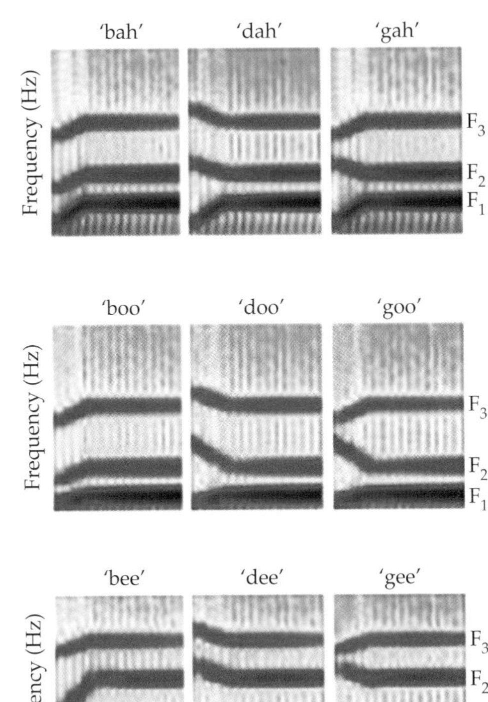

do many different things very quickly. However, articulators can move only so fast; mass and inertia keep articulators from getting all the way to the position for the next consonant or vowel. Experienced talkers also adjust their production in anticipation of where articulators need to be next. In these ways, production of one speech sound overlaps production of the next. This overlap of articulation in space and time is called **coarticulation**. As we turn from speech production to speech perception, we will find that although coarticulation does not cause much trouble for listeners understanding speech, it has made it harder for speech perception researchers to explain how we do it.

COARTICULATION AND LACK OF INVARIANCE To get a better sense of what coarticulation is, say the word *moody* a few times, and note the activity of your tongue as you form the 'd' sound. You will find that it starts in the back of your mouth, where it must be to form the 'oo' vowel sound. Then it touches the alveolar ridge just behind the teeth to form the 'd.' And finally it ends up toward the front of the mouth to form the 'ee.' Now say the nonsense word *eedoom*. Reversing the vowel sounds means sending the tongue on the opposite journey, from front to alveolar ridge to back. As a result of the very different path taken by the tongue in these two utterances, the acoustic qualities of the 'd' in the two utterances are quite different depending on the context of preceding or following tongue movements.

This context sensitivity is a signature property of speech. One might expect context sensitivity to cause a significant problem for speech perceivers, because it means there is no single diagnostic cue that we can count on to uniquely identify different speech sounds. For 'b,' 'd,' and 'g' in **FIGURE 11.14**, notice that the shape of the first formant (F_1) is pretty much the same for all three consonants when they precede the same vowel. F_1 is helpful in telling 'b,' 'd,' and 'g' apart from other speech sounds, but it does not help much in telling these sounds apart from one another. An F_1 like that shown in Figure 11.14 is necessary for a sound to be 'b,' but it is not sufficient to inform the listener that the sound is 'b,' and not 'd' or 'g.' F_2 is very important for telling 'b' from 'd' from 'g,' but what F_2 tells the listener depends on its relationship to F_3 and the formants of the following vowel.

Explaining how listeners understand speech despite all this variation has been one of the most significant challenges for speech researchers. Context sensitivity resulting from coarticulation also presents one of the greatest difficulties in developing computer recognition of speech. We cannot program or train a computer to recognize a speech sound—consonant or vowel—without also taking into consideration which speech sounds precede and follow that sound. And we cannot identify those preceding and following sounds without also taking into consideration which sounds precede and follow them, and so on. As it happens, this is pretty much what computers do to "understand" speech: they are trained across millions of slices of every speech sound, preceded and followed by slices of nearly every other speech sound.

CATEGORICAL PERCEPTION Shortly after World War II, researchers invented machines that could produce speechlike sounds and started testing listeners to try to determine exactly what the acoustic cues were that enabled them to distinguish

coarticulation The phenomenon in speech whereby attributes of successive speech units overlap in articulatory or acoustic patterns.

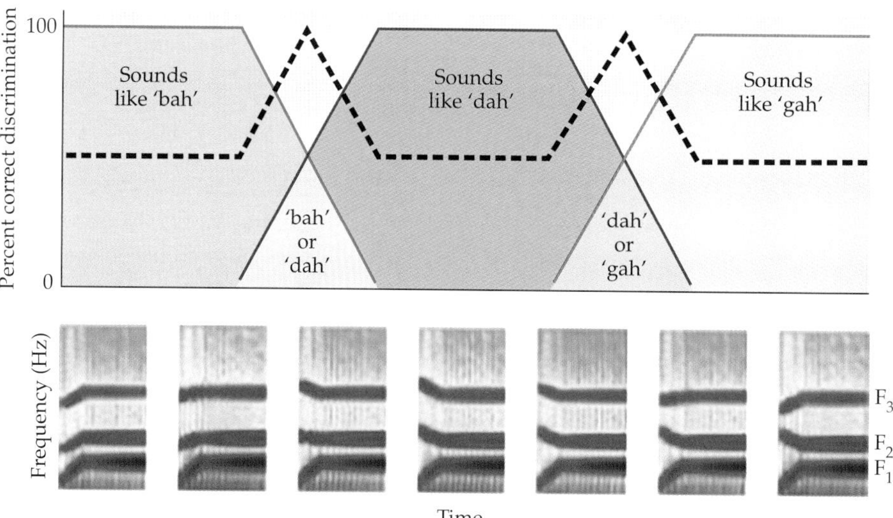

FIGURE 11.15 Categorical perception The sound spectrograms at the bottom of this figure indicate acoustic stimuli that change smoothly from a clear 'bah' on the left through 'dah' to a clear 'gah' on the right. As seen across the top of the figure, perception does not change smoothly. All the sounds on the left sound like a 'bah' (blue curve) until we reach a sharp 'bah'-'dah' border. Listeners are much better at discriminating a 'bah' from a "dah" than at discriminating two 'bah's or two 'gah's. The dashed black line indicates discrimination performance. The same is true for 'dah' (red curve) and 'gah' (green curve).

different speech sounds. They found, for example, that by varying the transitions of F_2 and F_3, they could produce sounds that listeners reliably reported hearing as 'bah,' 'dah,' or 'gah' (**FIGURE 11.15**).

These researchers knew that making small, incremental changes to simple acoustic stimuli such as pure tones leads to gradual changes in people's perception. For example, tones sound just a little higher in pitch with each small step in frequency. Surprisingly, speech sounds were not perceived in this way. When researchers started with a synthesized 'bah' and gradually varied the formant transitions moving toward 'dah' and then 'gah,' listeners' responses did not gradually change from 'bah' to 'bah'-ish 'dah' to 'dah' to 'dah'-ish 'gah' to 'gah' (Liberman et al., 1957). Instead, listeners identified these sounds as changing abruptly from one consonant to another.

Furthermore, listeners appeared incapable of hearing that much of anything was different when two sounds were labeled as the same consonant. In this second part of the experiments, researchers played pairs of synthesized speech sounds and asked listeners to tell them apart. Listeners performed almost perfectly when detecting small differences between two sounds if one was 'bah' and the other was 'dah.' But if both sounds were 'bah' or both were 'dah,' performance dropped to nearly chance levels (dashed line in Figure 11.15), even though the differences in formant transitions in the first and second pairs of stimuli were equally large.

This pattern of results has come to be called **categorical perception**. As illustrated in Figure 11.15, three qualities define categorical perception. The first two were just described: a sharp labeling (identification) function and discontinuous discrimination performance. The third definitional quality of categorical perception follows from the first two: researchers can predict discrimination performance based on the labeling data. In short, listeners report hearing differences between sounds only when those differences would result in different labels for the sounds, so the ability to discriminate sounds can be predicted by how listeners label the sounds.

Categorical perception of speech sounds is not limited to 'bah'/'dah'/'gah'; it has been shown for many different contrasts between sounds in English, as well as other languages. These findings, along with the failure to find invariants that distinguish speech sounds from each other, led many speech researchers to suspect that humans had evolved special mechanisms just for perceiving speech. One very influential version of the "speech is special" idea, called the "motor theory" of speech perception (Liberman and Mattingly, 1985; Liberman et al., 1967), held

categorical perception For speech as well as other complex sounds and images, the phenomenon by which the discrimination of items is little better than the ability to label items.

(A)

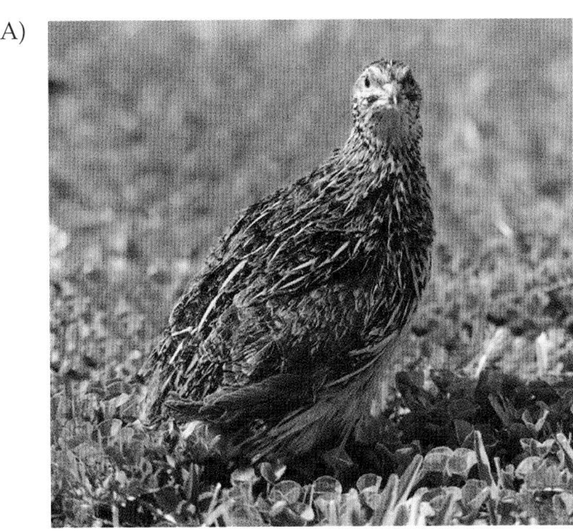

(B)

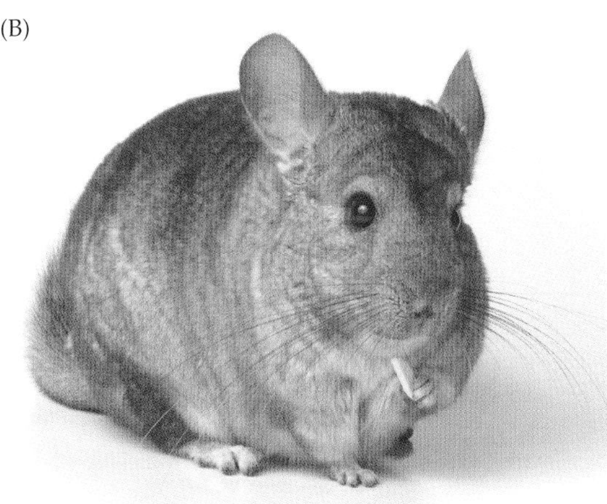

FIGURE 11.16 Speech perception by nonhumans (A) Japanese quail can learn to tell 'd' from 'b' and 'g' preceding different vowels, just as humans do. (B) Chinchillas have shown categorical perception of sounds varying from 'dah' to 'tah.'

that processes used to produce speech sounds can somehow be run in reverse to understand the acoustic speech signal.

Over time, however, problems with the motor theory cropped up. First, it turns out that speech production is at least as complex as speech perception, if not more so. Every aspect of the acoustic signal relates to a particular aspect of the vocal tract. So, if the acoustic signal is complex, this complexity must be the result of complexity in production. Trying to explain speech perception by reference to production is at least as difficult as explaining speech perception on the basis of acoustics alone.

A second reason to doubt that processes for perceiving speech are unique to humans is that numerous demonstrations have shown that nonhuman animals can learn to respond to speech signals in much the same way that human listeners do (Kluender, Lotto, and Holt, 2005; Kluender et al., 1998). For example, Japanese quail (**FIGURE 11.16A**) can be taught to tell 'd' from 'b' and 'g' across the same sort of acoustic variation depicted in Figure 11.14 (Kluender, Diehl, and Killeen, 1987). Chinchillas (**FIGURE 11.16B**) have also shown classic categorical-perception effects (Kuhl, 1981; Kuhl and Miller, 1978).

Furthermore, we now know that categorical perception, one of the defining characteristics of speech that was thought to be so unusual as to require a special processing mechanism, is not at all limited to speech sounds. Other types of auditory stimuli, such as musical intervals (J. D. Smith et al., 1994), are also perceived categorically, as are visual stimuli such as familiar objects (Newell and Bülthoff, 2002), human faces (Levin and Beale, 2000), and facial expressions (De Gelder, Teunisse, and Benson, 1997). People even perceive differences between familiar animals categorically (R. Campbell et al., 1997) (**FIGURE 11.17**), and monkeys learn to perceive images of cats versus dogs categorically (Freedman et al., 2001).

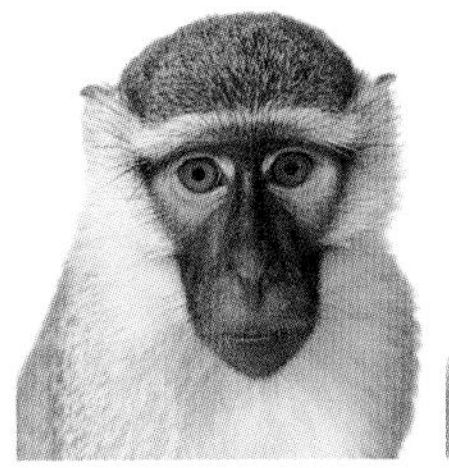
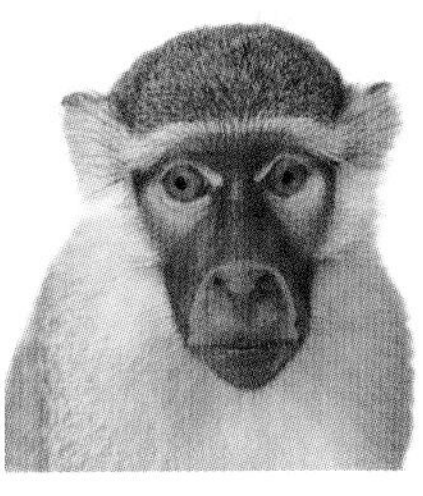
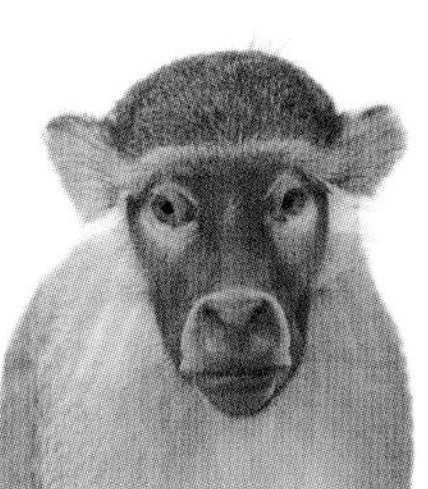
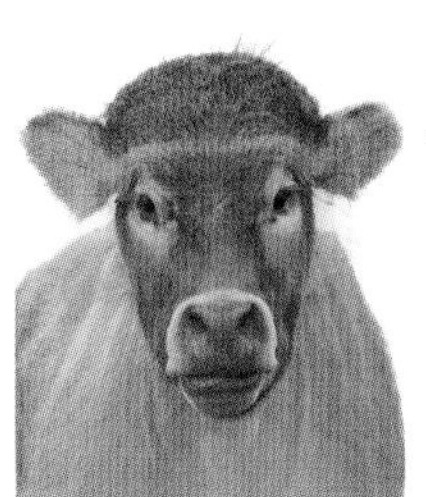
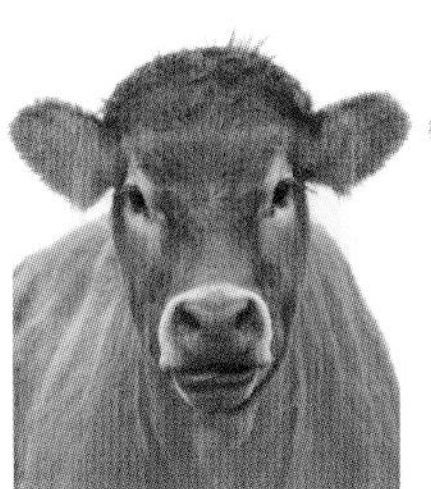
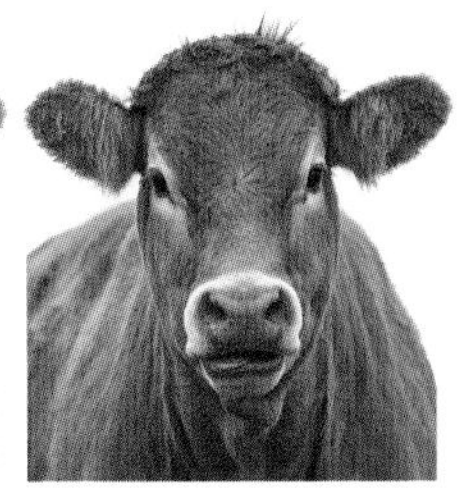

FIGURE 11.17 Categorical perception of familiar images People categorically perceive changes between images of familiar animals such as monkeys and cows. The labels that observers use shift abruptly between "monkey" and "cow" when they identify images like those in the series shown here. Observers also are better at discriminating two images when they label one as "monkey" and one as "cow."

We now understand that the pattern of results known as categorical perception depends on how one measures speech perception. Early studies relied on having listeners make discrete decisions (Was that a 'bah' or a 'dah'?) that produced coarse measures of perception. Simply allowing listeners to rate "How good of a 'bah' was that?" or using finer-grained measures like eye tracking or electroencephalographic measures of brain response reveals more graded—and less categorical—speech perception than we originally thought.

An example from vision can help to clarify. Penguins and robins are both birds, but most would say that a robin is a "better" example of a bird than a penguin. In a similar way, more sensitive speech perception methods have allowed us to discover that listeners find some instances of 'bah' to be better instances than others. This runs counter to the early claim that listeners could not differentiate among speech sounds that belong to the same category. Today, research focuses on how the many, redundant acoustic cues to speech sounds contribute to categorizing speech sounds. In this way, speech sounds are now thought of as *categorized* rather than *categorical* (Holt and Lotto, 2010). In an interesting twist, the categorical perception phenomenon that made speech seem like a special case of perception has developed to emphasize commonalities with other sensory modalities, like vision.

COARTICULATION AND SPECTRAL CONTRAST Contemporary research has turned increasingly to investigating how speech perception is explained by general ways that hearing, and perception more broadly, works. For example, the perception of coarticulated speech appears to be at least partially explained by some fundamental principles of perception that you've already read about. Let's turn again to our example of syllables such as 'bah' and 'dah' (see Figure 11.14). An acoustic feature that contributes to the perception of 'bah,' as contrasted with the perception of 'dah,' is the onset frequency and trajectory of the second formant (F_2). Because of coarticulation, production of one speech sound always affects production of the next sound; formants for one sound always are more like (assimilate to) the sounds that precede and follow. The onset of F_2 varies depending on whether 'bah' or 'dah' are preceded by vowels such as 'ee' (higher F_2) or 'oo' (lower F_2). Because of coarticulation, the F_2 of the consonant in 'eebah' and 'oodah' is nearly identical (Figure 11.18). Yet, listeners hear the consonant as 'bah' following 'ee' and 'dah' following 'oo.'

Why does perception work this way? Because coarticulation always causes a speech sound to become more like the previous speech sound, auditory processes that enhance the contrast between successive sounds undo this assimilation. Listeners are more likely to perceive 'bah' (low F_2) when preceded by 'ee' (high F_2) and to perceive 'dah' (high F_2) when preceded by 'oo' (low F_2). The auditory system exaggerates the change in F_2, undoing the assimilative effects of coarticulation. Preceding sounds do not even have to be speech. If, instead of playing 'ee' and 'oo' we present only a single small band of energy at the frequencies where F_2 would be in 'ee' or 'oo,' perception of the following syllable changes just as it does with the full 'ee' or 'oo' vowel sound

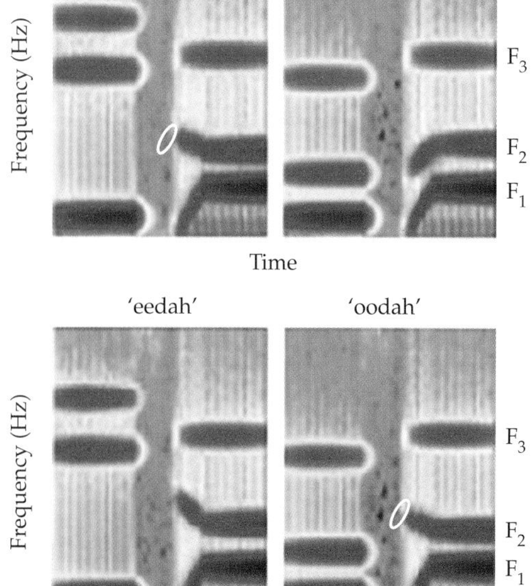

FIGURE 11.18 Coarticulation Because of coarticulation, consonant sounds such as 'bah' and 'dah' are acoustically very different, depending on the preceding vowel. Here, 'bah' is shown following 'ee' (top left) and 'oo' (top right), and 'dah' is shown following the same vowels (bottom). Note that F_2 in 'eebah' (top left) is acoustically identical to F_2 in 'oodah' (bottom right). Listeners hear the same consonant sound as 'b' following 'ee' and as 'd' following 'oo' because of the contrast between the spectrum of 'ee' and 'oo' and the spectrum of the following consonant.

(Holt & Lotto, 2002). The onset of F_2 for 'bah' and 'dah' is perceived relative to whether the preceding energy is lower or higher in frequency. We perceive syllables such as 'bah' and 'dah' in terms of the relative change in the spectrum—how the onsets contrast with the energy that precedes them.

You've encountered contrast effects several times before in this book. Remember that melodies are defined by changes between adjacent notes, not by the exact notes. While learning about vision, you saw many examples of contrast. Contrast plays a large role in the perception of brightness, color, and size, as well as line orientation, position, curvature, depth, and spatial frequency. Here, spectral contrast helps listeners perceive speech, despite the lack of acoustic invariance resulting from coarticulation. Underscoring how general these auditory contrast effects are in speech perception, Japanese quail trained to peck to a button when hearing speech show the same spectral contrast effects syllables precede the consonants (Lotto, Kluender, and Holt, 1997).

USING MULTIPLE ACOUSTIC CUES What do speech sounds and faces have in common? They are stimuli that people have a great deal of experience perceiving. We spend a large chunk of our waking lives listening to speech and identifying people by their faces. Another thing that makes distinguishing among individual speech sounds and individual faces similar is that many small differences must be used together, in coordination to discriminate different speech sounds and different faces (e.g., small changes in formant transitions and small changes in nose shape). For example, utterances of the syllables 'aba' and 'apa' can be distinguished from each other by at least 16 different characteristics of the acoustic signal (**FIGURE 11.19**) (Lisker, 1986). Listeners can make use of their experience with the co-occurrence of these multiple acoustic differences to understand speech. Similarly, you recognize friends based on your experience seeing their many features, such as eyes, nose, mouth, ears, and chin.

At the same time, other stimulus differences must be ignored so that multiple instances of the same speech sound or multiple images of the same face can be classified properly (e.g., acoustic variation introduced when different speakers utter the same speech sound, or image variation introduced when a face is viewed from different angles).

To the extent that perception depends heavily on experience, speech is special because (1) humans have evolved unique anatomical machinery for producing it and (2) we spend a great deal of time practicing the perception of speech, beginning even prenatally as we hear speech through the womb! The fact that there are no acoustic invariants for distinguishing speech sounds is really no different from many comparable situations in visual perception. For example, we saw in Chapter 6 that a single cue for depth perception may fail us, but by taking multiple cues into account, we rarely make large mistakes when calculating distance relations.

The comparison with face recognition may be even more apt. Sofia's nose may be quite similar to Jasmin's nose, Sofia's eyes may be exactly as far apart as Aria's eyes, and Sofia's mouth may be shaped just like Lakshmi's mouth. But given enough experience with all four faces (and enough experience with face recognition, in general), we can use the pattern of facial features to pick Sofia out from a lineup every time—even if she's covering her mouth with her hand.

To sum up, we don't need individual acoustic invariants to distinguish speech sounds; we just need to be as good at pattern recognition for sounds as we are for visual images. And one of the things that the billions of neurons in the brain do best is integrating multiple sources of information to recognize patterns.

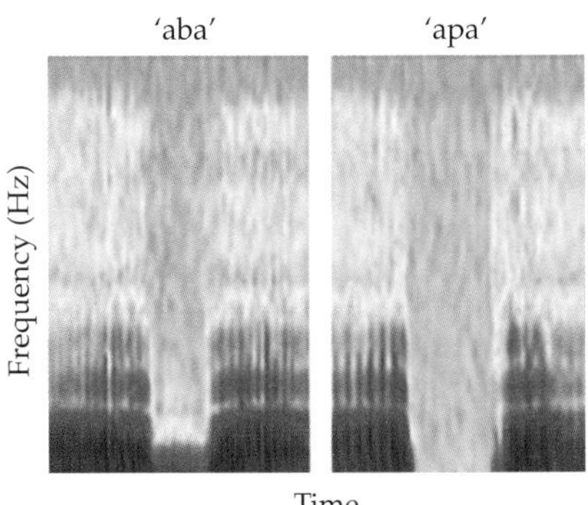

FIGURE 11.19 Multiple speech cues The simple distinction between 'aba' (left) and 'apa' (right) includes at least 16 acoustic differences. Some differences that are easy to see include duration of the first vowel, duration of the interval between syllables, and the presence of low-frequency energy in the middle of 'aba.'

Scientists at Work

Tickling the Cochlea

Question What speech sounds are most important? When reading, th* b*s*c d*m*nstr*t**n *s th*t t*xt *s st*ll m*r* *r l*ss l*g*bl* wh*n th* v*w*ls h*v* b**n r*m*v*d. Many experiments have been conducted to learn whether consonants, vowels, or combinations between consonants and vowels are most essential for understanding spoken language. The answer has been unclear. How much can we learn about understanding speech if we go back to what we learned in Section 9.3 about the basilar membrane within the cochleas?

Hypothesis The most important parts of the speech signal are those that change patterns of vibration across the basilar membrane the most.

Test Replace portions of sentences with either 80 or 112 milliseconds of noise during selected intervals. For some selected intervals, the pattern of stimulation along the basilar membrane did not change a lot (low change). Other intervals were selected because the pattern of stimulation changed a lot (high change). Finally, intervals were selected because they fell in between a little and a lot.

Results We can predict how well listeners will understand speech by measuring the amount of change occurring along the length of the basilar membrane in the cochlea (**FIGURE 11.20**) (Stilp and Kluender, 2010).

Conclusion Listeners are better at understanding sentences when intervals spanning less change in the pattern of stimulation along the basilar membrane are replaced by noise.

Future work The knowledge that the most important part of understanding speech is how the input changes across time can be used to increase the information conveyed by cochlear implant electrodes to listeners with hearing impairments (Stilp et al., 2016).

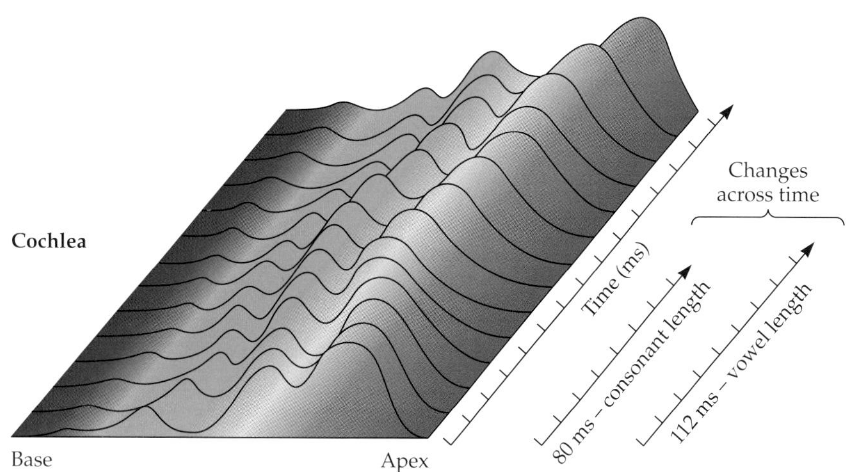

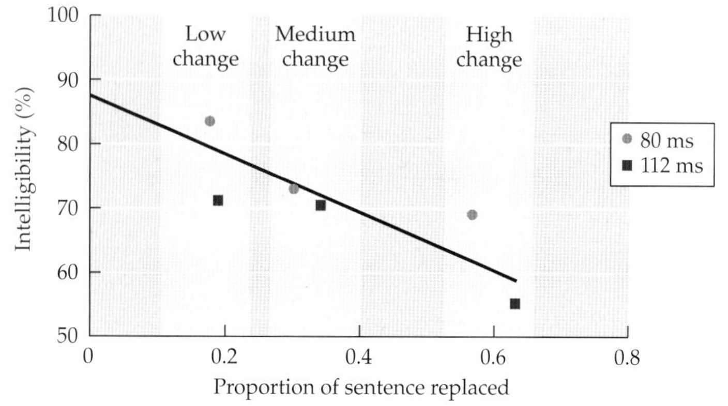

FIGURE 11.20 Patterns of cochlear change When speech sounds enter the ear, the pattern of stimulation along the basilar membrane changes nearly continuously across time—sometimes a lot and sometimes less. When intervals of sentences are removed and replaced with noise on the basis of how much the pattern of stimulation changes throughout an interval (80 or 112 milliseconds), the best way to predict how well listeners will understand speech is by measuring how much the basilar membrane changes shape. When noise replaces an interval when the pattern of stimulation along the basilar membrane changes more, people have more difficulty understanding the speech.

Learning to Listen

In our discussion of vision earlier in the book, we saw that experience is incredibly important for visual perception, particularly the higher-level perception of objects and events in the world. Experience is every bit as important for auditory perception, especially for perception of speech. Unlike vision, experience with speech begins very early in development. In fact, as we hinted above, fetuses gain significant experience with speech even before they're born.

Measurements of heart rate as indicators of the ability to notice change between speech sounds have revealed that late-term fetuses can discriminate between different vowel sounds (Lecanuet et al., 1986). Prenatal experience with speech sounds appears to have considerable influence on subsequent perception. For one thing, a newborn prefers hearing their mother's voice over other women's voices (DeCasper and Fifer, 1980). When 4-day-old infants in Paris were tested, they preferred hearing French more than Russian (Mehler et al., 1988). The "melodies" of newborn crying reflect this language preference. Swedish newborns cry with greater modulations in pitch than do German newborns, and these patterns reflect similar differences between the pitch variations for adult Swedish and German speakers (Prochnow et al., 2019). Perhaps most amazingly, newborns whose mothers had read *The Cat in the Hat* by Dr. Seuss aloud twice daily during the last trimester of pregnancy preferred to listen to this story compared to a control story (DeCasper and Spence, 1986). Even before birth, the fetal auditory system is learning about the patterns of speech spoken by the language community.

BECOMING A NATIVE LISTENER As we have seen, speech sounds can differ in many ways. Acoustic differences that matter critically for one language may be irrelevant or even distracting in another language. For example, the English language makes use of the distinction between the sounds 'r' and 'l,' whereas these two sounds are both very similar to only one sound (called a "flap") in Japanese. As another example, Spanish is one of many languages that uses only the five vowel sounds 'ee' (as in *beet*), 'oo' (as in *boot*), 'ah' (as in *bomb*), 'ay' (as in *bake*), and 'oh' (as in *boat*), whereas English employs up to ten additional vowel sounds.

Differences in the sounds used by languages can have a big influence in language learning, especially adult language learning. The inherent differences between English and Japanese make it difficult for native Japanese speakers to use the English 'r'/'l' distinction (**FIGURE 11.21**). Because the difference between 'l' and 'r' is irrelevant in Japanese, it is adaptive for native Japanese listeners to learn to ignore it and to focus on speech sound distinctions important in Japanese. When people have spent most of their lives listening to Japanese and not hearing the difference between 'r' and 'l,' we are not surprised that they have difficulty learning to produce the 'r' and 'l.' By the same token, a native Spanish speaker who claims that your dog just "beat" him is probably not claiming that Rover threw a punch; rather, the difference between 'ee' and 'ih' is less perceptible to the Spanish speaker, because both of these English sounds are similar to the Spanish 'ee.'

Interestingly, studies show that infants begin filtering out irrelevant acoustic differences long before they begin to utter speech sounds (even before their babbling stage). One study found that by 6 months of age, infants from Seattle were more likely to notice acoustic differences that distinguish two English vowels than to notice equivalent differences between Swedish vowels, and infants from Stockholm were more likely to notice the differences between two Swedish vowels than the differences between two English vowels (Kuhl et al., 1992). Tuning of perception for consonants appears to take a bit longer to develop, but by the time infants are

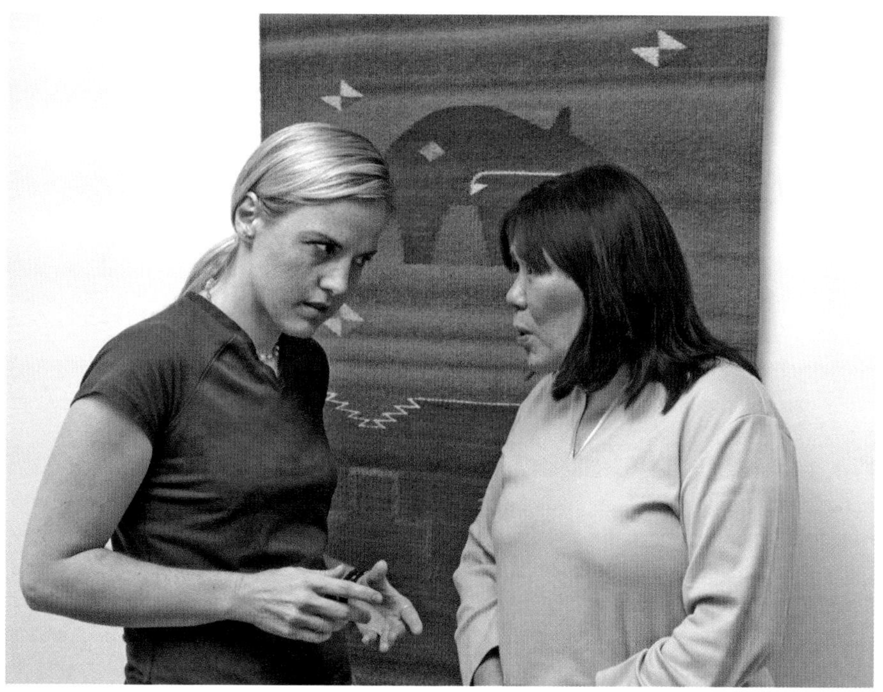

FIGURE 11.21 Experience shapes speech perception How we hear speech sounds depends on our experience with the speech sounds of our first language. Because of experience with one language, it is often difficult to perceive and produce distinctions in a new language. For example, most Japanese people learning English as a second language have trouble distinguishing between 'l' and 'r,' both when they listen and when they speak.

1 year old, infants have also begun to ignore consonant distinctions not used in their native language, just as their parents do (**FIGURE 11.22**).

It is possible, with much training, to learn to perceive and produce speech sound distinctions that you've spent most of your life ignoring. As you might expect, the longer a person uses only their first language, the longer it takes to learn to produce and perceive sounds from a second language (Imai, Flege, and Wayland, 2002). Many studies have been aimed at determining what makes new distinctions hard or easy for second-language learners to pick up. Learning is most difficult when both sounds in the second language are similar to a single sound in the first language (e.g., 'r' and 'l' for Japanese speakers learning English). Learning is easier if the two new sounds are both unlike any sound in the native language. For example, native English listeners have no problems distinguishing click sounds from Zulu because Zulu clicks are so unlike any English sounds (Best, McRoberts, and Sithole, 1988). Learning also is easier if two new sounds from a new language differ in the same way that two sounds from the first language differ.

Picking up on distinctions in a second language is easiest if the second language is learned at the same time as the first. This is why language immersion programs are popular in preschool and elementary curriculums of multicultural

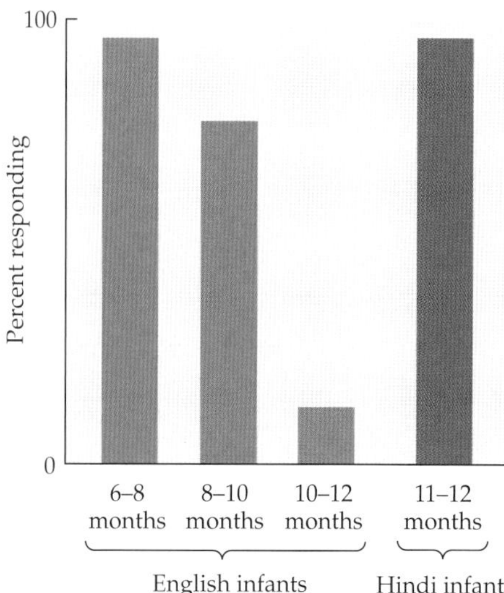

FIGURE 11.22 Infants lose the ability to discriminate non-native speech sounds Hindi has a dental stop consonant produced with the tongue tip touching the teeth and a retroflex stop consonant that requires the tongue to bend up and back in the mouth. Adult speakers of English hear both of these sounds as 't' because they are similar to the English 't.' When Werker and Tees (1984) tested infants from English-speaking families in Vancouver, the youngest (6–8 months old) reliably responded to the difference between these two Hindi sounds. By 1 year of age, however, the infants were mimicking their parents' behavior by ignoring the distinction between the two sounds.

countries. The downside to this strategy is that kids who learn multiple languages at the same time usually take a little longer to master each of the languages than do children learning only a single language (Bialystok and Hakuta, 1994; Haerazi, 2016). This is a natural consequence of having to learn not one but two sets of patterns of sounds (as well as learning two vocabularies, two sets of grammatical rules, and so on). On the upside, these children catch up and then are able use more than one language fluently.

LEARNING WORDS Thus far in this chapter, we've learned many things about the nature and complexity of speech sounds and about how listeners perceive consonants and vowels. But the whole point of producing and perceiving these speech sounds is to put them together to form words, which are the units of language that convey meaning. How do novice language learners (infants) make the leap from streams of meaningless speech sounds to the meaningful groups of speech sounds that we call words?

First, let's state the obvious. Just like strings of musical notes, no string of speech sounds is inherently meaningful. The string 'd'-'aw'-'g' becomes meaningful to English-speaking infants, but to French-speaking, Spanish-speaking, and German-speaking infants this string remains completely meaningless because their parents refer to their canine house companions as *chien*, *perro*, and *Hund*, respectively. Infants in different places in the world must learn the words that are specific to their native languages.

We've already seen how a series of consonants and vowels within a single word tend to "run into" one another because of coarticulation. It turns out that the situation is not much better for a series of words forming a sentence. This fact is easily seen in FIGURE 11.23: without the letters at the bottom of the figure, you would have no idea where the spoken word *where* ends and *are* begins.

Interestingly, perception usually seems at odds with this acoustic reality. When we listen to someone talking to us in our native language, individual words seem to stand out quite clearly as separate entities. But listening to someone speak an unfamiliar language can be a very different experience. If you have no experience with this language, it probably sounds as if it includes lots of long words—some as long as whole English sentences. It may also seem as if this speech is much faster than English. This is the situation faced by infants the world over. Of course, if you speak Chinese or Arabic fluently, these illusions disappear—as they do for English.

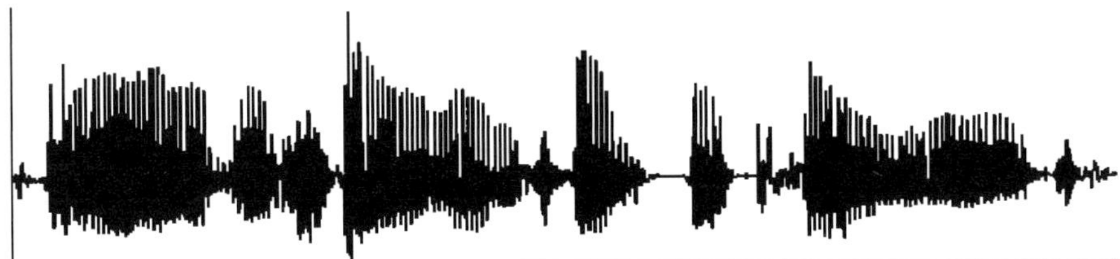

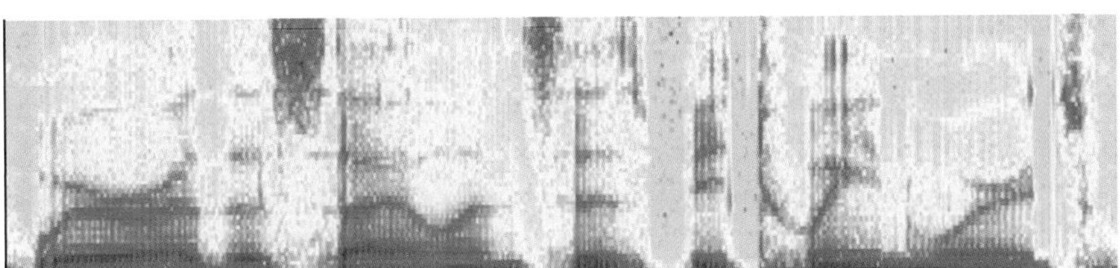
Wherearethe s i l e n c e s be t w een wo rd s ?

FIGURE 11.23 Spoken words run into one another In the sentence "Where are the silences between words?" we can see that there are no breaks between the sounds of one spoken word and the sounds of the next. Infants can use their experience with particular sequences of speech sounds to learn about boundaries between words.

(A)

tokibugopilagikobatipolutokibu
gopilatipolutokibugikobagopila
gikobatokibugopilatipolugikoba
tipolugikobatipolugopilatipolu
tokibugopilatipolutokibugopila
tipolutokibugopilagikobatipolu
tokibugopilagikobatipolugikoba
tipolugikobatipolutokibugikoba
gopilatipolugikobatokibugopila

(B)

tokibugopilagikobatipolutokibu
gopilatipolutokibugikobagopila
gikobatokibugopilatipolugikoba
tipolugikobatipolugopilatipolu
tokibugopilatipolutokibugopila
tipolutokibugopilagikobatipolu
tokibugopilagikobatipolugikoba
tipolugikobatipolutokibugikoba
gopilatipolugikobatokibugopila

FIGURE 11.24 Learning to separate words Saffran, Aslin, and Newport (1996) showed that 8-month-old infants can learn to pick out words from streams of continuous speech based on the extent to which successive syllables are predictable or unpredictable. (A) While sitting on their parents' laps, infants heard unbroken 2-minute sequences of syllables. (B) In the second part of the experiment, infants demonstrated familiarity with three-syllable sequences that they had heard before (e.g., "tokibu," "gopila," "gikoba," "tipolu"), but were aware that they had never heard syllable combinations that were not present in the original stream (e.g., "poluto," "bugopi," "kobati").

To study how infants learn words from the continuous streams of speech that they encounter in their environment, Saffran, Aslin, and Newport (1996) invented a novel "language" composed of just four words. Each of the words had three syllables—for example, *tokibu*, *gopila*, *gikoba*, and *tipolu*. Next, they strung these words together in a random order, with words running together just as they do in fluently produced sentences (**FIGURE 11.24**). A sample would sound like *tokibugopilagikobatipolugopilatokibutipolugikoba*. Eight-month-old infants listened to a 2-minute sequence of this novel language while sitting on their parent's lap. After this brief period of learning, infants heard either *tokibu* (one of the novel words) or *pabiku* (a new combination of the same syllables used to produce the "real" novel words). The infants listened longer to the nonwords than to the words, indicating that after just 2 minutes of exposure, they had begun to recognize the words in this new "language" enough to distinguish familiar from novel words. How did they do it?

Saffran and her colleagues suggest that the infants in their study learned the words by being sensitive to the statistics of the sequences of sounds that they heard in the first part of the experiment. In the real world of language, words are simply sequences of speech sounds that tend to occur together. Other sequences occur together less often. For example, think about the sequence 'p'-'r'-'ih'-'t'-'ee'-'b'-'ay'-'b'-'ee.' An infant will hear the sounds making up the word *pretty* in many different contexts ("pretty dress," "pretty good," and so on) and the sounds making up the word *baby* in other contexts (e.g., "good baby," "baby doll"). In contrast, the sequence 't'-'ee'-'b'-'ay' will almost never be heard in any other context, because no English words have this sequence of syllables. Saffran (2001, 2002) suggests that infants learn to pick words out of the speech stream by accumulating experience with sounds that tend to occur together; these are words (at least to babies). For example, infants eventually split the "word" *allgone* into two as they acquire more linguistic experience. When sounds that are rarely heard together occur in combination, that's a sign that there is a break between two words.

Speech in the Brain

Our earliest understanding of the role of cerebral cortex in the perception of speech and music was gained through unfortunate "natural" experiments in which people lost their ability to understand speech following stroke or other brain injuries. However, it is difficult to draw strong conclusions about brain processes from brain injuries. Brain damage from stroke—which results from damage to a blood vessel in the brain—follows patterns of blood vessels, not brain function. Damage from stroke might cover just part of a particular brain function, leaving some of the function undamaged; or damage could cover a wide region that includes some or all of a particular brain function, as well as all or part of other functions. Performance following brain damage, along with later experimental findings, has

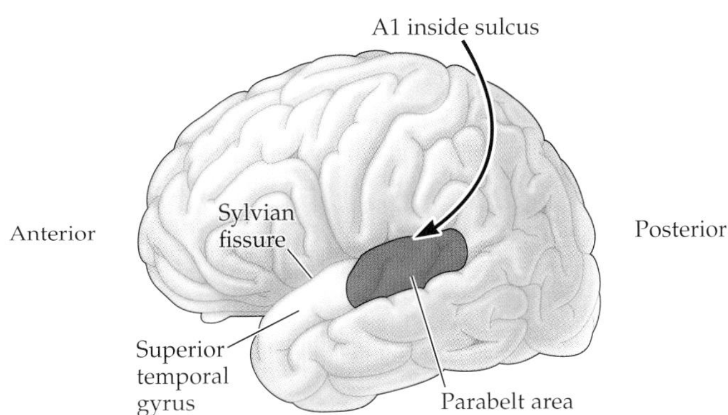

FIGURE 11.25 Higher-level auditory cortex The superior temporal gyrus extends along the upper surface of each temporal lobe. Primary auditory cortex (A1) and the adjacent belt area are hidden inside the Sylvian fissure (also known as the lateral sulcus; sulci are the deep grooves of the brain), with only the parabelt area exposed toward the posterior superior temporal gyrus. Portions of the superior temporal gyri (left and right) are active when we listen to complex sounds. (See also Figure 9.21.)

taught us that different hemispheres of the brain are better at doing some types of tasks. For most right-handed people, the left hemisphere is dominant for language processing. The development of techniques for brain imaging, such as functional magnetic resonance imaging, has made it possible for us to learn more about how speech is processed in the brain.

As we would expect based on what we learned in Chapter 9, hearing sounds of any kind activates the primary auditory cortex (A1). Further, we learned that the processing of complex sounds relies on additional areas of cortex adjacent to A1. These nearby areas of auditory cortex, called belt and parabelt areas, as shown in Figure 9.21 and **FIGURE 11.25**, often are referred to as secondary or association cortical areas. As one might expect, we see these areas activated when listeners hear speech and music. Even at this relatively early level of cortical processing, some areas are already more responsive to speech versus music versus other commonly heard natural sounds (Norman-Haignere, Kanwisher, and McDermott, 2015). Even for a simple speech utterance, some cortical areas differentiate voice (who is talking) versus message (what is said; Rupp et al., 2022).

Because we know that language is typically lateralized to one hemisphere—usually the left side for right-handed people—processing speech should become more lateralized at some point because perceiving speech is part of understanding language. One challenge for researchers is to create stimuli that have all the complex properties of speech without being heard as speech. We already learned that listeners are very good at understanding speech, even under adverse circumstances when some parts of the signal are missing or distorted, so this capability makes it difficult to construct stimuli that are complex like speech without being heard as speech.

Rosen et al. (2011) developed a particularly clever way to tease apart cortical responses to acoustic complexity from responses to speech per se. As **FIGURE 11.26** shows, the researchers played four types of sentences to listeners while their brains were being scanned using positron emission tomography. They began with presenting listeners complete sentences that included natural changes in both amplitude and frequency (Figure 11.26A), although they replaced voicing vibration with noise. Although using noise made the sentences sound whispered, they were perfectly intelligible. In the next presentation, the researchers eliminated changes in frequency, leaving only changes in amplitude (Figure 11.26B). Then they took away changes in amplitude, but left changes in frequency (Figure 11.26C). Finally, to match the amount of acoustic complexity in speech, they created hybrid "sentences" by adding the amplitude changes of one sentence (Figure 11.26E) to the frequency changes in another (Figure 11.26A). These hybrids (Figure 11.26D) were just as complex as the sentence in Figure 11.26A, but they were completely unintelligible.

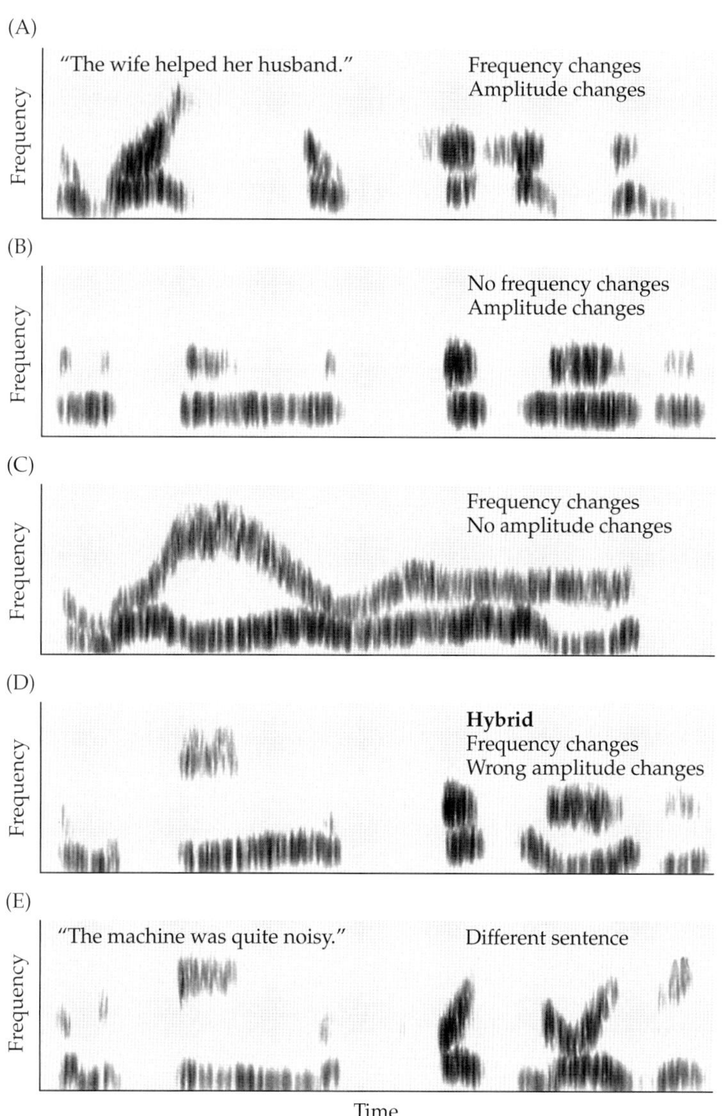

FIGURE 11.26 Hybrid sentences Stimuli created to measure cortical responses to acoustic complexity versus responses to speech. (A) This spectrogram represents an intact intelligible sentence with natural changes in frequency and amplitude. (B–E) In these spectrograms, the same sentence is now unintelligible because either frequency changes were removed (B) or amplitude changes were removed (C). The spectrogram in (D) has frequency changes from (A) but amplitude changes from (E). While (D) is equal to (A) in acoustic complexity, it is unintelligible because of the mismatch between changes in amplitude and frequency.

As **FIGURE 11.27** illustrates, neural activity in response to unintelligible hybrid "sentences" (see Figure 11.26D) was found bilaterally (in both hemispheres), with a little more activity along the superior temporal gyrus running along the top of the right temporal lobe. Responses in the left superior temporal gyrus became dominant only when sentences were intelligible because amplitude and frequency changes coincided properly (see Figure 11.26A). From these findings, it appears that language-dominant hemisphere responses depend on sound aligning with typical patterns of speech that convey linguistic understanding and are not caused by acoustic complexity alone.

A great deal of research is being conducted to further our understanding of how speech is processed in the brain on its way to becoming part of words and sentences (Holt et al., 2022). For now, the evidence suggests that as sounds become more complex, they are processed in more anterior and ventral regions of the superior temporal cortex farther away from A1 (R. D. Patterson and Johnsrude, 2008; Uppenkamp et al., 2006). This much appears to be true: when speech sounds become more clearly a part of language, they are processed more anteriorly (farther forward) in the left temporal lobe. However, this back-to-front path may not be all there is to speech perception in the brain; other brain regions are likely involved. Increasingly, researchers are documenting that speech perception engages much of the brain.

What could we learn if we could place electrodes right on top of, or even within, the human brain? Prior to performing brain surgery to remove a tumor or to reduce effects of severe epilepsy, neurosurgeons often place electrodes directly on the surface of the brain to localize

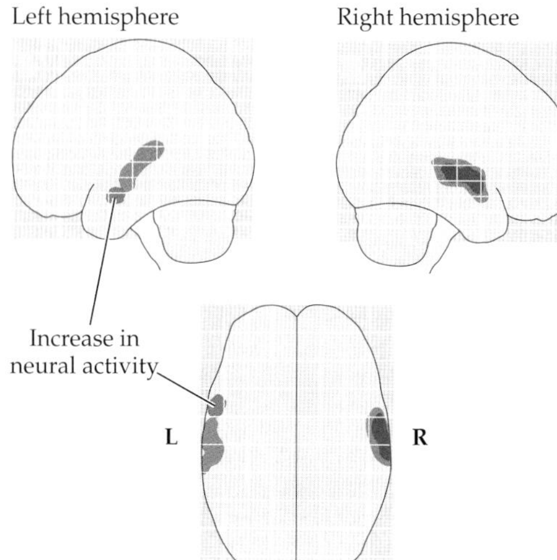

FIGURE 11.27 Where speech becomes language When listeners heard hybrid sentences such as the one shown in Figure 11.26D (for which amplitude and frequency changes came from different sentences), substantial neural activity (red) was observed in both left and right superior temporal lobes. An increase in activity (purple) was evident only in the language-dominant left anterior superior temporal lobe when the sentences were intelligible, like that in Figure 11.26A (with matching amplitude and frequency changes). ●

neural activity for clinical purposes. In Chapter 10, you were first introduced to an electrode grid placed over a region of left superior posterior temporal lobe (see Figure 10.27). Mesgarani et al. (2014) played 500 sentences spoken by 400 different people to 6 human participants while recording directly on the surface of their superior temporal gyri. At different single electrodes, responses were selective for certain classes of speech sounds such as fricatives, stop consonants, or vowels. In some cases, responses were even more selective. For example, responses to stop consonants might be selective for only voiceless stops ('p,' 't,' 'k') or for one place of articulation (e.g., 'd') versus others ('b' and 'g').

E. F. Chang et al. (2010) played a series of synthesized syllables varying incrementally from 'bah' to 'dah' to 'gah,' much like those in Figure 11.15, to patients who were awaiting surgery. The researchers found that, across populations of neurons recorded by surface electrodes, neural responses were much like listening data for the same syllables. Neural responses were very similar for pairs of stimuli that listeners would label as the same, as 'bah,' or 'dah,' or 'gah'; responses were quite distinct for pairs of syllables that were acoustically separated by the same extent but were labeled as different, as 'bah' paired with 'dah' or as 'dah' paired with 'gah.'

As with perception in general, cortical organization depends critically on experience, and the perception of speech sounds is tremendously experience-dependent. Because we know that English and Hindi speakers hear sounds like 'dah' differently, we know that the way listeners discriminate 'bah' and 'dah' depends on experience. Chang and colleagues (2010) have revealed places in the left temporal lobe where experience with English 'b' and 'd' shapes neural activity.

Cortical processes related to speech perception can be distinguished from brain processes that contribute to the perception of other complex sounds in two other ways. First, listeners have a wealth of experience simultaneously hearing speech and viewing talkers' faces. The famous McGurk effect is evidence of the profound effects that visual cues can have on the way speech sounds are perceived. Using the widely studied 'bah'–'dah'–'gah' phonemes (see Figure 11.15), McGurk and MacDonald (1976) demonstrated that what the listener saw while watching the speaker's face affected which *sound* they heard (**FIGURE 11.28**). Later neurological

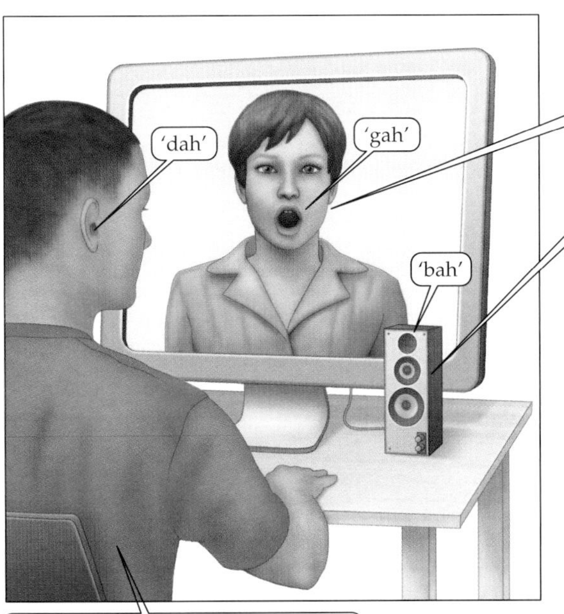
'dah'
'gah'
'bah'
1. A video shows a person repeating the sound 'gah.'
2. An audio track plays the sound 'bah.'
3. The subject hears the sound 'dah.'

FIGURE 11.28 The McGurk effect When most people hear the sound 'bah' repeatedly while watching a video of a person saying the syllable 'gah' at the same times, they frequently report hearing a third syllable, 'dah.' Participants do not hear 'bah' because the lips of the person they are watching do not close and open as they should if the person was saying 'bah.' This example of multisensory integration is so powerful that the illusion is maintained even when participants know they are being fooled (because they heard 'bah' when they closed their eyes). ●

work (Reale et al., 2007) used grids of electrodes on the surface of posterior temporal cortex (see Figure 10.27) to investigate cortical processing of audio and visual speech. The researchers found that neural responses to auditory speech stimuli in the language-dominant hemisphere were influenced substantially by simultaneous viewing of the lower half of the face of a person either producing audible speech or carrying out a meaningless mouth motion.

Because visual information combines with auditory experience when we're perceiving speech, you may wonder what happens for people who are deaf. Zatorre (2001) studied a group of people who previously had been deaf and had some hearing restored with a cochlear implant. These listeners exhibited increased brain activity in the visual cortex when listening to speech. Zatorre hypothesized that this activation of visual areas of the brain is the result of increased experience and ability with lip-reading for these formerly deaf individuals. •

In addition, when people talk, they both hear the sounds they're producing and experience the movements of speech production in their own vocal tracts. People have a lot of experience with the simultaneous activities of producing and perceiving our own speech, so one might expect to find brain regions where these related activities combine. As it happens, there are areas of the motor cortex (see Figure 1.15) that become active when listening to speech. As you might have anticipated from what you learned about the motor theory of speech perception, discovery of these areas of activity was taken by some investigators to be evidence that speech sounds are processed with reference to the motor activities engaged to produce them. This was a very controversial idea because motor theory had been abandoned by most investigators, so alternative explanations were developed (Lima, Krishnan, and Scott, 2016). While it is too soon to know exactly what the motor cortex is up to when a person is listening to speech, we have learned that responses in motor cortex and responses in the temporal lobe are organized similarly, and these responses are very different from brain responses recorded when people are talking (Cheung et al., 2016).

Summary

1. Musical pitch has two dimensions: tone height and tone chroma. Musical notes are combined to form chords. Notes and chords vary in duration and are combined to form melodies.
2. Melodies are learned psychological entities defined by patterns of rising and falling musical pitches, with different durations and rhythms.
3. Rhythm is important to music, and to auditory perception more broadly. The process of perceiving sound sequences is biased to hear rhythm.
4. Humans evolved to be able to produce an extremely wide variety of sounds that can be used in languages. The production of speech sounds has three basic components: respiration, phonation, and articulation. Speech sounds vary in many dimensions, including intensity, duration, periodicity, and noisiness.
5. In terms of articulation and acoustics, speech sounds vary according to other speech sounds that precede and follow (coarticulation). Because of coarticulation, listeners cannot use any single acoustic feature to identify a vowel or consonant. Instead, listeners must use multiple properties of the speech signal.

6. In general, listeners discriminate speech sounds only as well as they can label them. This is categorical perception, which also has been shown for the perception of many other complex familiar auditory and visual stimuli. But speech perception appears more graded and exhibits within-category differentiation with finer-grained measures; contemporary research thinks of speech as *categorized* rather than *categorical.*
7. How people perceive speech depends very much on their experience with speech sounds within a language. This experience includes learning which of the many acoustic features in speech tend to co-occur. Because of the role of experience in how we hear speech, it is often difficult to perceive and produce new speech sounds from a second language following experience with a first language.
8. One of the ways that infants learn words is to use their experience with the co-occurrence of speech sounds.
9. Speech sounds are processed in both hemispheres of the brain, much as other complex sounds are, until they become part of the linguistic message. Then, speech is further processed in anterior and ventral regions, mostly in the left superior temporal cortex, but also in posterior superior temporal cortex.

Chapter 12

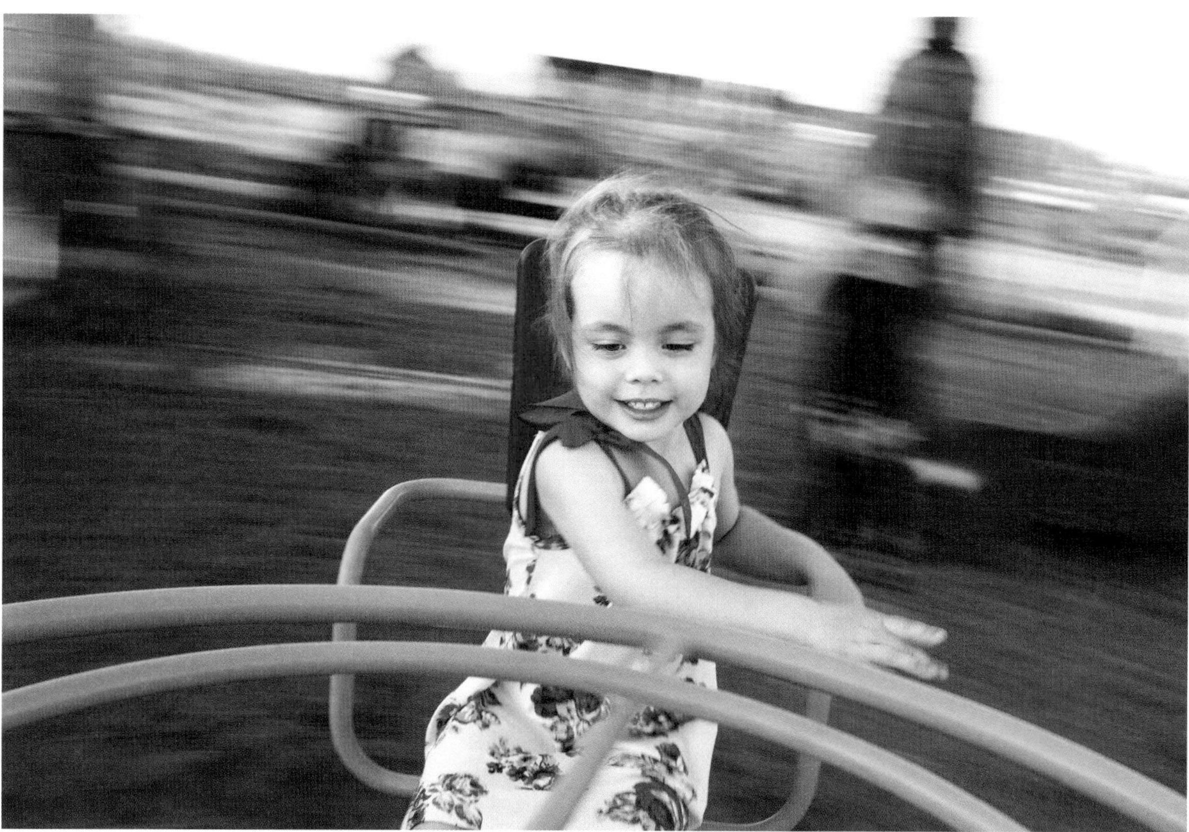

ILfoto, Little girl spinning on a children's carousel among the playground, 2020

Vestibular Sensation

Questions to Contemplate

Think about the following questions as you read this chapter.
By the chapter's end, you should be able to answer and discuss them.

- If you had to give up one sensory system, why would you not give up vestibular sensation?
- Can you identify at least four functional roles played by the vestibular system?
- Why can it be claimed that our tilt sense—often referred to as graviception—is among the most fundamental sensory modalities?
- Can you list at least three vestibular modalities?
- Why is it good that most contributions of the vestibular system are not usually consciously experienced?
- What does the vestibular system have to do with the motion sickness sometimes experienced with virtual reality?

Remember when you were a child and you used to spin around until you were dizzy and couldn't walk straight? Perhaps you even fell. Why were you dizzy? The sensations did not arise from one of the five senses that Aristotle recognized—vision, hearing, touch, taste, or smell. Your dizziness arose from contributions of your **vestibular organs** to your vestibular sense, which is also sometimes called your sense of equilibrium.

The vestibular organs are a set of specialized sense organs located in the inner ear right next to the cochlea (see Figure 9.8). Vestibular organs sense motion of the head, as well as the orientation of gravity, and make a predominant contribution to our sense of tilt and our sense of self-motion. Taken together, the senses of tilt and self-motion comprise a large part of our sense of **spatial orientation**.

FURTHER DISCUSSION of the cochlea can be found in Section 9.3.

You may be asking, "Wait a minute, why didn't I learn about the **vestibular system** and equilibrium when I first learned about the five senses?" Good question. Perhaps you should have. The vestibular "sixth sense" provides fundamental contributions that are often overlooked. For example, the vestibular system contributes to clear vision when we move, and it helps us maintain balance when we stand. And it is so crucial that some patients with vestibular dysfunction even report cognitive deficits when it fails. Yet, despite these essential contributions, the vestibular system toils in anonymity. Much of the time, we remain unaware of it until it stops working properly.

The fundamental nature of the vestibular system is emphasized by the fact that the vestibular organs appeared very early in evolutionary history and have remained relatively unchanged. The vertebrate fossil record shows the presence of distinct vestibular organs in fish at least 400 million years ago. The system is not only ancient but also largely automatic: vestibular perception is often relegated to

vestibular organs The set of five sense organs located in each inner ear that sense head motion and head orientation with respect to gravity.

spatial orientation A sense consisting of at least three interacting modalities: perception of linear motion, angular motion, and tilt.

vestibular system The vestibular organs as well as the vestibular neurons in cranial nerve VIII and the central neurons that contribute to the functional roles that the vestibular system participates in.

vertigo A sensation of rotation or spinning. The term is often used more generally to mean any form of dizziness.

vestibulo-ocular reflex (VOR) A short-latency reflex that helps stabilize vision by counterrotating the eyes when the vestibular system senses head movement.

the attentional background, and many responses evoked by the vestibular system are reflexive. Though we are all aware of the normal function of our eyes and ears, only when we experience problems such as dizziness, vertigo, spatial disorientation, imbalance, blurred vision, and/or illusory self-motion are we likely to become acutely aware of our vestibular sense.

We can no longer ask Aristotle—who is credited with first cataloging our sensory systems—why he did not include equilibrium or our vestibular sense among the specialized sensory systems, but we can speculate. It certainly is not because **vertigo** was unknown, since Aristotle himself described the vertiginous effects of alcohol. One explanation may be that it was not until the nineteenth century that scientists understood that the vestibular system is a specialized set of sense organs. Until then, the vestibular system had been considered an entrance to the cochlea. In fact, the name *vestibular* records this error for posterity, because *vestibule* means "entrance." But this explanation is not entirely satisfactory, since Aristotle had cataloged other senses without detailed anatomical or physiological knowledge. (See Wade [2000] for a historical review of vestibular knowledge prior to the nineteenth century.)

Another explanation may be the inconspicuous nature of our vestibular sense. In fact, as we'll see, many responses evoked by the vestibular system are reflexive. For example, the vestibular system helps us see clearly by reflexively rotating the eyeballs in the sockets to compensate for head rotation—thereby helping to keep visual images stable on the retina. This reflex is called the **vestibulo-ocular reflex (VOR)**.

To demonstrate this to yourself, move your hand a few inches back and forth in front of your face (**FIGURE 12.1A**). Start slowly and then speed up the movement. Focus on a fingertip and notice that it starts to appear more and more blurry as your hand moves at a higher frequency. This exercise demonstrates the limits of smooth pursuit, a form of visual tracking that you learned about in Chapter 8. Now hold your hand in front of your face and shake your head from side to side as if to say "no" (**FIGURE 12.1B**). Again, start slowly and gradually increase the speed. At higher frequencies of head rotation, you should notice that each fingertip stays in focus more readily when you move your head than when you move your hand. You can compensate for head movement more readily than hand movement because of a VOR that we will discuss in more detail later in this chapter.

(A)

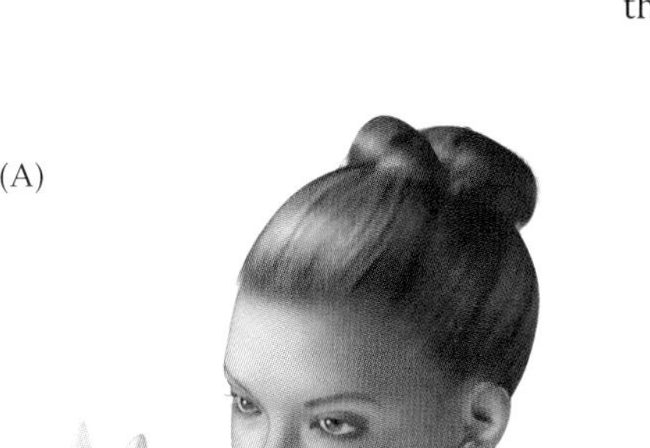

Individual's view

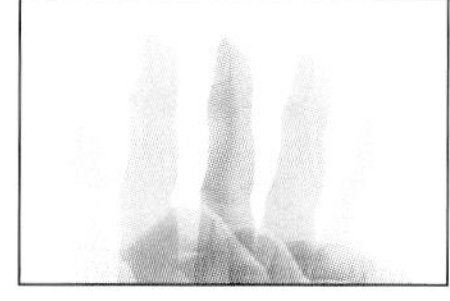

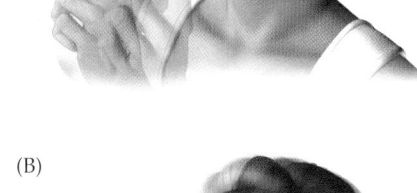

(B)

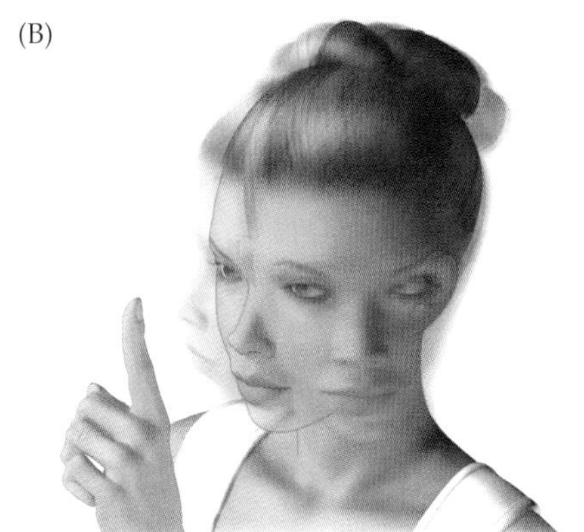

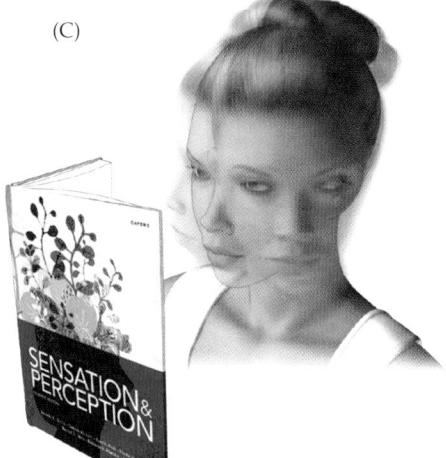

Individual's view

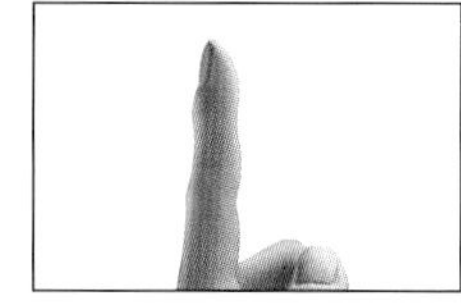

(C)

Individual's view

TEXT

FIGURE 12.1 Demonstration of the vestibulo-ocular reflex (A) As your fingertip moves faster and faster in front of your face, the fingertip begins to blur. (B) When you shake your head back and forth as if to say "no," the fingertip remains clearer. (C) Text also remains clearer during head shaking.

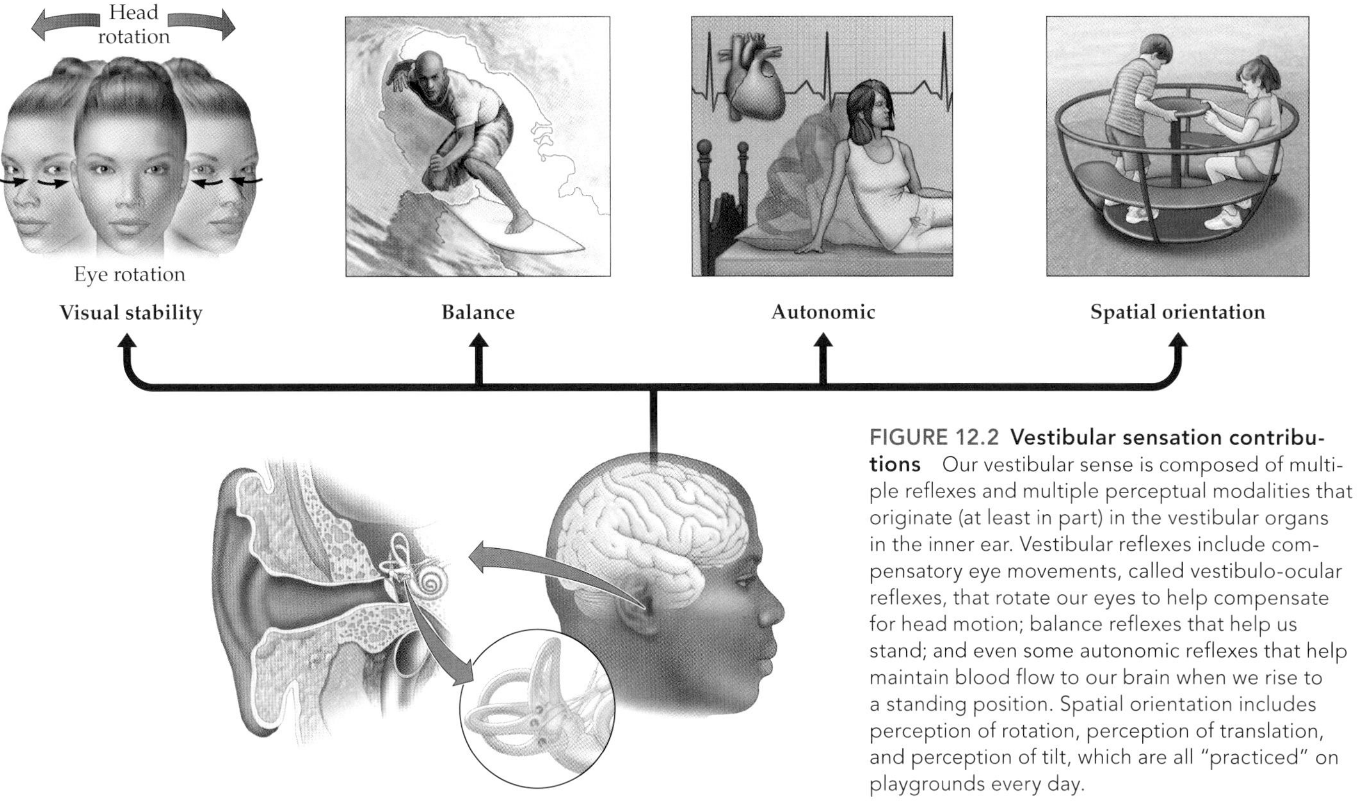

FIGURE 12.2 Vestibular sensation contributions Our vestibular sense is composed of multiple reflexes and multiple perceptual modalities that originate (at least in part) in the vestibular organs in the inner ear. Vestibular reflexes include compensatory eye movements, called vestibulo-ocular reflexes, that rotate our eyes to help compensate for head motion; balance reflexes that help us stand; and even some autonomic reflexes that help maintain blood flow to our brain when we rise to a standing position. Spatial orientation includes perception of rotation, perception of translation, and perception of tilt, which are all "practiced" on playgrounds every day.

Until now, you likely focused on what you saw. But now that we call your attention to head rotation, as you continue to shake your head and read this text (**FIGURE 12.1C**), you can perceive your head rotating, can't you? Thus, it is not that you are unable to perceive vestibular sensation, but rather that vestibular sensation is typically relegated to the attentional background (discussed in Chapter 7). Vestibular responses (**FIGURE 12.2**) are usually automatic. This is useful when you are multitasking, like when you are walking on rough terrain, thinking, and chewing gum all at the same time!

Your conscious awareness of vestibular sensation is typically evident only when you are dizzy or imbalanced; such awareness is especially useful when you need to regain stability to avoid falling!

12.1 Vestibular Contributions

The vestibular system provides the sensory foundation for spatial orientation, which includes perception of translation, rotation, and tilt. The vestibular system also makes crucial contributions to **balance**, but does not provide the sensory foundation for balance; **kinesthesia** does (see Chapter 13). While blind individuals and those without vestibular systems can stand, individuals lacking kinesthesia typically cannot stand. In addition, the vestibular system helps stabilize our eyes during head motion. In this role, the vestibular system makes crucial contributions to clarity of sight, but does not provide the sensory foundation; our eyes and visual system do (see Chapters 2–8). The vestibular system also helps maintain blood flow to the brain via contributions to cardiovascular regulation but is not foundational there either; somatosensation and interoception are (see Chapter 13).

balance The neural processes of postural control by which weight is evenly distributed, enabling us to remain upright and stable.

kinesthesia Perception of the position and movement of our limbs in space.

active sensing Sensing that includes self-generated probing of the environment. Besides our vestibular sense, other active human senses include vision and touch. Animal active sensing includes the use of echoes by whales and bats, the use of electrical signals by some fishes, and the use of whiskers/antennae by fishes, insects, and nocturnal rodents.

efferent commands Information flowing outward from the central nervous system to the periphery. A common example is motor commands that regulate muscle contraction. The copy of such motor commands is often called an efferent copy.

afferent signals Information flowing inward to the central nervous system from sensors in the periphery. Passive sensing would rely exclusively on such sensory inflow, providing a traditional view of sensation.

graviception The physiological structures and processes that sense the relative orientation of gravity with respect to the organism.

Also, as will be discussed in detail later in this chapter, our vestibular sense is active, not passive. By this we mean that our vestibular sense combines information flowing from our brain to our muscles with information flowing inward to the brain from various sensory systems, especially the kinesthetic, visual, and vestibular systems. For example, signals that tell our muscles to rotate our head provide information about head rotation just as vestibular signals do. Information from these various sources is combined to improve on vestibular sensation in isolation. More generally, **active sensing** balances information derived from **efferent commands** flowing outward from the brain to the periphery (e.g., to muscles) with information from various **afferent signals** flowing from sensors inward to the brain.

In summary, the vestibular system contributes to our sense of equilibrium, which is composed of many fundamental reflexes and perceptual modalities (Figure 12.2). The breadth of the vestibular system's contributions is pretty amazing (some might say it provides a "dizzying" array of contributions). When combined, these various perceptual and reflexive roles are referred to as our sense of equilibrium because they involve a balance of influences and/or a balance of forces—matching definitions of *equilibrium* you might find in a dictionary.

12.2 Evolutionary Development and Vestibular Sensation

Knowing up from down is crucial for us as humans, and this sensation provides a "stable permanent framework of the environment" for many perceptual processes that provides an "underlying and ceaseless awareness of what is permanent in the world" (Gibson, 1966). As just one fundamental example, the receptive-field orientation of simple visual cortical neurons (see Chapter 3) is affected by **graviception** (Tomko, Barbaro, and Ali, 1981) ● The fundamental nature and importance of this modality is even captured by the words we use to describe actions that define us as human (e.g., *stand up*). But tilt sensation, sometimes referred to as graviception, is not limited to humans. All mammals have vestibular labyrinths. In fact, all vertebrates, including fishes, amphibians, nonavian reptiles, and birds, have vestibular organs. Even the dinosaurs had vestibular organs. While crustaceans (e.g., crabs) and invertebrates (e.g., jellyfishes) do not have vestibular organs, some have dedicated graviceptors, and plants sense gravity (how else could trees grow up?) (**FIGURE 12.3**). Going further back along the

(A)

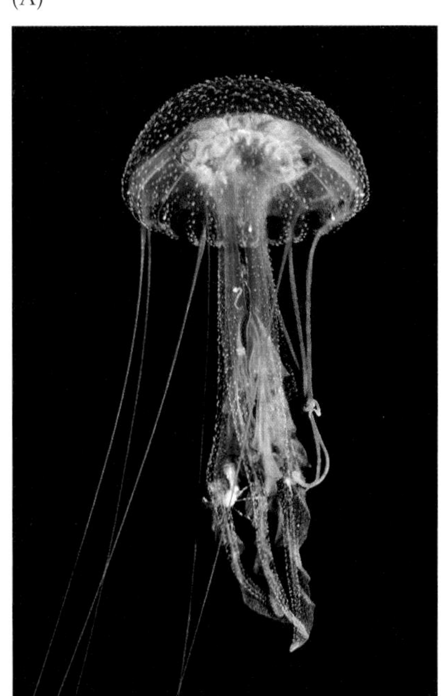

(B)

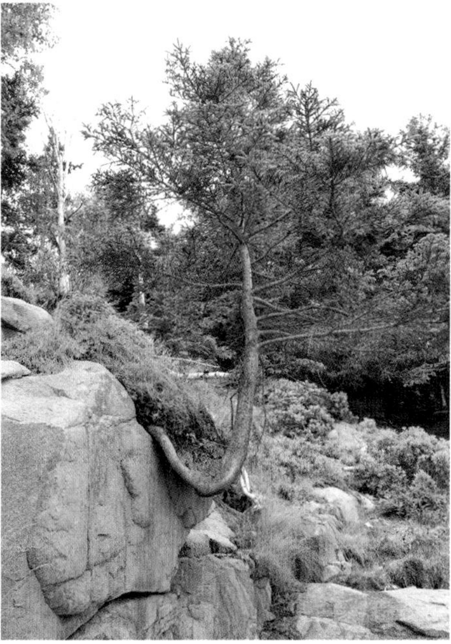

FIGURE 12.3 The fundamental nature of gravity sensation Even plants and invertebrates, such as jellyfishes, sense gravity. (A) Jellyfishes have what are called statoliths, which include calcium crystals that stimulate ciliated mechanoreceptors that are analogs to otoconia and hair cells of the otolith organs. (B) While plants don't have organs analogous to the otoliths, they too need to sense gravity for a root to grow downward and a shoot to grow upward.

evolutionary chain, even some bacteria need to know up from down. In summary, from an evolutionary perspective, graviception has been around awhile.

Furthermore, relative to the vestibular organs of all other vertebrates, the human vertical canals are relatively large. Larger canals contribute to higher sensitivity, which is believed to yield enhanced head and eye stabilization when we run (Spoor, Wood, and Zooneveld, 1994). This is believed to have contributed to enhanced exercise capacity (Bramble and Lieberman, 2004), which, in turn, is believed to have contributed to larger human brains (Raichlen and Gordon, 2011). In summary, vestibular sensation is fundamental to human behavior and likely even affected human evolution.

12.3 Modalities and Qualities of Spatial Orientation

Our perception of spatial orientation includes three sensory modalities: the senses of **angular motion**, **linear motion**, and **tilt**. Why do we call these "modalities," as though they were different senses, rather than calling them "qualities"? For example, vision and hearing are different modalities, but we would say that color and brightness are different *qualities*, not different modalities. The key lies in the energy **transduced**. Color and brightness are different interpretations of the same energy (light)—hence, *qualities*. Seeing and hearing involve different types of energy—light and pressure waves, respectively. For vestibular sensation, perceiving rotation, translation, and tilt requires that three different stimuli—angular acceleration, linear acceleration, and gravity, respectively—be transduced.

Sensing Angular Motion ("Rotation"), Linear Motion ("Translation"), and Tilt

These three stimulation energies are sensed by two types of vestibular sense organs: the semicircular canals and the otolith organs. The **semicircular canals** sense **angular acceleration**, which is a change in angular velocity; this signal makes a predominant contribution to our sense of angular motion. To experience your sense of angular motion, simply close your eyes and rotate your head from side to side as if to say "no." Because of contributions from your vestibular system, you should experience a perception of rotational motion that roughly matches the true motion of your head.

The **otolith organs** transduce both **linear acceleration**, which is a change of linear velocity, and **gravity**. The otolith organs provide a predominant contribution to your sense of head tilt and a predominant contribution to your sense of linear motion, which is also referred to as your sense of translation. To experience your sense of tilt, simply pitch your head forward as if to say "yes" and hold it there for several seconds; then pitch your head backward and hold it there. You should experience a perception of head tilt. Relatively pure linear motion is more difficult to achieve passively, but the experience of riding in a car, train, or bus provides an example. Try the following when you are a passenger in a vehicle. With your eyes closed, pay attention to your sense of motion as the driver backs the car out of the garage, brings the car to a stop, and then begins to accelerate forward. Initially, you should perceive backward translation (backward linear motion). You should also perceive the cessation of translation as the car comes to a stop and then forward translation as the car moves forward.

Two different types of sense organs—the semicircular canals and the otolith organs—establish at least two sensory modalities. But if we have only two types of sense organs, why do we say there are three modalities? As noted, the otolith organs

angular motion Rotational motion like the rotation of a spinning top or swinging saloon doors that rotate back and forth.

linear motion Translational motion like the predominant movement of a train car or bobblehead doll.

tilt To attain a sloped position like that of the Leaning Tower of Pisa.

transduce To convert from one form of energy to another (e.g., from light to neural electrical energy, or from mechanical energy to neural electrical energy).

semicircular canal Any of three toroidal tubes in the vestibular system that sense angular motion.

angular acceleration The rate of change of angular velocity. Mathematically, the integral of angular acceleration is angular velocity, and the integral of angular velocity is angular displacement. Angular acceleration, angular velocity, and angular displacement all mathematically represent angular motion.

otolith organ Either of two mechanical structures (utricle and saccule) in the vestibular system that sense both linear acceleration and gravity.

linear acceleration The rate of change of linear velocity. Mathematically, the integral of linear acceleration is linear velocity, and the integral of linear velocity is linear displacement, which is also referred to as translation. Linear acceleration, linear velocity, and linear displacement all mathematically represent linear motion.

gravity A force that attracts a body toward the center of the Earth.

Sensation & Perception in Everyday Life

The Vestibular System, Virtual Reality, and Motion Sickness

What does the vestibular system have to do with motion sickness experienced by some virtual reality gamers (**FIGURE 12.4**)? As noted earlier, visual cues combine with vestibular cues to yield our equilibrium sense. The brain learns to associate certain combinations of these cues. For example, if I rotate my head to the right, the vestibular system senses that head rotation, and my eyes see relative rotation of the visual field to the left. I don't expect relative motion of the visual field when my head is still (and vice versa). Any imperfections in these visual-vestibular interactions yield discrepancies relative to the normal sensory interactions that are expected by the brain. Such sensory discrepancies, often called **sensory conflict**, cause motion sickness. For example, when we are engaged with virtual reality, there is an inherent delay between sensing a head motion and the resultant virtual visual scene motion, because the calculations needed to move the image on the display cannot be performed instantaneously. When this delay is long enough, the brain senses discrepancies between the virtual visual motion experienced and the visual motion that would normally accompany the sensed head motion. This can (and often does) lead to motion sickness ●

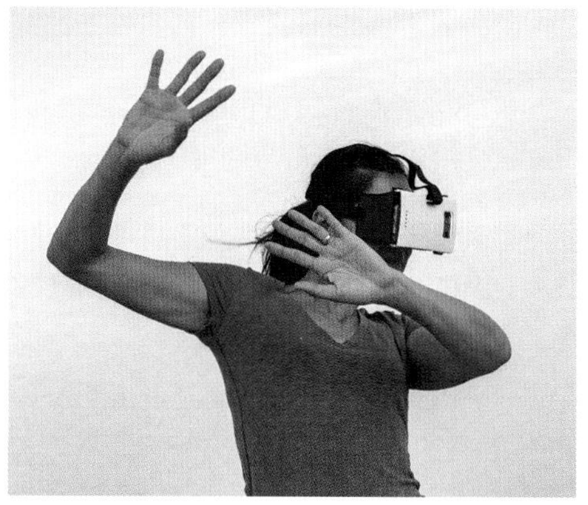

FIGURE 12.4 Vestibular sensation and virtual reality Virtual reality is becoming more popular. Motion sickness, believed to be caused by a mismatch between vestibular and visual cues, has limited the adoption of virtual reality as a standard visual display.

transduce both gravity and linear acceleration. The brain perceives tilt derived from the brain's estimate of orientation with respect to gravity and perceives translation from the brain's estimate of linear acceleration. Tilt perception seems fundamentally different from translation perception; these do not seem to be different sensory qualities like color and brightness.

Why is this so? This key question leads to the fundamental rationale for two modalities arising from otolith signals. Classical physics teaches that gravity and linear acceleration are distinct from one another, and the brain does its best to separate the signals from the otolith organs into signals representative of gravity and signals representative of linear acceleration (Angelaki et al., 1999; Merfeld, Zupan, and Peterka, 1999). Therefore, we assert three interacting sensory modalities—a **sense of angular motion**, a **sense of linear motion**, and a **sense of tilt**—paralleling the three different sources of stimulation energy—angular acceleration, linear acceleration, and gravity (Guedry, 1974; Young, 1984).

sensory conflict Sensory discrepancies that arise when sensory systems provide conflicting information. For example, vision may indicate that you are stationary while the vestibular system tells you that you are moving (or vice versa).

sense of angular motion The perceptual modality that senses rotation.

sense of linear motion The perceptual modality that senses translation.

sense of tilt The perceptual modality that senses head inclination with respect to gravity.

amplitude In reference to vestibular sensation, the size (increase or decrease) of a head movement (with angular velocity, linear acceleration, tilt, etc.).

direction The line one moves along (or faces), with reference to the point or region one is moving toward (or facing).

Basic Qualities of Spatial Orientation: Amplitude and Direction

Each of our three spatial orientation modalities includes two qualities: **amplitude** and **direction**. As an example of amplitude, the speed of our perceived motion can be large (as in a fast car on the freeway) or small (as in a car inching forward in a traffic jam). As an example of direction, perceived linear motion might be forward, up, or to the left.

AMPLITUDE For linear motion, we can perceive translation having high velocity (again, think of a fast car) or low velocity (again, think of a traffic jam). Similarly, we can perceive rotational velocity with high amplitude (think of

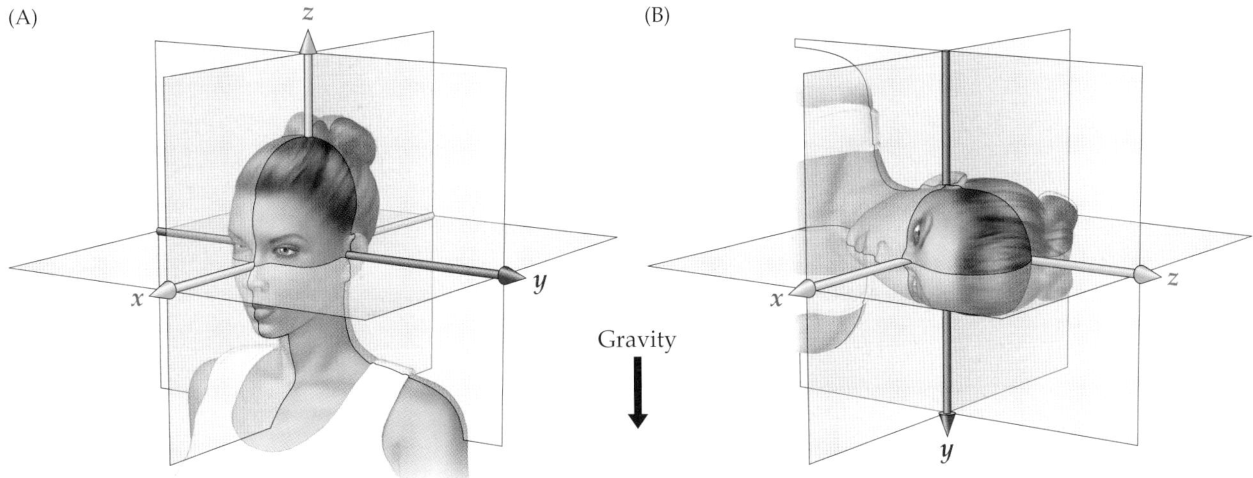

FIGURE 12.5 **Standard vestibular coordinate system** Movement of the head can be described using a head-fixed Cartesian coordinate system. (A) A positive *x*-axis points forward, a positive *y*-axis points out the left ear, and a positive *z*-axis points toward the top of the head. As (B) illustrates for a side-down position, this is a head-fixed coordinate system because it is stationary with respect to the head. For example, the *y*-axis always points out the left ear, independent of orientation relative to gravity.

vigorously shaking your head) or low amplitude (think of the slow rotation of minute or hour hands on a clock). Finally, tilt amplitude is also important. Tilt amplitudes can be small (as when you gently nod your head) or large (as when you lie down).

DIRECTION To help classify direction, we define a simple Cartesian coordinate system that moves with the head. Since the physical space that we move in is three-dimensional, we need three axes. In our head-fixed coordinate system, the *x*-axis always points forward, the *y*-axis always points out the left ear, and the *z*-axis always points out the top of the head (**FIGURE 12.5**).

There are three directions for our sense of linear motion. Imagine (1) stepping forward or backward along the *x*-axis (**FIGURE 12.6A**), (2) sliding from right to left along the *y*-axis (**FIGURE 12.6B**), and (3) translating up or down along the *z*-axis (**FIGURE 12.6C**). These three translation components can be combined to represent any three-dimensional linear motion.

FIGURE 12.6 **Translating bodies can move in three directions** The head can translate forward and backward along the *x*-axis (A), left and right along the *y*-axis (B), or up and down along the *z*-axis (C).

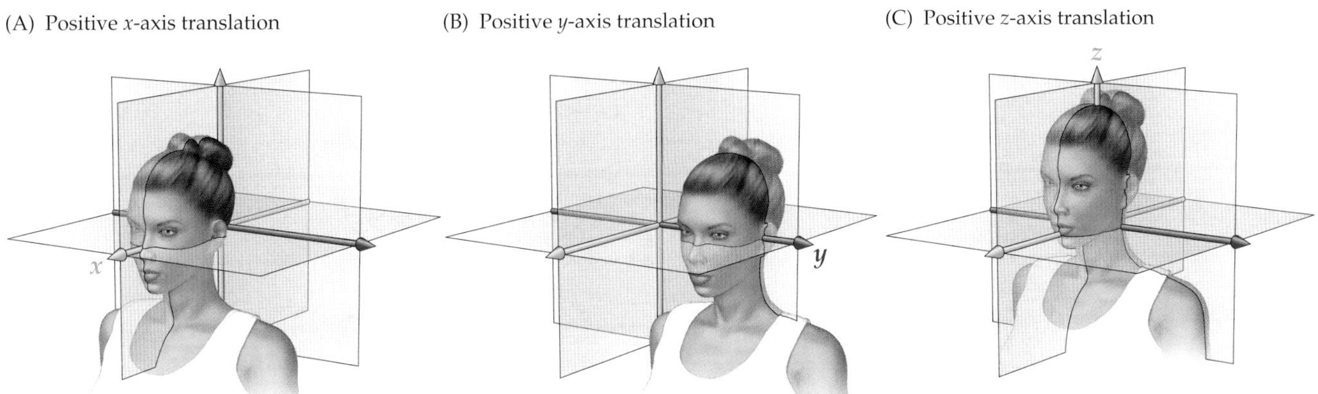

Similarly, three directions define our sense of angular motion (**FIGURE 12.7**). That is, the head can rotate in three independent ways, with the following representations:

1. *Roll angular velocity* (Figures 12.7A and 12.7B). Think of cartwheels or lying on your back with your nose at the center of a merry-go-round.
2. *Pitch angular velocity*. As when you nod "yes" (Figures 12.7C and 12.7D), but you might also think of somersaults or lying on your side with your ears at the center of a merry-go-round.

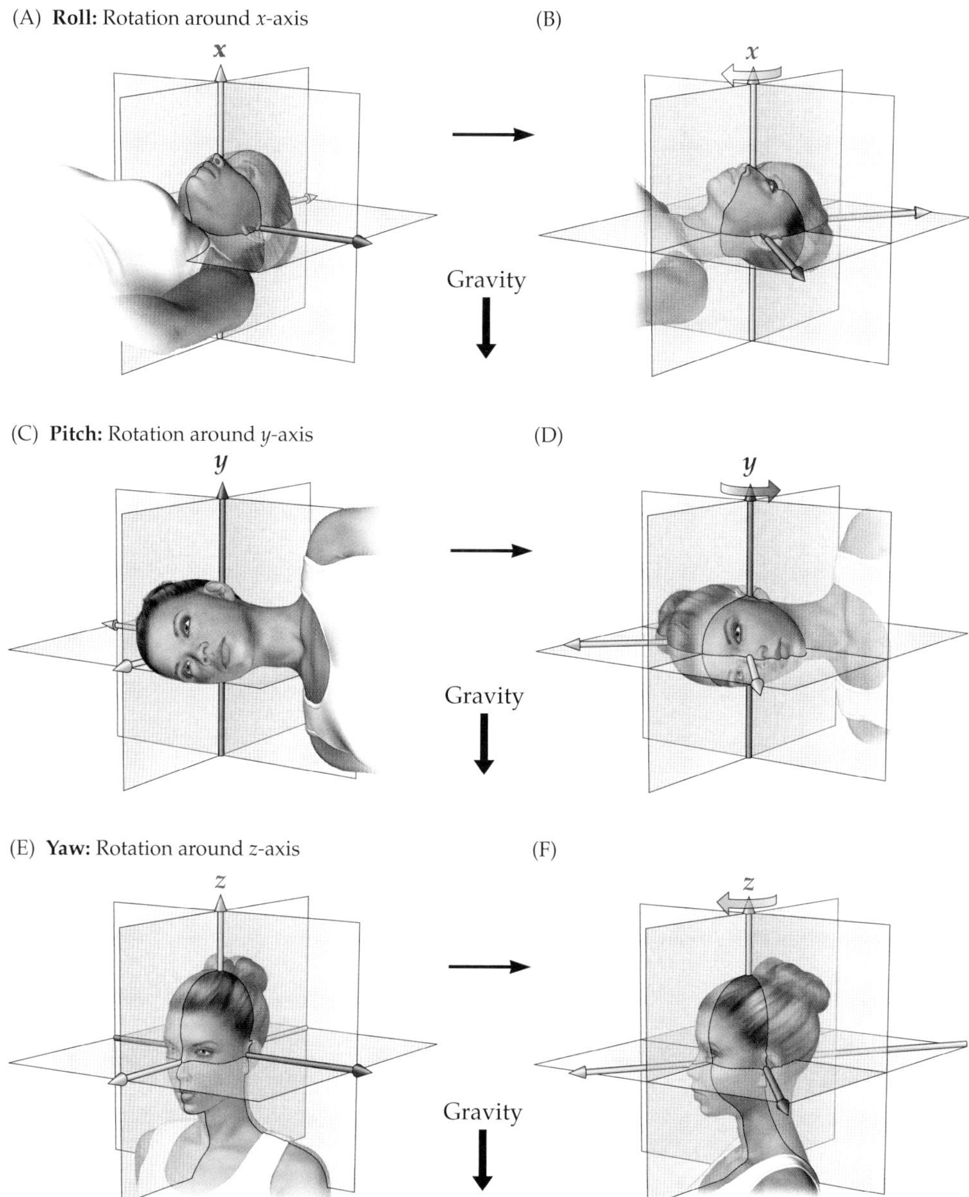

FIGURE 12.7 Bodies can rotate in three directions To illustrate each of these three "pure" rotations (that is, in the absence of any tilt), the head is prepositioned (left column) such that each of the three rotations illustrated in the right column yields no change in tilt (that is, the rotation axis is aligned with gravity). (For comparison, Figure 12.8 shows head tilts that result when rotation axes are not aligned with gravity.) When prepositioned to be supine (A), the head can turn with a pure roll rotation (represented by the curved blue arrow in the right column) around the *x*-axis with a change in roll orientation but no change in head tilt relative to gravity (B). When prepositioned to be right ear down (C), the head can turn with a pure pitch rotation (represented by the curved purple arrow in the right column) around the *y*-axis with a change in pitch orientation but no change in head tilt relative to gravity (D). When prepositioned to be upright (E), the head can turn with a pure yaw rotation (represented by the curved green arrow in the right column) around the *z*-axis with a change in yaw orientation but no change in head tilt relative to gravity (F).

3. *Yaw angular velocity*. As when you shake your head "no" (Figures 12.7E and 12.7F), but you might also think of a spinning skater or of sitting on a rotating barstool.

These three angular motions can be combined to represent any three-dimensional head rotation.

Finally, for any given head orientation, there are two tilt directions (**FIGURE 12.8**). For example, when you are upright, a pitch rotation would yield a pitch tilt forward or backward (Figure 12.8A)—again, think of somersaults—or a roll rotation would yield a roll tilt to the left or right (Figure 12.8B), as in a cartwheel. What happened to the third dimension? The third rotation direction would be a yaw rotation, but this would not yield a change in head tilt with respect to gravity (Figure 12.8C). When head rotations align with gravity, there is no change in head tilt. So, for any given head position, there are three directions for angular velocity and translation, but only two directions for tilt.

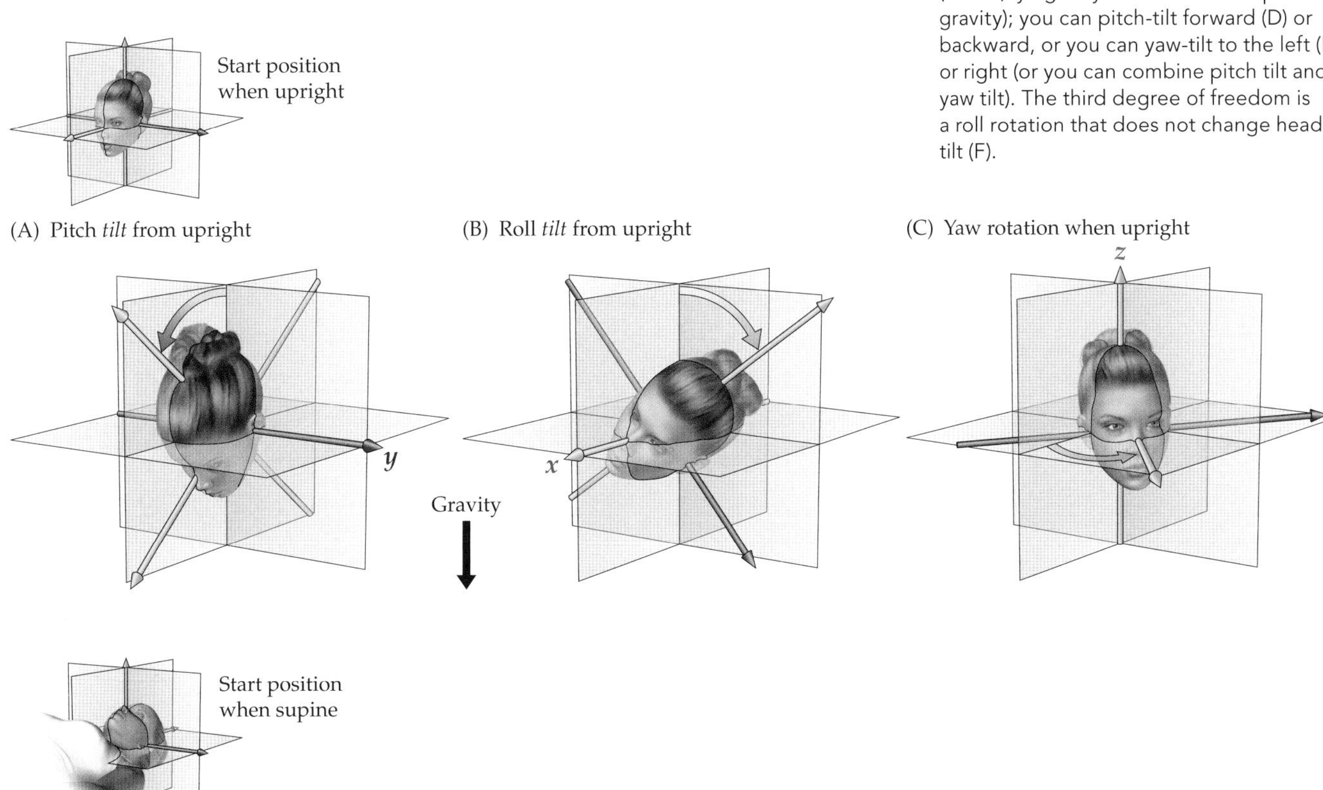

FIGURE 12.8 From any head orientation, two directions of head tilt are possible The top row shows the two possible tilt directions when you are initially upright with respect to gravity; you can pitch-tilt forward (A) or backward, or you can roll-tilt to the left (B) or right (or you can combine pitch tilt and roll tilt). The third degree of freedom is a yaw rotation that does not change head tilt (C). The bottom row shows the two possible tilt directions when you are initially supine (that is, lying on your back with respect to gravity); you can pitch-tilt forward (D) or backward, or you can yaw-tilt to the left (E) or right (or you can combine pitch tilt and yaw tilt). The third degree of freedom is a roll rotation that does not change head tilt (F).

velocity The speed and direction in which something moves. Mathematically, velocity is the temporal derivative of position. In words, linear velocity is distance divided by time to traverse that distance; angular velocity is rotation angle divided by time to traverse that angle.

acceleration A change in velocity. Mathematically, acceleration is the temporal derivative of velocity. In words, linear acceleration indicates a change in linear velocity; angular acceleration indicates a change in angular velocity.

hair cell Any cell that has stereocilia for transducing mechanical movement in the inner ear into neural activity sent to the brain. Some hair cells also receive inputs from the brain.

mechanoreceptor A sensory receptor that responds to mechanical stimulation (pressure, vibration, or movement).

12.4 The Vestibular Organs

The vestibular organs are each about the size of a large pea and can be found in the inner ear right next to the cochlea (**FIGURE 12.9A**). They respond primarily to head motion—both linear and angular—and head tilt with respect to gravity. Each inner ear has one vestibular labyrinth, and each vestibular labyrinth includes five sense organs (**FIGURE 12.9B**): three semicircular canals that sense rotational motion and two otolith organs that sense gravity and linear acceleration.

Note that neither the otolith organs nor the semicircular canals respond to constant **velocity**. Rather, they respond to *changes* in velocity—called **acceleration**. The sensitivity of the vestibular system to acceleration—angular acceleration for the semicircular canals and linear acceleration for the otolith organs—demonstrates that the vestibular system is principally sensitive to *changes* in motion. Constant motion, whether angular or linear, does not result in vestibular signals that directly indicate motion.

The otolith organs transduce both linear acceleration and gravity into a single neural signal sent to the brain. In fact, as Einstein asserted in his well-known equivalence principle, the impacts of gravity and linear acceleration are equivalent—meaning no device can measure a difference between gravity and linear acceleration. Separating the otolith measurement of gravity and linear acceleration into an estimate of gravity and an estimate of linear acceleration is not easy and must be important, since the brain expends energy and effort to do so (Angelaki et al., 1999; Merfeld, Zupan, and Peterka, 1999).

Hair Cells: Mechanical Transducers

Hair cells, which you read about in Chapter 9 when you began to learn about hearing (see Figures 9.9, 9.10, and 9.11 and associated text), act as **mechanoreceptors**

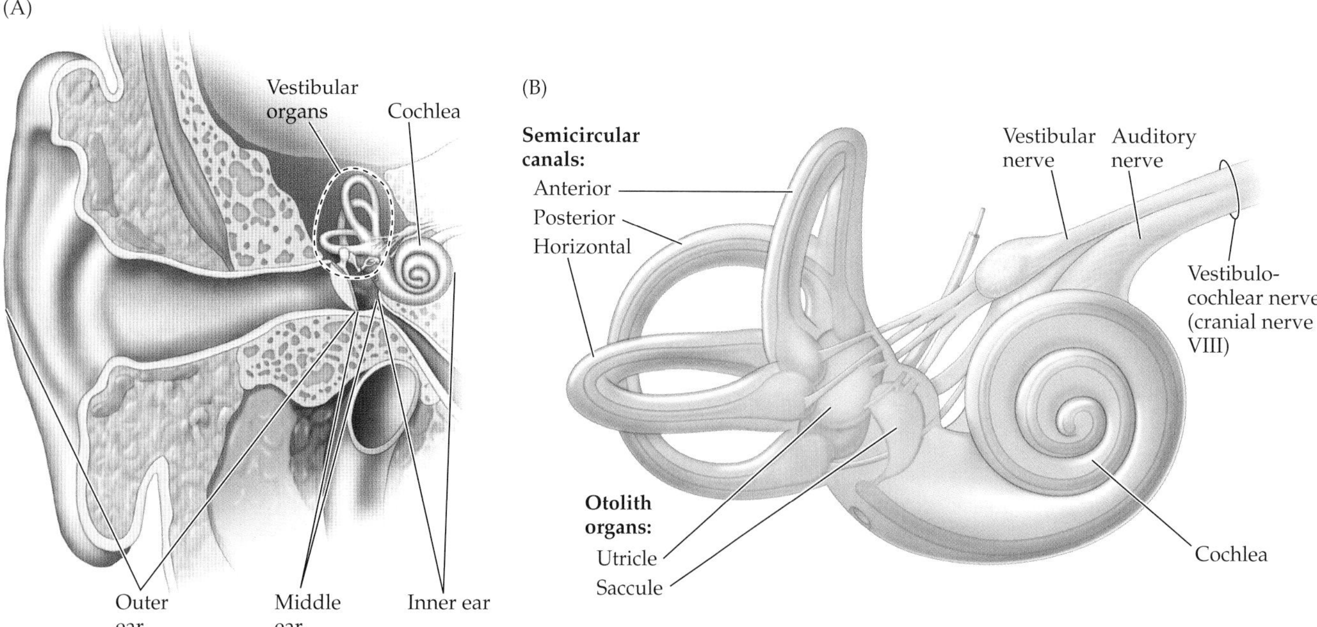

FIGURE 12.9 The vestibular labyrinth (A) The vestibular organs occupy a membranous, fluid-filled sac that is in a cavity in the temporal bone, near the cochlea, and is the nonhearing part of the inner ear. (B) The vestibular organs consist of three semicircular canals (anterior, posterior, and horizontal) and two otolith organs (utricle and saccule) on each side of the head. The vestibular organs are innervated by the vestibular nerve, which joins the auditory nerve to form cranial nerve VIII, called the vestibulocochlear nerve (see Figure 1.14).

in each of the five vestibular organs. Head motion causes hair cell stereocilia to deflect. Stereocilia deflection causes a change in the hair cell voltage, which alters neurotransmitter release, which, in turn, evokes action potentials in those vestibular-nerve fibers that have one or more synapses on the hair cell. These afferent neurons carry the action potentials to the brain.

receptor potential A change in voltage across the membrane of a sensory receptor cell (in the vestibular system, a hair cell) in response to stimulation.

Let's consider vestibular hair cell responses in a bit more detail. In the absence of stimulation, vestibular hair cells have a negative voltage and release neurotransmitters at a constant rate, evoking a constant rate of action potentials in the afferent neurons (**FIGURE 12.10A**). Changes in hair cell voltage—called the **receptor potential**—are proportional to the bending of the hair cell bundles and control the rate at which hair cells release neurotransmitters to the afferent neurons. When a hair cell bends toward the tallest stereocilia (**FIGURE 12.10**), the hair cell voltage becomes less negative. This voltage change is also called a depolarization because the hair cell becomes less polarized than the negative resting potential (see Figure 12.10A). The hair cell depolarization increases the release of neurotransmitter, causing an increase in the action potential rate (called excitation). However, if the hair cell is bent away from the tallest stereocilia, the cell potential becomes more negative (hyperpolarizes), causing a decrease in the release of neurotransmitter and a decrease in the action potential rate (called inhibition). In summary, the rate of

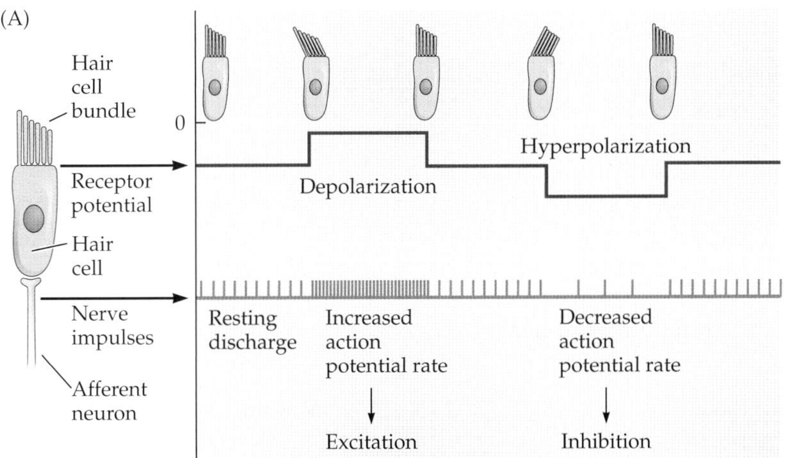

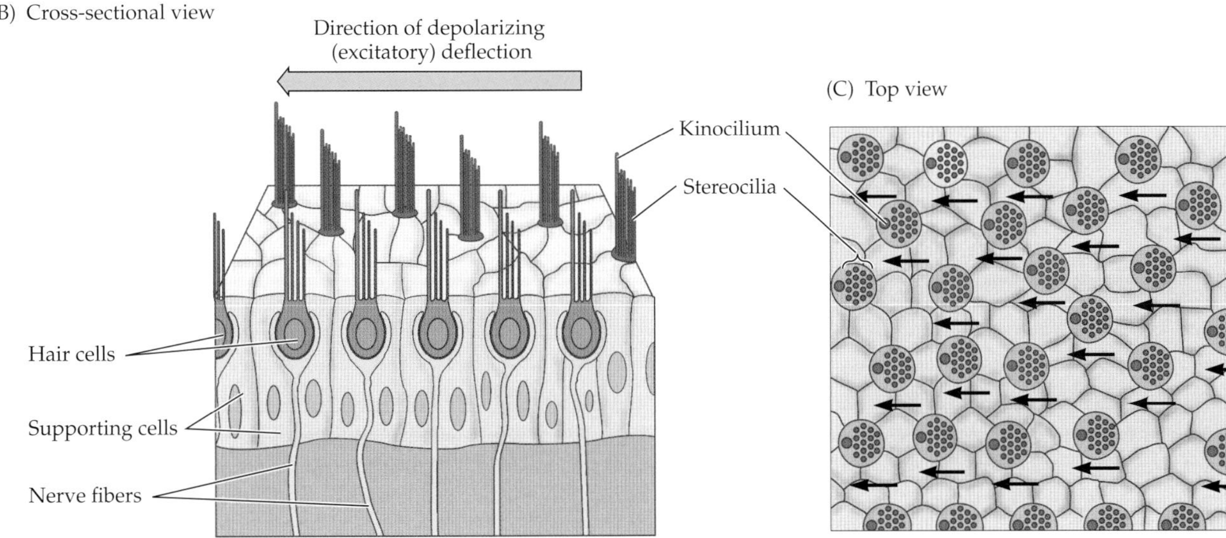

FIGURE 12.10 Hair cell responses (A) When not stimulated, the hair cells have a negative voltage and release neurotransmitter at a constant rate, evoking a constant rate of action potentials in the afferent nerves. When hair cell bundles bend toward the kinocilium and tallest stereocilia, the hair cells become depolarized and more neurotransmitter is released (excitation); when they bend away, they become hyperpolarized and less transmitter is released (inhibition). (B) This cross-sectional view of a hair cell array shows the direction of deflection that causes depolarization. (C) Top view of a hair cell array. The black arrows indicate the excitatory direction of hair cell deflection.

action potentials transmitted by afferent neurons increases or decreases following the hair cell receptor potential.

FURTHER DISCUSSION of the receptor potential of hair cells can be found in Section 9.3.

Thinking back to the fact that amplitude is one quality of our vestibular sense, we can begin to see how amplitude is encoded, since the rate of action potentials is proportional to the receptor potential, which in turn is proportional to the amount of hair cell deflection, which in turn is proportional to the amplitude of the motion.

The fact that the hair cells respond oppositely for deflections in opposite directions (see Figure 12.10A) is also crucial for the coding of vestibular stimuli. For example, as we'll discuss in detail in the following section, a yaw rotation to the left will increase the hair cell receptor potential for a hair cell located in the horizontal canal of the left ear, and a yaw rotation to the right will decrease the receptor potential for that same hair cell. A similar general principle applies for the otolith organs: acceleration in one direction increases the receptor potentials of some hair cells, while acceleration in the opposite direction decreases those receptor potentials.

Semicircular Canals

Each inner ear has three semicircular canals—horizontal (or lateral), anterior (or superior), and posterior (**FIGURE 12.11A**) (the anterior and posterior canals are sometimes called the vertical canals). These canals are roughly perpendicular (that is, at right angles to one another). The name *semicircular canal* loosely reflects the gross anatomy of this structure, which has the circular shape of an incomplete toroid or doughnut. Specifically, about three-fourths of a toroid is formed by a bony tube approximately 15 millimeters (mm) long, with a cross section about 1.5 mm in diameter. This space—called the osseous (meaning "bony") canal because it is a canal carved out of the mastoid bone—is colored tan in Figure 12.11A and is filled with a fluid called perilymph. The remaining length of the toroid passes through the vestibule, which is opened up in the figure to allow a glimpse inside. A second, smaller toroid, appearing bluish in the figure, is found inside the larger toroid. This smaller toroid is called the membranous labyrinth, because it is formed by a membrane filled with a fluid called endolymph. In cross section, the smaller toroid has a diameter of about 0.3 mm, which is just a little thicker than a very thick human hair.

The cross section for each canal swells substantially near where the canals join the vestibule. Each swelling is called an **ampulla** (plural *ampullae*) (**FIGURE 12.11B**). Within the endolymph space of each ampulla, the angular-motion detectors are assembled into a sensory epithelium called the **crista** (plural *cristae*). Each crista consists of a small ridge, which has an epithelium made up of about 7000 hair cells and is innervated by about 4000 nerve fibers. The kinocilium and stereocilia (singular *stereocilium*) of each hair cell project into a jelly-like cupula (plural *cupulae*) that forms an elastic dam extending to the opposite wall of the ampulla, with endolymph on both sides of the dam.

When the head rotates, the inertia of the endolymph causes it to lag behind the motion of the head (Breuer, 1874; Brown, 1874; Mach, 1875/2001), leading to deflection of the cupula and thereby to tiny deflections of the stereocilia in the crista. As mentioned earlier, such deflections evoke voltage changes in the hair cells, which in turn cause changes in the firing rate of afferent neurons (see Figure 12.10A). For each individual semicircular canal, all of the hair cells are aligned

ampulla An expansion of each semicircular-canal duct that includes that canal's cupula, crista, and hair cells, where transduction occurs.

crista Any of the specialized detectors of angular motion located in each semicircular canal in a swelling called the ampulla.

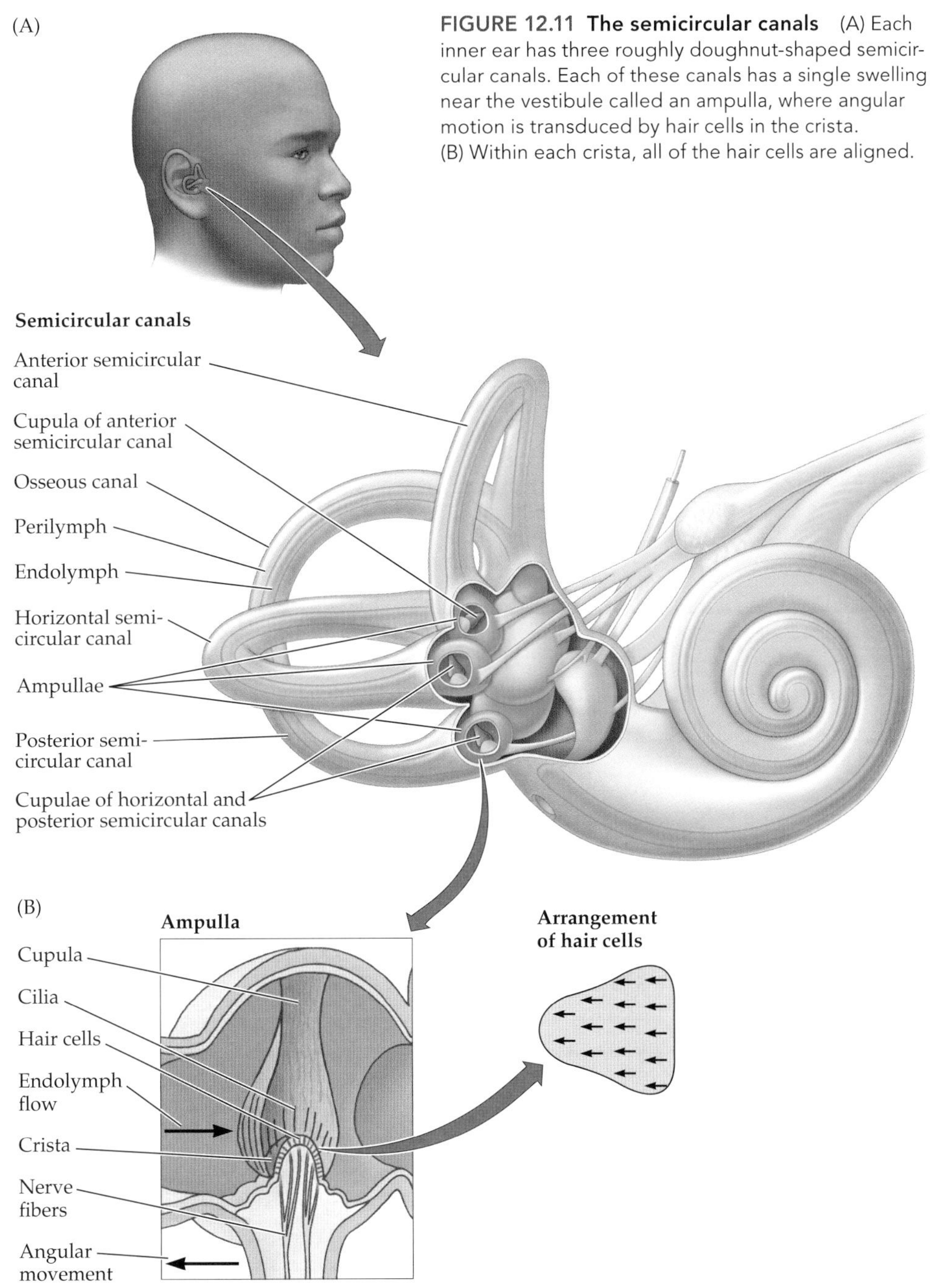

FIGURE 12.11 The semicircular canals (A) Each inner ear has three roughly doughnut-shaped semicircular canals. Each of these canals has a single swelling near the vestibule called an ampulla, where angular motion is transduced by hair cells in the crista. (B) Within each crista, all of the hair cells are aligned.

(see Figure 12.11). Thus, rotations in one direction yield increases in the receptor potential of all hair cells in that semicircular canal, as well as increases in the action potential rate for all neurons that innervate that semicircular canal. Rotations in the opposite direction yield decreases in the hair cell receptor potentials and decreases in the rate of action potentials.

The three semicircular canals are maximally sensitive to rotations in different planes, thus yielding direction coding for head rotation. Specifically, each canal is maximally sensitive to rotations about the axis perpendicular to it and is insensitive

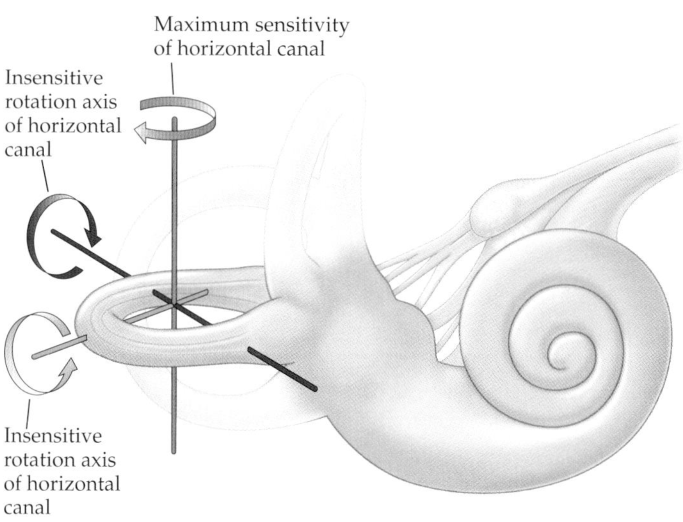

FIGURE 12.12 Maximal sensitivity of the semicircular canals Each semicircular canal is maximally sensitive to rotations perpendicular to the canal plane. Thinking of each semicircular canal as a wheel, we can see that the canals are maximally sensitive to rotations that align with the rotation axis (green) and are insensitive to rotations that fall in the plane of the semicircular canal (e.g., red and blue).

to rotations about axes that fall in its plane (**FIGURE 12.12**). Think of each canal as a wheel that can spin about the axle. The canal is maximally sensitive to rotations that match the normal rotation of a wheel and insensitive to rotations in other planes.

HOW AMPLITUDE IS CODED IN THE SEMICIRCULAR CANALS In the absence of any rotation, many afferent neurons from the semicircular canals respond with a nearly constant rate of action potentials (see Figure 12.10A); canal afferent firing rates at rest average nearly 100 action potentials ("spikes") per second (Goldberg and Fernandez, 1971), a rate that is high relative to spontaneous rates for nerve fibers for other sensory systems. For comparison, recall from Chapter 2 that retinal ganglion cells fire spontaneously at a rate of about one spike per second in the dark.

The relatively high spontaneous firing rate of vestibular afferent neurons allows these neurons to decrease the firing rate for rotations in one direction and increase the firing rate for rotations in the opposite direction. In addition, the semicircular canals are organized as functional pairs in what is called a push-pull arrangement. The two horizontal canals—one on the right side of the head and one on the left—lie roughly in the same plane and form one of the three functional canal pairs (**FIGURES 12.13A** and **12.13B**) (Curthoys, Blanks, and Markham, 1977; Wilson and Melvill Jones, 1979). The horizontal-canal afferent neurons on the right all increase their firing rate for yaw head turns to the right (shaking "no"), while those on the left decrease their firing rate. For head turns to the left, the pattern is reversed, with left-canal afferent neurons increasing their firing rate and right-canal neurons decreasing their firing rate. The anterior and posterior canals are minimally sensitive to these yaw rotations.

In contrast to the horizontal-canal arrangement, the mirror symmetry of the semicircular canals in the left and right ears yields functional pairs that involve different vertical canals (**FIGURE 12.13C**); the maximum-sensitivity axis of the anterior semicircular canal on one side roughly parallels the maximum-sensitivity axis of the posterior semicircular canal on the opposite side. So the right anterior and left posterior canals form one canal pair, as do the left anterior and right posterior canals. These canal pairs work in a push-pull manner like that previously described for the horizontal canals.

The change in the firing rate is larger for large changes in the angular velocity of the head than for small changes (Goldberg and Fernandez, 1971). Since the change in the firing rate is proportional to angular velocity, we can think of the

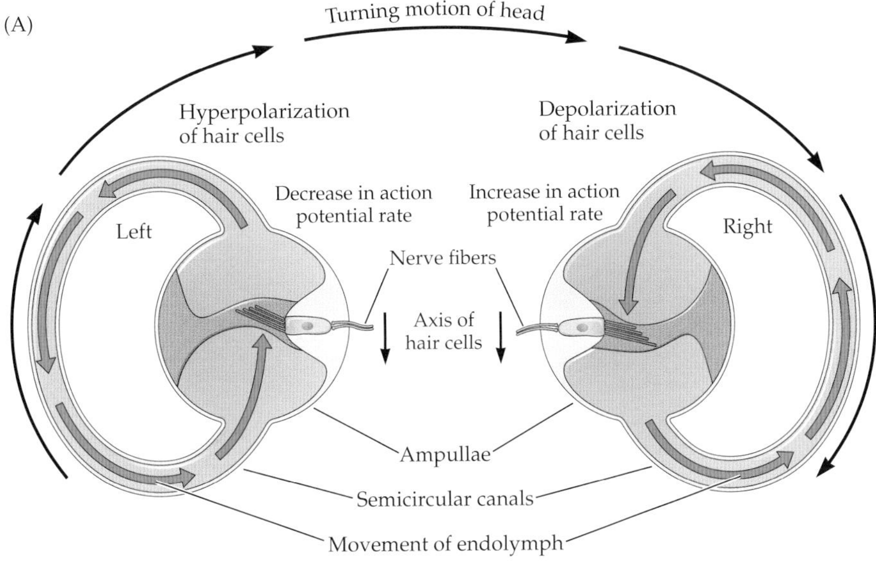

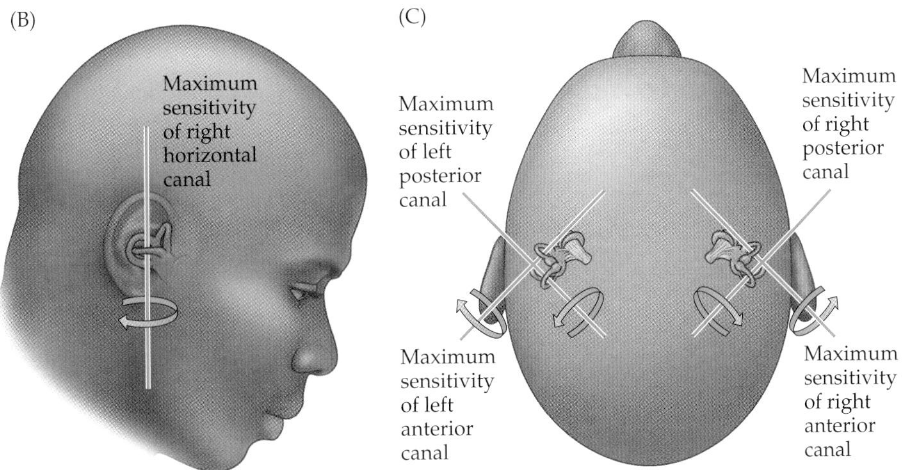

FIGURE 12.13 Push-pull relationship of the semicircular canals The semicircular canals function in pairs that have a push-pull relationship. (A) Bilateral stimulation of the horizontal semicircular canals as the head turns to the right (a yaw head rotation as shown in Figures 12.7E and 12.7F). This yaw rotation produces relative movement of the endolymph in the horizontal semicircular canals on both sides of the head. The movement of the fluid bends the hair cell bundles toward the tallest stereocilia on the right side, which depolarizes these hair cells and increases the rate of action potentials for neurons from the right side. The hair cell bundles move away from the tallest stereocilia on the left, hyperpolarizing the hair cells and decreasing the rate of action potentials for left-side neurons. This response—an increase on one side coupled with a decrease on the other side—is often called a push-pull response. The two horizontal canals form one push-pull pair. (B) The axis of maximum sensitivity for the right horizontal canal. (C) The right anterior canal and the left posterior canal form another pair. Note that the maximum-sensitivity axes for the right anterior and left posterior canals are parallel. This means that they maximally respond to rotations around the same axis. The push-pull nature of this canal pair is a consequence of the opposite directions of their maximum-sensitivity rotations, as shown by the green arrows.

canals as somewhat similar to the speedometer in a car, with the change in neural activity proportional to the angular velocity of the head. As a specific example, if the afferent neurons from a horizontal canal suddenly change their firing rate, we know that the rotation includes a change in the velocity component aligned with the sensitive axis of that horizontal canal. The same is true for the other canals.

HOW DIRECTION IS CODED IN THE SEMICIRCULAR CANALS As previously discussed, the three semicircular canals in each ear are maximally sensitive to rotations in different planes; the result is direction coding of head rotations. Specifically, the head can rotate about any arbitrary rotation axis made up of roll, pitch, and yaw rotational velocity components. Each canal transduces the component of head velocity perpendicular to its plane. The brain then combines these signals to sense the rotation direction of the head movement.

SEMICIRCULAR-CANAL DYNAMICS If you suddenly begin to rotate at a constant velocity, the semicircular canals sensitive to that rotation will respond by causing a sudden change in afferent neural activity. But as the rotation continues at a constant velocity, the afferent neural activity will decay back to near zero after about

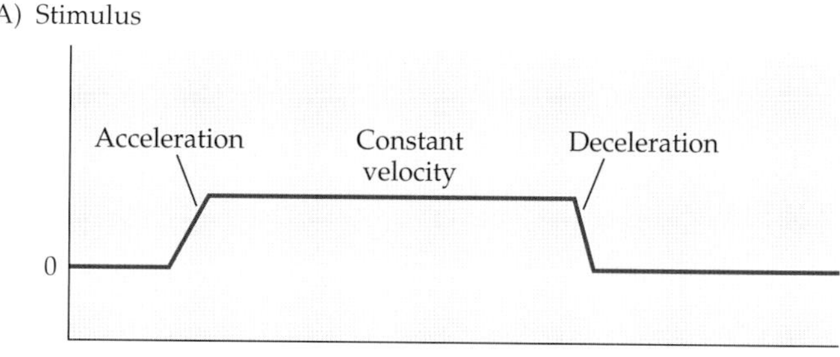

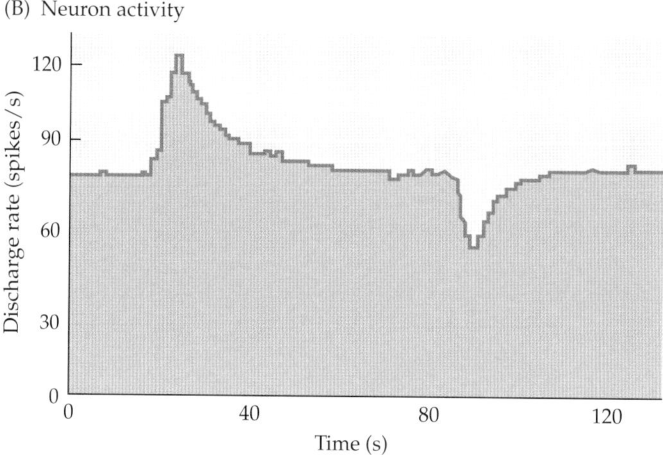

FIGURE 12.14 Response of a semicircular-canal neuron to constant-velocity rotation (A) The stimulus is a rotation that first accelerates to a constant angular velocity, then maintains that velocity, and then decelerates the head to a stop. (B) During the initial acceleration, the cupula deflects, causing the neuron activity to increase. During the constant angular velocity, the cupula returns to its nondeflected position, so the neuron activity returns to the baseline rate after about 15 seconds of constant-velocity rotation. During deceleration, the cupula is deflected in the opposite direction, causing a transient decrease in the firing rate.

oscillatory Referring to back-and-forth movement that has a constant rhythm.

sinusoidal Referring to any oscillation, such as a sound wave or rotational motion, whose waveform is that of a sine curve. The period of a sinusoidal oscillation is the time that it takes for one full back-and-forth cycle of the motion to occur. The frequency of a sinusoidal oscillation is defined as the numeral 1 divided by the period.

15 seconds. If you then suddenly decelerate to a stop, the canals will show a large response in the opposite direction (**FIGURE 12.14**). The afferent neural activity will then decay with a time course similar to that during the constant-velocity rotation (Goldberg and Fernandez, 1971).

What happens for **oscillatory** back-and-forth movement when you shake your head "no"? (If you don't have a solid understanding of frequency analysis, now may be a good time to review "Fourier analysis" in Section 3.1.) **FIGURE 12.15A** shows a **sinusoidal** motion trajectory at a frequency of 0.05 hertz (Hz)—a repeating back-and-forth motion that takes 20 seconds to complete (like slowly shaking your head). **FIGURE 12.15B** shows the oscillatory neural response in an afferent neuron evoked by that sinusoidal motion (Fernandez and Goldberg, 1971). The firing rate increases and decreases as the angular velocity of the head increases or decreases; that is, the change in firing rate has the same frequency as the head velocity. We can calculate an estimate of afferent neuron sensitivity by taking the peak-to-peak amplitude of the change in the firing rate (from Figure 12.15B) and dividing it by the peak-to-peak velocity (from Figure 12.15A). The maximum firing rate is about 170 spikes/second; the minimum is about 10 spikes per second. So the peak-to-peak amplitude of the change in the firing rate is about 160 spikes/second. The peak-to-peak amplitude of the change in motion is 160 degrees/second (80 degrees/second to the left and 80 degrees/second to the right). The result is a sensitivity of about 1 spike/second per degree/second of motion. Experimentally, this process is often repeated at several different head rotation frequencies, yielding a number representing the neural sensitivity at each frequency tested.

Semicircular canals are not equally sensitive to all frequencies of rotation. **FIGURE 12.15C** shows a plot of response sensitivity as frequency is varied for a typical neuron innervating a semicircular canal; this plot indicates how the magnitude of the canal afferent firing rate changes with head rotation frequency. The data show that the amplitude of the canal afferent neuron's response is nearly constant for

(A)

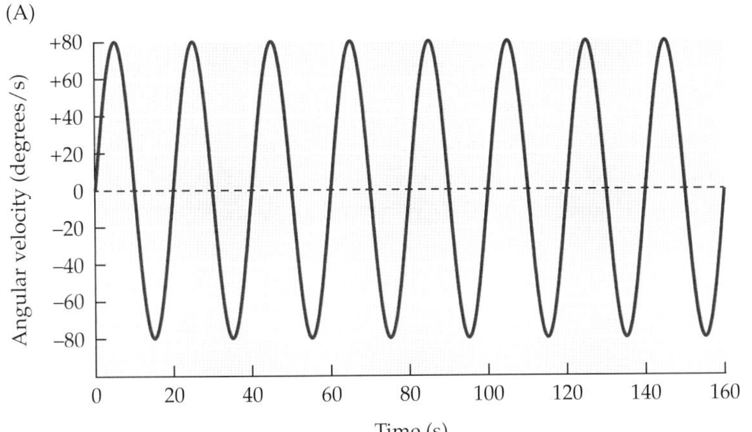

(B)

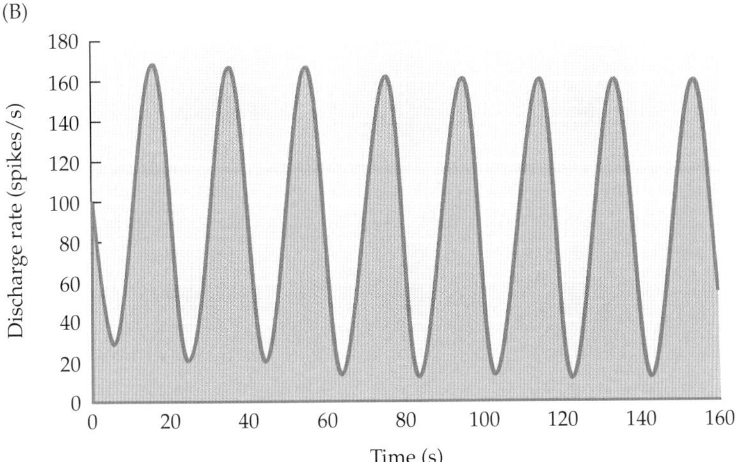

(C)

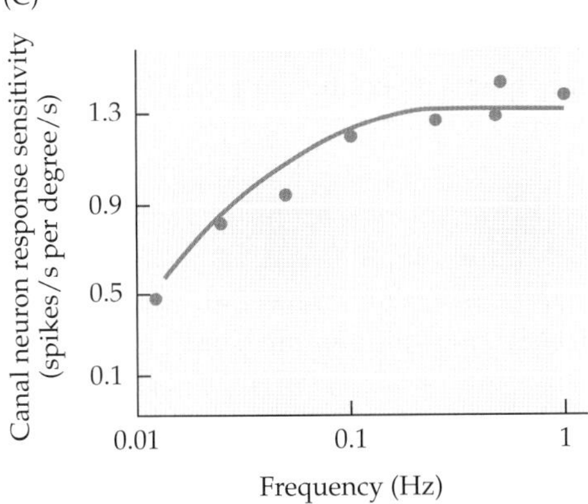

FIGURE 12.15 Sinusoidal motion trajectories Stimulus (A) and response (B) for a single semicircular-canal afferent neuron at 0.05 Hz. Note that the neural firing rate increases and decreases nearly in tandem with the oscillating stimulus. (C) Repeating the sensitivity calculation at different stimulus frequencies shows that the sensitivity of the neuron changes with frequency. For this semicircular-canal neuron, the response sensitivity averaged about 1.3 spikes/second per degree/second for frequencies above 0.1 Hz. The response sensitivity decreases substantially for frequencies below about 0.1 Hz.

rotation frequencies above about 0.1 Hz. But when the frequency is less than about 0.1 Hz, the neuron responds less and less. For example, the response sensitivity at a frequency of 0.02 Hz (one cycle in 50 seconds) is only about 0.5 spike/second per degree/second—more than a 50% reduction from that observed at 1 Hz (one cycle in 1 second).

WHY SINE WAVE MOTIONS? Now that we have described canal afferent responses to sinusoidal motion in some detail, you may wonder why anyone would care. We rarely experience perfect sinusoidal motion in the real world; we experience

Fourier analysis A mathematical procedure by which any signal—in this case, motion trajectories as a function of time—can be separated into component sine waves at different frequencies. Combining these sine waves will reproduce the original motion trajectory.

utricle One of the two otolith organs. A saclike structure that contains the utricular macula. Also called *utriculus*.

saccule One of the two otolith organs. A saclike structure that contains the saccular macula. Also called *sacculus*.

macula Any of the specialized detectors of linear acceleration and gravity found in each otolith organ.

otoconia Tiny calcium carbonate stones in the ear that provide inertial mass for the otolith organs, enabling them to sense gravity and linear acceleration.

complex motions that vary with time. What do responses to sinusoidal motion at different frequencies tell us about how we sense motion?

One answer is that, although "pure" sine wave motions may be rare in the real world, patterns of oscillatory motions that have a predominant frequency are quite common: think again of shaking your head to say "no" or nodding your head to say "yes." More generally, **Fourier analysis** tells us that any complex motion can be broken down into some number of single-frequency components. Therefore, if we know responses to single frequencies, we know a good deal about responses to more complex motion.

FURTHER DISCUSSION of Fourier analysis in vision can be found in Section 3.1.

Otolith Organs

As we mentioned earlier, the sensing of gravity and linear acceleration relies on two structures in each ear called the otolith organs: the **utricle** (or utriculus) and the **saccule** (or sacculus). Each of these organs consists of a small, oval-shaped, fluid-filled sac that is about 3 mm long in the longest direction and includes an area called the **macula** (plural *maculae*), which is where actual sensory transduction occurs (**FIGURE 12.16A**). Each human utricular macula contains about 30,000 hair cells; each saccular macula has about 16,000. The utricular and saccular maculae are innervated by about 4000 neurons each. Each macula is roughly planar and is primarily sensitive to shear forces—forces parallel to the macular plane. Perpendicular forces have little influence on neural response. Small movements caused by parallel shear forces, the result of gravity and/or linear acceleration, deflect the hair cells and produce changes in the firing rate of afferent neurons.

The cilia of the otolith hair cells are encased in a gelatinous structure (**FIGURE 12.16B**) that contains calcium carbonate crystals called **otoconia** (singular *otoconium*) (**FIGURE 12.16C**). There are literally millions of these otoconia in the utricle and saccule. These small stones give the otolith organs their name: *oto* means "ear," and *lithos* means "stone" in Greek, so *otolith* translates as "ear stone." The otoconia are denser than the surrounding fluid. Like any dense object, they are pulled by both gravitational force and inertial force as a result of linear acceleration. The resulting displacement of the otoconia drags the gelatinous layer, thereby moving the hair cell stereocilia, leading to changes in the hair cell receptor potential, which in turn cause changes in the rate of action potentials in the afferent neurons.

HOW AMPLITUDE IS CODED IN THE OTOLITH ORGANS As in the semicircular canals, one aspect of amplitude coding in the otolith organs can be found in the response of a single neuron or single hair cell. Recall that (1) hair cell receptor potentials increase when hair bundle tips move toward the largest stereocilia, (2) receptor potentials decrease for movements in the opposite direction (see Figure 12.10A), and (3) the direction of rotation is coded by excitation from a semicircular canal on one side and inhibition from the other side.

Similar mechanisms are at work in each otolith organ macula. Populations of hair cells on each macula have their stereocilia oriented in opposite directions (see Figure 12.16A). Both the utricle and the saccule include a central band called the striola (plural *striolae*). On opposite sides of the striola, hair cells are oriented in opposite directions. Remember that movement toward the tallest stereocilia excites the hair cells, and movement in the opposite direction inhibits the hair cells. Since the neuronal response arises from synapses to the hair cells, tilts

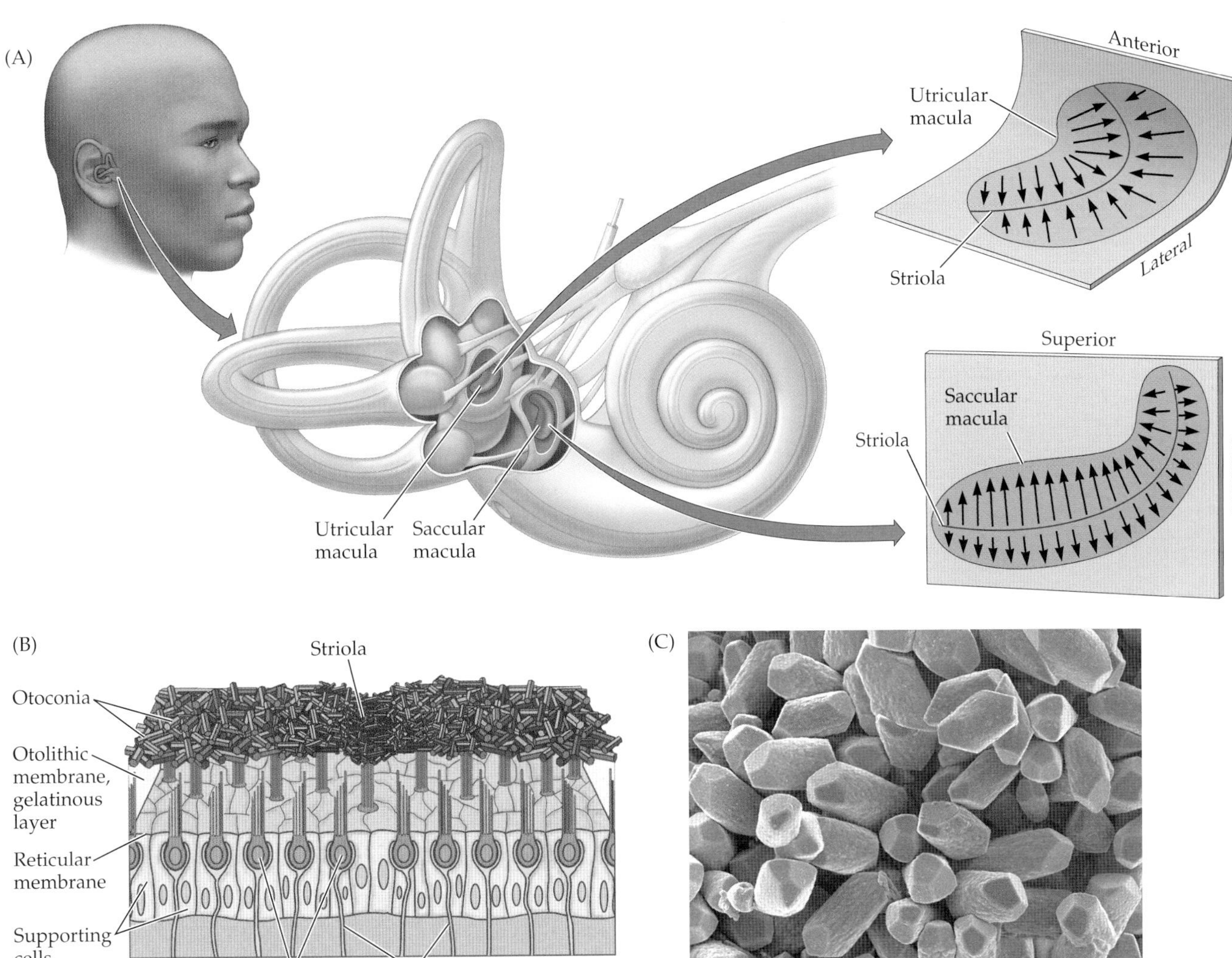

FIGURE 12.16 The otolith organs (A) Orientation of the utricular and saccular maculae in the head. The saccules are oriented more or less vertically; the utricles are more or less horizontal. The striola is a structural landmark that divides each otolith organ. The tallest stereocilia point toward the striola in the utricular macula and away from it in the saccular macula, as the arrows indicate. Because hair cells depolarize if they deflect toward the tallest stereocilia and hyperpolarize if they deflect away from them, the arrows also show the movement direction that causes maximal neural excitation at each location on the maculae. Note that, given one utricle and one saccule on each side of the head, there is a continuous representation of all directions for sensing gravity and linear acceleration. (B) Cross section of the macula of an otolith organ. Hair bundles project into a gelatinous layer. (C) The otoconia shown in this scanning electron micrograph (3000×) come from the utricular macula of a cat. Crystals are between 0.5 and 10 micrometers long.

(or linear accelerations) in opposite directions cause opposite changes in firing rate (**FIGURE 12.17**) (Goldberg and Fernandez, 1976). So a tilt or an acceleration that maximally excites a hair cell and afferent neuron near the striola on one side will maximally inhibit a hair cell and afferent neuron near the striola on the opposite side.

Larger accelerations (or larger gravitational shear forces) move the otolith organs' otoconia more. This movement, in turn, leads to greater deflection of the hair cell bundles, which causes larger changes in the hair cell receptor potentials. The receptor potential evoked in a given hair cell is proportional to the component

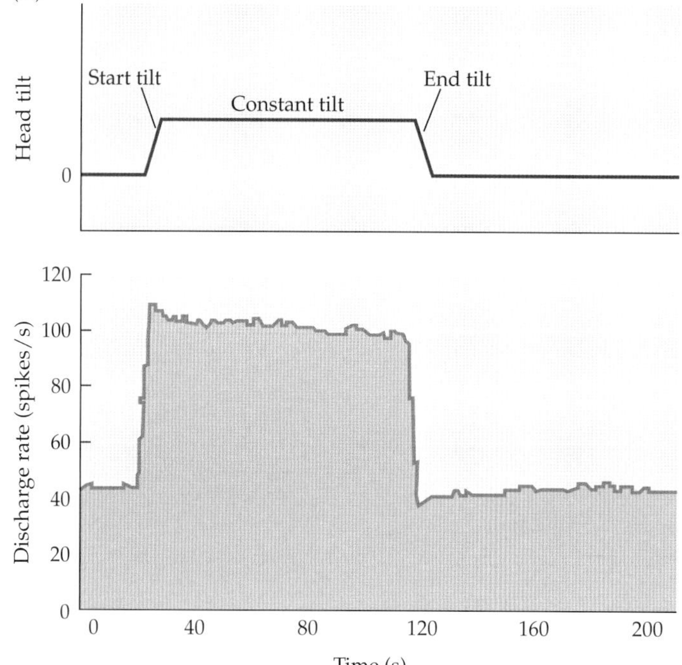

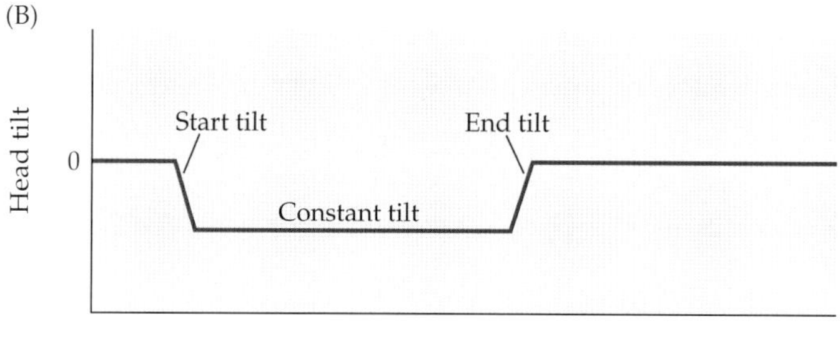

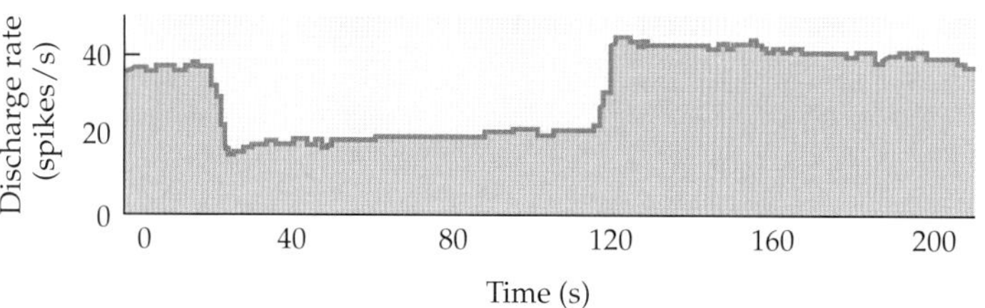

FIGURE 12.17 Activity of a vestibular neuron innervating the utricle (an otolith organ) (A) A change in head tilt is the stimulus (top). As shown in the histogram of the discharge rate (bottom), the neuron's activity increases in response to tilt in a particular direction. (B) The same neuron decreases its activity in response to tilt in the opposite direction.

of gravity or linear acceleration that is aligned with the sensitive axis of that hair cell. Larger changes in the hair cell receptor potential lead to larger changes in the rate of action potentials sent to the brain via afferent neurons.

HOW DIRECTION IS CODED IN THE OTOLITH ORGANS Direction coding in the otolith organs arises, in part, from their anatomical orientation. The plane of the utricular macula is horizontal; the plane of the saccular macula is vertical (see Figure 12.16A). The maculae are exquisitely sensitive to gravity and linear acceleration in the plane of the macula and insensitive to gravity and acceleration perpendicular to the macula. Therefore, with the head near upright, the utricle will be sensitive primarily to any Earth-horizontal linear acceleration, while the saccule will be sensitive to any Earth-vertical linear acceleration as well as forward/backward Earth-horizonal linear acceleration. (Note that both the utricle and the saccule sense forward/backward Earth-horizontal linear acceleration.)

The other component of direction coding arises from variations in the orientation of the hair cells (Figure 12.16A, far right). Different hair cells respond maximally to different movement directions, with the direction of maximal sensitivity varying systematically across the plane of each macula. For example, hair cells in one region of the utricular macula will be maximally sensitive to forward-backward acceleration, while cells in another region will be maximally sensitive to side-to-side linear acceleration. In between, cells will maximally respond to linear acceleration that has both forward-backward and side-to-side components.

12.5 Spatial Orientation Perception

Long after it was known that we see with our eyes and hear with our ears, the primary source for our perception of spatial orientation remained a mystery. In fact, in the eighteenth century, gross fluid shifts in the head were accepted as an explanation for the source of our sense of spatial orientation. Once it was established that this sense degrades when the vestibular system is damaged, it became clear that the vestibular system provides crucial information regarding spatial orientation. For example, when patients with vestibular loss are moved in the dark, they have a much more difficult time correctly perceiving their motion than do people with normal vestibular function.

Today, three different techniques are frequently used to investigate spatial orientation perception: thresholds, magnitude estimation, and matching. For a vestibular threshold study, a helpful question is, What is the minimum motion (the threshold) required to correctly perceive the direction we just moved? Note that this is different from simply reporting *whether* we've moved, since vibration can provide a motion cue without informing us about the direction of the motion. The vestibular system tells us more than whether motion is present; it actually informs us of the direction of motion—for example, whether we moved to the left or to the right.

In a magnitude estimation study, participants might be asked to give verbal reports of how much they tilted, rotated, or translated, using physical units like the number of degrees they rotated. Alternatively, magnitude estimation may utilize arbitrary scaling. For example, participants may be trained to rotate a knob in proportion to their perceived velocity or provide a verbal indicator of their velocity on a scale of 1 to 10.

In a matching task, participants might be asked to align a visual line with perceived Earth-vertical (Which way is "down"?). In such a task, called the subjective visual vertical task, the investigator could produce a vestibular stimulus by tilting the participant. That participant would be provided with a visible line in otherwise dark surroundings and with the ability to rotate the line to the perceived Earth-vertical. Alternatively, haptic sensation, which you will learn more about in Chapter 13, could be utilized instead of vision. For this technique, participants might be asked to use their sense of limb position to align a bar that they hold—but cannot see—with perceived vertical.

FURTHER DISCUSSION of similar matching tasks in connection with the sense of touch can be found in Section 13.3.

Rotation Perception

If you are spun on a barstool in the dark at a nearly constant velocity, you will initially perceive an angular velocity that is roughly the same as the actual rotation. However, if the constant-velocity rotation lasts more than a second or two, you will perceive that you are slowing down (**FIGURE 12.18**). If the constant-velocity rotation continues for more than 30 seconds or so, you will perceive that you are no longer rotating.

This description may remind you of the way the response of the semicircular canals decays during constant-velocity rotation (see Figure 12.14), and it is another example of how the vestibular system is attuned to *changes* in motion. Interestingly, though, the time course of the perceptual decay is more gradual than that of the semicircular-canal signal sent to the brain. This effect is sometimes called **velocity storage**

velocity storage Prolongation of a rotational response by the brain beyond the duration of the rotational signal provided to the brain by the semicircular canals, typically yielding responses that are nearer the actual rotational motion than the signal provided by the canals.

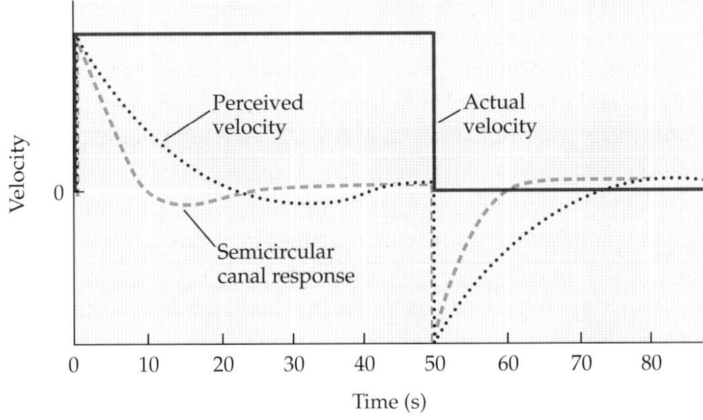

FIGURE 12.18 Time course of angular velocity perception The solid red line on this graph shows the angular velocity of a person who began at rest with eyes closed, was suddenly rotated at a constant speed for 50 seconds, and then was abruptly returned to rest. Initially, the participant's estimate of angular velocity was accurate (dotted purple line at time 0), but then the perceived velocity dropped to near 0 after nearly 30 seconds. When stopped, the participant perceived an abrupt velocity in the opposite direction, which mimicked the initial perception but in the opposite direction. For comparison, we show a representation of the canal response in the dashed blue line, similar to that shown in Figure 12.14. Note the faster return to baseline for the canal response.

dizziness A commonly used lay term that nonspecifically indicates any form of perceived spatial disorientation, with or without instability.

imbalance Lack of balance; unsteadiness; nearly falling over.

mathematical integration Computing an integral—one of the two main operations in calculus (the other, the inverse operation, is differentiation). Velocity is the integral of acceleration. Change of position is the integral of velocity.

because the perception of rotation persists after the afferent signal from the semicircular canals has dissipated. The velocity storage phenomenon is interesting and important because it shows that the brain has improved on the incoming sensory information to yield a rotation perception that—while far from perfect—is closer to the actual rotation than if the perception simply followed the time course of the semicircular-canal afferent signal (Bertolini et al., 2011).

Later, if you are abruptly brought to a stop following extended rotation, you will perceive an angular velocity opposite the one you experienced while rotating (see Figure 12.18). This rotation illusion is one that many of us played with as children when we would spin ourselves for a while and then suddenly stop spinning and try to stand or walk. (And some amusement park junkies still play with this illusion, as you'll see at the end of this chapter!) The **dizziness** and **imbalance** that we experienced when we stopped rotating were the result of an illusion of self-rotation caused by the semicircular-canal response. (You can view examples of this by searching YouTube for "people spinning and falling.")

One can develop an intuitive understanding of the reason for this illusion by considering the analogy of riding in a car. When you're riding at a constant velocity, you and the car are moving together. But when the car suddenly stops, you are thrown forward because you have momentum and keep moving even though the car has stopped. When you're rotating at a constant velocity, there is little or no hair cell deflection, because the endolymph and cupula are moving together. When the rotation is suddenly halted, however, the cupula stops moving quickly but the endolymph has momentum and tends to keep moving. The hair cells are therefore deflected, and the direction of the hair cell response is opposite the one measured when the constant-velocity rotation began.

How sensitive are we to rotation? Direction recognition thresholds for yaw rotation have been measured for rotational motion frequencies ranging from 0.05 Hz (one back-and-forth cycle of yaw acceleration in 20 seconds) to 5 Hz (five back-and-forth cycles of yaw acceleration in 1 second). For frequencies above 1 Hz (one back-and-forth acceleration cycle in 1 second), direction recognition thresholds are roughly constant; your head has to be moving at a speed of just a little below 1 degree per second, which at 5 Hz corresponds to a head angular displacement of just 0.1 degree or just 0.02 of a minute on a clockface! Clearly, we are very sensitive to rotation. For frequencies below 0.5 Hz (one back-and-forth oscillation in 2 seconds), thresholds increase with decreasing frequency (**FIGURE 12.19**) (Grabherr et al, 2008). The important point here is to recognize that rotation thresholds vary as the frequency of the angular acceleration stimulus varies. (Recall that hearing thresholds also changed with frequency [see Figure 9.22], though the causes of the variations with frequency are different for the two modalities.)

Translation Perception

When participants are passively translated short distances while seated in a chair in the dark and then asked, while still seated in the chair, to use a joystick to actively move the chair to reproduce the distance that they had been passively translated, they do so accurately. But even though not asked to do so, they also reproduce the *velocity* of the passive-motion trajectory (Berthoz et al., 1995). The unrequested replication of velocity suggests that the brain remembers and replicates the velocity trajectory. Earlier, we said that the otolith organs transduce linear acceleration, which is the change in linear velocity. Therefore, replication of the velocity trajectory means that the brain also seems to **mathematically integrate** the acceleration signal provided by the otolith organs to yield a perception of linear velocity. This apparent calculation suggests that while otolith organs sense linear acceleration, our brains turn this information into a perception of linear velocity.

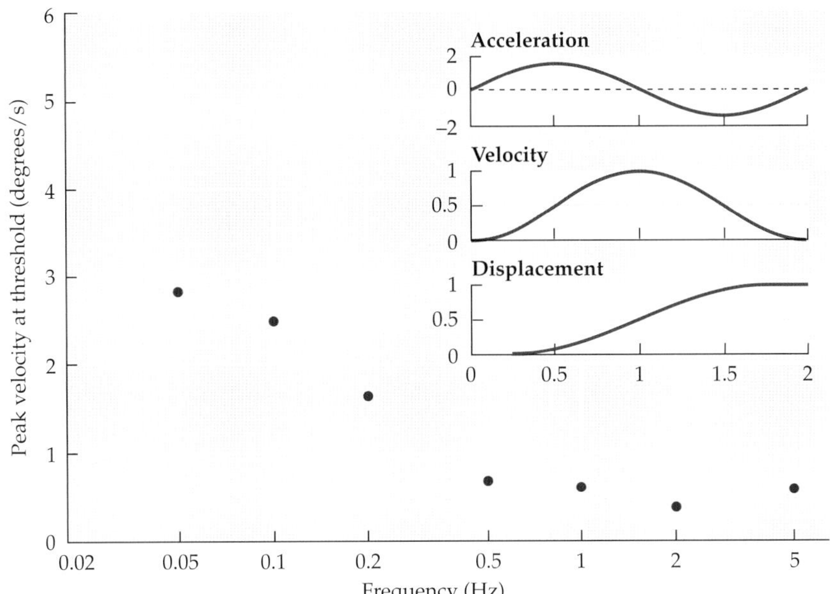

FIGURE 12.19 Mean velocity threshold (across N = 7 participants) at each of seven frequencies The angular velocity threshold was the peak angular velocity achieved during a single cycle of sinusoidal acceleration at which participants correctly recognized the direction of motion most of the time. The inset shows the angular acceleration, angular velocity, and angular displacement for a single cycle of sinusoidal acceleration at 0.5 Hz. For the example shown, the peak magnitude of the acceleration is 1.57 degrees/second^2, the peak velocity is 1 degree/second, and the peak displacement is 1 degree.

As for yaw rotation, direction recognition thresholds for side-to-side (y-axis) translation have been measured for motion frequencies ranging from 0.05 Hz (one back-and-forth cycle of acceleration in 20 seconds) to 5 Hz (five back-and-forth cycles of acceleration in 1 second). For frequencies above 1 Hz (one back-and-forth cycle in 1 second), direction recognition thresholds are roughly constant. To sense translation direction correctly, your head has to be moving at least at a speed of 5.0 mm per second, which at 5 Hz corresponds to a head angular displacement of just 0.5 mm! Clearly, we are also very sensitive to translation. As for yaw rotation, for frequencies below 0.5 Hz (one back-and-forth oscillation in 2 seconds), thresholds increase with decreasing frequency (Valko et al., 2012).

Tilt Perception

How well do we perceive our tilt when we are slanted away from true Earth-vertical? For tilt angles less than 90 degrees—that is, body orientations between standing up (0 degrees) and lying down (90 degrees)—we are pretty good, according to a variety of magnitude estimation techniques. Observers produce reliable and consistent answers if they indicate their perceived tilt verbally or if they align a handheld probe with perceived vertical (**FIGURE 12.20**) (Bortolami et al., 2006).

We are not perfect, though. Some consistent errors appear, especially in the subjective visual vertical task described near the beginning of Section 12.5. Back in 1861, Hermann Rudolf Aubert found that when he roll-tilted his head to the left or right while looking at a vertical streak of light, the vertical line appeared to tilt in the direction opposite his head tilt. For tilt angles less than 90 degrees, the illusory tilt error is typically about 10 degrees, but the apparent tilt of the visual line can be as large as 45 degrees when the head is tilted 135 degrees. You can investigate this illusion in a completely dark room by leaving the door open just a crack—just enough to see a line of light in the doorway without illuminating the room at all—while you hold your head in a tilted position. Does the line appear to tilt when your head is tilted? Does it move in the direction of your tilted head or in the opposite direction?

Thresholds for recognizing the direction of tilt show that healthy, asymptomatic individuals correctly report the direction of a static tilt when tilted about 1 degree off vertical in the dark. This sensitivity serves our ability to stand upright, because

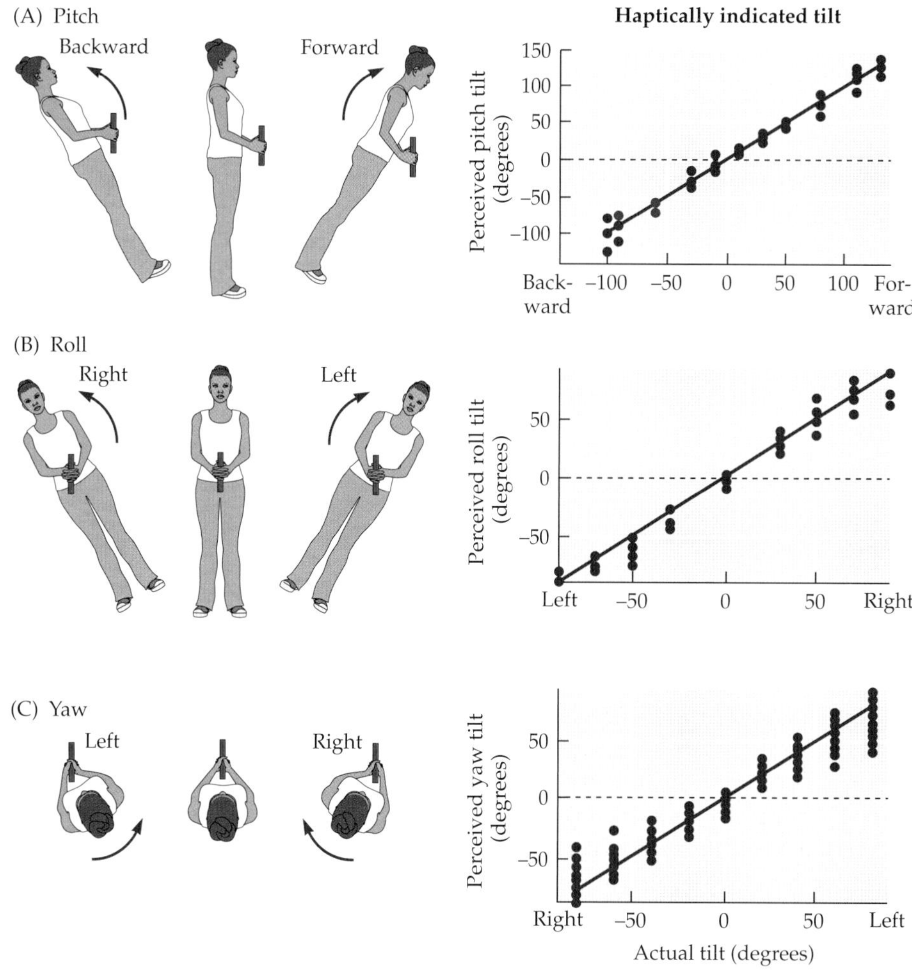

FIGURE 12.20 Tilt perception Participants are generally pretty good at indicating how much they are tilted. Data points show tilt perception provided by participants using a handheld haptic indicator (shown schematically at left) for static pitch (A), roll (B), and yaw (C) tilts. Perceived tilt roughly reflects the actual tilt (solid lines) for all three tilt directions.

the farther we are tilted from upright, the more difficult standing up is. For example, the amount of muscular effort required to maintain posture roughly doubles if we are tilted 2 degrees instead of 1 degree, so just imagine the effort of trying to stand tilted 20 degrees away from upright!

Spatial Orientation Cognition

Spatial orientation cognition and spatial navigation are important skills for any living creature. Without accurately remembering where food or water sources are and how to get there, our ancestors—both human and animal—probably would not have survived!

There are many different types of cells within the brain whose responses work together to aid in spatial orientation cognition, including place cells and head direction cells. These cells are in the hippocampus, which is vital for memory storage and retrieval. Place cells show increased firing when a living creature is in a specific location in the environment. Head direction cells display increased firing when the head is facing a specific range of directions. The brain is able to use these firing patterns to help create a cognitive map of the environment. In animals where we can make direct recordings of neural activity, removing or damaging the vestibular system leads to place cells and head direction cells no longer displaying location- or direction-specific changes in activity (Taube, 2007). Imaging of the brain in humans with vestibular dysfunction has revealed decreased volume of the hippocampus

(Brandt et al., 2005), suggesting that hippocampal structures, including place cells and head direction cells, may degrade when vestibular sensation degenerates. As described below, these anatomical changes are also accompanied by spatial cognition and spatial navigation behavioral changes.

Spatial Cognition

Spatial cognition is a broad term to describe how the brain organizes and understands three-dimensional space, including spatial memory and mental rotation. Spatial memory is our ability to be able to recall multiple facets of the environment, such as relative distance, size, and orientation. Mental rotation is the ability to manipulate and rotate two-dimensional or three-dimensional visual representations of objects in the mind.

One of the first studies to assess spatial memory in humans with vestibular dysfunction used the virtual Morris water maze task. For this test, participants sat at a computer and used a controller to "swim" around in a virtual tank of water to find a specific goal location. In general, after completing the task several times, people are able to find the goal more quickly and use a more direct path, demonstrating a memory of platform location. In comparison to age- and gender-matched healthy adults, ten patients with vestibular loss showed worse performance (Brandt et al., 2005). Of note, these changes in performance were seen even though the patients were stationary at the computer and the vestibular system was not sensing motion!

Similarly, mental rotation is a spatial cognitive task linked to vestibular function. This is true even when mental rotation is assessed while stationary and the vestibular system is not stimulated. To assess mental rotation ability, people are asked to judge if two similar objects are identical or mirror images of each other. These objects may be hands, blocks, or any other two- or three-dimensional image. Adults with vestibular disorders have been found to show more errors and take longer on mental rotation tasks in comparison to healthy adults (Grabherr et al., 2011). As a whole, these studies suggest that our ability to accurately perceive and remember spatial cues is reliant on a healthy vestibular system.

Spatial Navigation

Spatial navigation refers to the ability to move throughout the environment and is also linked to vestibular function. Navigation is typically assessed by asking subjects to move toward memorized targets or along memorized paths while blindfolded, thus not being able to see the environment. This is something we regularly do, such as when getting up in the middle of the night to get a glass of water. While most healthy adults can safely and accurately perform this task, in adults with vestibular loss, clear decrements in spatial navigation are seen. When asked to walk along a memorized path when blindfolded, older adults (Xie et al., 2017) and individuals with vestibular dysfunction (Glasauer et al., 2002) take longer to complete the task and make more errors.

Nonspatial Cognition

While vestibular function is important particularly for skills reliant on understanding how we or other objects are oriented in space, vestibular input also has been associated with aspects of nonspatial cognition (Bigelow and Agrawal, 2015; Bosmans et al., 2021). Those who have worked with patients with vestibular disorders have not been surprised by these findings because reports of "brain fog" and changes in memory are very common complaints in the clinic. Associations between vestibular loss and general cognition are most commonly seen for nonspatial memory, such

multisensory integration The process of combining different sensory signals. Typically, combining several signals yields more accurate and/or more precise information than can be obtained from individual sensory signals. This is *different from* the mathematical process of integration learned in calculus (e.g., the integral of acceleration is velocity).

vection An illusory sense of self-motion caused by moving visual cues when one is not, in fact, actually moving.

as remembering a list of words, or executive function, such as our ability to plan ahead and follow multiple-step directions.

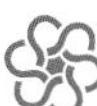

12.6 Multisensory Integration

The senses do not operate independently. Instead, the brain combines signals from different sensory systems via neural processes of **multisensory integration**. For example, visual cues influence sound localization—an effect used by ventriloquists. Vestibular signals combine with information from numerous sensory systems to provide us with an understanding of the position and movements of the head and body.

FURTHER DISCUSSION of a remarkable example of multisensory integration—the McGurk effect on speech perception—can be found in Section 11.2.

Visual-Vestibular Multisensory Integration

Most of us have experienced illusions of self-motion caused by moving visual cues. Perhaps you've perceived self-motion while watching an IMAX movie. Or perhaps you've felt as if you were moving backward when you were stationary but the car (or train or bus) next to you began to move forward. Or perhaps you felt unsteady when standing on a bridge looking at the water flowing beneath. All of these situations can lead to perceptions of illusory self-motion called **vection**. Vection can be very compelling. For example, drivers stopped in traffic often press harder on the brake pedal when they perceive that they and their stationary car are moving, even when it is the cars around them that are moving.

To consider how vection contributes to spatial orientation, imagine a person standing upright while viewing the inside of a sphere rotating about an Earth-horizontal axis (**FIGURE 12.21A**). At first, subjective perceptions match reality; humans initially perceive that they are stationary and that the sphere is rotating. But if they continue to observe the rotating visual display for 10 seconds or so, they usually begin to perceive that they're rotating in the direction opposite the sphere rotation (**FIGURE 12.21B**). This illusory rotational vection demonstrates the crucial contributions of vision to our sense of self-rotation. In fact, signals related to vision converge with the semicircular-canal signals in the vestibular nuclei, which is the first place in the brain that vestibular information reaches.

Paradoxically, individuals experiencing such rotational vection almost never report that they are tumbling head over heels as they would if they truly were rotating to the extent that they perceive. In fact, individuals typically experience a simultaneous illusory sensation of tilt that gradually builds up to a relatively constant level (**FIGURE 12.21C**). These perceptions—experienced as a sensation of motion without getting anywhere—are contradictory, since we cannot be rotating relative to gravity (as suggested by the visual cues) while also maintaining a constant orientation with respect to gravity (as indicated by the otolith organs). In addition to exemplifying multisensory integration, this sensation of motion without getting anywhere demonstrates that spatial orientation perception is not constrained to combinations of motion and orientation that are physically possible.

In this example, the role played by the vestibular system is to put the brakes on visually induced vection. Individuals suffering from severe vestibular damage generally report greater vection than do individuals with healthy vestibular function. Astronauts experiencing rotational vection in space—in the absence of gravitational

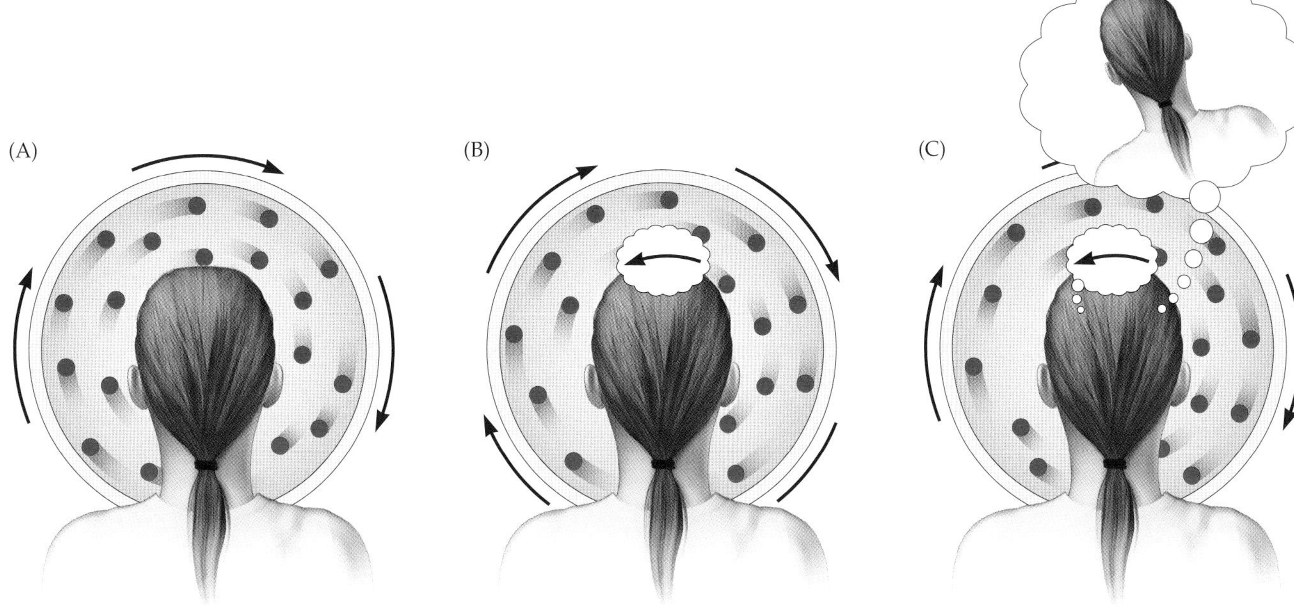

FIGURE 12.21 **Rotational vection** An individual views a visual display rotating in roll. For demonstration purposes, the visual display is shown here as transparent. (A) Initially, the individual correctly senses that she is stationary and the visual display is rotating. (B) The individual begins to perceive vection, a sense of self-rotation in the direction opposite the rotation of the visual display. (C) Roll vection is often accompanied by an illusion of roll tilt that is induced by the perceived roll rotation. The direction of the perceived tilt is consistent with the tilt direction that would occur if the individual were truly rotating in roll.

signals—report a head-over-heels tumbling sensation that is absent on Earth. These findings are explained by the fact that neither the individuals with vestibular damage nor the astronauts receive normal gravitational cues from the otolith organs to contradict their visual rotational cues. Since illusory motion is greater when there are no otolith cues to contradict the visual cues, we can infer that, under normal circumstances, information from the vestibular system is combined with visual information to yield a "consensus" about our sense of spatial orientation ●

Vestibulo-interoceptive Multisensory Integration

As introduced in Chapter 1 and described in more detail later (Section 13.2), interoception refers to sensory information arising from the internal organs. There is evidence that interoceptive signals arising from our cardiovascular system (i.e., the heart and blood vessels) and possibly the digestive system (i.e., the stomach) contribute to spatial orientation. An interesting example of this comes from a study described by Carriot and colleagues (2011), who utilized bending one's legs as a manipulation to displace blood toward one's head and clearly showed that this manipulation of interoceptive cues influenced perceived self-tilt.

FURTHER DISCUSSION of interoception can be found in Section 13.2.

This suggests that interoceptive signals interact with the vestibular system to help inform us where our body is relative to gravity. This has potentially important implications for flight and space flight, where exposure to different gravitational environments can impact the function of internal organs and the interoceptive

sensory reafference Change in afference caused by self-generated activity. For the vestibular system, vestibular afference evoked by an active self-generated head motion would yield sensory reafference.

sensory exafference Change in afference caused by external stimuli. For the vestibular system, vestibular afference evoked by passive head motion would yield sensory exafference.

efference copy A neural copy of an efferent command sent from the central nervous system to the periphery. One example pertinent to spatial orientation is a copy of the efferent command sent to muscles; this muscle efferent copy transmits information about expected motion resulting from the anticipated muscle activation.

signals arising from them. Indeed, in both of these environments becoming spatially disoriented is relatively common and can have fatal consequences. This example also highlights an opportunity to contribute to our understanding of something as fundamental as graviception (see Section 12.2), since much remains to be learned about how sensory information from the vestibular system is combined with interoceptive cues.

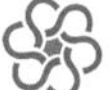

12.7 Beyond Multisensory Integration: Active Sensing

Our sensory systems are simultaneously activated as the result of our own actions and changes in the external world. Indeed, most of our sensory experiences are gained by active exploration of the world resulting from locomotion, eye movements, touching, and other interactive activities. Our brain's ability to distinguish sensory events that are self-generated, sometimes called **sensory reafference**, from those that arise externally, sometimes called **sensory exafference**, is essential for perceptual stability and accurate motor control. For example, when our eyes move, the image of the world moves across our retinas, yet we do not perceive the image of the world as moving.

To avoid responding to sensory inputs that arise from self-generated actions, the sensory system needs to know what the motor system has done. Based on their observations, Von Holst and Mittelstaedt (1950) proposed the principle of reafference. In today's version of this principle (FIGURE 12.22A), a copy of motor commands, called an **efference copy**, is generated to help the brain predict the expected sensory results of motor commands. This predicted sensory activity is called sensory reafference, and the brain's estimate of sensory reafference is subtracted from the sensory afferent signal to eliminate reafferent information. In certain model systems, including the electrosensory systems of electric fish, self-generated sensory information is selectively suppressed at the level of afferent fibers.

Signals from the vestibular afferent neurons do not distinguish between active and passive head movements; vestibular afferent neurons respond identically to self-generated and externally applied self-motion (FIGURES 12.22B and 12.22C). But differential processing of vestibular signals is evident at the next stage of processing in the vestibular nuclei. The modulation of some vestibular nuclei neurons, which receive direct inputs from the vestibular afferents, is dramatically attenuated in response to vestibular inputs that result from self-generated movements (Cullen, 2011). The dramatic difference between the responses of these vestibular nuclei neurons demonstrates a clear example of active sensing, since this brain signal directly depends on whether the motion is self-generated (active) or not (passive). We emphasize that this distinction between self-generated neural activity and externally generated neural activity arises at the first central synapse in the vestibular nuclei for those vestibular pathways that contribute to balance and perception. This shows that this distinction occurs very early in the processing of some vestibular information, which suggests that the ability to distinguish between self-generated and externally generated neural activity is fundamental ●

12.8 Reflexive Vestibular Responses

As mentioned earlier, some crucial contributions of the vestibular system are automatic, or reflexive, doing their work outside conscious awareness. For example, there is a set of automatic responses called vestibulo-ocular reflexes—VORs for short. We started the chapter with one of these. Remember looking at your finger

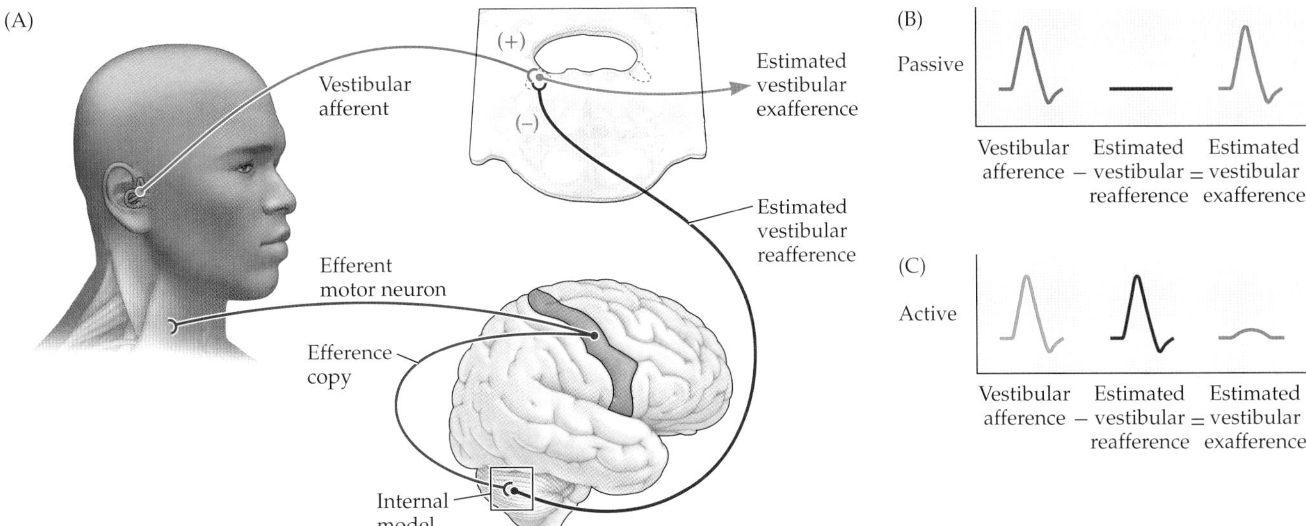

FIGURE 12.22 Simplified representation of the active vestibular sensing network (A) When a command is sent to the neck muscle to rotate the head via efferent motor neurons, a copy of those motor command signals—called an efference copy—is sent in parallel to the brain. This signal is processed by a neural network, called an internal model, that predicts the expected vestibular afference resulting from the self-generated motion, which is called estimated vestibular reafference. This estimated reafference is subtracted from the signals from the vestibular afferent neurons to yield estimated vestibular exafference, the component of the afferent signal that is not caused by self-generated motion. (B) When the head undergoes passive rotation, the head rotation is accurately encoded by the vestibular afference (blue). No neck motor command is generated during passive rotation, so the passive expected vestibular reafference signal is flat, corresponding to no self-generated motion. The difference between these is the estimated vestibular exafference, which, for passive motion, is identical to the vestibular afferent signal. (C) When the head is actively rotated, the head rotation is accurately encoded by the vestibular afference. In this case, a neck motor command is generated to evoke the head rotation, so a motor command is sent to the neck muscles, and a copy is sent to an internal model that predicts the vestibular afference anticipated for the active head rotation being generated. For some vestibular nuclei neurons, the difference between the vestibular afference and the estimated reafference yields estimated exafference, which is nearly flat.

as you shook your head? (If not, now might be a good time to go back and try this demonstration again; see Figure 12.1.) This task illustrates how the VOR contributes to visual stability by counterrotating the eyes in the head during head motion sensed by the vestibular system.

There is also a set of vestibulo-autonomic reflexes that contribute to autonomic responses like those that regulate blood pressure and help maintain adequate blood flow to the brain. Other vestibulo-autonomic reflexes lead to motion sickness. Finally, vestibulospinal reflexes contribute to postural control via the **balance system**. To demonstrate vestibular contributions to balance, try standing on one foot with your eyes closed. (When you start to feel unsteady, immediately open your eyes and put both feet on the ground!) Most people with a healthy balance system—including healthy vestibular function—can do this for at least 5 seconds and often much longer. Patients without vestibular function, however, cannot stand on one foot in the dark for more than an instant.

balance system The sensory systems, neural processes, and muscles that contribute to postural control. Specific components include the vestibular organs, kinesthesis, vestibulospinal pathways, skeletal bones, and postural control muscles. Because of the vestibular system's crucial contributions to balance, some even informally refer to the vestibular system as the "balance system" and the vestibular organs as the "balance organs." But the balance system is much more than just the vestibular system, and the vestibular system contributes to much more than just balance.

Vestibulo-ocular Responses

The angular VOR, the eye rotation that helps compensate for angular rotations of the head, is a robust reflex. In fact, this reflex is so robust that it is a standard part of clinical examinations of vestibular function. Furthermore, the VOR is certainly among the best-studied reflexes, dating as far back as the late 1700s with reports by William Charles Wells (1792).

The angular VOR is the compensatory eye rotation evoked by the semicircular canals when they sense head rotation. For example, when the head rotates (yaws) to the left, the reflex pathways cause the eyes to rotate to the right with respect to the head, to compensate—at least in part—for the head turn. When observing the eyes, we see this eye rotation as movement of the pupils to the right. Of course, since the eyeball is roughly a spherical ball, it is really rotating in the eye socket, not moving laterally.

Recall that six ocular muscles—called oculomotor muscles—rotate the eyeball (see Figure 8.16). Muscles can only pull; they cannot push. Muscles are paired to pull in opposite directions and are therefore called agonist-antagonist muscle pairs. For example, moving the left eye horizontally requires a coordination of the lateral rectus that pulls the eye to the left and the medial rectus that pulls the eye to the right. To make an eye movement to the right, the lateral rectus is inhibited and thus relaxes its pull, while the medial rectus is excited and thus increases its pull. The six oculomotor muscles are organized in three pairs that rotate the eye in each of three directions. Eye movements result from a coordinated inhibition and excitation of the eye muscles.

When the VOR is working effectively, it actively rotates the eyes in the head such that the rotation of the eyes roughly compensates for the rotation of the head in space. **FIGURE 12.23** demonstrates this with a simple example. In Figure 12.23A, the eyes rotate with the head; they do not counterrotate in the head. In Figure 12.23B, the eyes counterrotate in the head, which helps stabilize the visual field on the retina. If the eyes do not counterrotate in the head, the retinal image tends to blur during head rotation. (Remember how your fingers blurred when you rapidly moved them back and forth?) The counterrotation of the eye in the head helps reduce this blur by reducing the motion of the image of an object

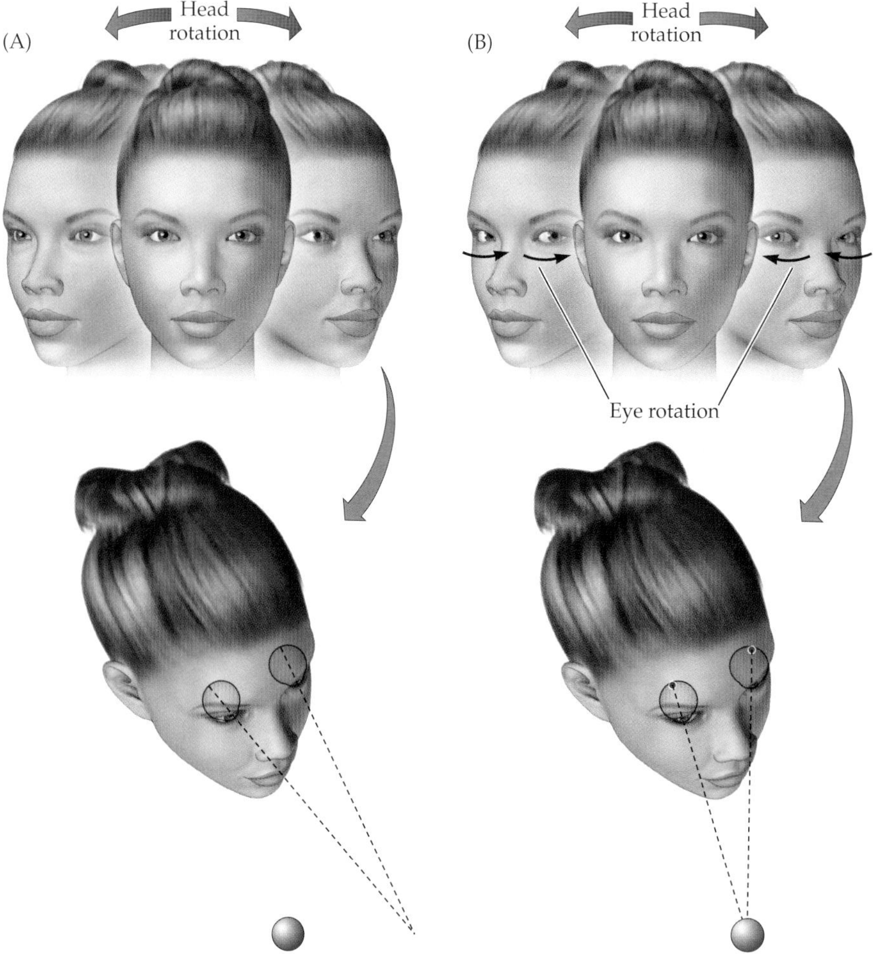

FIGURE 12.23 Contribution of the angular vestibulo-ocular reflex (VOR) to visual stability (A) When the eyes do not counterrotate, the image of the object moves across the retina during head rotation, causing blurred vision. (B) When the eyes counterrotate during head rotation—with the amount of eye rotation roughly equal to the amount of head rotation—the image of an object can remain stationary on the retina even during head rotation. Because the eyes counterrotate in the head in (B) but not in (A), they continue to look at you in (B) but not in (A). This effect demonstrates how the angular VOR contributes to visual acuity, by helping to keep object images stationary on the retina, thereby reducing blurring.

across the retina. Note that because of eye counterrotation, the actual rotation of the eyes with respect to the external world is much less than that of the head.

The most direct neural path for the VORs consists of an arc of three neurons that yields reflexive eye responses with a latency of less than 10 milliseconds between the start of head motion and the eye movement. (That is really fast. Try doing anything else in less than 10 milliseconds!) The first neurons in the arc are the afferent neurons (shown in blue on the bottom right in **FIGURE 12.24**); these neurons transmit information from the vestibular organs to the vestibular nuclei. There, the afferent neurons synapse on interneurons (shown in green). The interneurons synapse on efferent oculomotor neurons (shown in red) in the ocular motor nuclei. These oculomotor neurons synapse with the oculomotor muscles to rotate the eyes with respect to the head.

As you rotate your head from side to side, the angular VOR has properties similar to the characteristics that were discussed earlier for the semicircular canals, as illustrated in **FIGURES 12.25** and **12.26**. The VOR demonstrates a constant, relatively high amplitude at high frequencies, but it gets smaller and smaller as the

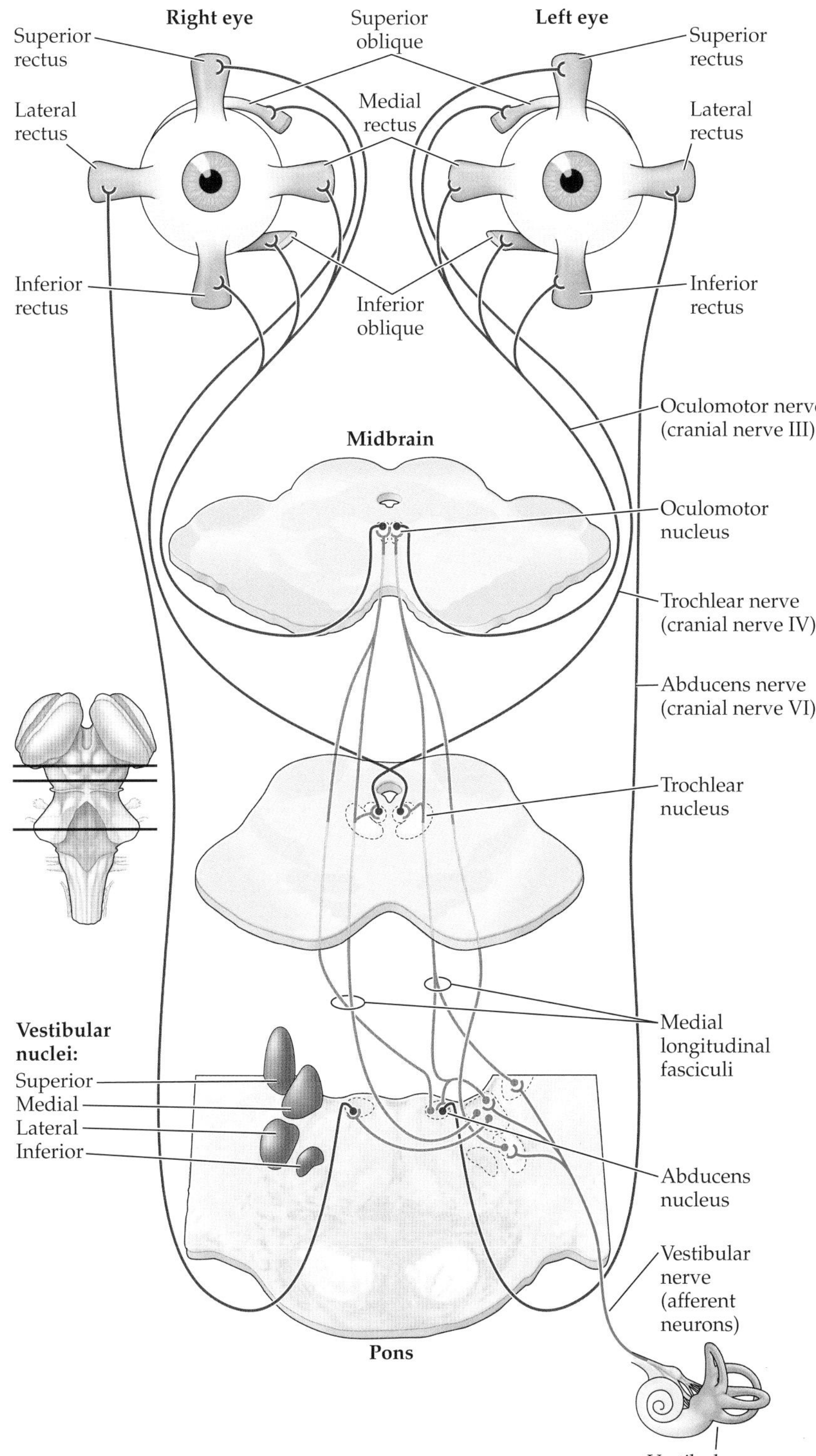

FIGURE 12.24 Neural pathways for the three-neuron arc of the angular vestibulo-ocular reflex While the circuitry may appear complex, the primary point here is that a sequence of just three neurons (blue to green to red) convey rotation information from the semicircular canals to the oculomotor muscles! Each type of neuron is depicted using a different color. Each of the vestibular afferent neurons (blue)—one branch for each of the three canals—projects to one of three vestibular nuclei: superior, medial, or lateral. Neurons that connect afferent to efferent neurons, called interneurons (green), project from the vestibular nuclei to the three ocular motor nuclei: abducens, trochlear, and oculomotor. (Only the oculomotor nucleus, which is one of the three ocular motor nuclei, is shown.) The six efferent oculomotor neurons (red) project from these three ocular motor nuclei to the six oculomotor muscles: inferior oblique, superior oblique, inferior rectus, superior rectus, lateral rectus, and medial rectus. Recall that you previously were introduced to the oculomotor muscles in Figure 8.16. The inset on the left indicates the location of each of the three brainstem slices shown.

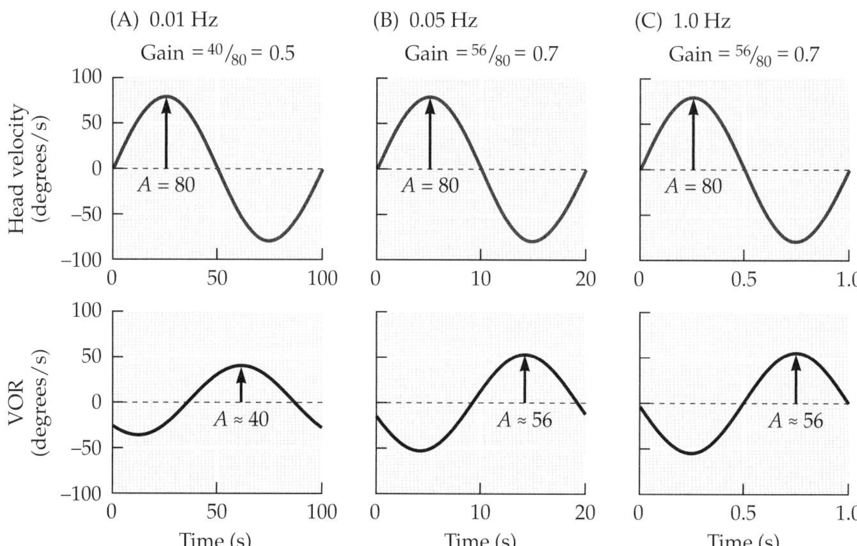

FIGURE 12.25 Vestibulo-ocular reflex (VOR) responses in the dark at three frequencies The stimulus (sinusoidal head rotation; top row) is shown for (A) 0.01 Hz, (B) 0.05 Hz, and (C) 1.0 Hz. Sinusoidal motion evokes an oscillatory VOR (bottom row), which opposes the head rotation such that head rotations to the right are accompanied by eye rotations to the left. If the VOR were perfect, it would have the same peak amplitude (labeled *A* in the figure) as the head rotation, meaning that the eye rotated at the same velocity as the head rotation. However, the peak compensatory eye velocity shown for 0.05 and 1.0 Hz in the dark is about 70% of the peak head velocity. We would say that this has a gain of about 0.7, where gain is a dimensionless ratio of the eye velocity divided by the head velocity. A gain of 0 would indicate that the eyes did not rotate with respect to the head, as in Figure 12.23A. A gain of 1 would indicate that the eyes were counterrotating with the same amplitude as the head motion, as suggested by Figure 12.23B. The remaining 30% is usually made up by visual contributions. At lower frequencies, the VOR is smaller; for example, at 0.01 Hz it is only about 50% of the peak head velocity (a gain of about 0.5).

frequency drops below about 0.05 Hz (see Figure 12.25). Though the frequency characteristics of the VOR and canal afferents are qualitatively similar, there is an interesting difference. As Figure 12.26 shows, the response of canal afferent neurons declines for frequencies below 0.2 Hz. In comparison, the VOR declines for frequencies below 0.05 Hz.

That difference is interesting because it means that, in some sense, the VOR response is more accurate than a simple reading of its input signal would provide. This effect is analogous to what we saw earlier for rotation perception (see Figure 12.18) and is called velocity storage. It shows that the brain is not simply a relay station that passes sensory information to the muscles that yield the reflexive action. Instead, the brain helps shape the reflexes to be as effective as possible, given the available sensory information. In this specific case, central processing increases the effective VOR frequency range (Raphan, Matsuo, and Cohen, 1977; Robinson, 1977; Merfeld et al., 1993).

We also have a translational VOR that is evoked when the otolith organs sense head translation, especially high-frequency head translation. This translational VOR helps us keep our eyes pointed at an object when the head translates in one direction or the other.

Vestibulo-autonomic Responses

The vestibular system also makes contributions to responses of the **autonomic nervous system**. Perhaps the most vivid of these responses is motion sickness, a vestibulo-autonomic ordeal that many of us wish we had never experienced. Severe symptoms of motion sickness include nausea and vomiting. Motion sickness typically results when there is a disagreement between the motion and orientation signals provided by the semicircular canals, otolith organs, and vision (Reason and Brand, 1975; Oman, 1990). For example, if you are below deck on a boat, your vestibular system will accurately record the motion of the boat while vision suggests no relative motion of the world, since you and the boat are moving together.

autonomic nervous system The part of the nervous system that is responsible for regulating many involuntary actions and that innervates glands, heart, digestive system, etc.

What is this response good for? One of several hypotheses is that it is a defense against some classes of poisons (Treisman, 1977). If you have been poisoned, you want to get rid of the poison before it gets rid of you. But how do you know if

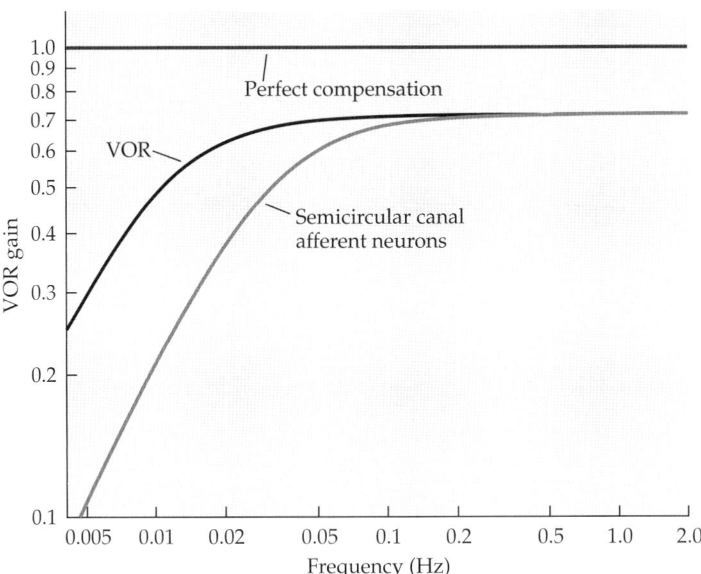

FIGURE 12.26 Vestibulo-ocular reflex (VOR) dynamics Dynamics of the VOR (black curve) are such that the response has a nearly constant gain—roughly a gain of 0.7—at frequencies between about 0.05 and 2.0 Hz. VOR gain is defined as the amplitude of the response ("VOR") divided by the amplitude of the stimulus, as shown in Figure 12.25. In fact, while not shown in this figure, the VOR gain remains nearly constant for frequencies up to 25–30 Hz (Huterer and Cullen, 2002; R. Ramachandran and Lisberger, 2005). Perfect compensation—having a gain of 1—is shown in red. See Figure 12.25 for examples of how this gain is calculated at each frequency. Below 0.05 Hz, the gain of the VOR decreases. For comparison, the normalized frequency response of semicircular-canal neurons that we saw in Figure 12.15 is indicated by the green curve. Since the green curve represents the information provided to the brain and the black line represents the VOR response at different frequencies, the difference between the black and green curves represents neural compensation performed by the brain. Data are plotted on a logarithmic scale along the *y*-axis.

you have been poisoned? If the poison is a neurotoxin, disruption of the sensory systems is a good hint. How do you know that your senses have been disrupted? One way is to check whether senses that normally agree with one another have stopped doing so. Normally, if you move, your visual system and your vestibular system both register that fact. If the vestibular system says one thing and the visual system says another, the brain may decide that it is time to rid the body of a possible cause of the disagreement. This response could be a lifesaver if you just ate a bad mushroom. It is less desirable when you have to pull out the motion sickness bag during turbulence at 35,000 feet.

Other vestibulo-autonomic responses are less familiar and generally take the form of compensatory contributions (Yates, Bolton, and Macefield, 2014). For example, consider the problem of regulating blood pressure. The heart pumps blood throughout the body, but maintaining oxygenation of the brain via blood flow is especially critical because you will black out in just a few seconds if your brain does not receive adequate oxygen. Gravity pulls blood downward, so in the normal upright posture your heart has to work to maintain blood flow to the brain. When you're lying down, it takes much less work to pump blood to the brain. Now suppose you rapidly stand up. The cardiovascular system has to suddenly change the regulation of blood flow to maintain adequate oxygen supply to the brain. If these mechanisms fail, you will experience light-headedness or, in extreme cases, blackout. By informing the relevant parts of the autonomic nervous system about

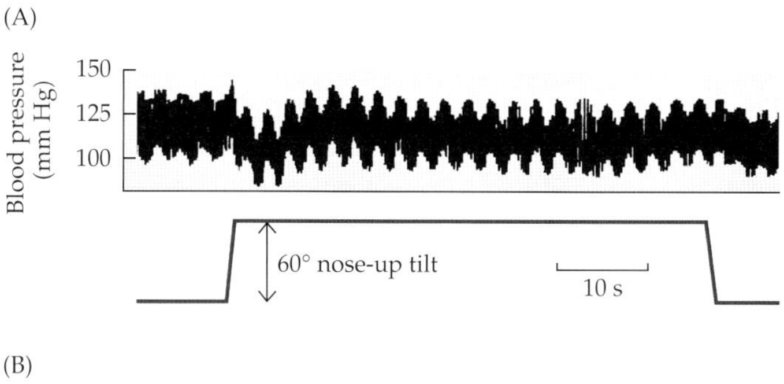

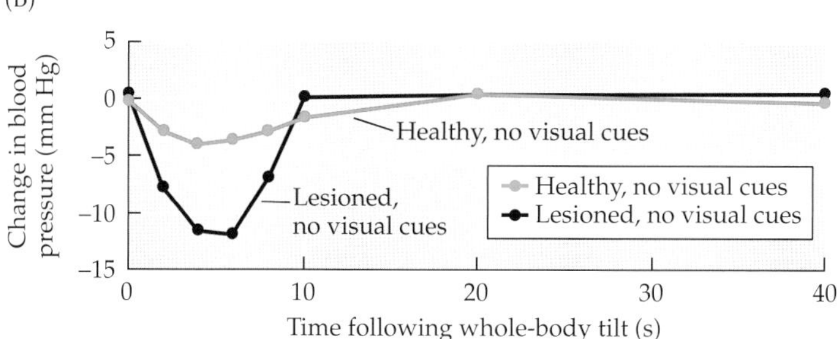

FIGURE 12.27 Vestibular influences on blood pressure (A) The trace represents blood pressure in the head versus time in response to a nose-up tilt in an animal with a lesioned vestibular system. In the absence of vestibular contributions, a transient decrease in blood pressure can be observed immediately after the tilt. (B) Change in blood pressure is much greater for the animal without a functional vestibular system (lesioned) than for the animal with a healthy vestibular system, demonstrating that the vestibular system helps maintain more constant blood pressure during whole-body tilts.

the position and motion of the head, the vestibular system contributes to the regulation of blood flow to the brain. As a result, one consequence of destructive lesions of the vestibular organs is that blood pressure regulation during whole-body tilts becomes much less stable (**FIGURE 12.27**) (Yates and Miller, 1998).

Vestibulospinal Responses

In the early 1800s, the French physiologist Jean Pierre Flourens reported abnormal head movements in pigeons after he had cut individual semicircular canals. The head movements he reported were in the plane of the lesioned canal. These studies demonstrated the presence of what we today consider to be the vestibular influences on posture control, and they initiated the formal study of vestibular influences on balance.

Vestibular reflexes keep us from falling over. Without vestibulospinal reflexes, our balance (**FIGURE 12.28**) would be severely degraded. We would be unable to stand in the dark. Part of the reason is that when we stand, we are inherently unstable. As two-legged creatures, we can be thought of as being composed of a series of inverted pendulums—pendulums in which the mass is above the pivot point. A pencil or broom balanced on your palm demonstrates a simple inverted pendulum. Such challenging tasks can be mastered with practice, but imagine trying to stabilize a series of at least four brooms or pencils on top of one another. At its essence, this is the task faced by our balance system, which works to keep the head, torso, thighs, and calves—each an inverted pendulum—upright with respect to gravity.

A thorough discussion of the dynamics of the entire posture control system is beyond the scope of this book. To study the postural system experimentally, investigators have simplified the dynamics by strapping the head and body to a rigid board that converts the complex multijoint body into a single inverted pendulum pitching forward and backward about the ankle joint (**FIGURE 12.29**). When the foot plate that the participant stands on is gently rocked forward and backward while the participant's eyes are closed, healthy, asymptomatic participants demonstrate body

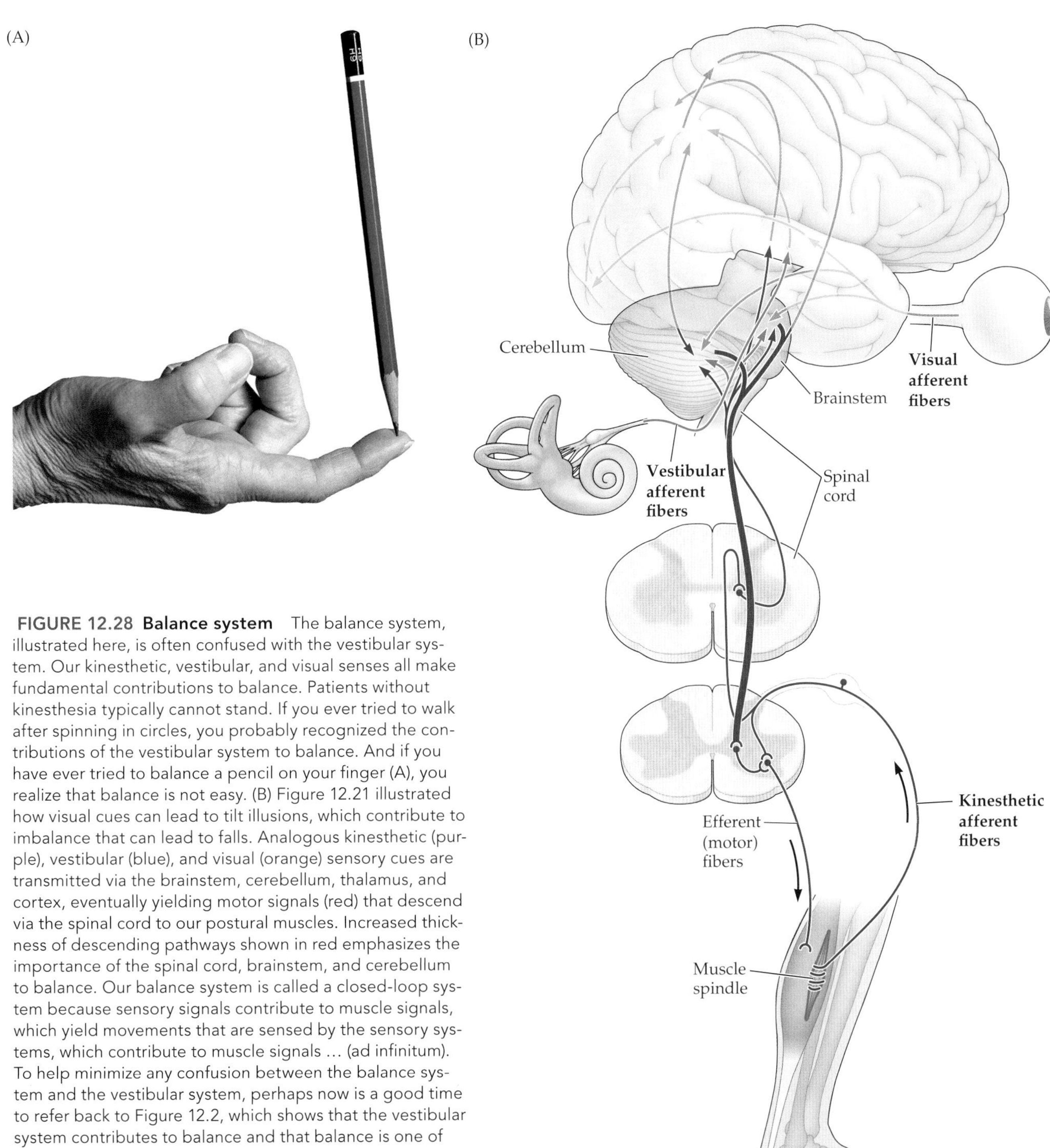

FIGURE 12.28 **Balance system** The balance system, illustrated here, is often confused with the vestibular system. Our kinesthetic, vestibular, and visual senses all make fundamental contributions to balance. Patients without kinesthesia typically cannot stand. If you ever tried to walk after spinning in circles, you probably recognized the contributions of the vestibular system to balance. And if you have ever tried to balance a pencil on your finger (A), you realize that balance is not easy. (B) Figure 12.21 illustrated how visual cues can lead to tilt illusions, which contribute to imbalance that can lead to falls. Analogous kinesthetic (purple), vestibular (blue), and visual (orange) sensory cues are transmitted via the brainstem, cerebellum, thalamus, and cortex, eventually yielding motor signals (red) that descend via the spinal cord to our postural muscles. Increased thickness of descending pathways shown in red emphasizes the importance of the spinal cord, brainstem, and cerebellum to balance. Our balance system is called a closed-loop system because sensory signals contribute to muscle signals, which yield movements that are sensed by the sensory systems, which contribute to muscle signals ... (ad infinitum). To help minimize any confusion between the balance system and the vestibular system, perhaps now is a good time to refer back to Figure 12.2, which shows that the vestibular system contributes to balance and that balance is one of four fundamental contributions of the vestibular system. ●

sway between 0.1 and 1 Hz that is about the same as the applied rocking movement (Peterka, 2002); this is shown in Figure 12.29A as an amplitude ratio of about 1, which means that body tilt relative to gravity is about the same as the platform tilt. In contrast, patients with severe vestibular loss demonstrate body sway that exceeds the amplitude of the disturbance by a factor of 5 or so (shown in Figure 12.29A

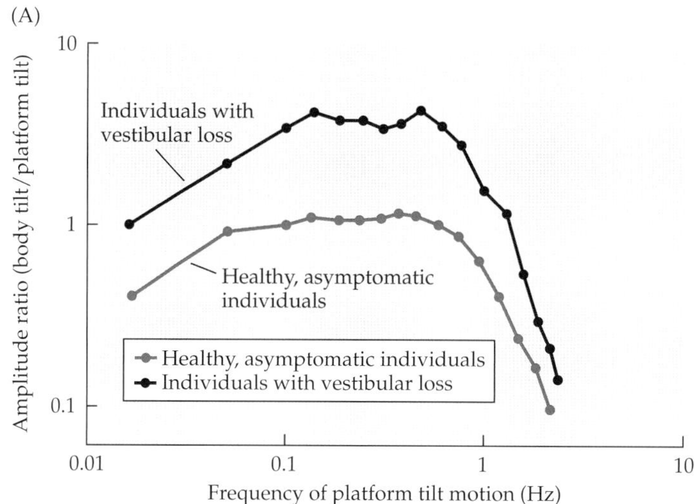

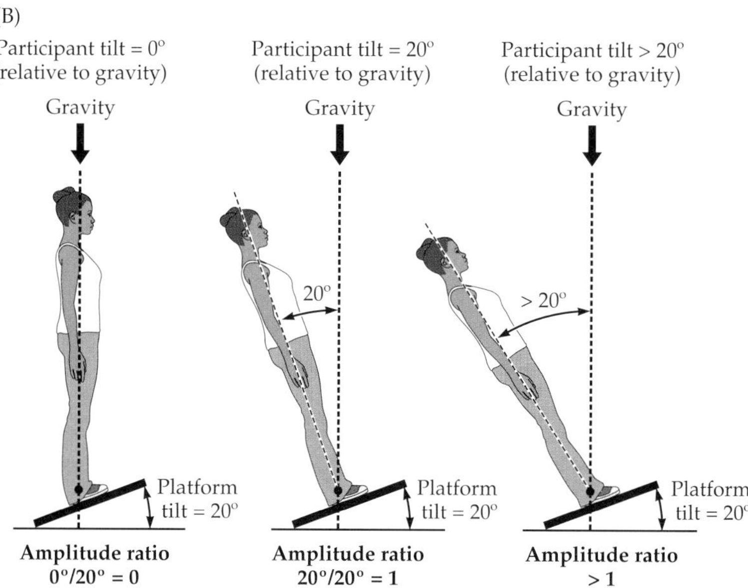

FIGURE 12.29 Vestibular function contributes to balance The contributions of the vestibular system to balance are demonstrated by the comparison of postural responses of individuals with healthy, asymptomatic vestibular function to responses of individuals suffering severe bilateral vestibular loss. With eyes closed, participants were asked to maintain themselves upright in the presence of an input disturbance—small, angular displacements of their feet that were designed to challenge their balance. To help demonstrate the concept, the platform disturbance illustrates a tilt of 20 degrees; however, in typical experiments the tilt would be much smaller (otherwise participants would fall off!). (A) The values on the *y*-axis represent an amplitude ratio (that is, participant's tilt divided by the platform tilt). (B) If the participant remained perfectly upright, the resulting amplitude ratio would be 0 (0/20). If the participant remained perpendicular to the platform, the amplitude ratio would be 1 (20/20). If the participant tilted more than the platform, that ratio would be greater than 1. Amplitude ratios for healthy, asymptomatic individuals were always near or below 1. However, individuals with vestibular loss had response ratios that often far exceeded 1, indicating that body tilt far exceeded platform tilt. In other words, a platform tilt of 2 degrees might yield a body tilt of 10 degrees or more! In summary, individuals with vestibular loss exhibited much greater sway than normal individuals, clearly demonstrating the fundamental contributions of the vestibular system to balance control.

spatial disorientation Any impairment of spatial orientation. More specifically, any impairment of our sense of linear motion, angular motion, or tilt.

as an amplitude ratio far exceeding 1 across a broad range of frequencies). This difference between postural responses of people with normal vestibular function and those of patients with vestibular loss is a clear indication of the importance of the vestibular system to balance and posture control—showing that the vestibular system is helping to respond to the applied-movement disturbance to reduce body sway. A little later in the chapter, we'll discuss mal de debarquement syndrome, an unusual disorder that causes imbalance and/or **spatial disorientation**.

The vestibulospinal response can be thought of as a whole family of reflexes (**FIGURE 12.30**). In the vestibular nuclei, the primary afferent neurons synapse on descending interneurons that carry information through the lateral and medial vestibulospinal tracts. How far these neurons carry information down the spinal cord depends on their contribution to the balance system. If the interneuron synapses onto a neuron that controls a leg muscle, the information is transmitted beyond the bottom of the spinal cord. If the information contributes to postural control of the head, it is transmitted only as far as the neck.

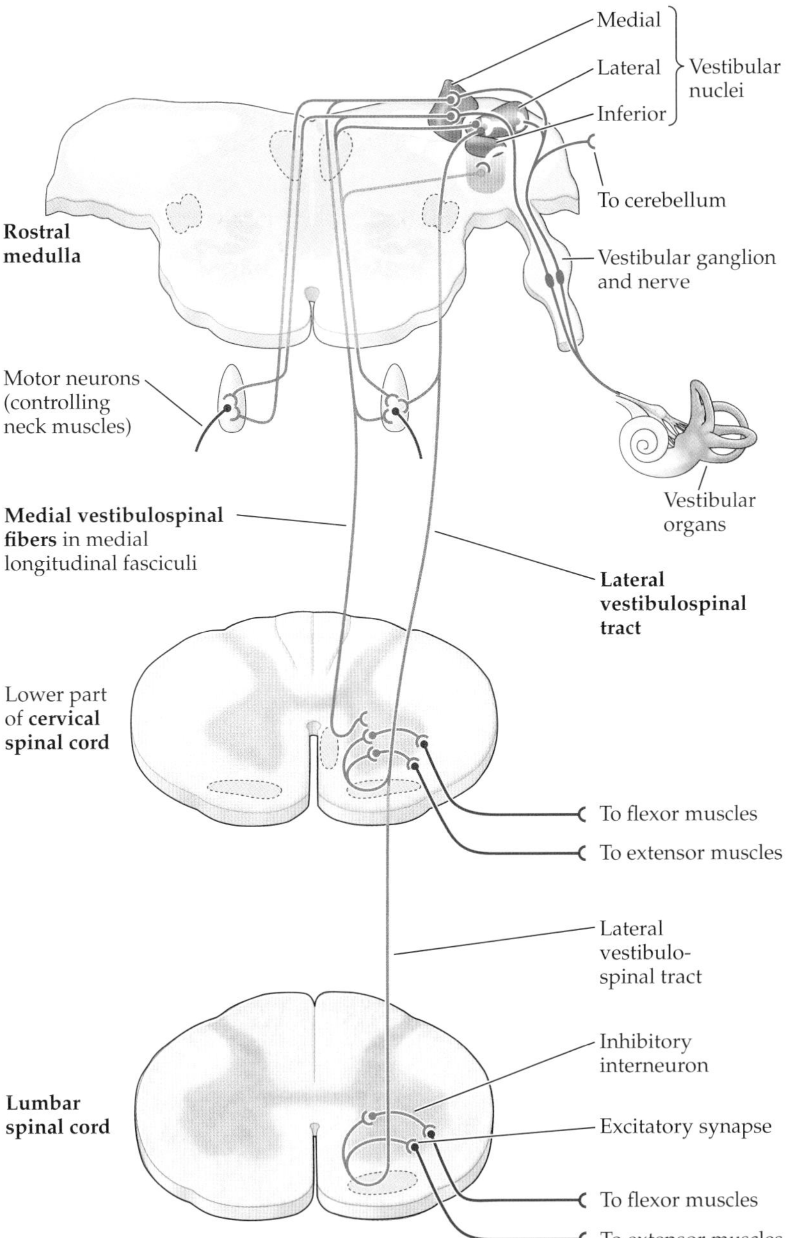

FIGURE 12.30 Neural pathways for vestibulospinal reflexes Most vestibular afferent neurons (blue) synapse in one of the vestibular nuclei, but some project to the cerebellum. From the vestibular nuclei, descending interneurons (green) carry the information via vestibulospinal tracts downward through the brainstem and spinal cord until they synapse on efferent neurons (red) that activate the muscles that control balance.

12.9 Multisensory Spatial Orientation Cortex

We have visual cortex and auditory cortex. Do we have vestibular cortex? Some areas of the cortex certainly do respond to vestibular input, but these areas include a variety of sensory and motor signals. There does not appear to be an area of the cortex exclusively dedicated to vestibular signals. This is not shocking, since we learned earlier that perception of body motion and tilt result from multisensory convergence, including predominant contributions by the vestibular system and vision.

It may be that there is simply no good reason for the cortex to process vestibular information in isolation when other sensory information is available. For example, the visual system is responsive to constant-velocity visual motion—like that experienced during rotation in the light as you see the room spin around you—while the vestibular system responds primarily to changes in velocity and is relatively insensitive to constant-velocity motion. More specifically, recall that when rotated at a constant velocity in the dark, after about 30 seconds humans perceive that they are not rotating (see Figure 12.18). Therefore, when you are rotating with a nearly constant velocity in the light, it seems reasonable that your brain would utilize the visual information indicating motion to better estimate self-motion. It thus makes sense that areas of the cortex related to the perception of tilt and self-motion demonstrate a convergence of visual and vestibular information, as well as information from other sensory systems that contribute to spatial orientation.

Vestibular Thalamocortical Pathways

Vestibular information reaches the cortex via thalamocortical pathways (**FIGURE 12.31**). This means simply that the vestibular information, like most other sensory information, reaches the cortex via the thalamus. Neurons from the vestibular nuclei carry vestibular information to the thalamus, where that information is processed and relayed to the cortex. Compare this, for example, to the visual system, where the retinal ganglion cells synapse in the lateral geniculate nucleus of the thalamus (see Figures 3.14 and 3.15 and Section 3.3). There the information is processed and passed on to visual cortex.

Evidence suggests that the temporo-parieto-insular cortex is involved in spatial orientation perception. This area of the cortex receives input from both the semicircular canals and the otolith organs. Furthermore, many patients with lesions to this part of the cortex caused by a stroke report illusory tilts and/or illusory translation. Though more rare, rotational vertigo—an illusory sense of spinning—is reported by some of these patients.

Though more direct vestibular projections may exist, there is a vestibular pathway that leads to the hippocampus through the cortex, and neurons in the hippocampal formation respond to vestibular stimuli (Horii et al., 2004). These include "head direction cells," a set of neurons that tend to spike vigorously when an animal's head is pointed toward a specific direction (Taube, 2007).

Cortical Influences

The areas of the cortex that receive projections from the vestibular system also project back to the vestibular nuclei. The existence of these pathways suggests that feedback from areas of the cortex that respond to vestibular stimulation likely modulates low-level vestibular processing in the brainstem. A specific role for these projections has not been proven, but it is known that higher cognitive knowledge can affect both perceptions and reflexive responses. For example, imagining whether an unseen visual target rotates with you alters the VOR evoked by rotation. As is appropriate, the VOR is suppressed when participants imagine that the target moves with them, but is relatively large when participants imagine that the target is Earth-fixed (Barr, Schultheis, and Robinson, 1976).

As another example of higher-order cortical influences, knowledge can influence motion perceptions (Wertheim, Mesland, and Bles, 2001; Rader, Oman, and Merfeld, 2011). Complex motions (as one example, think of a car on a cloverleaf freeway exit) are experienced differently if you have no idea what the motion will be than if you know what the motion will be (for example, think of the same car but traveling a route that you traverse often). The vestibular stimuli can be the same, but your knowledge and expectations—both of which are cognitive—will impact your perceived spatial orientation ●

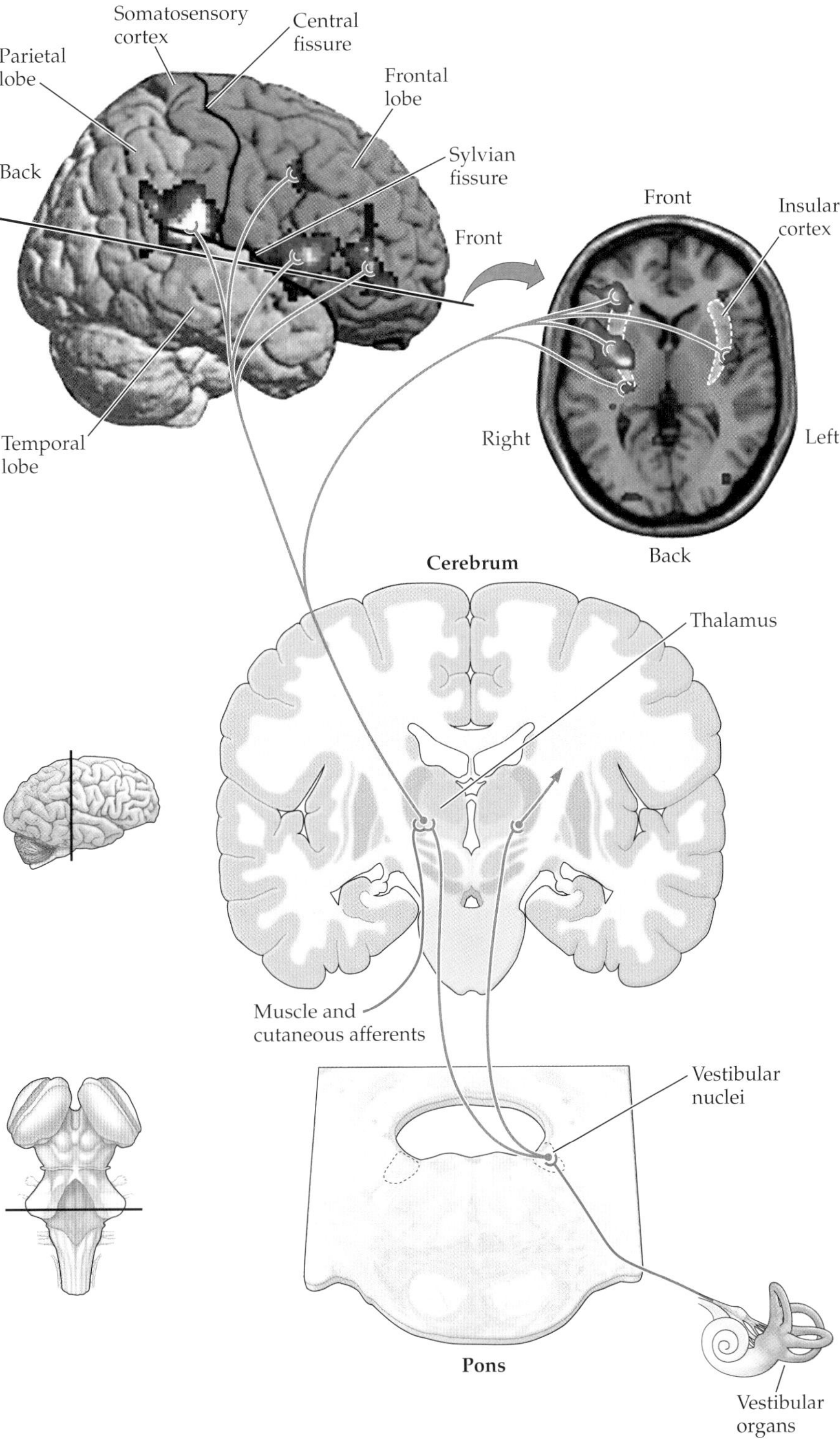

FIGURE 12.31 Neural pathways for spatial orientation perception Ascending vestibular (thalamocortical) pathways pass from the vestibular nuclei to the thalamus on their way to the cortex. The brain is viewed from the right side. Cortex activation patterns shown at the top are positron emission tomography scans (the one on the left is colorized) obtained during stimulation of the vestibular system on the right side. Red and yellow indicate activation, which occurs in the temporo-parieto-insular areas of both hemispheres. Unlike activation in most other sensory systems, much of the vestibular activation is not visible on the outermost surface of the cortex but is found deeper in the brain, in the insular cortex.

12.10 When the Vestibular System Goes Bad

We have learned that the vestibular system makes fundamental contributions to our sense of spatial orientation and contributes to a number of reflexive responses. What happens when the vestibular system fails? Reflecting the widespread

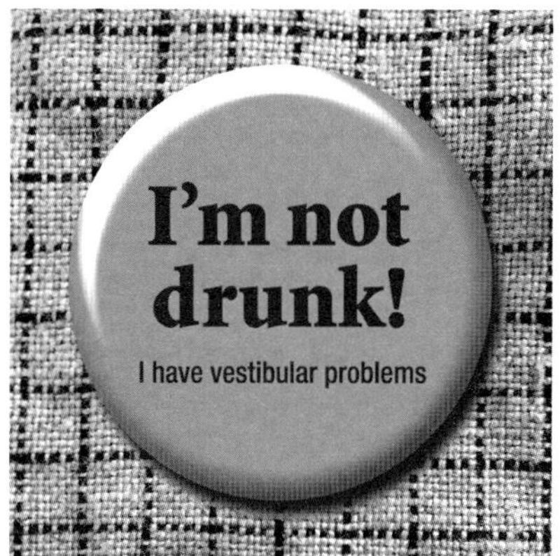

FIGURE 12.32 Vestibular dysfunction can be difficult to recognize Some symptoms of vestibular dysfunction, like imbalance causing falls, mirror the effects of alcoholic beverages. This button highlights how unaware observers might misinterpret the symptoms of vestibular disorders. Even the best-trained clinicians have difficulty diagnosing some forms of vestibular dysfunction.

influence of the vestibular system, the bad news is that a lot of problems develop (Baloh and Halmagyi, 1996). Many patients with vestibular dysfunction develop spatial disorientation. Many experience imbalance. Many cannot see clearly unless they make an effort to hold their heads absolutely still. Many develop motion sickness that can lead to nausea or even vomiting. Some even develop cognitive problems. Because we are usually unaware of the vestibular system's contributions, it is possible to misinterpret the actions of people suffering from vestibular disorders (**FIGURE 12.32**).

The good news is that most patients with vestibular dysfunction partially adapt to the situation. For example, many patients with vestibular dysfunction quickly learn to curtail activities that lead to problems. This strategy is effective, but curtailing one's lifestyle is not an entirely satisfactory solution. Fortunately, in addition, most patients with vestibular dysfunction also learn to utilize other sensory information. As with the exquisite sense of hearing that is sometimes reported in patients with blindness, other sensory systems fill in to help reduce behavioral deficits caused by vestibular problems. This adaptation, coupled with physical rehabilitation and a curtailing of motion-related activities, yields an altered lifestyle that helps patients with vestibular dysfunction acclimate to their disability.

Falls and Vestibular Function

Fall risk increases with age, and falls are a leading cause of accidental death. Moreover, balance data correlate with falls, and vestibular dysfunction impacts balance (e.g., Horak, Nashner, and Diener, 1990). Recent data show that higher roll tilt thresholds in the dark are significantly correlated with failure to complete the vestibular condition of a standard balance test (Bermúdez Rey et al., 2016). Furthermore, an analysis of more than 5000 Americans showed that failure to complete this same balance test condition was correlated with substantially higher odds of having fallen in the past year (Agrawal et al., 2009). These findings together indicate that substandard vestibular sensation, including declines with age, might contribute to the death of 50,000 Americans each year (Bermúdez Rey et al., 2016).

Mal de Debarquement Syndrome

Most travelers feel a little unbalanced after disembarking from a large ship following an extended cruise. This imbalance is sometimes accompanied by motion sickness and by swaying, rocking, or tilting perceptions. You may have experienced these sensations after spending just a few hours on a boat. After disembarking, as you lay in your bed, you may have felt the gentle rocking of the waves, even though you knew you were perfectly still. These symptoms are bothersome but typically dissipate within a few hours. It is generally believed that these perceptions are an aftereffect of adaptation. Specifically, you adapt to the rocking motion experienced while on the boat. This adaptation—"getting your sea legs"—is appropriate while you're onboard the boat, but it is inappropriate once you're back on land, where it leads to transient perceptions of disorientation, imbalance, and rocking when you first disembark that eventually dissipate as you readapt to firm ground.

Relatively rarely, people are unable to readily readapt, and the condition sometimes leads to a clinical syndrome called mal de debarquement (meaning "disembarking sickness"). For these patients with mal de debarquement syndrome, the symptoms of spatial disorientation, imbalance, and rocking last a month or more after they disembark (Dai et al., 2017). In extreme cases, the symptoms can last for years and can be very debilitating. It remains a mystery why some individuals are unable to readapt when they leave the ship. Many believe that mal de debarquement syndrome results from a misadaptation to multisensory integration ●

Scientists at Work

Vestibular Aging

Question How does vestibular function vary with age?

Hypothesis Vestibular thresholds will increase as part of the aging process.

Test Direction discrimination thresholds (the smallest motion that individuals can reliably perceive) were measured in 105 people between the ages of 18 and 80 (Bermúdez Rey et al., 2016; **FIGURE 12.33**). Each was strapped into a chair that moved within a completely dark room. For the *z*-translation curve in the graph, in which perceptual thresholds are plotted versus age, participants were translated along their *z*-axis either upward or downward, with each movement taking 1 second. The participants performed a forced-choice perceptual task in which they were required to respond "up" or "down." Thresholds were determined by fitting a psychometric function—like that shown in Figure 1.3 to each participant's perceptual responses.

Results Thresholds for up/down *z*-axis translations were constant between the ages of 18 and 40, but increased at a rate of 84% on average every 10 years above the age of 40. Four other motions (including *y*-translation, yaw rotation, and roll tilts at motion durations of 1 and 5 seconds) yielded similar degradation patterns with age.

Conclusion Vestibular thresholds showed no evidence of aging prior to the age of about 40. After age 40, vestibular thresholds increased relatively rapidly. For example, the *z*-axis translation thresholds shown in Figure 12.33B roughly doubled between the ages of 42 and 54 and continued to increase at the same rapid rate above age 54.

Future work Might this degradation in vestibular function be a contributor to the increased risk of falling as we age? How would you design a study to investigate this question?

(A)

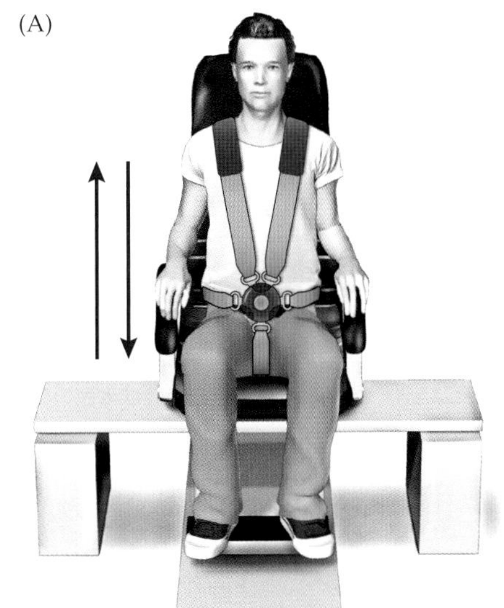

(B)

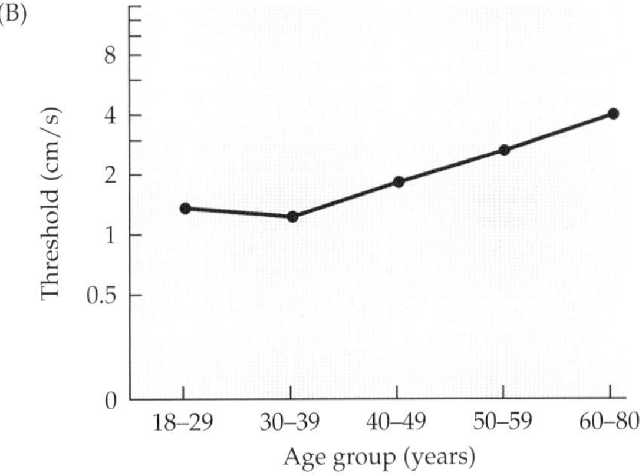

FIGURE 12.33 Aging of vestibular sensation Vestibular function declines markedly after the age of 40. (A) Experimental setup. (B) Vestibular thresholds to discriminate up translation from down translation were relatively constant until age 40, when they increased a little more than 80% every 10 years. Data are plotted on a logarithmic scale along the *y*-axis.

Ménière's Syndrome

Imagine suddenly experiencing dizziness, imbalance, and spatial disorientation so severe that either you have to lie down (quickly!) or you fall down. Imagine that severe motion sickness ensues and leads to repeated vomiting. Now imagine that these symptoms can occur suddenly and more or less unexpectedly at any time. This is the plight experienced by some patients with Ménière's syndrome, named after Prosper Ménière, the French physician who first described the syndrome in 1861.

Ménière's syndrome afflicts about one in 500 people. It may strike at any age, but typically the syndrome first occurs in mid-adulthood. Other symptoms include tinnitus (an illusory ringing sound), hearing loss, and a feeling of pain or fullness in the ear—making this an inner-ear disorder and not just a vestibular disorder.

The vestibular symptoms of dizziness, imbalance, and disorientation are so debilitating that patients often are incapacitated when experiencing a Ménière's attack. Furthermore, the concern that these symptoms might return at any time can be terrifying; some patients become afraid to leave their homes even when they are symptom-free. Making matters worse, although the vestibular system is known to be the source for the spatial disorientation suffered, the specific cause of

Sensation & Perception in Everyday Life

Amusement Park Rides—Vestibular Physics Is Fun

The semicircular canals are not very good transducers of low-frequency rotations—an effect that amusement park rides use to great advantage. What makes playground and amusement park rides fun? Clearly these are designed to be sensory experiences. Certainly hearing, taste, and smell are not the predominant sensory contributors, and while vision may play a role in the overall experience, most of these rides do not require vision to create the sensations people feel. In fact, some roller coaster patrons enjoy the experience more with their eyes closed! Playground and amusement park rides are designed, in large part, to stimulate the vestibular system. In fact, much of the enjoyment from a good amusement park ride derives from tricking the vestibular system in some way; typically, the designer of a good amusement park ride is playing with one or more of the fundamental characteristics of the vestibular system.

As a first example, let's consider the simple child-powered merry-go-round found in playgrounds (see Figure 12.2). These devices typically have a great deal of mass, especially compared with the mass of the children. The large device mass means that it takes a substantial amount of time—say 10 seconds or more—for it to speed up or slow down. Such gradual changes have low-frequency components that trick the semicircular canals into incorrectly sensing angular velocity. At the same time, the combination of both the radius (from the rotation axis at the center of the ride to the edge) and the angular velocity at the edge yield a centripetal acceleration with low-frequency components that is sensed by the otolith organs. Low-frequency accelerations trick the brain into perceiving self-tilt even in the absence of actual tilt. This divergence of perception from reality is the definition of an illusion. Such illusions seem to yield at least some of the fun experienced when riding playground and amusement park rides, but can also lead to motion sickness.

Now let's consider the roller coaster (**FIGURE 12.34**). Although part of the fun of a roller coaster comes from the thrill of moving at a high speed, the twists and turns of a roller coaster minimally change the speed of the carriage. These twists and turns are there primarily to yield vestibular stimulation well beyond that typically experienced in normal life. Usually, the turns are located where the carriage travels with nearly maximal speeds—thereby yielding high angular velocities transduced by semicircular canals and high linear accelerations transduced by the otolith organs. These extreme vestibular stimuli add to the thrill experienced during roller coaster rides.

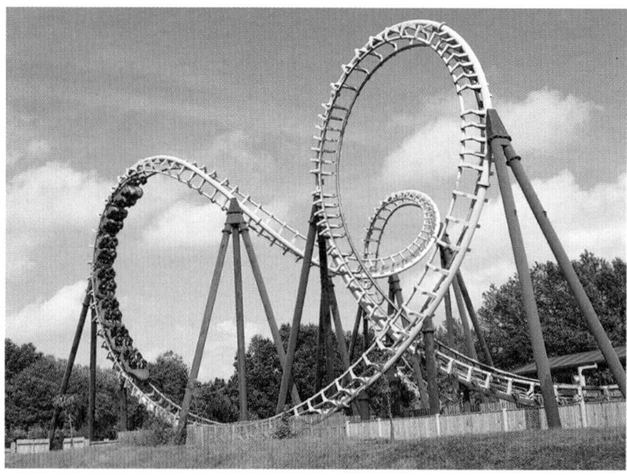

FIGURE 12.34 The thrill of vestibular sensation Many, but not all, enjoy the thrill of vestibular stimuli. Much of the thrill (or fear) experienced while riding a roller coaster results from vestibular stimulation.

the symptoms remains elusive. While some think that excess fluid in the inner ear causes Ménière's syndrome, others think that several different inner-ear disorders yield this constellation of symptoms.

Treatments of the disease include medications to lower pressure in the inner ear, implanted devices that provide transtympanic micropressure pulses, and sometimes procedures that destroy the vestibular apparatus. Stop for a moment and imagine that! The transient Ménière's syndrome symptoms are so severe that patients (and their physicians) are willing to induce a permanent disability just to be rid of transient symptoms. For those of us lucky enough to have never experienced severe vestibular problems, this provides a small hint at how disabling the symptoms can be when the vestibular system malfunctions, as well as a glimpse at the fundamental contributions provided by the vestibular system.

Summary

1. The vestibular organs are the inner-ear organs that sense head motion and gravity and contribute to our equilibrium sense.
2. The vestibular organs include three semicircular canals (horizontal, anterior, and posterior), which sense angular motion, and two otolith organs (utricle and saccule), which sense both gravity and linear acceleration.
3. Vestibular hair cells are the mechanoreceptors that convert both orientation with respect to gravity and head motion into signals that are sent to the brain.
4. Spatial orientation includes three perceptual modalities: linear motion, angular motion, and tilt. Direction and amplitude are qualities that define each of these three perceptual modalities.
5. We are exquisitely sensitive to head motion even in the dark, recognizing the directions of rotation, linear motion, and tilt at very low thresholds.
6. We do not have vestibular perception isolated from the other senses. Spatial orientation perception combines information from multiple sensory systems (i.e., multisensory integration)—with the vestibular and visual systems making predominant contributions.
7. The brain processes the vestibular information to yield perceptions that differ substantially from the signals found on the afferent neurons.
8. In addition to their contributions to spatial orientation perception, the vestibular organs contribute to postural, vestibulo-autonomic, and vestibulo-ocular reflexes. Vestibular-evoked postural reflexes help us maintain balance. Vestibulo-autonomic reflexes help regulate blood flow, especially to the brain. Vestibulo-ocular reflexes are compensatory eye movements that helps us see clearly even when the head moves.
9. Vestibular problems are widespread, and treatments are limited. For patients with Ménière's syndrome, for example, the symptoms may become so disabling that these patients accept treatments that yield permanent disability just to be rid of the symptoms.

Chapter 13

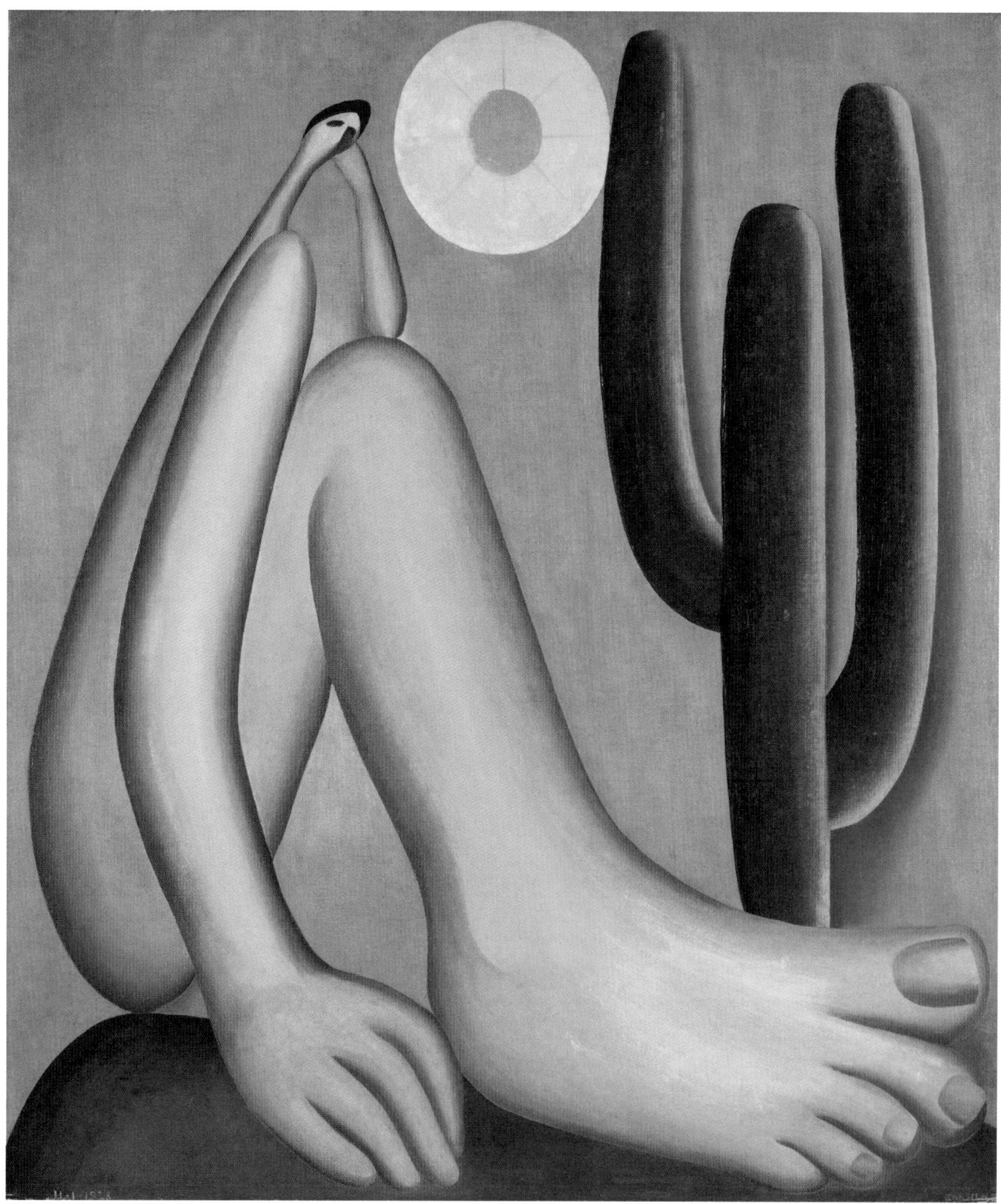

Tarsila do Amaral, *Abaporu*, 1928

Touch

Questions to Contemplate

Think about the following questions as you read this chapter.
By the chapter's end, you should be able to answer and discuss them.

- What physical stimuli trigger this sense?
- What are the limitations of touch perception without movement?
- If someone strokes your arm, you might feel it as pleasant, informative, or painful—what would determine the perceptual result?
- Should babies be petted, like cats and dogs?
- If you had to give up one sensory modality, why would you not give up the sense of touch?

This chapter provides a broad overview of perception through the sense of **touch**. It begins with the first question above, namely, how this perceptual modality is activated by physical stimulation. Answering that question leads to a discussion of receptor populations that underlie touch sensing and the associated neural fibers that carry receptor signals to interactions in the spinal cord (which might remind us of the retina in the visual system) and further to the brain. The chapter then turns to higher-level perceptual phenomena, such as recognizing objects by touch, feeling pain, and communicating social messages. The chapter concludes with **haptic perception**, which uses active exploration to enhance our ability to mentally represent the physical world and our place within it. Along the way, multisensory interactions involving touch are highlighted.

In answer to the last question raised above, you would *not* want to give up the sense of touch. It is difficult to conceive of our species surviving without it. Touch is sometimes referred to as the "proximal" sense, to indicate its role in telling us about our interactions with nearby surfaces and objects. (Perception of far objects like the sun still relies on their effects proximal to our body!) Temperature sensations contribute to our perception of materials and play the important role of enabling us to seek or create a thermally safe environment. Pain serves as a sophisticated warning system that alerts us when something might be internally wrong or when an external stimulus might be dangerous, enabling us to defend our bodies as quickly as possible. Social touch provides a powerful means of communicating thoughts and emotions nonverbally and is a calming influence in the face of stress.

Touch is fundamental to the most casual activities of everyday life. We use it to identify and manipulate objects without the need to look at them directly. You don't typically use vision, or any sense other than touch, for many routine tasks (e.g., buttoning your shirt, brushing your teeth). What's more surprising, perhaps, is that you can accomplish many tasks that are normally visually guided without sight. Blindfold yourself for a few minutes and try some routine activity like making a sandwich. You will discover that touch can be an effective substitute for vision:

touch The sensations caused by stimulation of the skin, muscles, tendons, and joints.

haptic perception Perceptual processing of inputs from discriminative touch in the context of active information-seeking: the haptic perceiver explores the world rather than passively receiving it.

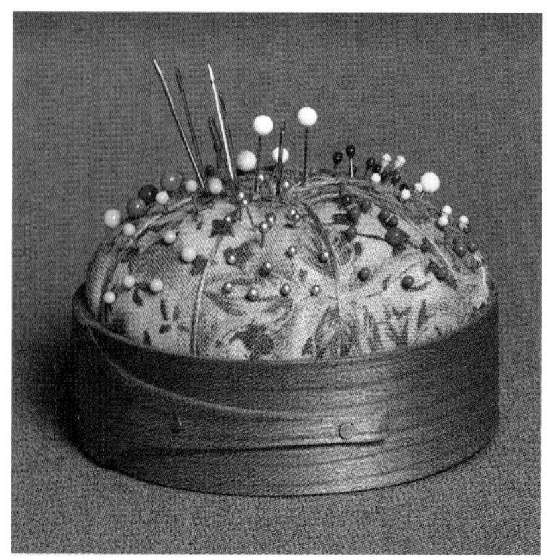

FIGURE 13.1 **What would this feel like?** Shaker-style pincushion.

you won't have as much trouble distinguishing the peanut butter jar from the jelly jar as you might think, and you will easily open it.

There is one more thing you may become acutely aware of during your experiment with the blindfold: we use active contact to learn about the world through touch. The pincushion in FIGURE 13.1 invites us to press our palms on the pins to detect their collective motion. We might also run our fingers along the interesting raised contour of the container or enclose the beaded tops to feel their smoothness and contrast their different sizes. It is only when we pick up the object that we become aware how the pins make it top-heavy. In sum, touch involves action, arguably to a greater degree than any of our other senses do.

13.1 Neural Pathways of Touch: From Physics to Brain

Let's next consider in detail the first question raised above, about what physical stimulation is perceived by the modality of touch. This sensory system encompasses multiple "submodalities," conveying different kinds of physical information for distinct functions. One submodality, **discriminative touch**, operates as we contact objects and surfaces. It includes what we might think of as touch in the narrowest sense: the sensations caused by mechanical displacements of the skin. These occur any time you grasp, wield, or otherwise make contact with an object, as when you pick up a spoon or fist-bump your friend. We will use the term **tactile** (the adjective form of *touch*) to refer to these mechanical interactions with skin. We will expand the definition of discriminative touch to include other "channels," or specialized information-processing avenues: the perception of temperature changes (thermal sensation) and the sensations arising from muscles, tendons, and joints that inform us of the positions and movements of our limbs in space, technically called **kinesthesia**. All these components operate together. If we wrap our fingers around a glass of milk, discriminative touch conveys information about its roundness, coolness, and smoothness, and even how full it is. Another **submodality of touch** collects the negative aspects of touch: pain and itch (and sometimes tickle). The **affective** submodality includes pleasant effects of being stroked and more complex patterns of social touch. **Interoception** processes sensory input from locations internal to the body, like your stomach.

Other terms arise in connection with the sensory modality of touch, varying in inclusiveness. **Proprioception** (from the Latin for "one's own") combines interoception and kinesthesia. **Somatosensation** (*soma* is the Greek word for "body") puts input from the skin together with the proprioceptive system. As was noted in Chapter 12, the vestibular system adds to proprioceptive information in controlling balance and to somatosensation in controlling the autonomic nervous system.

discriminative touch Relies on mechanical and thermal sensations for information about surfaces and objects with which we are in contact.

tactile Referring to the result of mechanical interactions with the skin.

kinesthesia Perception of the position and movement of our limbs in space.

submodality of touch A specialized domain of psychological functions, such as perceptual discrimination, social-emotional consequences, perceived unpleasantness, and interoception.

affective touch Submodality related to emotional and social functions.

interoception Sensory input from locations internal to the body, such as your stomach.

proprioception Perception mediated by kinesthetic and internal receptors.

somatosensation Collectively, sensory signals from the skin, muscles, tendons, joints, and internal receptors.

Neural Fibers, Receptors, and End Organs

The sites of our sensing equipment for vision, audition, olfaction, and gustation are all located in organs (the eyes, ears, nose, and mouth, respectively) that are more or less dedicated to sensory processing. Some other animals have analogous appendages: antennae. You might think that, for touch, humans do not have a readily apparent sense organ. To the contrary, the site of touch sensing includes the most obvious organ of all!

In fact, the human sense of touch is mostly housed in what is actually the largest and heaviest of the sense organs, the skin, which covers an area of approximately 1.8 square meters and weighs about 4 kilograms. Some skin, like that on our lips and fingertips, is without hair, or **glabrous**. Most skin, in contrast, is hairy. Touch receptors are embedded all over the body, in both glabrous and hairy skin. They are also found within our mouths and our muscles, tendons, and joints, as well as in internal organs. Just as the eye has its rods and three types of cones, the sense of touch has several types of receptors. These receptors form the basis for the multiple submodalities and the specialized channels that contribute to the overall perceptual experience.

SOMATOSENSORY FIBERS A touch receptor is connected to a "nerve fiber" composed of its axon and myelin sheath, if present. Four types of nerve fibers carry information about somatosensation, as shown in FIGURE 13.2. These types differ in the fiber's diameter and in whether a myelin sheath is present, resulting in different conduction speeds. **A-alpha fibers** carry information from proprioceptive receptors in muscles and tendons. Their relatively wide diameters permit very fast neural conduction. **A-beta fibers**, moderately thick and myelinated, are connected to receptors that respond to pressure and vibration. The thinner **A-delta fibers** and **C fibers**, the latter without myelin, carry information about temperature, pain, and itch, as well as interoception and a special sensation called pleasant touch. FIGURE 13.3 shows a cross section of hairy and glabrous skin with the embedded fibers. We will next discuss the receptors and fibers for various channels and submodalities in detail.

TACTILE RECEPTORS Although the external quality of the skin varies across different parts of the body (it is thicker in some parts and thinner in others, smoother in some regions and coarser in others, and so on), most skin includes tactile receptors called **mechanoreceptors** because they respond to mechanical stimulation or pressure. The tactile receptors are embedded in both the outer layer, called the **epidermis**, and the underlying layer, known as the **dermis**. Their nerve fibers all fall into the myelinated type called A-beta. The fiber of a tactile mechanoreceptor extends from its ending within the skin all the way to the spinal cord, and it can sometimes be very long (stretching from the sole of your foot to your backbone, for example).

glabrous In reference to skin, lacking hair.

A-alpha fiber A wide-diameter, myelinated sensory nerve fiber that transmits signals from proprioceptive receptors in muscles and tendons.

A-beta fiber A wide-diameter, myelinated sensory nerve fiber that transmits signals from mechanical stimulation.

A-delta fiber An intermediate-sized, myelinated sensory nerve fiber that transmits pain and temperature signals.

C fiber A narrow-diameter, unmyelinated sensory nerve fiber that transmits pain and temperature signals.

mechanoreceptor A sensory receptor that responds to mechanical stimulation (pressure, vibration, or movement).

epidermis The outer of two major layers of skin.

dermis The inner of two major layers of skin, consisting of nutritive and connective tissues, within which lie the mechanoreceptors.

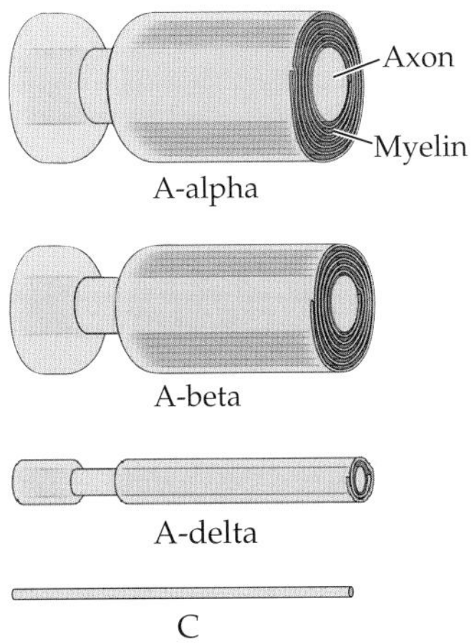

Associated receptor	Fiber type and structure	Diameter (micrometer)	Conduction speed (m/s)
Proprioceptor	A-alpha (Axon, Myelin)	13–20	80–120
Mechanoreceptor	A-beta	6–12	35–75
Pain and temperature	A-delta	1–5	5–30
Pain, temperature, itch	C	0.2–1.5	0.5-2

FIGURE 13.2 Neural fibers of the somatosensory receptors The figure represents the structure, diameter, and conduction speed of these fibers.

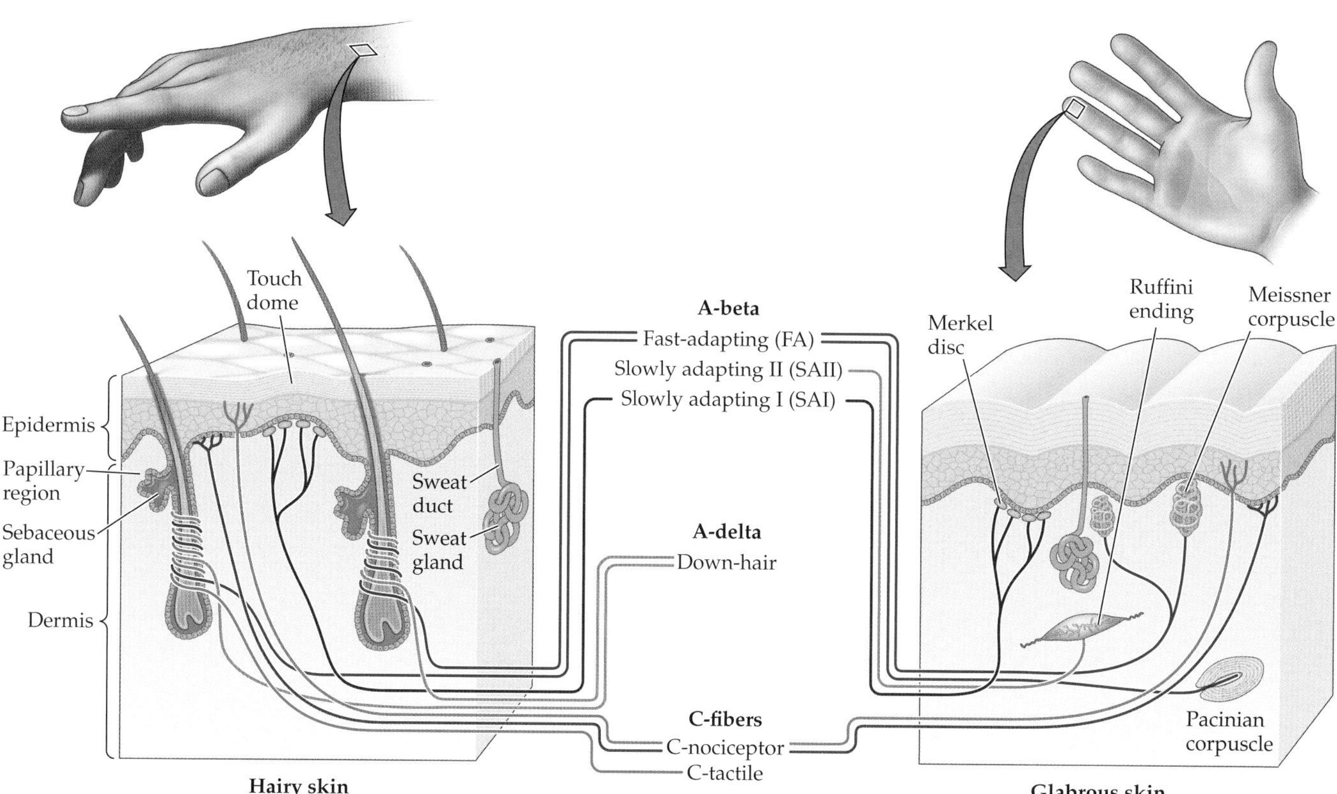

FIGURE 13.3 Cross section of skin Left: The types of fibers found in hairy skin, including A-delta fibers specifically associated with down-hair; skin layers are also identified. Right: The fibers found in glabrous skin, with the mechanoreceptors identified. Additional A-delta fibers found within the epidermis of both hairy and glabrous skin are not illustrated.

Based on responses from individual A-beta fibers when the skin is probed, four distinct classes of mechanoreceptor have been identified. These represent combinations of two attributes describing how they function:

1. *Size of the receptive field.* Recall that a cell in the visual system will have a receptive field, a region of the visual world where a stimulus can produce a response in the cell. Tactile receptors have receptive fields too. Indeed, the concept is, if anything, more straightforward here. The tactile receptive field is the patch of the body where a stimulus will produce a response. The size of a tactile receptive field depends to some extent on the stimulation applied to the skin, but fields are generally classified as small (around 10–20 square millimeters [mm^2]) or large (from 60 mm^2 to the size of an entire finger).

FURTHER DISCUSSION of receptive fields as they relate to vision can be found in Section 2.3 and throughout Chapter 3.

2. *Rate of adaptation (fast versus slow).* A fast-adapting (FA) receptor responds with bursts of action potentials, first when its preferred stimulus is applied and then again when the stimulus is removed. It does not respond during the steady state between stimulus onset and offset. In contrast, a slowly adapting (SA) receptor remains active throughout the period during which the stimulus is in contact with its receptive field.

These two dimensions lead to the four classes of mechanoreceptor listed in **TABLE 13.1**, which also shows how each is particularly sensitive to certain features of mechanical stimulation, rendering it suitable for particular functions.

TABLE 13.1 The four mechanoreceptor populations: Response characteristics, feature sensitivity, and associated function

Mechanoreceptor type	Size of receptive field	Adaptation rate	Maximum feature sensitivity (Hz = cycles per second)	Primary perceptual functions
SA I (Merkel)	Small	Slow	Sustained pressure, very low frequency (<~5 Hz)	Coarse texture and pattern
FA I (Meissner)	Small	Fast	Temporal changes in skin deformation (~5–50 Hz); skin slip	Low-frequency vibration; grasp stability
SA II (Ruffini)	Large	Slow	Sustained downward pressure; lateral skin stretch (~5–50 Hz)	Finger position
FA II (Pacinian)	Large	Fast	Temporal changes in skin deformation (~50–700 Hz)	High-frequency vibration; fine texture

Note: FA I = fast-adapting type I; FA II = fast-adapting type II; SA I = slowly adapting type I; SA II = slowly adapting type II. The terminal ending associated with each type of tactile nerve fiber is shown in parentheses.

- Slowly adapting type I (SA I) receptors respond best to steady downward pressure, as well as very-low-frequency vibrations. They are especially important for texture and pattern perception. We use these receptors to decode raised surface features like Braille symbols or to feel the slot on the head of a screw when we figure out how to align the screwdriver. When a single SA I neural fiber is stimulated, people report feeling "pressure."
- Slowly adapting type II (SA II) receptors respond to sustained downward pressure and particularly to skin stretch, as occurs when we grasp an object. As you reach to pick up your coffee cup, the SA II receptors help shape your fingers appropriately. SA II receptors terminating in the folds of skin around the nails convey forces on the fingertips as they interact with objects (Birznieks et al., 2009). When a single SA II fiber is stimulated, people report no tactile sensation at all; for stimulation to be detectable, more than one SA II fiber must be stimulated.
- Fast-adapting type I (FA I) receptors respond best to low-frequency vibrations. If your coffee cup begins to slip across your fingers, this motion across the skin will cause just such vibrations, and FA I receptors will help you correct your grip before your coffee spills all over you. When a FA I fiber is stimulated, people report a very localized sensation that they describe as "wobble" or "flutter."
- Fast-adapting type II (FA II) receptors respond best to high-frequency vibrations. These occur when an object makes contact with the skin, as, for example, when a mosquito lands on your arm or your hand accidentally brushes against the wall. They are transmitted to the skin when you hold your pen and tap it on the table. Stimulating a SA II fiber leads to a diffuse sensation in the skin that people report as like a "buzz."

Although mechanoreceptors can be classified by how the neural fibers respond to stimulation, another part of the story is that the neurons in glabrous skin terminate in conjunction with specialized structures called end organs, as shown in Figure 13.3. They have come to be named after the anatomists who first described them: **Meissner corpuscles**, **Merkel discs**, **Pacinian corpuscles**, and **Ruffini endings**. As listed in Table 13.1, each of the four receptor types, as defined by adaptation rate and receptive-field size, is associated with a particular ending.

Meissner corpuscle A specialized nerve ending associated with fast-adapting (FA I) fibers that have small receptive fields.

Merkel disc A specialized nerve ending associated with slowly adapting (SA I) fibers that have small receptive fields (also known as Merkel cell neurite complex).

Pacinian corpuscle A specialized nerve ending associated with fast-adapting (FA II) fibers that have large receptive fields.

Ruffini ending A specialized nerve ending associated with slowly adapting (SA II) fibers that have large receptive fields.

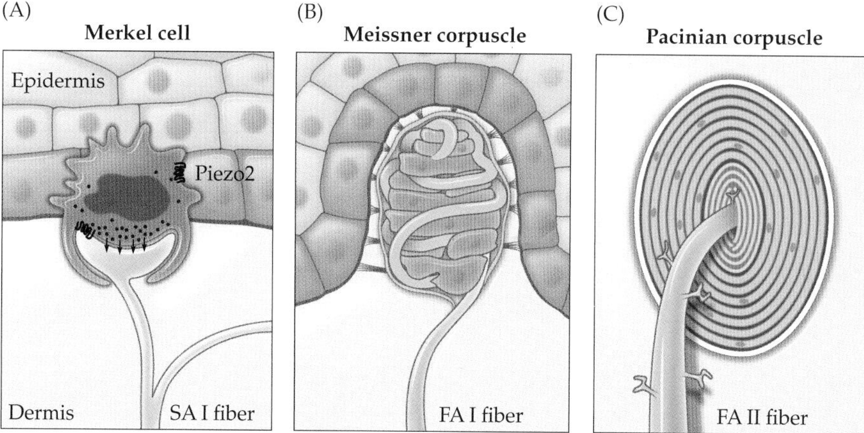

FIGURE 13.4 Anatomical connections between specialized end organs found in human glabrous skin and the neural fibers associated with them. Piezo2 is the ion channel associated with the Merkel cell.

The end organs differ with respect to their structure and location within the skin. The Meissner corpuscles and Merkel discs are found at the junction of the epidermis and dermis, in specific relation to the ridges found in the fingertip. As shown in Figure 13.3, counterparts of the ridges and troughs on the fingertip are found in indentations and protrusions of the epidermis at its junction with the top of the dermis, an area called the papillary dermis. Merkel discs are found at the tips of protrusions, while Meissner corpuscles lie between them. The Pacinian and Ruffini end organs, associated with FA II and SA II receptors, respectively, are embedded more deeply in the dermis and underlying subcutaneous tissue. It should be noted that there is some doubt as to whether the SA II fibers in human skin actually terminate in Ruffini endings or may instead simply lack specialized terminal structures.

FIGURE 13.4 shows more details of the structure of the Merkel, Meissner, and Pancinian end organs and how they connect to neural fibers. Each Merkel cell forms something like a handshake with an ending of the corresponding SA I fiber. Meissner corpuscles take the form of a stack, which the FA I fiber encircles and penetrates like a snake. The Pacinian structure is a layered cylinder that is cleaved at its center by the associated FA II fiber. These intriguing structural relationships have led to the question of which member of the pair, end-organ or neural fiber, is actually receiving a sensory signal from mechanical interaction with the skin, and in particular, whether the end organs merely act as accessories to enhance the neuron's response. The Meissner and Pancinian corpuscles appear to function as mechanical assistants, conveying vibrations from the skin to the fiber that penetrates them, although this may not be their only role. The Merkel cells form a synapse with the associated SA I fiber, and the two act as partners in neural signaling, with the fiber producing an initial response to touch and the Merkel component sustaining the response under continued pressure (Woo, Lumpkin, and Patapoutian, 2015).

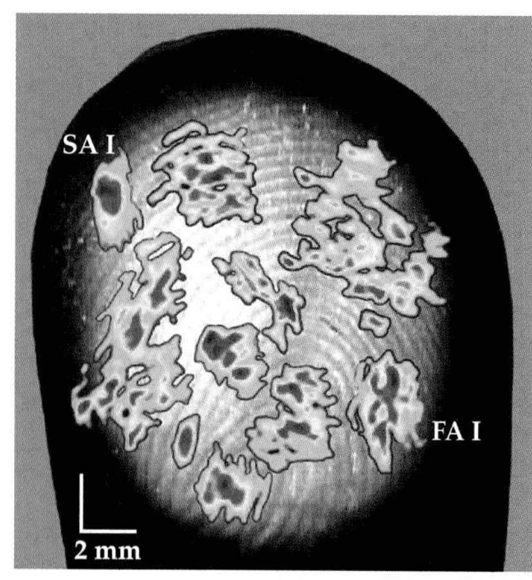

FIGURE 13.5 Subfields of type I fibers Each outlined patch depicts a receptive field's subfield structure; the fields are superimposed on a fingertip to show the scale in relation to the fingerprint ridges. Fields of both SA I and FA I receptors are shown (two are labeled). There would be about 500 densely overlapping receptive fields in an actual finger.

Closer examination of the responses of neural type 1 receptors (Merkel and Meissner), which terminate close to the surface of the skin and have small receptive fields, reveals that the response to stimulation within the receptive field shows positional variation. That is, locations within the receptive field, or *subfields*, lead to more or less firing when stimulated, as can be seen by the color-coded patches in FIGURE 13.5 (Jarocka, Pruszynski, and Johansson, 2021). The entire receptive field of a neuron encompasses several of the ridges in the finger surface (which form our fingerprint), whereas the size of a subfield is approximately the width of a single fingertip ridge. The explanation for the subfield variations lies in the fact that type I fibers exhibit a branching pattern, such that a single SA I fiber connects to multiple, spatially separated Merkel cell complexes, and likewise, a single FA I fiber connects with multiple Meissner corpuscles (as shown in Figure 13.3). Each individual Merkel or Meissner end organ lies in close proximity to a fingertip ridge, and it is particularly stimulated by contact with that ridge. Accordingly, the associated neural fiber fires more when skin contact is near the ridge above a connected end organ and less when skin contact moves away. The result is "hot" and "cold" spots across the fiber's receptive field, which essentially form a map of its connections to end organs.

Like glabrous skin, hairy skin contains sensory fibers with distinct functionality, but the sole specialized endings found in substantial number are the Merkel cells, which lie in regions of epidermis called touch domes. Receptors are also located near the follicles of the hair itself, as shown in Figure 13.3, left. In humans, hairy skin appears to play a unique and important role in pleasant touch, to be discussed below.

Although we can identify four distinct types of mechanoreceptors, they tend to be working together in everyday manual activity. The SA I and FA I receptors, in particular, are analogous to cones and rods, respectively, in their functions: one affording acuity and the other sensitivity to low-intensity stimulation. K. O. Johnson (2002) gave the example of opening a door with a key. Feeling the shape of your key in your pocket requires the SA I channel. Shaping your fingers to grasp the key involves the SA II channel. As you insert the key into the lock, your grip force increases so that the key does not slip, thanks to your FA I channel. Finally, your FA II channel tells you when the key hits the end of the keyhole.

KINESTHETIC RECEPTORS In addition to the tactile mechanoreceptors in the skin, other types of mechanoreceptors lie within muscles, tendons, and joints. These receptors, which are served by the A-alpha and A-beta fiber populations, are collectively referred to as **kinesthetic** receptors, and they play an important role in sensing where our limbs are and what kinds of movements we are making (Clark and Horch, 1986; L. A. Jones, 1999). The angle formed by a limb at a joint is perceived primarily through muscle receptors called muscle spindles (**FIGURE 13.6**), which convey the rate at which the muscle fibers are changing in length. Receptors in the tendons, called Golgi tendon organs, provide signals about the tension in the muscles attached to the tendons, and receptors directly in the joints themselves come into play particularly when a joint is bent to an extreme angle (in which case pain fibers described below come into play).

The importance of kinesthetic receptors is illustrated by a neurological patient named Ian Waterman. The nerves connecting Waterman's kinesthetic and tactile mechanoreceptors to his brain were destroyed at age 19 by a viral infection. Waterman became completely dependent on vision to tell him where his limbs were. If the lights went off, he could not navigate stairs or even clap his hands, because he had no idea where his hands and feet were! Caught in an elevator when the lights went out, he he could not remain standing.

THERMORECEPTORS **Thermoreceptors** located in both the epidermal and the dermal layers of the skin inform us about changes in skin temperature. There are two distinct populations of thermoreceptors (**FIGURE 13.7**): **Warmth fibers** fire when the temperature of the skin surrounding the fibers rises. **Cold fibers** (which outnumber warmth fibers by a ratio of about 30:1) fire in response to decreases in skin temperature. The neural fibers that mediate cold and warmth include the unmyelinated, and hence relatively slowly conducting, C fibers and the faster-conducting, myelinated A-delta fibers. These both have **free nerve endings**; that

kinesthetic Referring to perception involving sensory mechanoreceptors in muscles, tendons, and joints.

thermoreceptor A sensory receptor that signals information about changes in skin temperature.

warmth fiber A sensory nerve fiber that fires when skin temperature increases.

cold fiber A sensory nerve fiber that fires when skin temperature decreases.

free nerve ending The terminus of a neural fiber without a specialized ending.

FIGURE 13.6 A muscle spindle The spindle is embedded in main (extrafusal) muscle fibers and contains inner (intrafusal) fibers. When the inner fibers contract, a sensory response from the spindle is sent back to the central nervous system, conveying information about muscle length and thus regulating muscle tension.

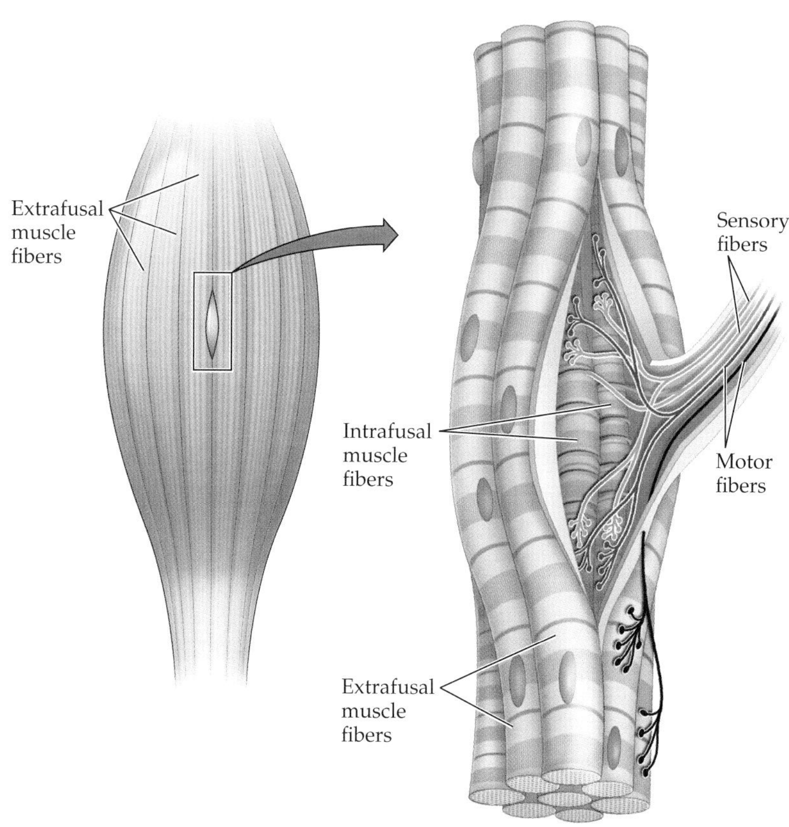

thermoTRP channel Thermally sensitive transient receptor potential ion channel found in sensory neurons.

is, the nerve endings are bare, rather than having specialized end organs like the fibers from mechanoreceptors. Thermally sensitive transient receptor potential ion channels, or **thermoTRP channels**, found in these neurons play a role in thermally induced pain, as discussed below.

Our bodies are constantly working to regulate their internal temperature, so under normal conditions the skin is kept between 30°C and 36°C, and neither cold nor warmth fibers respond much while skin temperature remains within this range. If you bundle up in a blanket but then sit inside in front of the fire, your skin temperature will probably rise above 36°C, and your warmth fibers will begin to fire. If you remove the blanket and walk out into the snow, your skin temperature will rapidly begin to fall, and as soon as it goes below 30°C, your cold receptors will start firing.

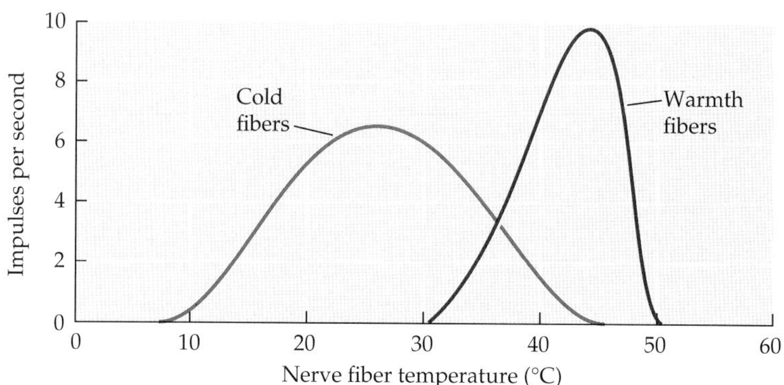

FIGURE 13.7 Thermal receptivity functions These graphs show the response of warmth and cold fibers to different temperatures.

nociceptor A sensory receptor that responds to painful input, such as extreme heat or pressure.

Thermoreceptors also kick in when we make contact with an object that is warmer or colder than our skin. Objects in the environment are typically cooler than 30°C, so it is usually the cold fibers that tell us about the object. For example, steel conducts heat more efficiently than stone. Your cold fibers will thus fire less rapidly and for a shorter period of time when you touch a steel object than when you touch a stone object (because the steel object will warm more quickly to match your skin temperature). If you've had prior experience with steel and stone, you can make use of the different thermoreceptor responses to make this material distinction. As we will see in the following discussion of pain, receptors that respond to extreme temperature changes also respond to foods that we associate with thermal sensations, like chili (warmth) and menthol (cold).

NOCICEPTORS AND PRURICEPTORS Pain is the realm of touch that has the dubious honor of being home to the sensations we like the least. We may find some visual stimuli revolting and some olfactory or gustatory stimuli disgusting, but of all the sensations, it is pain that we take the most drastic actions to avoid. Pain itself is the unpleasant sensory and emotional consequence of signals from **nociceptors**, touch receptors that have bare nerve endings and that respond to various forms of tissue damage or to stimuli that have the potential to damage tissue (including extreme skin temperatures lower than 15°C or higher than 45°C). Pain receptors are found throughout the body, including in some internal organs.

Like thermoreceptors, nociceptors in the skin lack specialized endings and can be divided into two types by their nerve fibers. The myelinated A-delta fibers respond primarily to strong pressure or heat, and the unmyelinated C fibers respond to intense stimulation of various sorts: pressure, heat or cold, or noxious chemicals. Many painful events seem to occur in two stages: a quick, sharp burst of pain, followed by a throbbing sensation. These two stages may reflect the onset of signals first from the A-delta fibers and then from the C fibers (Price et al., 1977).

How do nociceptive neurons detect the thermal and chemical stimulation that produces pain? A critical role appears to be played by the thermoTRP ion channels, which regulate the flow of charged atoms and molecules across the membrane of a cell (Julius, 2013). **FIGURE 13.8** illustrates the range of temperatures associated

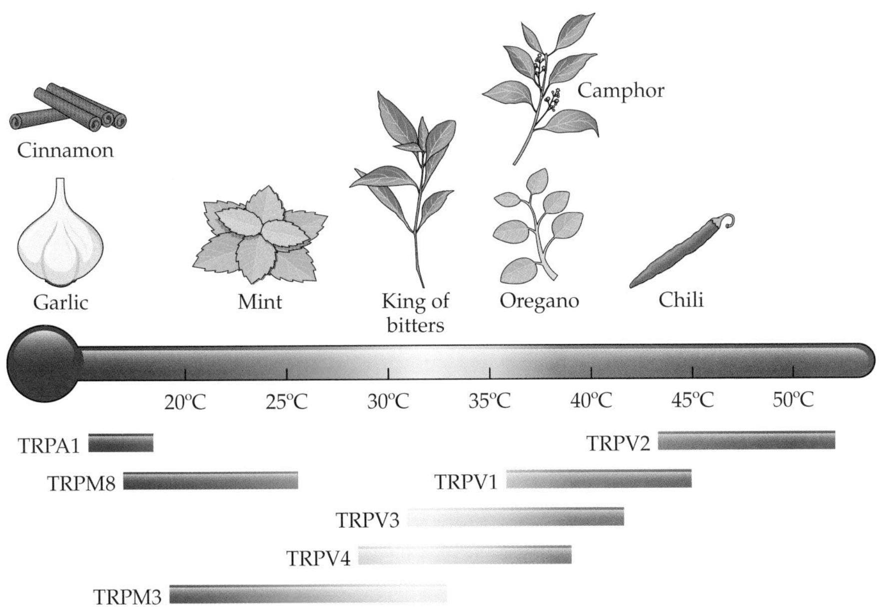

FIGURE 13.8 ThermoTRPs Natural plant compounds activate TRP channels that operate across distinct ranges of thermal stimulation (thermoTRPs), as shown. These channels operate in normal thermal sensation and at extremes of painful cold and painful hot.

pruriceptor A neural fiber that carries the sensation of itchiness

C tactile (CT) afferent A narrow-diameter, unmyelinated sensory nerve fiber that transmits signals from pleasant touch.

with various TRP channels also activated by natural foodstuffs, which span from noxious cold to noxious heat. Chili pepper and wasabi mustard (sushi, anyone?) are two foods that, at extreme levels, lead to pain. Each is associated with a thermoTRP channel (TRPV1 and TRPA1, respectively). When we say that food like chili feels hot, we are implicitly recognizing that the TRPV1 channel responds to intense thermal heat as well as spiciness. Mice lacking the TRPV1 channel are insensitive to heat at levels that normally cause pain. TRPV1 is also implicated as a channel for the induction of itch, which might cause you to wonder whether losing this channel would be such a bad thing (Ross, 2011)! Conversely, there is a TRP channel (TRPM8) associated with the sensation of noxious cold, and lack of this channel makes animals insensitive to a painfully cold surface contacting the skin.

When unpleasant consequences of somatosensation are considered, itch has been neglected relative to pain, despite the fact that chronic itch plagues a sizable segment of the population. It may be argued that itchiness is as great a pain as pain itself. In one extreme case, Mary Ellen Nilsen, over a period of a year after experiencing an outbreak of shingles (the same virus that causes chicken pox), scratched her scalp so intensively that she broke through the bone and damaged brain tissue. Researchers have now identified itch-specific receptors, or **pruriceptors**, in the form of a C fiber responsive to histamine, a molecule known to induce itchiness (Schmelz et al., 1997). Further, they have traced neural pathways that carry itch signals from the skin to the brain (Andrew and Craig, 2001). The separation of itch pathways from touch is demonstrated by mice whose itch neurons in the spinal cord were eliminated. They didn't scratch, even when injected with a substance that drove normal mice into scratching frenzies; the animals' response to pain, in contrast, was unaffected (Y.-G. Sun et al., 2009). Although we can identify distinct neural pathways for pain and itch, we will soon see that their signals intersect at the spinal cord, allowing one channel to influence the other.

PLEASANT TOUCH RECEPTORS Affective, or emotional, properties of non-painful bodily touch have been associated with a class of unmyelinated (and thus relatively slow) C fibers known as **C tactile (CT) afferents** (McGlone et al., 2007). This type of C fiber preferably responds to mechanical stimulation in the form of slowly moving, lightly applied forces (like petting!). The optimal stroke rates to produce firing in CT afferents are in the range of 1 to 10 centimeters (cm) per second. These correspond to speeds of stroking that people select as more pleasant (Perini, Olausson, and Morrison, 2015). CT afferents have been located only in hairy skin.

Isolating attributes of the pleasant touch system is rather difficult because, ordinarily, stimulation of the CT fibers also induces responses from the myelinated A-beta fibers that respond to general mechanical stimulation. This isolation has been made possible, however, by studies of individuals who lack A-beta fibers because of a rare disorder. One such individual, GL, feels no sensation of touch below the nose and cannot feel pleasant touch when stimulated on hairless skin. Yet when stroked on hairy skin with a brush, she can detect and coarsely localize the source, which she finds vaguely pleasant (Olausson et al., 2008; Björnsdotter et al., 2009). It has been suggested that the CT afferents form part of a neural subsystem that integrates the body with its sensory and social environment, inducing emotional, hormonal, and behavioral responses to skin-to-skin contact, as will be discussed further in Section 13.2 when submodalities of touch are introduced in detail.

Pathways from Skin to Brain

Initially, the axons of various tactile receptors are combined into single nerve trunks, in much the same way that retinal ganglion axons converge in the optic nerve (see

Chapter 2) and cochlear hair cells converge in the auditory nerve (see Chapter 9). This analogy omits important differences, however: First, whereas there are only two optic nerves and two auditory nerves, there are a number of somatosensory nerve trunks, arising in the hands, arms, feet, legs, and other areas of the skin. Second, the tactile nerves must carry their messages considerably farther. Because the receptors for sights, sounds, tastes, and smells are all located in the skull, the pathways that deliver information from these receptors to the brain are connected directly to the brainstem, rather than to nerves that have to travel up the spinal cord. Touch messages, however, must travel as far as 2 meters to get from the skin and muscles of the feet to the brain.

To cross this distance, the information must move up through the spinal cord. The cord is far more than a handy transmission pipe; its neural structure makes important contributions to the perceptual outcomes of touch. As described thus far, the nerve fibers arising from the skin might seem to constitute **labeled lines**; that is, each fiber type codes a particular touch sensation. Beyond the peripheral neural layer, however, the lines become interconnected, making it possible for complex patterns to emerge. The spinal cord is the site at which this cross communication is initiated.

The cell bodies associated with the tactile neural fibers are bundled into a cascade of ganglia, lumpy bodies that lie just outside the cord. The axons themselves enter the spinal cord at the **dorsal horn**, which is toward the back of the spinal column. The horn is organized into multiple layers, or laminae, as shown in FIGURE 13.9. Here again, a distinction is made between the different channels of somatosensation, with the pain and pleasant touch fibers entering the uppermost laminae of the horn and the A-beta fibers from mechanoreceptors entering more deeply. Every skin mechanoreceptor projects into the horn, although that may not be its only projection. The inputs to the cord are organized in a **somatotopic** manner. Somatotopy is analogous to the topographical spatial representation of events on the retina found in vision (see Chapter 3); adjacent areas on the skin are ultimately

labeled lines A theory of sensory coding in which each nerve fiber carries a particular stimulus quality.

dorsal horn A region at the rear of the spinal cord that receives inputs from receptors in the skin.

somatotopic Referring to spatial mapping in the somatosensory cortex in correspondence to spatial events on the skin.

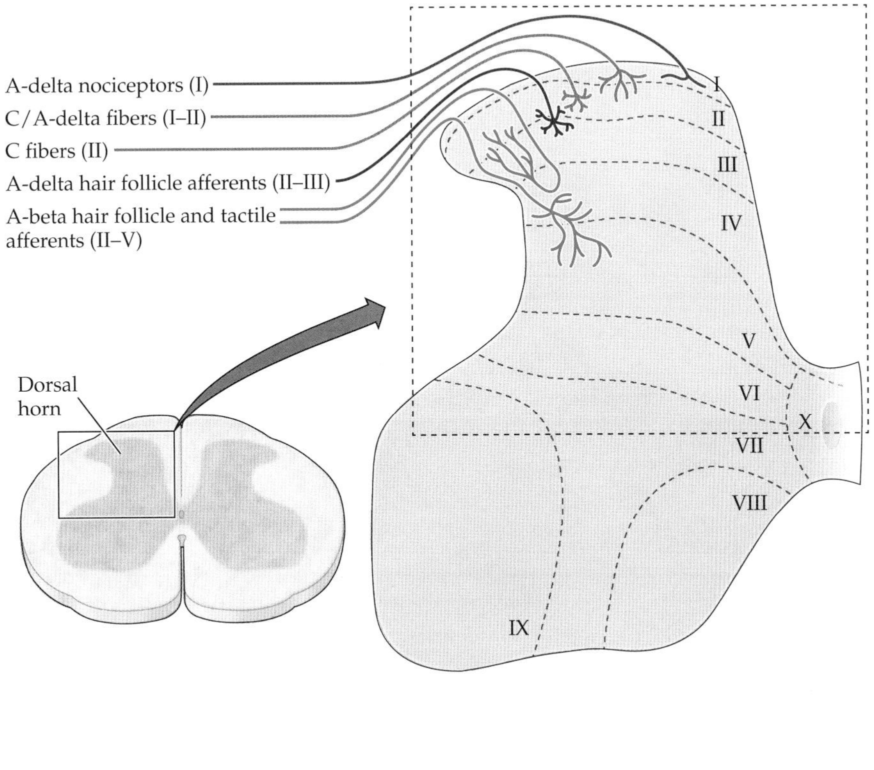

FIGURE 13.9 **Neural projections to the spinal cord** Neural projections to the dorsal horn of the spinal cord, based on the cat, rat, and monkey. The horn is divided into layers (laminae—of which layer II is the substantia gelatinosa). Afferent types terminate within the horn in a regular pattern, as shown.

spinothalamic pathway The route from the spinal cord to the brain that carries most of the information about skin temperature and pain.

dorsal column–medial lemniscal (DCML) pathway The route from the spinal cord to the brain that carries signals from skin, muscles, tendons, and joints.

connected to adjacent areas within a region of the cord. What may be surprising is that these inputs constitute only a small part of the neural structure of the dorsal horn. The axons and dendrites of most of the horn's neurons lie entirely within the spinal cord and serve as local connections, like the intermediate layers of the retina. In a review of dorsal horn function, Abraira and Ginty (2013) propose that it is this connectivity that provides the sense of touch with its rich canvas of effects, from caresses to pokes.

Once in the spinal cord, touch information proceeds upward toward the brain via two major pathways, as shown in FIGURE 13.10. The evolutionarily older **spinothalamic pathway** (FIGURE 13.10A) is the slower of the two and carries most of the information from thermoreceptors and nociceptors. The **dorsal column–medial lemniscal (DCML) pathway** (FIGURE 13.10B) includes wider-diameter axons and fewer synapses and therefore conveys information more quickly to the brain. Tactile and kinesthetic information carried along this pathway is used for planning and executing rapid movements, where quick feedback is a must. The DCML pathway not only includes fibers ascending directly from the mechanoreceptors, but also is densely populated by fibers from neurons originating in the dorsal horn, presumably conveying the output of the neural activity within the spinal cord.

Neurons in the DCML pathway first synapse in the cuneate and gracile nuclei, near the base of the brain (see Figure 13.10B). These synapses are not just waypoints; they are sites of complex information processing. The cuneate nucleus, in particular, contains neurons that selectively respond to features extracted from touched objects, like the orientation or direction of movement of an edge (Suresh et al., 2021). In this regard, they function more similarly to neurons found in somatosensory

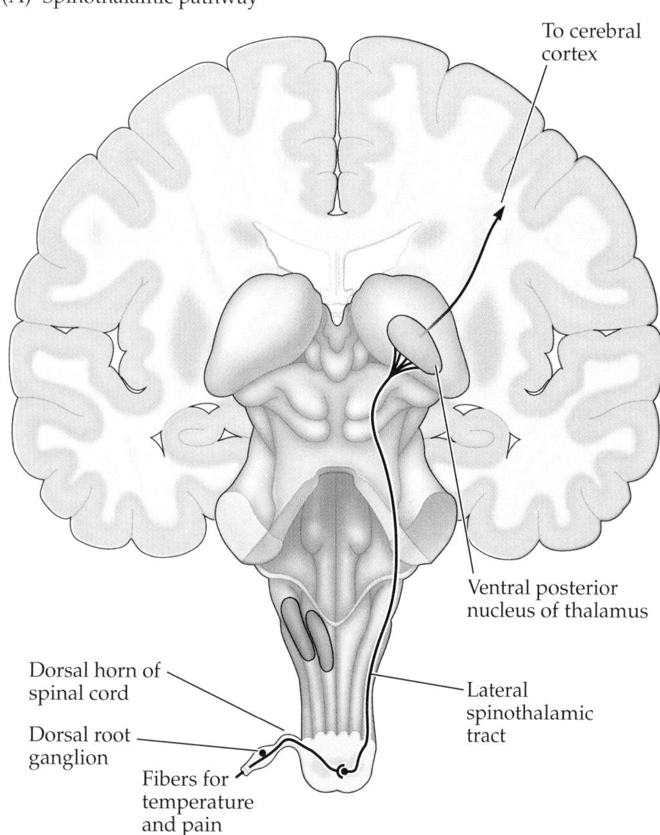

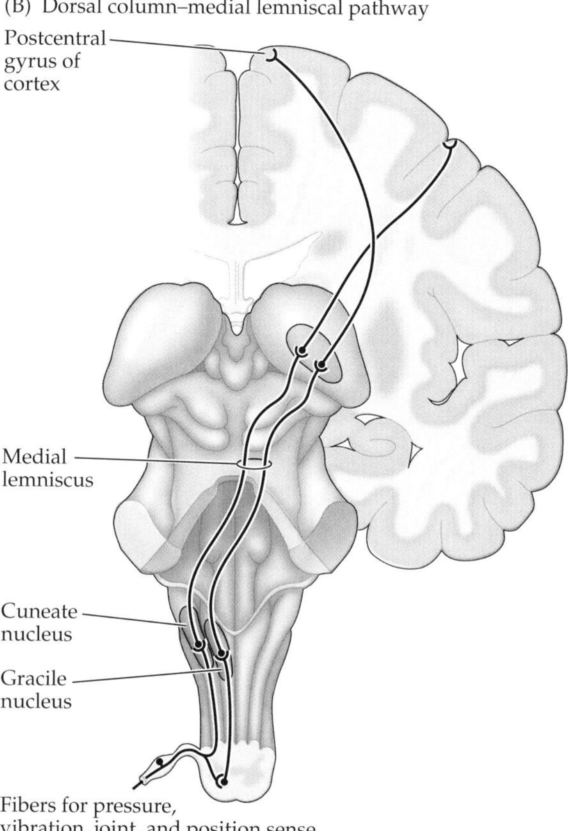

FIGURE 13.10 Pathways from skin to cortex (A) Spinothalamic pathway. (B) Dorsal column–medial lemniscal pathway.

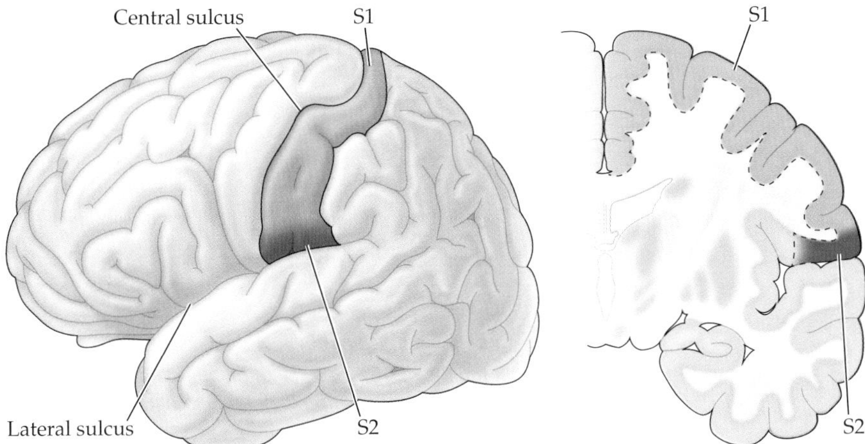

FIGURE 13.11 Primary somatosensory receiving areas in the brain Somatosensory area 1 (S1) includes multiple areas identified by the famous anatomist Brodmann on the basis of their cellular structure: 1, 2, 3a, and 3b. (Brodmann areas are not shown in this figure.) Somatosensory area 2 (S2) lies within the lateral sulcus.

areas of the brain (coming up next!) than to those in the skin. From these nuclei, activity is passed on to neurons that synapse in the ventral posterior nucleus of the thalamus. Recall from Chapters 3 and 9 that the visual and auditory pathways also pass through the thalamus, each synapsing in its own modality-specific nucleus.

From the thalamus, much of the touch information is carried up to the cortex (**FIGURE 13.11**) into **somatosensory area 1 (S1)**, located in the parietal lobe just behind the postcentral gyrus. In terms of its position in the transmission chain from the periphery to the brain, S1 is analogous to V1 (primary visual cortex) in vision (see Chapter 3). The receptive fields of neurons in this area maintain the analogy. Similar to the neurons in V1 that are selective to particular edge orientations, about half the neurons in S1 respond to bars pressed into or scanned over the skin at a particular orientation (Bensmaia et al., 2008). Neurons in S1 communicate with **somatosensory area 2 (S2)**, which lies in the upper bank of the lateral sulcus, and with other cortical areas. The motor areas of the cortex, which control movements of body parts, are located just in front of the central sulcus. This adjacency facilitates communication between the somatosensory and motor control systems.

Touch sensations that result from stimulation of the skin are represented in S1, and to some extent beyond, **somatotopically**. Similar to the skin's projection to the spinal cord, adjacent areas on the skin have a connection to adjacent areas in the brain (**FIGURE 13.12A**). As a result, the somatosensory cortex is organized into a spatial map (or, as we will see below, multiple maps) of the layout of the skin. Each map has been called a sensory **homunculus** (plural *homunculi*) (**FIGURE 13.12B**) and actually has a twin homunculus, because there are corresponding spatial maps in the left and right hemispheres.

The sensory homunculus was initially derived largely from the work of Canadian neurosurgeon Wilder Penfield, who charted the somatotopic map with the aid of patients undergoing brain surgery to alleviate epilepsy. Because there are no pain receptors in the brain, the patients did not need to be anesthetized and could remain responsive. During the operation, Dr. Penfield systematically stimulated different parts of a patient's somatosensory cortex with an electrode. As the probe was moved from one location in S1 to another, the patient reported feeling sensations in the arms, legs, face, and so on. The correspondence between the stimulation and the sensation gave rise to a map of the body in the brain. Newer tools now exist for associating body locations to brain areas using precise control of cortical stimulation (McMullen et al., 2021) and noninvasive imaging methods described in

somatosensory area 1 (S1) The primary receiving area for touch in the cortex.

somatosensory area 2 (S2) The secondary receiving area for touch in the cortex.

somatotypical Referring to normal somatosensation.

homunculus A maplike representation of regions of the body in the brain.

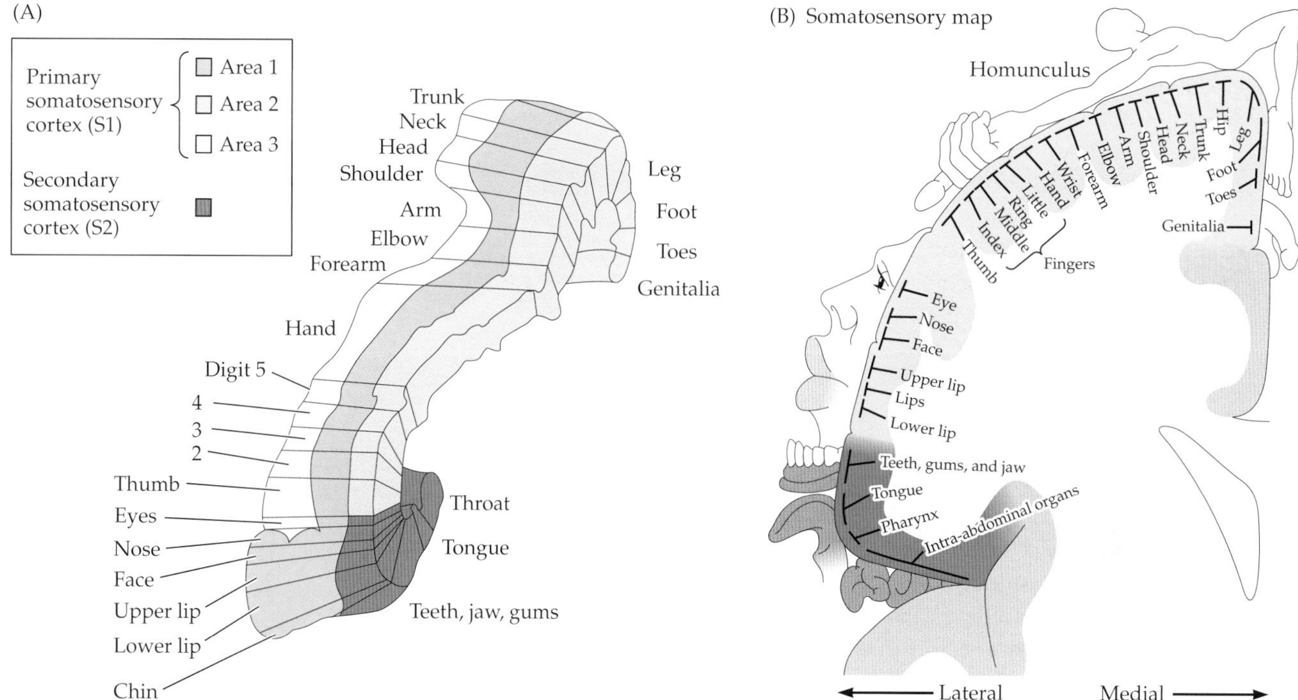

FIGURE 13.12 The sensory homunculus Brain regions respond to stimulation of different parts of the body. (A) Multiple maps exist in primary (S1) and secondary (S2) somatosensory areas, three of which are shown within S1 and one within S2. (B) A schematic of the relative distribution of body parts in S1.

Chapter 1. In fact, the brain contains multiple sensory maps of the body. Separate maps exist in the different subareas of S1, and additional maps exist in secondary areas, as shown in Figure 13.11A.

Like the retinotopic map in V1 (see Figure 3.18, Penfield's somatotopic map in S1 is distorted. The thumb, for example, grabs a big piece of cortical real estate relative to its physical size. In contrast, sensations from the leg are processed in a relatively small portion of S1. In the visual system, the foveal area is overrepresented in V1 (cortical magnification; see Chapter 3) because there are many more photoreceptors in the fovea than in peripheral parts of the retina. Similarly, a larger chunk of S1 is dedicated to processing information from the lips than from the neck because tactile receptors are much more heavily concentrated in the lips than they are in the neck.

Projections from S1 form the basis for further analysis of objects and surfaces by the cortex of the brain. Like vision (see Chapter 4), the sense of touch shows a division between *what* and *where* systems in higher cortical centers. People with unique touch impairments help to demonstrate this division. A patient studied by Reed, Caselli, and Farah (1996) had **tactile agnosia**—impairment in her ability to recognize objects by touch (*what*), but she showed no deficit in her spatial ability (*where*). In contrast, another patient could locate and manipulate objects by touch without recognizing them (Rossetti, Rode, and Boisson, 1995). Activation of the brain, observed with functional magnetic resonance imaging (fMRI; see Chapter 1), has been found in different areas, depending on whether the task is to locate an object or to recognize it tactually. And, as in vision, there is relatively more dorsal activation for locating objects and more ventral activation for recognizing objects (Reed, Shoham, and Halgren, 2004; Reed, Klatzky, and Halgren, 2005). A ventral area called the lateral occipital complex responds specifically to objects presented visually and haptically, which Lacey and Sathian (2012) have attributed

tactile agnosia The inability to identify objects by touch.

to a modality-independent representation of shape (*what*) in that region. In contrast, electroencephalography recordings (Chapter 1) implicate posterior parietal cortex, a dorsal region, in enabling people to determine *where* a handheld tool has been tapped, which they can do remarkably well without sight of the tool (L. E. Miller et al., 2019). When a patient who lacked proprioceptive neurons in her right upper arm felt the same taps on a tool, her ability to locate them, and the corresponding electroencephalography signals, resembled those of unimpaired participants, indicating that skin vibrations on the hand, not inputs from muscles and tendons, were used to determine where the taps occurred.

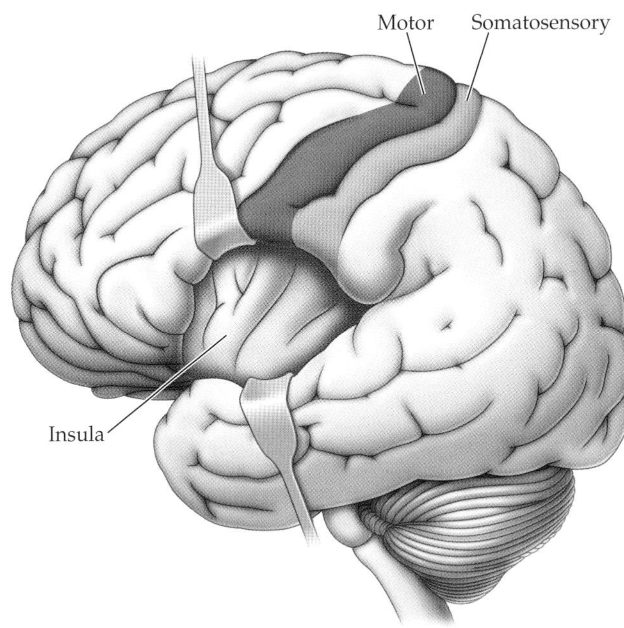

FIGURE 13.13 The insula Its location is beneath the surface of the brain, in proximity to sensory and motor areas.

Thus far, we have described the pathways of mechanical, thermal, and unpleasant touch signals to the brain. Pleasant touch, however, follows a different trajectory. Whereas primary somatosensory cortex is activated by the physical aspects of the stimulus (e.g., by the pressure it produces on the skin or a change in skin temperature), the CT system is associated with another brain area, the **insula**, which lies beneath the surface of the brain, in proximity to sensory and motor areas, as shown in FIGURE 13.13. The insula plays a role in regulating the body and linking sensory to emotional systems (Uddin et al., 2017). When GL, who has CT fibers but lacks input from tactile mechanoreceptors, was stimulated by brushing hairy skin, brain activation was found in the insula but not the somatosensory areas (Björnsdotter et al., 2009). Another area of the frontal lobes known to be involved in emotion—the orbitofrontal cortex—is also activated by pleasant mechanical stimulation (D. Francis et al., 1999). As described in Chapter 15, both insula and orbitofrontal cortex receive direct projections from the taste receptors.

A study by Case et al. (2016) shows a remarkable separation between the brain's processing of the stroking sensations and the pleasantness that results from stimulating CT fibers. Using fMRI, the researchers recorded brain activity while participants rated the pleasantness and intensity of stroking on hairy and glabrous portions of the hand at slow or fast rates (3 versus 30 cm per second). The results are shown in FIGURE 13.14. Intensity ratings corresponding to slow stroking of hairy skin were related to brain activity in the primary and secondary somatosensory cortices as well as the insula. Pleasantness ratings, however, were found to be related to brain activity in another area, the **anterior cingulate cortex (ACC)**, which we will soon encounter in the discussion of pain. The researchers then applied magnetic stimulation to the scalp to momentarily suppress activity in S1. This suppression resulted in reduced ratings of perceived stroke intensity, but no change in ratings of the degree to which pleasantness was experienced. The findings clearly implicate the ACC as a processor for the pleasantness of the CT stimulation, separately from the perception of the skin sensations from stroking, which is mediated by activation of S1.

insula A cortical area lying beneath the surface of the brain, which plays a role in regulating the body and linking sensory to emotional systems.

anterior cingulate cortex (ACC) A region of the brain associated with the perceived unpleasantness of a pain sensation.

Neural Plasticity of Somatosensation

So far, we have laid out the neural organization of touch from sensory receptors to brain as if it was unvarying. But before you reach that conclusion, consider an experiment performed by Pascual-Leone and Hamilton (2001). These neuroscientists deprived normal, sighted volunteers of visual stimulation by having them wear a

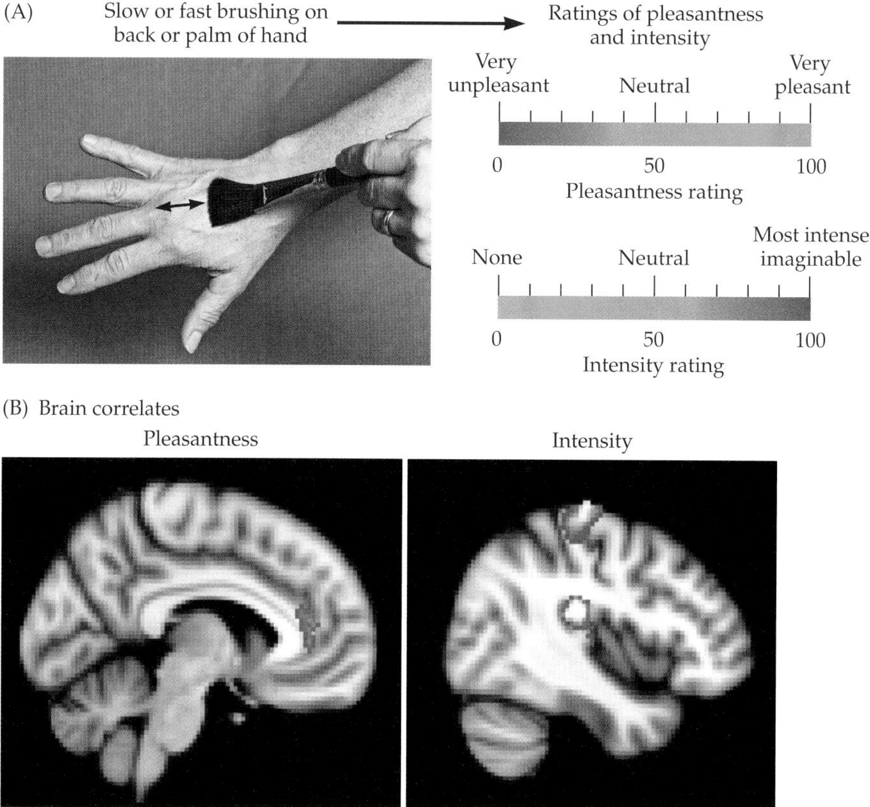

FIGURE 13.14 Intensity versus pleasantness of stroking Brain areas correlated with ratings of intensity versus pleasantness of stroking stimulation on hairy skin. Intensity ratings are related to brain activity in S1, S2, and insula. Pleasantness ratings are related to brain activity in the anterior cingulate.

blindfold for 5 days. Each day, the volunteers participated in an fMRI study during which Braille patterns were presented to the right index finger. Participants were required to judge whether two patterns were the same or different. Brain imaging found that on the first day, the Braille task activated only S1 on the left side of the brain (which, because of the neural pathways from the skin, is activated by touching the right side of the body). But as the days progressed, the amount of activation declined in S1 while increasing in V1. Apparently, area V1, which we think of as dedicated to vision, took over processing the spatial patterns introduced through the sense of touch. This change in V1 was transient: removing the blindfold resulted in a full return to the neural functioning that had been observed before blindfolding.

Such results reveal the remarkable **neural plasticity** of the somatosensory system. Plasticity is a recurring theme in sensory systems. We saw something very similar at the end of Chapter 3 in the discussion of visual development and strabismus, in which abnormal experience alters the wiring of the visual system. Note that the example we're discussing here shows that plasticity is a property of the adult brain and is not limited to the immature nervous system.

The philosopher William Molyneux was probably not thinking about neural plasticity when, in 1688, he posed the question to John Locke about whether a blind person who was suddenly able to see would recognize objects previously known only by touch (**FIGURE 13.15**). Medical interventions eventually made it possible to answer this question by providing sight to congenitally blind individuals. It was demonstrated that although visual objects like spheres and cubes are not connected immediately to their touched equivalents, only a few days of visual experience are needed to make the connection (Held et al., 2011). This surprising finding, given the individuals' long-term experience without vision, underscores

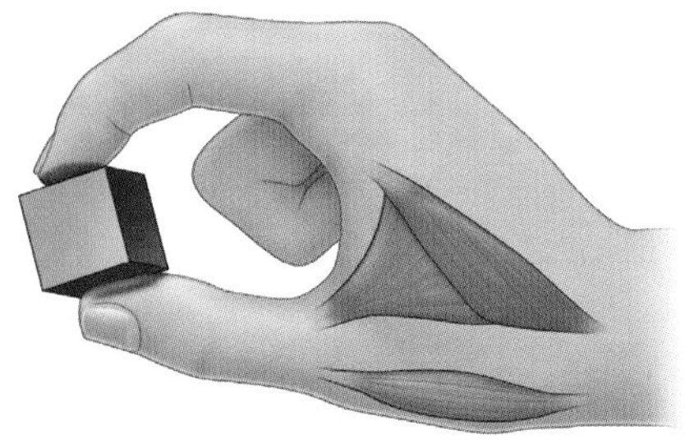

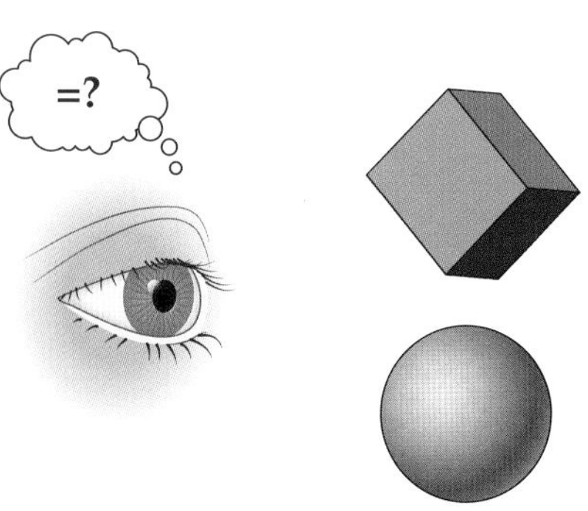

FIGURE 13.15 Molyneux's problem Would a person suddenly given sight, who previously sensed a cube only through cutaneous (skin) and kinesthetic (muscle/tendon/joint) receptors, be able to match it to its visual equivalent?

the plastic nature of the perceptual system. Bumblebees may even beat humans in making cross-modal connections: when raised in total darkness, where they were rewarded for discriminating cubes from spheres by touch, the creatures could instantly tell the shapes apart in a lighted environment while prevented from touching their outsides (Solvi, Gutierrez al-Khudhairy, and Chittka, 2020). ●

Some of the most remarkable consequences of neural plasticity in touch can be seen in cases where a limb has been lost. An unfortunate side effect reflects the correspondence between body parts and areas of S1. If an amputee's left arm is missing, obviously no receptors are sending touch signals from that arm to the corresponding maps in the right S1 area of the brain. However, sporadic activity can continue in the area corresponding to the arm, leading to the perception of a **phantom limb**. At times, individuals may perceive their phantom limbs to be in uncomfortable positions, leading to persistent (and very real) pain. The psychologist Vilayanur Ramachandran made the astonishing observation that amputees often report feeling sensations in their phantom arms and hands when their faces or remaining limbs are touched (**FIGURE 13.16**). The source of this somatosensory confusion can be traced to an idiosyncrasy in the homunculus. Note in Figure 13.12 that the area responding to the face is located (somewhat arbitrarily) adjacent to the area responding to the hand and arm. Apparently, the hand and arm areas of S1 are, to some extent, "invaded" by neurons carrying information from touch receptors in the face. However, other parts of the brain listening to the hand and arm areas are not fully aware of these altered connections, and therefore they attribute activity in these areas to stimulation from the missing limb.

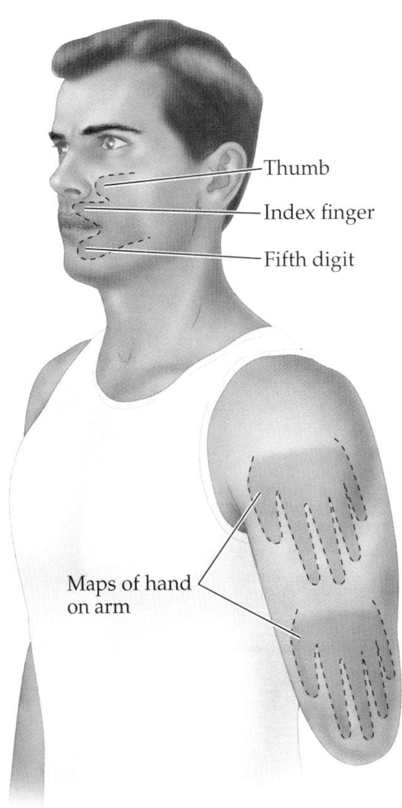

FIGURE 13.16 Phantom limbs Amputated limbs may be perceived on the face and stump subsequent to removal. Amputees report feeling the amputated hand when their face or remaining limbs are stimulated.

Plasticity following amputation is not entirely negative, however; it opens the door to novel interventions intended to enable a useful limb. A number of people have received transplants of whole hands from cadavers to the remaining portion of their forearm, which involves reconnecting blood vessels and nerves and bridging bone (**FIGURE 13.17A**). Frey et al. (2008) reported the case of a 54-year-old man who received a transplant 35 years after his own hand was lost in an industrial accident. Four months later, stimulating the palm of the transplanted hand evoked activity in the S1 on the opposite side of the brain, at a level that matched normal controls. Two years later, the patient was able to wield a hammer, throw a baseball, and open doors. The story doesn't end here, however. Other transplant cases have been less successful on a functional level, and complications can result from the drugs needed to prevent rejection of the hand by the recipient's body. Some patients have even elected to have the transplant removed.

Another approach to aiding amputees is less biologically invasive but again exploits neural plasticity. This promising avenue to rehabilitation is the "bionic" hand. The version shown in **FIGURE 13.17B** (George et al., 2019) allows a closed-loop form of control that attempts to closely mimic biological signals, called **biomimetic feedback**. The user's forearm muscles control the prosthetic hand, which is capable of dexterous interaction with the world. The resulting contact events are signaled back to the remaining sensory nerves in the stump of the arm. In experiments, the researchers compared different types of feedback: (1) turning on a signal whenever the sensors indicated the prosthesis was in contact with a surface, (2) turning on a signal at contact and increasing its magnitude directly with the sensed force, or (3) an algorithm designed to resemble natural neural activation, in the form of strong

neural plasticity The ability of neural circuits to undergo changes in function or organization as a result of previous activity.

phantom limb Sensation perceived from a physically amputated limb of the body.

biomimetic feedback A system that attempts to closely mimic biological signals.

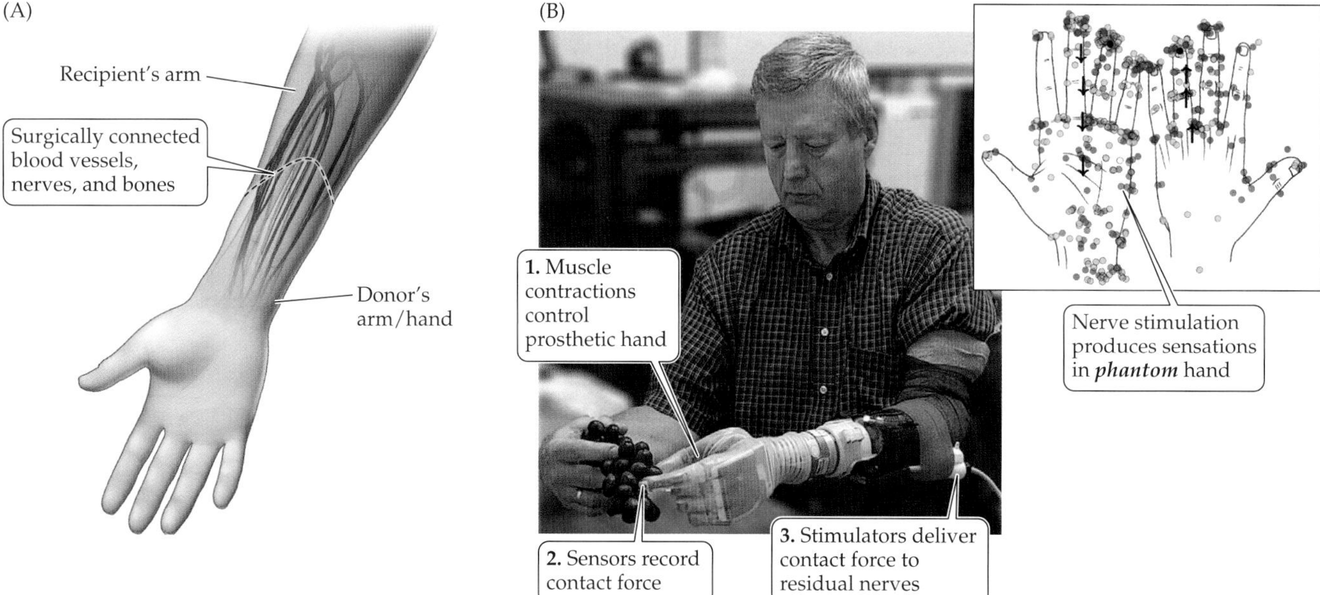

FIGURE 13.17 Two versions of alleviating sensory loss (A) Transplants from a cadaver hand and forearm to a recipient involve reconnecting blood vessels, nerves, and bridging bone. Recipients have acquired sensory responses and motor function even when the transplant occurred years after the loss of their natural limbs. (B) A biomimetic prosthetic limb controlled through arm muscles enables fine manipulation and (inset) leads to the experience of phantom sensations when the limb is touched.

stimulation at initial contact that decreased as the pressure on the prosthesis became steady. The user shown in Figure 13.17B could interact with fragile objects and discriminate properties like size and softness by the neural signals provided, most effectively when the feedback was biomimetic (option 3). In addition, stimulation of the residual nerves led the user to experience sensations that were described as tactile events—vibration, pressure, and even pain—*apparently originating from locations on the bionic hand!* Essentially, the bionic limb acted as a phantom, but functional, limb.

The distortion in the brain's map is echoed in how people perceive their own bodies, or their **body image**. Fuentes, Longo, and Haggard (2013) had people draw maps of their own bodies on a computer by clicking on locations of body parts relative to the on-screen image of a head. People's body image proves to be systematically distorted toward top-heaviness, with expanded shoulders and upper arms, but with lower arms and legs reduced in size (**FIGURE 13.18**). The body representation can be changed by experience, even by something as mundane as wielding a tool (**FIGURE 13.19**). After blindly wielding a tool to retrieve objects arranged on the floor, wielders were asked to indicate the location of their elbow and wrist under an occluding box, thereby indicating the subjective length of the forearm. Like Pinocchio's nose after lying, it grew! For a tool that was 100 cm in length, the increase in perceived arm length amounted to over 1 cm, suggesting that about 1% of the tool had been incorporated into the mental representation of the arm (Canzoneri et al., 2013).

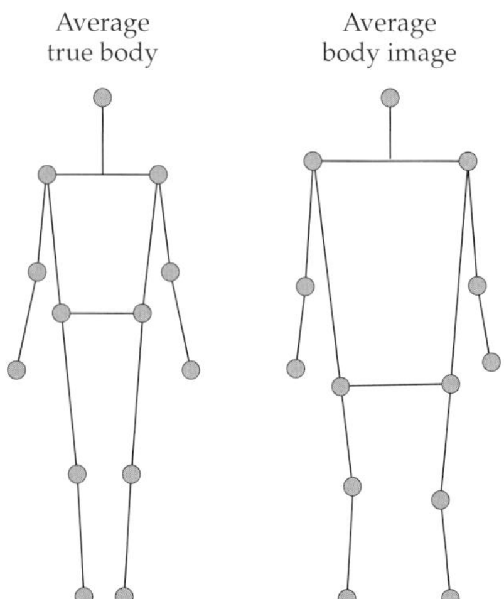

FIGURE 13.18 The body image Shape of the body as determined from locations of parts (dots) for people's true body (left) and locations they report relative to the head, which form their body image (right). Multiple maps are averaged by scaling each one relative to the person's body height.

The body image changes with direct transformation of the body itself, as was shown by the results of a surgical procedure to elongate arms shortened by dwarfism (Cimmino et al., 2013). Within 6 months, the patient's body image of her upper limbs changed from being shortened to being congruent with normal controls, while the lower portion of her body image remained unchanged.

The pathways from the skin to the brain tell just one part of the story of the transmission of signals in touch. Downward pathways from the brain can alter the sensations that stimulating the periphery produces. We will see such effects when considering the submodalities of touch.

(A)

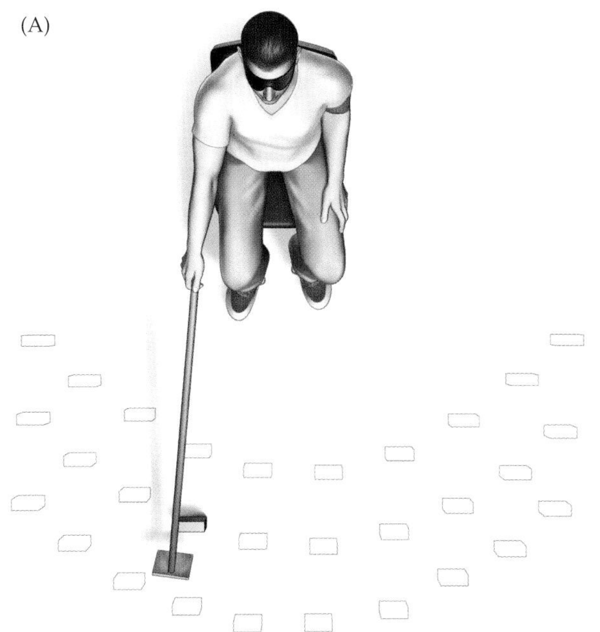

(B)

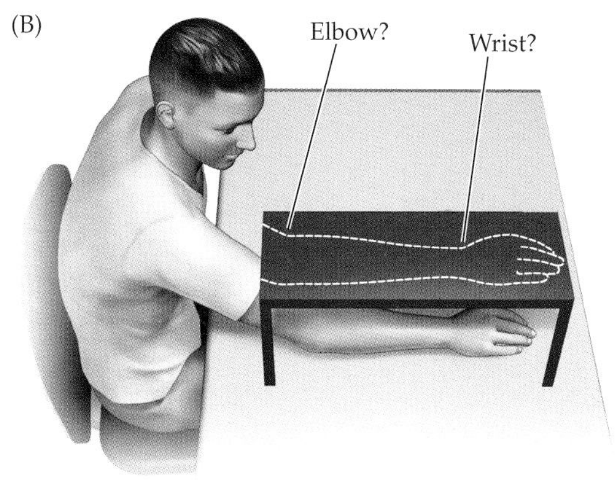

FIGURE 13.19 Distortion of the body image after tool use (A) The participant wields a tool to find targets. (B) Subsequently, the participant identifies the location of hidden joints at the elbow and the wrist, revealing an illusory increase in arm length.

13.2 Submodalities of Touch

Now that we've covered the physiological substrate of the touch system, we can focus on psychological aspects, ranging from the sensory limits that we can measure with psychophysical techniques to complex perceptual, cognitive, and emotional responses. As noted previously, touch psychology encompasses multiple submodalities, corresponding to different types of information that are delivered by the neural receptors, along with distinct contexts in which that information is interpreted and used. Discriminative touch is the submodality that may come to mind first. As described previously, this component of touch relies on mechanical and thermal sensations for information about surfaces and objects with which we are in contact. Pain and itch are closely connected submodalities, each having aversive sensory consequences. Affective touch, which comprises emotional and social components, constitutes yet another submodality. We'll take a look at tickle here as well.

body image The mental representation of how our bodies appear in space.

The Submodality of Discriminative Touch

Perception of objects and surfaces begins with the mechanical stimulation from pressure against the skin. Scientific understanding of this submodality begins with questions about its most basic capabilities: How sensitive are we to mechanical stimulation? What are the limits on tactile acuity in space and time? Put a bit differently, what are the smallest details that we can feel?

SENSITIVITY TO MECHANICAL PRESSURE To measure the minimum pressure that can be reliably sensed by a particular region of skin, we need a way to present well-defined amounts of pressure over and over again. In the nineteenth century, Max von Frey (1852–1932) developed an elegant and simple way to do this using carefully calibrated stimuli, including horse and human hairs. Modern researchers typically use nylon monofilaments (e.g., fishing lines) of varying diameters. The smaller the diameter, the less force the line applies to the skin before it buckles.

To replicate von Frey's method yourself, touch different parts of your skin with a hair from your head and a bristle from a hairbrush to reveal the relative skin sensitivity to these two different forces. With the thinner hair, you will probably find that you can feel it on the more sensitive areas, such as your lips and perhaps some parts of your hand. You probably will not feel it pushing into your thigh or upper arm. With the bristle, however, you should discover that your skin is sensitive to mechanical pressure all over, but not uniformly so. For example, if you explore the skin on the back of your hand, you should be able to convince yourself that there are spots of greater and lesser sensitivity (Geldard, 1972).

Data from more controlled pressure sensitivity studies reveal that thresholds vary across different sites of the body (a high threshold means that that part of the body is less sensitive). In general, tactile pressure sensitivity is highest on the face, followed by the trunk and upper extremities (arms and fingers) and then the lower extremities (thigh, calf, and foot) (Weinstein, 1968). The pattern for males and females is very similar, except that women tend to be more sensitive to pressure than men. Sensitivity to temperature changes, as well as to pain, also varies markedly as a function of body site.

Another approach to measuring sensitivity is to ask what the smallest raised element is that we can feel as an otherwise completely smooth surface is passed over the skin. Like the storied princess who detected a pea under a pile of mattresses, we appear to be very sensitive to the pressure difference caused by a raised dot on a smooth surface. At a criterion of 75% detection, people can detect a dot only 1 micrometer high—that's a millionth of a meter, or 39 millionths of an inch! The dot seems to trigger detection by the FA I receptors, which also help us detect and correct for an object slipping as we grasp it. Even more impressive, when a texture that is made of many raised dots only a very small fraction of a micrometer high moves across the skin, the resulting vibrations trigger the FA II receptors deep within the skin, enabling us to distinguish the dots from a perfectly smooth surface (LaMotte and Srinivasan, 1991). How sensitive the skin is measured to be depends on the precision of measurement, it appears, as much as on the skin. Advanced techniques have allowed wrinkles scaled in nanometers (nm = one billionth of a meter) to be manufactured, and the smallest wrinkle height that can be detected by rubbing the surfaces is approximately 10 nm (Skedung et al., 2013)!

People are also sensitive to changes in pressure over time—that is, to tactile vibration. **FIGURE 13.20** shows the absolute vibratory threshold (the minimum

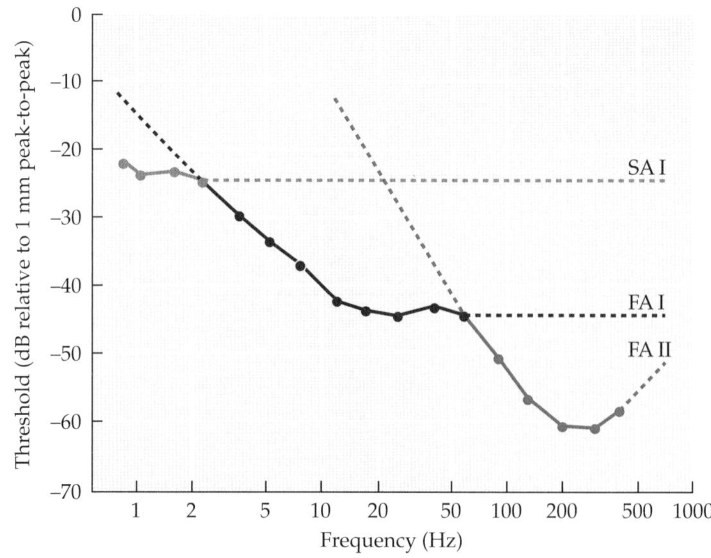

FIGURE 13.20 Vibratory thresholds Results of an experiment measuring the minimal (threshold) amplitude of vibration at the fingertip that people can detect, as a function of the vibratory frequency. As labeled on the *y*-axis, the threshold is measured on a decibel (dB) scale relative to a reference vibration (see Chapter 9). The experimentally obtained function, portrayed by the solid line, is believed to reflect the contribution of three different mechanoreceptor populations (SA I, FA I, and FA II), which are shown as different-colored segments. Each population is assumed to control the threshold in the limited frequency range where it is most sensitive. For comparison, the dashed lines in different colors show the vibratory thresholds for the corresponding mechanoreceptor populations across the entire range of frequencies tested. These lines cannot be obtained from the experiment portrayed here but, rather, are based on the results of neurophysiological studies of single-unit mechanoreceptor responses. Researchers have proposed that SA I units mediate our threshold for vibrations below about 5 Hz; FA I fibers, for frequencies from about 5 to 50 Hz; and FA II units, for frequencies above about 50 Hz.

amount that a vibrating stimulus displaces the skin in order to be detected) as a function of the frequency presented to the fingertip (Löfvenberg and Johansson, 1984). In this study, people could detect the presence of vibrations from below about 5 Hz up to about 400 Hz, the highest frequency that was tested. Other studies have confirmed that people can detect vibrations up to 700 Hz (Verrillo, 1963).

Although people can detect vibrations over a wide frequency range, they are not equally sensitive to all frequencies, as Figure 13.20 clearly shows. Since the various mechanoreceptor populations are sensitive to different frequencies, the overall psychophysical function for the detection of vibration reflects the contributions of different mechanoreceptor populations at different levels of vibration. Take a look at the corresponding vibration sensitivities of SA I, FA I, and FA II mechanoreceptor populations at frequencies from under 5 to 400 Hz, also shown in Figure 13.20. The SA I receptors seem to mediate our absolute vibratory thresholds for frequencies below about 5 Hz; the FA I receptors for frequencies from about 5 to 50 Hz; and the FA II receptors for frequencies above about 50 Hz.

RESOLUTION OF SPATIAL DETAILS Pressure detection is the tactile equivalent of detecting a spot of light, where the basic question is whether you can see or feel anything at all. For the tactile equivalent of visual acuity (can you make out the pattern of what you see or feel?), try measuring your **two-point touch threshold**. As the name suggests, this is the smallest separation at which we can tell that we're being touched by two points and not just one. This experiment is best done with a partner, although it will work to some degree if you test yourself. A compass (the kind that draws circles) is a useful stimulator, but you can use anything that enables you to vary the separation between two points, such as a bent paper clip. Pick one of your own or your partner's body regions, and see if you can distinguish between a single point and two points. Then repeat the procedure with different separations of the two points (e.g., 0.5, 2, and 4 cm) and at different places on the skin (**FIGURE 13.21**).

Like sensitivity to pressure, spatial acuity varies across the body. Systematic studies of two-point touch thresholds as a function of body site demonstrate that the extremities (hands, face, feet) show the highest acuity (Weinstein, 1968; Mancini et al., 2014) (**FIGURE 13.22**). On the fingertips, we are capable of resolving a separation of only about 1 mm (Loomis, 1981). These results place tactile acuity

two-point touch threshold The minimum distance at which two stimuli (e.g., two simultaneous touches) are just perceptible as separate.

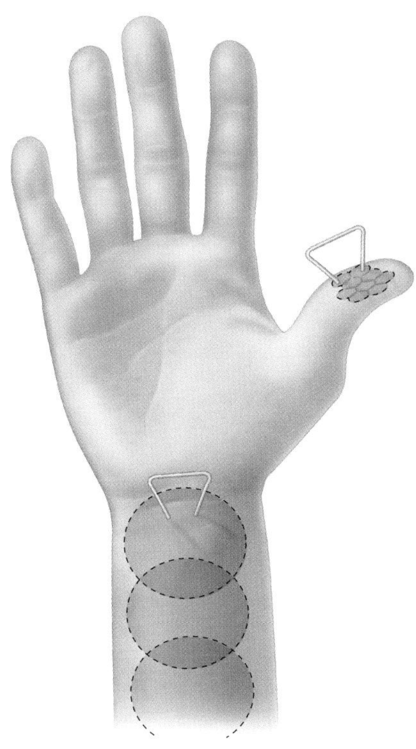

FIGURE 13.21 Measuring two-point touch thresholds The ability to separate two points depends primarily on the concentration and receptive-field sizes of tactile receptors in an area of the skin. The triangles represent point stimulators, and the circles represent the areas of skin that would respond to a single stimulation.

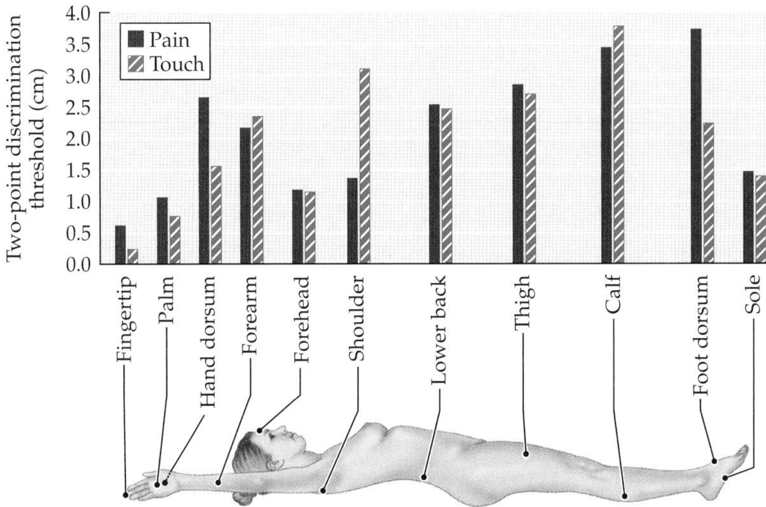

FIGURE 13.22 The two-point discrimination threshold for pain and touch The threshold is the minimal separation between two stimulated points on the body needed to perceive them as separate.

somewhere between vision and audition: it is worse than visual acuity, but better than auditory spatial resolution.

After looking at the two-point threshold for spatial acuity with pressure stimulation, we might ask, How does this compare to spatial acuity for pain? A stumbling block on measuring pain acuity is the difficulty of constructing pinpoint-sized painful stimuli that people can be asked to differentiate. By delivering very small pulses of radiant heat, the laser has made it possible to determine the threshold distance between two pain locations that can be resolved as distinct (Mancini et al., 2014). Figure 13.22 compares the two-point threshold between pain and touch at various body sites. The skin of the hand and forehead shows the greatest sensitivity (lowest threshold) for both, and at these locations, spatial acuity for pressure is slightly superior to that for pain. On other parts of the body, however, pain and touch diverge, and touch is not always the winner. For example, the shoulder differentiates points of pain better than it does points of mechanical pressure.

Note the general correspondence between the pattern of two-point touch thresholds across the body in Figure 13.22 and the relative distortion of different body parts in the sensory homunculus of Figure 13.12. This match is not coincidental. The determination that two closely spaced points instead of just one are touching your skin requires that your brain receive two separate signals. This means that at the skin there must be a sufficient concentration of receptors, each with a small enough receptive field that the two contact points will elicit different responses. An additional constraint is that as the signals are sent to the cortex, they must not converge. A chunk of cortical real estate large enough to receive them separately is necessary. In short, the two-point threshold is low (that is, the ability to discern two very close points as separate is high) only when the density of receptors is relatively high, the receptive fields are small, and cortical convergence does not occur. Tactile spatial acuity thresholds are mediated by the SA I (and possibly FA I) tactile receptors, which have relatively small receptive fields and high receptor densities. Where pain and tactile sensitivity differ, as in the relative acuity of the shoulder versus the forearm seen in Figure 13.22, the patterns follow the density of the receptor populations for touch versus pain in those regions of the body.

Although useful, the traditional two-point touch test has some drawbacks, as you may see when you try your own experiment. Even if the two stimulated points feel like one, it is not quite the same as stimulating the skin with a single continuous contact. Therefore, asking people whether they are really being touched by one point or two yields quite a different answer than does asking them if it *feels like* one point or two, especially in sensitive areas such as the fingertip. Alternatives that are more objective have been suggested, including accuracy of judging whether an edge has a gap or indicating how a grating (a surface with alternating grooves and ridges) applied to the skin is oriented—along versus across the finger (Craig and Johnson, 2000).

RESOLUTION OF TEMPORAL DETAILS After discussing spatial acuity, let's consider the temporal equivalent—how well people can detect small timing differences in tactile stimulation. Various psychophysical methods have been used to address this question. One requires participants to decide whether two tactile pulses delivered to the skin are simultaneous or separated in time. With this method, participants can resolve a temporal difference of only 5 milliseconds (ms) (Gescheider, 1974). Touch proves to be better than vision (which is 25 ms) but worse than audition (0.01 ms) (Sherrick and Cholewiak, 1986). As with spatial acuity, you will notice that touch falls somewhere between vision and audition; in this case, however, audition is best and vision worst.

INDIVIDUAL DIFFERENCES IN TACTILE SENSITIVITY If you are a sighted person reading this book conventionally, your tactile sensitivity in 10 years is likely not to be what it is today; a decline with age is to be expected. Studies of blind people who read Braille reveal an exciting exception to this trend, however: Legge and colleagues (2008) tested the ability of blind and sighted people to identify raised three-dot patterns derived from Braille symbols, displayed at different scales. They found that sighted adults lost about 1% per year in their acuity levels between their teens and their 80s, but blind Braille readers showed essentially no age-related decline (**FIGURE 13.23**). There is an unfortunate implication of this trend for people who lose their sight late in life (a sizable proportion of the blind population). The zero point on the left vertical axis is set to the standard spacing between Braille dots; once the threshold-level font size passes above it (at around 74 years of age), fingertip sensitivity is not sufficient to read Braille. But wait! Is it blindness per se that preserves tactile acuity, or might it be the day-to-day practice of attending to tactile stimulation on the fingers? To answer this question, Legge et al. (2019) examined another population that pays attention to touch, namely, experienced pianists. When applied to the musicians, the same dot-pattern tests previously used on the blind revealed some decline in acuity with age, but far less than the loss evident in the previously tested sighted population. Another tactile acuity test found the older pianists performing as well as the blind. It appears that tactile acuity can be maintained across a lifetime, as long as it is a lifetime of close attention to touch.

Aside from practice, another factor that affects your tactile sensitivity is, apparently, your genes. Both tactile spatial acuity and vibratory sensitivity are more correlated in identical than in nonidentical twins, pointing to a genetic contribution (Frenzel et al., 2012). The same study asked whether genes that influence one sense organ that responds to pressure, the skin, might also influence

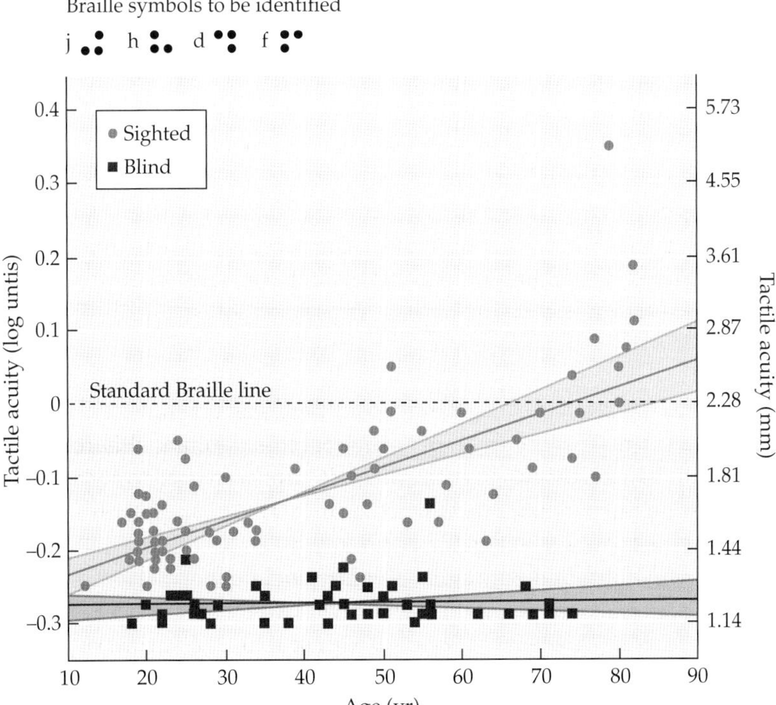

FIGURE 13.23 Tactile acuity versus age Acuity is measured by the accuracy of symbol identification when using the index finger, across different scales. The left vertical axis uses a log measure, where the spacing of dots in a standard Braille character is set to zero (dashed line). On the right vertical axis, the measure is the distance between dot centers within the identified characters in millimeters (mm). The bands around the lines that are fit to the data represent 95% confidence intervals.

another, the ear. They found that hearing acuity was significantly correlated with both tactile spatial acuity and the threshold for warmth; moreover, individuals who had genetic mutations leading to early deafness showed reduced spatial and vibratory sensitivity in touch. Thus, common genes appear to be expressed in multiple sensory forms.

In contrast to the reduced sensitivity associated with early deafness, individuals diagnosed with autism spectrum disorder display heightened sensitivity to a broad range of touch stimulation: thermal and vibratory, and in glabrous and hairy skin. These responses are so intense that they have been described as overwhelming (Tomchek and Dunn, 2007). A possible genetic basis for this sensitivity has been identified by modifying the genes of mice so as to affect their processing of touch afferents (Orefice et al., 2016). Relative to controls, the modified mice were more sensitive to an air puff on the skin but, conversely, showed less discrimination between textures when exploring them with the hairless skin on their paws—which they were induced to do by removing their whiskers. In conjunction with these sensory deficits, the genetically modified mice showed deficits in social behaviors. They explored the world around them less and failed to habituate to repeated noise, indicators of anxiety. They constructed nests of lower quality and didn't approach another mouse any more than an empty cup, indicators that they were less sociable. These social deficits appear to be specific to animals whose touch is altered early in development. This was shown by comparing the genetically modified strain to a set of controls in which corresponding somatosensory abnormalities were chemically induced during adulthood. While the controls showed alteration similar to that of the genetically modified mice on tactile sensitivity tests, they were not afflicted by the same anxiety and social nonresponsiveness. The specificity of these latter effects to mice whose sensory systems were affected at birth suggests that the altered sensations of early experience played a critical role in engendering the deficits in personality (or should we say, "mouseness") observed in the adult. A counterpart to these results can be found in humans with autism spectrum disorders, who show multimodal sensory differences. The mouse genetic model suggests that a developmental pathway encompassing not only touch, but also multiple sensory modalities could contribute to the social phenomena associated with the condition.

The Submodality of Affective Touch

Touch can act as the "feel-good" sense. Feeling good arises from a pat on the back (which is such a positive experience it has become a metaphor for praise), being stroked on the arm, hugging, or, in some cultures, rubbing noses. The functioning of neural fibers called C tactile (or CT for short), which were previously described as pleasant touch receptors, is central to these experiences. Recall that CT fibers are activated when hairy skin is stroked at a particular rate, around 1 to 10 cm per second.

The influence of CT activation begins with adult-infant interactions. Caregivers tend to spontaneously stroke at the appropriate rate for pleasant touch when touching a real baby, but not when petting an artificial arm (Croy, Fairhurst, and McGlone, 2016). The importance of parental skin contact for the welfare of premature infants has been demonstrated by analyzing hormones related to well-being and stress. During contact by mothers and fathers, levels of oxytocin (a hormone associated with childbirth and social bonding) increase, and levels of cortisol (a stress-related hormone) decrease, as do measures of anxiety (Cong et al., 2015). Fairhurst, Loken, and Grossmann (2014) stroked 9-month-old infants with a soft brush at a preferred speed for pleasant touch of 3 cm per second or at faster or slower speeds (30 and

0.3 cm per second, respectively) (**FIGURE 13.24**). They found that during periods of stroking at the moderate speed, infants' heart rates declined, whereas at speeds slower or faster, they slightly increased. Individual infants' responsiveness to optimal brush stroking was correlated with reports of how much their parents liked to give, receive, and observe touch.

Adults as well as infants show beneficial effects of activating the CT system. Experiments that involve stroking hairy skin at appropriate speeds have revealed a remarkable range of positive effects. Optimal stroking elicits activity in smile muscles that is not evident at other speeds (Pawling et al., 2017). Electroencephalography recordings indicate that CT-targeted stroking makes people more attentive to the emotional content of voices (Schirmer and Gunter, 2017). Another important effect demonstrates interactions between the pleasant touch and pain channels; stroking hairy skin reduces the experienced pain from thermal heat. This analgesic effect of pleasant touch does not extend to people with damage to C fibers, further implicating the specific role of the CT fibers in reducing discomfort (Habig et al., 2017).

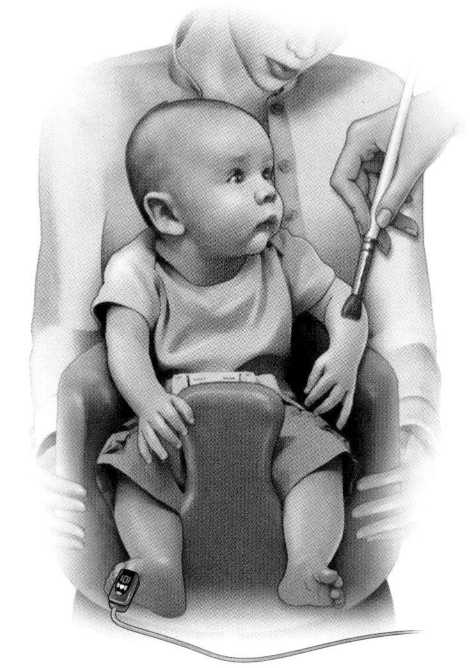

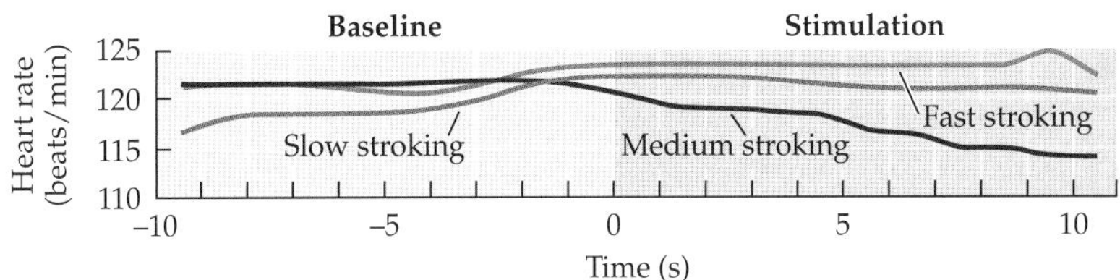

FIGURE 13.24 Effects of pleasant touch Baby being stimulated by brushstrokes and resulting change in heart rate for three different speeds of stroking.

Although the CT fibers are called the pleasant touch receptors, social contact occurs in broader contexts than stroking hairy skin. Accordingly, an overarching concept of "social touch" has been invoked to recognize that multiple neural pathways interact to influence the well-being we experience from physical interactions. Patterns of touch associated with specific social messages have been identified, as shown in **FIGURE 13.25** (McIntyre et al., 2022). Receivers of a touch pattern on the arm from an unseen partner were able to pick the intended message from a list with above-chance accuracy. Social touch further prominently involves what was introduced in Chapter 1 as "top-down" processing, whereby knowledge and context enhance our ability to interpret sensory input. While the physical patterns shown in Figure 13.25 can be confusing (like mistaking calming for love), context would make the sender's intention clear. Social top-down influence emerges early in life, as shown by 9-month-old infants, whose heart rate is lowered more by optimal stroking from a known caregiver than from a stranger (Aguirre et al., 2019).

Variations in caregiving environments mean that infants and children will have different experiences with social touch, which appear to have long-term consequences (Cascio, Moore, and McGlone, 2019). In addition to effects of an individual's history of touch-related behaviors, there may also be a genetic component to how people respond to contact. It has been found that touch affects social interactions through individual characteristics that we think of as genetically determined, like personality. Work in the field of epigenetics has led to a model describing how the expression of genes related to social interaction is controlled by touch in the rat. Mother rats that lick and groom their pups produce

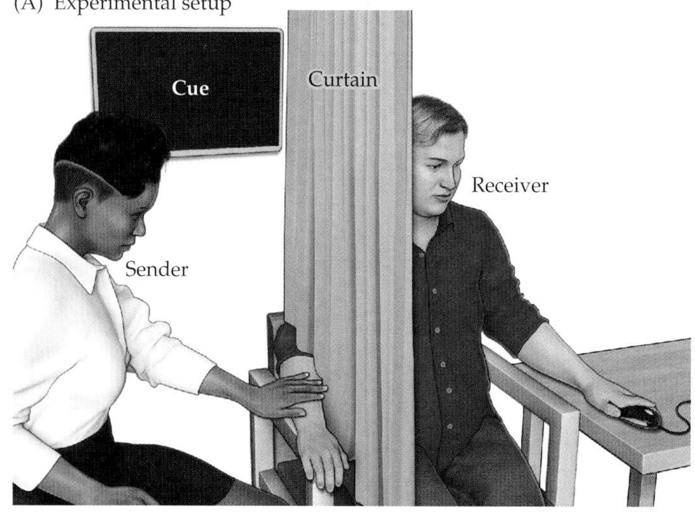

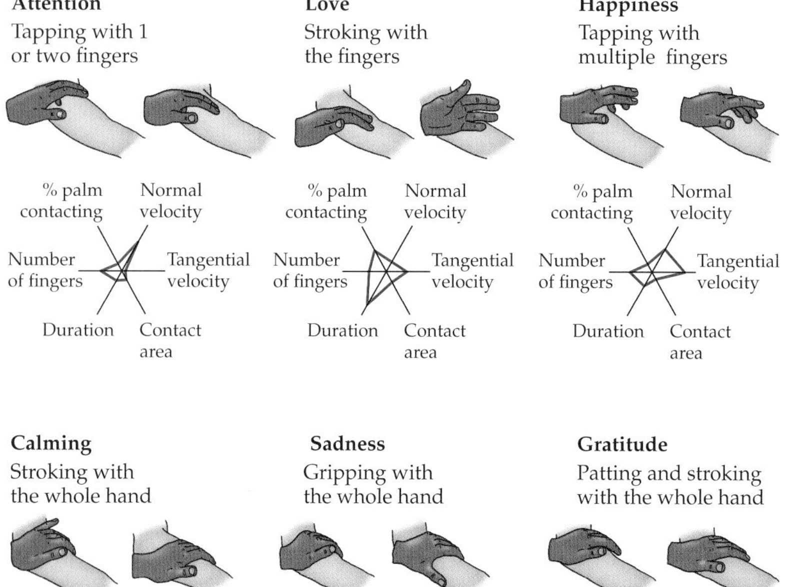

FIGURE 13.25 **Social touch patterns** Top: Experimental task: The sender attempts to send a message to the receiver by a touch on the arm. The receiver selects the intended message from a list. Bottom: Stereotyped patterns of touch that emerged from the senders' successful messages for the six social categories tested.

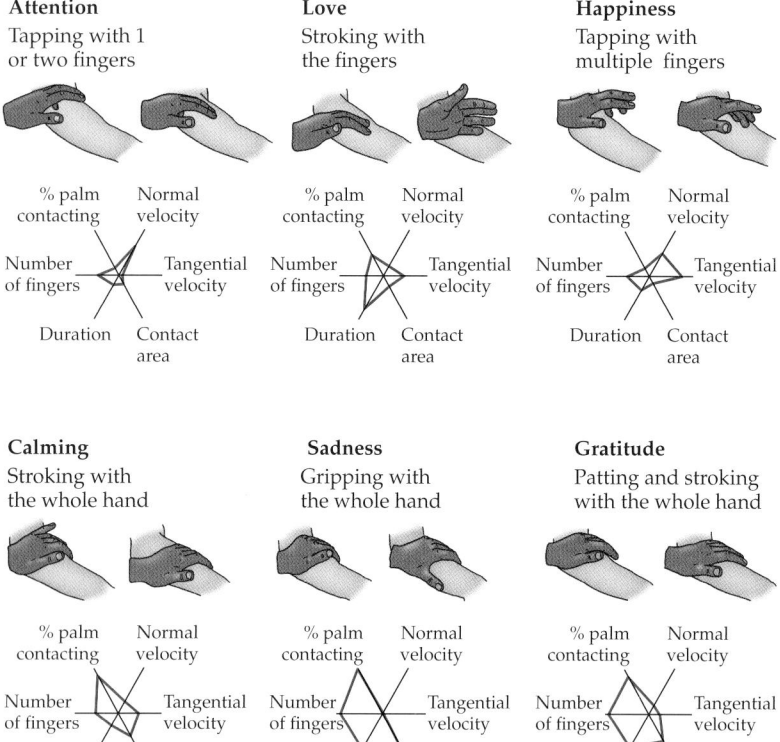

offspring that tend to lick and groom their own pups as well. "Aha!" we might say, there must be a licking-and-grooming gene that is passed from one generation to the next. But to complicate matters, if pups from attentive and remote rat moms are switched at birth, as in the old fable, they "inherit" the behaviors of their adoptive, rather than biological, mothers (D. Francis et al., 1999). Their maternal behavior is governed not by their genetic makeup, but by the grooming behavior they have experienced.

Have the pups learned from their experience, then, to lick and groom? The mechanism for passing on the behavior is not what we normally think of as learning by association. There is instead an epigenetic process that turns licking-and-grooming genes off or on, according to the pup's experience with the same behaviors, by regulating neuroendocrine systems (Champagne, 2008). Complex behaviors are transmitted from one rat generation to the next by regulation of the genes, not control of their component DNA. Evidence for a similar mechanism in humans has been obtained (McGowan et al., 2009). The rat mother's contact has consequences well beyond the maternal care exhibited by the offspring when they, in turn, have pups. Offspring of licking-and-grooming mothers turn out to be less timid than those of remote mothers.

Croy, Fairhurst, and McGlone (2022) propose that the reinforcing power of the CT response to being stroked during infancy opens the door to more general acceptance of social interaction. Once the door is ajar, diverse forms of contact that activate the myelinated fibers associated with discriminative touch, as well as the pleasant touch receptors, serve a reward function. Thus, we feel good when we are hugged, contact another person with the glabrous (nonhairy) skin on our lips, or have a friend lay their head on our shoulder. Affectionate touch between adults promotes the health of the individuals and their relationship (Jakubiak and Feeney, 2017). Deep pressure, as occurs during massage, has been suggested to be another distinct form of social touch that, by activating receptors in muscles and tendons, reduces anxiety and pain (Elias and Abdus-Saboor, 2022).

The Submodality of Pain and Itch

There is no fixed rule for what constitutes a submodality, so here we will pair the aversiveness of pain and itch together. We tend to think of pain as an inevitable consequence of stress on, or damage to, our bodies, flowing upward from sensory levels to the conscious feeling of "ouch." The scientific study of pain, however, reveals it to be a highly subjective state with distinguishable components. What we think of as pain arises at multiple levels—sensory, emotional, and cognitive—which interact to create a conscious experience, one that is subject to multiple psychological and physical influences. Itching is not so easy to ignore, but as we all know, the experience can be lessened, at least temporarily, by scratching. Other interventions also do the job of itch reduction, including causing pain!

substantia gelatinosa A region of interconnecting neurons in the dorsal horn of the spinal cord.

gate control theory A description of the pain-transmitting system that incorporates modulating signals from the brain.

MULTIPLE LEVELS OF PAIN Pain sensations are triggered by the nociceptors. Neurons carrying nociceptive signals arrive at the dorsal horn of the spinal cord in its outermost layers, particularly the second layer called the **substantia gelatinosa** (see Figure 13.9). Neurons there receive information from the brain, and they form synapses with the neurons that are conveying sensory information from nociceptors to the brain (see Figure 13.10). According to the very influential **gate control theory** (Melzack and Wall, 1988), the bottom-up pain signals from the nociceptors can be blocked via a circuit located in the spinal cord. Neurons in the dorsal horn of the cord actively inhibit pain transmission, and what is transmitted to somatosensory areas in the brain is the combined output of pain excitation from the nociceptors and this inhibition. To further complicate matters, the inhibitory neurons in the dorsal horn receive input signals from two quite disparate sources: the large-diameter A-beta fibers coming from the skin, which respond to benign touch rather than pain, and the top-down pathways from the brain. Gate control theory gets its name from the idea that the transmission of the pain acts like a gate that is pushed open by excitatory pain signals but closed by inhibitory inputs. The theory is supported by the identification of neural circuits that could act as the mechanism to open and close the gate (Peirs and Seal, 2016).

Pain signals arising at S1 and S2 don't tell the whole story, however. Imaging methods identify other areas of the brain that correspond to the emotional aspects of painful experiences. The complex cluster of brain areas that respond to the emotion and discriminative aspects of noxious touch is shown in **FIGURE 13.26**. Among those we have previously discussed are the thalamus and insula. Another area, the ACC mentioned previously, responds differentially to hypnotic suggestions of increased or decreased pain unpleasantness, while S1 and S2 consistently respond to the painful stimulation regardless

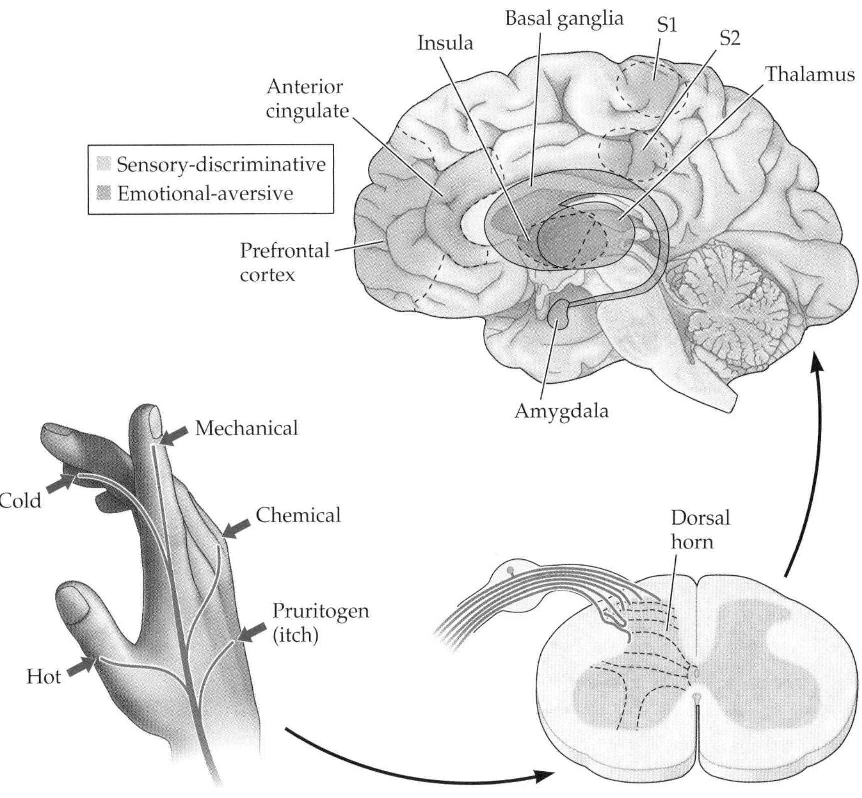

FIGURE 13.26 Organization of pain circuits Nociceptive and tactile afferents project to the dorsal horn of the spinal cord and from there to brain centers that process sensory-discriminative or emotional-aversive touch.

of suggestions to the contrary (Rainville et al., 1997). Yet another region involved in pain circuitry is the prefrontal cortex, an area concerned with cognition and executive control that may represent what Price (2000) called "secondary pain affect," the emotional response associated with long-term suffering that occurs when painful events are imagined or remembered.

It might seem that pain has no upside, but documented cases of people without pain perception, either congenitally or acquired (for example, from leprosy), indicate otherwise. People who lack nociceptive signals are vulnerable to self-harm and may even die as a result. A more benevolent version of this situation, however, is indicated by the case of Joanne Cameron, who not only fails to feel normal levels of pain but also responds to tragic life events, like the death of a parent, with equanimity and even ebullience. Genetic analyses have traced Cameron's profile to mutations in genes labeled FAAH and FAAH OUT (the latter a bit of a pun on the tendency toward bliss it seems to produce) (Habib et al., 2019). This remarkable case illustrates the close connection between physical pain and emotional distress and points to genetic factors affecting them in common.

MODERATING PAIN AND ITCH Pain experiences are the complex result of sensory signals interacting with many other factors that have moderating effects. Damping of pain sensations (without losing consciousness) is called **analgesia**. Responses to noxious stimulation can be affected by analgesic drugs, of course, but perhaps more surprising are the attenuating effects of anticipation, religious belief, controlled thought, or excitement. Studies also highlight the importance of interpersonal and broader social influences on the emotional component of pain.

Pain can be moderated to some extent by benign counterstimulation—for example, rubbing the skin near a stubbed toe. This results from interactions at the level of the spinal cord between the large-diameter fibers and the nociceptors, as described by the gate control model. Although it won't work for all types of pain, crossing your fingers eliminates the pain induced by the thermal grill illusion, where a pattern of warm-cold-warm across the middle fingers of the hand makes you feel like the middle (cold) finger is burning (Marotta, Ferre, and Haggard, 2015)! A more drastic measure is counterirritation or "diffuse noxious inhibitory control"—extreme pressure, cold, or other noxious stimulation applied to another site distant from the source of the pain. For example, pain from electrically stimulating a tooth can be reduced by noxious stimulation of the hand (Motohashi and Umino, 2001).

There are many stories of soldiers in battle who did not feel painful wounds until the stress was over. The analgesic effect in such cases is probably caused by **endogenous opiates**, chemicals released by the body that block the release or uptake of neurotransmitters necessary to transmit pain sensations to the brain. Differences between individuals with respect to pain responsiveness (that is, pain "thresholds") may reflect differences in their baseline levels of these substances, although other causes have been implicated, such as genetically caused differences in nociceptive pathways. Manufactured substances such as morphine, heroin, and codeine are similar in chemical structure to these endogenous opiates, and thus they have similar analgesic effects. Other drugs, such as acetaminophen and ibuprofen, alleviate pain at its source by counteracting chemicals that would otherwise start the nociceptors firing.

What about pain reduction by a simulated intervention? The **placebo effect** is the reduction of pain when people merely think they are being treated, for example, when they take a surrogate for an analgesic drug. The subjective reduction of pain by placebos is well documented, and imaging of the spinal cord with fMRI reveals that placebos actually inhibit nociceptive processing as early as the dorsal

analgesia Decreasing pain sensation during conscious experience.

endogenous opiate A chemical released by the body that blocks the release or uptake of neurotransmitters necessary to transmit pain sensations to the brain.

placebo effect Decreasing pain sensation when people think they're taking an analgesic drug but actually are not.

horn (Eippert et al., 2009). Placebos can enhance positive effects as well as reduce negative ones: When people who used an inert nasal spray were told that it would heighten their responses to pleasant touch, their brains showed relatively greater activation under the appropriate stroking stimulation. The locations of these effects encompassed somatosensory cortex and emotional sites, including the same areas that were attenuated by analgesic placebos under painful stimulation (Ellingsen et al., 2013).

Research has shown that contact with those we love reduces brain activation in areas that regulate our emotions and bodily arousal responses to the threat of painful stimulation. In an fMRI study by Coan, Schaefer, and Davidson (2006), women experienced the threat of electric shock under three conditions. A woman could hold her husband's hand, the hand of a male with whom she was unacquainted, or no hand at all. The neural pain response was reduced by touching another's hand, and this effect increased with the closeness of the relationship.

Individuals who suffer from chronic pain may benefit from training on how to control it cognitively. As reviewed in Driscoll et al. (2021), varied approaches have been tried, including relaxation training, biofeedback, hypnosis, conditioning, and mindfulness meditation. Asher and associates (2022) reported that when patients with chronic back pain participated in 4 weeks of "pain reprocessing therapy," which aims to change thoughts about the origins of pain and self-appraisals of its intensity, benefits were evident even a year later. Relative to placebo and conventional-treatment groups, the trained patients reported less chronic pain, and brain imaging while their chronically painful backs were aversively stimulated showed lower activation in pain-related areas like the ACC.

We've seen that pain can be moderated by physical, social, and cognitive influences. Itch too can be moderated, and one way to do this is with pain. Recall that C fibers that constitute pruriceptors (itch) and nociceptors (pain) can be differentiated. Their trajectories intersect at the spinal cord. With the inhibitory circuit shown in **FIGURE 13.27**, painful stimulation can suppress the sensation of itch, although you might prefer the itchiness. This mechanism resembles the type of inhibition proposed by the gate control model of pain regulation.

Scratching is the more familiar way to alleviate itch, and despite what you may have been told about "making it worse," it beneficially decreases activation at itch sites as early as the spinal cord (S. Davidson et al., 2009), acting through an inhibitory circuit like the suppression of itch by pain. At the level of the brain, scratching regulates responses of the ACC and the insula, which, you may recall, respectively respond to emotional pain and pleasant touch (Papoiu et al., 2013). And unlike tickling, which is more effective when done by someone else (more about this to come!), scratching yourself is more pleasurable and itch relieving than being scratched (Papoiu et al., 2013). Older people tend to itch and scratch more than

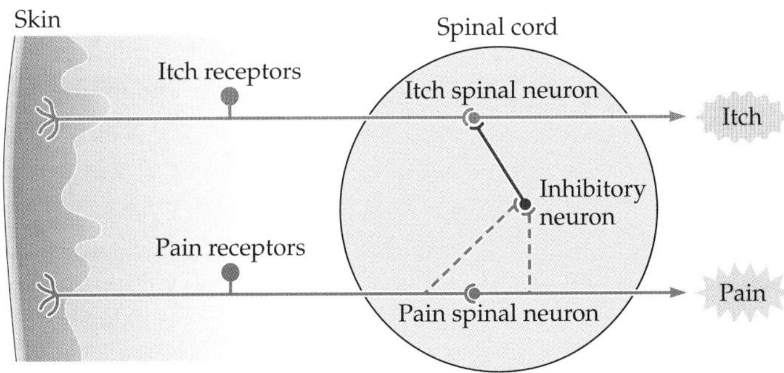

FIGURE 13.27 Pain and itch interactions Nociceptive and pruriceptive stimulation are initially transmitted by separate "labeled lines." In the spinal cord, pain neurons connect to an itch-inhibiting neuron, with the result that painful stimulation inhibits itch.

hyperalgesia An increased or heightened response to a normally painful stimulus.

nocebo effect Increasing pain sensation when people expect pain.

younger ones, and a rather surprising explanation for this phenomenon has been found (Feng et al., 2018), namely, that it results from a reduction in the population of Merkel cells (end organs of SA I receptors) with age. While you might think that losing tactile receptors would make people feel less, in this case it makes them itch more. A normal function of the Merkel cells, it appears, is to inhibit itch signals through the same spinal circuitry that makes scratching effective. The age-related loss of Merkel cells depletes these inhibitory circuits, and as a result, older adults are itchier.

PAIN SENSITIZATION Nociceptors provide a signal when there is impending or ongoing damage to the body's tissue. This is called nociceptive pain. When pain surpasses normal expectations, the experience is **hyperalgesia**. An increased or heightened pain response to a normally painful stimulus is called inflammatory, and it usually goes away once the tissue heals, although chronic pain can persist after healing. Pain can also arise in the absence of immediate trauma, because of damage to or dysfunction of the nervous system. The resulting pain is called neuropathic. Some neuropathic pain reflects changes in the sensory fibers at the skin that do not normally produce pain but now become pain inducers (a phenomenon known as allodynia); other neuropathic pain arises from changes in the dorsal horn of the spinal cord. The mechanisms by which neuropathic pain arises are increasingly understood at the cellular and molecular levels. An important implication of this research is that no single medication will alleviate all types of pain.

Just as placebos can reduce pain without analgesia, the **nocebo effect** can enhance pain in the absence of physical intervention. The magnitude of the effect is closely calibrated by expectations. Patients in one study were told that an itch-reducing cream could produce pain as a side effect. When people purchased a more costly cream, the greater price led them to expect larger side effects, so they would "pay the price" not only financially, but also in the pain they experienced! The difference between cheaper and more expensive creams was evidenced not only in reported pain, but also in several neural sites, including the ACC (Tinnermann et al., 2017).

TICKLE Where do we put tickle among submodalities? Should it be placed with affective touch or consigned to the aversive pole of pain and itch? Is tickle a sensation at all? No dedicated receptor population or sensory afferent has been found to carry a tickle signal, but we have evidence that tickle is distinguished from other forms of touch in the brain. In an experiment that sounds like a lot of fun (Ishiyama and Brecht, 2016), researchers tickled rats on their trunk (tummy). They assessed behavioral responses that might indicate the sensation of tickle and recorded the activity in the somatosensory area that represents the trunk. Behaviorally, tickled rats produced laugh-like vocalizations and chased after the experimenter's hand between bouts of tickling. As well, cells in the trunk area of the somatosensory cortex fired at higher rates during tickling as compared with gentle touch, and rats that demonstrated higher cortical firing rates also exhibited more playful behavior like hand chasing.

This leaves us with the question about whether tickle should be assigned to the affective-touch submodality or, alternatively, grouped with pain or itch. The answer depends partly on which type of tickle we are discussing. There are two types, called knismesis and gargalesis, corresponding to lighter or more forceful touch, respectively (Varlamov and Skorokhodov, 2022) (**FIGURE 13.28**). It is gargalesis that makes us (and presumably, rats) laugh, serving a social function. This form of tickle necessitates social contact, as we can see when we try to do it to ourselves and fail. Self-induced tickling not only produces less laughter, but also produces less

(A)

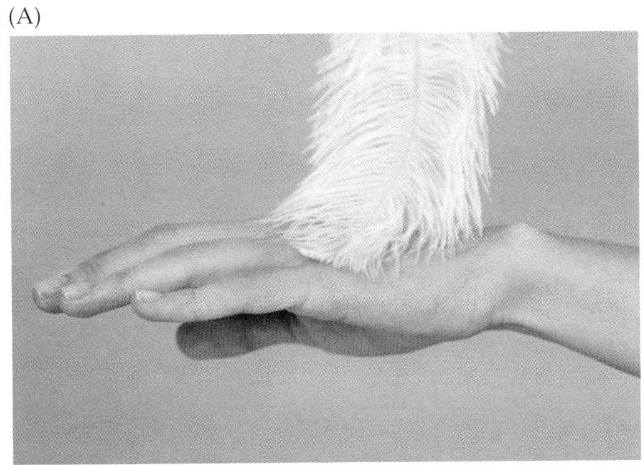

(B)

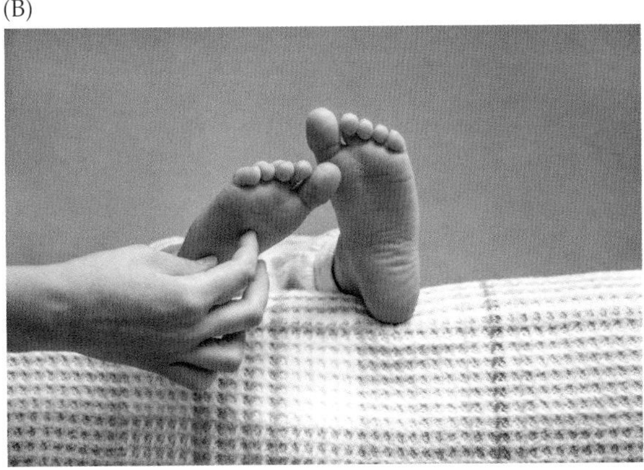

FIGURE 13.28 **Types of tickle** Knismesis (A) is the response to very light touch that disturbs the skin hairs, whereas gargalesis uses more robust touch. Although gargalesis (B) may make us laugh, both types can be aversive.

activity in the somatosensory cortex, because of canceling signals from other brain areas that know where the tickling stimulation is coming from (S.-J. Blakemore, Wolpert, and Frith, 1998).

On the unpleasant side, gargalesis can quickly become socially intrusive and lead the victim to protest. The knismesis version of tickle seems to be entirely a negative sensation with no laughable upside. Knismesis arises when receptors in hair follicles are activated by the hairs' movement under very light touch (so light we could not feel it on glabrous skin). The resulting neural response ultimately stimulates itch-related neurons in the spinal cord, leading to an itchy sensation that, it has been suggested, once served the function of alerting our ancestors to parasitic insects trying to penetrate the skin. Whatever its evolutionary value, people generally don't like tickle in the form of knismesis and don't find it funny.

The Submodality of Interoception

Interoception processes sensory input from locations internal to the body. Mechanoreceptors play an important role here. They are not confined to the tactile and kinesthetic components of touch, as described previously in this chapter, but are also found in the "gut," which technically includes everything in your body along the tubular structure between your mouth and your anus. Sensing of forces along this pathway—as the tube expands, contracts, or is subjected to flow-through—is essential to the functioning of your digestive system. The gut contains two distinct neural systems, called intrinsic (or enteric) and extrinsic (as reviewed in Blackshaw et al., 2007). The intrinsic component is not of particular interest to readers of a book on perception, because it mutely runs its course independent of the central nervous system. Signals from the extrinsic system have broad functions, among them to produce conscious sensations of pressure (my stomach is full) and pain (my stomach is *too* full!).

Mechanoreceptors in the gut, like those under the skin, have been found to have specialized end organs (some called intraganglionic laminar endings and others similar to the Merkel cells found below the skin surface). The gut communicates sensed mechanical forces and pain signals to the central nervous system by connections through the spinal cord or, particularly for signals originating in the gut's upper portion, directly via the vagus nerve. The vagus nerve carries bidirectional messages between gut and brain, leading to its being called an information superhighway (Mercado-Perez and Beyder, 2022).

Pressure signals along that highway appear to be potent regulators for feelings of hunger. Bai et al. (2019) found that stimulating neurons in a mouse's

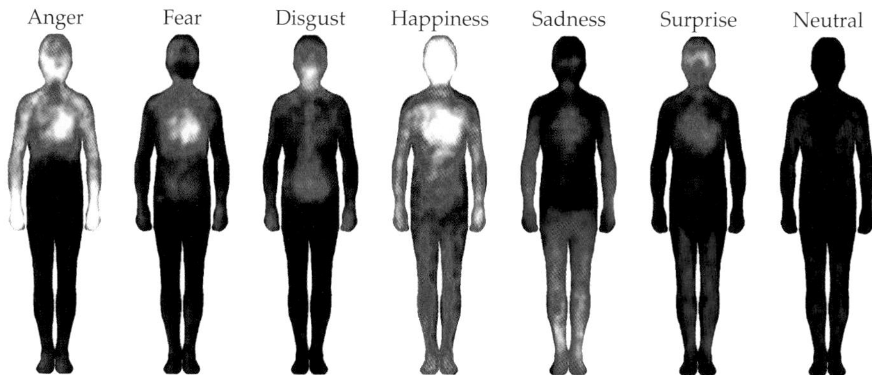

FIGURE 13.29 Association between emotional states and the body Topographical maps reported by participants as they experienced each of a set of basic emotions. Relative to neutral black, cool colors (blue range) indicate less activation and warm colors (red to yellow range) indicate more activation.

vagus nerve that were linked to mechanoreceptors in the intestine caused the animal to eat less and inhibited hunger-related circuitry in its brain, whereas stimulation of vagal neurons responsive to nutrients in food did not have the same effect. That is, for aspects of hunger regulated by the vagus nerve, effects of pressure from food intake appeared more potent than the food's nutritional value! These findings may help explain why surgery to reduce the size of the stomach, which would increase pressure sensations from eating, has been successful in promoting weight loss beyond what might be expected from the nutritional reduction alone.

Broadly conceived, interoception includes access to sensations throughout the body, like the beating of your heart or the heat in your face when you are aroused. Nummenmaa et al. (2014) asked whether people experience sensations at specific body sites in association with emotions. They first elicited emotions in European and Asian participants by showing them arousing texts, films, or faces and then asked them to indicate, on a body map, where they felt increased or decreased sensation. The topography they extracted from these reports is shown in FIGURE 13.29. The upper chest (site of heart rate and breathing) and the head were reported to be active across all emotions. Happiness made the whole body tingle, while the legs and arms were numbed by sadness. The gut was hit from top to bottom by disgust.

13.3 Haptic Perception: Linking Touch with Action

With physiology and basic psychophysics of the touch system in mind, we turn to how control of our body is employed to expand the information from thermoreceptors, muscle spindle fibers, Pacinian corpuscles, and the like. The term **haptic perception** refers to perceptual processing of inputs from discriminative touch in the context of active information-seeking: the haptic perceiver explores the world rather than passively receiving it.

Perception for Action

As mentioned earlier, touch relies on action to get information from the world. Expanding on this point a bit more, we can say that touch is active in two complementary ways. Using our hands to actively explore the world of surfaces and objects outside our bodies is *action for perception*. Using sensory input to prepare us to interact with objects and surfaces around us involves *perception for action*.

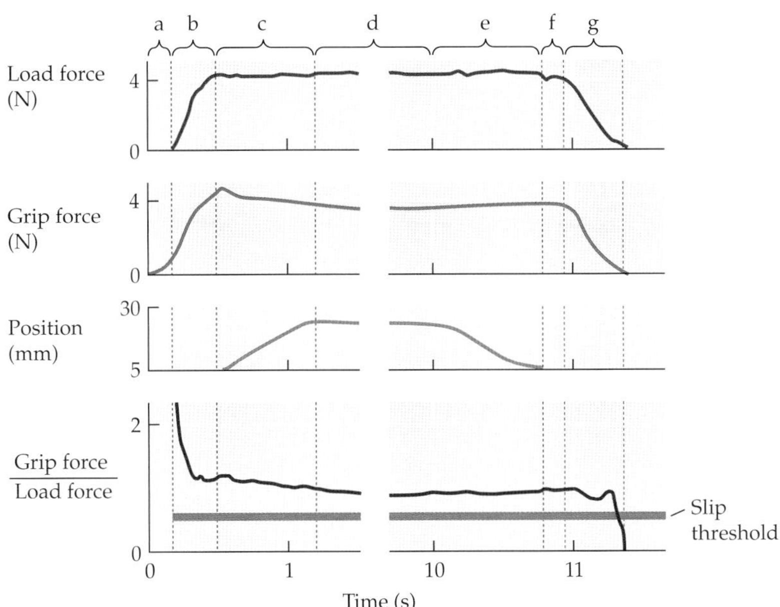

FIGURE 13.30 Profiling active touch Force and position during lifting, grasping, and replacing a cube. Region a = grasping; b and c = lifting; d = holding; e = lowering; f and g = releasing. The load force (in newtons [N]) is in the gravitational direction, the grip force is imposed by the fingers pinching the cube, and the position is the height of the cube relative to its starting position on the table. The ratio of grip force to load force is set such that it just prevents the cube from slipping.

Preparation for action starts well before contact when an object is in view. Vision allows us to plan the approach to manipulation, slowing our reach to a slippery object, for example. This advance planning is evidenced by fMRI imaging not only in visual areas of the brain, but also in somatosensory areas: Area S2 responds differently to objects that *look* slippery (have glossy surfaces) versus rough (matte surfaces), and the differences mimic those found when smooth and rough objects are touched. These results suggest an information-processing network that proceeds from visual analysis to somatosensory areas, preparing people for the expected consequences of action before an object is even touched (H.-C. Sun et al., 2016). ●

Once we touch an object, somatosensation controls our impressive ability to grasp and manipulate it. In our discussion of kinesthetic receptors, we talked about how the loss of these internal tactile receptors leads to a devastating inability to know (without looking) where our limbs are positioned. Westling and Johansson (1984) showed that mechanoreceptors in the skin also play critical roles when we're interacting with objects (**FIGURE 13.30**). After these investigators anesthetized the skin on volunteers' hands, the volunteers could no longer maintain a stable grasp of objects that they could see perfectly well. Feedback from the mechanoreceptor populations in the skin appears to provide crucial information about when an object is about to slip on the skin. You may know this yourself from trying to unlock a door when your fingers are very cold!

Action for Perception

Let's now consider the action-for-perception side of haptic processing. Lederman and Klatzky (1987) coined the term **exploratory procedure** for a particular way of feeling an object to learn about one or more of its properties (**FIGURE 13.31**). Each exploratory procedure is optimal for obtaining precise details about one or two specific properties. For example, to find out how rough an object is, the best exploratory procedure is lateral motion—moving the fingers back and forth across the surface. This is the exploratory procedure that people freely choose when they

exploratory procedure A stereotyped hand movement pattern used to touch objects in order to perceive their properties. Each procedure is best for determining one or more object properties.

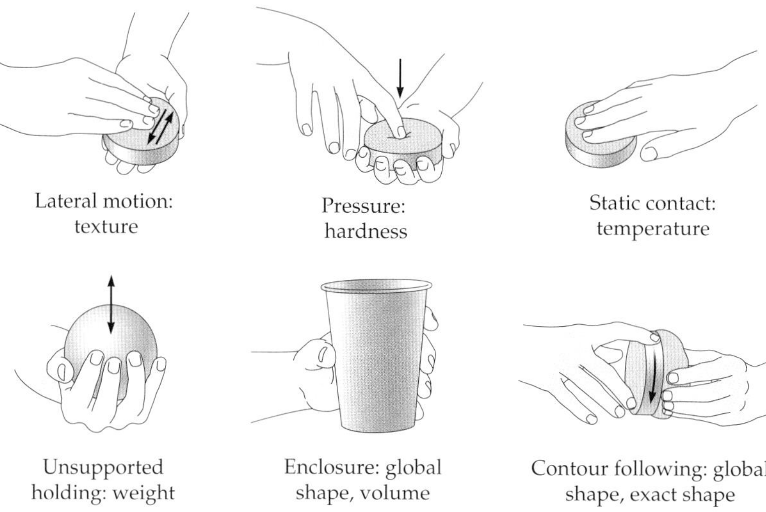

FIGURE 13.31 Haptic exploratory procedures Lederman and Klatzky (1987) described hand postures and motions that were associated with the perception of specific object properties by touch, as shown.

wish to learn about roughness, and research indicates that it is also the one that works best.

A closer look within these general patterns reveals that people fine-tune exploration according to expectations and goals. People apply more force and move more quickly when discriminating surfaces by roughness than when they are merely told to explore (Tanaka et al., 2014). When they expect to probe a soft surface, they

Scientists at Work

Haptic Exploratory Procedures Used by Sea Lions

Question Does a whiskered species use its exploratory appendages in a pattern specific to its perceptual goal?

Hypothesis It has been demonstrated that whiskered species use their hairy appendages as sensors. Here, it is proposed that they might adjust whisker movements in response to a specific perceptual goal, more specifically, that they would exhibit exploratory procedures analogous to those humans exhibit with their hands.

Test Lo, a 15-year-old sea lion, was trained to find a target fish shape that differed from distractor fish shapes on a single dimension at a time: texture, size, or brightness. She was videotaped in the course of training, and the movements of two whiskers and her nose and time to respond were extracted from the records (**FIGURE 13.32A**).

Results By the end of training, Lo achieved 100% correct performance on each task within less than 1 second. Her whisker movements were larger when judging size than texture, and she hardly used whiskers at all to judge brightness (**FIGURE 13.32B**). The time she spent exploring varied correspondingly: slowest for size and fastest for brightness. In all these respects, her behavior looked much like those of humans in comparable tasks, except that Lo was faster to reach an answer!

Conclusion Lo the sea lion exhibits active exploration that resembles human behavior, in that it is efficient and linked to particular perceptual goals. Presumably, Lo's specialized exploratory patterns are driven by the same constraints that humans must deal with: the appropriate receptors in our sensory apparatus must be activated to deliver the information required for our task. Lo uses whiskers and we use our fingers, but we all optimize action in the service of perception.

Future work Given Lo's adaptation of exploration to suit her goal of perceiving texture versus size, how do you think she might use her whiskers to detect a target with a particular level of *softness*? Might there be limits in the usefulness of whiskers for this purpose? (Think about how von Frey hairs buckle when they are too weak to measure the human pressure threshold!)

Scientists at Work (continued)

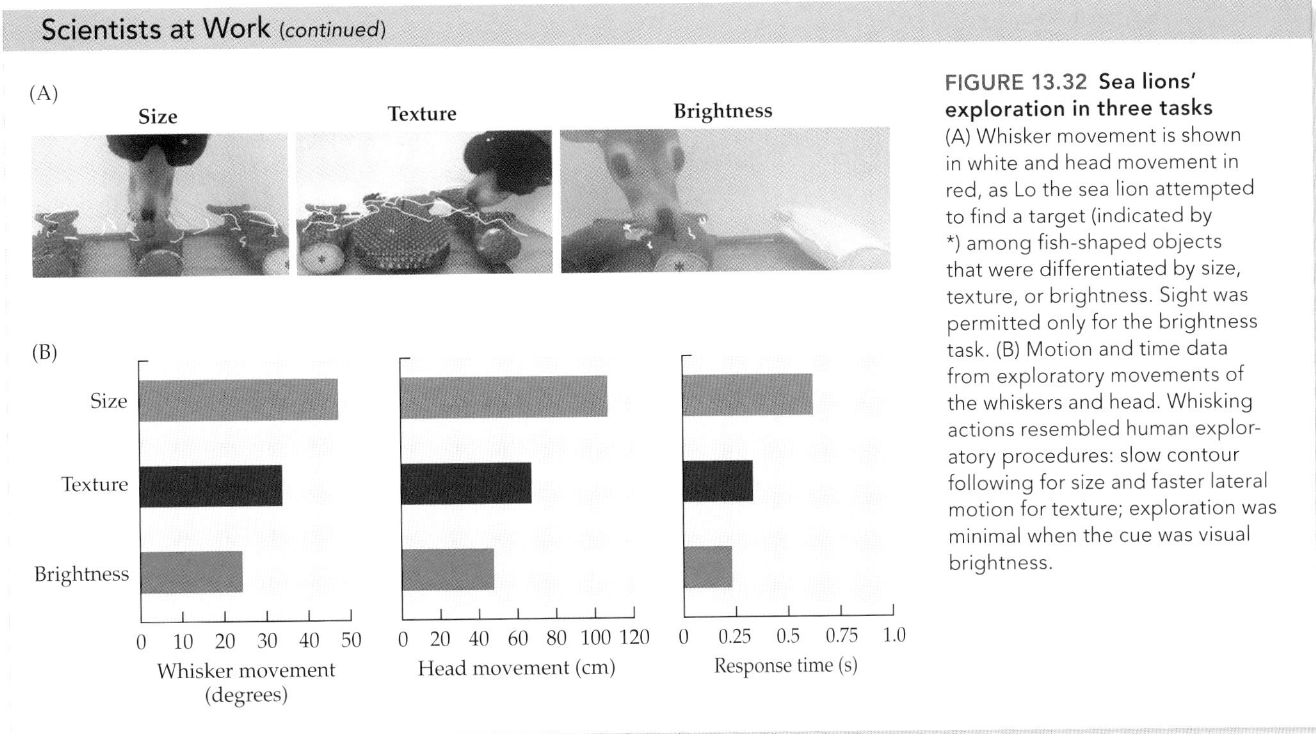

FIGURE 13.32 Sea lions' exploration in three tasks (A) Whisker movement is shown in white and head movement in red, as Lo the sea lion attempted to find a target (indicated by *) among fish-shaped objects that were differentiated by size, texture, or brightness. Sight was permitted only for the brightness task. (B) Motion and time data from exploratory movements of the whiskers and head. Whisking actions resembled human exploratory procedures: slow contour following for size and faster lateral motion for texture; exploration was minimal when the cue was visual brightness.

move more quickly, but less forcefully, than when they expect a rigid surface (Kaim and Drewing, 2009). Variations are observed according to the specific material that is being explored and whether people are asked to judge it as soft, wobbly, or fluffy (Cavdan, Doerschner, and Drewing, 2021).

To explain why each exploratory procedure is linked to a specific object property, we must consider both the neural structures that transduce information and the processes that operate on that information. Why do we rub, for example, in order to perceive surface roughness? The answer is that relevant receptors become more active. For roughness, two neural populations are relevant. K. O. Johnson (2002) has shown that the activity of slowly adapting mechanoreceptors (the SA I fibers) is a principal basis for the perception of surfaces that are at least moderately rough; these receptors are ten times as responsive when there is relative motion between the skin and the surface (rubbing) as when the fingers rest against the surface. When surface variations are very fine, the mechanoreceptors responsive to high-frequency vibrations (the FA I and FA II fibers) appear to encode surface roughness; again, stroking with the fingers is needed to set up the vibration (see Hollins, 2002).

The activity of the receptors is sent on for processing that further differentiates coarse and fine textures. As your finger sweeps across a coarsely varying surface like rough sandpaper, the pattern of force varies with the hills and troughs on the object's surface, providing a spatial map of the variations in skin deformation that is sensed by the SA I fibers. This map is passed on to higher-level neural structures, which integrate the lower-level information into an overall measure of the amount of variation that the brain then uses to estimate the roughness of the surface. Whereas coarse textures are perceived over space, fine textures are processed as pressure variation over time. Now the skin may act less like a map and more like the ear. Just this argument was made by Saal, Wang, and Bensmaia (2016), using

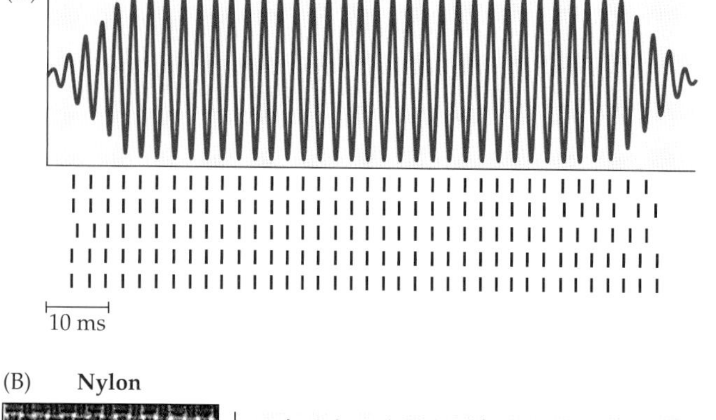

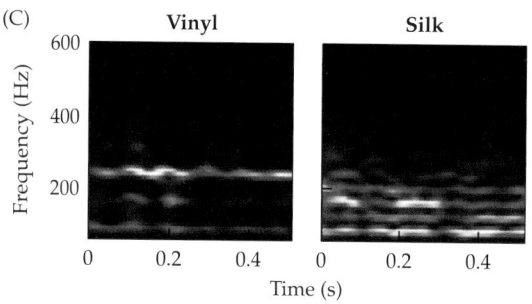

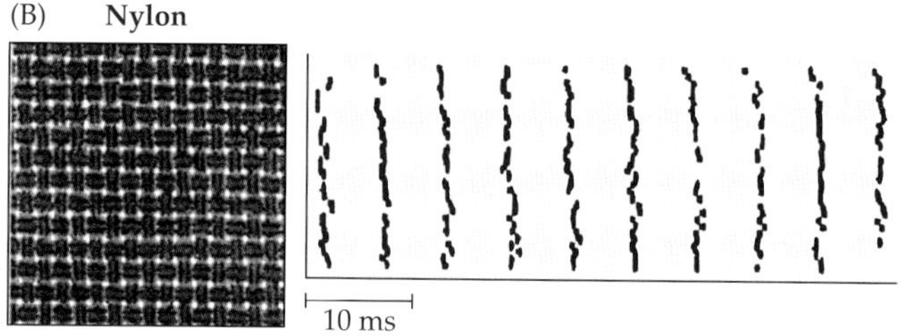

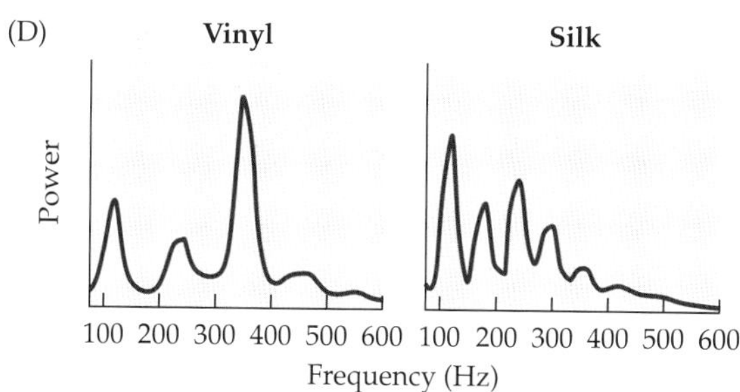

FIGURE 13.33 Skin and neural responses to vibration Effects from a vibrating stimulus on the skin and rubbing fabric are measured at two locations: on the skin itself and by the responses of neural afferents. (A) Trace of a vibrating stylus pressing on the skin at a rate of 400 Hz. Just below it are points in time where an FA II afferent fired as the skin was vibrated; each row depicts firing to a different presentation of the stimulus. All presentations produce a firing pattern that is directly coupled with the vibration over time. (B) Similarly synchronized firing of FA II afferents for a nylon patch (illustrated at left). (C) The spectrogram (frequency versus time) obtained from measurement of skin oscillation as a fabric (vinyl or silk) is scanned over the skin at 80 Hz. (D) The power at different frequencies in the spectrograms for the two fabrics; vinyl and silk demonstrate distinct fabric "timbres."

data like that shown in **FIGURE 13.33**. Figure 13.33A shows that FA II afferents fire in synchrony with vibrating pressure applied to the skin. Figure 13.33B shows a similar pattern produced when the skin rubs a fabric texture. The analogy between hearing and tactile texture perception becomes even more compelling when we see that the equivalent of a sound spectrogram can be obtained for fabrics passed over the fingertip, in this case showing the frequency of oscillation on the skin rather than sound waves acting on the tympanic membrane (Figures 13.33C and 13.33D). Different fabrics, like instruments, produce different "timbres," which can be measured both from vibrations at the skin and from the FA II neural code that is coupled with it.

FURTHER DISCUSSION of timbre can be found in Section 10.2.

The What System of Touch: Perceiving Objects and Their Properties

Chapter 4 described the processes that underlie visual object recognition. We need somatosensation to control simple actions such as standing or grasping and to warn of danger through pain, but how much value does the sense of touch have as an object recognition system? You know that touch alone can function quite well to identify objects if you have ever gotten out of bed in the dark to use the bathroom. The introduction to this chapter invited you to try the simple exercise of doing a familiar task like making a sandwich with your eyes closed, which should have convinced you (if you tried it!) that even when you habitually use vision, you can rely on touch to recognize objects and their parts. However, object recognition by touch has its limits: the designers of coins know that it is imperative to be able to tell one from another in your pocket, but the Susan B. Anthony version of the US dollar nonetheless failed soon after its introduction in 1979, because it felt too similar to the quarter.

PERCEIVING MATERIAL VERSUS GEOMETRIC PROPERTIES People can perform haptic object recognition very well. Klatzky, Lederman, and Metzger (1985) asked expeirmental participants to identify each of 100 common objects (e.g., a fork, a brush, a paper clip) placed in their hands. Not only did they perform almost perfectly without looking at the objects, but also they generally responded in less than about 2 seconds. These exploratory experiences can lead to enduring representations in long-term memory. One experiment (Hutmacher and Kuhbandner, 2018) reported approximately 80% accuracy at remembering which of two objects from the same class (e.g., which of two pens) was explored a week earlier, even when the memory test was unexpected (compare this to the rates of visual picture and scene perception reported in Chapter 7).

The information used in haptic object identification is quite different, however, from that used in visual object recognition. Consider the difference between material properties—those that do not depend on the structure of a particular object, like its surface roughness—and geometric properties like size and shape. In haptic perception, the observer is in contact with the object being observed, so material properties of the object (Is it soft? cold? fuzzy?) are easy to perceive, and they play a crucial role in the recognition process. In vision, there is no physical contact, so thermal and textural properties of objects, as determined by their material, are much more difficult to perceive.

Therefore, the geometric properties of objects are the most important for visual recognition. Indeed, sparse line drawings may be quite easy to recognize visually, but they are hard to recognize when presented haptically as raised contours (**FIGURE 13.34**). To determine the overall shape of an object haptically, we usually must explore the object by tracing along its contours with our fingers. Integrating tactile information over time is possible but not very efficient, which is why the instantly recognizable material properties tend to be much more important in haptic recognition.

THE HAPTIC ALGORITHM FOR CURVATURE Although determining the overall shape of an object by touch may involve tedious exploration to follow its contours, the curvature in a relatively small region can quickly be determined with the fingertip. Much as visual perception identifies curves by applying heuristics and algorithms to sensory data (as described in Chapter 4), haptic contour perception appears to apply heuristics and algorithms to data from exploratory procedures. Take a look

FIGURE 13.34 Can we recognize drawings by touch? Examples of common objects that are easy to recognize visually in two-dimensional form but that when raised for haptic presentation are not easily recognized by touch.

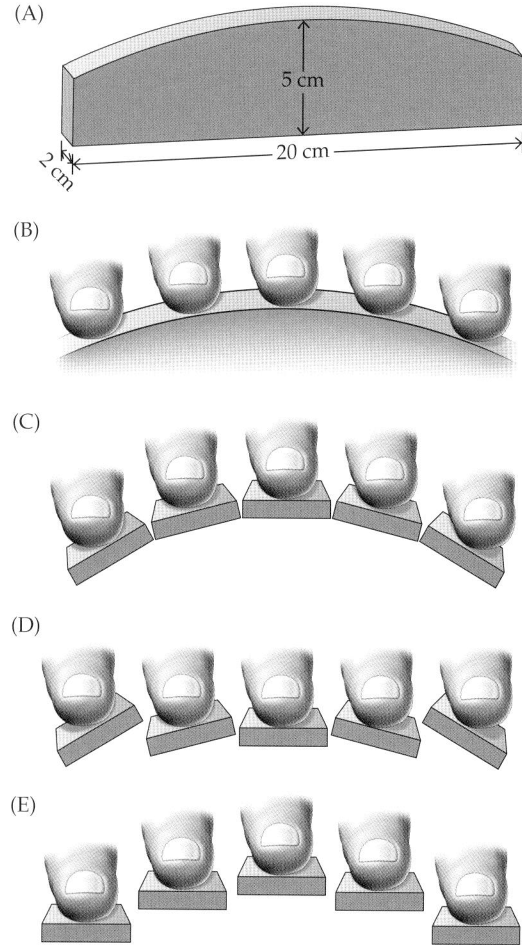

FIGURE 13.35 Illusory contours in touch (A) A physical curved surface; (B) position and height as a fingertip explores the surface; (C) equivalent changes to those in (B) but induced by a platform that rotates and changes height depending on spatial position; (D) a curve induced entirely by rotation of the platform; (E) a curve induced entirely by height changes in the platform.

at FIGURE 13.35A, which depicts the kind of curved contour you might feel on a computer mouse. As shown in FIGURE 13.35B, running your finger over this curve would change both your finger's height in space and the slant of the surface pressing against your finger at successive contact locations. Using a clever mechanical device, researchers were able to simulate these effects, as in FIGURE 13.35C, or manipulate the two cues independently (slant in FIGURE 13.35D, height in FIGURE 13.35E), to determine which cue produces the perception of a curved surface (Wijntjes et al., 2009). They found that discrimination between levels of curvature relied almost entirely on the momentary variation in slant, rather than the up-and-down movement of the finger. In fact, it is possible to produce the illusion of a curved surface simply by changing the slant of the surface against the finger as it makes a horizontal pass, without lifting it up and down. Thus, haptic curvature perception favors a skin slant algorithm over one using finger height.

HAPTIC SEARCH As we saw in Chapter 7, a number of so-called preattentive features in the visual domain are presumed to be critical in the visual object recognition process. These features can be identified by the extent to which they "pop out" in a visual search task. For example, if you are searching for a red object, you will be equally fast at finding it regardless of how many green objects are presented along with it. This result implies that the "redness" of an object is available to recognition processes before attentional mechanisms examine the objects in the display and integrate the various features of each one.

Does the sense of touch also support preattentive feature detection? To find out, Lederman and Klatzky (1997) constructed something like a tactile slot machine with one slot for each of six fingers. The subject's right hand is shown in FIGURE 13.36A. Stimulus patches were mounted on planes cut into each of six stimulus wheels. On each trial, the wheels were rotated until the desired stimulus patches were facing upward to form the haptic display. The entire display was then moved up to contact different combinations of the middle three fingertips of each hand. Using this apparatus, Lederman and Klatzky found that a number of haptic features do indeed pop out. As FIGURE 13.36B shows, participants in these experiments were just as fast at detecting a rough surface when there was no smooth surface in the tactile "display" as when there were as many as five smooth surfaces. Similarly, a hard surface popped out of a group of soft surfaces, a cool surface popped out of warm surfaces, and a surface with an edge popped out of perfectly flat surfaces.

Plaisier et al. (2009) developed a three-dimensional version of the haptic search paradigm in which clusters of objects were grasped in the hand, as shown in FIGURE 13.36C. Objects with different shapes had corresponding differences in the locations of edges, surface curvature, surface area, and height-to-width ratio. By means of a single grasp, participants exhibited highly efficient search when targets and distractors differed in the type of shape; for example, a sphere grasped within a handful of cubes tended to pop out.

However, not every haptic difference supports efficient search. For example, response times increased with the number of distractors when the task was to find a target with a horizontally oriented edge among distractors having vertical edges. Note that horizontal targets do pop out of vertical distractors in visual search tasks. This distinction fits nicely with the previous observation that haptic recognition

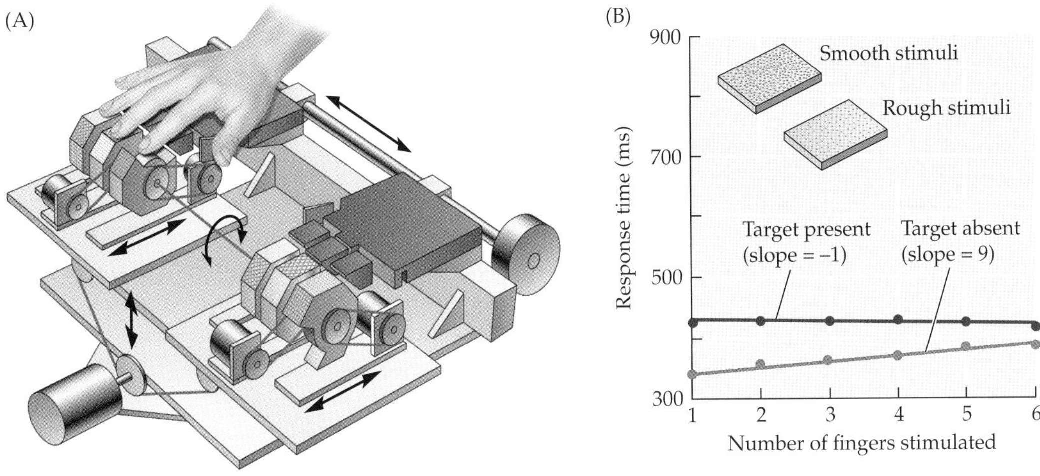

FIGURE 13.36 Preattentive feature detection in touch (A) To test the haptic equivalent of visual search, an experimental apparatus displays targets to the fingertips. The rotating drums bring either a stimulus patch or a cutout (no stimulus) to the upper surface, and then they rise as a whole to contact the middle three fingers of both hands (only one hand is shown). (B) The amount of time required to detect a rough target among smooth distractors as a function of the number of fingers stimulated. (C) A three-dimensional version, where a target object (sphere among cubes in the example shown) is detected among objects grasped in the hand (inset).

relies extensively on material properties but that the tactile system does not appear to be set up to efficiently differentiate object contours by their spatial layout.

PERCEIVING PATTERNS WITH THE SKIN Even if pattern perception by touch is not terribly efficient, it can be done, especially if the patterns are small enough to be perceived by a single fingertip. Loomis (1990) suggested that, to some extent, touch acts like blurred vision when the fingertip explores a raised pattern. (Note the contrast with the previous argument, that the skin acts like an ear when perceiving a fine texture!) He tested people's ability to identify a set of patterns including Braille symbols, English and Japanese letters, and geometric forms—a few of which are shown in FIGURE 13.37. Sometimes the patterns were presented to the fingertips as raised elements. Other times they were presented visually behind a blurring screen that matched the resolution of the eye with the more limited acuity of fingertip skin. Interestingly, Loomis found very similar patterns of visual and tactile confusion errors—that is, responses in which one pattern was confused for another. This finding suggests that a common decision process operates on both haptically and visually perceived patterns.

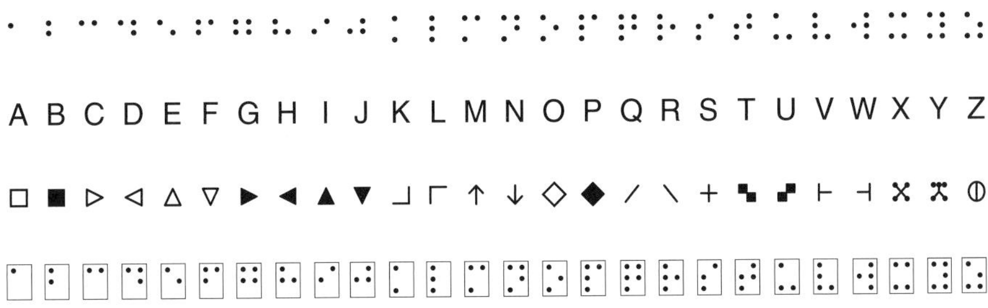

FIGURE 13.37 Tactile acuity testing Selected character recognition sets used by Loomis (1990), including Braille (top).

frame of reference The coordinate system used to define locations in space.

egocenter The center of a reference frame used to represent locations relative to the body.

In the Braille alphabet, shown in the first row of Figure 13.37, each letter is formed by raising some of the dots in a two-by-three array. For the letter *A*, for example, a single dot is raised in the top left position; and for the letter *Q*, all dots except for the one in the lower right position are raised. This design reflects a compromise between the skin's acuity and its "field of view," the area of skin that we can take in all at once. It would be nice to include more than six dots in the array, but because of the spatial blurring imposed by the skin, denser patterns would be difficult to resolve and discriminate (remember that two-point touch thresholds on the fingertips are about 1 mm). Spreading a greater number of dots across a larger contact area would not work either, because then the pattern would extend beyond the fingertip. Unfortunately, people are unable to "read" more than one finger at a time, suggesting that our tactile field of view is very narrow.

The *Where System of Touch: Locating Objects*

As with other sensory modalities, knowing *what* a haptic stimulus might be is only part of the perceptual problem. We also need to know *where* that stimulus is located, because we often want to do something with it. If you are already touching an object, you obviously know where it is relative to your body: it is at the point of contact! If you are not yet touching the object but can see it, your sense of vision can work out where the object is and guide your reaching behavior. But what about groping for your bedside light when your eyes have not yet opened for the day? As mentioned already, there is evidence that touch, like vision, has a specialized neural pathway for dealing with questions of where objects are located, as compared with knowing what they are like.

(A) Top view

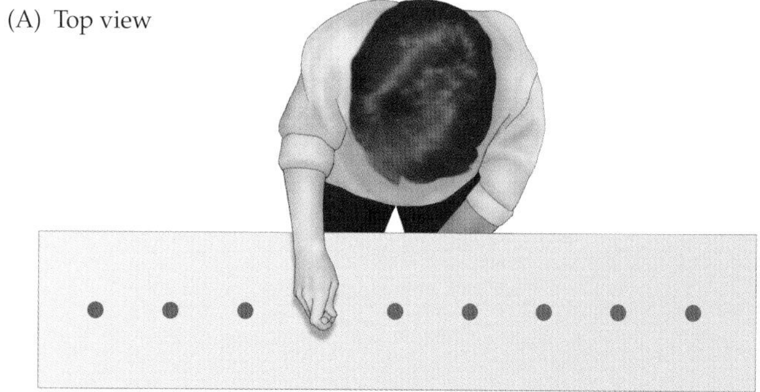

(B) Front view

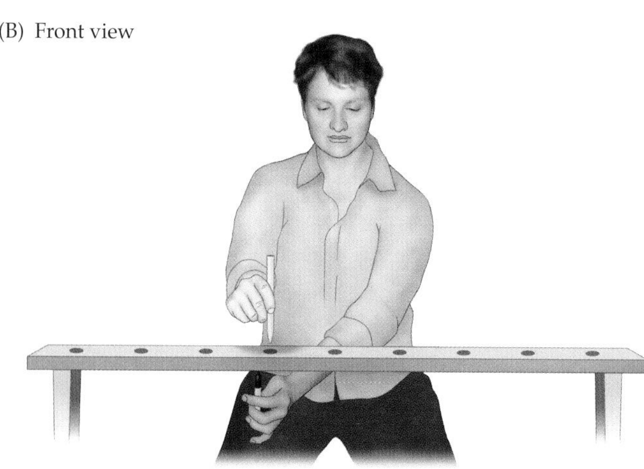

FIGURE 13.38 Locating the haptic egocenter One hand places a stylus on the target on the upper table surface, and the other hand attempts to match up underneath the table in the corresponding location.

HAPTIC OBJECT LOCALIZATION BEYOND THE BODY Like visual and auditory localization, haptic object localization first requires that we establish a **frame of reference**. For vision, the center of the reference frame—the **egocenter**—is located near the bridge of the nose, between the two eyes; the auditory egocenter is at a point smack in the middle of the head (between the two ears). One way to pinpoint your haptic egocenter is to place your left index finger on top of the edge of a desk or table in a natural position on the left side of your body, close your eyes, and try to match this location by placing your right index finger on the bottom of the desk. If you do this many times, you may find that you consistently go too far to the left. Conversely, if you try to match the location of your right index finger with your left, you will be more likely to err too far to the right. **FIGURE 13.38** shows a version of this task using a stylus in each hand instead of the index finger. A careful analysis of errors in a task of this type led Haggard et al. (2000) to conclude that there is, in fact, no single, fixed frame of reference for the haptic perception of locations. In the case of the index finger reaching task, the egocenter appears to be located at the shoulder of the arm doing the reaching. In other tasks, the egocenter may move to other positions on the body. Wherever the egocenter may be, it provides a frame of reference for returning to nearby objects you have touched previously. When you put your coffee cup down on the desk, you can quickly reach and find it without interrupting whatever activities occupy your vision at the time (social media? gaming? studying this book?).

HAPTIC OBJECT LOCALIZATION ON THE BODY When a bug lands on your arm, you are likely to give it a slap in an instant. Think for a moment, however, about the complexity of this action. First, the sensation you feel on your arm must be mapped into a body frame of reference like the homunculus in S1, so you know where the bug landed. The identification of the source location on the body must then initiate an appropriately directed action. But while you may know the bug resides on a particular site on your arm, the arm itself may be positioned in various ways, which means that an accurate slap requires linking the body site of tactile stimulation to a target location for reaching with another limb. Whew—this is more complicated than it first appeared! Yet, babies seem to accomplish a version of this problem early in life, when they manage to direct objects (as parents know, not just food!) toward their mouths while turning their heads. To discover how the ability to reach to a touched location on the body develops with age, experimenters placed vibrators on the heads, arms, and hands of young children and cajoled them into reaching for them if they did not do so spontaneously (Leed, Chinn, and Lockman, 2019). The infant in FIGURE 13.39A is doing just that for a vibrator placed behind the ear. Analyses of the rate of success at various body sites and ages revealed a gradual progression in body-to-action mapping over the period of 7 to 21 months of age, as shown in FIGURE 13.39B. Infants' earliest successes occurred when reaching for the mouth. Accurate contact-directed touching then progressed to the ear and forehead, and eventually the hand was mastered, then the arm. Vision helped the infants accomplish their task, but touch alone was eventually sufficient for touch-initiated action. The youngsters also proved to be highly efficient at reaching; for example, they used the right hand to touch their right ear, but never tried an impossible reach of the right hand to a target on the right arm.

HAPTIC PERCEPTION IN THE PRESENCE OF VISION This chapter began by noting that we perform many everyday tasks without using sight. That does not mean we perform tasks in the same way as when we can see. When discussing perception for action, we noted that vision allows us to plan manipulation in advance of contacting an object. We might feel for the keyhole when unlocking a door in the dark, but in daylight we smoothly guide the key to the lock. The specialized

(A)

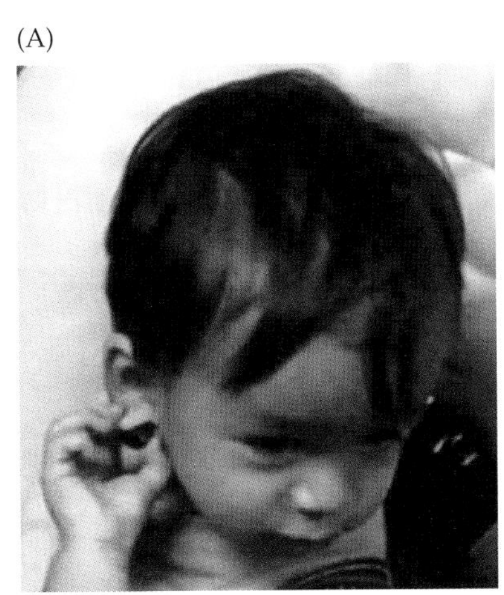

(B)

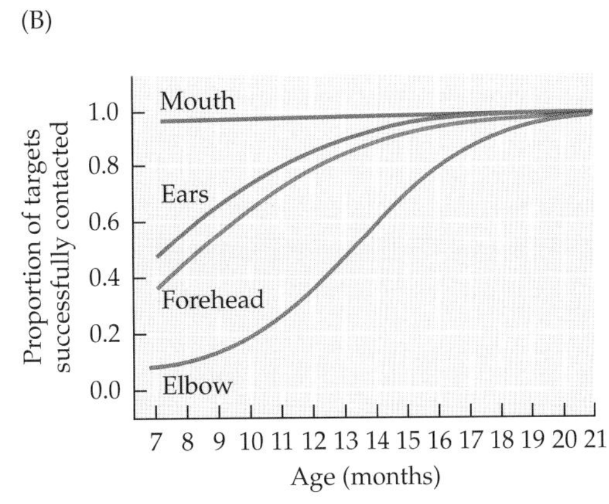

FIGURE 13.39 Development of ability to locate touches on the body (A) A child reaches to a vibrator placed out of sight behind his ear, successfully mapping the site of the skin sensation to an action-directed location in space. (B) As shown by the rate of success at contacting targets, touches to different body sites are achieved at different ages.

intersensory integration The use of information from multiple senses to arrive at a single perceptual estimate.

exploratory procedures used to perceive object properties like texture or size likewise change when vision is available. When a property of some object is clearly evident from vision (coarse sandpaper looks rough) or is well known by association with the object's identity (we know marshmallows are soft without looking at them or touching them), people tend to be content with looking, and specialized haptic exploration is not observed (Klatzky, Lederman, and Matula, 1993). Exploratory procedures emerge particularly when desired information is difficult to determine by sight, for example, when we rub a sanded surface to see if there is any grit left behind.

Vision and touch have the potential to cooperate when both senses offer information about the same physical property. The contribution of multiple senses to a single perceptual outcome is called **intersensory integration**. Integration is not the rule; sometimes one modality may dominate instead. In a classic study pitting vision against touch, Rock and Victor (1964) had people grasp a square while looking at it through a distorting lens. What these participants perceived that they felt was pretty much what they saw: a rectangle with sides of unequal length. That is, feeling that the sides of the shape were equal in length had essentially no influence on the perceptual outcome. A more general model is that people integrate the signals from two modalities, producing a weighted average. That is, they use x% of the information from one modality and $(100 - x)$% from the other. The relative weighting reflects the quality of the signal from each modality.

Ernst and Banks (2002) demonstrated such integration with an apparatus that simultaneously created touch and sight of the same virtual display. The display consisted of a plane with a raised bar across the middle (**FIGURE 13.40**). The virtual visual display was produced with stereo glasses and an appropriate pair of random dot stereograms, one presented to each eye (see Figure 6.37, creating the visual illusion of a bar stepping up from a plane. The corresponding virtual touch display was created with a device that generated forces that pushed back on the hand whenever contact was made with the simulated surface. When the bar heights presented to the two modalities did not match (the touched bar was higher than the viewed bar, or vice versa), the perceived height of the bar was a weighted compromise between them, with vision more strongly weighted than touch. When the investigators made the information from vision less reliable by randomly changing the apparent height of some of the surface dots, the weight assigned to touch increased, and it played a greater role in determining the perceived height of the bar.

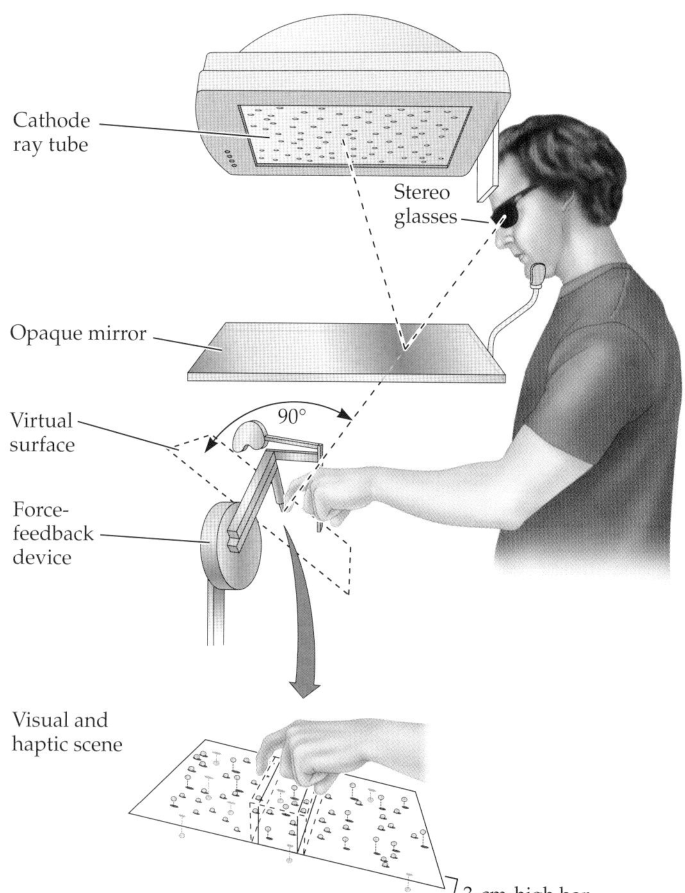

FIGURE 13.40 Testing the integration of sensory modalities The observer could see a virtual surface of dots through stereo goggles, which gave the appearance of a raised bar across the surface, and could touch the virtual surface and receive resisting forces consistent with the surface height.

Multiple modalities may further collaborate by signaling different, but complementary, sources of information about an object. Our discussion of object perception emphasized that vision and touch are intrinsically supportive: one is well suited to convey an object's geometry and the other its material. Vision quickly tells us the noodle is flat; touch tells us it is cooked. Perhaps the philosopher Molyneux had this complementarity in mind when he asked his famous question about whether a blind person who gained sight would recognize familiar objects with this new sense. ●

Sensation & Perception in Everyday Life

A Brain-Computer Interface with a Cortical Loop

Spinal cord injury is an unfortunate event that happens to more than 15,000 individuals per year (*Spinal Cord Injury Facts*, 2020). Over half of those affected show partial or complete tetraplegia; that is, they cannot voluntarily move the upper and lower parts of their body. Brain-computer interfaces aim to provide movement functionality for people with spinal cord injury by enabling them to control a robot. A brain-computer interface senses the neural responses in the brain that occur when a person intends to act and translates them into movement commands that are sent to an active agent. The most direct way to sense a person's intention to move is by means of small electrodes implanted into the areas of the brain that command movement. Research shows that this approach can be made even more effective by bringing the somatosensory cortex into the loop.

Flesher and associates (2021) developed and tested the system depicted in **FIGURE 13.41A**. A tetraplegic participant's brain was implanted with arrays of tiny electrodes in both motor cortex and the primary somatosensory cortex, S1. The electrodes in the motor area were placed in regions known to send commands to the hand and arm. The electrodes in S1 were placed in areas known to represent the four fingers of the hand (see previous discussion of the somatosensory homunculus). When the robot hand moved and contacted objects, the resulting torque (rotational force) on each robotic finger was translated into activation of the corresponding electrodes in the participant's S1 area.

Experiments compared the participant's ability to control the robot with and without feedback to S1 (vision was always present). Results from one task, called

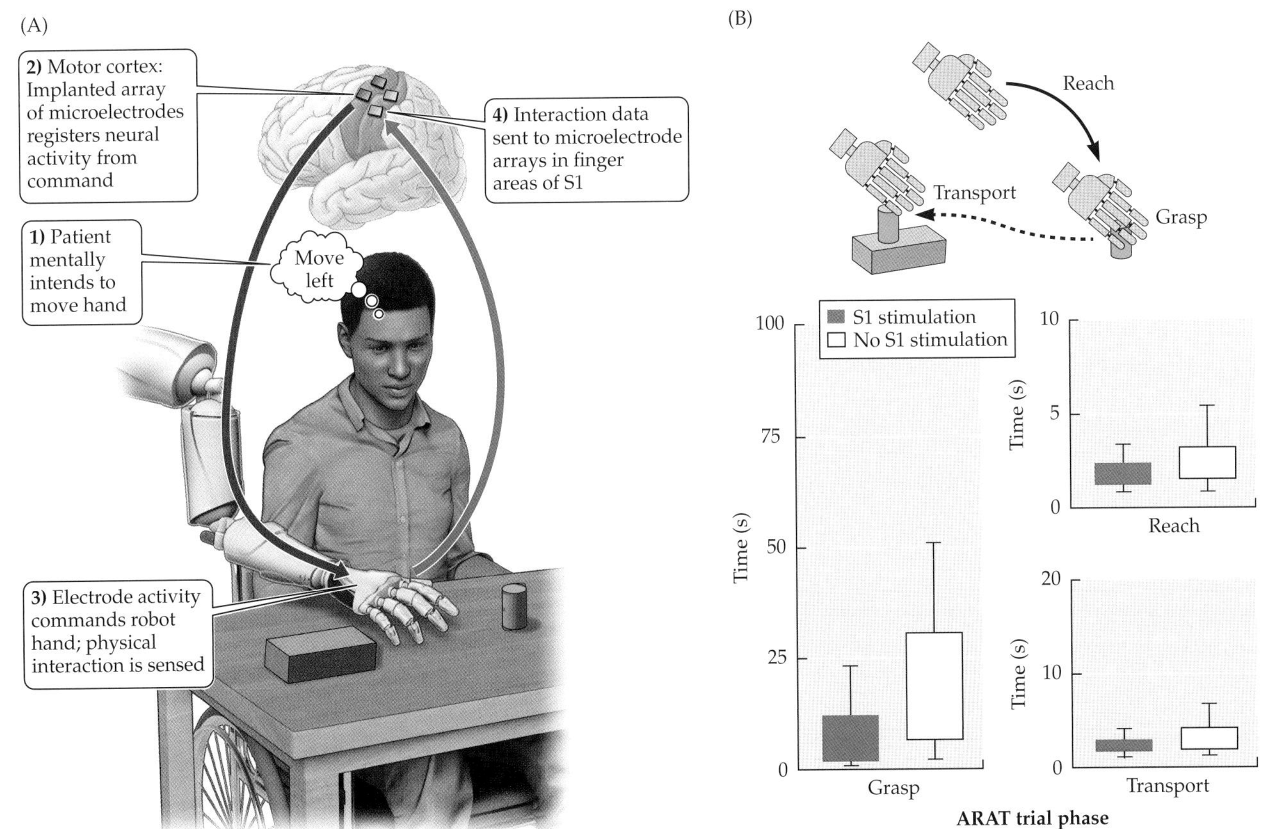

FIGURE 13.41 Brain-computer interface (A) Flow of control from the participant's intention to the feedback from the robotic interaction. (B) Data from the Action Research Arm Test (ARAT): time for each phase of the action when the somatosensory feedback to S1 is on versus off.

(Continued)

Sensation & Perception in Everyday Life *(continued)*

the Action Research Arm Test (ARAT), are shown in **FIGURE 13.41B**. The goal here is to control the robot so as to pick up an object and place it on a platform. Movements of the robot are measured in each of three phases: reach (from the start of movement to contacting the object), grasp (from first contact to lifting the object), and transport (bringing the lifted object to the platform). The S1 feedback cut the time to grasp the object in half and shortened the other phases as well.

Why should adding touch signals have such a dramatic effect? Flesher and associates (2021) note that a training period does not seem to be required to use the feedback to S1. This participant had years of prior experience with the experimental task, and he showed immediate improvement when the S1 link was turned on, which vanished when it was turned off. It appears that the biological link between movement and its somatosensory consequences exploits a natural avenue for the brain to control the robot. Although brain-computer interfaces are not everyday technology at present, it is hoped that they will become available for many of the thousands of people whose lives are suddenly changed as a result of spinal cord injury.

Summary

1. The sense of touch is vital to our experience of the world and to our very existence. Perception by touch begins as neural receptors sense the consequences of physical contact in many forms: mechanical pressure, vibration, noxious stimulation, thermal change, itchy stimulation, or stroking. Signals from these neural receptors pass to the brain via the spinal cord and ultimately lead to the rich representations of the world we touch.
2. Four classes of pressure-sensitive (mechano-) receptors have been found within hairless skin, and others are found within hairy skin. These receptors consist of neural fibers, some of which connect to specialized end organs that enhance neural function. Other receptors at muscles, tendons, and joints sense limb position and movement. Thermoreceptors respond to changes in skin temperature; nociceptors signal tissue damage (or its potential) and give rise to sensations of pain; pleasant touch receptors respond to stroking.
3. Two major pathways from skin to brain have been identified: a fast one (the dorsal column–medial lemniscal pathway), which carries information from mechanoreceptors, and a slower one (the spinothalamic pathway), which carries thermal and nociceptive information. Both enter the dorsal horn of the spinal cord, which itself has dense neural connectivity. The pathways project to the thalamus and from there to the primary somatosensory area, located in the parietal lobe just behind the central sulcus. This area contains several somatotopically organized subregions, in which adjacent areas of the body project to adjacent areas of the brain. The neural organization of the brain for touch has been shown to be remarkably plastic, even in adults.
4. The complex perceptual functions enabled by the physiology of touch can be organized into submodalities, including *discriminative* touch, which enables us to perceive vibratory patterns and the spatial distribution of contact; the aversive sensations of *pain and itch*; and affective touch, which comprises emotional and social components. Interoception constitutes another submodality, with unique mechanoreceptors and pathways to the brain.
5. To assess discriminative touch, investigators determine pressure thresholds and spatial acuity of the skin by measuring responses to points of touch or

patterns applied to the skin. These measures vary with body site, reflecting differences in mechanoreceptor density; similar (but not identical) variations are found with pain. The minimum depression of the skin needed to feel a stimulus vibrating at a particular rate (frequency) provides a measure of vibration sensitivity.

6. Downward pathways from the brain play an important role in the perception of pain. According to the gate control theory, signals along these pathways interact at the spinal cord with those from the periphery of the body. Such interactions can block the pain signals that would otherwise be sent forward to the brain. The sensation of pain is further moderated by other methods, including thought control and interactions with itch.
7. Touch provides a means of social signaling. The interpretation of social touch depends both on its physical characteristics, such as the rate of stroking, and on our knowledge of the world and the immediate context, which act top-down to disambiguate social intentions.
8. The sense of touch is intimately related to our ability to perform actions. Signals from the mechanoreceptors are necessary for simple actions such as grasping and lifting an object. Conversely, our own movements or exploratory procedures determine how touch receptors respond and, hence, which properties of the concrete world we can feel. Touch is better adapted to feeling the material properties of objects than it is to feeling their geometric features (e.g., shape), particularly when an object is large enough to extend beyond the fingertip.
9. Like other sensory modalities, touch gives rise to internal representations of the world, which convey the positions of objects using the body as a spatial reference system. Touch-derived representations are inputs to higher-level functions like allocation of attention and integration with information from other modalities.

Chapter 14

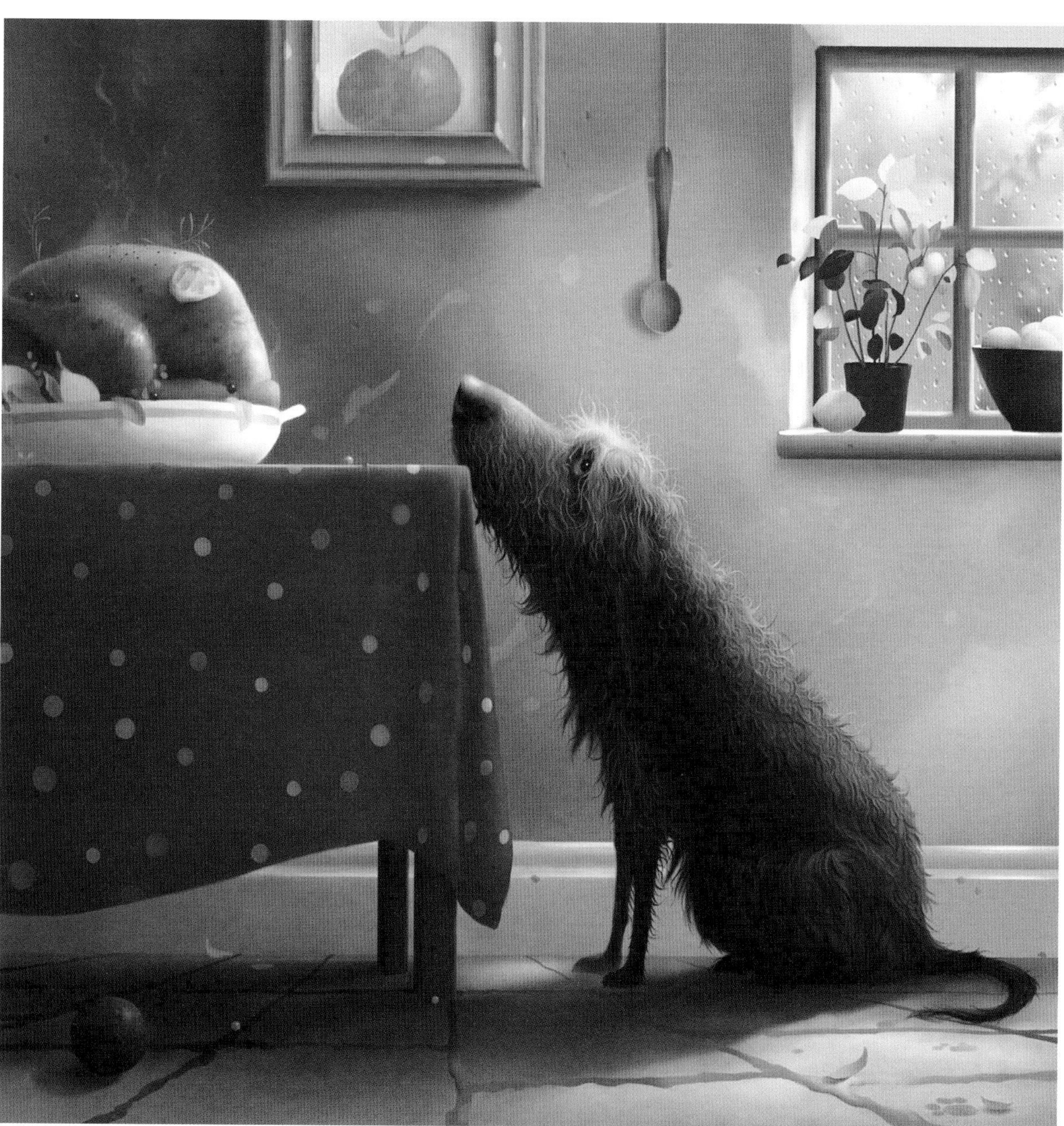

Stephen Hanson, *Sunday Roast*, 2017

Olfaction

Questions to Contemplate

Think about the following questions as you read this chapter.
By the chapter's end, you should be able to answer and discuss them.

- If you had to give up one sensory modality, why would you not want to give up your sense of smell?
- How are odor liking and odor perception influenced by emotion and experience?
- What are some of the individual difference characteristics that influence olfactory sensitivity and perception?
- Is there any scientific basis to aromatherapy? If so, what is it?
- What are some ways in which olfaction is not like any of our other senses?

The story of the next two chapters begins at the dawn of life itself. When single-celled organisms first appeared on Earth, their basic purpose in life was to take in some substances (nutrients) and avoid others (toxins). As these organisms evolved into multicellular creatures, detecting chemicals in the environment continued to be crucial for survival. Systems to detect and analyze environmental molecules were thus the first senses to evolve. Today, from the most complex of life-forms to the simplest, the basic principles—to approach chemicals that elicit pleasure and/or aid survival and to avoid chemicals that elicit aversion and/or hasten demise—remain the primary functions of the chemical senses.

Humans have two main chemical detection systems: one for molecules floating in the air and another for molecules that enter our mouths. The technical names for these two systems are **olfaction** and **gustation**, respectively. The former, more commonly known as "smell," is the subject of this chapter. Gustation, which you probably know as "taste," will be explored in Chapter 15. Another chemical-sensing system that is important for our experiences of both smells and tastes is the trigeminal system, innervated by the trigeminal nerve. The trigeminal system enables us to feel gustatory and olfactory experiences, like burning and cooling.

Our sense of smell is critically involved in our experience of food. The reason is because there are two routes through which we perceive odors. **Orthonasal olfaction**, the primary topic of this chapter, occurs when we sniff odorant molecules through our nostrils and they travel up our nose and onto the olfactory epithelium—as happens when we smell a rose. The second route is **retronasal olfaction**, which occurs when we exhale odorant molecules in our mouth and they travel up from the back of our mouth into our upper nasal cavity and onto the olfactory epithelium. Retronasal olfaction occurs when we are eating and drinking, and it produces the sensation of "flavor," as will be detailed in Section 15.1.

olfaction The sense of smell.

gustation The sense of taste.

orthonasal olfaction Sniffing in and perceiving odors through our nostrils, which occurs when we are smelling something that is in the air.

retronasal olfaction Perceiving odors through the mouth while breathing and chewing. This is what gives us the experience of flavor.

odor The translation of a chemical stimulus into the sensation of an odor percept. For example, "The cake has a chocolate odor."

odorant A specific molecule defined by its physicochemical characteristics that can be translated by the central nervous system into the perception of an odor. For example, "The odorant methyl salicylate has the odor of wintergreen mint."

volatile A molecule that is buoyant in air and therefore can be inhaled. Odorants are volatile molecules.

14.1 Olfactory Physiology

According to the American Lung Association (2018), we inhale about 21,000 times per day, and with each breath comes the opportunity to experience the world around us through smell. But what is it that we are experiencing?

Odors and Odorants

Olfactory sensations are called **odors**. The stimuli for odors are chemical compounds called **odorants**. An analogy can be made with vision, where wavelengths of light are the stimuli and colors are the visual sensations. However, not every chemical is an odorant. To be smelled, odorant molecules must be **volatile** (able to float through the air), small (between 25 and 300 daltons), and hydrophobic (repellent to water). FIGURE 14.1A shows the chemical structures of two odorant molecules. However, not all molecules that would seem to meet the basic requirements for being odorants have a smell; two examples are natural gas (methane) and a by-product of methane, carbon monoxide (FIGURE 14.1B). Our evolutionary ancestors would have had no reason to detect these substances, which are not dangerous in the concentrations found in nature. But because the buildup of methane in enclosed spaces such as homes with gas furnaces can be fatal, gas companies add a compound (tertiary-butyl mercaptan) that we smell as rotten eggs, to act as a warning signal when a pilot light goes out. We also can't smell the molecules that make up the air we breathe, such as oxygen, helium, and nitrogen. Conceptually, the air is a blank canvas upon which the odorants we can smell are painted.

The Human Olfactory Apparatus

Unlike the visual and auditory systems, but like the systems of touch and taste, the human olfactory system is "tacked on" to an organ that serves another purpose. The primary function of the nose (FIGURE 14.2) is to filter, warm, and humidify the air that carries oxygen to our lungs. In addition to this life-sustaining task, the inside

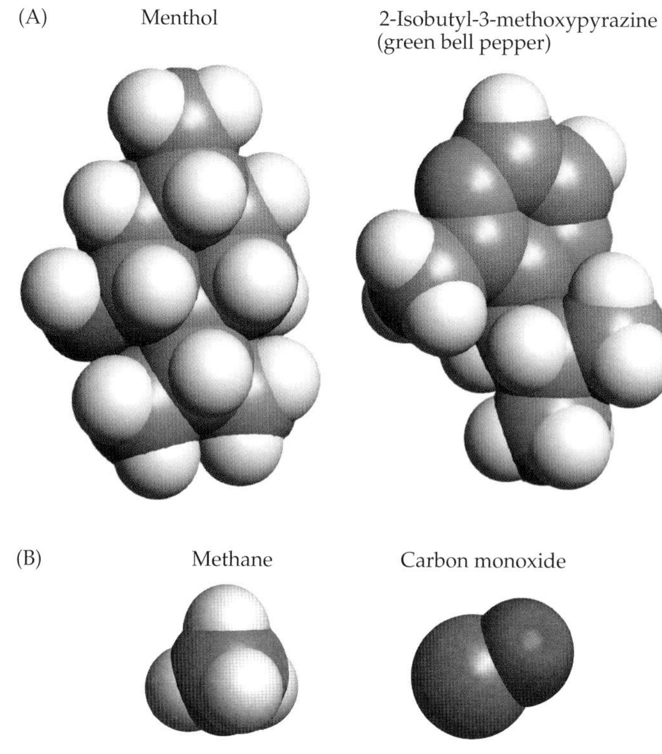

FIGURE 14.1 **Odorants** (A) Most small, volatile, and hydrophobic molecules activate the sense of smell, but there are notable exceptions. (B) Methane and carbon monoxide molecules are odorless in the natural state.

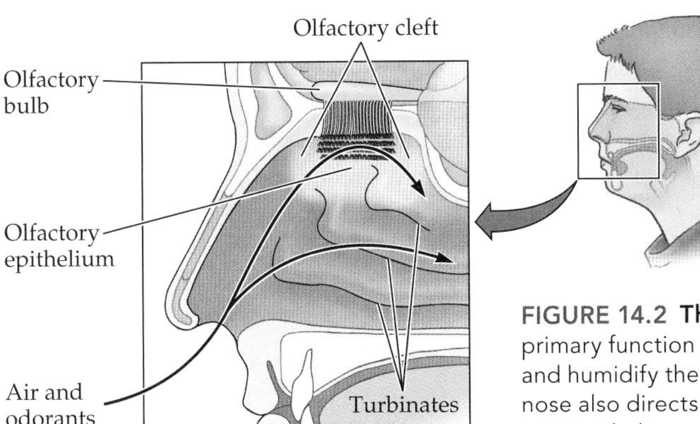

FIGURE 14.2 **The nose** Although the primary function of the nose is to warm and humidify the air that we breathe, the nose also directs odorants onto the olfactory epithelium.

of the nose has small ridges called **turbinates** that add turbulence to incoming air, causing a small puff of each breath to rise upward, pass through a narrow space called the **olfactory cleft**, and settle on a yellowish patch of mucous membrane called the **olfactory epithelium** (FIGURE 14.3). Individual differences in the size of the olfactory cleft can affect olfactory sensitivity. The bigger the cleft, the more air containing odorants can reach the olfactory epithelium, and therefore the more intense things may smell. In addition, our two nostrils take in different amounts of air, and this **nasal dominance** alternates between our nostrils throughout the day. This means that, as a function of the amount of air inhaled, the two nostrils continually vary in their sensitivities to odorants.

The olfactory epithelium is the "retina of the nose." We have an olfactory epithelium at the back of each nasal passage, about 7 centimeters (cm) up from the nostril. Each epithelium measures about 2.5 to 5 cm^2 (depending on the size of the nose) and contains three types of cells: **sustentacular cells** (also called **supporting cells**), **basal cells** (also called **stem cells**), and **olfactory sensory neurons (OSNs)**.

turbinates Curved bony protrusions inside the nasal cavity. The small ridges of the turbinates create turbulence to incoming air, causing a small puff of each inhalation to rise and pass through the olfactory cleft, facilitating the ability to detect odorants.

olfactory cleft A narrow space at the back of the nose into which air flows and where the olfactory epithelium is located. It can vary in size.

olfactory epithelium A mucous membrane in the nose whose primary function is to capture odorants in inhaled air. Located on both sides of the upper portion of the nasal cavity (the olfactory clefts), the olfactory epithelium contains three types of cells: sustentacular cells, basal cells, and olfactory sensory neurons.

nasal dominance The asymmetry characterizing the intake of air by the two nostrils, which leads to differing sensitivity to odorants between the two nostrils. Nasal dominance alternates nostrils throughout the day, but there is no predictability for when the nostrils alternate.

sustentacular or supporting cell One of the three types of cells in the olfactory epithelium. Sustentacular cells provide metabolic and physical support for the olfactory sensory neurons.

basal cell or stem cell One of the three types of cells in the olfactory epithelium. Basal cells are the precursor cells to olfactory sensory neurons.

olfactory sensory neuron (OSN) One of the three cell types—the main one—in the olfactory epithelium. OSNs are small neurons located within a mucous layer in the epithelium. Cilia on the OSN dendrite contain receptor sites for odorant molecules.

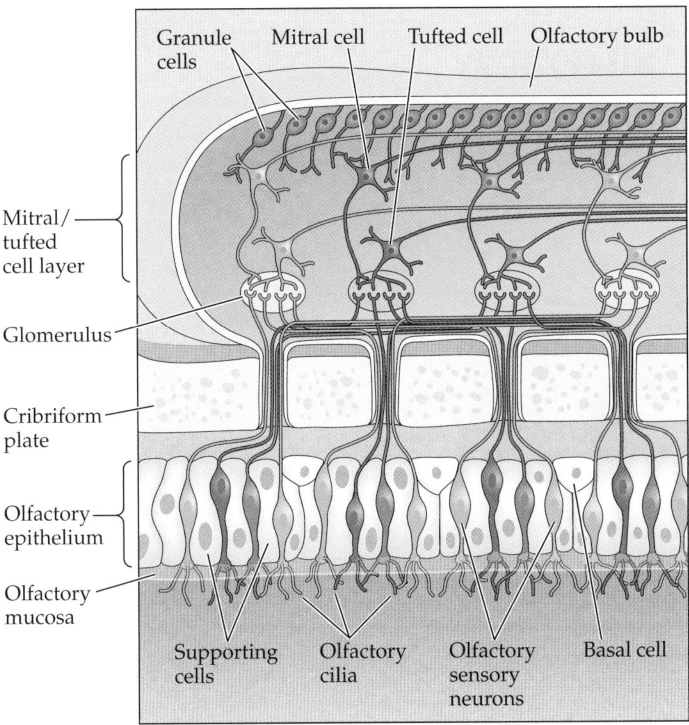

FIGURE 14.3 **The "retina of the nose"** The olfactory epithelium contains three types of cells: olfactory sensory neurons (OSNs), basal cells, and sustentacular cells. The OSNs are located within a watery mucous layer on the epithelium; the hairlike olfactory cilia of the OSN dendrite project into the mucus, and within them are the receptor sites for odorant molecules. The different colors of the OSNs in this illustration indicate the glomeruli onto which they converge. All blue OSNs connect to blue glomeruli, all purple to purple, and so on. This schematic illustrates the fact that different OSNs expressing the same receptors converge on the same type of glomerulus, no matter where they are in the olfactory epithelium.

cilium Any of the hairlike protrusions on the dendrite of olfactory sensory neurons. The receptor sites for odorant molecules are in the cilia, which are the first structures involved in olfactory signal transduction. Plural, *cilia*.

odorant receptor (OR) The region in the cilia of olfactory sensory neurons where odorant molecules bind.

glomerulus Any of the spherical conglomerates containing the incoming axons of the olfactory sensory neurons. Each OSN converges onto two glomeruli (one medial, one lateral). Plural, *glomeruli*.

G protein–coupled receptor Any of a class of receptors that are present on the cilia of olfactory sensory neurons. All G protein–coupled receptors are characterized by a common structural feature of seven membrane-spanning helices. Binding of a substrate molecule to the receptor transmits a signal across the membrane to a G protein, which then initiates a cascade of biochemical events.

Importantly, it is the through the basal, and especially sustentacular, cells that the spike protein, which is unique to the SARS-CoV-2 virus (responsible for the COVID-19 pandemic), enters the body and causes the olfactory loss that is both a critical early marker and a long-term symptom of COVID-19 infection (Butowt and von Bartheld, 2021). Though you might think destruction of the OSNs is necessary to produce olfactory loss, with COVID-19 the route is indirect. The SARS-CoV-2 virus causes disruption and inflammation to the sustentacular cells, which has the effect of damaging the OSNs, and this leads to impaired olfactory function (Brann et al., 2020). This underscores how important and supportive these "supporting" cells truly are.

OSNs are small neurons that have hairlike **cilia** (singular, *cilium*) protruding into the mucus covering the olfactory epithelium. Note that OSNs are bipolar neurons and have one axon and one dendrite at opposite ends of the neuron (**FIGURE 14.4A**). The cilia are at the tip of the OSN dendrite and their membranes are spanned by **odorant receptors (ORs)** (**FIGURE 14.4B**).

The basic rule of olfactory sensory physiology is "one to one to one": each OSN expresses only one type of OR, and all OSNs expressing the same type of OR project to the same type of **glomerulus** (see Figure 14.3). Odorant receptors belong to a class of proteins known as **G protein–coupled receptors.** When an odorant binds to the receptor on the cilium, it transmits a signal through the membrane to a G protein (guanine-nucleotide binding protein) in the cilium interior (see Figure 14.4B). This interaction between an odorant and its receptor stimulates the G protein and initiates a cascade of biochemical events, ultimately producing an action potential (see Section 14.3) that is transmitted along the axon of the OSN

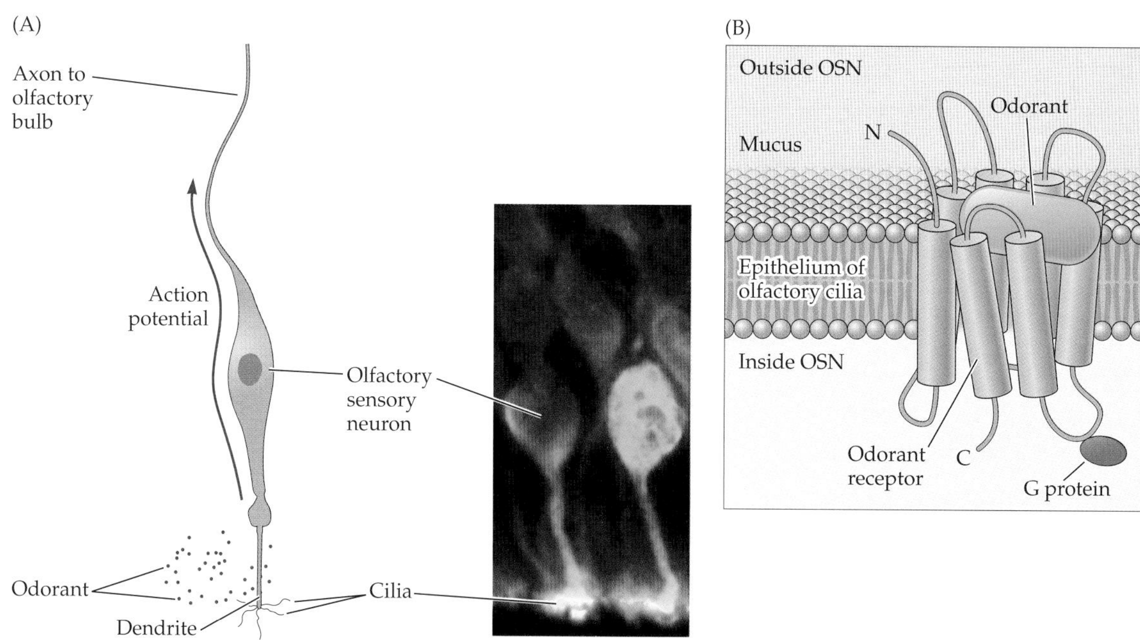

FIGURE 14.4 Olfactory sensory neurons (OSNs) respond to odorants The OSN collects odorant molecules via receptors on the cilia of its dendrite and sends an action potential to the brain through its axon. (A) A fluorescence image of an olfactory sensory neuron with schematic. (B) An odorant makes its way from the mucus layer of the olfactory epithelium to where the olfactory cilia reside. The binding of the odorant to an olfactory receptor embedded in the cilium activates a G protein–coupled receptor signaling pathway that will trigger an action potential.

to the **olfactory bulb**—an extension of the forebrain (Schild and Restrepo, 1998). To initiate an action potential, about seven or eight odorant molecules must bind to a receptor, and it takes about 40 of these nerve impulses for a smell sensation to be registered by the olfactory bulb, which processes this information, as we will describe in Section 14.2.

The OSN axons carrying the action potential are on the ends of OSNs opposite the dendrite and cilia. Axons pass through the tiny sieve-like holes of the **cribriform plate**, a bony structure at the level of the eyebrows that separates the nose from the brain (see Figure 14.3). A hard blow to the front or back of the head can cause the cribriform plate to be sharply jarred or fractured, slicing off the fragile olfactory axons and consequently inducing **anosmia** ("smell blindness"), the total absence of a sense of smell. Stem cells in the olfactory epithelium can form new OSNs; indeed, all of our OSNs continually die-off and regenerate. However, fractured cribriform plates tend to scar over, preventing new OSN axons from passing into the brain, and this leads to permanent smell loss.

olfactory bulb (OB) A blueberry-sized extension of the forebrain just above the nose, where olfactory information is first processed. There are two olfactory bulbs, one in each brain hemisphere, corresponding to the right and left nostrils.

cribriform plate A bony structure riddled with tiny holes that separates the nose from the brain at the level of the eyebrows. The axons from the olfactory sensory neurons pass through the holes of the cribriform plate to enter the brain.

anosmia The total inability to smell, most often resulting from sinus or viral illness.

How Well Do We Smell?

You might be wondering, How many odors can humans detect? The latest research suggests that the number is at least 40 billion (Mayhew et al., 2022)! This is far more stimuli than we can detect in any other modality. For example, the number of colors we can see is about 7.5 million, and the number of tones we can hear is approximately 340,000. Without knowing an exact number, the main point is that we can detect any and all "smellable" molecules. Amazing as this is, there are some constraints on our smell-ability, as you will discover throughout this chapter.

The number of OSNs in the human olfactory epithelia has never been counted. The current best estimate is that we have between 10 and 20 million OSNs split between the epithelia of our right and left nostrils. The range depends on a person's age (aging will lead to fewer OSNs) and the environment (exposure to environmental toxins will lead to fewer OSNs). Whatever the exact number, we know that vision is the only sensory system that has more sensory neurons than olfaction. Despite this large number, we are not the extreme sniffers of the animal kingdom. Dogs have at least 100 times more OSNs than humans. Humans can likely smell the same number of scents as dogs (the bloodhounds aren't talking, so we can't be sure), but dogs can sense odors at concentrations nearly 100 million times lower than the concentrations humans can detect (Krestel et al., 1984; Willis et al., 2004). Other "super smellers" include pigs, which can smell truffles (the mushroom, not the chocolate) under 15 cm of soil, and salmon, which use smell to find the water they were born in from hundreds of miles away (Dittman and Quinn, 1996).

But the most extreme sniffer of all appears to be the elephant, with approximately 2000 functional ORs (more than five times as many functional ORs as humans) and the longest nose in the animal kingdom (Niimura, Matsui, and Touhara, 2014). Their incredible proboscis allows African elephants to distinguish, with just a whiff, two ethnic groups with whom they share their habitat: the Masai, whom they fear (to show their virility, young Masai men spear them), and the Kamba, whom they ignore (the Kamba are farmers and do not bother the elephants) (Bates et al., 2007). Elephants can even calculate quantity with their noses. In one study, Asian elephants at a sanctuary in Thailand were offered two buckets containing different quantities of sunflower seeds (a favorite snack). Even though the buckets were covered, with only tiny holes bored into the lid (so they could sniff but not see), the pachyderms correctly chose the bucket containing the larger quantity of sunflower seeds up to 82% of the time (Plotnik et al., 2019). Even dogs can't do this!

Sensation & Perception in Everyday Life

Anosmia and the Effects of Olfactory Dysfunction

Anosmia ("smell blindness") is total smell loss—in other words, you can't perceive smells at all. Hyposmia is a significantly reduced sense of smell—you can still smell, but you perceive scents as being much weaker that other people do. Parosmia is a distorted sense of smell. Things that normally smell good, like vanilla, smell strange or bad. Phantosmia is when you perceive a scent (usually an unpleasant one) that is not objectively there. That is, the chemical you think you smell is a phantom.

Smell loss is much more prevalent than most people think. Prior to the COVID-19 pandemic, the National Institutes of Health estimated that 1.4% of the US population suffered from anosmia (Scangas and Bleier, 2017), and as many as 14 million Americans over the age of 55 had a severely compromised sense of smell. Since COVID-19, it is estimated that at least several million more Americans across all adult age groups are suffering from varying degrees of olfactory dysfunction. Currently, the number of people afflicted is inexact, but more precise data are expected soon. It is conservatively estimated that ~15 million people worldwide are currently suffering from persistent smell loss as a result of COVID-19. People with persistent smell loss from COVID-19, known as "smell long-haulers," may end up experiencing a multitude of cognitive and emotional deficits because of long-term disruption of their olfactory function (L. M. Kay, 2022). Even though many people have either experienced or are now aware of the hardships of olfactory dysfunction, olfactory loss is still given little attention by the medical community and the general public.

In terms of disability compensation, the American Medical Association values the loss of smell as being between 1–5% of person's net worth, whereas loss of vision is valued at 85%. With regard to public opinion, a large survey study administered to both college students and adults in their 40s that compared the value of the senses of smell, hearing, and vision to each other and in relation to nine common commodities (e.g., cell phone, 10,000 dollars, dream vacation, hair, social media, streaming service, pet, little left toe), found that the sense of smell was vastly underappreciated compared to hearing and vision (Herz and Bajec, 2022). These findings are probably not very surprising. However, what was shocking were the results comparing the value of each sense to the various commodities. For example, 25% of college students would rather give up their sense of smell than their cell phones—no college students would give up vision for their cell phones; and over 40% of all women surveyed would give up their sense of smell to keep their hair (approximately 27% of men would give up smell to keep their hair). Only 2% of those surveyed would give up their vision for their hair. Although hair is an important physical feature, it is not a critical mode through which we navigate the world—like our senses are. Of interest, this survey was conducted in the spring of 2021—during the height of the COVID-19 pandemic when awareness about the sense of smell and issues related to smell loss were widespread; nevertheless, the sense of smell was still highly undervalued.

Unfortunately, anosmia can cause great suffering. In one report comparing individuals who became blind versus those who had lost their sense of smell from an accident, the trauma of being blinded was initially far worse than losing olfaction, but a year later, blind people were coping much better, whereas the quality of life of the anosmics was becoming progressively worse (Herz, 2007).

Losing one's sense of smell can negatively affect nearly every aspect of life, ranging from the obvious inability to enjoy food aroma and flavor or detect environmental hazards that don't have visual cues (e.g., methane accumulation) to the less well-known consequences of decreased learning, memory, spatial and cognitive abilities, compromised social and sexual relationships, and an overall decline in mental health. If anosmia is untreatable, worsening quality of life is often progressive.

The functioning of our sense of smell is also a bellwether for our physical health and mortality. Americans over the age of 55 who experience smell loss are four times more likely to die in a 5-year span than their same-age peers with a functioning sense of smell—and this finding takes into consideration preexisting adverse health and lifestyle factors (Pinto et al., 2014). A similar, more recent study that examined people aged 40 and older also found that smell loss predicted all-cause mortality over a 5-year period regardless of the individual's demographics or health comorbidities (Choi et al., 2021). Interestingly, this

Sensation & Perception in Everyday Life *(continued)*

study found no association between self-reported olfactory dysfunction and mortality, which underscores the importance of objective smell testing. You may not know that your sense of smell is compromised, so it should become part of routine health care screening.

There are several explanations for the connection between olfactory health and mortality: (1) olfactory is directly exposed to the environment, therefore smell loss can be a marker for injuries to various organs or a general indicator of physiological health. (2) Smell loss may be an indicator of premature aging. (3) Smell loss may signal increased inflammation and/or decreased mental and cognitive functioning. All of these conditions increase the risk of earlier death.

Being born anosmic (referred to as **congenital anosmia**) is rare, affecting less than 0.06% of the population, and in itself is not associated with decreased life span or health span. Becoming anosmic through life's insults (referred to as **acquired anosmia**) is far more common. The causes of acquired anosmia include sinus and viral infections (sudden smell loss is a very important early indicator of COVID-19 infection, especially for some variants of the virus; Eliezer et al., 2020); nasal obstructions such as polyps; and physical injury to the olfactory system. Prior to COVID-19, about 30% of anosmia cases were caused by head trauma, which can occur in sports like football or boxing or through car or bicycle accidents—this percentage is probably lower now since the relative proportion of viral-induced anomia is higher.

Many everyday toxins, including gasoline and hairdressing chemicals, can cause either temporary or permanent smell dysfunction (W. M. Smith, Davidson, and Murphy, 2009). Air pollution is also bad for olfactory function. People who live in unpolluted environments generally have greater olfactory sensitivity than people who live in industrialized communities (Sorokowska, Sorokowski, and Frackowiak, 2015). Certain medications can also cause smell loss or disturbance. This is particularly true of drugs used in chemotherapy, but many common medications—including antibiotics, antidepressants, and even some antihistamines—can impair olfactory function (Doty and Bromley, 2004). Long-term excessive alcohol consumption also reduces olfactory function (C. I. Rupp et al., 2003). By contrast, marijuana may have enhancing effects.

Smell loss can also be the first warning sign of several neurological disorders—in particular, Alzheimer's disease and Parkinson's disease—and olfactory symptoms often appear years before any other signs of the illness are present (see "Scientists at Work: A New Test to Diagnose Parkinson's Disease" later in this chapter). If you know someone over 40 who has suddenly started having trouble identifying familiar smells, you may want to recommend a visit to a neurologist.

On the other end of the spectrum, children and adolescents with attention deficit hyperactivity disorder often have heightened olfactory sensitivity (Romanos et al., 2008; Lorenzen et al., 2016). But this advantage goes away once drug treatment begins. Since drugs for attention deficit hyperactivity disorder target dopamine dysregulation, dopamine function appears to underlie this effect. Contrary to what might be expected, no reliable olfactory differences have been found between people with autism spectrum disorder and matched controls.

Currently, there is no "cure" for smell loss. However, if the olfactory sensory epithelium and neural interconnections are intact (e.g., as in the case of COVID-19 and other viral infections), "smell training" can be a successful treatment. Smell training typically involves smelling four common odors twice daily for 12–24 weeks. Encouraging results in all aspects of olfactory function have been seen, especially if treatment is begun within the first year of loss (Jiang, Twu, and Liang, 2017; Sorokowska et al., 2017). Olfactory training can also enhance olfactory and cognitive function in people with a healthy sense of smell (Al Aïn, 2019), especially over the course of aging. The downside of smell training is that it can take months before benefits are seen, and people often give up before completing the regimen.

Many smell and taste clinics throughout the country administer simple tests to determine the causes and treatment possibilities for olfactory loss and dysfunction. However, smell loss is widespread and has far-reaching implications. Scientists and patient advocates are now working hard to make routine olfactory screening part of your annual visit to the doctor's office.

congenital anosmia. Having no sense of smell from birth on, and thus never experiencing scent. This condition is rare.

acquired anosmia. Possessing a sense of smell and then losing it sometime after birth. The most common causes of acquired anosmia are illness and head trauma.

orbitofrontal cortex (OFC) The part of the frontal lobe of the cortex that lies behind the bone (orbit) containing the eyes. The OFC is responsible for the various aspects in the conscious experience of olfaction, as well as the integration of pleasure and displeasure from food. The OFC is also involved in many other functions, and it is critical for assigning affective value to stimuli—in other words, determining hedonic meaning. It is also referred to as the secondary olfactory cortex and the *secondary taste cortex.*

hippocampus A region of the brain involved in spatial mapping, associative learning and memory, and processing olfactory information. It is adjacent to the amygdala, which processes emotion.

It has long been assumed that humans are not very good at using their noses. But, despite having comparatively few functional OSNs, human olfactory ability is actually very good. In one study, humans were able to follow a 10-meter-long scent track of chocolate aroma while on all fours in an open grass field (Porter et al., 2007), and the tracking pattern that they used was strikingly similar to that of a dog (**FIGURE 14.5**). Another recent study showed that humans, like homing pigeons, can use odors located in different places in a room to form a spatial map and then navigate accurately to specific points in that room (Jacobs et al., 2015). Indeed, it has recently been established that spatial navigation and olfactory ability are linked. For example, people who are better at navigating through a virtual town and forming cognitive maps are better at identifying odors, and they have a larger **orbitofrontal cortex (OFC)** and **hippocampus** regions than people who perform less well at navigating (Dahmani et al., 2018). These same researchers also found that patients with damage to the OFC performed worse than control subjects on odor identification and spatial memory tasks.

And, as with vision and hearing, it turns out that our olfactory navigation abilities are based on stereo perception. Wu and colleagues (2020) found that a difference in the concentration of the few odorants that don't activate the trigeminal nerve—phenylethyl alcohol (rose scent) and vanillin (vanilla scent)—simultaneously presented to each nostril biased participants to move their head toward the nostril exposed to the stronger intensity, even though the participants did not register a difference in odorant potency (when asked which nostril was presented with the stronger intensity, their responses were at chance). The findings further showed that the intensity orienting effect was a result of the ratio of concentration difference between the odorants presented to each nostril, not absolute intensity. That is stereo odor perception!

(A)

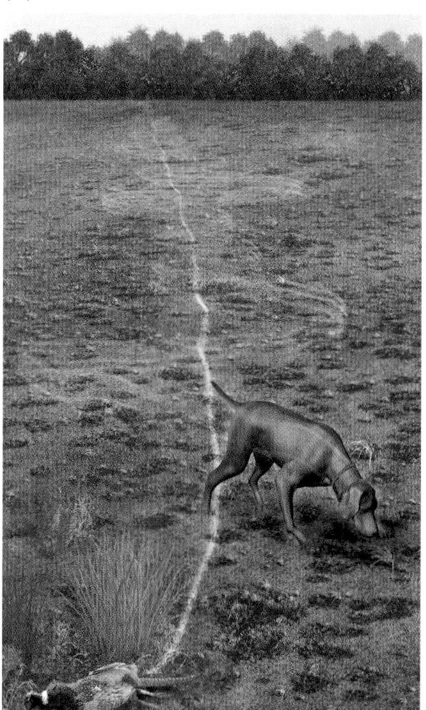

(B)

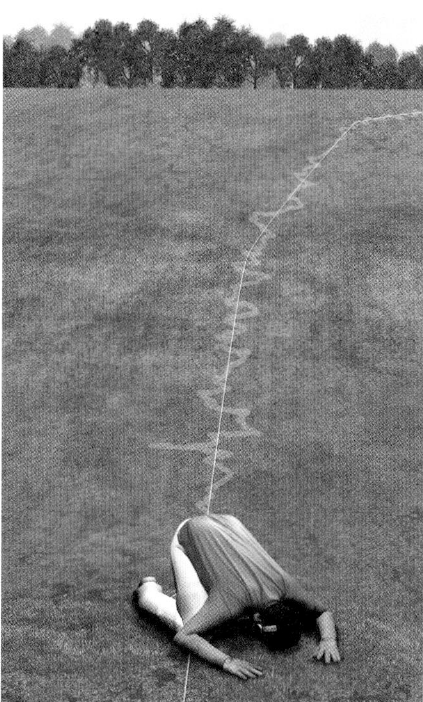

FIGURE 14.5 Tracking scents (A) The path (red) of a dog following the scent trail (yellow) of a pheasant dragged through a field. (B) The path (red) of a human following a scent trail (yellow) of chocolate essential oil through a field.

We are also good at using olfactory landmarks to navigate through space when no visual cues are available. In a virtual maze, participants performed well with only odors as cues after learning how to directionally navigate through the labyrinth with them (turn right at the maze intersection that smells like lemon, turn left at the scent of vanilla, go straight when you smell aftershave, and so on) (Hamburger and Knauff, 2019) (**FIGURE 14.6**). Moreover, just as with the exceptional duration of our olfactory memory—as you'll learn in Section 14.4—the participants' ability to remember how to navigate the maze with the specific odor landmarks was intact one month after learning them—the researchers did not test any longer durations (Arena and Hamburger, 2023). This exciting new finding has important implications for using odors to help blind people navigate. Additionally, as new research on the connection between spatial and olfactory abilities accrues, it will help clinicians diagnosing and working with patients with various neurological disorders, including Alzheimer's disease.

Compared to other animals, how good we are at smelling seems to depend on the odorant in question. In a test using six sulfur-containing compounds, humans were able detect two of the compounds better than mice, whereas mice were better than humans at detecting the other four (Sarrafchi et al., 2013; McGann, 2017). The absolute size of the human olfactory bulb is also much greater than that of the mouse (**FIGURE 14.7A**), even though 200 times more of a mouse's brain is devoted to the sense of smell. In fact, the number of neurons in the olfactory bulb is relatively conserved across mammals compared to the variability of other physical

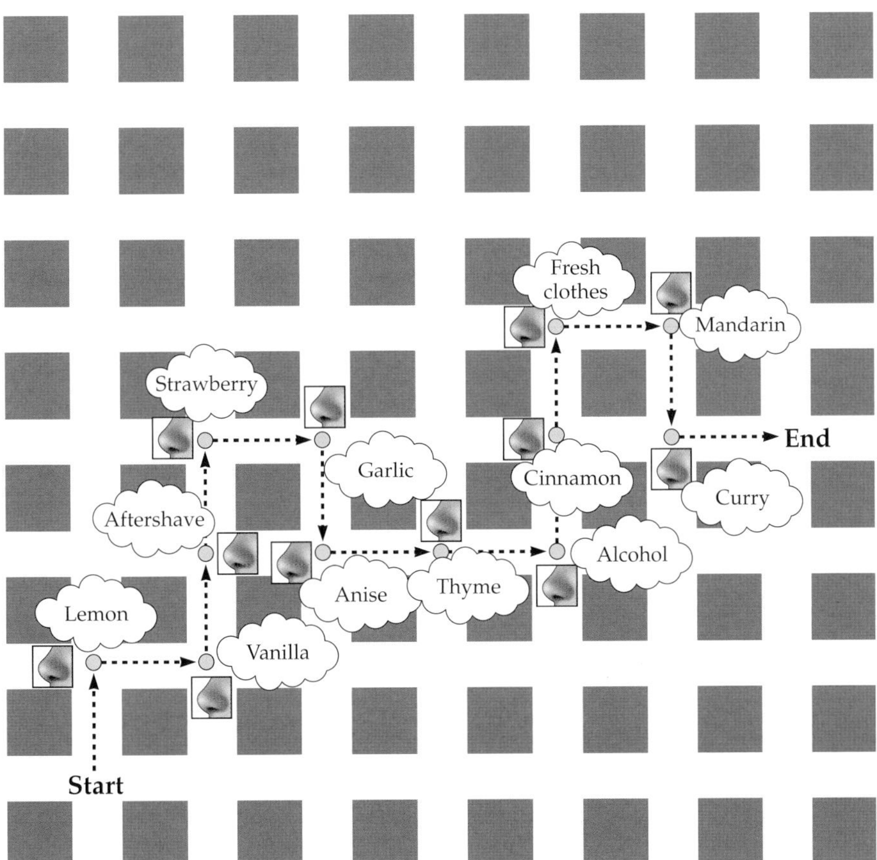

FIGURE 14.6 Humans can use odors as landmarks to navigate through a virtual reality maze

olfactory nerve The first cranial nerve. The axons of the olfactory sensory neurons bundle together after passing through the cribriform plate to form the olfactory nerve, which conducts impulses from the olfactory epithelium in the nose to the olfactory bulb. Also called *cranial nerve I*.

ipsilateral Referring to the same side of the body (or brain).

juxtaglomerular neurons The first layer of cells surrounding the glomeruli. They are a mixture of excitatory and inhibitory cells and respond to a wide range of odorants. The selectivity of neurons to specific odorants increases in a gradient from the surface of the olfactory bulb to the deeper layers.

features, such as size and weight (**FIGURE 14.7B**). Therefore, absolute differences in the neural hardware for olfaction across species is much less than previously assumed. A reexamination of the literature has revealed that the belief that humans are poor smellers arose as a result of pressures from nineteenth-century religious and philosophical doctrine and is not based on scientific evidence. The truth is that humans can smell very well (McGann, 2017)!

14.2 Neurophysiology of Olfaction

The axons of the OSN's pass through the cribriform plate and form the **olfactory nerve** (cranial nerve I) as they enter the olfactory bulb (**FIGURE 14.8**). We have two olfactory bulbs, one in each brain hemisphere. Unlike the other senses we've studied, olfaction is **ipsilateral**, meaning that the right olfactory bulb gets information from the right nostril, and the left olfactory bulb gets information from the left nostril.

The chemical methyl salicylate has an odor that we identify as wintergreen mint. Like other odorants, methyl salicylate can activate several different types of ORs, and it does so with different degrees of "weighting," depending on the receptor's affinity to the wintergreen molecule. Humans have between 350 and 400 different types of functioning ORs. Most of these receptors won't be activated by methyl salicylate; a few will be weakly activated, and one or two will be strongly activated; this will become clearer as you read the following sections.

Despite a recent study (Weiss et al., 2020) reporting that some women have a normal sense of smell even though they apparently have no olfactory bulbs, the first relay for the OSNs in the brain is in the olfactory bulb, where the sensory nerve endings gather together to form tiny spheres called glomeruli. Molecular genetic

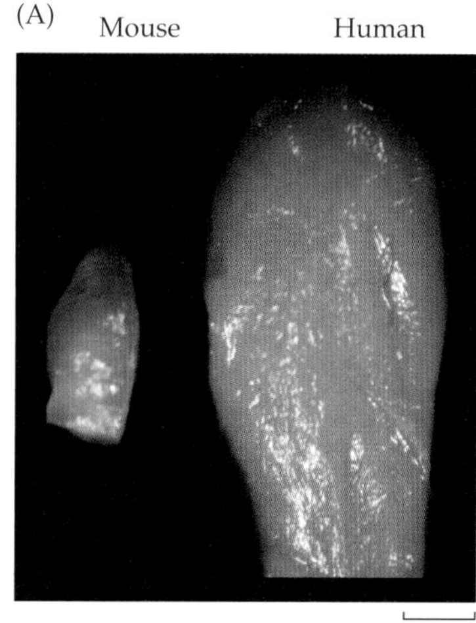

FIGURE 14.7 Olfactory bulb (A) Comparison of the mouse and human olfactory bulb. (B) The number of olfactory bulb neurons differs across mammalian species, but is much less variable than the differences in other physical features across those same species.

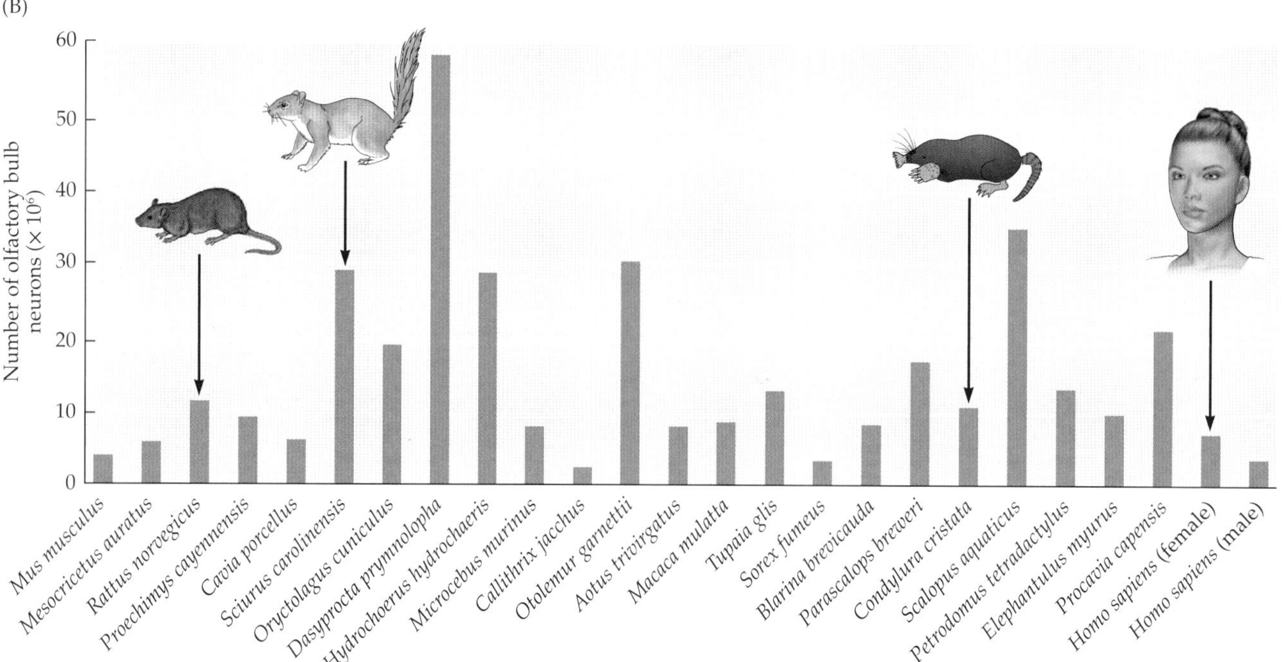

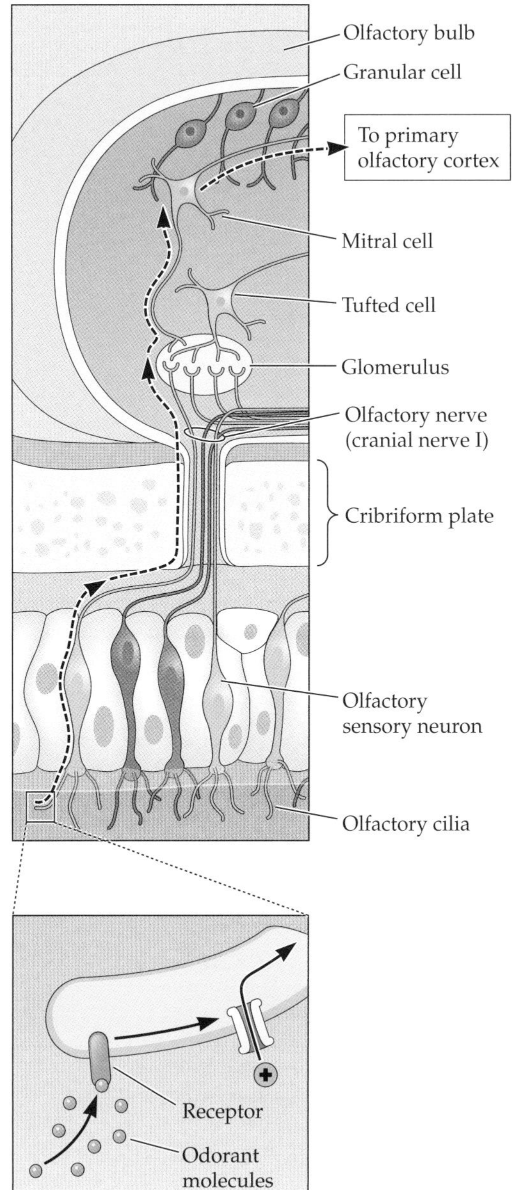

FIGURE 14.8 From odorant to odor perception The pathway of olfactory perception starts with the binding of odorant molecules to receptors on the cilia of olfactory sensory neurons (see Figure 14.4). Action potentials generated by G protein–coupled reactions in the olfactory sensory neuron travel to the olfactory bulb and then to the primary olfactory cortex.

studies in mice have shown that all neurons expressing a particular OR type, no matter where they are on the nasal epithelium, send their axons to the same glomerulus pair (consisting of one medial and one lateral glomerulus) in the olfactory bulb (Mombaerts et al., 1996). The distinct pattern of OR activation for a specific odorant is then translated into a specific pattern of spatial activity across the glomeruli. Methyl salicylate, for example, will activate a particular set of ORs and consequently produce a specific pattern of glomerular activity. The chemicals that produce rose scent will initiate a different activation pattern, and so on. The specific pattern of glomerular activity is then interpreted by the brain as indicating a specific odor (see Section 14.3).

This relatively simple picture is complicated by the fact that each glomerulus may receive axons from several different receptor types. Moreover, our personal experience with an odor can actually change the pattern of activity produced by the glomeruli in the olfactory bulb. For example, if you liked wintergreen mints (i.e., methyl salicylate) but one day became ill after eating them—thereafter finding the scent very unpleasant (illustrating what is known as a learned taste aversion, discussed further in Section 14.5)—the pattern of activity produced by the scent of methyl salicylate in the olfactory bulb would become different from what it was when you liked wintergreen mints. Astonishingly, this means that there is no fixed code for odor perception; rather, our personal experience with an odor and its meaning to us determines how it will be processed by the olfactory system and its neurologically coded valence (see Section 14.6) (D. A. Wilson, Best, and Sullivan, 2004; Gadziola et al., 2019).

Immediately surrounding each glomerulus is a mixed population of excitatory and inhibitory cells called **juxtaglomerular neurons**. These cells respond to a much wider range of odorants than the next layer of neurons, the **tufted cells**, which in turn respond to more odorants than the next layer comprising **mitral cells**. In other words, the selectivity of neurons to a specific odorant is increasingly sharpened in a gradient from the surface of the olfactory bulb to the deeper layers (Kikuta et al., 2013). Recent work in mice further suggests that mitral cells play a critical role in boosting the detection of important smells. That is, tufted cells enable greater odorant intensity and identity detection in general, and mitral cells help prioritize the scent of meaningful odors, such as the smell of food or predators (Chae et al., 2022). In fact, the latest research suggests that finely tuned interactions between mitral cells and the OB are critical for fully understanding how the sense of smell works (Chen and Padmanabhan, 2022). We now need to wait for further research to confirm the details. Stay tuned! At the deepest level of the olfactory bulb are **granular cells**, an extensive network of inhibitory neurons that integrate input from all the earlier projections and are thought to function as higher-order feature detectors, capable of detecting and learning specific combinatorial patterns of mitral and tufted cell activation and thus responding specifically to different odorants (Koulakov and Rinberg, 2011).

tufted cells The next layer of cells after the juxtaglomerular neurons. They respond to fewer odorants than the juxtaglomerular neurons, but more than neurons at the deepest layer of cells.

mitral cells The deepest layer of neurons in the olfactory bulb. Each mitral cell responds to only a few specific odorants.

granular cells Like mitral cells, granular cells are at the deepest level of the olfactory bulb. They comprise an extensive network of inhibitory neurons that integrate input from all the earlier projections and are thought to be the basis of specific odorant identification.

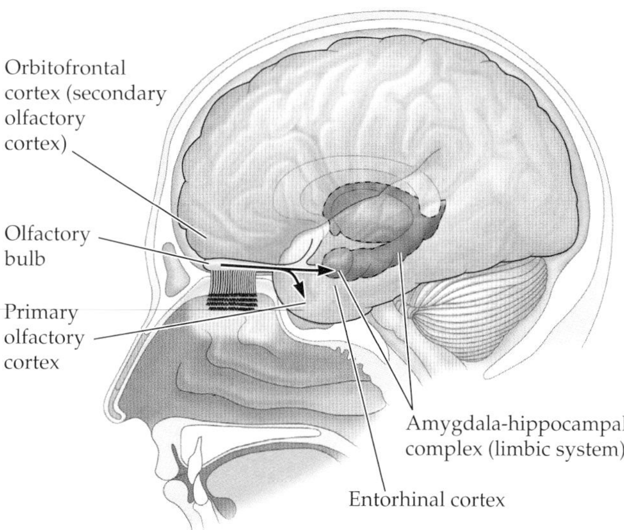

FIGURE 14.9 The neuroanatomy of olfaction A cross-sectional view of the neural organization of olfaction. Olfactory information is transmitted from the olfactory bulb to the primary olfactory cortex comprising the amygdala-hippocampal complex of the limbic system in the first stages of olfactory processing. The orbitofrontal cortex is considered the secondary olfactory cortex.

Axons of the mitral and tufted cells of each bulb combine to form the **olfactory tract**, one in each hemisphere of the brain, that conveys odor information ipsilaterally to the **piriform cortex**, also known as the **primary olfactory cortex**. The primary olfactory cortex comprises the amygdala, the parahippocampal gyrus, and the interconnected areas known as the **amygdala-hippocampal complex**, and it intimately interacts with the **entorhinal cortex** (FIGURE 14.9). The primary olfactory context is where our first conscious perception of smell takes place. The "secondary olfactory cortex" is the orbitofrontal cortex (OFC). The OFC is involved in various aspects of olfactory perception, taste perception, and in coding the valence of experiences—that is, our hedonic responses to a wide range of stimuli (R. J. Davidson, Putnam, and Larson, 2000) (see Figure 14.8). This will be discussed in more detail in Section 14.5.

Though they number in the millions, OSNs converge onto a relatively small number of glomeruli. The mouse, whose brain and OR physiology is much more devoted to olfaction than are those of humans, has 3600 glomeruli (Richard, Taylor, and Greer, 2010). It was therefore speculated that humans, with far fewer functioning ORs, would have about 700 glomeruli. However, immunohistochemistry research from Charles Greer's laboratory at Yale University has revealed that humans have around 5500 glomeruli—almost twice as many as the mouse for only a third the number of functioning receptors (Maresh et al., 2008; Zapiec et al., 2017). This discovery was quite a surprise and suggests that the wiring must be different in the two species: either humans have many more glomeruli devoted to a single OR than mice do, or the molecular specificity of human glomeruli is not equivalent to that of the mouse. In any case, this is a cautionary tale for directly applying findings from mouse models to human olfaction.

The central brain structures that process olfactory information are part of a network of structures known as the **limbic system** that is involved in many aspects of emotion and memory. As we will see in Section 14.6, these connections are key to the unique associative learning and emotional properties of olfaction. It may be surprising, but paleontological research has shown that mammalian brain evolution was precipitated by an increase in olfactory ability (Rowe, Macrinin, and Luo, 2011). That is, the first structures in mammalian brains to increase in size and complexity were those associated with the sense of smell. One theory is that increased olfactory capacity enabled our 200-million-year-old ancestors to hunt at night, giving them the evolutionary edge they needed to develop further and eventually evolve our current brains.

The OSNs are different from all other sensory receptor cells in that they are not mediated by a protective barrier, but instead connect directly from inside the nose to the brain. By contrast, visual receptors are protected by the cornea, receptors for hearing are protected by the eardrum, and taste buds are buried in papillae. Lack of protection from environmental assault makes OR regeneration crucial (neural regeneration is a special feature of olfactory perception)—if ORs did not regenerate, we would all lose our sense of smell as children.

Despite their direct linkage into the brain, OSN axons are among the thinnest and slowest in the body. Therefore, even though the nose connects directly to the brain, the time it takes to process the sensation of an odor is long, compared with our

olfactory tract The bundle of axons of the mitral and tufted cells within the olfactory bulb that sends odor information to the primary olfactory cortex.

piriform cortex (the primary olfactory cortex) The neural area where conscious olfactory perception takes place. It comprises the amygdala, parahippocampal gyrus, and interconnected areas, and it interacts closely with the entorhinal cortex.

amygdala-hippocampal complex The conjoined regions of the amygdala and hippocampus, which are key structures in the limbic system. This complex is critically involved in the unique emotional and associative properties of olfactory cognition.

entorhinal cortex A phylogenetically old cortical region that provides the major sensory association input to the hippocampus. The entorhinal cortex also receives direct projections from olfactory regions.

limbic system A group of neural structures that includes the primary olfactory cortex (piriform cortex) and the entorhinal cortex. The limbic system is involved in many aspects of emotion and memory. Olfaction is unique among the senses for its direct integration with the limbic system.

other sensory experiences. The lag time between sniffing and the brain registering a scent varies, averaging approximately 400 milliseconds (ms)—almost half a second. Compare this with the 45 ms it takes for the visual cortex to register an image presented to the retina. On top of the half-second duration for odor registration is the time it takes to react to a scent, which effectively doubles the perceptual time, making olfaction a particularly slow sense. You have probably observed that smells seem to emerge gradually, rather than flashing into your awareness.

FURTHER DISCUSSION of how long it takes the brain to register a sound or a touch can be found in Section 9.4 and Section 13.2, respectively.

These distinctions bring up the subtle differences between sensation and perception in olfaction. *Sensation* occurs when an odor is neurally registered; *perception* occurs when we become aware of detecting a scent. Odor clearance is also slow, and you may have noticed that odors tend to linger. This is because of both ambient air currents (e.g., a breeze versus still air) and the time it takes ORs to clear an odorant. The relatively slow speed and lingering features of olfaction have been central obstacles in attempts to develop movie theater technologies like "smell-o-vision."

The Genetic Basis of Olfactory Receptors

In 1991, molecular biologists Linda Buck and Richard Axel (who were awarded a Nobel Prize in 2004 for their efforts) showed that the mammalian genome contains at least 1000 different odorant receptor genes, depending on the species (elephants have the most), each of which codes for a single type of OR. The OR genome is the largest gene family known in mammals. All mammals appear to have pretty much this same set of OR genes, but some genes in each species are nonfunctional "pseudogenes"—that is, the genes are present on the chromosomes, but the proteins coded for by the genes do not get made. For example, dogs have 811 functional OR genes (Niimura, Matsui, and Touhara, 2014), and about 25% of their OR genes are pseudogenes. In humans, the OR genome contains less than 1000 genes, and the proportion of pseudogenes is approximately 52% (**FIGURE 14.10**). Importantly, it has been suggested that the large number of pseudogenes in humans may operate as a regulatory network that affects what genes are turned on or off depending on the olfactory environment (Cadiou et al., 2014). The proportion of functional OR genes differs considerably across mammals. This is in contrast to the number of neurons in the olfactory bulb, where there is relative consistency across mammalian species.

We don't have a precise percentage of pseudogenes for humans, because there is enormous diversity in the repertoire of functional OR genes among different people; in olfaction, everybody has a unique nose (McRae et al., 2013; Menashe et al., 2003). This reflects both which genes are expressed as functional receptors and how many copies of a specific receptor a person has. The more copies of a specific receptor you have, the more sensitive you will be to certain odorants (that is, specific chemicals will smell stronger to one person than they do to another because of the number of receptor copies they have). Whether you have a pseudogene or a functional gene for a given receptor also alters odor perception (Keller et al., 2007). For example, people who "hate" the aroma of cilantro (also known as coriander) have a nonfunctional gene for detecting the herbal floral component of this aroma and therefore only detect the soapy note (Kurz, 2008). Similarly, people who think that beets "taste" like dirt (it is really beet flavor, not taste) have a mutation on an OR that enables them to detect the strong earthy note of 2-ethylfenchol—a compound in beets. People without this mutation don't smell dirt and are more likely to enjoy

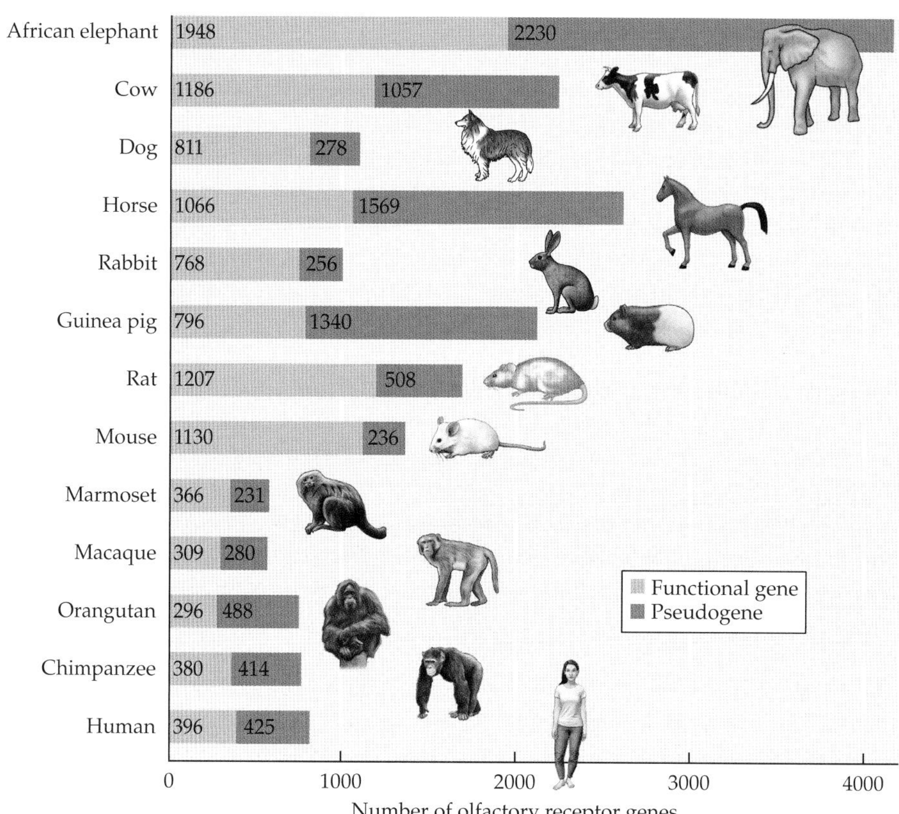

FIGURE 14.10 Olfactory receptor (OR) genes by species Comparison of the number of OR genes in selected mammalian species. Note that these are rough estimates.

eating beets (Trimmer et al., 2019). The genes associated with the OR expression that determines our sensitivity to four other food-relevant odors—banana, beer, blue cheese, and violets—have also been identified (McRae et al., 2013). Even more recently, a major genome-wide association study in Iceland found that specific genetic variants were responsible for differences in the sensitivity and naming accuracy capabilities of chemicals responsible for fishy, licorice, and cinnamon odors (Gisladottir et al., 2020). Depending on the allele variant, Icelanders detected fishy odor (trimethylamine) as either weaker or stronger, which corresponded to their pleasantness rating and naming ability for the fishy smell. As discussed in the next paragraph, the more intense an odor is perceived to be, the higher the potential for it to be experienced as unpleasant. Two other genetic variations were found to be related to the intensity and ability to identify cinnamon and licorice aromas. Beyond variation among people within the same population (i.e., Icelanders), the frequency of gene variants differs between ethnicities. For example, people of East Asian descent are much more likely to have the allele variant with high sensitivity to the main aromatic compound in licorice (trans-anethole) than people of European descent (Gisladottir et al., 2020). Beyond these findings, the specific genetic basis for our perception of most other scents is currently unknown. However, with continued research we will continue to learn more about the genetic basis of odorant detection and perception.

The number of particular receptors people express can modulate their liking for an odor, because having more receptors leads to a more intense smell, and strong scents in general tend to be perceived as less pleasant than the same scents at a lower intensity (see Section 14.5). We see this relationship with intensity in all our senses. Very bright lights and loud sounds are more aversive than moderate-intensity lights and sounds, and our relative sensitivity to light and sound will affect how much each of us can tolerate (see Chapters 5 and 9). Having few receptors of a given type can lead us to perceive a scent only weakly, and if we like an aroma, we may expose ourselves to more of it to get the same "bang for our buck" than someone with more ORs sensitive to that odorant would.

When it comes to eating, the more intense our perception of the retronasal aroma of the food (see Chapter 15 for more on retronasal aroma), the less we tend to consume (Ruijschop et al., 2008). For example, if our OR expression for the odorant that contributes to the banana aroma in banana cream pie is low, we may eat more pie than someone who can perceive the banana aroma strongly, and this may lead us to consume more dessert than we might have intended. These findings demonstrate the subtle but important ways by which OR variation can influence our food choices as well as our food intake. It should, however, be noted that many psychological factors mediate our food consumption as well as our odor preferences (see Section 14.5). Therefore, our genetic makeup does not predestine our response to any given odor or food.

There are also factors that can temporarily increase our sensitivity to odors. For example, even though heavy alcohol consumption (e.g., three drinks per hour) impairs olfactory sensitivity, having only one drink (blood alcohol level less than 0.06%) improves olfactory acuity (Endevelt-Shapira et al., 2014). This may be a benefit to having a glass of wine with dinner, because with one glass of wine the flavor aromatics of your meal will be enhanced. But beware that the more you pour, the less flavor you'll perceive.

Another popular recreational drug, marijuana, also boosts olfaction. It was found that activating cannabinoid receptors (the receptors that respond to the active component in marijuana) in the brains of fasted mice increased their smell sensitivity and induced the mice to eat more (Soria-Gómez et al., 2014). Extrapolating to humans, the reason for the "munchies" that come with a marijuana buzz may be that food aroma and flavor perception is intensified, and thus food is more enticing.

Indeed, stimulating appetite is one of the main reasons marijuana is prescribed for patients undergoing chemotherapy. However, the picture gets more complicated because it has also been found that, although in low doses tetrahydrocannabinol, the main psychoactive ingredient in marijuana, stimulates appetite, high doses decrease food consumption. There are also complicated findings surrounding the correlation between body weight and cannabis use. Higher blood levels of naturally circulating endocannabinoids (our body's natural version of cannabis) are associated with decreased olfactory perception and higher body mass index among women (Pastor et al., 2016). At the same time, frequent marijuana use in healthy adults is associated with a lower incidence of obesity. Although the relationship between olfaction, marijuana, food intake, and body weight is not yet fully understood, marijuana holds promise for therapies targeting weight management and olfactory function (Tarragon and Moreno, 2019). Stay tuned. ●

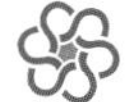

The "Feel" of Scent

As mentioned at the start of this chapter, our experience of odors often has a feel to it, as well as a smell. This is because most odorants stimulate the somatosensory system to some degree through polymodal nociceptors (touch, pain, and temperature receptors) inside the nose. For example, menthol feels cool and ammonia feels burning. These sensations are mediated by the **trigeminal nerve** (cranial nerve V), which responds to stimuli in and around the mouth, nose, and eyes (**FIGURE 14.11A**). In many cases it is impossible to distinguish between the sensations traveling up cranial nerve I from ORs and those traveling up cranial nerve V from somatosensory receptors. For example, the nasal cooling (cranial nerve V) and specific scent

trigeminal nerve The fifth cranial nerve. It transmits information about the "feel" of an odorant (e.g., mint feels cool, cinnamon feels warm), as well as pain and irritation sensations (e.g., ammonia feels burning). Also called *cranial nerve V*.

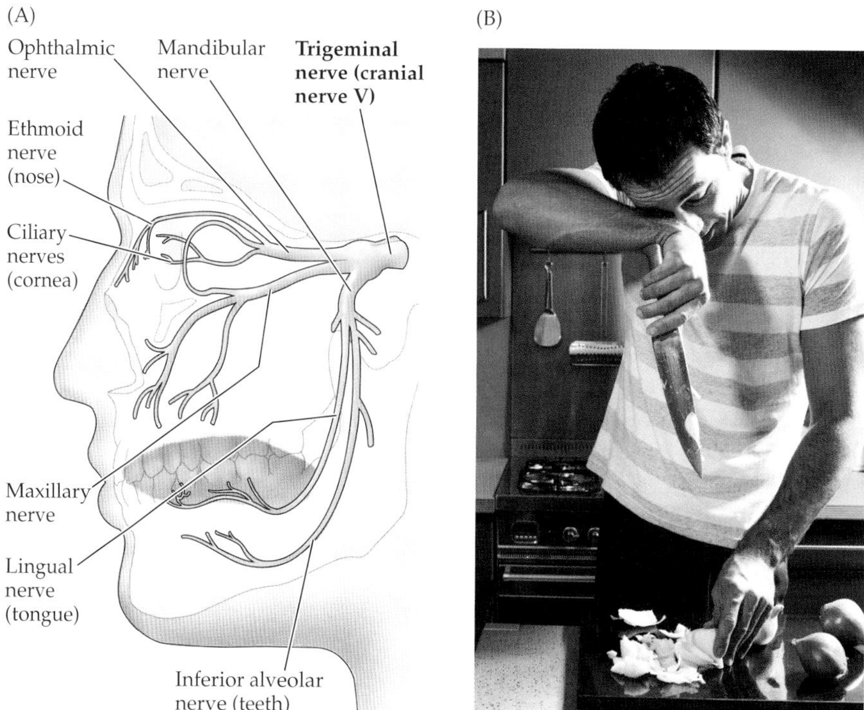

FIGURE 14.11 The trigeminal nerve's role in the perception of odors (A) The trigeminal nerve carries information from somatosensory receptors in the nose and other areas of the face to the thalamus and then on to the somatosensory cortex. (B) Your eyes tear when you chop onions because volatiles released from the onion stimulate the trigeminal nerve.

(cranial nerve I) associated with the smell of peppermint fuse to produce a holistic sensory experience. Trigeminal stimulation also accounts for why our eyes tear when we chop onions (**FIGURE 14.11B**) and why we sneeze when we sniff pepper. High levels of trigeminal stimulation can produce a severe burning sensation, and trigeminal activity has been linked to the facial and head pain felt in migraine headaches. Smelling salts (made from ammonia combined with eucalyptus oil) revive us because of their trigeminal activation. ●

FURTHER DISCUSSION of the trigeminal nerve can be found in Section 15.6.

14.3 From Chemicals to Smells

Now that we know something about the physiological basis of olfaction, we can ask the following crucial question: How does the biochemical interaction between an odorant and an OR, as well as subsequent neurological processing in the olfactory bulbs and later brain structures, result in the psychological perception of a scent such as wintergreen mint? L. Buck and Axel's (1991) seminal discovery of olfactory receptor genes has prompted an explosion of research surrounding this question over the past three decades, but a comprehensive theory of how we perceive scents is not yet fully resolved.

Theories of Olfactory Perception

At present, the best-accepted biochemical theory (first proposed in its modern form in the 1950s by the British scientist John Amoore) is based on the match

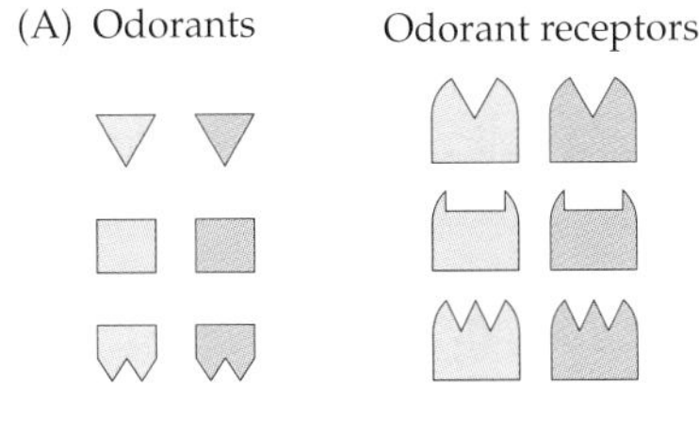

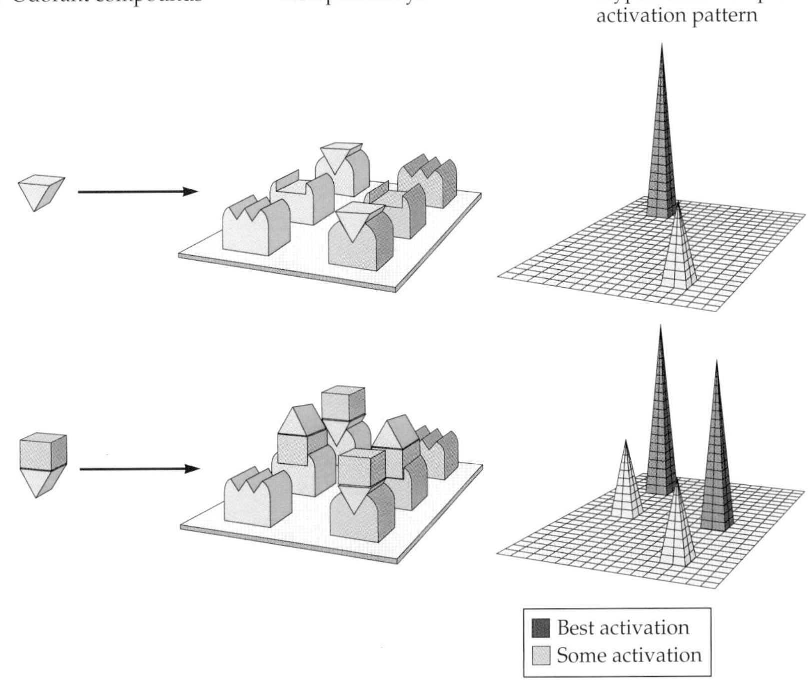

FIGURE 14.12 Shape-pattern theory account of odorant-receptor binding and activation (A) Odorants (chemicals) fit receptors with shapes that best accommodate them. (B) The specific pattern of activity elicited by a given set of receptors determines the specific scent perceived.

between the shapes of odorants and ORs. It was dubbed "shape theory," but is better denoted as shape-pattern theory. In a nutshell, **shape-pattern theory** contends that odorant molecules have different shapes and ORs have different shapes, and an odorant will be detected by a specific OR to the extent that the odorant's molecules fit into that OR (**FIGURE 14.12**). Gordon Shepherd and his students at Yale University pioneered the idea that when a given odorant is sniffed, a particular pattern is generated across the glomeruli. Differences in those spatial patterns provide the basis for the array of odors that we perceive. Among the evidence for shape-pattern theory are findings from in vitro experiments using cloned ORs that have revealed chemical-receptor interactions of specific odorants binding with specific receptors.

According to shape-pattern theory, scents are detected by means of a combinatorial code, where one odorant may bind to several different receptors and one receptor may bind several different odorants to varying degrees (see Figure 14.12). This means that different scents activate different arrays of ORs in the olfactory epithelium, producing specific glomerular activity in the olfactory bulb. The specific pattern of glomerular activity in the olfactory bulb then determines the particular scent we perceive, with different patterns elicited for the perception of rose, mint, urine, and skunk (for example). That is, the perception of rose starts with a chemical analysis of the molecules that make up the rose scent, with specific ORs recognizing various chemical features. This feature information is then transmitted to the olfactory bulb, where a unique spatial-temporal pattern of activity consisting of second-order neurons and mitral and tufted cells occurs.

Within the olfactory bulbs, inhibitory networks enhance the contrast between the various spatial-temporal patterns that different odors produce and modulate the patterns according to both the physical and the contextual states of the individual (see Kontaris, East, and Wilson, 2020). That is, the olfactory bulb response to chocolate and cheese odors will change as a function of both how hungry or full you are and what you interpret these odors as being (Palouzier-Paulignan et al., 2012). This theory was implied in Section 14.2. However, there are also alternative explanations of how olfaction works, because shape-pattern theory has problems explaining how molecules with very different shapes can produce very similar smells. For example, the single chemical phenylethyl alcohol and a chemical mixture composed of more than 1000 different chemicals both produce a scent we perceive as "rose."

The strongest alternative to shape-pattern theory is **vibration theory**, championed most recently by Luca Turin (Franco et al., 2011; Turin, 1996; Turin et al., 2015). In essence, vibration theory proposes that, because of atomic structure,

shape-pattern theory The current dominant biochemical theory for how chemicals come to be perceived as specific odors. Shape-pattern theory contends that different scents—as a function of the fit between odorant shape and olfactory receptor shape—activate different arrays of olfactory receptors in the olfactory epithelia. These various arrays produce specific firing patterns of neurons in the olfactory bulbs, which then determine the particular scent we perceive.

vibration theory An alternative to shape-pattern theory for describing how olfaction works. Vibration theory proposes that every odorant has a different vibrational frequency and that molecules that produce the same vibrational frequencies will smell the same.

specific anosmia The inability to smell one specific compound amid otherwise normal smell perception.

every odorant has a different vibrational frequency, and molecules that produce the same vibrational frequencies have the same smell. Turin reported that various chemicals that have predictably similar vibrations because of their molecular composition also have similar smells. For example, all citrus odors fall into the same vibrational-frequency class. In support of this theory, fruit flies are capable of distinguishing between two molecules that are identical in shape but have different vibrational frequencies (Franco et al., 2011).

A number of researchers have argued against the vibration theory (e.g., Block et al., 2015; Keller and Vosshall, 2004), while others are trying to bridge the gap and are working to show how receptors influence the vibrational properties of odorants (Reese et al., 2016). Nevertheless, vibration theory has problems explaining various aspects of odor perception, in particular, specific anosmias and the different scents produced by stereoisomers, which shape-pattern theory can explain.

A **specific anosmia** is the inability to smell one specific compound amid otherwise normal smell perception. Specific anosmias are caused by faulty OR interactions or the lack of (or different variants of) specific ORs, not odorant vibrations. Most specific anosmias are to steroidal musk compounds, and the condition appears to be genetic. The most studied specific anosmia is an inability to smell the compound androstenone, which is found in armpit sweat and pork. A large proportion of the population has a specific anosmia to androstenone; estimates range from 11% to 75%, but between 20% and 40% is more typical (Bremner et al., 2003). Interestingly, among those who can smell androstenone, the majority find it to be unpleasant and "urinous," while the rest describe it as a "sweet musky-floral" scent. A cloning study of human ORs showed that the variability in detection of the odorant androstenone, as well as its perceived quality, is a result of genetic differences in OR expression between individuals (Keller et al., 2007). Similarly, the different anosmia rates obtained for androstenone in different studies most likely reflect the fact that the gene governing the ability to smell androstenone varies randomly within any given sample of participants.

FURTHER DISCUSSION of specific sensory deficits amid otherwise normal perception—in this case vision (agnosias)—can be found in Section 4.2.

Non-musk odorants for which specific anosmias have been found include the sulfur compound in asparagus—this is the "funny" smell in urine that many people detect after eating it—but in addition to variation in the ability to smell this compound, the amount of the compound that is excreted in urine varies genetically among individuals. Therefore, if you don't smell something funny after eating asparagus, it may be because you don't excrete the sulfur metabolite, not because you're missing the receptor to detect the odorant (Pelchat et al., 2011). If you really want to check whether you're among the approximately 6% of Americans who are anosmic to asparagus pee, you'll need to take a sniff after a friend who can smell it in her own urine and ate asparagus with you goes to the bathroom. Approximately 10% of the population is anosmic to the scent of freesia flowers, and sensitivity to the sweaty-sock aroma of isovaleric acid also varies vastly among people, with about 6% of the population unable to detect it at all (Vockley and Ensenauer, 2006).

These examples illustrate how individual genetic variability in receptor expression determines each of our own unique olfactory experiences. Although the differences in perception may be small, everyone does indeed have a different nose. This complication—that the same stimulus is perceived differently by different individuals—is not unique to olfaction. People who are color-blind perceive the same visual stimulus differently from standard observers; however, in olfaction the difference between individuals is much more complex. Vibration theory cannot explain the presence of specific anosmias or why the same odorant produces different scent sensations in different people, but shape-pattern theory can: these phenomena could arise from differing OR interactions or the absence of or variance in certain receptors.

Another mark in favor of shape-pattern theory comes from the study of stereoisomers. **Stereoisomers** are molecules that are mirror-image rotations of one another, and although they contain all the same atoms, they can smell completely different. For example, D-carvone (the right-handed isomer; **FIGURE 14.13A**) smells like caraway, and L-carvone (the left-handed isomer; **FIGURE 14.13B**) smells like spearmint. According to shape-pattern theory, this difference arises because the rotated molecules do not fit the same receptors (as if you were trying to put your right hand into your left-hand glove); thus, these two molecules activate different receptors, causing different scents to be perceived. Vibration theory cannot explain why stereoisomers smell different, because their vibrations should be the same. Even though a fully understood or agreed-on explanation for odor perception has yet to be determined, the benefit of scientific controversy is that it motivates continued research to solve the problem.

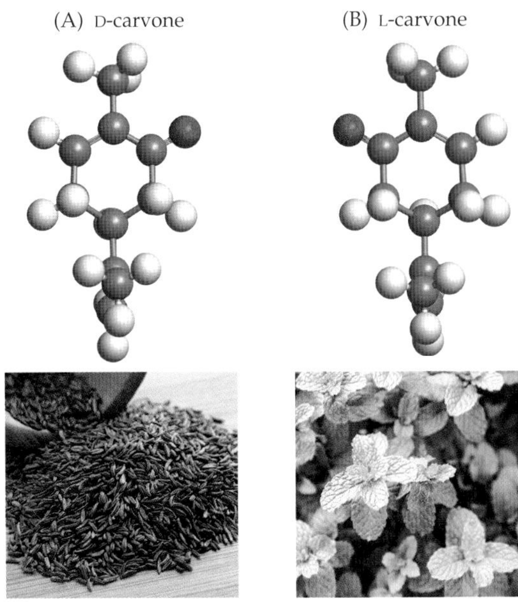

FIGURE 14.13 Stereoisomers smell different The stereoisomers D-carvone (A) and L-carvone (B) contain the same atoms, yet they smell completely different: D-carvone smells like caraway; L-carvone smells like spearmint. Shape-pattern theory can account for this fact.

stereoisomers Isomers (molecules that can exist in different structural forms) in which the spatial arrangements of the atoms are mirror-image rotations of one another, like a right and left hand.

Recently, there have been several attempts to apply machine learning (ML) algorithms to predict the relationship between odorant chemistry and odor perception (Keller et al., 2017)—Google has even gotten involved (B. K. Lee et al., 2022). These attempts have had varying degrees of success, but in the best case to date demonstrate only about 50% correlation between an odorant's chemical structure and what it is typically reported to smell like (**FIGURE 14.14**). There are several explanations for why ML hasn't had more success, including that more data are needed for the artificial intelligence models to learn how different people respond to different odorants. However, the most meaningful explanation for the lack of robust artificial intelligence capabilities in olfaction is that the current ML approach in olfaction relies on verbal descriptors, which are themselves learned and can be highly variable across people, as you will see in Section 14.4, and that ML is overly reliant on odorant chemistry and largely ignores odorant biology. Odorant biology considers the neurophysical response of the sensory neurons to specific odorants (which you now know is not identical between any two people) and is focused on causal as opposed to correlational relationships between odorants and responses. (For an excellent discussion and review of this topic, see Barwich and Lloyd, 2022.) Some biological research into how specific ORs respond to selected odorants has been undertaken (Poivet et al., 2016, 2018), but more work is needed. In the future, ML that integrates olfactory chemistry, biology, and the responses of the organism to specific odorants could indeed crack the code!

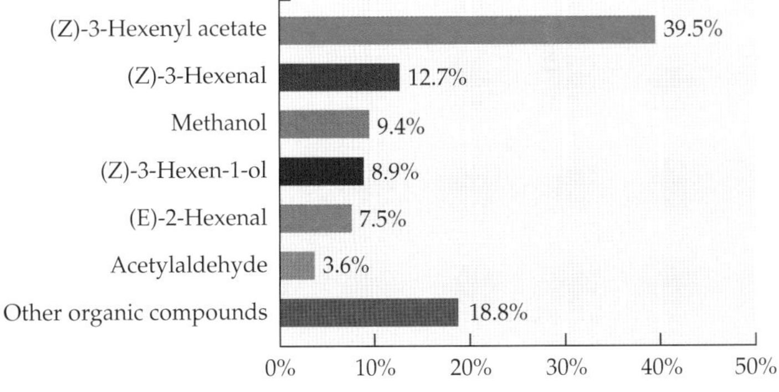

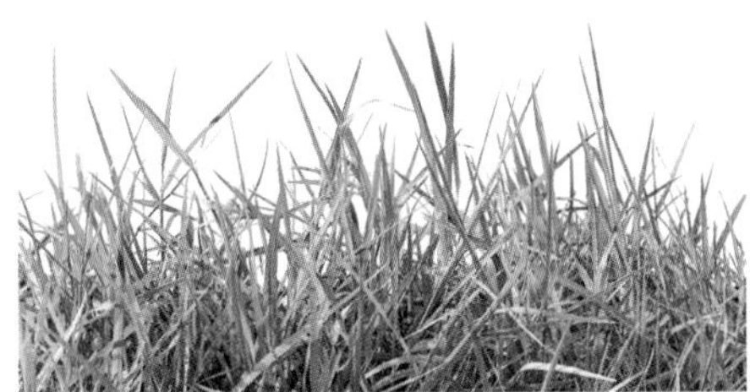

FIGURE 14.14 What is the scent of freshly cut grass? These chemicals describe the scent mixture in freshly cut grass. However, this chemical recipe is not necessarily a predictor of the perceptual experience. That is, knowing the chemical recipe in machine learning does not ensure what it will smell like to a given individual.

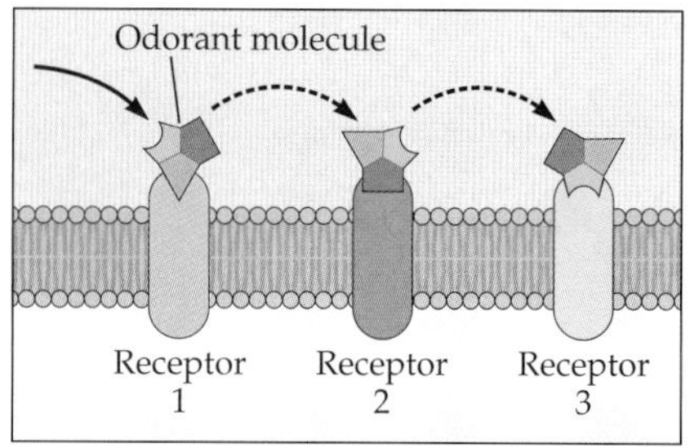

FIGURE 14.15 The hypothetical role of olfactory receptor activation timing and order A single molecule binds first to receptor type 1, an instant later to receptor type 2, and then to receptor type 3. Brains are especially well suited to recognizing patterns of responses such as this, so the number of odors we can recognize greatly exceeds the number of receptor types available.

The Importance of Patterns

You may have noticed a potential discrepancy in our account of odor perception. As noted, we can detect an enormous number of odors, yet our genes code for only about 1000 ORs, and 600–650 of these are nonfunctional. How can we detect so many different scents? To see a way out of this conundrum, recall that in vision we can tell the difference between thousands of different colors, even though we have only three types of cones. Each type of OR responds to the structure of certain molecules only; however, a molecule may have features that stimulate several different receptors. Moreover, each receptor has various feature detectors that contribute to further specificity in OR activation. Thus, in addition to differences in OR activation, a different set of feature detectors will be activated when we smell chocolate or wintergreen or rose.

As with color detection, we detect odors by the pattern of activity across different receptor types. The intensity of an odor also changes which receptors (and hence patterns) will be activated, which is why weak and strong concentrations of an odorant do not smell quite the same. The fact that receptor activation is affected by odorant concentration likely explains why dogs with many more functional receptors than we have can perceive odorants at considerably lower concentrations.

The timing of OR activation is also important. As described earlier in this section, an odorant that activates several receptors will also stimulate them in a specific temporal sequence (order) and at a particular rate (speed). Therefore, two odorants may activate the same ORs, but do so in a different order and/or speed, each of which (or taken together) would lead to different perceptions (**FIGURE 14.15**). Thus, the perception of different odors is a result of complex factors that include different OR firing patterns and firing of the same receptors at a different speeds and/or in different sequences.

The flip side of the pattern perception mechanism is that if two odorants, one molecularly simple and the other complex, activate the same receptors in the same way, we end up smelling the same thing. For example, the feature detectors for the single-molecule odorant phenylethyl alcohol (an artificial rose scent) and for the odorants of a living rose (a scent composed of more than 1000 different molecules) both yield essentially the same pattern of OR activation and hence the same perception of "rose" (this phenomenon should be reminiscent of metamers in color vision, discussed in Section 5.3).

Patterns are also important for odor processing at early stages in the olfactory cortex. Specific patterns of activity are produced by specific odors in the piriform cortex, and odors that are perceived as smelling similar produce similar patterns. For example, "minty" odors like wintergreen and spearmint typically produce patterns of activity that have a lot of overlap, but the pattern produced by a "citrus" odor like lemon does not tend to overlap with the pattern elicited by wintergreen. The fact that configural representations of odors (e.g., citrusy, minty) occur in the piriform cortex (the primary olfactory cortex) suggests that the piriform cortex is the olfactory analog of visual associative areas in the ventral temporal cortex. Notably, however, these areas differ substantially in their connectivity to emotion and language. As you will read about in Sections 14.4 and 14.5, the piriform cortex is intertwined with limbic areas that process motivation and emotion but is poorly connected to areas that process language—which is one reason why odors are so difficult to name. Moreover, consistent patterns of activity by specific categories of odors are *not* seen farther downstream in olfactory processing, such as in the amygdala or OFC (J. D. Howard et al., 2009). Consistency may be absent in these regions of the brain because at these later stages of processing, personal and emotional associations mediate activity patterns. Even in the piriform cortex, patterns of activity to specific odorants vary between people as a function of the meaning and experience they have with the odorant, and within the same person depending on their state (e.g., hungry versus full), as well as what they are doing (e.g., level of attention to smelling). This is further evidence that olfaction is an extremely dynamic system and it will be very difficult to find a fixed code.

Is Odor Perception Synthetic or Analytical?

Just as we rarely hear pure tones outside auditory perception experiments, we rarely smell "pure odorants" outside of an olfactory perception lab. Almost all of the olfactory stimuli that we encounter in the real world are mixtures, like the 1000-molecule scent emanating from a rose bush mentioned earlier. How do we process the components in an odorant mixture? There are two broad possibilities: analysis and synthesis. Auditory mixtures provide the classic example of analysis: a high note and a low note played simultaneously on a piano each can be analyzed out of the mix and perceived separately (**FIGURE 14.16A**). Color mixtures provide the classic example of synthesis: if we mix red and green lights, we perceive the resulting light as yellow (**FIGURE 14.16B**). Red and green cannot be analyzed out, because the two lights have been synthesized into something else. Is olfaction (**FIGURE 14.16C**) an analytical or a synthetic sense?

It seems that the answer is "both." Olfactory perception can be both analytical and synthetic, although the synthetic aspect is what we are more likely to perceptually experience. The analytical qualities of olfaction are evident in **binaral rivalry**. As you read in Chapter 6, when a different object is presented to each eye simultaneously, binocular rivalry occurs, and rather than a blend of objects, you see the two objects alternating. A similar phenomenon occurs in hearing when discrepant sounds are presented to each ear. It was found that binaral rivalry also occurs in olfaction: when two different odors are presented, one to each of our nostrils, we alternate in our ability to smell one odor or the other (W. Zhou and Chen, 2009; J. Chen, Zhou, and Chen, 2012). For example, when researchers presented a rose scent to one nostril and simultaneously an odor that smelled like marker pens to the other nostril, participants alternated back and forth between saying that they smelled "markers" or "rose." The marker scent was perceived as more intense and was usually

binaral rivalry Competition between the two nostrils for odor perception. When a different scent is presented to each nostril simultaneously, we perceive each scent to be alternating back and forth with the other, and not a blend of the two scents.

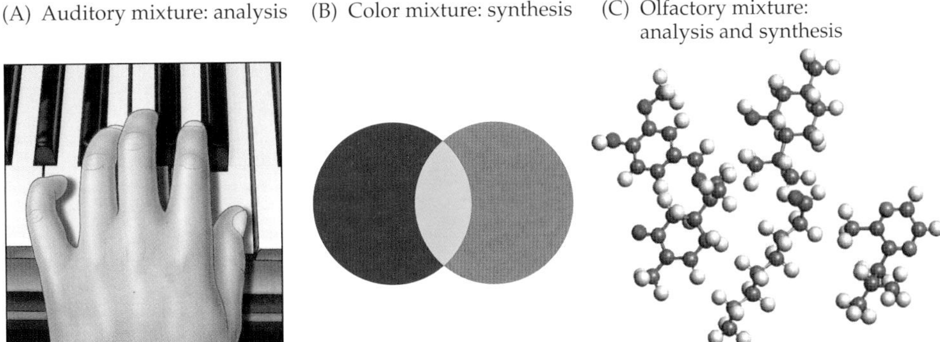

FIGURE 14.16 The roles of analysis and synthesis in sensory perception We can separately perceive the three tones of the musical chord being played in (A), but not the high- and medium-wavelength light rays mixing in the center of (B). When we mix odorants (C), we perceive the mixture primarily synthetically, but some degree of analytical perception is possible. Analytical ability varies with prior training and with the odorants that constitute the mixture.

olfactory white The olfactory equivalent of white noise or the color white. When at least 30 odorants of equal intensity that span olfactory physiochemical and psychological (perceptual) space are mixed, they produce a resultant odor perception that is the same as that of every other mixture of 30 odorants meeting the same span and equivalent intensity criteria, even though the various mixtures do not share any common odorants.

perceived first (as also occurs in binocular rivalry, where the "stronger" image tends to dominate). Interestingly, when the same participants were later presented with a scent mixture of both rose and markers to both nostrils simultaneously, most of them reported smelling first markers and then rose and then markers again, and so on. Moreover, binaral rivalry persists even when visual or verbal cues are simultaneously presented; it didn't matter whether participants saw a picture or the word for rose or marker at the same time as sniffing. These observations indicate that binaral rivalry is inherently a stimulus-driven process.

Although we are capable of discriminating thousands of different odors, intuition tells us that most mixtures are perceived as unitary wholes. For example, the smell of bacon is distinctive, and most people would perceive it to be a unitary sensation. But, as with natural rose aroma, there is no single "bacon" odorant, and the sensation we recognize as bacon is made up of a combination of approximately 150 different volatiles (**FIGURE 14.17**).

To test the synthetic/analytical nature of olfactory perception, Laing and his colleagues (Laing and Francis, 1989; Laing and Glemarec, 1992) conducted a classic series of experiments in which they asked (1) untrained participants, (2) participants who had received preliminary "odor training," and (3) experienced perfumers and flavorists to identify the constituents of mixtures containing between one and five common odorants. The average analytical ability from all the participants combined was no more than three components in a five-component mixture. Though the more training the participants had the better they did, when there were more than five components in a mixture, even professional perfumers' analytical ability broke down. Thus, it appears that olfaction is primarily a synthetic sense, but a certain amount of analytical ability can be developed.

The predominantly synthetic quality of odor mixture perception was also supported by a more recent experiment demonstrating the existence of **olfactory white**. Like white noise, where various mixtures of many different frequencies all are perceived as sounding like the same kind of meaningless buzz, or white in vision, where different mixtures of many different wavelengths all produce the perception of "white," olfactory white is produced by many different odorants.

Researchers found that when at least 30 odorants that span olfactory, physiochemical, and psychological (perceptual) space and that are of equal intensity are mixed, they produce an odor that is the same as the odor produced for every other mixture of 30 odorants meeting the same span and intensity criteria, even though the various mixtures do not share any common odorants (Weiss et al., 2012). That is, three different mixtures of 30 different odorant molecules will smell the same

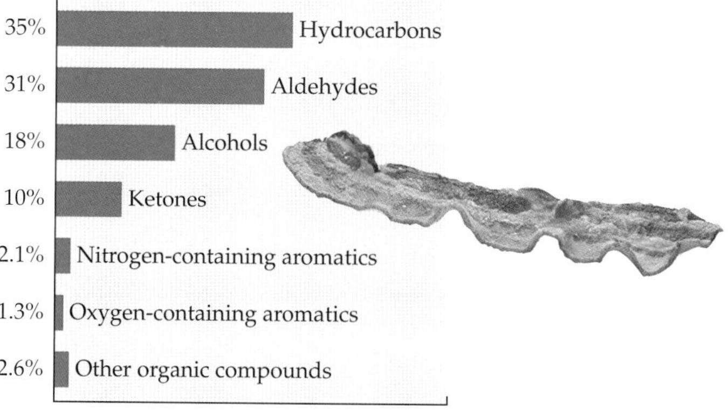

FIGURE 14.17 Bacon aroma There is no single scent that is "bacon." Rather the aroma of bacon is composed of approximately 150 different aromatic compounds.

if the contributing odorants have the same intensity and are distributed across the range of olfactory stimulus space. The more odorants in the mixture, the more indistinguishable the mixtures become, and 30 seems to be the tipping point. There isn't clear consensus on what olfactory white smells like, though some describe it as floral and it is consistently rated as being of neutral pleasantness. This exciting finding suggests an underlying commonality between olfaction, vision, and audition: a uniform perceptual experience can arise from large mixtures.

You may now be wondering why the complex odorant mixtures that produce the perceptions of bacon or rose do not instead all smell the same. The answer is that the component odorant molecules in bacon and rose aroma do not span the range of olfactory stimulus space, nor are they of equal intensities; rather, the odorants with dominant intensities and certain blends stand out, producing the specific perceptions of rose, bacon, coffee, and all the other specific odor sensations we can perceive.

FURTHER DISCUSSION of color mixture synthesis can be found in Section 5.3.

Another fascinating feature of olfactory perception is that the whole is not the same as the sum of its parts. New research has shown that *fewer* OSNs respond to a mixture of two odorants than to each odorant by itself (Xu et al., 2020). That is, less is used for more. It seems that some molecules within a mixture act to either enhance and/or inhibit the responding of various OSNs. This helps to explain how we perceive a "new" odor sensation when odorants are mixed together that can't be predicted from what we expect based on the odorants in the mix—and why creative perfumers won't be replaced by artificial intelligence (yet). The fact that certain molecules within a mixture either inhibit or enhance the responses of various OSNs also means that a simple combinatorial code does not fully explain how we perceive odors. Stay tuned.

Nasal Power

When you smell something passively, you are simply inhaling air containing odorant molecules and detecting those molecules. By contrast, when you sniff, you are consciously and forcibly pulling bursts of air into your nostrils, and this increases your ability to detect odorants. But sniffing can do more than just enhance odor perception. Inhaling with precise types of sniffs can assist people who are completely paralyzed or quadriplegic with using technology to help them interact with their environment both physically and socially, including maneuvering wheelchairs and using text-writing software (Plotkin et al., 2010). Research has also shown that nasal breathing improves everyone's learning and memory abilities (Arshamian et al., 2018). When participants learned 12 different odors and then breathed through their nose for an intervening hour, they remembered more of the odors than if they breathed through their mouth for that hour (**FIGURE 14.18**). Other research has shown that nasal, but not mouth, respiration cycles lock in neural oscillations that enhance transfer between sensory information and learning and memory (Zelano et al., 2016). Now you have a good reason to

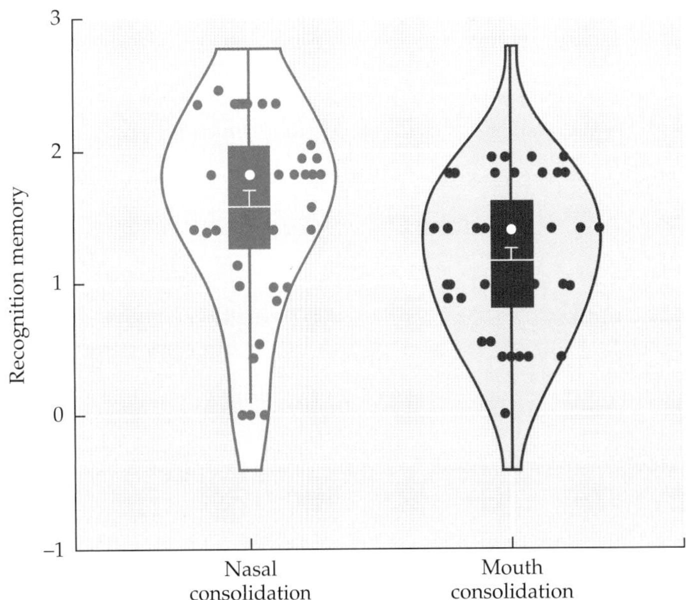

FIGURE 14.18 Learning through the nose Participants remembered more odors when they breathed through their nose during the hour between odor presentation and an odor memory test than if they breathed through their mouth.

try some deep nose-breathing exercises during study breaks when preparing for your next exam!

Odor Imagery

Imagery is one area where olfaction diverges from our other senses. We know that visual and auditory imagery is readily accessible and, though in somewhat different ways, imagery is also evident in touch (e.g., shivers, tingles, phantom limbs) and taste (e.g., the sour salivation reaction). By contrast, humans appear to have little or no ability to conjure "odor images." For example, you can probably see the visual image of a Hershey's chocolate kiss in your mind's eye. But can you reproduce the smell of chocolate in your "mind's nose"? Brain-imaging studies (e.g., Kosslyn et al., 1995) have shown that many parts of the brain that would be involved in actually seeing the kiss are also involved in visually imaging it; however, similar studies suggest that the degree of overlap between actually smelling an odor and "imaging" it is much weaker (Djordjevic et al., 2005). Dreams with olfactory sensations are also very rare (Carskadon et al., 1989; Zadra, Nielsen, and Donderi, 1998).

Animals such as rodents, that rely predominantly on their sense of smell to negotiate the world, may well think and dream in odors. However, because we do not think in odor terms, it is not necessary to have stored representations of olfactory experiences. Nevertheless, functional neuroimaging research suggests that, although odor imagery among average people is weak, expert perfumers may be able to acquire the ability to image odors through training. Functional magnetic resonance imaging revealed that perfumers produced activation in their piriform cortex when asked to image odors, and the greater their perfumery experience, the more their brains appeared to be reorganized to accommodate this skill (Plailly, Delon-Martin, and Royet, 2012). This is another example of how the olfactory system is extremely flexible and capable of neural reorganization on the basis of experience and learning.

14.4 Olfactory Psychophysics, Identification, and Adaptation

The subfield of psychology called **psychophysics** was introduced in Section 1.2. The goal of a psychophysicist is to quantify the psychological experience of our sensory world. In this section, some of the nuts-and-bolts questions addressed by olfactory psychophysics are discussed, and then we'll go on to consider how we identify and adapt to odors.

Detection

Although we may theoretically be able to detect billions of odorants, various factors limit our detection ability in reality, including how much stimulation is required before we perceive something and characteristics of the odorant molecules. For instance, odorant molecules with longer carbon chains, such as vanillin (vanilla scent), are easier to detect (have lower detection thresholds) than those with shorter carbon chains, such as acetone (nail polish remover). Other limitations have to do with individual difference factors (see Section 14.4).

The ability to detect an odorant can also be manipulated by experience. Serendipitous observation revealed that through repeated testing, sensitivity to androstenone (the steroidal musk compound for which many people have a specific anosmia, discussed in Section 14.3) can be induced in about half of the people who are initially unable to detect it (Wysocki, Dorries, and Beauchamp, 1989). That is, a proportion of the people who are anosmic to this particular chemical

psychophysics The science of defining quantitative relationships between physical and psychological (subjective, perceptual) events.

develop an ability to smell androstenone through repeated exposure to it. Other studies have shown that increased sensitivity to some common odorants, such as benzaldehyde (cherry-almond aroma) and citralva (lemon-orange scent), can also be induced through repeated exposure to these chemicals, particularly among females (Dalton, Doolittle, and Breslin, 2002; Diamond et al., 2005). Indeed, overall olfactory detection abilities can be generally enhanced with deliberate odor exposure. Smell training, where people are exposed to a set of familiar odors, typically twice a day for at least 12 weeks (see "Sensation and Perception in Everyday Life: Anosmia and the Effects of Olfactory Dysfunction"), has been shown to improve anyone's olfactory abilities—from young children to adult professional beer and wine tasters (see Majid et al., 2017).

It is not definitively known how these enhancements take place, but cognition, neuroplasticity, and gene expression all appear to be involved (Reichert and Schöpf, 2018). For example, we know from other areas of biology that genes can be "turned on" by external factors, and because each olfactory receptor is coded for by a specific gene, it is conceivable that the receptors for detecting chemicals can be activated through repeated exposure to them. Neuroplasticity and modulation from the environment and experience are basic principles in olfaction.

Odor detection is also influenced by attention. Neuroimaging research has shown that paying attention to odors alters brain activity and increases odor detection ability (Plailly et al., 2008; Zelano et al., 2005). We use more of our brain and can smell more acutely when we consciously focus on smelling than when we don't. Likewise, when our attention is taken away from smelling, our ability to perceive odors becomes drastically reduced.

We can even experience "inattentional anosmia," just as we experience inattentional blindness when our mental resources are co-opted by a demanding task. When participants were distracted from the ambient aroma of coffee by having to do a complex visual search task, most of them barely perceived the smell of coffee even when directly asked about it (Forster and Spence, 2018). This shows that a visual task can interfere with olfactory perception. Another important finding from this study was that adaptation to the odor took place even though the participants were distracted from the coffee scent and were not aware of smelling it in the first place: after 20 minutes of odor presentation, participants could not perceive the coffee aroma, even when they were no longer distracted. There are important implications from this finding. For example, if you are highly distracted by a captivating visual experience (e.g., an intense movie sequence), you might not notice an odor signaling danger (e.g., smoke), and then, after the intense scenes are over, not be able to smell the smoke because you have adapted to it. ●

Discrimination and Recognition

A healthy person can discriminate—tell the difference between—a huge number of odors. Note that *discrimination* is not the same thing as *recognition* (the ability to remember whether we've smelled an odor before). We need up to three times as many odorant molecules to recognize an odor as we do to simply detect its presence. You've probably experienced this phenomenon yourself: you register that you smell something before you know what the smell is. Interestingly, we don't need to know what a smell is, or be able to name it, to recognize it or even to have a memory triggered by it. The only requirement is that we have previously encountered the scent and have a past experience with it (Cleary et al., 2010; Herz and Cupchik, 1992). This is different from other sensory experiences among cognitively healthy adults. For example, we wouldn't be able to say that we recognize, respond appropriately to, or have a memory elicited by something that we see without having

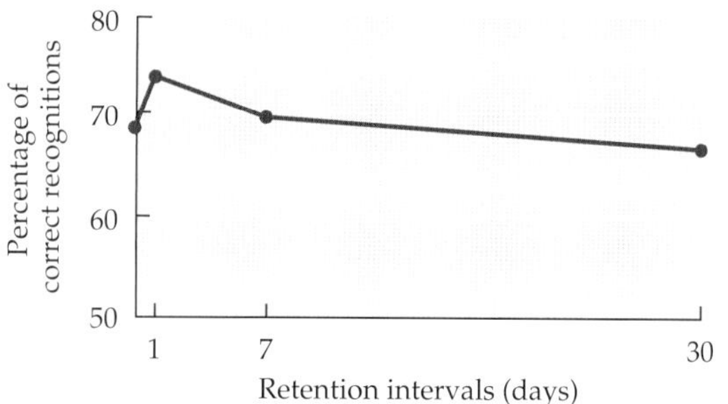

FIGURE 14.19 Long-term memory for odors The first point on this graph, at about 70%, indicates odor recognition accuracy with only a 30-second delay from learning. Note, however, that this accuracy level is the same after a week and has dropped only about 3% after a month. This retention rate remains relatively constant over intervals at least as long as a year.

some kind of label for it, even if the label is very vague or idiosyncratic, such as "food" or "my uncle's weird hat." Brain-damaged patients with visual agnosia are the exception, in that they often know how to use an object even if they don't know what the object is called.

Another interesting feature of odor recognition is its durability. In controlled experiments, a 30-second delay between odor presentation and testing produces a precipitous drop in recognition accuracy, but what we remember after 30 seconds is very close to what we remember after 3 days, a month, or even a year (**FIGURE 14.19**) (Arena and Hamburger, 2023; Engen, Kuisma, and Eimas, 1973; Engen and Ross, 1973; C. Murphy et al., 1991; Rabin and Cain, 1984). Again, you probably know this phenomenon from your own life. If you smelled a certain perfume in a meaningful situation only once and then came upon that perfume 15 years later, you would likely say that the odor was familiar. Our memory for odors is even more resilient if the initial exposure is accompanied by emotion (Herz, 1997).

Psychophysical Methods for Detection, Discrimination, and Recognition

Researchers wanting to measure how perceptually sensitive people are to odors (*detection*), whether they can tell the difference between one odorant and another (*discrimination*), or whether a person knows whether they have smelled an odor before (*recognition*) use various psychophysical methods. A common olfactory technique for determining someone's *detection* threshold is the **staircase method** (also called the reverse staircase method), an example of what are known as methods of limits (see Section 1.2). There are various versions of the staircase method. In a typical procedure, an odorant is presented in ever-increasing concentration increments until the participant reports being able to "smell something" for several repeats of a concentration (**FIGURE 14.20A**). Then the odorant's concentration is decreased incrementally until the participant reports no detection. These reversals are repeated a number of times, and the concentrations at the point where reversals occur are averaged to determine the approximate concentration needed for that person to detect the odorant. Staircase methods can be used to determine a general benchmark for someone's olfactory sensitivity. They can also be used to determine an individual's detection thresholds for a range of different odorants, because the detection threshold for one odor may not be the same as for another.

staircase method A psychophysical method for determining the concentration of a stimulus required for detection at the threshold level. The staircase method is an example of a *method of limits*. A stimulus (e.g., odorant) is presented in an ascending concentration sequence until detection is indicated, and then the concentration is shifted to a descending sequence until the response changes to "no detection." This ascending and descending sequence is typically repeated several times, and the concentrations at which reversals occur are averaged to determine the threshold detection level of that odorant for a given individual. Also called *reverse staircase method*.

triangle test A test in which a participant is given three odorants to smell, of which two are the same and one is different. The participant is required to state which is the odd odor out. Typically, the order in which the three odorants are given (e.g., same, same, different; different, same, same; same, different, same) is manipulated and the test is repeated several times for greater accuracy.

The most common psychophysical test used to determine whether someone can *discriminate* between two odorants is called the **triangle test**: A participant is presented with three odorants, of which two are the same and one is different. The participant is required to state which is the "odd odor out" (**FIGURE 14.20B**). Typically, the order in which the three odorants are given (e.g., same, same, different; different, same, same; same, different, same) is alternated, and the test is repeated several times to establish accuracy.

Odor *recognition* is typically measured by presenting an odorant and providing a choice of several labels in a multiple-choice format and having the participant pick the label corresponding to what they think the odor is (**FIGURE 14.20C**). A more difficult task is asking the participant to come up with the correct name for the odor themselves by free recall. This is odor identification. (**FIGURE 14.20D**).

Identification: Olfaction and Language

Coming up with a verbal label for an odor is a step beyond odor recognition. Olfaction has been called the "mute sense" because we are so often at a loss for words

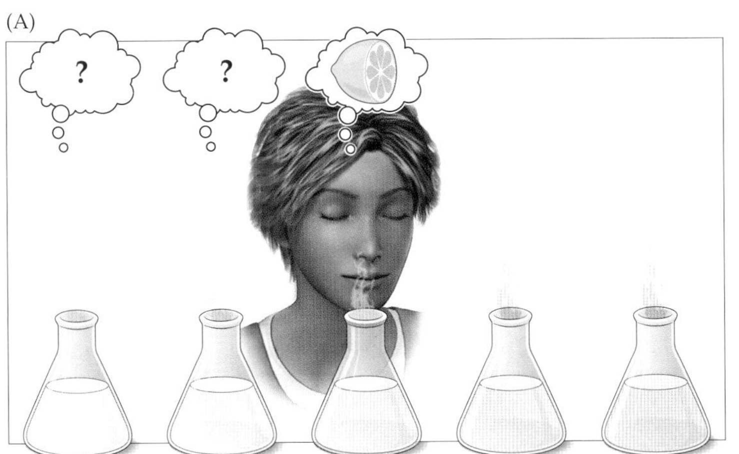
(A)
?
?

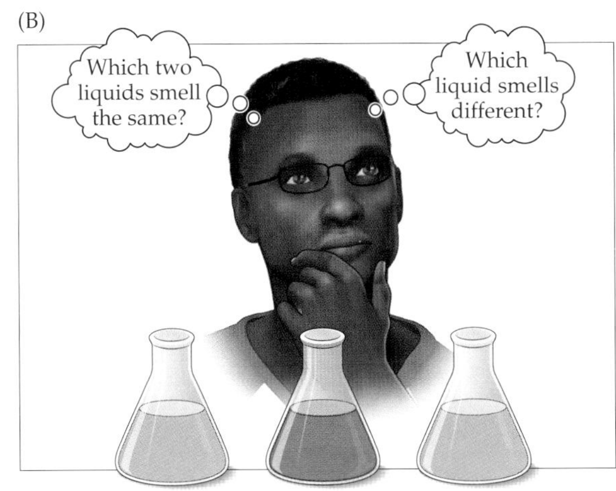
(B)
Which two liquids smell the same?
Which liquid smells different?

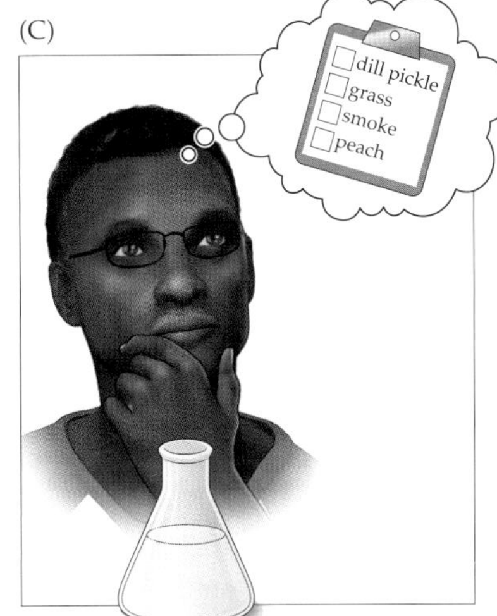
(C)
dill pickle
grass
smoke
peach

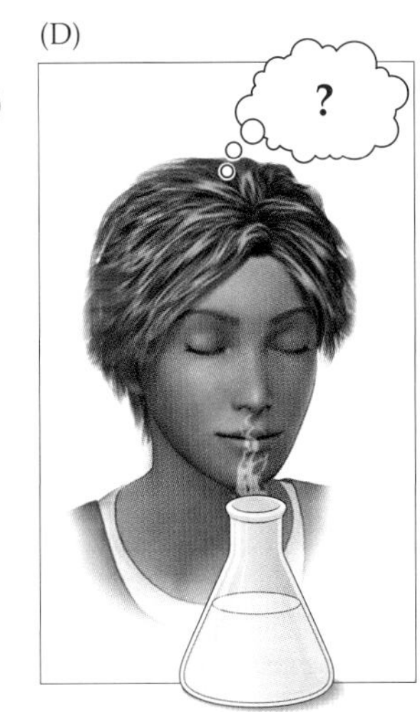

FIGURE 14.20 **Detection, discrimination, and recognition** (A) Staircase method of increasing odorant concentrations to determine the threshold concentration where odor detection occurs. (B) Triangle test for odor discrimination. (C) Recognition of an odor from a list of verbal descriptors. (D) Odor identification by free recall of the correct name for the odor.

to describe our olfactory experiences (D. Ackerman, 1990). All of us have had the experience of not being able to come up with the name of something we know; for example, what was the name of your fourth-grade teacher? This experience is known as the tip-of-the-tongue phenomenon. In the olfactory domain, it occurs when you take a sniff of something where there are no visual clues to what it is and immediately know that the scent is extremely familiar, but you can't come up with the name for it. Borrowing from the verbal scenario, we call this experience the **tip-of-the-nose phenomenon** (Lawless and Engen, 1977), and it can be very frustrating.

There are some important differences between the tip-of-the-nose state and the tip-of-the-tongue state. For one, in the tip-of-the-tongue state, even though we don't know the exact word we're looking for, we typically have some semantic information, such as its first letter, its general word configuration, the number of syllables in the word, and so on. ("Starts with a *K*, two syllables, sounds like a sandwich roll ... aha, my fourth-grade teacher was Mrs. Kaiser!") By contrast, in the tip-of-the-nose state, we typically know nothing about the label we're searching for.

Until very recently, anthropologists thought that in all languages there were fewer words that referred exclusively to our experience of smells than there were for any other sensation (Classen, Howes, and Synnott, 1994). In English, *aromatic*, *fragrant*, *redolent*, and *stinky* pretty much exhaust the list of adjectives that specifically describe olfactory stimuli and nothing else. People typically use words

tip-of-the-nose phenomenon The inability to name an odor, even though it is very familiar. Contrary to the tip-of-the-tongue phenomenon, one has no lexical access to the name of the odor, such as first letter, rhyme, number of syllables, and so on, when in the tip-of-the-nose state. This is an example of how language and olfactory perception are deeply disconnected.

referring to the perceived source of the scent, like *lemony*, or category terms, like *floral* or *fruity*, or commercial products we are familiar with, like *soapy*. We also borrow terms from other senses (cake smells "sweet," grass smells "green," and so on). As you might expect, the more familiar we are with a scent, the easier it is for us to describe it. New evidence, however, suggests that although an impoverished olfactory vocabulary is the case for most languages, there are at least a few languages whose speakers name various odors as easily as they name colors. In particular, hunter-gatherer groups, such as the Jahai and Semaq Beri who live in the mountainous rain forest of Southeast Asia's Malay Peninsula, have a rich vocabulary of 12–15 terms for olfactory properties that have important meanings. For example, the Jahai word *pus* (pronounced "pa-oos") describes what dead branches and some types of fur and feathers smell like (Majid and Burenhult, 2014).

To investigate if there is something that makes the Jahai and Semaq Beri particularly adept at naming odors, researchers compared the color- and odor-naming abilities of the hunter-gatherer Semaq Beri with those of the Semelai, pastoral rice farmers who live near the Semaq Beri and speak a very similar language (Majid and Kruspe, 2018). Both groups were given a commonly used Western odor identification test comprising 16 odors and a color naming test where they had to name 20 colors out of 80 Munsel color hue chips. The Semaq Beri used specific words describing particular odors 86% of the time and specific terms to describe color hues 80% of the time. However, the Semelai rice farmers used specific words for odors only 56% of the time, a performance similar to that of typical Westerners, whereas their use of color words was about the same as that of the Semaq Beri.

Hunter-gatherers need to know and use specific odors to effectively hunt and avoid danger. The Semaq Beri even use their noses to determine if a prey animal is pregnant (so as to avoid killing it in order not to threaten the prey population). By contrast, odor differentiation does not play a vital survival role for the agricultural Semelai (or for most Westerners). Necessity is the mother of invention, and the need for understanding various odor meanings plays a large role in determining our linguistic fluency with odors.

Nonetheless, when we do need to communicate something important about odors, it is still more difficult to name odors than other sensory experiences. It is not yet entirely understood why, though both neuroanatomy and neural processing mechanisms appear to play a role. For example, the majority of olfactory processing occurs in the right hemisphere of the brain, whereas language processing is known to be dominated by the left hemisphere (see Royet and Plailly, 2004), and the association area for olfaction (the piriform cortex) is not anatomically linked to language-processing networks. Additionally, brain-imaging studies have shown that conscious odor perception interferes with language processing. That is, processing odors and processing words compete for the same cortical resources. This means that naming something at the same time as smelling an odor is much more difficult than with no odor present, and processing words at the same time as smelling diminishes the perceptual quality of the odor and the odor smells weaker (Lorig, 1999; Parr, Heatherbell, and White, 2002; Walla et al., 2003; Walla, 2008). The ability to discriminate between odors is also affected by human sounds. In a test of how background noise affected odor discrimination ability, it was found that background "crowded party sounds" and the sound of someone reading an audio book decreased participants' ability to discriminate the odd odor out from a set of three (triangle test)—the clear human voice (audio book) had the most determinantal effect. However, being exposed to nonspeech background sound (e.g., a Mozart piano sonata) did not impact odor discrimination ability—either positively or negatively. This further shows that the cognitive processing of language in particular, and not complex sound in general, interferes with odor perception (Seo et al., 2011).

Research even suggests that olfaction can affect visual perception. When participants smelled an apple odor while they were exposed to a nearly subliminal image of either an apple or a banana (around critical flicker fusion frequency, which is the frequency at which an intermittent [flickering] light appears to be constantly visible), they detected the apple image faster than a picture of a banana. What's more, the presence of an odor that matched the visual image (congruent) made the visual image appear to last longer, even though it wasn't presented for any more time (B. Zhou et al., 2018). In other words, odor input warps visual time. This is not science fiction! ●

Individual Differences

Not everyone perceives all odors the same way or equally acutely. One of the reasons for the differences is individual variation in how many and which OR genes are expressed in our olfactory epithelia (see Section 14.2). Genetic variability accounts for differences in perception among people with a "normal" sense of smell and those with a specific anosmia. However, there are two other major individual difference factors that affect our overall olfactory capabilities: sex and age.

Sex differences are reliably demonstrated in odor perception, with women at all ages outperforming men on odor identification and also, although less consistently, on odor detection and discrimination (Boesveldt et al., 2011; Doty and Cameron, 2009; Hedner et al., 2010). During a woman's reproductive years, it seems that female superiority is mediated by hormonal fluctuations, with women being especially sensitive to odors during ovulation but no different from men during menses (Doty et al., 1981). However, a female advantage is also seen before puberty and after menopause, and postmortem brain analyses have found more neurons in the olfactory bulbs of women than in men (Oliveira-Pinto et al., 2014). It has been speculated that endocrinologic effects exert an organizing influence on the nervous system during early development such that baseline sex differences in olfactory sensitivity persist throughout the life span (Doty and Cameron, 2009). Contrary to popular belief and many new-mom declarations, extensive research has revealed that olfactory sensitivity is *not* heightened during pregnancy or shortly after giving birth (Cameron, 2007; Fornazieri et al., 2019; Hummel et al., 2002; Laska et al., 1996). (See "Adaptation" section for further discussion.)

Our ability to detect odorants declines with age, because as we age, the number of ORs that die off begins to rise beyond the number that are regenerated (Kern et al., 2004). This ratio continues to worsen in favor of cell death as we grow older, such that after the age of 85 it is estimated that about 50% of that population has effectively become anosmic (Hummel et al., 2007; J. C. Stevens and Cain, 1987). It has also been found that healthy older adults (65+ years) give lower pleasantness ratings to typically pleasant odorants such as methyl anthranilate (smells like grape juice) than 20-somethings do, although their ratings of unpleasant odorants such as thioglycolic acid (smells like rotten eggs) are comparable to those of young adults (Joussain et al., 2013). Aging may take a greater toll on olfactory receptors that are responsive to fruity and floral odorants, though this has not yet been systematically tested.

Trigeminal perception also declines with age and seems to be directly related to loss in olfactory function (Hummel et al., 2003). Sensitivity to tastants decreases as we get older too, but not all tastes suffer to the same extent; sweet seems to be least affected (Yoshinaka et al. 2016). These declines in chemosensory function

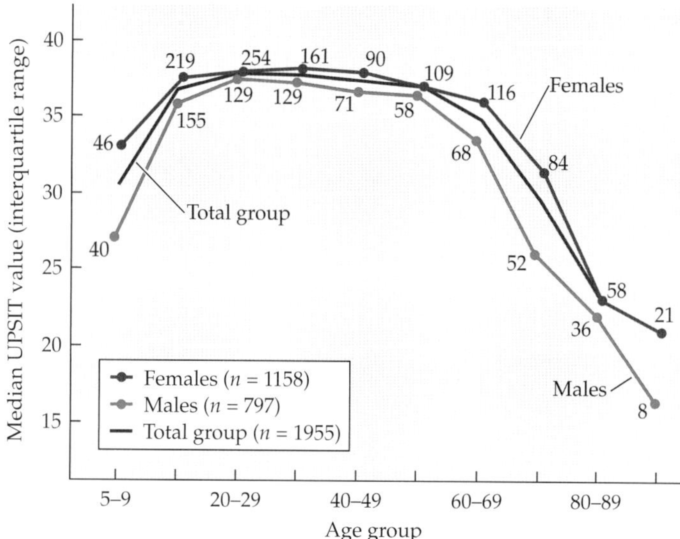

FIGURE 14.21 Olfactory identification ability by age and sex Our ability to correctly identify odors peaks in our 20s and stays relatively constant until our mid-50s, when it starts to decline. Males tend to have slightly lower scores than females at all ages. However, there is a great deal of individual variability, and a number of octogenarians still have high function.

explain the increased use of condiments among the elderly (especially salt, which may produce unhealthy outcomes).

Similar to detection, our ability to identify odors is best between our teenage years and our 40s, but starts to decline fairly precipitously when we reach our 50s, such that by age 65, about half of the population have noticeably impaired olfactory identification ability. For people age 80 or older, about 75% suffer from major impairments in odor identification (Doty et al., 1984) (**FIGURE 14.21**). A main reason for this sharp decline is that odor identification is strongly influenced by verbal and semantic processing; it is well established that as we age, our ability to name everything gets worse (Au et al., 1995). It should also be noted that odor sensitivity in young children is at least as good as, if not better than, that of adults (Solbu et al., 1990), but the ability to name odors does not attain proficiency until our teenage years. For aging adults, the already weak connection between language and olfaction means that any increase in the vulnerability of our naming ability is most readily observed in olfactory identification. That is, "senior moments" may be most obvious with olfaction because it's always been harder to identify the scent in the spice jar as "rosemary" than to say that the name of that guy in the movie is "Tom Cruise."

Notably, people with higher education levels (more years of postsecondary schooling) have better odor identification ability as they age than people with less education (Boesveldt et al., 2011). The correlation is presumably the result of an association between more education and greater naming ability (vocabulary and verbal fluency), which buffers the odor identification declines of aging. Age-related declines in ability are not nearly as pronounced for odor detection and discrimination as they are for odor identification, because they rely much less on semantic processing (Hedner et al., 2010). It is also the case that, as with hearing and vision, there is considerable individual variability in age-related declines in odor perception, and many octogenarians have excellent olfactory ability.

Many people wonder if having a deficit in one sense makes a person more acute in another sense. One example is the common anecdotal that people with blindness have enhanced olfactory abilities. But is this true? In fact, the overwhelming majority of research indicates that there are no olfactory detection differences between the blind and sighted (e.g., Cornell Kärnekull et al., 2016; Sorokowska et al., 2019), although some studies find better odor *naming* ability by blind people (Cuevas et al., 2010), and other studies show that blind people can determine emotions based on body odor better than their sighted peers (Iversen et al., 2015). Blind people also pay more attention to odors (Ferdenzi et al., 2010), which itself can increase olfactory perception, as noted earlier in this section. Consistent with the greater attentional effects among the blind, it was recently found that blind people are more susceptible than sighted people to olfactory illusions elicited by verbal labeling, such as presenting an odor and labeling it either Parmesan cheese or vomit and believing the scent to be what the label states it is (Cornell-Kärnekull et al., 2021). Importantly, these enhanced capabilities show up in tasks that rely on cognitive attentional resources, not odor perceptual mechanisms. In the one controlled laboratory study to date that has examined olfactory acuity in deaf people, these individuals showed olfactory *impairments* compared to both blind and sighted individuals (Guducu et al., 2016). It is not currently known why this is the case.

Odor naming and olfactory identification can be important in diagnosing certain neurological diseases at their earliest stages. This is particularly true of Alzheimer's disease (AD), which is characterized by loss of memory, especially of semantic memory (memory for the names of things and factual information). Because naming odors (compared with naming anything else) is most vulnerable to slight cognitive perturbations, it will show up as a deficit at the earliest stages of semantic loss. Testing for such a deficit is crucial because the sooner people are correctly diagnosed and treated for AD, the better their quality and duration of life will be. Parkinson's disease (PD) is also typically foreshadowed by a loss of odor-identification abilities, and the same benefits from early intervention apply (see "Scientists at Work: A New Test to Diagnose Parkinson's Disease").

Scientists at Work

A New Test to Diagnose Parkinson's Disease

Background and aim Parkinson's disease (PD) is a neurodegenerative disorder characterized by various motor and cognitive disturbances. The motor symptoms are the result of degeneration of dopaminergic neurons in the basal ganglia. This degeneration produces deposits of a protein in the olfactory system that impedes odor perception. Importantly, olfactory loss can precede the observable motor symptoms in PD by years, and as with Alzheimer's disease, the sooner treatment can be started, the better the long-term outcome. In addition to having impaired odor detection, discrimination, and identification, people with PD perceive odors overall as less pleasant. Odor identification tests can differentiate people with PD from healthy peers, but these tests rely on cognitive ability and language, which can also become impaired in PD. Evaluating odor pleasantness requires only minimal effort and therefore could be highly useful. The aim of this study was to determine whether a new tool called the New Test of Odor Pleasantness (NTOP) could distinguish people with PD from healthy controls and whether it would be suitable for use with PD patients.

Test Researchers asked 30 PD patients and 30 healthy control participants to perform two previously established olfactory perception tests and the NTOP, which involved smelling 32 odorants and then categorizing them for pleasantness.

Results Lower hedonic ratings on the NTOP were strongly correlated with lower identification scores on the other tests and successfully differentiated PD patients from controls. That is, the PD patients exhibited significantly lower odor pleasantness ratings than controls did on the NTOP (**FIGURE 14.22**).

Conclusions The NTOP is a promising new tool for distinguishing individuals with PD from healthy controls, and it is well accepted in this patient group.

Future work Developing a pleasantness test that has fewer odorants and is therefore faster and more efficient to administer would be a beneficial avenue for further research.

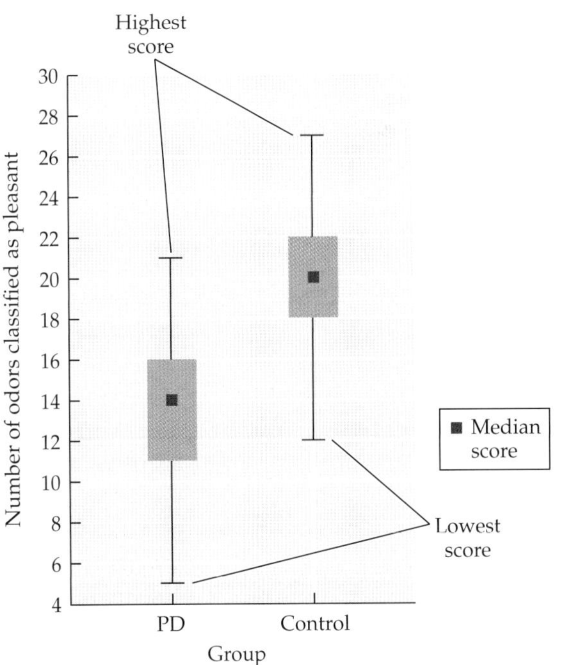

FIGURE 14.22 Odor pleasantness test for Parkinson's disease The boxplot shows the number of odors classified as pleasant by individuals in the Parkinson's disease (PD) group and in the control group.

(For reviews of olfactory impairment in AD and PD, see Mesholam et al. [1998] and Ruan et al. [2012].) Research during the COVID-19 pandemic also revealed that sudden loss of smell is a signal of COVID-19 infection among otherwise asymptomatic individuals (Eliezer et al., 2020).

In addition to differences between individuals, new evidence indicates that our ability to detect odors varies throughout the day. A study with adolescents, in which the effect of circadian rhythms was separated from the influence of how long someone had been awake, found that olfactory acuity was never best during the circadian phase that approximately maps onto the clock time between 2:00 AM and 10:00 AM (Herz et al., 2018b). In addition, the longer the teenagers had been awake, the worse their olfactory sensitivity became, and the deleterious effect of staying up late was most pronounced for females. After being awake for more than 15 hours, girls performed substantially worse on an odor threshold test than they had earlier in the day. Boys showed a more minor decrement in sensitivity (Herz et al., 2018a). This has important implications for staying up late and snacking—lower olfactory acuity has been shown to lead to less satisfaction from food and increased body mass index (Aschenbrenner et al., 2008; Pastor et al., 2016). Moreover, research has shown that sleep deprivation increases the brain's sensitivity to food aromas (Bhutani, Gottfried, and Khant, 2017) and the consumption of high-calorie treats like doughnuts and pizza (Bhutani et al., 2019). With insufficient sleep, the piriform cortex encodes food smells more strongly, and at the same time the connection between the piriform cortex and the insula, a key brain region involved in taste and food intake is reduced (see Section 15.2). This means that when we're sleep-deprived, the aromas of tasty treats are more alluring and we are less able to evaluate our food intake in relation to these tantalizing odor cues. The fact that one in three people in the United States is chronically sleep-deprived provides insight into the various ways in which olfactory function is involved in the current obesity epidemic.

Adaptation

Have you ever had a coworker or classmate who seems to pour cologne over their head every morning, leaving you choking on the overpowering aroma? Can't they smell anything? Or perhaps you've noticed that, after using a perfume for a few months, you can't smell the fragrance in the bottle anymore. Or you've gone away on vacation and returned home to find that your house seems to have a "funny" smell that it didn't have when you left. What's going on? The answer has two parts: the first involves the nose, and the second involves the mind.

Among its many functions, the sense of smell is a change-detection system. When a new chemical comes along, your olfactory receptors fire in response to it and you perceive a scent. For example, when you first enter a bakery, you notice the mouthwatering aromas of cakes, cookies, pies, and pastries. But if you stand inside for a while, you may find that by the time you've picked out the cake you want for dessert, you can no longer smell it; the odorant molecules that make up the bakery aroma have bound to the corresponding olfactory sensory neurons in your nose. When this happens, the ORs retreat into the cell body (Firestein, 2001) and are no longer physically available to respond to the bakery scent molecules. This response is a process in "receptor recycling." Specifically, an odorant binding to an OR causes the OR to be internalized into its cell body, where it becomes unbound from the odorant and is then recycled through the cell and emerges again in a number of minutes if that same odorant doesn't block it. Receptor recycling is a mechanism common to all G protein–coupled receptors, the class to which ORs belong (see Section 14.1).

FURTHER DISCUSSION of parallels to visual adaptation can be found in Section 2.3.

This process is called **receptor adaptation**. The precise length of time required for adaptation varies as a function of both the individual (Dalton, 2002) and the odorant (Pierce et al., 1996). Generally, it takes about 15–20 minutes of continuous exposure to an odorant for the molecules to stop eliciting an olfactory response, but adaptation can also occur in less than a minute. Receptor adaptation can also be undone relatively quickly. Stepping outside the bakery for a few minutes gives unbound olfactory receptors a chance to accumulate on the cell surface again, so when you go back in you can enjoy the appetizing scents once more. The magnitude of adaptation is also affected by odor intensity (Kadohisa and Wilson, 2006). As the concentration of an odorant increases, the length of time for adaptation to occur decreases. For example, it takes less time to adapt to the aroma wafting from an apple pie baking in the oven than to the scent emanating from a cool pie on the kitchen counter. This is because there are more volatile molecules of apple pie aroma available to activate ORs when the pie is hot and steaming than when it is cold.

receptor adaptation The biochemical phenomenon that occurs after continual exposure to an odorant, whereby receptors are no longer available to respond to the odorant and detection ceases.

cross-adaptation The reduction in detection of one odorant following exposure to a prior odorant. Cross-adaptation is presumed to occur because the components of the odorants in question share one or more olfactory receptors for their transduction, but the order in which odorants are presented also plays a role.

One way to prolong the effect of smelling a scent before adaptation kicks in is to dispense an odor intermittently. For example, bursts of air freshener alternated with no scent will draw out the time before your receptors are smothered by the air freshener molecules and duck for cover. A potential benefit of receptor adaptation is that when you are being exposed to an odor you don't like, you can take solace in knowing that in less than 20 minutes you'll barely be able to smell it.

Another benefit of OR adaptation is that it enables us to filter out stable background odors, which OSNs do via moment-to-moment interactions with the olfactory environment (Tsukahara et al., 2021). This filtering ability can also be enhanced through active sniffing—taking deliberate, quick inhalations (Kepecs, Uchida, and Mainen, 2007). Sniffing makes OR neurons less responsive to stable odors and more responsive to new odorants (Verhagen et al., 2007). For example, if we're at a car dealership and think we smell something burning, we typically engage in active sniffing to (1) see if we're right and (2) determine which car is smoldering. In vision and hearing, perceptual stimuli in the foreground can be segregated from stimuli in the background through spatial analysis. In olfaction, spatial analysis is compromised because background and foreground odors merge in the air. However, provided that background and foreground odors are at least briefly separated in time (new-car smell first, then the scent of burning plastic), sniffing enables us to separate components of an olfactory scene. Also, the faster sniffing is, the better and more efficiently mice (and presumably we) are at finding the source of an odor (Shusterman, 2019). So the next time you're trying to find where an odor is coming from, take quick, deliberate sniffs.

In some cases, exposure to one odorant can raise the odor detection threshold for a second, completely different odorant. For example, after sniffing several perfumes in a department store, your nose may become fairly useless at differentiating the fragrances, despite the salesperson's insistence that the perfumes are quite different from each other (**FIGURE 14.23**). This phenomenon is called **cross-adaptation**, and it is presumed to occur when components of the odorants in question rely on similar sets of ORs. However, this simple explanation is complicated by the fact that most cross-adaptation relationships are nonreciprocal. For example, smelling pentanol (a chemical used in some paints) seems to have a strong cross-adapting effect on next smelling propanol (an antiseptic and solvent), whereas smelling propanol first has only a minor cross-adapting effect on then smelling pentanol (Cain and Engen,

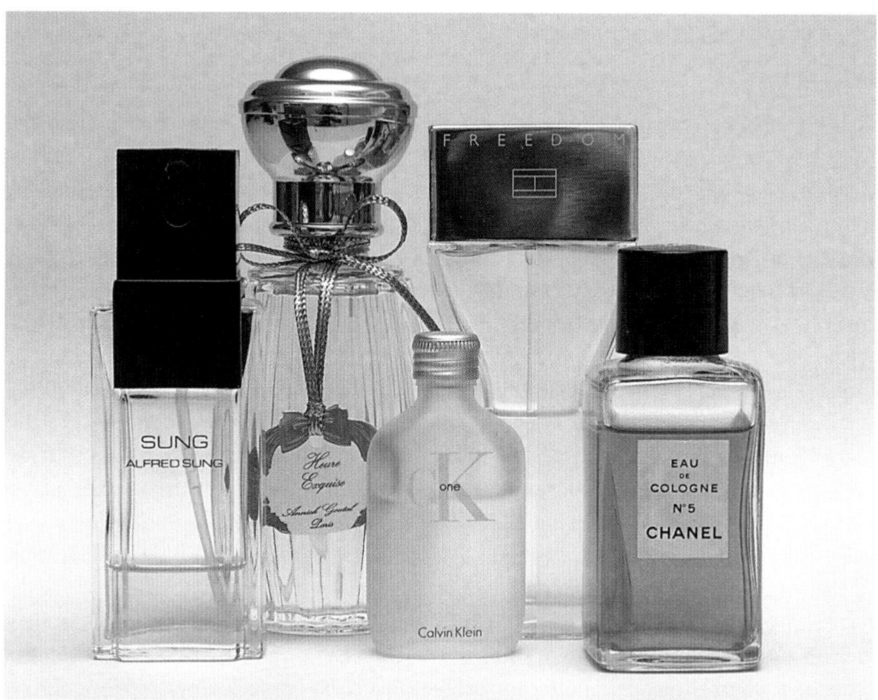

FIGURE 14.23 **Cross-adaptation can numb your nose** These five fragrances all smell different, but because of olfactory cross-adaptation, as you go through smelling them it becomes harder to tell them apart.

1969). Indeed, exposure to the first odorant can sometimes enhance sensitivity to the second odorant.

Regardless of why they occur, cross-adaptation effects usually go away after a few minutes. Professional perfumers, who may have to smell hundreds of scents a day and thus don't have a few minutes to spare, use a trick of sniffing their bare arm or cotton shirtsleeve between smelling odorants; doing this effectively clears the nose, even at a fast pace of odorant presentation. Nobody knows exactly why this works, but it does. The next time you find yourself suffering from numb nose at a perfume counter, try it.

Notably, the mind can control *perceived* odor adaptation, and believing that an odor is dangerous can influence perceived odor intensity. This was demonstrated in an experiment where half the participants were told that an odor they were being exposed to was "healthful," while the other participants were told the odor was "hazardous" (Dalton, 1996). Twenty minutes after initial exposure, the participants smelling the supposedly healthful odor had adapted to it, whereas the participants who thought they were smelling a hazardous chemical reported the smell as even more intense after 20 minutes than at the start of the experiment. However, when these participants were given a psychophysical test of odor detection, it was found that they had adapted just like the people who were told that the odor was healthful had adapted. Fear of odor exposure can even make people perceive an odor that does not exist (Engen, 1972). For example, people who believe that a factory is emitting dangerous chemicals frequently complain that they can smell a malodor coming from the facility, regardless of what the factory produces or whether it is even operating.

Psychological factors may explain why physical reality can be subverted in odor perception. For example, when we are anxious, initially neutral odors become perceived as unpleasant, and these now-negative odors correspondingly elicit augmented responses in higher-order olfactory and emotional processing centers in the brain—the OFC and pregenual anterior cingulate cortex (Krusemark et al., 2013). Moreover, anxiety strengthens the connection between olfactory processing in the OFC and emotional processing in the amygdala (see Section 14.6). The link between perceived increased olfactory sensitivity and anxiety may also explain why pregnant women can feel as though certain odors smell very intense. If we are worried an odor may harm us, we perceive it as more intense and unpleasant, and it elicits greater emotional processing, which potentiates further negative emotional responses to that odor. Therefore, if you're a first-time mom and feeling generally anxious and hypervigilant to your surroundings, various odors may smell especially intense and unpleasant. Emotional hypersensitivity can also create olfactory illusions, and you may believe that you are smelling a "bad" odor by merely *seeing* the feared source—for example, seeing a smokestack that you're worried is emitting dangerous chemicals. In general, people who consider themselves extra sensitive at detecting smells tend to have more negative emotional and perceptual responses to scents than people who self-evaluate as normal smellers (Knaapila and Tuorila, 2014). Individuals who objectively score higher on odor sensitivity tests tend to have more gray matter volume in the hippocampus—part of the primary olfactory cortex. Interestingly, recent work has found that self-rated supersensitive smellers (irrespective of their actual olfactory sensitivity) have greater gray matter volume in several brain areas that are involved in the cognitive aspects of odor processing, including the hippocampus (Han et al., 2020). This illustrates again how powerful emotional and cognitive involvement is in our perception of odors.

Cognitive Habituation and Odor Consciousness

Receptor adaptation explains why you stop detecting the delicious aroma of the bakery after you've been in the store for a while, but can smell it again after a short break outside. If you took a job at a bakery, however, a different process would take place. This is the phenomenon that your friend who can't smell their own cologne is experiencing, and it's the reason why you don't smell the ambient scent of your own home unless you go out of town for a couple of weeks. It is a psychological effect called **cognitive habituation**; simply put, when we live with an odor, we no longer react to the smell or have a very diminished response to it. For example, textile workers exposed daily to acetone exhibited acetone detection thresholds that were eight times higher (i.e., they were eight times less sensitive) than those of a comparable group of control subjects. However, thresholds to another chemical (butanol), to which neither group had been regularly exposed, were no different for the two groups (Wysocki et al., 1997).

We habituate (that is, our receptors adapt) to some degree to stimuli presented to all our senses (e.g., you stop hearing a ticking clock after being in the room for a while), but attention can bring us out of habituation with every sense except smell. Unlike receptor adaptation, which can be undone in a few minutes, cognitive habituation requires weeks to reverse, even for pungent trigeminal stimulants like acetone (Dalton et al., 1997; Wysocki et al., 1997). For example, if you stopped wearing your cologne for 5 days, you would still not be able to smell it well when you used it again. But if you abstained for 2 weeks or more, it would likely smell as strong as when you first wore it. What accounts for the long duration of odor habituation is not fully understood, but a mix of cognitive and physiological factors are involved (Dalton, 2002).

Another feature of olfactory perception that highlights the importance of conscious perception is that we do not respond to odors while we're asleep

cognitive habituation The psychological process by which, after long-term exposure to an odor, one no longer has the ability to detect that odor or has very diminished detection ability.

(Carskadon and Herz, 2004). Unlike what happens with auditory stimuli, when trigeminally activating odorants such as menthol and pyridine (also a chemical component of smoke) were presented, even at high concentrations, to participants in slow-wave sleep (deep sleep) or rapid-eye-movement sleep, they did not awaken or show any electroencephalogram (EEG) sleep pattern changes. More recently, it was found that exposing sleepers to artificial smoke during all stages of sleep had no effect on arousal frequency or EEG activity (Heiser et al., 2012). These findings underscore the need for auditory smoke detectors and why our sense of smell cannot protect us from smoke inhalation and consequent disasters while we are asleep.

Neurological research in rodents has also shown that the piriform cortex (the primary olfactory cortex) is hyporesponsive to odors during slow-wave sleep (see Courtiol and Wilson, 2017). However, there is some evidence that odors presented during other stages of sleep may be able to modify our behavior. A study testing whether odors could be used to curb smoking found that using a conditioning procedure where a noxious odor was paired with the smell of cigarette smoke while the participants were awake had no effect on the number of cigarettes they later smoked (Arzi et al., 2014). However, the same conditioning procedure presented during rapid-eye-movement sleep and, especially, stage 2 sleep significantly reduced the number of cigarettes smoked, and the effect lasted for several days. This was the case even though there were no arousals from sleep, there were no EEG changes during the odor presentations, and the waking ratings of the pleasantness of cigarette smoke pre- and postconditioning were the same. It has also been found that when smokers smell an odor that is pleasant to them it reduces their urge to smoke a cigarette for at least 5 minutes—which is often sufficient for the craving state to diminish (Sayette et al., 2019). Odors may be especially well suited for modulating addictive behaviors because of their unique connectivity to emotion and reward centers in the brain.

Also fascinating is how our ability to respond to odors may be an indicator of our general state of consciousness. In a study conducted by Noam Sobel's group at the Weizmann Institute in Israel, patients who were in a coma after severe brain damage were exposed to the pleasant scent of shampoo and the unpleasant odor of rotting fish and the patient's sniffing behavior was then observed. It was found that the patients whose sniffing rate differed as a function of what scent they were exposed to—by taking shorter sniffs to the rotten fish smell (an indicator of avoidance) than to the pleasantly scented shampoo differentiated between people who were in a vegetative state with "unresponsive wakefulness syndrome" (i.e., a potentially permanent condition) and those who were minimally conscious (Arzi et al., 2020). Additionally, among patients who were in a vegetative state, the patients who showed some degree of variable sniff response all transitioned to a minimally conscious state and then either recovered or transitioned into a higher level of consciousness. Although the discovery of a sniff test to assess consciousness is amazing, brain injuries often also involve trauma to the olfactory system, which causes anosmia, and a prognosis based on a sniff test would not be meaningful for these patients (see "Sensation & Perception in Everyday Life: Anosmia and the Effects of Olfactory Dysfunction"). Moreover, some people may have had some olfactory dysfunction prior to their brain damage. Therefore, although the connection between olfactory function and consciousness is tantalizing, relying solely on a sniff test to determine who will recover from a coma (and who will not) is not medically or ethically advisable.

14.5 Olfactory Hedonics

odor hedonics The liking dimension of odor perception, typically measured by ratings of an odor's perceived pleasantness, familiarity, and intensity.

The most immediate and basic response we have to an odor is whether we like it or not. This evaluation is known as **odor hedonics**. In tests of odor hedonic evaluation, people are typically asked to rate how pleasant, familiar, and intense a given odor is. These measures are then used to determine the overall hedonic value of a specific scent.

Pleasantness

The pleasantness of a scent is traditionally defined in terms of approach-avoidance behavior. We want to get closer to odors that we perceive as pleasant (and sniff more), and we want to get away from odors that we perceive as unpleasant from (sniff less). A more general way of conceiving of odor pleasantness is how much we "like" a scent. The factors that determine odor pleasantness have been the subject of debate, as will be discussed further in the next section. Nevertheless, it is generally agreed that perceived odor pleasantness is modulated by the odor's familiarity and intensity, learning, context, genetic factors, and various individual difference characteristics such as age and sex (Shanahan and Kahnt, 2022).

A sizable proportion of the population evaluates the brands and products that they buy based on how they smell. In the fragrance industry, these people are called "scent seekers." Most of us are at least moderate scent seekers and prefer consumer products to have some added scent, though what the product is used for (cleaning the floor versus cleaning your face) strongly affects whether and what scents are preferred. Interestingly, during times of social upheaval such as the months following the 9-11 terrorist attacks and the acute phase of the COVID-19 pandemic, purchasing of scented products and fine fragrance skyrocketed (Herz et al., 2022). The emotional comfort and personal meaning that people can obtain from scents, especially when isolated from loved ones, is a major driver for scent seeking overall. It is obvious that perceived pleasantness is related to our liking for an odor. But how are familiarity and intensity related?

Familiarity and Intensity

As with many other facets of life, we tend to prefer the familiar over the unfamiliar—that is, we like odors that we've smelled many times before. Moreover, we often perceive pleasant odors as being more familiar than unpleasant odors, regardless of how familiar we truly are with them (Moskowitz, Dravnieks, and Klarman, 1976; Sulmont, Issanchou, and Koster, 2002). Thus, ratings of odor pleasantness and familiarity show a linear relationship with odor liking.

The perceived intensity of a given chemical is dependent both on how many molecules reach the ORs (i.e., the concentration) and on how those molecules interact with the ORs (i.e., how those ORs are activated). That is, concentration alone does not necessarily predict how intense an odorant will smell. Intensity has a more complex relationship to odor liking and is often represented by an inverted-*U* function, but this depends on the odorant. A rose scent like phenylethyl alcohol may be evaluated as more positive with increasing intensity—up to a point; then the function reverses, and as the scent becomes stronger, it is judged to be more disagreeable (**FIGURE 14.24A**). This is why an overdose of cologne is unpleasant. By contrast, a fishy odor (e.g., trimethylamine) may be acceptable at low concentrations, but as intensity increases, its perception becomes steadily more negative (**FIGURE 14.24B**). Note also that individual differences in the number and type of receptors expressed, as well as the size of one's olfactory cleft, may influence one's

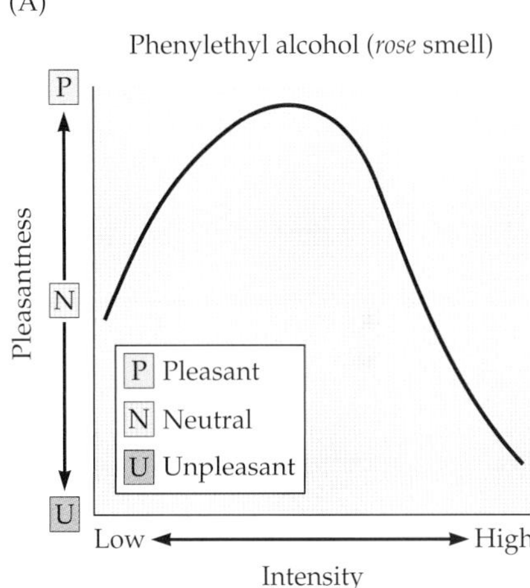

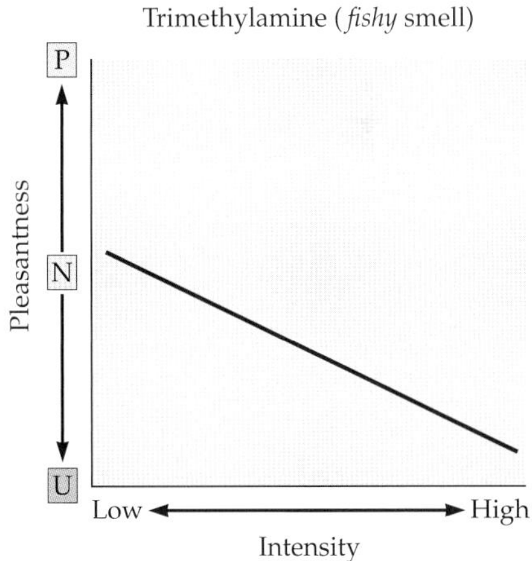

FIGURE 14.24 Pleasantness ratings of odorants plotted against intensity (A) The relationship between odor intensity and pleasantness is often described by an inverted-*U* function if the odorant is initially considered pleasant, as the synthetic rose scent (phenylethyl alcohol) usually is. (B) For an odorant that is initially considered tolerable (but not necessarily pleasant), such as fishy-smelling trimethylamine, the relationship is typically described by a linear function.

sensitivity (intensity perception) and hence the predisposition to experience the intensity of specific odorants along a pleasantness continuum.

Nature or Nurture?

An ongoing debate in the field of olfaction is the degree to which hedonic responses to odors are innate or learned. Researchers on the innate side of the debate to varying degrees claim that we are born with a predisposition to like or dislike various smells. Researchers taking the view that hedonic responses are learned hold that we are born merely with a predisposition to *learn* to like or dislike smells and that whether a smell is liked or not is determined by the emotional value (good or bad) of the experiences that have been associated with it. That is, if we like rose and dislike skunk, it is because we have a good and a bad association, respectively, with these two scents. Note that we do not need to have direct contact with a skunk to form such an association because cultural learning gives us meanings for many unencountered stimuli. For instance, you opinion of skunk scent may be based on Pepé Le Pew cartoons rather than personal experience.

If you were asked to take a position on the sole basis of your own personal experiences, perhaps you would come down on the innate side of the debate. After all, who could like the smell of skunk, and who wouldn't like the smell of a rose? In fact, however, the preponderance of evidence points to odor hedonics being learned.

A good place to start looking for such evidence is with infants. If odor preferences are innate, then newborns should display them. However, researchers have repeatedly found that infants and children often display very different preferences from those of adults. For instance, infants do not find the smells of sweat and feces unpleasant (Engen, 1982; M. Stein, Ottenberg, and Roulet, 1958), and toddlers typically do not hedonically differentiate between odors that adults find either offensive (e.g., butyric acid, which smells like dirty socks) or pleasing (e.g., amyl acetate, which smells like bananas).

One difficulty with these types of studies is that the olfactory system is fully functional by the third month of gestation (6 months before the baby is born) (Schaal, Marlier, and Soussignan, 1995, 1998; Winberg and Porter, 1998), and odorant molecules from what a mother consumes are present in amniotic fluid in the womb. So it is difficult to know exactly how much exposure even a newborn infant has had to an odorant. But exposure to odors in utero has led to yet another line of evidence in support of the learned view of hedonics: Mennella and colleagues found that when mothers consumed distinctive-smelling volatiles (e.g., garlic, alcohol, cigarette smoke) during pregnancy or breastfeeding, their infants showed greater preferences for these odors than did infants who had not been exposed to these scents (Mennella and Beauchamp, 1991, 1993; Mennella, Johnson, and Beauchamp, 1995). What we learn about odors prenatally and during infancy and early childhood can also go on to influence our food and flavor preferences in adulthood. For example, it was found that adults who had been fed a strongly vanilla-flavored milk formula as infants preferred vanilla-flavored ketchup over regular ketchup (Haller et al., 1999). This correlation suggests that it might be a good idea for women to eat lots of broccoli, salmon, and other healthful, flavorful foods during pregnancy and breastfeeding.

Cross-cultural data provide further support for the idea that associative learning, and not hardwired reactions, is responsible for olfactory preferences. For one, there is very little agreement cross culturally as to what odors people find pleasant or unpleasant (Ayabe-Kanamura et al., 1998; Schleidt, Hold, and Attila, 1981). Food aromas are a classic case in point. For example, Asians typically consider the smell of cheese to be disgusting, yet most Westerners consider it anything from comfort food to an indulgence. In contrast, many Japanese enjoy a breakfast of *nattō*, a fermented soybean dish that most Westerners wouldn't bring near their mouths (some say it smells like burning rubber). Both cheese and *nattō* are high in protein and nutritious; the cultural preference has to do with the respective differences in the learned associations to their scents (**FIGURE 14.25**).

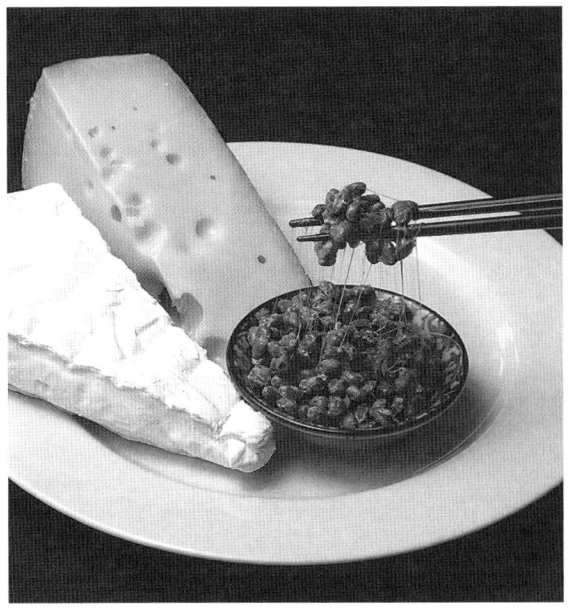

FIGURE 14.25 Cross-cultural differences in odor liking Many Japanese regularly eat *nattō* (shown at right) for breakfast, but Westerners do not associate its smell with food. In contrast, cheese, which most Westerners enjoy, is considered disgusting by most Japanese.

One recent study on the innate side of the argument has suggested that there is some universality in odor liking based on the physiochemical characteristics of certain scent molecules (Arshamian et al., 2022). Interestingly, the odor found to be most pleasant across cultures was vanillin, which is the key compound of vanilla and is present in breast milk and baby formula. This fact alone actually supports a learning theory explanation, rather than an odor chemistry explanation, because vanillin is first experienced for everyone during cuddling, nurturing, sustenance, and warmth. Beyond infancy, vanillin is also most often paired with the taste of sweet, which, as you'll see in the next chapter, is an innately positive sensation (see Section 15.3).

In case you're thinking that the examples of odors we've given so far aren't really that bad and that there must be consensus on really horrid stenches, this also doesn't seem to be the case. Indigenous peoples of the Bering Strait (between Alaska and Russia) *prefer* rotten-smelling fish and meat (Yamin-Pasternak et al., 2014) (**FIGURE 14.26**). The Masai of Kenya dress their hair with cow dung as a cosmetic color treatment. And in a study undertaken by the US military to create a stink bomb to be used instead of tear gas to disband riots, it was impossible to find an odor (including "US Army–issue latrine scent") that was unanimously considered repellent across ethnic groups (Dilks, Dalton, and Beauchamp, 1999).

Laboratory studies directly aimed at testing the learning theory account have shown that a novel odor can be made to be perceived as good or bad as a function of associating good or bad experiences with it (Herz, Beland, and Hellerstein, 2004). Other studies have shown that simply the name given to an odorant (and hence the meaning of the odor that is extrapolated) can dramatically alter hedonic responses to it (de Araujo et al., 2005; Herz and von Clef, 2001). For example, the chemical combination of isovaleric and butyric acid labeled "vomit" in one case and "Parmesan cheese" in another produced the illusion that the odorant was not the same and elicited completely opposite hedonic responses. Neurobiological evidence also shows that how an odor is coded as pleasant or unpleasant is a result of our experience with it (see Section 14.6).

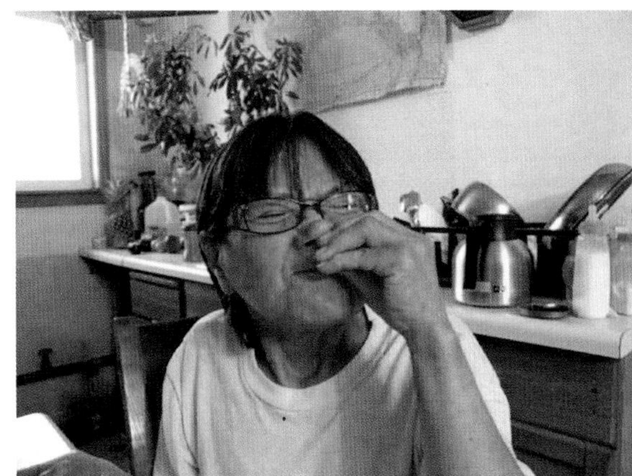

FIGURE 14.26 Deliciously smelly! Indigenous people from the Bering Strait indicate how much they like smelly, rotted foods by inhaling deeply and waving their fingertips in front of their nose.

As noted above, researchers who argue for an innate foundation to odor hedonics look for a physiochemical (molecular) basis for odor pleasantness. One study showed that the more oxygen atoms there are in a chemical, the more pleasant it is perceived to be (Keller and Vosshall, 2016). However, even the most recent data arguing for a molecular basis to odor hedonics have shown that individual differences in odor preferences are the most important factor for determining odor pleasantness (Arshamian et al., 2022). Importantly, the way that we and other species interact with the environment can help explain the innate versus learned controversy, as we'll discuss next.

(A)

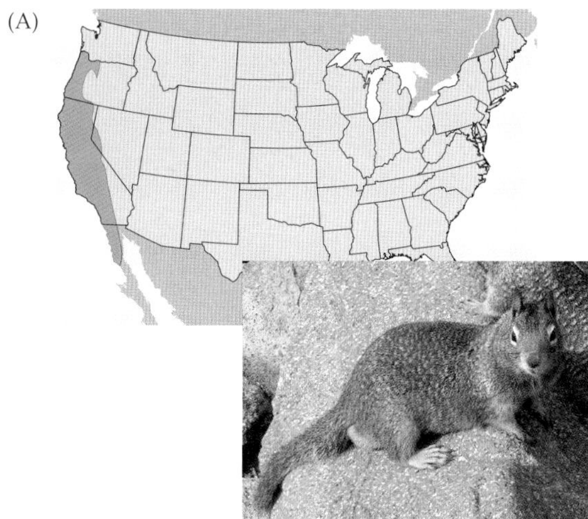

(B)

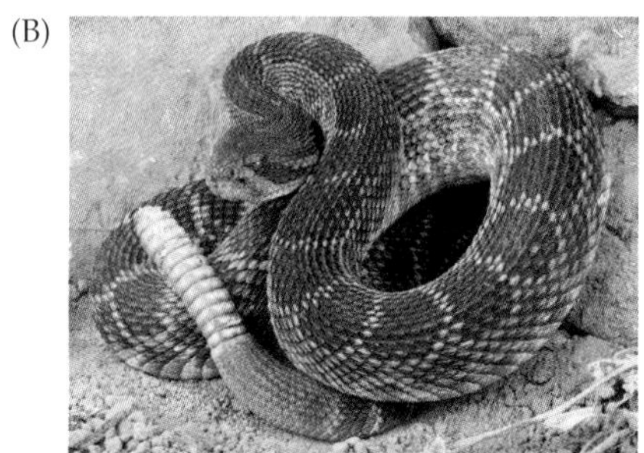

FIGURE 14.27 Specialist animal species The California ground squirrel lives in a restricted habitat (A), so it has only a few natural predators, including the Pacific rattlesnake (B). Studies have shown that, unlike humans, specialist species such as the California ground squirrel exhibit innate odor responses, in this case to avoid the scent of the animal that will try to eat them.

An Evolutionary Argument

Specialist animal species live in very specific habitats and have a limited number of food sources and predators. For such species, innate responses to particular odors are adaptive. California ground squirrels, for example, exhibit an instinctive defensive response the first time they are exposed to the odor of their natural predator, the Pacific rattlesnake, but they don't show the same response to the scent of Pacific gopher snakes, which are not their natural predators (**FIGURE 14.27**) (Coss et al., 1993; Poran and Coss, 1990). By contrast, generalist species (including humans, rats, and cockroaches) exploit many different habitats. For generalists, the available resources and potential predators vary widely across environments, so it would not be adaptive for these species to have predetermined olfactory responses to a particular odor. For example, a certain odor in one locale may signal poisonous mushrooms, but in another environment that same odor may mean nutritious food.

Clear evidence that learning is a critical mechanism by which generalists acquire odor responses is shown by **learned taste aversions**. Rats and humans can be made to avoid a flavor by being made sick after consumption (see Section 15.1 for an explanation of the critical role of olfaction in flavor perception). For example, presenting a rat with a sweet-tasting, banana-smelling drink and then injecting the rat with lithium, which causes nausea, creates a conditioned avoidance of the banana flavor in the future. Similarly, a pioneering experiment in humans testing the phenomenon of learned taste aversions showed that children who had chemotherapy (which made them nauseous) after ingesting a novel flavor of ice cream (dubbed "mapletoff") subsequently refused to eat mapletoff ice cream but had no problem enjoying a different novel-flavored ice cream (Bernstein, 1978). For both rats and humans, the central feature of the conditioned aversion is to the substance's smell (flavor), not its taste (Bartoshuk and Wolfe, 1990; Capaldi, Hunter, and Privitera, 2004; Chapuis et al., 2007; also see Miranda, 2012, for review).

The one-trial learning seen in taste aversions is clearly adaptive. If poison is ingested, it is best to learn to immediately avoid it, rather than repeating the mistake until it kills you. The special importance of first associations in odor learning was further shown in a functional magnetic resonance imaging study, where it was found that the original association made to an odor is etched into the brain and produces a unique neural signature in the amygdala-hippocampal complex (see Section 14.6), which predicts later memory for that odor association. After the first association is made, subsequent associations do not produce a new unique neural signature for that odor (Yeshurun et al., 2009). The bottom line is that the olfactory systems of generalists are not preprogrammed, but rather are geared to effectively learn the meaning of smells based on experience, especially first experiences.

learned taste aversion The avoidance of a novel flavor after it has been paired with gastric illness. The smell, not the taste, of the substance is key for the learned aversion response in humans.

The defining characteristic of generalists is the ability to adapt to the local environment. From an olfactory perspective, one way this is witnessed is in heightened ability to distinguish and determine edible foods from available resources. In exciting new research, De March and colleagues (De March et al., 2023) performed a genetic analysis using a database of OR genes from our extinct relatives—Neanderthals and Denisovans who migrated from Africa ~750,000–450,000 years ago—and compared them with ORs from modern humans, who emerged ~65,000 years

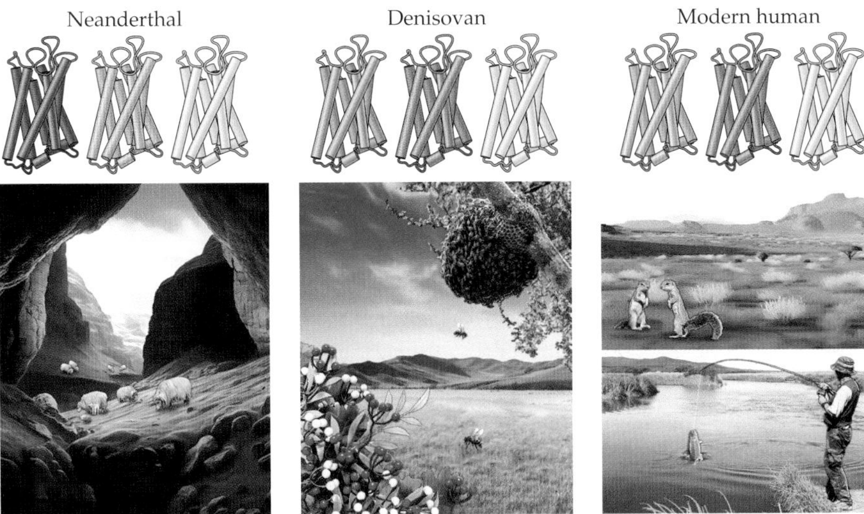

FIGURE 14.28 **At least some hominid OR receptors evolved in adaptation to environmental conditions and food sources**

ago.[1] A high degree of overlap in OR genes was observed between Neanderthals and Denisovans, who both primarily inhabited Eurasia (though Denisovans may have also lived further north). However, interesting differences were found in the sensitivity of certain ORs to specific odorants that are relevant for food and foraging (FIGURE 14.28). Neanderthal ORs were the least sensitive of the three groups to green, spicy, and floral odorants. Archaeological and geographical evidence suggests that the Neanderthal diet mainly comprised meat, so the need to sniff out plants to eat was likely low. By contrast, Denisovans, who from archaeological evidence appear to have had a more plant-based diet than Neanderthals, had ORs that were more sensitive than those of modern humans (and Neanderthals) to sweet and spicy vegetation aromas like honey, vanilla, cloves, and herbs. These differences speak to the differences in the local ecology and survival pressures that these different groups faced and illustrate that the evolution of hominid ORs has been influenced at least in part by environmental food conditions. Most important, this same genetic analysis showed that modern humans have much more variability and diversity in their OR gene repertoire than our extinct relatives did. This reflects how we are able to exploit all habitats on Earth and the enormous diversity in food possibilities that this presents. It also points to the evolutionary benefits that maximal variability in ORs confers and might even suggest that our olfactory genetic diversity has played a role in the global success of our species.

The Importance of Emotional Associative Learning

The central role of emotional associative learning as the basis for the formation of odor preferences has been shown through various findings. One compelling anecdotal example is the difference between how people in the United Kingdom and people in the United States respond to the scent of methyl salicylate (wintergreen mint). In North America, wintergreen mint is typically perceived as a pleasant flavor and aroma, and it is found in candy, mint, and gum. In Britain, however, it

[1] Note that dates of evolutionary emergence are estimates, because in the genus *Homo* they are not yet fully known.

is a very disliked odor and is found only in toilet cleaning products and medicinal balms. Taking a step back to empirical findings supporting this, in the mid-1960s in Britain, adult respondents were asked to provide hedonic ratings for a battery of common odors (Moncrieff, 1966). A similar study was conducted in the United States in the late 1970s (Cain and Johnson, 1978). Both studies included the odorant methyl salicylate (wintergreen). In the British study, wintergreen was given one of the lowest pleasantness ratings; in the American study, it was rated as the most pleasant scent tested. There is a historical reason for this difference. In Britain, the smell of wintergreen is associated with medicine; in particular, wintergreen was added to analgesics popular during World War II, a time that the adults in the 1966 study would not have remembered fondly. But in the United States, the scent of wintergreen is associated with candy, so it has sweet, positive connotations. It is thus the meaning of wintergreen scent in these two cultures that determines how it is perceived (Bartoshuk, 1991; Engen, 1991; Herz, 2006). Perceived odor pleasantness is most often a function of the learned association between an odor and the emotions involved when the odor was first encountered. For more discussion, see "Sensation & Perception in Everyday Life: Odor-Evoked Memory and the Truth behind Aromatherapy."

Neuroanatomy further supports the proposition that our olfactory system is especially prepared to learn the emotional significance of odors. The amygdala, which synapses directly with the olfactory nerve, is critical for emotional associative learning and emotional memory. The hippocampus is also involved in odor-associative learning and memory, as well as spatial mapping. Furthermore, the most ancient part of the brain, the rhinencephalon—literally, the "nose brain"—which comprises the piriform cortex, developed first from neural tissue that was dedicated only to processing chemicals (e.g., odorants). It wasn't until later in evolution that limbic structures such as the amygdala and hippocampus emerged.

It is interesting to consider that our hedonic and emotional reactions to stimuli in general may have their origin in our sense of smell. The most immediate responses we have to odors are simple binary opposites: like or dislike, approach or avoid. Emotions convey similar messages: approach what is good, safe, and joyful; avoid what is bad, dangerous, or liable to cause grief. Thus, emotions and olfaction are functionally analogous. Both enable an organism to react appropriately to its environment, maximizing its chances for basic survival and reproductive success. Viewed in this context, the human emotional system can be seen as a highly evolved, abstract cognitive version of the basic behavioral motivations instigated by the olfactory system in other animals (Herz, 2000, 2004).

Caveats

Although a great deal of evidence suggests that odor hedonics are learned, we must note two caveats. First, trigeminally irritating odorants may elicit pain responses, and all humans will innately avoid pain. But when it comes to food, even this response can be overcome by social and cultural influences, as attested by the popularity of chili peppers in many ethnic cuisines. Second, as has been mentioned several times, the variability of OR genes and pseudogenes that are expressed across individuals influences odor intensity, and consequently the perceived pleasantness, of odors. For example, people who like the scent of skunk may exhibit this response in part because they are missing or have very few receptors for detecting some of the more pungent volatiles, whereas people who are particularly repulsed by this smell may be endowed with many ORs that are keenly attuned to the mercaptan and sulfide components of this bouquet. That is, detection of the full complement of chemicals that make up an odor (whether skunk or cilantro) and how strong or weak an odor is perceived to be play a role in its perceived (un)pleasantness. Recall that for many odors, an inverted-*U* function describes the relationship between liking and intensity (see Figure 14.24A). Genetic differences in OR expression have also been found to extend to ethnicities (Menashe et al., 2003) and are especially connected to perceived odorant intensity (Trimmer et al., 2019), which may help explain why it has not been possible to develop a universally effective stink bomb. As this example demonstrates, the key to olfactory associative learning is the experience connected to the odor and, in particular, the emotional connotation of that experience (Bartoshuk, 1991; Engen, 1991; Herz, 2001).

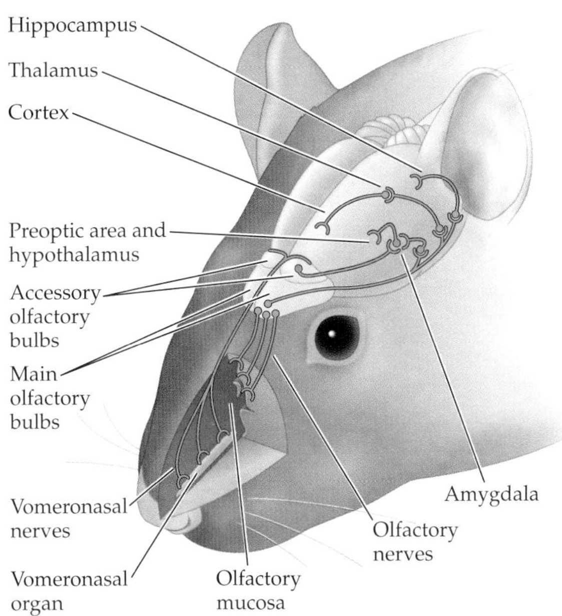

FIGURE 14.29 The olfactory system of the hamster The hamster has a main olfactory system and secondary olfactory system comprising the vomeronasal organ and accessory olfactory bulbs. Note that no functional vomeronasal organ or accessory olfactory bulbs have been found in humans.

14.6 The Vomeronasal Organ, Human Pheromones, and Chemosignals

In some vertebrates that rely on smell for survival, the olfactory system consists of two subdivisions: the **main olfactory bulb (MOB)** and the **accessory olfactory bulb (AOB)** (FIGURE 14.29). The AOB is attached to the back of the MOB. Just as each hemisphere of our brain has an olfactory bulb, in animals that possess them each hemisphere has an MOB and AOB. Neurons from the MOB and the AOB do not interconnect, and the two systems function separately in the integration of specific chemicals. For the AOB to be activated, a structure different from the nose needs to be engaged. This structure is called the **vomeronasal organ (VNO)**, sometimes also referred to as Jacobson's organ, after the Danish anatomist who discovered it.

The VNO is found in some amphibians, most reptiles (but not birds), and many mammals, including New World primates. When a snake opens its mouth and appears to be licking the air, it is moving chemicals from the air into the VNO. The VNO can respond to some olfactory stimuli, but it responds primarily to chemicals that are too high in molecular weight to be detected by the olfactory sensory neurons, as well as to chemicals that are nonvolatile. It also detects chemicals dissolved in water (as opposed to only in air). Whether humans possess a functioning VNO has been the focus of much debate, but it is now generally accepted that although human embryos may have a VNO, this tissue is not neurally connected and disappears shortly after birth. Moreover, humans do not have an AOB for VNO neurons to connect to in the brain.

In animals that possess a VNO, its primary function is to detect **pheromones**. Pheromones are not odors. They are chemicals that may or may not have a smell. The word *pheromone* is derived from the Greek *pherein*, meaning "to carry," and *hormon*, meaning "to stimulate." It was first coined in 1959 by Peter Karlson (a German biochemist) and Martin Lüscher (a Swiss entomologist) to describe a chemical substance that carries a message about the physiological or behavioral state of one insect to another, and in turn leads to a specific reaction in the receiver insect. That is, pheromones are a means of chemical communication. Today, the more generalized definition of a pheromone is "a chemical compound produced by one animal that elicits a specific behavioral or physiological response in another animal of the same species."

main olfactory bulb (MOB) The rounded extension of the brain just above the nose that is the first region of the brain where smells are processed. In humans, we refer simply to olfactory bulb(s); in nonhuman animals with accessory olfactory bulbs, we distinguish between main and accessory.

accessory olfactory bulb (AOB) A neural structure found in nonhuman animals that is smaller than the main olfactory bulb and located behind it. The AOB receives input from the vomeronasal organ.

vomeronasal organ (VNO) Found in nonhuman animals, it is a chemical-sensing organ at the base of the nasal cavity with a curved tubular shape. The VNO evolved to detect chemicals that cannot be processed by olfactory receptors, such as large and/or aqueous molecules, the types of molecules that constitute pheromones. Also called *Jacobson's organ*.

pheromone A chemical emitted by one member of a species that triggers a physiological or behavioral response in another member of the same species. Pheromones are signals for chemical communication and may or may not have any smell.

Pheromones are most important for communication among the social insects, like ants, termites, and bees, but they also convey important information for many noninsect species, including mammals. There are many examples of this form of chemical communication. Pheromones are used to identify territory. For example, a tiger will rub a tree with glands from its cheeks to claim it—just as a cat rubs your leg with its eyebrow and rump glands to mark you as its territory! Pheromones also initiate alarm or defense reactions. When a honeybee stings us, the chemical released from the stinger (which happens to smell like banana) is a signal to other bees to join in—unfortunately for us. Most important, for many animals, pheromones are critically involved in communication about reproductive behavior. They can provide signals to males about when a female is fertile and provide signals to females to initiate sexual behavior. For example, a male rhesus monkey will ignore a female rhesus in heat if his nose is blocked, and a female pig will not go into lordosis (the position necessary for impregnation) if she isn't exposed to the male pig pheromone androstenone.

Pheromones have two kinds of effects, known as **primer pheromones** and **releaser pheromones.** Primer pheromone effects are slow and produce a physiological change in the recipient over time. For example, female rodents that are housed together will come into estrus at the same time after several cycles. Releaser pheromone effects are fast and always produce behavioral responses. The consequence of the banana aroma from a bee sting is one example. Sexual cues and behavioral responses to those cues, such as lordosis, are other examples of releaser pheromone effects.

The most frequently mentioned example of a primer pheromone effect in humans is known as the McClintock effect after the psychologist Martha McClintock, who identified this phenomenon in college while pursuing her undergraduate degree. McClintock reported that when women are in physical proximity (e.g., live together) over time, they start to have menstrual cycles that coincide (McClintock, 1971). That is, women who move into college dormitories together at the beginning of the school term often find that by the end of the semester they're having their periods in sync with one another, and this was not due to chemicals that could be smelled. Subsequent research, however, has refuted the validity of human pheromones (Doty, 2010), and the McClintock effect has been explained as an artifact of mathematical and social phenomena (Ziomkiewicz, 2006). Moreover, we do not have a functioning VNO or AOB, and therefore it is unknown how pheromones could be processed. That said, humans do respond to perceptible scents that are emitted by the body and the term used here is **chemosignal**. Chemosignals are chemicals emitted by humans that are detected by the olfactory system and that may have some effect on the mood or behavior of other humans.

The chemical androstadienone is a steroid derivative of the male sex hormone testosterone (it is chemically related to androstenone, which was mentioned earlier), and it is present in body fluids (e.g., sweat) at higher concentrations in males than in females. In several studies, androstadienone has been observed to improve women's mood, but only when women are in the presence of men (Jacob, Hayreh, and McClintock, 2001; Lundstrom and Olsson, 2005). In the presence of a female experimenter, androstadienone had no effect on female participants' mood. With regard to sexual desire, there is no reliable evidence that sex hormone steroids have any effect on sociosexual responses for either men or women (Hare et al., 2017).

However, human chemosignals may exert some interesting effects on mood, behavior, and physiology. It was recently found that after women had been highly

primer pheromone A pheromone that triggers a physiological (often hormonal) change among conspecifics. This effect usually involves prolonged pheromone exposure.

releaser pheromone A pheromone that triggers an immediate behavioral response among conspecifics.

chemosignal Any of various chemicals emitted by humans that are detected by the olfactory system and that may have some effect on the mood, behavior, hormones, and/or sexual arousal of other humans.

stressed by a laboratory task, the scent of their male romantic partner reduced their self-reported stress levels, while the scent of a male stranger elevated their cortisol levels (the hormonal indicator of stress) (Hofer et al., 2018). This finding dovetails nicely with research showing that the scent of a loved one (romantic or otherwise) can provide emotional comfort (Shoup, Streeter, and McBurney, 2008). Additionally, a study with professional exotic lap dancers found that the dancers earned almost twice as much in tips (averaging $335 a night versus $185) when they performed during the ovulatory phase of their menstrual cycles compared with the menstrual phase of their cycles (G. Miller, Tybur, and Jordan, 2007). By contrast, dancers who were taking birth control pills (and were thus hormonally infertile) showed no change in tip earnings over time and earned less overall than did dancers who were not using hormonal contraception (averaging $193 versus $276). Since the dancers all claimed that they performed the same way every day and their behavior to the patrons was consistent, the explanation offered is that the women were perceived as more attractive by the male patrons when they were most fertile, through some mechanism other than behavioral or visual cues. This other mechanism is proposed to be chemical. Another study found that when men smelled T-shirts that had been worn by ovulating women, their testosterone levels were higher than they were after they sniffed T-shirts worn by nonovulating women or a clean unworn T-shirt (S. L. Miller and Maner, 2010).

Not all chemosignals increase sexual desire. Indeed, Noam Sobel's lab found that chemicals present in the tears of women dampen the sexual desire of men (Gelstein et al., 2011). When men were exposed to a solution containing emotional tears from women (collected from crying elicited by sad movie scenes), though they knew nothing about the source of the solution, a significant decrease was observed in self-rated sexual desire, rated sexual attractiveness of female faces, testosterone level, and brain activity associated with sexual arousal. Are the tears of a distressed woman a turnoff, or is the effect caused by something else? The authors suggested that the drop in testosterone and sexual arousal may be a by-product of a drop in aggression, which is also manifested by lowered testosterone, and there are good evolutionary reasons to hope for a decrease in testosterone from potential aggressors when they are exposed to your tears. With that in mind, the authors speculated that the effect would also be seen if the tears came from a man. However, this has not yet been tested, nor has sexual orientation been examined as a variable in these effects. Interestingly, recent research from the Sobel lab (Mishor et al., 2021) showed that smelling an odorant expressed in human sweat and breath (hexadecanol), even when masked by eugenol (smells like clove), increased aggressive responses toward a selfish and unethical online game partner (really a computer algorithm) among women, but decreased aggressive responses in the same scenario among men. This suggests that, like tears, hexadecanol is a social signal that has different social-behavioral impacts on men versus women. Chemosignals may also increase our ability to distinguish human faces from nonface visual stimuli. In a new study (Rekow et al., 2022), participants were shown pictures of human faces, cars, face-like objects (also called "peridiole stimuli," e.g., a rock with suggestive indentations at locations for the eyes and mouth), and random objects that did not look like faces. The images were presented at a very fast rate (12 images per second) while the participants were exposed to human body odor (a composite from 16 male and female sweat donors), gasoline, or an unscented control, and their neural activity was recorded with EEG. It was found that body odor affected the processing of

Sensation & Perception in Everyday Life

Odor-Evoked Memory and the Truth behind Aromatherapy

You have probably had the experience where an odor triggered a specific and special past personal (autobiographical) memory. These occurrences are often referred to as Proustian memories, after the literary anecdote described by Marcel Proust where the aroma of linden tea and a madeleine cookie suddenly triggered the recollection of a long-forgotten event (Proust, 1928). Proustian memories have been shown to differ from episodic memories triggered by other cues in several important ways.

Compared with visual and verbal cues, odors elicit more emotional, evocative, old, rare, and intense personal memoires, as well as greater activity in the amygdala, than memories elicited by verbal or visual representations of the same cue (Arshamian et al., 2013; Chu and Downes, 2000; de Bruijn and Bender, 2018; Herz and Schooler, 2002; Herz et al., 2004; Hinton and Henley, 1993; Larsson and Willander, 2009; Rubin, Groth, and Goldsmith, 1984; Willander and Larsson, 2007; Zucco et al., 2012). Odors even evoke more emotional memories than musical or tactile cues (Herz, 1998). Herz (1998, 2004) compared recollections stimulated by a familiar smell—for example, popcorn—with memories evoked by the sight of popcorn, the sound of popcorn popping, the feel of popcorn kernels, or simply the word *popcorn* (**FIGURE 14.30**). Consistently, memories that were triggered by odors were experienced as more emotionally intense, and participants felt more transported back to the original time and place of the event, than when memories were triggered by cues in any other modality. These effects have now been replicated many times. (e.g., Larsson et al., 2014).

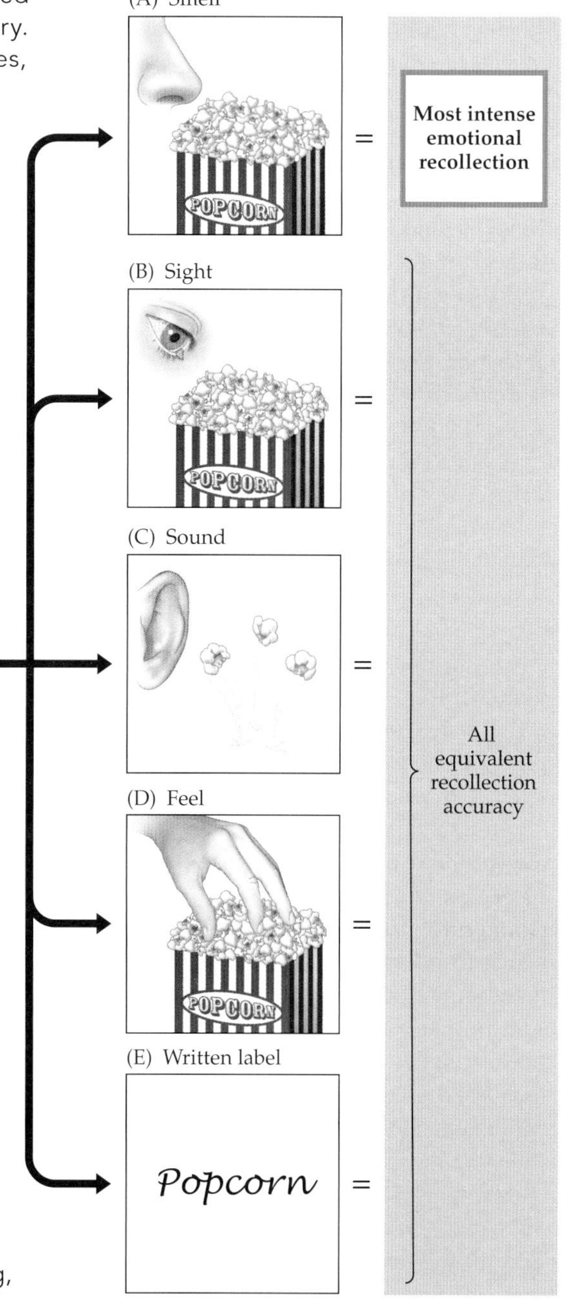

FIGURE 14.30 Cross-modal episodic memory paradigm The smell (A), sight (B), sound (C), feel (D), and written label (E) of popcorn elicit memories that are equivalent in terms of their accuracy. However, odor-induced recollections are more intensely emotional, and this quality has earned odors a reputation as particularly good cues for memory.

The distinctive emotional features of odor-evoked memory are explained by the uniquely direct connection between the neural substrates of olfaction, emotion, associative learning, and memory (Cahill et al., 1995). Only two synapses separate the olfactory nerve from the amygdala, critical for the expression and experience of emotion and emotional memory, and only three synapses separate the olfactory nerve from the hippocampus, which is involved in associative learning and memory. The amygdala has also been shown to play a major role in stimulus reinforcement association learning in primates

Sensation & Perception in Everyday Life *(continued)*

(B. Jones and Mishkin, 1972; F. A. W. Wilson and Rolls, 2005), and neuroimaging studies in humans have shown a direct neurobiological correlation between recall of significantly emotional odor-evoked memories and activity in the amygdala (Arshamian et al., 2013; Herz et al., 2004; Vermetten et al., 2007).

Notably, although memories evoked by odors have many unique and special characteristics, they are not more accurate than memories elicited by other cues. Nevertheless, odors have earned the reputation of being the "best cues" to memory. Part of this can be explained by the same mechanisms that make eyewitness testimony so fraught. When there is a high degree of emotion experienced during recollection, people are much more confident that their memories are correct, even though they are often shown to be inaccurate (Herz, 1998). However, it is also the case that, as Proust experienced, odors can remind one of memories that might otherwise be forever forgotten. That is, odors may unlock memories whose only "mental tag" was the odor that was present when the memory was encoded. The reason for the special capacity of odors to do this may be twofold: (1) the low frequency that certain odors are encountered, rendering minimal interference from multiple associations, and (2) resistance to being overwritten—there are very strong proactive interference effects in olfaction, so the first association you acquire to an odor is extremely hard to undo, and subsequent associations are very hard to make. Unfortunately, it is not possible to test whether odors can retrieve memories that would otherwise never be remembered, but anecdote suggests that this may indeed be the one feature that makes odors "better" memory cues (Herz, 2007).

Odors that elicit specific emotional associations can also produce concomitant changes in behavior. For example, it has been shown that an odor that was associated with a frustrating experience led to reduced motivation and performance when later smelled (Epple and Herz, 1999; Herz, Schankler, and Beland, 2004), and odors that have acquired connotations of being energizing, such as peppermint, cinnamon, and grapefruit, can lead to heightened physical and mental performance when participants are later exposed to them (Raudenbush, Corley, and Eppich, 2001; Raudenbush et al., 2009). These findings also have important applications. A recent study found that the scent of peppermint helped drivers become more alert after being awoken from a light sleep (Tang et al., 2020). The bidirectional interactions between our mind and body enable odors to affect our physiology and physical well-being. For example, research has shown that a scent that evokes a pleasant personal memory also enhances immune system responding (Matsunaga et al., 2011, 2013; see Herz, 2016). Some of the most exciting opportunities for odor therapy are in health conditions where emotion contributes to the experience. Pain is a perfect example. Indeed, several studies have found that the negative emotionality of pain can be substantially reduced when people smell a preferred scent and that painful experiences overall become better tolerated in the presence of a well-liked odor (see Herz, 2021a for review).

Many practitioners of **aromatherapy** contend that odors alter mood, performance, well-being, and the physiological correlates of emotion (e.g., heart rate, blood pressure, and sleep) in a drug-like automatic manner. There is, however, no evidence for pharmacological effects of odors in humans. Instead, so-called aromatherapeutic effects can all be explained by the emotions associated with the scent (Herz, 2009, 2016). The scent of peppermint can indeed make you feel invigorated, but only if you have uplifting and energizing associations to this aroma. Emotions in general have downstream effects on our physiology and performance. Therefore, an odor associated with an exhilarating experience (e.g., pine trees) can increase your heart rate and may also make you run faster. However, if you have never smelled pine trees before, or if you dislike the scent, it will produce either no effect or a negative one (Herz, 2009).

face-like stimuli such that neural responses to peridoles became more similar to the EEG responses elicited by actual faces. The presence of body odor did not affect processing of the other visual images, nor did gasoline have any effects. In other words, the scent of human body odor biased the processing of ambiguous face-like images to seem more human face-like. This shows that olfactory information affects visual processing and underscores the social information imparting capabilities of human body odor.

aromatherapy The manipulation of odors to influence mood, performance, and well-being, as well as the physiological correlates of emotion such as heart rate, blood pressure, and sleep.

In sum, chemicals present in human body fluids appear to be able to modulate social behavior to some extent. However, this is not the same as the pheromonal effects observed in other animals. More research is needed to discern the underlying mechanisms for these human responses.

14.7 The Future of Scent

Digitizing Scent

Have you ever wished you could share or post the scent of the beach where you're relaxing—and do it through just a tap on your phone? As mentioned in Section 14.3, some of the most cutting-edge research in olfactory science today is trying to map the physical chemistry of odorants to conscious odor perception using ML approaches, and as this becomes more advanced, it will assist with fulfilling these digital wishes (Keller et al., 2017; D. S. Lee et al., 2022). However, given the enormous variety of scents—not to mention diversity in our perception of them—the ability to do in-the-moment scent sending of the exotic food aroma you're experiencing in Vietnam won't be available tomorrow. However, what you will be able to do very soon is use preprogrammed scent emojis and create your own novel and personalized fragrance mixtures that can be shared through new olfactory technology, wearables, and social media platforms. Stay tuned for your new scent app and nose-piece coming soon.

Olfactory Virtual Reality

Virtual reality (VR) is a computer-simulated multidimensional environment in which the user wears a headset that eliminates most input from the outside setting and creates new experiences within an inner landscape. Because the headset provides its own sensory and psychological environment, it creates the experience of "presence"—the illusion of "being there" in a world that exists outside the self (Steuer, 1992), where the external physical environment disappears from the user's phenomenal awareness (Lombard and Ditton, 1997; Riva and Waterworth, 2003; Riva et al., 2007). The condition of "presence" is the sought-after state in VR and constitutes a complex psychological experience formed through the multifaceted interaction between sensory stimulation and ensuing cognitive responses (Spagnolli and Gamberini, 2005).

Until recently, immersive VR applications were limited to visual and auditory stimulation and the omission of olfaction was a recognized shortcoming (for a review, see Baus and Bouchard, 2017). It is now accepted that olfaction is an especially important dimension to incorporate into VR because scents evoke such uniquely emotional and visceral psychological states. Studies have directly shown that including scent in VR environments (olfactory virtual reality—OVR) substantially increases presence compared to VR without olfaction (Munyan et al., 2016). Devices through which one can experience OVR are currently available. In addition to scent being a new special feature of the gaming and entertaining side of VR, OVR can be a beneficial adjunctive treatment in psychological therapies for a range of conditions. For example, there is tremendous potential for OVR to be used effectively in both the treatment and the prevention of posttraumatic stress disorder (Herz, 2021b).

Summary

1. Olfaction is one of the two chemical senses; the other is taste. The primary function of olfaction is to detect volatile chemicals in order to respond to the environment most effectively. These responses include safety, social, and navigational dimensions. To be perceived as a scent, a chemical must possess certain physical properties.
2. Contrary to long-standing beliefs that human olfactory capabilities are poor compared to those of other animals, recent research indicates that human odor detection is similar to that of many other mammalian species. Human olfaction also has some unique physiological properties, one of which is that only 35% to 40% of the genes that code for olfactory receptors in humans are functional. Another unusual feature is that most odorants also stimulate the somatosensory system via the trigeminal nerve, and it is often impossible to distinguish the contribution of olfactory sensation from trigeminal stimulation.
3. Anosmia is the complete absence of a sense of smell. It is most frequently caused by sinus disease, which can often be treated. However, if anosmia is caused by head trauma, it is likely to be permanent. Anosmia can lead to severe disturbances in an individual's quality of life. Gradual loss of olfaction is a normal consequence of aging; however, sudden olfactory loss can be the first sign of various diseases, including COVID-19, and warrants examination. Smell testing is an important addition to health assessment and should become standard practice.
4. The dominant biochemical theory of odor perception—shape-pattern theory—contends that the fit between a molecule and an olfactory receptor and the spatial and temporal combinatorial code that is then activated determines the scent that is perceived. However, this theory is not entirely accepted, and alternate explanations exist (e.g., vibration theory).
5. Researchers have demonstrated close connections between the visual system and olfaction. Two examples are binaral rivalry and the discovery of "olfactory white." Recent evidence further suggests that smelling odors that are congruent with what we see alters visual perception.
6. There is a difference between active sniffing and passive inhalation of odors at both neurological and functional levels. Active sniffing may have therapeutic applications for individuals suffering from extreme physical disabilities and may also help distinguish between people in varying states of consciousness following serious brain injury. There are also new olfactory therapies to help recovery from anosmia.
7. Almost all the odors that we encounter in the real world are mixtures, and we are generally not very good at analyzing the discrete chemical components of scent mixtures. Olfaction is thus primarily a synthetic, as opposed to analytical, sense. True odor imagery is also weak (or nonexistent) for most people, but training, as in the case of odor experts (e.g., perfumers), appears to facilitate this ability.

8. The psychophysical study of smell has shown that features of odorant intensity and various cognitive functions are required for odor detection, discrimination, and recognition. Identification differs from odor recognition in that, in the former, one must come up with a name for the olfactory sensation. It can be difficult to name even familiar odors. This state is known as the tip-of-the-nose phenomenon—one of several indications that linguistic processing is disconnected from olfactory experience. However, at least some cultures possess an enhanced verbal connection with odors, which seems to be a result of their need to use olfactory information. Regardless, unlike with other sensory experiences, we do not need to access semantic information to respond to an odor appropriately, as long as the odor is familiar.
9. Another important discrepancy between the physical and the psychological experience of odors is the difference between receptor adaptation and cognitive habituation. Receptor adaptation occurs after continuous odorant exposure over a number of minutes, can be undone after a few minutes away from the odorant, and is explained by a basic biochemical mechanism. Cognitive habituation occurs after long-term exposure (e.g., in a living or work environment) to an odor, takes weeks away from the odor to undo, and has not been conclusively defined in terms of mechanism. Psychological influences can have strong effects on both perceived odor adaptation and habituation.
10. The most immediate and basic response to an odor is whether we like it or not; this is called hedonic evaluation. Odor hedonics are measured by pleasantness, familiarity, and intensity ratings. Pleasantness and familiarity are linearly related to odor liking; odor intensity has a more complex relationship with hedonic perception. Substantial evidence suggests that hedonic responses to odors are learned, even for so-called stenches, though there are certain caveats. That we learn to like or dislike various odors rather than being born with hardwired responses is evolutionarily adaptive for generalist species such as humans. The key to olfactory associative learning is the emotional meaning of the situation or context in which the odor is first encountered. If the emotional context is good, the odor will be liked; if it is bad, the odor will be disliked. Previously acquired emotional associations with odors also underlie "aromatherapy" effects. Emotional potency and evocativeness distinguishes odor-evoked memories from memories triggered by other sensory cues. The neuroanatomy of the olfactory and limbic systems and their neuroevolutionary development illustrate how emotional processing and olfactory processing are uniquely and intimately interrelated.
11. Pheromones are chemicals emitted by individuals that affect the physiology and/or behavior of other members of the same species; they may or may not have any smell. In all mammals that have been shown to use pheromones for communication, detection is mediated through the vomeronasal organ (VNO) and processed by the accessory olfactory bulb (AOB). Humans do not possess a functional VNO or AOB, and empirical evidence for human

pheromones is lacking. Nonetheless, human chemosignals that are processed through the olfactory system appear to have some influence on hormonal and social responses.

12. The latest discoveries from scent technology are on the verge of entering daily life. New apps and features to experience olfaction in multiple domains will soon be available that have the potential to alter a host of human experiences, from entertainment to therapy.

Chapter 15

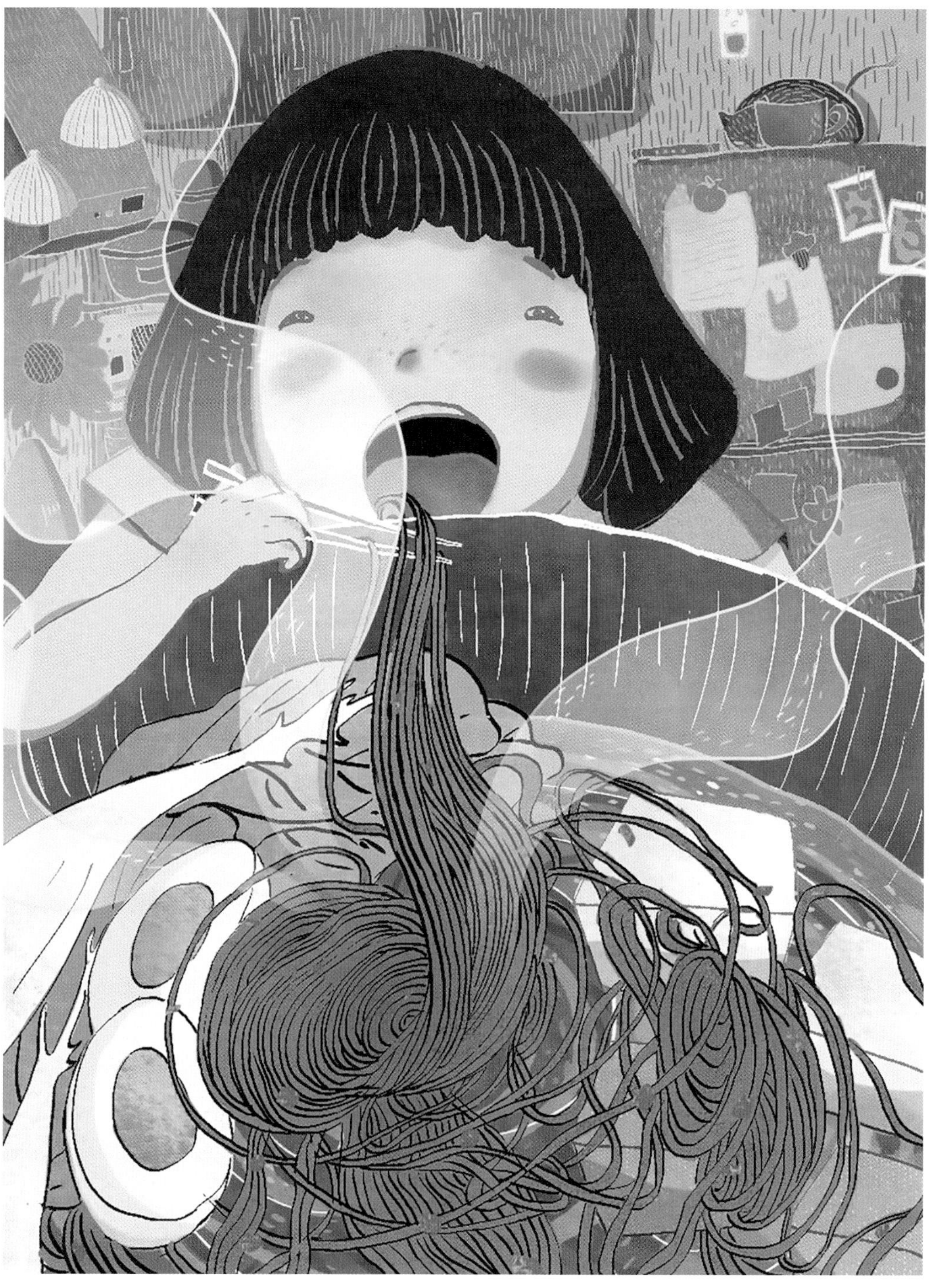

Jing J, *Soba Love*, 2014

Taste

Questions to Contemplate

Think about the following questions as you read this chapter.
By the chapter's end, you should be able to answer and discuss them.

- If you had to give up one sensory modality, why would you not give up the sense of taste?
- How are taste and flavor linked to survival?
- Why is the pleasure you experience from sweet special?
- Do we all live in the same taste worlds?

In her autobiographical novel *Heartburn*, the writer and film director Nora Ephron wrote about living in New York City, "I look out the window and I see the lights and the skyline and the people on the street rushing around looking for action, love, and the world's greatest chocolate chip cookie, and my heart does a little dance" (Ephron, 1983, p. 35). Why do we love chocolate chip cookies? Is it the smell, the taste of sweet, the flavor of the chocolate?

Chemicals create the smell, taste, and flavor of chocolate chip cookies. These three chemical senses in some ways are quite similar, but they make very different contributions to why we love cookies. The many chemicals we taste in food have already entered our mouths and are about to move even farther into our bodies. Thus, **taste** serves the most specific function of any of the senses: discerning which chemicals we need to ingest because they are nutritious and which we need to spit out because they may be poisonous. Our liking for the sweet taste of the cookie is hardwired in our brains; we are *born* liking the sensation of sweet. However, we *learn* to like the chocolate flavor of the cookie based on experience. As we grow up, we eat chocolate paired with sugar, fat, and starch, all of which are sources of energy. Our brain tells us that energy sources are good for us, and we learn to like chocolate. But if you were to become nauseated after eating chocolate chip cookies, you might dislike them for the rest of your life. That nausea associates with the flavor of the cookie. Liking or disliking tastes and flavors seems to be very different from the liking or disliking that one might associate with the color red or the sound of middle C on the piano. Nature has equipped us to care passionately about taste and flavor because that passion holds the key to our survival.

15.1 Taste versus Flavor

Before delving any further into the taste system, we need to clear up a very old misunderstanding. According to Aristotle (384–322 BCE), there are five types of sensations: seeing, hearing, and touching (touch to Aristotle included irritation/pain and temperature), as well as smelling and tasting. Imagine Aristotle with an apple (apples were a favorite in ancient Greece). When he sniffed it, he sensed apple odor: smelling. When he bit into it, chewed it, and swallowed it, he tast-

taste Sensations evoked by solutions in the mouth that contact receptors on the tongue and the roof of the mouth that then connect to axons in cranial nerves VII, IX, and X.

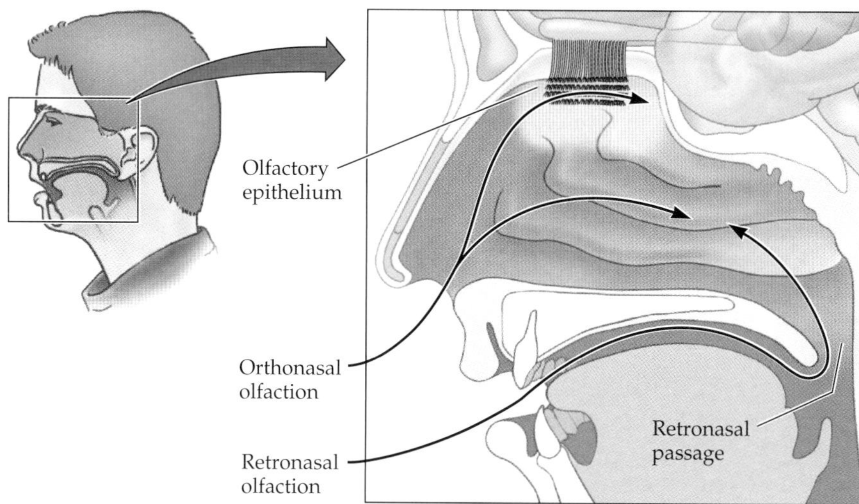

FIGURE 15.1 Orthonasal versus retronasal olfaction Orthonasal olfaction is the detection of odorant molecules inhaled through the nose (see Chapter 14). Retronasal olfaction is produced when volatiles released in our mouths as we chew and swallow food travel up through the retronasal passage into the nose, where they contact the olfactory epithelium.

ed sweetness (and perhaps sourness, depending on the apple), and he perceived apple flavor. The sweetness, sourness, and apple flavor all seemed to come from his mouth; not surprisingly, he lumped them together as tasting. However, if he had plugged his nose when he ate the apple, the apple flavor would have disappeared, leaving only sweetness and sourness. That might have convinced Aristotle that the apple flavor should have been considered a different sensation. But Aristotle did not understand **retronasal olfaction** (**FIGURE 15.1**). Odorants emitted by foods are in fact volatiles (see Chapter 14) that rise up behind the palate and enter the nose from the rear of the mouth. These volatiles produce flavor sensations. Aristotle's failure to distinguish between taste and flavor was not corrected until 1812 by a student at Edinburgh University in Scotland who noted that sensations from substances like nutmeg were abolished by plugging the nose. That student concluded that the sensation evoked by nutmeg should be called "flavor" rather than "taste." Incidentally, that student published his essay anonymously in the *London Medical and Physical Journal*. More than 150 years later, a historian ultimately identified the student as William Prout, who later became a distinguished chemist and physician. Prout's contributions to chemistry led Rutherford (Nobel Laureate in chemistry) to suggest that the hydrogen ion be called a "prouton," but the simpler "proton" won out.

In fact, there are remnants of that confusion today. For example, we don't have a verb to describe experiencing flavor. "I taste food" and "I smell food" make sense; however, consider what happens when we try to use "flavor" as a verb: "I flavor food" means that we add flavoring to food, not that we perceive the flavor of food. Since we don't have a verb to describe experiencing flavor, we borrow "taste." "I taste the salt in that casserole" and "I taste the cinnamon in that roll" describe the distinct perceptions of taste (salt) and flavor (cinnamon), respectively.

As if this confusion were not bad enough, in the early nineteenth century, food companies began defining the word "flavor" to describe the aggregate of sensations produced when we eat, and this is reflected in many dictionary definitions of flavor today. We are left with two different usages of flavor. In this chapter, flavor is used to denote retronasal olfaction.

retronasal olfactory sensation The sensation of an odorant that is perceived when chewing and swallowing force that odorant in the mouth up behind the palate into the nose. Such odor sensations are perceived as originating from the mouth, even though the actual contact of odorant and receptor occurs at the olfactory mucosa.

Plugging the nose prevents the airflow that carries odorants through the retronasal passage. Children do it all the time when they hold their noses while eating something with a flavor they don't like (such as spinach), and you've probably noticed that flavor is impoverished when you have a stuffy nose. Try the following experiment—you can use a piece of strawberry candy if you're not crazy about spinach. Plug your nose before putting the candy in your mouth, and then chew it and note the sensations (only sweet and maybe a little sour if your nose is really plugged). Then swallow and release your nose. The volatile molecules responsible for the strawberry sensation will flow up behind your palate and into the nasal cavity, you will suddenly perceive strawberry, and you will understand the difference between taste and flavor.

If you are a careful observer, you will notice something else that happens when you do this retronasal olfaction demonstration: the sweetness of the candy increases when you perceive the strawberry sensation. This occurs because some odorants perceived retronasally enhance the taste of sweet. Strawberries contain more than 30 odorants that can enhance sweetness (see "Sensation & Perception in Everyday Life: Volatile-Enhanced Taste: A New Way to Sweeten Foods").

Foods are also perceived by the somatosensory system (see Chapter 13) via touch, temperature, and pain receptors in the tongue and mouth. Some of these sensations have protective functions: the burn of acid (which might damage your stomach if swallowed), the heat pain from scalding coffee, the pain of biting the tongue, and so on. Somatosensations also provide information about the nature of foods and beverages. For example, we get information about the fat content of foods from tactile sensations such as oily, viscous, thick, and creamy. ●

Localizing Flavor Sensations: The Role of Taste

You may have realized something else when you plugged your nose and performed the experiment described in the previous section: even though you now know that the strawberry sensation originates from the olfactory receptors in your nose, you probably still perceived the flavor as coming from your mouth. Taste causes this mislocalization. Because you taste the food in your mouth, your brain localizes the retronasal olfactory sensations to your mouth.

Now consider the following curious case. A patient with normal olfaction but damaged taste reported that she could smell lasagna, but when she ate it, it had no flavor. A similar effect was produced in a laboratory using lidocaine anesthetic and blueberry yogurt. Participants in this study had their left **chorda tympani**—a branch of cranial nerve VII that carries information from taste receptors to the brain (see Figure 15.7)—anesthetized with lidocaine while they tasted the yogurt. In this situation, participants reported that the blueberry sensation, which is entirely a result of retronasal olfaction, seemed to come only from the unanesthetized side of the mouth. Moreover, the intensity of the blueberry sensation was reduced, and this intensity was reduced even further when both taste nerves were blocked (D. J. Snyder et al., 2001). In both the patient and the experimental participants, the pathway from the mouth to the nasal cavity was completely intact, but when taste was reduced, retronasal olfaction was reduced as well.

Brain-imaging research by Dana Small (Small et al., 2005) was key to unraveling the way the brain processes flavor and taste. Olfactory input goes to different areas of the brain depending on whether it comes from the mouth (flavor) or through the nostrils (smell). This distinction makes good sense functionally, because the significance of odorants within the mouth is very different from that of odorants inhaled from the outside world. Without the proper cues to tell us where an odorant

chorda tympani The branch of cranial nerve VII (the facial nerve) that carries taste information from the anterior, mobile tongue (the part that can be stuck out). The chorda tympani exits the tongue with the lingual branch of the trigeminal nerve (cranial nerve V) and then passes through the middle ear on its way to the brain.

Sensation & Perception in Everyday Life

Volatile-Enhanced Taste: A New Way to Sweeten Foods

We love sweet, but we worry about the effects on health of consuming too much sugar or using artificial sweeteners. When the first hints arose in the 1970s that adding a small amount of an odorant (volatile) to sugar could make it sweeter, the effects seemed too small to be practical. However, a serendipitous finding during a tomato (botanically, a fruit) experiment showed that volatile-enhanced sweetness could be quite intense.

The tomato experiment was aimed at a problem food shoppers are well aware of: it's hard to find a good-tasting tomato in a supermarket. Recently, heirloom tomatoes have been finding their way into markets. Why do these tomatoes taste better? The answer is that intensive breeding to give tomatoes characteristics that are desirable to marketers (uniform ripening time, fruit size, firmness, and so on) have in some cases led to a deterioration in flavor. Heirloom tomatoes are genetically more diverse because they come from a time prior to the intensive breeding (**FIGURE 15.2A**). But diversity does not guarantee flavor; although some heirloom tomatoes have the fine flavors remembered from earlier days, others are not palatable.

Collaboration between plant biologists and psychologists at the University of Florida led to an experiment utilizing 80 different heirloom tomatoes grown on university farmland (Tieman et al., 2012). After harvesting, half went to a chemistry lab where the sugars, acids, and volatile components were measured; half went to a psychophysics lab where taste, flavor (retronasal olfaction), and preference were measured. Regression analyses identified the components responsible for the sensory properties of the tomatoes, as well as how much they were liked. Some tomato constituents correlated positively with liking; that is, the more of that constituent that was in the tomato, the more it was liked. Some did the reverse (that is, they correlated with disliking), and some did not matter. So the solution turned out to be simple: to make a better tomato, increase the constituents contributing to liking and decrease those contributing to disliking. Knowing what to aim for, crossbreeding can give us better tomatoes (**FIGURE 15.2B**).

The serendipitous result came from *multiple regression*, a technique widely used in the social sciences to examine the impacts of multiple sources on a

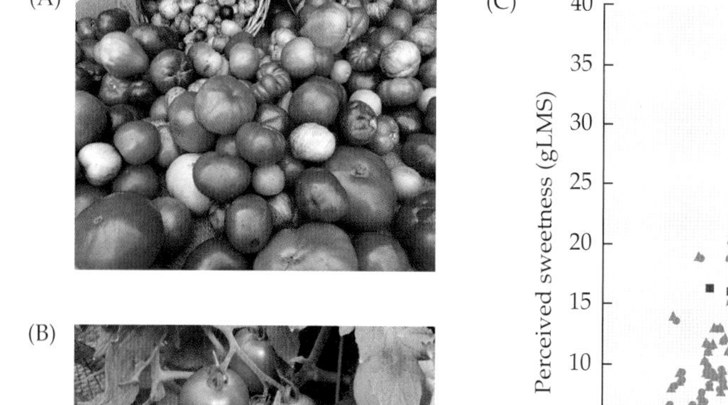

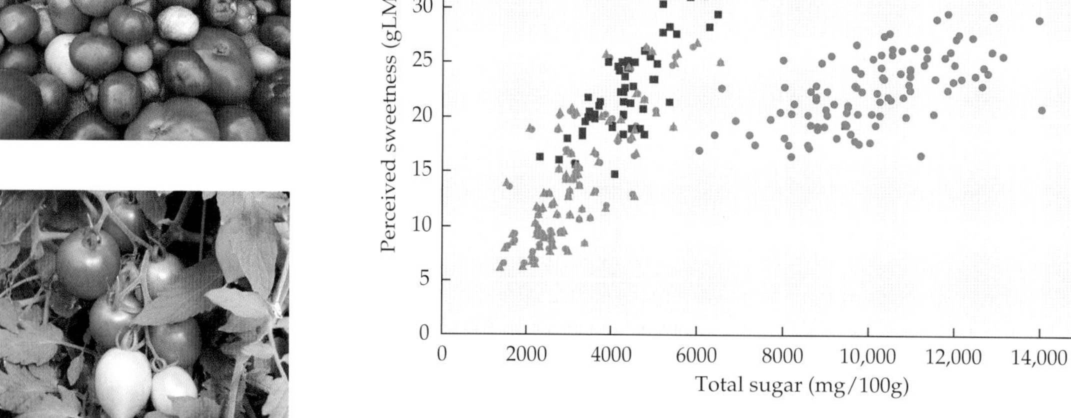

FIGURE 15.2 Some volatiles enhance sweetness (A) Heirloom tomatoes are genetically diverse and come in a variety of shapes, sizes, and colors. Some heirlooms are perceived as having better (sweeter) taste than modern monocultured strains. (B) Garden gem tomatoes are a hybrid created by Harry Klee using insights about taste from the University of Florida tomato study (Tieman et al., 2012). (C) Plotting sweetness as a function of sugar concentration shows that sweetness depends on volatiles as well as sugars.

Sensation & Perception in Everyday Life *(continued)*

given effect. For example, an investigator might want to look at contributions to IQ from a variety of sources (age, health, income, education, and so on). Multiple regression was applied to the tomato data to see if any constituents other than sugars were contributing to sweetness. The result was startling. A considerable amount of the sweetness of tomatoes was coming from volatiles that enhanced the sweet taste of the sugars. The right volatiles could double the sweetness of the tomato.

The group went on to study strawberries, blueberries, oranges, and peaches. The combination of all of these fruits led to the identification of about 100 volatiles that enhance sweetness. Interestingly, blueberries proved to be an exception (**FIGURE 15.2C**). They contain few volatiles that enhance sweetness; when you taste the sweetness of a blueberry, you are tasting the sugar in the blueberry.

The implications for sugar reduction are clear: adding the correct volatiles can reduce the amount of sugar needed to sweeten foods and beverages. However, the potential goes even further. A different group of volatiles can enhance saltiness. Are these effects hardwired in the brain? Are they acquired somehow from experience? The original thinking about the volatiles that enhanced sweet was that these would be limited to fruity flavors, because we so often experience fruit and sweet together. However, one of the tomato volatiles that enhanced sweet was isovaleric acid, which smells like sweaty socks. Sweaty socks and sweet do not seem to be a combination that would be experienced together very often!

Incidentally, this work was possible because of the new insights from psychophysics that let us compare taste sensations across individuals—a reminder about the practical value of basic research.

is coming from (sniffing for smell, taste for flavor), the brain would not be able to send the olfactory information to the right areas.

Understanding the interactions between taste and retronasal olfaction owe much to an early observation of Rosemary Pangborn, a pioneer in the sensory studies of foods. She showed that adding sugar to apricot juice intensified the apricot sensation (Pangborn, Simone, and Platou, 1957). The increase in sweetness (a pure taste sensation) enhanced the retronasal olfactory sensation produced by apricots. Only more recently have we begun to focus on the reverse interaction, retronasal olfactory intensification of taste. Consider the health implications: the addition of the appropriate volatiles could allow a manufacturer to reduce the amount of sugars and artificial sweeteners in foods and beverages.

Mixtures of Taste and Flavor

We experience foods as combinations of taste and flavor. Thus, the way mixtures are processed is very important. First, we note that taste mixtures have very different characteristics than do the olfactory mixtures described in Chapter 14. Olfactory mixtures (smell or flavor) show synthesis, but taste mixtures do not. Taste mixtures are analytic; in taste mixtures, the identities of the taste qualities of the components are not lost. However, the perceived intensities of the components in taste mixtures are reduced. The components of taste mixtures taste less intense than when unmixed. If some of the components of a taste mixture are very weak, they may disappear altogether.

When tastes and flavors are mixed, they retain their qualities, but the perceived intensities tend to be reduced. Imagine what your food world would be like if the perceived intensities of each ingredient in a food simply added linearly. The suppression that occurs in taste/flavor mixtures prevents complex foods from getting much more intense than simple foods.

taste bud A globular cluster of cells that has the function of creating neural signals conveyed to the brain by the taste nerves. Some of the cells in a taste bud (receptor cells) have specialized sites on their apical projections that interact with taste stimuli. Receptor cells that mediate sourness form synapses with taste nerve fibers. Receptor cells that mediate sweetness and bitterness do not form synapses; rather, they communicate with nearby taste fibers chemically.

papilla Any of multiple structures that give the tongue its bumpy appearance. From smallest to largest, the papilla types that contain taste buds are fungiform, foliate, and circumvallate. Filiform papillae are the smallest and most numerous, but do not contain taste buds.

taste receptor cell A cell within the taste bud that contains sites on its apical projections (microvilli) that can interact with taste stimuli. These sites fall into two major categories: those interacting with charged particles (e.g., sodium and hydrogen ions) and G protein–coupled receptors that interact with sweet and bitter stimuli.

filiform papillae Small structures on the tongue that provide most of the bumpy appearance. Filiform papillae have no taste function.

15.2 Anatomy and Physiology of the Gustatory System

Taste perception consists of the following sequence of events (the structures involved are illustrated in FIGURE 15.3): Chewing breaks down food substances into molecules, which are dissolved in saliva. The saliva-borne food molecules flow into taste pores that lead to the **taste buds** housed in structures called **papillae** (singular *papilla*) that are located mostly on the tongue in a rough oval (if the olfactory epithelium is the retina of the nose, the tongue is the "retina" of the mouth). Taste buds, in turn, contain multiple **taste receptor cells**, each of which responds to a limited number of molecule types. When a taste receptor cell comes in contact with one of its preferred molecules, it creates a message that travels along one of the cranial nerves to the brain.

Papillae give the tongue its bumpy appearance and come in four major varieties: filiform, fungiform, foliate, and circumvallate. The last three of these contain taste buds.

Filiform papillae, the ones *without* any taste function, are located on the anterior portion of the tongue (the part we stick out when giving someone a "raspberry") and come in different shapes in different species. In cats, filiform papillae are backward-pointing spikes with a spoonlike cavity at the tip. They aid in licking and grooming and help the cat deposit saliva near its skin to aid in cooling (Noel and Hu, 2018).

Fungiform papillae, so named because they resemble tiny button mushrooms, are also located on the anterior part of the tongue. They are larger than filiform papillae; blue food coloring swabbed onto the tongue makes the fungiform papillae particularly easy to see (FIGURE 15.4). Fungiform papillae vary in diameter, but the maximum is about 1 millimeter. On average, about six taste buds are buried in the surface of each fungiform papilla, although there is a large amount of variation.

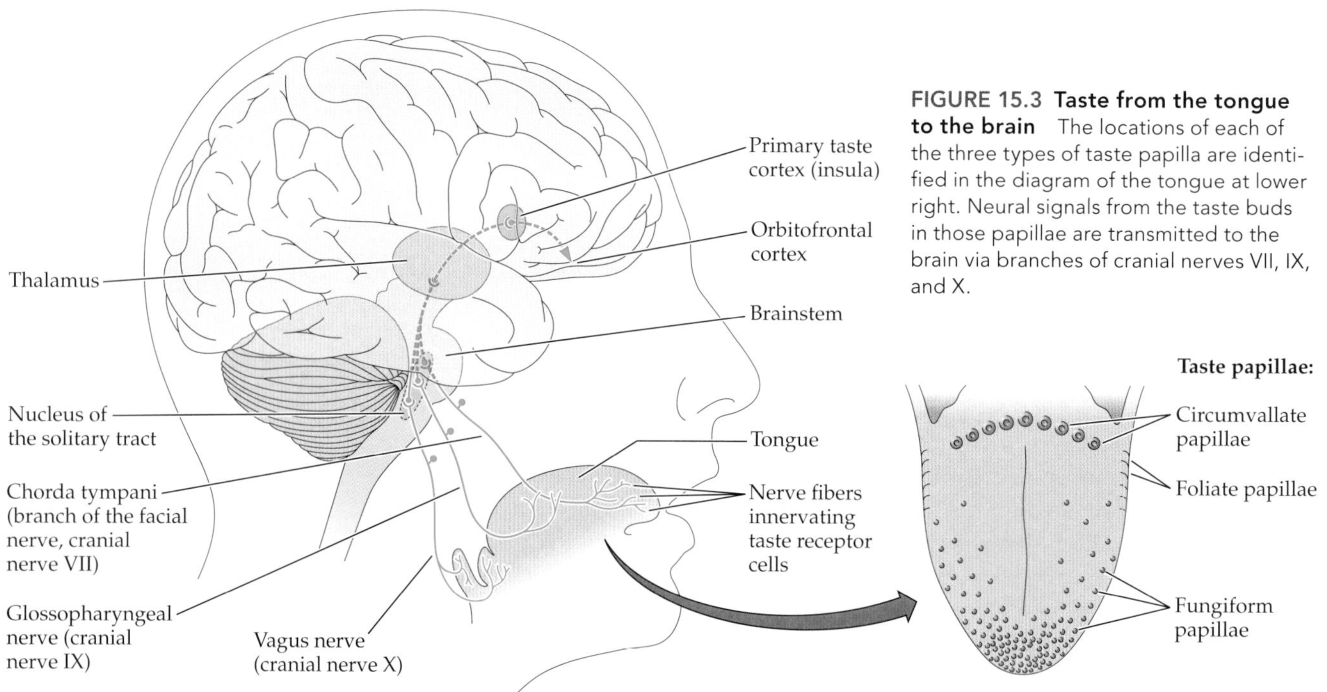

FIGURE 15.3 **Taste from the tongue to the brain** The locations of each of the three types of taste papilla are identified in the diagram of the tongue at lower right. Neural signals from the taste buds in those papillae are transmitted to the brain via branches of cranial nerves VII, IX, and X.

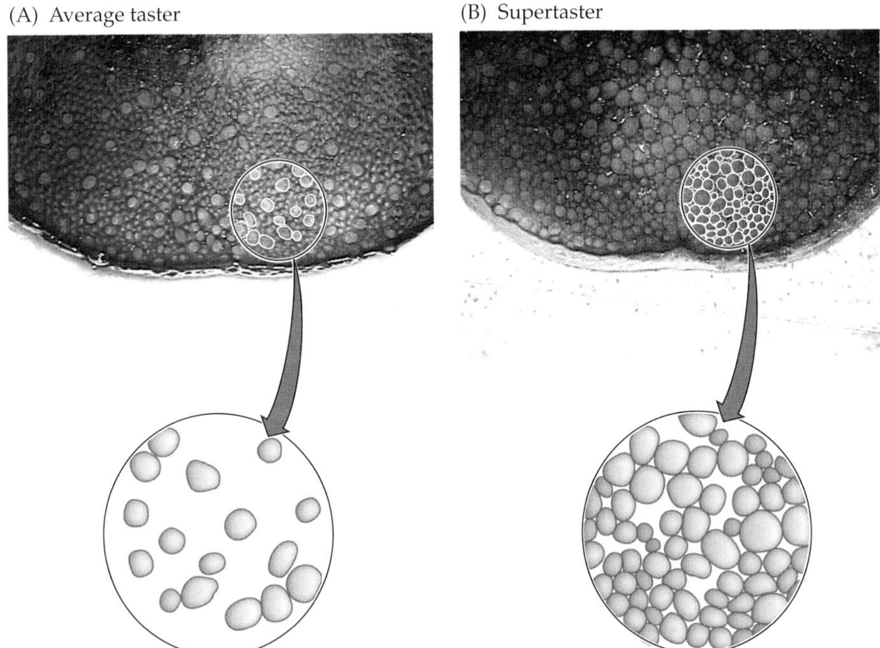

FIGURE 15.4 Average and supertaster tongues Examples showing typical variability in the density of fungiform papillae from one individual to the next. The circles show the 6-millimeter template area used for counting fungiform papillae on tongues stained with blue food coloring. Because blue food coloring does not stain fungiform papillae as deeply as the rest of the tongue tissue, the papillae appear as light circles against a darker blue background. (A) The template area of this "average" taster has 16 fungiform papillae. In extreme cases, individuals may have as few as 5 fungiform papillae. (B) This supertaster's tongue (supertasters are discussed in Section 15.5) has 60 fungiform papillae in the template area.

Some people have so few fungiform papillae that their stained tongues appear to have polka dots on them. Other tongues—those of **supertasters**—have so many that there is little space between them.

Foliate papillae are located on the sides of the tongue at the point where the tongue is attached. Under magnification, they look like a series of folds. Taste buds are buried in the folds.

Circumvallate papillae are relatively large, circular structures forming an inverted *V* on the rear of the tongue. These papillae look like tiny islands surrounded by moats. The taste buds are buried in the sides of the moats.

Although most people don't realize this, there are also taste buds on the roof of the mouth where the hard and soft palates meet. To demonstrate these, wet your finger and dip it into salt crystals. Touch the roof of your mouth and move your finger back until you feel bone (the margin between the hard and soft palates). You will experience a flash of saltiness as you move the salt crystals onto the taste buds arrayed on that margin.

In sum, the taste buds are distributed in a line across the roof of the mouth and in papillae distributed in an oval on the tongue. Fungiform papillae make up the front of the oval, and foliate and circumvallate papillae make up its rear. Note that we have no subjective awareness of this distribution of taste buds.

fungiform papillae Mushroom-shaped structures (maximum diameter 1 millimeter) that are distributed most densely on the edges of the tongue, especially the tip. Taste buds (an average of six per papilla) are buried in the surface.

supertasters Those individuals whose perception of taste sensations is the most intense. A variety of factors may contribute to this heightened perception, including density of fungiform papillae.

foliate papillae Folds of tissue containing taste buds. Foliate papillae are located on the rear of the tongue lateral to the circumvallate papillae, where the tongue attaches to the mouth.

circumvallate papillae Circular structures that form an inverted *V* on the rear of the tongue (three to five on each side, with the largest in the center). Circumvallate papillae are moundlike structures, each surrounded by a trench (like a moat). They are much larger than fungiform papillae.

Taste Myth: The Tongue Map

In 1901, D. P. Hänig published a paper (in German) of work done in the laboratory of Wilhelm Wundt (Wundt's laboratory was the first dedicated to psychology). Hänig measured taste thresholds for bitter, sweet, salty, and sour all around the perimeter, as well as at the base of the tongue. Hänig's paper was translated by Edwin Boring, a famous psychologist at Harvard, and described in his classic book, *Sensation and Perception in the History of Experimental Psychology* (1942). This contributed to one of the most widely disseminated "facts" about taste.

Hänig provided tables of thresholds measured from five participants for each of the four classic taste qualities (see Section 15.3). (Incidentally, Hänig listed

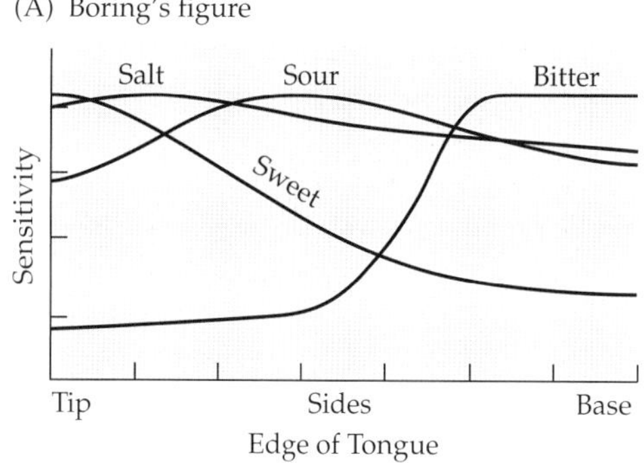

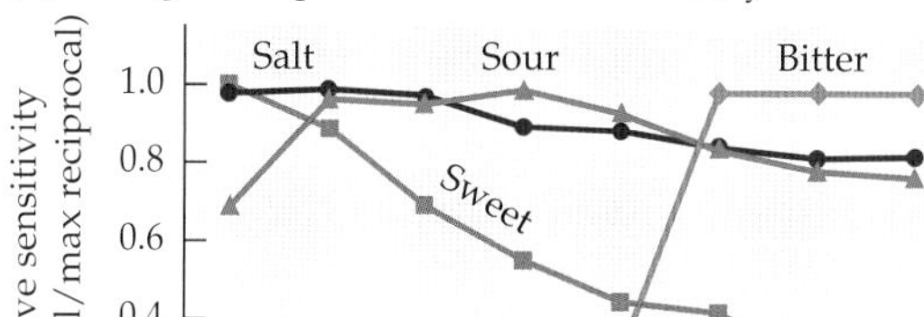

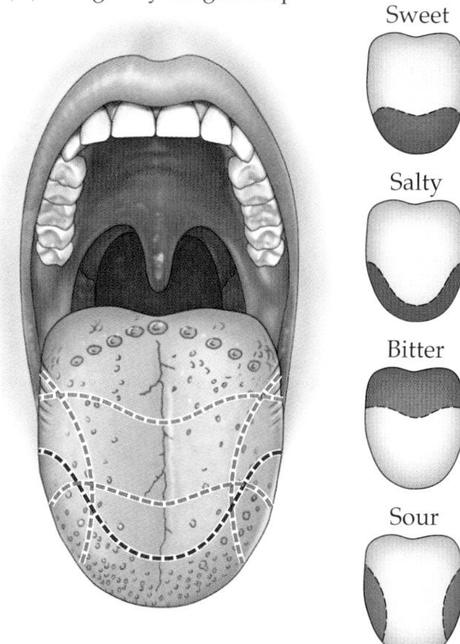

FIGURE 15.5 Origin of the tongue map myth (A) Boring's figure shows his version of Hänig's data. (B) Hänig's actual data are plotted and labeled more clearly. (C) One example of the imagined tongue maps.

his participants by name, a common practice of the era, which would violate our modern rules of participant confidentiality.) Boring calculated the reciprocals of those thresholds (1/threshold). He called these transformed values "sensitivity" and plotted somewhat smoothed curves that seemed to show a picture of how the classic taste qualities varied across tongue locations (**FIGURE 15.5A**). For comparison, **FIGURE 15.5B** plots Hänig's actual data, unsmoothed and correctly labeled. Over the years, various authors transferred these data into "tongue maps," such as the one shown in **FIGURE 15.5C**.

THE MAP IS BOGUS Figure 15.5C is one of many renditions of the imagined tongue map as it became enshrined in texts. But such maps are misleading to the point of being bogus. Taste thresholds do vary across different tongue locations, but that variation is quite small. Boring plotted *relative*, not *absolute*, variation. His label "sensitivity" obscured this. However, there is an even more profound error involved. Thresholds only reflect the lowest detectable taste concentrations; they do not predict taste intensities in the real world. One reason that taste thresholds fail to predict real-world perceived intensities has to do with characteristics of individual taste nerve fibers. Thresholds are determined by the most sensitive of the fibers. Real-world taste intensities are produced by the summation across fibers with varying thresholds.

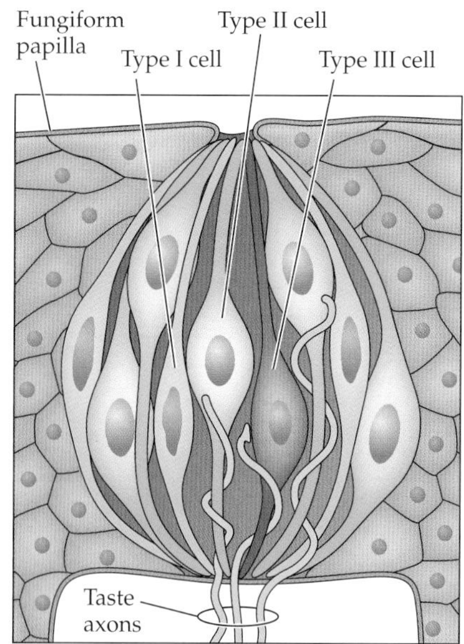

FIGURE 15.6 Taste bud A taste bud buried in the tissue of a fungiform papilla has three types of cells. Type I cells have housekeeping functions. Type II cells are the receptor cells for sweet, bitter, and amino acid stimuli. They secrete adenosine triphosphate, which excites taste axons. Type III cells are excited by sour stimuli and transmit signals to the brain via synapses.

Taste Buds and Taste Receptor Cells

Each taste bud is a cluster of elongated cells, organized much like the segments of an orange (**FIGURE 15.6**). The tips of some of these cells (the taste receptor cells) end in slender **microvilli** (singular *microvillus*) containing sites that bind to taste substances. In an earlier era, these microvilli were mistakenly thought to be tiny hairs.

Some years ago, taste receptor cells were thought to have sites stimulated by taste stimuli at the tip and synapses with peripheral taste axons at the other end.

But more recent work shows that not all receptor cells synapse with taste nerve fibers. How is information from these receptor cells conveyed to the brain?

Recent work describes an intricate network of connections among cells in taste buds (Roper and Chaudhari, 2017; Roper, 2021). Anatomically, taste bud cells fall into three groups with different functions (see Figure 15.6). Most are type I cells; these appear to have primarily housekeeping functions. What we know so far suggests that type II cells express G protein–coupled receptors (GPCRs) that wind back and forth seven times across the microvillus membrane. When a particular **tastant** molecule "key" is fitted into the "lock" portion of a GPCR on the outside of the membrane, the portion of the GPCR inside the cell starts a cascade of molecular events. Type II cells express GPCRs either for sweet or for bitter. These receptor cells do not have synapses; however, they secrete chemicals (such as the neurotransmitter adenosine triphosphate), which can activate nearby taste axons. The smallest number of cells, type III cells, do have synapses and appear to mediate sour taste. We are still not sure about salty.

The discovery of chemical and electrical connections between cells in taste buds not only explains how cells without conventional synapses can transmit information, but also introduces feedback mechanisms. For example, type III cells can secrete inhibitory transmitters like gamma-aminobutyric acid that can inhibit type II cells.

This updated view of taste buds shows a complex structure with communication among the cells that suggests considerable processing before the taste messages are sent to the brain. What does this processing do to the message? We still are not sure.

FURTHER DISCUSSION of the lock-and-key metaphor in relation to other sensory modalities can be found in Sections 4.5 and 14.3.

Taste receptors have a limited life span. After a matter of days, they die and are replaced by new cells. This constant renewal enables the taste system to recover from damage, and it explains why our taste systems can remain robust even into old age. It appears that the nerve fibers are somehow able to select the taste receptors that they contact so that the message they convey remains stable, even though the receptor cells are continually replaced.

Nonoral Locations for Taste Receptors

When we think of taste receptors, we naturally think of the mouth. However, as far back as Ivan Pavlov, there was speculation about receptors that could sense chemicals in the gastrointestinal tract (commonly called the gut). The taste receptors in the mouth produce conscious sensations, while those in the gut play other roles. We will discuss these roles at greater length in Section 15.4.

In addition, the GPCRs that mediate sweet and bitter sensations have been found in an amazing array of places outside the mouth and gut. For example, in the upper airways, bitter compounds can cause cilia to beat and clear bacteria from airways (R. J. Lee et al., 2014). In the stomach, bitter compounds can slow absorption of toxins that are not successfully rejected at the mouth (Jeon et al., 2008).

FURTHER DISCUSSION of GPCRs in the context of olfaction can be found in Section 14.4.

Taste Processing in the Central Nervous System

Taste information travels to the brain in branches of three **cranial nerves**: chorda tympani and greater superficial petrosal (two branches of the facial nerve, CN VII),

microvilli Slender projections of the cell membrane on the tips of some taste bud cells that extend into the taste pore.

tastant Any stimulus that can be tasted.

cranial nerves Twelve pairs of nerves (one set for each side of the body) that originate in the brainstem and reach sense organs and muscles through openings in the skull.

insular cortex The primary cortical processing area for taste—the part of the cortex that first receives taste information. Also called the *insula* or the *gustatory cortex*.

orbitofrontal cortex The part of the frontal lobe of the cortex that lies behind the bone (orbit) containing the eyes. It is involved in many functions and is responsible for the conscious experience of olfaction, as well as the integration of pleasure and displeasure from food, and has been referred to as the *secondary olfactory cortex* and *secondary taste cortex*. It is also critical for assigning affective value to stimuli—in other words, determining hedonic meaning.

glossopharyngeal (CN IX), and vagus (CN X). Taste information travels through the medulla and thalamus before reaching the **insular cortex**, also referred to as the gustatory cortex (**FIGURE 15.7**) (Pritchard and Norgren, 2004). The **orbitofrontal cortex** receives projections from the insular cortex. Some orbitofrontal neurons are multimodal; that is, they respond to temperature, touch, and smell, as well as to taste, suggesting that the orbitofrontal cortex may be an integration area. Notice in Figure 15.7 that taste projects ipsilaterally (i.e., axonal projections remain on the same side) from the periphery (i.e., outside the brain) to the cerebral cortex. An injury to the central nervous system (e.g., a stroke in an area of the brain mediating taste) will result in loss of taste on the tongue on the same side as the stroke (Pritchard, Macaluso, and Eslinger, 1999).

The functional separation of the taste qualities suggested to early investigators that there would likely be a gustotopic map in the cortex, but evidence for this has been elusive (Di Lorenzo, 2021). Earlier studies stimulating the tongue with taste solutions while simultaneously recording electrical activity from individual neurons in the cortex failed to find a gustotopic map. Optical imagery, a newer method that visualizes changes in light reflectance from the surface of the brain (produced by metabolic events like blood flow), has found "distinctive spatial patterns" with some overlap for the four classic taste qualities (Accolla et al., 2007). However, this is not the simple gustotopic map that early investigators expected to find. More recently,

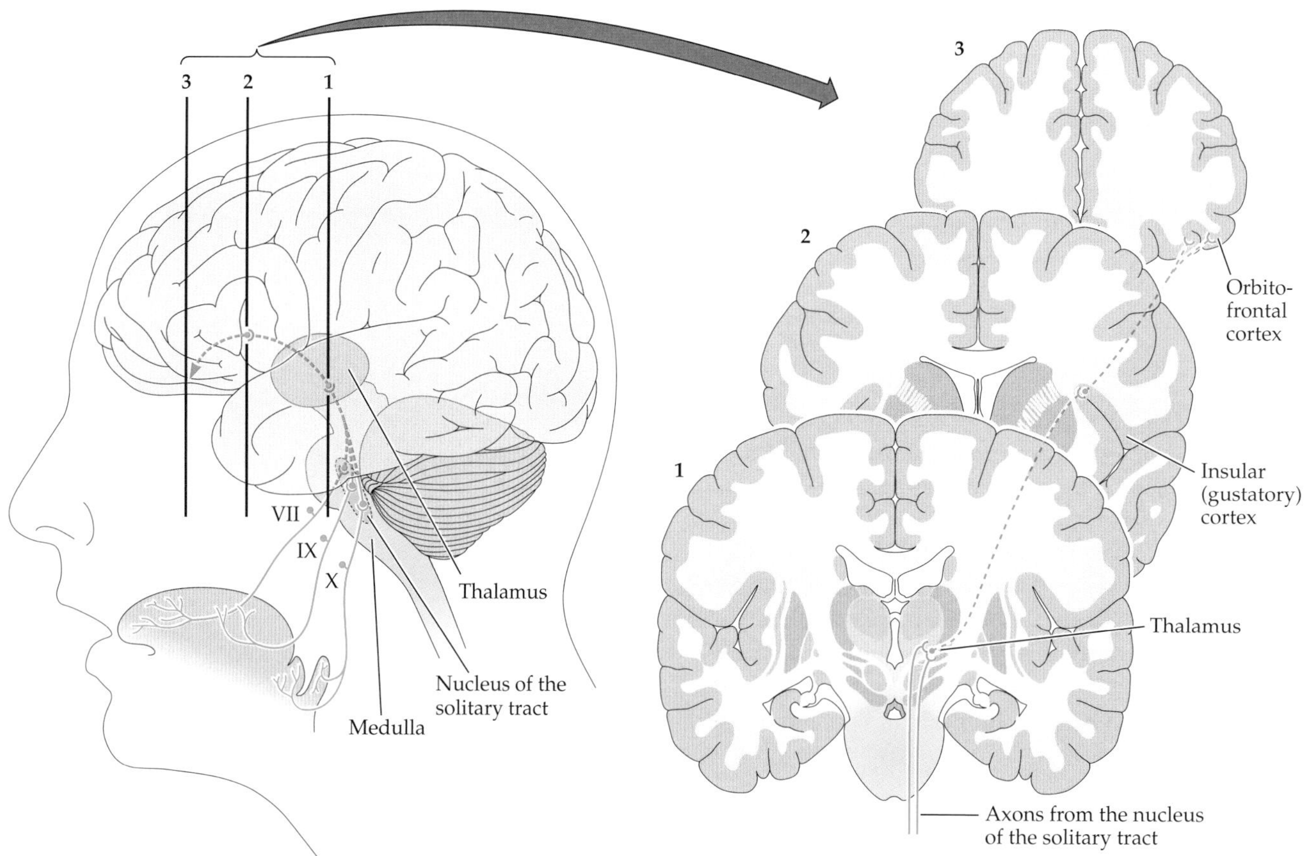

FIGURE 15.7 Projection of the cranial nerves for taste Branches of cranial nerves VII, IX, and X carry taste information from the tongue to a cluster of cells in the medulla of the brain; this cell cluster is the nucleus of the solitary tract, sometimes called the gustatory nucleus. From the medulla, the information projects to the thalamus (shown in cross section 1 of the cerebral cortex), then to the insular (gustatory) cortex (cross section 2), and finally to the orbitofrontal cortex (cross section 3).

some investigators have argued that the early studies were done with anesthetized animals. Newer work recording from awake, behaving animals has failed to show a clear gustotopic map, and so the debate goes on (Chen, Kogan, and Fontanini, 2021). However taste quality turns out to be coded in the brain, our taste sensations remain analytic.

Inhibition plays an important role in the processing of taste information in the brain. One of the functions of this inhibition may be to protect our whole-mouth perception of taste in the face of injuries to the taste system. Our brains receive taste input bilaterally from three cranial nerves. Damage to one of these nerves diminishes its contribution to the whole; however, that damage also releases the inhibition that is normally produced by the damaged nerve. The result is that whole-mouth taste intensities are relatively unchanged. Unfortunately, in some cases this preserved whole-mouth perception comes at a cost. Localized taste damage is often accompanied by "phantom taste" sensations (recall the phantom limbs experienced by many limb amputees, described in Section 13.1), as if the release of inhibition permits even noise in the nervous system to be perceived as a taste.

Descending inhibition from the taste cortex to a variety of other structures may also serve other functions. For example, mouth injuries that lead to oral pain make it harder to eat. The inhibition of such pain perceptions by taste-processing parts of the brain would make eating easier and thus increase the likelihood of survival (because no matter how much the mouth hurts, we still have to eat). Consistent with this principle, patients with a serious oral pain disorder known as burning mouth syndrome were shown to have localized taste damage as well (Grushka and Bartoshuk, 2000). Furthermore, women who have taste damage are more likely to suffer from severe nausea and vomiting during pregnancy (Sipiora et al., 2000); and patients with cancer, whose chemotherapy and radiation therapy is known to damage the taste system, are more likely to experience coughing, gagging, hiccups, and oral pain. In all these cases, inhibitory signals from the taste cortex that normally help prevent eating-disruptive symptoms (oral pain, vomiting, hiccupping, and so on) may have been turned off because of the damage to the taste system.

15.3 The Four Basic Tastes?

We learned in Chapter 14 that we are able to distinguish many different odorants. Thus, when we understand that flavor comes from olfaction, much of the complexity of the sensations evoked by foods vanishes. The number of true taste qualities is small. In fact, the current universally accepted list includes only the four **basic tastes** mentioned in the "tongue map" discussion in Section 15.2: **salty**, **sour**, **bitter**, and **sweet**. As we discuss these in the sections that follow, remember that one of the most important features of the basic tastes is that our liking (or disliking) for them is hardwired in the brain—that is, we are essentially born liking or disliking these tastes. This hardwired affect is very important for their biological purposes. This is very different from the way we learn to like or dislike flavors.

The number of basic tastes has been the subject of argument that goes back even before Aristotle (see Bartoshuk, 1978). Various investigators have suggested adding to the list of basic tastes; the two most recent contenders (umami and fatty) are important because of their special association with learned preferences. There is no universal definition of "basic taste"; however, the authors of this text prefer to reserve the term for those sensations that produce hardwired affect, since this affect is arguably the characteristic of taste that most distinguishes it from the other senses. Some argue that any chemicals for which there are receptors in the mouth produce basic tastes. However, as we noted at the end of Section 15.2, receptors for

basic taste Any of the four taste qualities that are generally agreed to describe human taste experience: sweet, salty, sour, bitter.

salty One of the four basic tastes; the taste quality produced by the cations of salts (e.g., the sodium in sodium chloride produces the salty taste). Some cations also produce other taste qualities (e.g., potassium tastes bitter as well as salty). The purest salty taste is produced by sodium chloride (NaCl), common table salt.

sour One of the four basic tastes; the taste quality produced by the hydrogen ion in acids.

bitter One of the four basic tastes; the taste quality, generally considered unpleasant, produced by substances like quinine or caffeine.

sweet One of the four basic tastes; the taste quality produced by some sugars, such as glucose, fructose, and sucrose. These three sugars are particularly biologically useful to us, and our sweet receptors are tuned to them. Some other compounds (e.g., saccharin, cyclamate, aspartame) are able to stimulate the major sweet receptor and so we have "artificial sweeteners."

chemicals are now known to be throughout the body, and we certainly would not argue that these mediate basic tastes. As we will discuss in Section 15.4, umami and fatty appear to be examples of stimuli for which there are receptors that function to regulate the palatability of protein and fat, but this appears to occur in the gut, not in the mouth.

For many years we have known that taste stimuli can be divided into two major groups: salty and sour, mediated by ion channels (small openings in the membranes of the microvilli in taste bud receptor cells), and bitter and sweet, mediated by protein receptors (which we now know to be GPCRs in the membranes of the microvilli).

Salty

Salts are made up of two charged particles: a cation (positively charged) and an anion (negatively charged). For example, common table salt is NaCl; the sodium is the cation (Na^+), and the chloride is the anion (Cl^-). The source of the salty taste is the cation (**FIGURE 15.8A**). Although all salts taste at least a little salty to humans, pure NaCl is the saltiest-tasting salt around. Sodium must be available in relatively large quantities in the body to maintain nerve and muscle function, and loss of too much body sodium leads to a swift death.

Our ability to perceive saltiness is not static. Gary Beauchamp and his colleagues showed that diet can affect the perception of saltiness (Bertino, Beauchamp, and Engelman, 1982). Our liking for saltiness is not static either. For example, when we lose water and salt through exercise, we return to equilibrium in three stages that involve changes in the palatability of NaCl. First, thirst makes us drink water, but salty taste is aversive. We drink water, but having lost NaCl, we cannot hold enough water to rehydrate completely. Second, salty taste becomes palatable again and we replace the lost NaCl, permitting the body to hold more water. Third, we drink an additional amount of water that rehydrates us completely (Takamata et al, 1994).

Sour

As you may remember from high school chemistry, a solution containing hydrogen ions (H^+) and hydroxide ions (OH^-) in equal proportions produces water (HOH, or H_2O). As the relative proportion of H^+ increases (decreasing the pH level), the solution becomes more *acidic*. Why do you need to be reminded of all this? Because sour taste is produced by hydrogen ions (**FIGURE 15.8B**). Hydrogen ions enter the receptor cell through ion channels; however, an additional mechanism for sour taste allows undissociated acid molecules (intact molecules that have not split into two charged particles) to enter as well. The undissociated acid molecules dissociate inside the receptor. Ultimately, the stimulus that triggers sour taste is the hydrogen concentration inside the receptor cell (DeSimone et al., 2011). For this

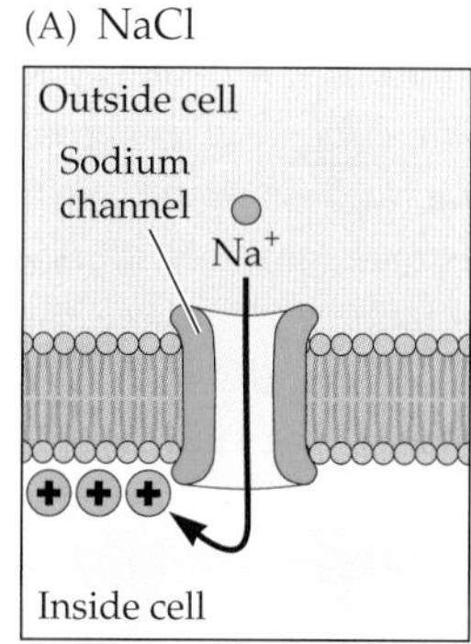

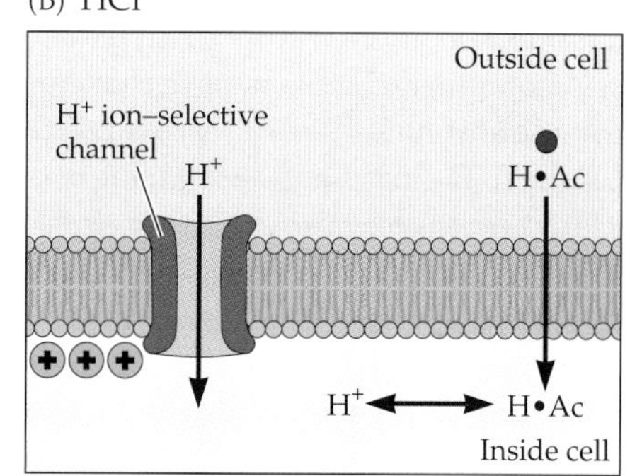

FIGURE 15.8 Ionic tastes: salty and sour Diagram of a taste receptor cell, illustrating the different receptor mechanisms for ionic stimuli (salty and sour). (A) Salty taste is produced by the cation (the positively charged ion) in a salt. In NaCl, the sodium cation (Na^+) is admitted to the receptor cell by sodium ion channels. (B) Sour taste is produced by hydrogen ions (H^+), which enter the cell through ion channels (left). In addition, undissociated hydrogen ions (H•Ac) can cross the membrane and dissociate inside the cell (right).

reason, organic acids, which do not completely dissociate, are more intensely sour than their pH values would suggest.

Some individuals like the sourness of acids in relatively low concentrations. Many adults enjoy pickles and sauerkraut, both of which get their sour tastes from acids. In addition, many children in particular like sour candies (Liem and Mennella, 2003). At high concentrations, however, acids will damage both external and internal body tissues.

Bitter

There are 25 different bitter receptor proteins, and they face a formidable task. Wolfgang Meyerhof, one of the world's experts on bitter, estimates that there are thousands of bitter molecules, many coming from plants that protect themselves from predators by tasting bitter (Meyerhof et al, 2010). How can only 25 bitter receptors handle the job? Part of the answer is that some of the bitter receptors respond only to specific compounds, whereas others are "generalists" that respond to many compounds. The studies identifying the compounds that stimulate the bitter genes have been summarized on a website (www.bitterdb.agri.huji.ac.il/dbbitter.php). For example, denatonium benzoate (marketed as Bitrex) is a very bitter compound that is sometimes added to dangerous household products to prevent children from ingesting them; Bitrex stimulates 8 bitter receptors. Limonin is a bitter compound that is increased in oranges attacked by the HLB bacteria ("greening disease," which is decimating the citrus industry). Limonin stimulates only 1 bitter receptor. Quinine, which gives tonic water its bitter taste, stimulates 9 of the 25 bitter receptors.

Tonic water was originally formulated as a treatment for malaria; now, however, we know that tonic water does not contain enough quinine for that purpose. However, tonic water does contain enough quinine to taste very bitter, and for this reason lots of sugar was added to make tonic water palatable. This approach works because of mixture suppression (different taste qualities suppress one another): tonic water tastes much less bitter than the quinine content alone would, and it also tastes much less sweet than the sugar content alone would. Tonic water actually contains about the same amount of sugar as sodas.

Although a great many different compounds taste bitter, we generally do not distinguish between the tastes of these compounds—we simply avoid them all. The diversity of receptors for bitterness enables species or even individuals in a given species to have varying responses to an array of bitter compounds. One of the most famous of these is human "taste blindness" to phenylthiocarbamide (PTC)—a phenomenon we will revisit in Section 15.5.

Although bitter taste usually signals toxicity, some bitter stimuli are actually good for us. For example, bitter compounds in some vegetables help protect against cancer. We would like to be able to "turn off" these bitter sensations to make it easier for people to eat their vegetables. In pursuit of this goal, Robert Margolskee, a pioneer in studies of bitter transduction, used his understanding of the bitter system to identify a substance that can inhibit some bitter sensations: adenosine monophosphate (AMP) (Ming, Ninomiya, and Margolskee, 1999). AMP may function as a natural bitter inhibitor in mother's milk. A number of compounds in milk, such as casein (milk protein) and calcium salts, taste bitter, and aversions to bitter tastes are present at birth. The presence of AMP in mother's milk may suppress those bitter tastes enough to allow milk to be palatable to babies who are particularly responsive to them (e.g., supertaster babies).

Bitter perception is also affected by hormone levels in women. Sensitivity to bitterness intensifies during pregnancy and diminishes after menopause

(Duffy et al., 1998). These differences make sense in the context of the function of bitterness as a poison detection mechanism. Intensifying the perception of bitter early in pregnancy, when toxins exert their maximum effects, has clear biological value. Consistent with this correlation, some of the aversions common during pregnancy occur with foods or beverages that have bitter tastes (e.g., coffee).

Sweet

Glucose and fructose are simple sugars. Sucrose is the combination of a molecule of glucose and a molecule of fructose. Glucose is the principle source of energy in humans, as well as nearly every other living thing on Earth. Unfortunately, glucose often turns up in nature in the form of sucrose (e.g., in sugar cane, sugar beets, corn). When we consume sucrose, an enzyme breaks the molecule into its constituents, glucose and fructose. The glucose speeds away, providing energy to all the cells in our bodies. The fructose goes to the liver, where some of it is converted to glucose, but the rest of it has a variety of fates that are not necessarily good for us. High-fructose corn syrup (HFCS) is increasingly used as a sweetener. HFCS is made by breaking the sucrose in corn into glucose and fructose, but in addition to this, some of the glucose is converted to fructose. Why? Because fructose is sweeter than glucose. Since we love sweet, we love HFCS. Agave syrup has been touted as a healthy alternative to sucrose. But the fructose content of agave syrup varies depending on the source, and it can be even higher than the fructose content of HFCS.

heterodimer A chain of two molecules (a *dimer*) that are different from each other (hence *hetero*).

The biological function of sweet is different from that of bitter, and the way taste receptors are tuned supports that biological difference. Many different molecules taste bitter. Our biological task is not to distinguish among them, but rather to avoid them all. Thus, we have multiple bitter receptors to encompass the chemical diversity of poisons, but they feed into common lines leading to rejection. With regard to sweet, some biologically useless sugars have structures very similar to those of glucose. In this case, then, the task of the taste system is to tune receptors such that the biologically important sugars stimulate sweet taste, but the others do not. Why aren't our sweet receptors tuned to glucose only? Perhaps because one of the best ways to get glucose is from the sucrose in nature.

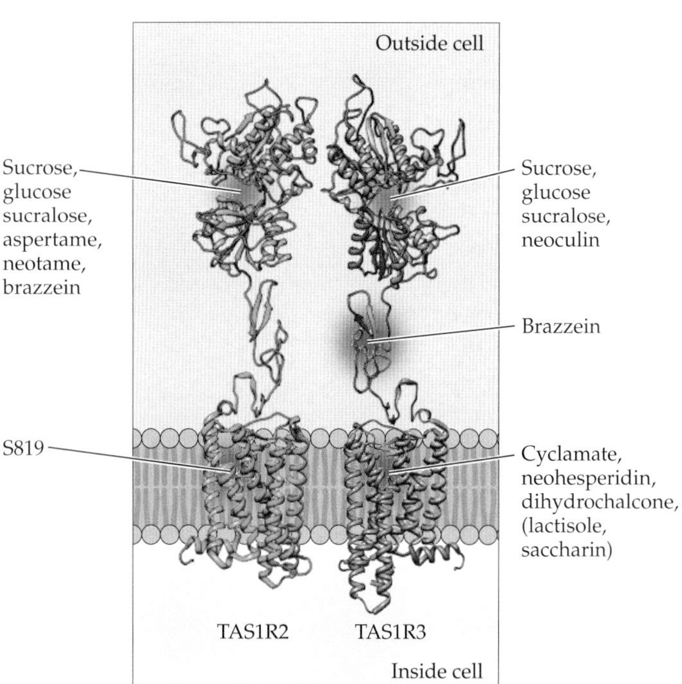

FIGURE 15.9 Sweet heterodimer receptor The sweet heterodimer is made up of two slightly different proteins, designated TAS1R2 (left) and TAS1R3 (right). Some examples of different locations on the receptor that can bind various compounds are shown by the green areas on the receptor. The compound S819 is a synthetic sweetener, as is neotame (an analog of aspartame). Brazzein and neoculin are sweet-tasting proteins extracted from plants.

Consistent with the biological purpose, only two GPCRs are involved with sweet taste. These two GPCRs combine to form a single receptor called a **heterodimer** ("hetero" because the two GPCRs are different from one another, and "dimer" because there are two) (**FIGURE 15.9**). The sweet heterodimer binds sucrose, glucose, and fructose, but also binds a variety of other compounds on different sites. Those other compounds are what we call "artificial sweeteners." Initially, the heterodimer was thought to be responsible for all sweetness, but it introduced a new puzzle: No matter how the heterodimer is stimulated, the receptor cell produces only one signal. Therefore, we would expect all sweeteners—sugars and artificial sweeteners alike—to produce the same sweetness. However, artificial sweeteners like saccharin, cyclamate, and aspartame do not taste exactly like sugar; if they did, there would be no need to continually search for better artificial sweeteners. Some claim that artificial sweeteners produce additional tastes that account for the difference. For example, saccharin tastes bitter as well as sweet to many. But some of us (the author included) do not taste the bitterness of saccharin at all; we are quite convinced that the nature of the sweetness differs. One possible solution to this comes from another sweet receptor. This one is formed by doubling one of the GPCRs found in the heterodimer (and so it is called a "homodimer"). This homodimer appears to respond only to high concentrations of sugars (Zhao et al., 2003). This receptor would help the brain tell the difference between sugars and artificial sweeteners.

Artificial sweeteners exist because they accidentally stimulate the sweet heterodimer. Are artificial sweeteners medically useful? Certainly they enable people with diabetes to enjoy sweet taste without the dangers of sugar, but the early claims that artificial sweeteners would be a panacea for weight loss now appear to be wrong.

Saccharin was discovered in 1879 when the chemist Ira Remsen, working on coal tar derivatives, failed to wash up before dinner and subsequently noticed that the tar residue on his hands tasted sweet. Similarly, another artificial sweetener, cyclamate, was discovered in 1937 by a graduate student who tasted sweet while smoking a cigarette and realized that some compound in the lab must be responsible. Cyclamate was popular for a few years, but suspicions were raised that it caused cancer. Although those suspicions were challenged and cyclamate remains legal in a number of countries, the Food and Drug Administration banned it in the United States. Ironically, saccharin has also been associated with cancer in animals, but remains legal in the United States.

Artificial sweeteners are attractive to dieters because their sweet taste comes with essentially no calories, but a 1986 epidemiological study showed that women who consumed artificial sweeteners actually gained weight (Stellman and Garkinkel, 1988). Also in 1986, John Blundell, an English expert on weight regulation, published a provocative article suggesting that aspartame (the artificial sweetener sold as NutraSweet) increases appetite (Blundell and Hill, 1986). Was the benefit of the reduced calories lost when individuals using aspartame actually increased their caloric intake in subsequent meals? Terry Davidson and Susan Swithers elaborated on this kind of thinking with studies using rats (T. L. Davidson and Swithers, 2004). The earlier work with humans was discounted by many; after all, those with weight problems may be the individuals who choose to consume artificial sweeteners and it is not surprising that they gain weight. However, the same criticism could not apply when rats fed artificial sweeteners gained weight. Davidson and Swithers point to the fact that the "obesity epidemic" occurred over the same years as the introduction of low-calorie foods into the American market. They argue that the uncoupling of the sensory properties of these diet foods from their metabolic consequences disrupts regulation, leading to weight gain.

15.4 Are There More Than Four Basic Tastes? Does It Matter?

Historically, the qualitatively distinct sensations that characterize each sense were identified by introspection. As more and more sensory receptors were discovered, investigators sought to link specific receptors to these distinct sensations. However, it is worth remembering that not all responses to stimuli produce conscious sensations. Proteins and fats provide examples. Proteins and fats are large molecules—too large to stimulate either taste or olfaction. Fats do produce conscious sensations, but they are somatosensations (e.g., thick, oily, viscous, creamy) mediated by neurons that respond to touch. Both fat and protein are broken into their constituent parts by digestion, and some of those constituents stimulate receptors

umami The taste sensation produced by monosodium glutamate.

monosodium glutamate (MSG) The sodium salt of glutamic acid (an amino acid).

in the gut. This stimulation does not produce conscious taste sensations. Rather, this stimulation appears to contribute to the palatability of the foods containing proteins and fats through learning.

Protein: The Umami Question

Umami arose as a candidate for a fifth basic taste as part of advertising claims by manufacturers of **monosodium glutamate (MSG)**, the sodium salt of glutamic acid. Identified by Japanese chemists in the early 1900s, MSG was initially marketed as a flavor enhancer, said to suppress unpleasant tastes and enhance pleasant ones. Taste experts expressed skepticism. MSG manufacturers then went on to claim that MSG was a fifth basic taste, speculating that it signaled protein and thus played an important role in nutrition. Unfortunately, although having special receptors for proteins might be nutritionally helpful, protein molecules are too large to stimulate taste or olfaction.

A protein is a chain of amino acids. One of these is glutamic acid, which turns into glutamate by losing a hydrogen atom. Although a small amount of protein may be broken into its constituent amino acids in the mouth, most protein molecules are broken down by digestion in the gut. Glutamate does not produce a universally liked sensation in the mouth. However, because glutamate is an important neurotransmitter, receptors for this molecule are common throughout the body. The argument that some of these receptors might have been harnessed by the taste system to signal umami gained respectability when neuroscientists Nirupa Chaudhari and Steve Roper identified a version of a glutamate receptor in rat taste papillae. There is now evidence for multiple receptors for umami (Roper and Chaudhari, 2017).

Robert Margolskee (whose pioneering studies focused on not only the bitter receptor but also the sweet receptor) was an early advocate for the importance of taste receptors in the gut. Glutamate receptors can signal the brain that protein has been consumed, but the signal comes from the gut, not the mouth. Consistent with this finding, John Prescott (a cognitive psychologist who studies the chemical senses) showed that consuming a novel-flavored soup with MSG added to it produces a conditioned preference for the novel flavor, while simply holding the soup in the mouth does not (J. Prescott, 2004). Note that using glutamate receptors in the gut to signal protein makes biological sense. This allows many different proteins (that do not taste of umami) to evoke pleasure—not hardwired pleasure, but learned pleasure.

Because glutamate is a neurotransmitter, concerns have been raised about its safety in the human diet. MSG became particularly notorious in the 1960s. First, it became associated with "Chinese restaurant syndrome"—a constellation of symptoms including numbness, headache, flushing, tingling, sweating, and tightness in the chest—that was reported by some individuals after consuming MSG (Kwok, 1968). Then, Dr. John Olney, a toxicologist, suggested that MSG might induce brain lesions, particularly in infants (Olney and Sharpe, 1969). In response to these concerns, MSG was removed from baby foods in the 1970s. The final conclusion (see Walker and Lupien, 2000) is that MSG in large doses may be a problem for some sensitive individuals, but apparently it does not present a serious problem for the general population.

Fat

Like protein, fat is an important nutrient. Also like protein, fat molecules are too large to stimulate either taste or olfaction, but are broken into their constituent parts by digestion in the gut. Fat molecules are made up of fatty acids attached to a support structure. A few fat molecules may be partially digested while still in the mouth, thus releasing fatty acids that could be tasted; however, we now know that fatty acid receptors are found throughout the gut, so it appears that nature uses a more general method to ensure that we love fat-containing foods. Anthony Sclafani (a learning theorist who is an expert on conditioned food preferences) showed that fat in the gut produces conditioned preferences for the sensory properties of the food containing the fat (Sclafani, 1997). Once we understand the role of conditioning in food preferences, we should have a healthy skepticism about the value of so-called diet foods. Mimicking the sensory properties of normal foods but reducing the caloric content disrupts normal regulatory mechanisms.

nontaster (of PTC/PROP) An individual born with two recessive alleles for the PTC/PROP gene who experiences little or no taste from the compounds phenylthiocarbamide (PTC) and propylthiouracil (PROP).

taster (of PTC/PROP) An individual born with one or two dominant alleles for the PTC/PROP gene and able to taste the compounds phenylthiocarbamide (PTC) and propylthiouracil (PROP). PTC/PROP tasters who also have a high density of fungiform papillae tend to be supertasters.

15.5 Genetic Variation in Bitter

In 1931, a chemist named Arthur Fox discovered that we do not all live in the same taste worlds (A. L. Fox, 1931). Fox was synthesizing the compound PTC when some spilled and flew into the air. A colleague nearby noticed a bitter taste, but Fox tasted nothing. A test of additional colleagues revealed a few more **nontasters** like Fox who tasted little bitterness in the compound, but most were **tasters**; that is, they perceived it as bitter. The next year, Albert Blakeslee (a famous geneticist of the day) and Fox took PTC crystals to a meeting of the American Association for the Advancement of Science and set up a voting booth for attendees to register their perceptions (Blakeslee and Fox, 1932). About one-third of those polled found the crystals to be tasteless, while two-thirds found them to be bitter. These proportions captured the imagination of many researchers, and for several years the *Journal of Heredity* sold papers impregnated with PTC for further studies. Family studies eventually confirmed that taster status is an inherited trait. Nontasters carry two recessive alleles, whereas tasters have either one or two dominant alleles.

Initially, individuals were simply classified according to whether they could taste PTC, but eventually threshold studies came into vogue. In a threshold method invented specifically for PTC studies, participants were given eight cups, four containing plain water and four containing water with a given concentration of PTC. Correct sorting determined the threshold. The distribution of thresholds was bimodal, with nontasters showing very high thresholds and tasters showing low thresholds. This distribution varied by sex and race: women had lower thresholds than men, and Asians had lower thresholds than Caucasians.

In the 1960s, Roland Fischer shifted studies to a chemical relative of PTC that was safer to test—propylthiouracil (PROP)—and focused on the nutritional implications of the genetic variation in taster status (Fischer and Griffin, 1964). Fischer suggested that tasters were more finicky eaters: because bitter tastes are more intense to these individuals, they tend to dislike foods high in bitter compounds. Fischer also related taster status to body type (e.g., weight) and health. Populations of alcoholics and smokers were found to contain a lower proportion of tasters than would be expected by chance, presumably because unpleasant sensations (e.g., bitterness) produced by alcoholic beverages and tobacco act as deterrents to tasters. The effect of genetic variation in taste can even be related to cancer risk (mediated by diet), as will be described at the end of this section.

In 2003, Dennis Drayna and his colleagues discovered the location of the gene that expresses PTC/PROP receptors (U. K. Kim et al., 2003). This gene is a member of the bitter family discussed earlier. Individuals with two recessive alleles are nontasters; those with either one or two dominant alleles are tasters.

cross-modality matching The ability to match the intensities of sensations that come from different sensory modalities. This ability allows insight into sensory differences. For example, supertasters will match tastes to louder sounds than will those who are not supertasters.

Supertasters

By the 1970s, the "direct" psychophysical methods introduced by Harvard's S. S. Stevens led to a new look at genetic variation in taste. Instead of measuring thresholds—the dimmest sensations—investigators could look at suprathreshold taste and plot the psychophysical functions showing how perceived taste intensity varies with concentration. You may remember from Section 1.2 that Stevens and his students documented what is now known as Stevens's power law. It holds that perceived sensations rise as the stimulus raised to some power. Written as an equation, this is

$$S = I^b$$

where *S* is sensation, *I* is stimulus intensity (concentration of a solution in taste), and *b* takes on different values for different sensory modalities (Stevens and Galanter, 1957). If we take the logarithm of each side of the equation above, we get

$$\log S = b \times \log I$$

which is the formula for a straight line of slope *b*. Of special interest for our present purposes, *b* takes on different values for different taste qualities. **FIGURE 15.10** shows plots of HCl (sour), sucrose (sweet), NaCl (salty), and QHCl (quinine hydrochloride, bitter). Note that the slope is highest for HCl and lowest for QHCl. That is, sourness grows much more rapidly with concentration than does bitterness.

Unfortunately, knowing how taste intensity grows with concentration does not permit comparisons of perceived taste intensity across individuals; *b* can be equal for two people even if one experiences taste intensities twice as great as the other. Fortunately, two of S. S. Stevens's students—Joseph Stevens and Lawrence Marks—made another fundamental discovery (J. C. Stevens, 1959). As we discussed in Section 1.2, humans are surprisingly good at **cross-modality matching** (see Figure 1.7). For example, we can match the loudness of a sound to the brightness of a light, and we can match either of these to the intensity of a taste. We can use this cross-modality matching to see if some individuals experience more intense sensations than others. First, we need to select a control modality that is not related to taste. As far as we know, our experiences of loudness or brightness are not related to our experiences of taste, so either of these could be our control modality. For this example, let's match our taste sensations to loudness. Give our subjects a sweet stimulus (e.g., Coke or Pepsi) and instruct them to select a sound whose loudness, measured in decibels (dB), matches the sweetness of the beverage; this is cross-modality matching of loudness and sweetness. Some participants match the sweetness to a sound of 90 dB (the loudness of a train whistle). Others match

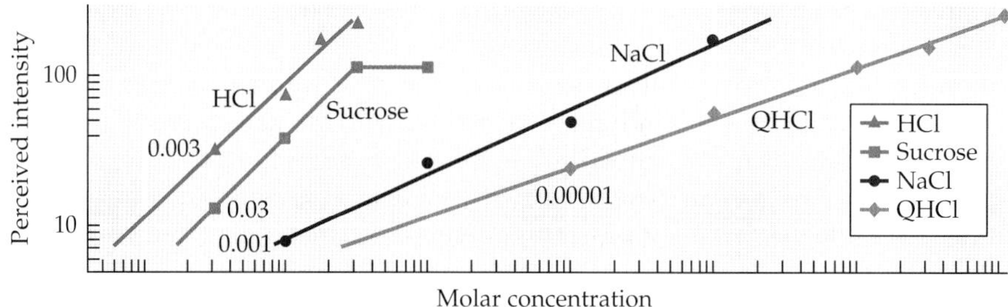

FIGURE 15.10 The growth of perceived taste intensities with concentration Psychophysical functions for sour (HCl), sweet (sucrose), salty (NaCl), and bitter (quinine hydrochloride, QHCl) tastants. The logarithm of the perceived taste intensity is plotted against the logarithm of the tastant's concentration. The lowest concentration of each tastant is indicated. The slopes (*b*) of the functions are as follows: HCl, 0.89; sucrose, 0.94 (for the lower portion); NaCl, 0.43; and QHCl, 0.32.

it to a much weaker sound, 80 dB (the loudness of a telephone dial tone). Because every 10 dB doubles loudness, we know that 90 dB is twice as loud as 80 dB. This tells us that some participants perceive a beverage to be twice as sweet as do other participants. Those in the first group, who experience the more intense sweetness, are called supertasters.

What causes supertasting? There are probably several factors, but one of them is anatomy. If we look at the tongues of the subjects in our cross-modality matching experiment, we find that those who experienced the beverage as twice as sweet tend to have the most fungiform papillae (and thus the most taste buds; see Figure 15.4B). However, the association between tongue anatomy and taste perception can be obscured by pathology. For example, damage to taste neurons that is central to their nuclei will cause degeneration into the brain, affecting taste perception while leaving tongue anatomy intact.

This association between supertasting and tongue anatomy causes more differences between supertasters and others. Supertasters experience the most intense sensations of oral burn (e.g., from chili peppers) and oral touch (from fats or thickeners in foods), presumably because fungiform papillae are innervated by nerve fibers that convey burn and touch sensations as well as those that convey taste sensations. Thus, the more fungiform papillae you have, the more nerve fibers that carry oral pain and oral touch. In addition, because of interactions between taste and retronasal olfaction, those who experience the most intense taste sensations also perceive more intense retronasal olfaction (flavor) sensations. So, for example, if a group of supertasters and a group who are not supertasters each sniff a bowl of chocolate pudding, they will experience, on average, the same chocolate smell. However, if they then sample the pudding, the supertasters will experience more intense chocolate flavor.

Pathology adds yet another source of variation in our oral sensations. Surprisingly, removing input from one of the taste nerves (by anesthesia or damage) can actually *intensify* whole-mouth taste sensations (Bartoshuk et al., 2012). This intensification happens because inputs from the different taste nerves inhibit one another in the brain. Loss of input from one nerve releases others from inhibition. In some cases, the release of inhibition is greater than the loss of input and the result is actual intensification of whole-mouth taste. When damage is more widespread, not surprisingly, taste perception diminishes.

In sum, the intensities of our taste experiences result from genetic variation, pathology, and interactions among all of the cranial nerves innervating the mouth.

Health Consequences of Variation in Taste Sensations

With these insights, the potential links between responsiveness to PROP and health have become the focus of considerable interest. The new psychophysical methods permitted nutrition expert Valerie Duffy to show that variation in the sensory properties of foods and beverages affects food preferences and thus diet. Because diet is a major risk factor for a variety of diseases, genetic variation in taste plays a role in these diseases. For instance, some vegetables produce unpleasant sensations (e.g., bitter) to medium tasters and supertasters, leading these individuals to eat fewer of them. Reduced vegetable intake is a risk factor for colon cancer.

Sure enough, Duffy and her colleagues found that, in a sample of older men getting routine colonoscopies, those tasting PROP as most bitter had the most colon polyps, a precursor to colon cancer (Basson et al., 2003). However, fats can also produce unpleasantly intense sensations in supertasters, leading them to eat fewer high-fat foods and thereby lower their risk of cardiovascular disease (Duffy et al., 2004). Sensory links to behavior that affects health are not limited to diet.

Fischer's early suggestion that nontasters are more likely to smoke and consume alcohol has proved correct (Duffy et al., 2004; D. J. Snyder et al., 2005).

More generally, variation in the sensory properties of foods and beverages is linked to health because that variation affects what we like to eat, and diet affects health. In addition to variation resulting from genetic differences, there is taste damage caused by common pathologies. The pathways of the taste nerves from the tongue to the brain are vulnerable to damage. The chorda tympani taste nerve passes through the middle ear, where it is vulnerable to middle-ear infections (otitis media). The glossopharyngeal taste nerve is physically near the tonsils. A layer of muscle can protect the glossopharyngeal nerve during tonsillectomy, but that muscle is lacking in some individuals. Both the chorda tympani and the glossopharyngeal nerves can be damaged by head injuries, even if they are relatively mild. Taste damage can have unexpected consequences because of inhibitory connections between taste nerves and nerves that carry other oral sensations. Individuals with histories of middle-ear infections (usually occurring in infancy or childhood), tonsillectomy, or head injury were found to weigh more in their 40s than those without those histories (Bartoshuk et al., 2012, 2013). Sensory testing revealed a likely scenario. The localized taste damage released inhibition on undamaged nerves such that whole-mouth taste, perception of touch (fats in foods), and retronasal olfaction all increased. These sensory changes were associated with enhanced palatability of high-fat foods, which could potentially lead to weight gain.

COVID-19 As you read in Chapter 14, the COVID-19 pandemic can cause smell loss and dysfunction, which can be persistent. The confusion between flavor and taste means that many patients report a loss of taste when they have really experienced loss of flavor. However, a few studies that tested genuine taste did find some losses. The coronaviruses might behave as do some upper respiratory viruses (like those that cause middle-ear infections). The eustachian tubes connect the back of the throat to the middle ear. The eustachian tube is a conduit that allows pressure equalization between the middle ear and the mouth (think of the pop you feel when the pressure changes in an airplane). Viruses can move through that conduit from the mouth/nose to the middle ear, where they have access to the chorda tympani taste nerve. This kind of damage can be detected by a spatial taste test. Patients lose taste only on the area innervated by the chorda tympani nerve: the anterior, mobile part of the tongue. The rear of the tongue is spared. This is the pattern of damage seen in patients with middle-ear infections. Will taste loss in COVID-19 be associated with enhanced palatability of high-fat foods and weight gain? Time will tell.

15.6 How Do Taste and Flavor Contribute to the Regulation of Nutrients?

Bentham said, "Nature has placed mankind under the governance of two sovereign masters, pain and pleasure. It is for them alone to point out what we ought to do, as well as to determine what we shall do" (Bentham, 1876). Bentham would not have been surprised to learn that the pleasure associated with taste and flavor guides our food choices (see "Scientists at Work: The Role of Food Preferences in Food Choices"). Some species have few food choices to make; for example, koala bears eat primarily leaves from the eucalyptus tree. However, humans (and rats) are omnivores; we are confronted with an array of choices, and we must select safe foods and avoid poisons to survive. Paul Rozin described this as the *omnivore's dilemma* (E. Rozin and Rozin, 1981). Michael Pollan subsequently borrowed the term to apply to the modern human's need to find a healthy diet amid the dizzying choices available to us today (Pollan, 2006). How does the pleasure associated with taste and flavor solve this dilemma?

Taste

The taste system responds to a small set of molecules that we encounter in nature. This precise tuning is consistent with the role of taste as a system for detecting nutrients and "antinutrients" (substances that are either helpful or harmful, respectively, to our bodies).

Each of the four basic tastes is responsible for a different nutrient or antinutrient and has evolved according to its purpose. For example, the bitter taste subsystem is nature's poison detector. In terms of chemical structure, poisons are quite diverse. Thus, the bitter receptors must be diverse as well. However, given that we don't really care if we can discriminate among poisons—we just want to avoid them all—we could hook all of those receptors up to a few common lines to the brain. As we saw earlier, this is how the bitter subsystem is set up. Similarly, the sour subsystem is configured to reject any highly acidic solution without identifying its source. The other two taste subsystems enable us to detect, and therefore selectively ingest, foods that contain nutrients that our bodies need: sodium (salty) and sugars (sweet).

● Scientists at Work

The Role of Food Preferences in Food Choices

Question Do our food preferences determine how much we weigh? Our diets have a great deal to do with risk for cardiovascular disease (i.e., heart attacks, strokes). A great deal of effort has been put into devising measures of dietary intake, but this has proved difficult because of recall problems and biases (e.g., people who are overweight tend to underestimate fat intake). Valerie Duffy and her colleagues looked at this problem in a new way, using a psychophysical measure of food preference (Duffy et al., 2007).

Hypothesis We are not very good at recalling what we eat accurately. However, we are good at describing what we like to eat. Thus, our food preferences may be a good way to assess dietary risk.

Test Duffy recruited 422 men from a manufacturing company to participate in a health risk appraisal survey. Their adiposity (e.g., waist circumference as well as body mass index, which is weight corrected for height) was assessed, and they (1) reported the number of times per week that they consumed high-fat foods and (2) rated their liking for high-fat foods.

Results The degree to which these men liked high-fat foods correlated significantly with body mass index and waist circumference; the frequency with which they said they ate high-fat foods did not. There are two reasons why an affective measure (liking) mapped onto adiposity better than dietary recall did. First, memory experts know that it is harder to recall facts than it is to recall feelings. For example, think about how hard it is to remember how often you have consumed chocolate cake. Now think about how much easier it is to remember how much you like chocolate cake. Second, the investigators asked participants to rate their liking for high-fat foods on a special rating scale. The key to that special scale was the context. Participants rated how much they liked high-fat foods in the context of all kinds of pleasures (e.g., enjoying music, spending time with friends, watching a favorite TV show). The pleasure from the nonfood items served as a kind of standard that was not related to adiposity and thus could be assumed to be roughly equal for all participants. Thus, the pleasure experienced by the heavier individuals from the high-fat foods could be seen as higher relative to the nonfood pleasures.

Conclusion Food preferences can predict adiposity. Jeremy Bentham, an eighteenth-century philosopher, argued for the primacy of pleasure in determining what we do. The pleasure associated with eating is an example of this.

Future work Assessing food preferences is much easier than assessing dietary intake. Would you recommend adding food preference assessment to health risk appraisals?

Some of the most impressive evidence for this hardwired affect with taste came from the work of Jacob Steiner on facial expressions in newborn infants (Steiner, 1973). Steiner found that infants responded with stereotyped facial expressions when sweet, salty, sour, and bitter solutions were applied to their tongues. Sweet evoked a "smile-like" expression followed by sucking (**FIGURE 15.11A**). Sour produced pursing and protrusion of the lips (**FIGURE 15.11B**). Bitter produced gaping, movements of spitting, and, in some cases, vomiting movements. Even infants born without cerebral hemispheres (a condition known as anencephaly) showed the same facial expressions, suggesting that these expressions are mediated by very primitive parts of the brain.

The fact that the basic tastes provide both information and pleasure (affect) enables organisms to solve critical nutritional problems immediately, without having to learn (which takes time). The newborn baby can nurse because the sweet taste of mother's milk is pleasurable. The baby can also reject poisons because the bitter tastes they evoke are aversive. The athlete who sweats or the new mother who loses blood can replace lost sodium because the taste of salt is pleasant and often becomes more pleasant when salt is needed.

Flavor

Taste affect guides us very effectively for the few nutrients discussed above. However, olfactory affect becomes critical when nutrients are not conveniently labeled by taste. When we eat foods, we experience retronasal olfactory stimulation. Specific features of the olfactory molecules interact with receptors tuned to them. All receptors of a given type project to individual glomeruli in the olfactory brain. The pattern across the glomeruli creates a "picture" of the chemical structure of a molecule (or a mixture of molecules). These pictures are stored in the brain and can be associated with positive or negative affect, depending on the consequences of what we eat. If we get sick, the pictures acquire negative affect. If our brains judge the consequences as good (e.g., calories, positive mood states), the pictures acquire positive affect. Our like or dislike of foods is made up of the hardwired affect of taste along with the learned affect of retronasal olfaction.

This view of nutrient regulation owes much to the work of Paul Rozin, who debunked an important early idea, "wisdom of the body." The phrase *wisdom of the body* dates back to a famous lecture by E. H. Starling (1923) and a subsequent

(A)

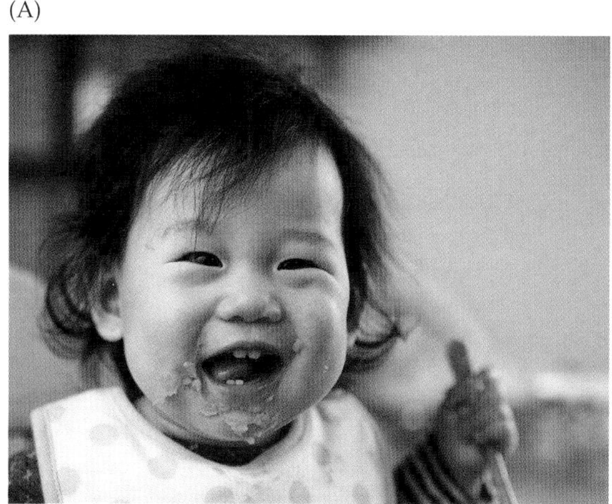

(B)

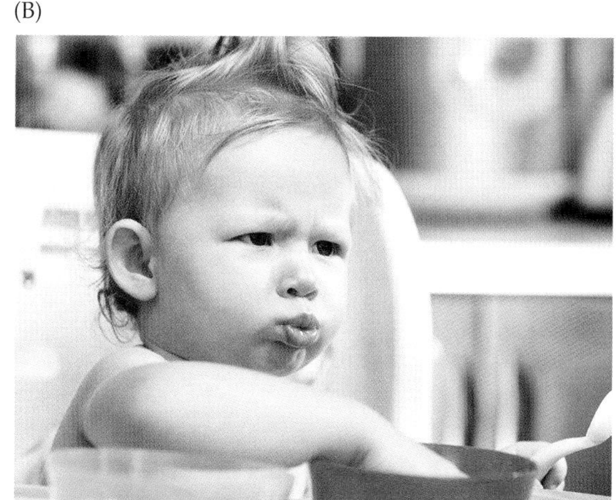

FIGURE 15.11 Facial expressions for sweet and sour The two toddlers' facial expressions reveal the taste qualities that they're experiencing. (A) Sweet potato produces the typical smile associated with the acceptance of sweet. (B) The toddler eating green apples produces the puckery face associated with sour.

book by Cannon (1939) on homeostasis, the body's ability to maintain constancy (as in the regulation of blood sugar by insulin). However, Curt Richter extended this thinking to behavior with his **specific hungers theory**. Richter suggested that animals can recognize a need for a specific nutrient, find and consume it, and so restore the body to its normal condition. The evidence for wisdom of the body at first looked impressive. For example, a 3½-year-old boy with an intense craving for salt died when his salt intake was restricted during a hospital stay. An autopsy revealed a tumor of his adrenal gland that had caused his body to lose sodium. His salt craving had enabled his body to retain enough sodium to keep him alive when he was home and had access to all the salt he wanted (Wilkins and Richter, 1940).

specific hungers theory The idea that deficiency of a given nutrient produces craving (a specific hunger) for that nutrient. Curt Richter first proposed this theory and demonstrated that cravings for salty or for sweet are associated with deficiencies in those substances. However, the idea proved wrong for other nutrients (e.g., vitamins).

Another source of support for specific hungers was a treatment for schizophrenia that was popular in the 1940s. At the time, some experts believed that the brain, which depends on glucose for fuel, could be forcibly rested if blood glucose were driven to very low values with insulin. Intense cravings for sweet were an unexpected by-product of the therapy. Richter concluded that ingestion of a nutrient reduces craving and brings the body back to baseline: homeostasis. Even more support for the idea of specific hungers seemed to come from the work of a pediatrician, Clara Davis. She allowed a group of 6-month-old infants to eat whatever they liked, to see if they would choose wisely (C. M. Davis, 1928). The infants thrived, leading Davis to conclude that, when allowed to choose among a variety of healthy foods, infants had the ability to select a healthy diet.

The specific hungers theory came to a screeching halt when investigators tried to extend it to vitamins. In one of the early studies, rats were fed a diet deficient in vitamin B_1, which made them sick (in humans, B_1 deficiency is called beriberi.) When the rats were offered a choice of remaining on the same diet or switching to a different diet that contained B_1, they immediately switched. But Rozin conducted a crucial control: he let rats choose between the original diet and a diet that was also deficient in B_1 but had a different flavor. These rats switched to the differently flavored diet even though it did not contain B_1. Thus, the rats in the original study had not specifically sought B_1; they had simply learned to avoid the flavor of the diet that made them sick (P. Rozin, 1967).

Rozin's work ended belief in specific hungers as an explanation of dietary regulation for anything beyond sugar and salt. In retrospect, we can see that the theory lacked an important ingredient. For craving to cause an animal to seek out and take in a needed nutrient, a sensory cue would have to be unambiguously associated with the nutrient. The saltiness of salt and the sweetness of sugar could serve as such cues, but the B_1 molecule does not produce a detectable cue in food (**FIGURE 15.12**).

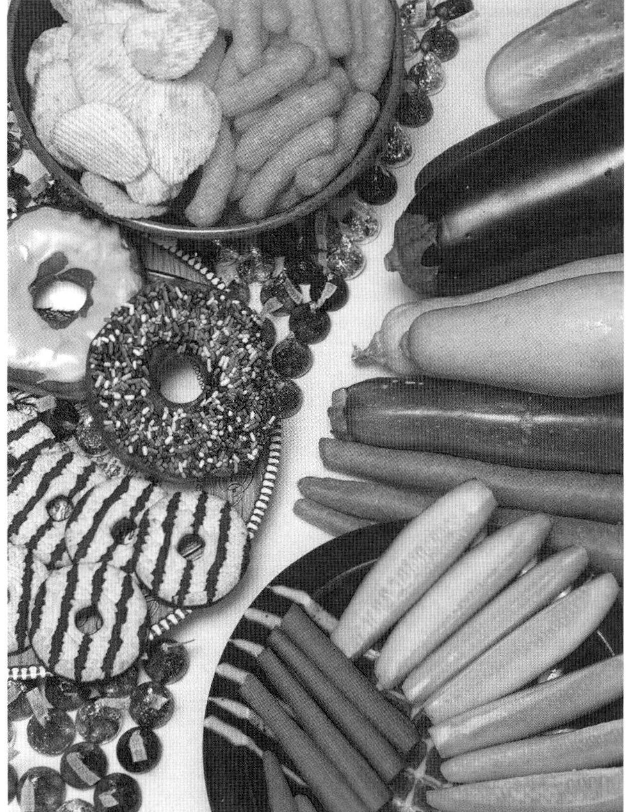

FIGURE 15.12 **Micronutrients (vitamins and minerals) in foods are not detectable** In our evolutionary past, when food was scarce and we had to expend considerable physical effort to get it, specific hungers for sugar and salt were adaptive. In the current era, in which foods are plentiful and easily obtained, these specific hungers (combined with the profit motive for the food industry) lead many to consume too much junk food. The nutrients in vegetables are, alas, largely undetectable, so we cannot develop specific hungers for them.

We were then left with a problem: How did Clara Davis's infants know how to select a healthy diet if specific hungers do not operate for all nutrients? It turned out that they were not selecting a healthy diet at all. They were simply eating a variety of the foods presented because they got bored eating any single food. This phenomenon is called *sensory-specific satiety*

(Rolls, 1986). Because all of the choices were healthy, all the infants needed to do was eat a variety. In the modern world, eating whatever we like will not produce good health, because too many of the available foods are not healthy. In fact, the specific hungers that are genuine can do us considerable harm—just think about our love for sweet and salty junk foods.

Rozin's work ended the belief that the brain was hardwired to tell us what to eat. But he offered us a much more flexible guide: learning. We come to like or dislike foods based on the consequences of consuming them. When the consequences are negative (e.g., nausea), we dislike the food and avoid it (conditioned aversion); when the consequences are positive (e.g., calories), we like the food and consume it (conditioned preference). As we saw in Section 14.5, olfactory likes and dislikes are not hardwired as those for taste are.

The association of negative or positive affect with a neutral experience is called *evaluative conditioning*. The phenomenon has received remarkably little attention, given the powerful role that affect plays in our lives. The experience of value is important in our social worlds (e.g., in religion, politics), as well as in our food worlds. A classic example of evaluative conditioning is the transfer of affect from a positive stimulus (sugar) to a neutral stimulus (tea). Debra Zellner and Paul Rozin (Zellner et al., 1983) conducted an experiment ostensibly about preference for teas. Participants were asked to rate the palatability of a variety of teas; some had sugar added, some did not. Tested a second time, the teas that had originally been paired with sugar were rated as more positive. The hardwired affect associated with the sweetness of sugar transferred to the neutral tea flavors.

Let's go back to our beloved chocolate chip cookies. Why are they so universally loved? They contain sugar, which we are hardwired to love, and they contain chocolate, which we have learned to love because it has been paired with fat and starch (calories).

Is All Olfactory Affect Learned?

The evidence that all olfactory affect is learned is still provisional. One- and two-year-old children appear to lack affect to odors that are unpleasant to their mothers (Engen and Engen, 1997). However, the number of odorants tested on young children is limited by the difficulty of doing these experiments. Could there be a few odorants that, like taste, have hardwired affect? One suggestion makes considerable evolutionary sense. Certain odorants are derived from important nutrients in fruits and vegetables and are thus cues to those nutrients. Hardwired liking for these odorants would lead to a healthier diet (Goff and Klee, 2006).

Another reason to consider the possibility of hardwiring of the pleasure associated with some odorants is the evidence for hardwired olfactory aversions in some species. Once we consider the possibility that some odorants are innately disliked, it is reasonable to reevaluate the possibility that some are innately liked. The problem with innate aversion to odors is that studies claiming this must provide a crucial control. Since pain and its milder cousin, irritation, are innately disliked, any odorant claimed to be innately disliked must be shown to lack irritation sensations. For example, consider sniffing ammonia. Ammonia has an odor, but it also burns the nose. The burn is mediated by the trigeminal nerve. With humans, there is an easy way to identify an odorant that also stimulates the trigeminal nerve through the localization of sensation. If a pure odorant is introduced to just one nostril but both nostrils are stimulated, the odor cannot be localized to the appropriate nostril. If the odorant contains trigeminal stimulants, the sensation can be localized. There are no final answers yet. Stay tuned.

15.7 The Nature of Taste Qualities

Although we take for granted that sweet, salty, sour, and bitter are different taste qualities within the modality of taste, historically that was not always the case. Hermann von Helmholtz, a physician and physicist of note in the nineteenth century (see Chapter 1), first argued that *modality* and *quality* should be distinguished: if two sensations are so different that there are no transitions between them, then they should be considered separate modalities. Two students of Helmholtz (Wilhelm Wundt and Frithiof Holmgren) in turn produced students (Friedrich Kiesow and Hjalmar Öhrwall) who saw Helmholtz's view differently. Kiesow saw the different taste sensations as analogous to colors and so concluded that different taste sensations are different qualities within the taste sense. However, Öhrwall saw taste qualities as independent of one another and so as separate modalities. The details of their research duels (see Bartoshuk, 1978) actually supported Öhrwall, but Kiesow obviously won the battle. One important factor was that Wundt's lab hosted a variety of prominent psychologists, among them many Americans. The proximity of Kiesow to Americans who wrote influential texts may have contributed to that victory.

Reminiscent of this old debate is a modern debate over how taste quality is coded. A major source of historical controversy in the taste literature revolved around whether tastes are coded mainly via **labeled lines**, in which each taste neuron unambiguously signals the presence of a certain basic taste, or via patterns of activity across many different taste neurons. We've seen examples of both types of coding in other senses. For example, color vision and olfaction use pattern coding. A single type of cone cannot tell us the wavelength of a light ray, but the pattern of activity across our three cone types can give us this information. Hearing, however, uses a mechanism more akin to the labeled-line approach: certain neurons always respond best to 1000 hertz (Hz) tones, others always respond best to 2000 Hz tones, and so on. Which scheme is used in the gustatory system?

FURTHER DISCUSSION of the coding of colors, sounds, and odors can be found in Chapters 5, 9, and 14, respectively.

Given what we've already learned about the functions of the four basic tastes, it is easy to construct an evolutionary argument for labeled-line coding. Recall that in olfaction, which uses pattern coding, identity of components can be lost in a mixture. Taste components do not lose their identities in mixtures. Loss of taste identity would be disastrous in taste. Imagine not being able to identify a bitter poison in a food.

The historical controversy arose because initial research seemed to indicate that most neurons coming from taste buds responded to more than one of the four basic tastes. How could such a system code sweet, sour, salt, and bitter without confusion? Carl Pfaffmann initially concluded that taste qualities must be coded by a pattern across taste fibers, but behavior in squirrel monkeys changed his mind (Pfaffmann, 1974a, 1974b). Pfaffmann was fascinated by what he called a "paradox": Squirrel monkeys prefer sucrose to fructose, but recordings from their intact chorda tympani nerves showed greater responses to fructose than to sucrose. Why, then, didn't the monkeys prefer fructose? The answer came from recordings from single-taste nerve fibers. Fibers that responded best to sucrose were very specific to sugars. However, a group of fibers that responded better to fructose than to sucrose actually responded best to salt. Pfaffmann concluded that the sucrose-best fibers were conveying a sweet taste, while the fibers responding better to fructose than

labeled lines A theory of taste coding in which each taste nerve fiber carries a particular taste quality. Thus, a fiber that responds best to sucrose but also responds with small responses to other stimuli mediates only sweet sensations.

to sucrose were actually conveying a salty taste. The monkeys preferred the pure sweet sucrose to the sweet-salty taste of fructose.

No matter how neural data are interpreted, the coding debate between labeled lines and pattern coding cannot be resolved by looking only at neural data. Any neural coding theory must be able to account for the observation that taste qualities maintain their integrity in mixtures.

Taste Adaptation and Cross-adaptation

As we've seen throughout this book, all sensory systems show adaptation effects, in which constant application of a certain stimulus temporarily weakens subsequent perception of that stimulus. In taste, our constant adaptation to the salt in saliva affects our ability to taste salt; in addition, adaptation to certain components in one food can change the perception of a second food. You've experienced cross-adaptation yourself if you've ever noticed that a beverage like lemonade tastes too sour after you eat a sweet dessert. The sugar in the dessert adapts the sweet receptors so that the subsequent lemonade tastes less sweet and more sour than normal.

The Pleasure of the Burn of Chili Peppers

Capsaicin produces the burn associated with chili peppers. As you learned in Section 1.3, capsaicin stimulates both fibers that mediate warmth and those that mediate burn, but there is one important difference between the tongue and outer body skin: the tongue is more sensitive. For example, if you use chilis in cooking, you have probably gotten capsaicin on your hands. Your hands may feel fine, but if you lick your fingers, you will burn your tongue, and if you rub your eyes, you will be very sorry! The skin on your hands is a pretty good barrier to capsaicin, but the mucous membranes in our mouths and eyes are not.

Many people experience pleasure from the burn of capsaicin, but we are not born liking this burn. Rozin (P. Rozin and Schiller, 1980) studied the acquisition of chili pepper preference in Mexico and found that the process depends on social influences. Chili is gradually added to the diet of young children beginning at about age 3, and the children observe their family members enjoying it. By age 5 or 6, children voluntarily add chili to their own food. At some point, the chili is liked for its own sake.

A variety of arguments based on presumed health benefits have been introduced to account for our love of chili peppers. For example, some have argued that chilis kill microorganisms in food, thus acting as a preservative. Others have argued that chilis contain vitamins A and C, which give them adaptive value (in other words, the pain of the chili serves as a cue for the presence of the vitamins). The pleasure that some people experience from chilis has also been linked to the idea that the resulting burn leads to the release of endorphins, the brain's endogenous morphines.

One of the most interesting features of the liking for the burn of chili peppers is its near-total restriction to humans. Rozin has documented a few cases on record of animals showing a liking for chilis, but in all cases these were pets fed chili pepper by their human companions. When Rozin tried to produce liking for chilis in rats, he failed (P. Rozin, Gruss, and Berk, 1979). But one of Rozin's students, Bennett Galef (Galef and Wigmore, 1983), was finally able to get rats to like a diet seasoned with a mild level of cayenne pepper by exposing the rats to a "demonstrator" rat that had just eaten the diet. It seems that growing to like chili peppers is a social phenomenon for rats as well.

The burn that we experience from chili peppers is highly variable across individuals (**FIGURE 15.13**). The variability has two sources. First, as noted earlier, individuals with the largest number of fungiform papillae (supertasters) have the most fibers mediating oral pain, and thus they perceive the most intense oral burn from chilis. Second, capsaicin, the chemical that produces the burn in chilis, desensitizes pain receptors. This means that individuals who consume chilis quite often (once every 48 hours is sufficient) are chronically desensitized. Chili peppers produce considerably less burn in those who are desensitized.

Incidentally, you may see your favorite chilis rated in terms of Scoville units. For example, the jalapeño pepper you can buy in supermarkets is rated at 3500–10,000 Scoville units, while the habanero and Scotch bonnet peppers (you may have to grow these yourself since they are too hot for most consumers) are rated at 100,000–350,000 Scoville units. A Scoville unit is a strange sort of unit: it is the number of times you have to dilute the dry pepper until the burn can no longer be detected. If you would like your peppers described in terms of capsaicin content, you can express this in parts per million (1 part per million equals 1 milligram of capsaicin per liter of water). However, since the burn of chili peppers is not the same for everyone, these units will not tell you how much the pepper will burn to you.

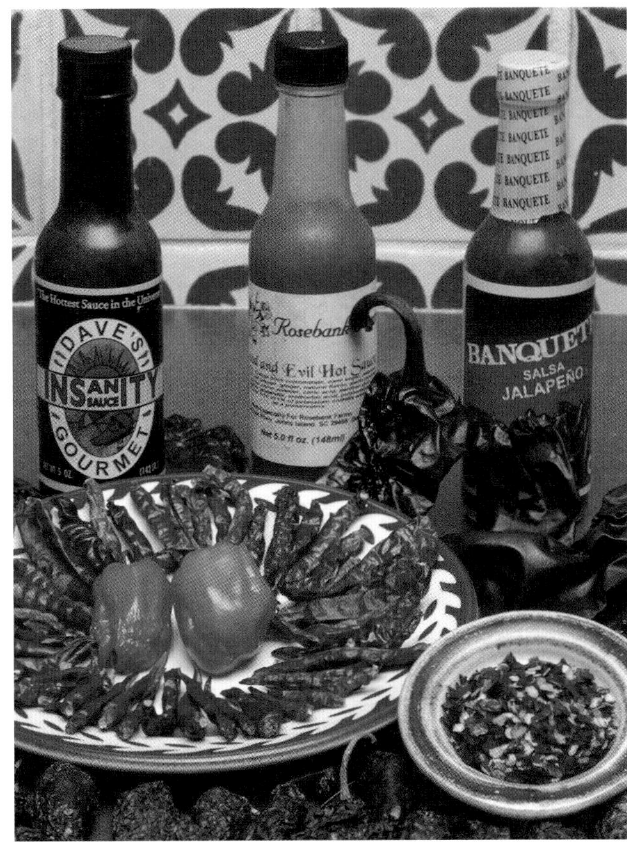

FIGURE 15.13 Chili peppers (capsaicin) Do these images inspire fear or delight?

Desensitization can come to your rescue if you accidentally order a meal that burns more than you like. After the first mouthful, wait until the burn has subsided. The mistake many diners make is to keep eating. As long as the capsaicin continues to be applied, desensitization does not occur. Desensitization occurs only during the decline of the burn (Green, 1993). Once the initial burn has faded, the rest of the meal can be consumed with relative comfort.

Capsaicin desensitization has important clinical value. The ancient Mayans used a concoction made of chilis to treat the pain of tongue piercings, done as part of ceremonial rituals. In the 1990s, Wolffe Nadoolman, then a medical student at Yale working in Bartoshuk's laboratory, created a similar remedy by adding cayenne pepper to a recipe for taffy. People with cancer often develop painful mouth sores from chemotherapy and radiation therapy. If patients suck on the capsaicin candies and then let the burn diminish, their pain receptors are desensitized, and the pain is dramatically reduced for several hours (Berger et al., 1995). Although capsaicin can be used to reduce pain at any body site, the skin is a potent barrier that prevents capsaicin from contacting pain receptors. Thus, capsaicin remedies for disorders like arthritis are rarely very satisfactory. In the mouth, the mucous membrane permits capsaicin to easily contact pain receptors, so in the mouth desensitization is fast and powerful.

In case you would like to try the candy, you can find the recipe in Berger et al. (1995), but you can also turn ordinary caramels into capsaicin caramels by melting a pound of them and adding 1/2 teaspoon of McCormick cayenne pepper. Why McCormick? The company was kind enough to tell us how much capsaicin is in their cayenne pepper so that we could make the candy contain 5–9 ppm capsaicin, an amount that will desensitize most lesions.

Summary

1. Flavor is produced by retronasal olfaction (olfactory sensations produced when odorants in the mouth are forced up behind the palate into the nose by swallowing). Flavor sensations are perceptually localized to the mouth, even though the retronasal olfactory sensations come from the olfactory receptors.
2. Taste buds are globular clusters of cells (like the segments in an orange). The tips of some of the cells (microvilli) contain sites that interact with taste molecules. Those sites fall into two groups: ion channels that mediate responses to salts and acids, and G protein–coupled receptors that bind to sweet and bitter compounds as well as amino acids.
3. The tongue has a bumpy appearance because of structures called papillae. Filiform papillae (the most numerous) have no taste buds. Taste buds are found in the fungiform papillae (front of the tongue), foliate papillae (rear edges of the tongue), and circumvallate papillae (rear center of the tongue), as well as on the roof of the mouth.
4. Taste projects ipsilaterally from the tongue to the medulla, thalamus, and cortex. It projects first to the insula in the cortex and from there to the orbitofrontal cortex, an area where taste can be integrated with other sensory input.
5. Taste and olfaction play very different roles in the perception of foods and beverages. Taste is the true nutritional sense; taste receptors are tuned to molecules that function as important nutrients. Bitter taste is a poison detection system. Sweet taste enables us to respond to the sugars that are biologically useful to us: sucrose, glucose, and fructose. Salty taste enables us to identify sodium, a mineral crucial to survival because of its role in nerve conduction and muscle function. Sour taste permits us to avoid acids in concentrations that might injure tissue.
6. Umami, the taste produced by monosodium glutamate, has been suggested as a fifth basic taste that detects protein. However, umami lacks one of the most important properties of taste: hardwired affect. Some individuals like umami, but others do not. Taste receptors are not only in the mouth, but also in the gut. Digestion breaks down proteins into their constituent amino acids, and the glutamate released stimulates gut glutamate receptors, leading to conditioned preferences for the sensory properties (largely retronasal olfaction) of the foods containing protein.
7. The importance of taste to survival requires that we be able to recognize each taste quality independently, even when present in a mixture. Labeled-line coding preserves this independence.
8. Foods do not taste the same to everyone. We carry 25 genes for bitter taste. The most studied bitter receptor responds to PROP and shows allelic variation in humans, leading to the designations "PROP nontaster" for those who taste the least bitterness and "PROP taster" for those who taste the most. In addition, human tongues vary in the number of fungiform papillae (and thus taste buds) they possess. Those with the most taste buds are called supertasters and live in a "neon" taste world; those with the fewest taste buds live in a "pastel" taste world. Psychologists discovered these differences by testing people's ability to match sensory intensities of stimuli from different modalities. For example, the bitterness of black coffee

matches the pain of a mild headache to nontasters but resembles a severe headache to supertasters. The way foods taste affects palatability, which in turn affects diet. Poor diet contributes to diseases such as cancer and cardiovascular disease.

9. For basic tastes, unlike olfaction, liking and disliking are hardwired: babies are born liking sweet and disliking bitter; salty taste is liked when its receptors mature a few weeks after birth. When we become deficient in salt or sucrose, liking for them increases. Junk foods are constructed to appeal to these preferences. Liking the burn of chili peppers, however, is acquired and, with the exception of some pets, is essentially limited to humans. Taste buds are surrounded by pain fibers; thus, supertasters perceive greater burn from chilis than do nontasters. In addition, fungiform papillae, structures that house taste buds, are innervated by touch fibers; thus, supertasters perceive greater touch sensations from fats (e.g., creamy, viscous, thick) in foods.

Glossary

Numbers in brackets refer to the chapter(s) where the term is introduced.

A

A-alpha fiber A wide-diameter, myelinated sensory nerve fiber that transmits signals from proprioceptive receptors in muscles and tendons. [13]

A-beta fiber A wide-diameter, myelinated sensory nerve fiber that transmits signals from mechanical stimulation. [13]

A-delta fiber An intermediate-sized, myelinated sensory nerve fiber that transmits pain and temperature signals. [13]

abducens (VI) nerves The sixth pair of cranial nerves, which innervate the lateral rectus muscle of the eyeballs. [1]

absolute disparity The difference in the angular distance of the images of an object from the foveas of the two eyes. [6]

absolute metrical depth cue A depth cue that provides quantifiable information about distance in the third dimension (e.g., his nose sticks out 4 centimeters in front of his face). [6]

absolute pitch (AP) A rare ability whereby some people are able to accurately name or produce notes without comparison to other notes. [11]

absolute threshold The minimum amount of stimulation necessary for a person to detect a stimulus 50% of the time. [1]

absorb To take up something—such as light, noise, or energy—and not transmit it at all. [2]

acceleration A change in velocity. Mathematically, acceleration is the temporal derivative of velocity. In words, linear acceleration indicates a change in linear velocity; angular acceleration indicates a change in angular velocity. [12]

accessory olfactory bulb (AOB) A neural structure found in nonhuman animals that is smaller than the main olfactory bulb and located behind it and that receives input from the vomeronasal organ. [14]

accidental viewpoint A viewing position that produces some regularity in the visual image that is not present in the world (e.g., the sides of two independent objects lining up perfectly). [4]

accommodation The process by which the eye changes its focus (in which the lens gets fatter as gaze is directed toward nearer objects). [2, 6]

achromatopsia An inability to perceive colors that is caused by damage to the central nervous system. [5]

acoustic reflex A reflex that protects the ear from intense sounds via contraction of the stapedius and tensor tympani muscles. [9]

acoustic startle reflex The very rapid motor response to a sudden sound. Very few neurons are involved in the basic startle reflex, which can also be affected by emotional state. [10]

active sensing Sensing that includes self-generated probing of the environment. Besides our vestibular sense, other active human senses include vision and touch. Animal active sensing includes the use of echoes by whales and bats, the use of electrical signals by some fishes, and the use of whiskers/antennae by fishes, insects, and nocturnal rodents. [12]

acuity The smallest spatial detail that can be resolved at 100% contrast. [3]

acquired anosmia Possessing a sense of smell and then losing it sometime after birth. The most common causes of acquired anosmia are illness and head trauma. [14]

adaptation A reduction in response caused by prior or continuing stimulation. [3]

adapting stimulus A stimulus whose removal produces a change in visual perception or sensitivity. [5]

additive color mixture A mixture of lights. If light A and light B are both reflected from a surface to the eye, in the perception of color the effects of those two lights add together. [5]

affective touch Submodality related to emotional and social functions. [13]

afferent fiber A neuron that carries sensory information to the central nervous system. [9]

afferent signals Information flowing inward to the central nervous system from sensors in the periphery. Passive sensing would rely exclusively on such sensory inflow, providing a traditional view of sensation. [12]

age-related macular degeneration A disease associated with aging that affects the macula. It gradually destroys sharp central vision, making it difficult to read, drive, and recognize faces. There are two forms: wet and dry. [2]

agnosia A failure to recognize objects despite the ability to see them. Agnosia is typically a result of brain damage. [4, 5]

akinetopsia A rare neuropsychological disorder in which the affected individual cannot perceive motion. [8]

altered tuning An effect of attention on the response of a neuron in which the neuron responds differently to the features of an attended versus an unattended stimulus. For example, a neuron that responds strongly to lines with orientations from −20 degrees to +20 degrees might shift to respond strongly to −10 to +30-degree lines. [7]

amacrine cell A retinal cell found in the inner nuclear layer that makes synaptic contacts with bipolar cells, ganglion cells, and other amacrine cells. [2]

ambiguous figure A visual stimulus that gives rise to two or more interpretations of its identity or structure. [4]

amblyopia A developmental disorder characterized by reduced spatial vision in an otherwise healthy eye, even with proper correction for refractive error. Also known as *lazy eye*. [3]

amplitude In reference to vestibular sensation, the size (increase or decrease) of a head movement (with angular velocity, linear acceleration, tilt, etc.). [12]

amplitude or intensity In reference to sound, the magnitude of displacement (increase or decrease) of a pressure wave. Amplitude is perceived as *loudness*. [9]

ampulla An expansion of each semicircular-canal duct that includes that canal's cupula, crista, and hair cells, where transduction occurs. [12]

amygdala-hippocampal complex The conjoined regions of the amygdala and hippocampus, which are key structures in the limbic system. This complex is critically involved in the unique emotional and associative properties of olfactory cognition. [14]

analgesia Decreasing pain sensation during conscious experience. [13]

anamorphosis or anamorphic projection Use of the rules of linear perspective to create a two-dimensional image so distorted that it looks correct only when viewed from a special angle or with a mirror that counters the distortion. [6]

anchor objects Typically, a relatively big object that provides information about the location of other objects. For instance, the toilet provides information about the location of the toilet paper. [7]

angular acceleration The rate of change of angular velocity. Mathematically, the integral of angular acceleration is angular velocity, and the integral of angular velocity is angular displacement. Angular acceleration, angular velocity, and angular displacement all mathematically represent angular motion. [12]

angular motion Rotational motion like the rotation of a spinning top or swinging saloon doors that rotate back and forth. [12]

anisometropia A condition in which the two eyes have different refractive errors (e.g., one eye is farsighted and the other is not). [3]

anomia An inability to name objects despite the ability to see and recognize them (as shown by usage). Anomia is typically a result of brain damage. [5]

anosmia The total inability to smell, most often resulting from sinus illness or head trauma. [14]

anterior cingulate cortex (ACC) A region of the brain associated with the perceived unpleasantness of a pain sensation. [13]

aperture A windowlike opening that allows only a partial view of an object. [8]

aperture problem The fact that when a moving object is viewed through an aperture (or a single receptive field), the direction of motion of a local feature or part of the object may be ambiguous. [8]

apparent motion The illusory impression of smooth motion resulting from the rapid alternation of objects that appear in different locations in rapid succession. [8]

aqueous humor The watery fluid in the anterior chamber of the eye. [2]

aromatherapy The manipulation of odors to influence mood, performance, and well-being as well as the physiological correlates of emotion such as heart rate, blood pressure, and sleep. [14]

articulation The act or manner of producing a speech sound using the articulators—vocal tract structures including the mouth, tongue, soft palate, and jaw. [11]

artificial neural networks Also referred to as *connectionist models*, these are computational methods that consist of networks of nodes with weighted connections between them. Connection weights increase and decrease following experience in ways that resemble the organization of biological neural networks. [1]

astigmatism A visual defect caused by the unequal curving of one or more of the refractive surfaces of the eye, usually the cornea. [2]

attack The part of a sound during which amplitude increases (onset). [10]

attention Any of the very large set of selective processes in the brain. To deal with the impossibility of handling all inputs at once, the nervous system has evolved mechanisms that are able to bias processing to a subset of things, places, ideas, or moments in time. [7]

attention deficit hyperactivity disorder (ADHD) A quite common childhood disorder that can continue into adulthood, symptoms of which include difficulty focusing attention and problems controlling behavior. [7]

attentional blink (AB) The tendency not to perceive or respond to the second of two different target stimuli amid a rapid stream of distracting stimuli if the observer has responded to the first target stimulus 200–500 milliseconds before the second stimulus is presented. [7]

audibility threshold The lowest sound pressure level that can be reliably detected at a given frequency. [9]

auditory nerve (AN) A collection of neurons that convey information from hair cells in the cochlea to the brainstem (afferent neurons) and from the brainstem to the hair cells (efferent neurons). [9]

auditory scene analysis Processing an auditory scene consisting of multiple sound sources into separate sound images. [10]

auditory stream segregation The perceptual organization of a complex acoustic signal into separate auditory events for which each stream is heard as a separate event. [10]

autonomic nervous system The part of the nervous system that is responsible for regulating many involuntary actions and that innervates glands, heart, digestive system, etc. [12]

azimuth The angle of a sound source on the horizontal plane relative to a point in the center of the head between the ears. Azimuth is measured in degrees, with 0 degrees being straight ahead. The angle increases clockwise toward the right, with 180 degrees being directly behind. [10]

B

balance The neural processes of postural control by which weight is evenly distributed, enabling us to remain upright and stable. [12]

balance system The sensory systems, neural processes, and muscles that contribute to postural control. Specific components include the vestibular organs, kinesthesis, vestibulospinal pathways, skeletal bones, and postural control muscles. Because of the vestibular system's crucial contributions to balance, some even informally refer to the vestibular system as the "balance system" and the vestibular organs as the "balance organs." But the balance system is much more than just the vestibular system, and the vestibular system contributes to much more than just balance. [12]

Balint syndrome A disorder where everything except the current object of attention seems to be blocked from conscious perception. [7]

basal or stem cell One of the three types of cells in the olfactory epithelium. Basal (or stem) cells are the progenerator cells that give rise to olfactory sensory neurons. [14]

basic color terms Color words that are single words (like *blue*, not *sky blue*), are used with high frequency, and have meanings that are agreed on by speakers of a language. [5]

basic taste Any of the four taste qualities that are generally agreed to describe human taste experience: sweet, salty, sour, bitter. [15]

basilar membrane A plate of fibers that forms the base of the cochlear partition and separates the middle and tympanic canals in the cochlea. [9]

Bayesian approach A way of formalizing the idea that our perception is a combination of the current stimulus and our knowledge about the conditions of the world—what is and is not likely to occur. The Bayesian approach is stated mathematically as Bayes' theorem: $P(A|O) = P(A) \times P(O|A)/P(O)$, which enables us to calculate the probability (P) that the world is in a particular state (A) given a particular observation (O). [4, 6]

Bayesian models Theoretical and/or computational models that employ Bayesian statistical methods to generate an internal model of the source of sensory inputs based on prior experience. [1]

belt area A region of cortex, directly adjacent to the primary auditory cortex (A1), with inputs from A1, where neurons respond to more complex characteristics of sounds. [9]

binaral rivalry Competition between the two nostrils for odor perception. When a different scent is presented to each nostril simultaneously, we perceive each scent to be alternating back and forth with the other, and not a blend of the two scents. [14]

binding problem The challenge of tying different attributes of visual stimuli (e.g., color, orientation, motion), which are handled by different brain circuits, to the appropriate object so that we perceive a unified object (e.g., red, vertical, moving right). [7]

binocular Referring to two eyes. [6]

binocular depth cue A depth cue that relies on information from both eyes. Stereopsis is the primary example in humans, but convergence and the ability of two eyes to see more of an object than one eye sees are also binocular depth cues. [6]

binocular disparity The differences between the two retinal images of the same scene. Disparity is the basis for stereopsis, a vivid perception of the three-dimensionality of the world that is not available with monocular vision. [6]

binocular rivalry The competition between the two eyes for control of visual perception, which is evident when completely different stimuli are presented to the two eyes. [6]

binocular summation The combination (or "summation") of signals from both eyes in ways that make performance on many tasks better than with either eye alone. [6]

biological motion The pattern of movement of living beings (humans and animals). [8]

biomimetic feedback A system that attempts to closely mimic biological signals. [13]

bipolar cell A retinal cell that synapses with either rods or cones (not both) and with horizontal cells and then passes the signals on to ganglion cells. [2]

bitter One of the four basic tastes; the taste quality, generally considered unpleasant, produced by substances like quinine or caffeine. [15]

Bloch's law The detection threshold for a brief flash of light (<0.1 second) is the product of the luminance of the light and its duration. [1]

blood oxygen level–dependent (BOLD) signal The ratio of oxygenated to deoxygenated hemoglobin that permits the localization of brain neurons that are most involved in a task. [1]

body image The mental representation of how our bodies appear in space. [13]

border ownership When one object is in front of another, there will be a visual border formed between the object and the background. That border is "owned" by the object. It is the edge of the object, not a property of the background. [4]

C

C fiber A narrow-diameter, unmyelinated sensory nerve fiber that transmits pain and temperature signals. [13]

C tactile (CT) afferent A narrow-diameter, unmyelinated sensory nerve fiber that transmits signals from pleasant touch. [13]

cataract An opacity of the crystalline lens. [2]

categorical perception For speech as well as other complex sounds and images, the phenomenon by which the discrimination of items is no better than the ability to label items. [11]

change blindness When one scene is replaced by another version of the same scene, observers may be unable to report what changed between the two versions. [7]

characteristic frequency (CF) The frequency to which a particular auditory nerve fiber is most sensitive. [9]

chemosignal Any of various chemicals emitted by humans that are detected by the olfactory system and that may have some effect on the mood, behavior, hormonal status, and/or sexual arousal of other humans. [14]

chord A combination of three or more musical notes with different pitches played simultaneously. [11]

chorda tympani The branch of cranial nerve VII (the facial nerve) that carries taste information from the anterior, mobile tongue (the part that can be stuck out). The chorda tympani exits the tongue with the lingual branch of the trigeminal nerve (cranial nerve V) and then passes through the middle ear on its way to the brain. [15]

chromophore The light-catching part of the visual pigments of the retina. [2]

cilium (pl. cilia) Any of the hairlike protrusions on the dendrites of olfactory sensory neurons. The receptor sites for odorant molecules are in the cilia, which are the first structures involved in olfactory signal transduction. [14]

circumvallate papillae Circular structures that form an inverted *V* on the rear of the tongue (three to five on each side, with the largest in the center). Circumvallate papillae are moundlike structures, each surrounded by a trench (like a moat). They are much larger than fungiform papillae. [15]

CO blobs Regular arrays of "blobs" spaced about 0.5 millimeter apart in the striate cortex (V1), so named because their presence is visualized by staining with the enzyme cytochrome oxidase. They may function in color perception. [3]

coarticulation The phenomenon in speech whereby attributes of successive speech units overlap in articulatory or acoustic patterns. [11]

cochlea A spiral structure of the inner ear containing the organ of Corti. [9]

cochlear nucleus The first brainstem nucleus at which afferent auditory nerve fibers synapse. [9]

cochlear partition The combined basilar membrane, tectorial membrane, and organ of Corti, which are together responsible for the transduction of sound waves into neural signals. [9]

cognitive habituation The psychological process by which, after long-term exposure to an odor, one no longer has the ability to detect that odor or has very diminished detection ability. [14]

cold fiber A sensory nerve fiber that fires when skin temperature decreases. [13]

color-anomalous A better term for the commonly used term *color-blind*. Most "color-blind" individuals can still make discriminations based on wavelength. Those discriminations are different from the norm—that is, anomalous. [5]

color assimilation A color perception effect in which two colors bleed into each other, each taking on some of the chromatic quality of the other. [5]

color constancy The tendency of a surface to appear the same color under a fairly wide range of illuminants. [5]

color contrast A color perception effect in which the color of one region induces the opponent color in a neighboring region. [5]

color space The three-dimensional space, established because color perception is based on the outputs of three cone types, that describes the set of all colors. [5]

column A vertical arrangement of neurons. Neurons within a single column tend to have similar receptive fields and similar orientation preferences. [3]

common fate Gestalt grouping rule stating that the tendency of sounds to group together will increase if they begin and/or end at the same time. [10]

comparator An area of the visual system that receives one copy of the command issued by the motor system when the eyes move (the other copy goes to the eye muscles). The comparator compares the image motion signal with the eye motion signal and can compensate for the image changes caused by the eye movement. [8]

complex cell A cortical neuron whose receptive field does not have clearly defined excitatory and inhibitory regions. [3]

computational model The use of mathematical language and equations to describe steps in psychological and/or neural processes (often implemented on a computer). [1]

conductive hearing loss Hearing loss caused by problems with the bones of the middle ear. [9]

cone A photoreceptor specialized for daylight vision, fine visual acuity, and color. [2]

cone monochromat An individual with only one cone type. Cone monochromats are truly color-blind. [5]

cone of confusion A region of positions in space where all sounds produce the same time and level (intensity) differences. [10]

cone-opponent cell A cell type—found in the retina, lateral geniculate nucleus, and visual cortex—that, in effect, subtracts one type of cone input from another. [5]

congenital anosmia Having no sense of smell from birth on, and thus never experiencing scent. This condition is rare. [14]

congenital prosopagnosia A form of face blindness apparently present from birth, as opposed to acquired prosopagnosia, which would typically be the result of an injury to the nervous system. [4]

conjunction search Search for a target defined by the presence of two or more attributes (e.g., a *red*, *vertical* target among *red* horizontal and blue *vertical* distractors). [7]

continuity constraint In reference to stereopsis, the observation that, except at the edges of objects, neighboring points in the world lie at similar distances from the viewer. This is one of several constraints that have been proposed as helpful in solving the correspondence problem. [6]

contralateral Referring to the opposite side of the body or brain. [3]

contralesional field The visual field on the side opposite a brain lesion. For example, points to the left of fixation are contralesional to damage in the right hemisphere of the brain. [7]

contrast The difference in luminance between an object and the background or between lighter and darker parts of the same object. [2, 3]

contrast sensitivity function (CSF) A function describing how the sensitivity to contrast (defined as the reciprocal of the contrast threshold) depends on the spatial frequency (size) of the stimulus. [3]

contrast threshold The smallest amount of contrast required to detect a pattern. [3]

convergence The ability of the two eyes to turn inward, often used to place the two images of a feature in the world on corresponding locations in the two retinal images (typically on the fovea of each eye). Convergence reduces the disparity of that feature to zero (or nearly zero). [6]

cornea The transparent "window" into the eyeball. [2]

correspondence problem 1. In reference to binocular vision, the problem of figuring out which bit of the image in the left eye should be matched with which bit in the right eye. The problem is particularly vexing when the images consist of thousands of similar features, like dots in random dot stereograms. 2. In reference to motion detection, the problem faced by the motion detection system of knowing which feature in frame 2 corresponds to a particular feature in frame 1. [6, 8]

corresponding retinal points Two monocular images of an object in the world are said to fall on corresponding points if those points are the same distance from the fovea in both eyes. The two foveas are also corresponding points. [6]

cortical magnification The amount of cortical area (usually specified in millimeters) devoted to a specific region (e.g., 1 degree) in the visual field. [3]

cranial nerves Twelve pairs of nerves (one set for each side of the body) that originate in the brainstem and reach sense organs and muscles through openings in the skull. [1, 15]

cribriform plate A bony structure riddled with tiny holes that separates the nose from the brain at the level of the eyebrows. The axons from the olfactory sensory neurons pass through the holes of the cribriform plate to enter the brain. [14]

crista Any of the specialized detectors of angular motion located in each semicircular canal in a swelling called the ampulla. [12]

criterion In reference to signal detection theory, an internal threshold that is set by the observer. If the internal response is above criterion, the observer gives one response (e.g., "Yes, I hear that"). Below criterion, the observer gives another response (e.g., "No, I hear nothing"). [1]

critical bandwidth The range of frequencies conveyed within a channel in the auditory system. [9]

critical period 1. A phase in the life span during which abnormal early experience can alter normal neuronal development. 2. A period of time during development when the organism is particularly susceptible to developmental change. There are critical periods in the development of binocular vision, human language, and so on. [3, 6]

cross-adaptation The reduction in detection of one odorant following exposure to a prior odorant. Cross-adaptation is presumed to occur because the components of the odors (or odorants) in question share one or more olfactory receptors for their transduction, but the order in which odorants are presented also plays a role. [14]

cross-modality matching The ability to match the intensities of sensations that come from different sensory modalities. This ability allows insight into sensory differences. For example, a listener might adjust the brightness of a light until it matches the loudness of a tone. [1, 15]

crossed disparity The sign of disparity created by objects in front of the plane of fixation (the horopter). The term *crossed* is used because images of objects located in front of the horopter appear to be displaced to the left in the right eye and to the right in the left eye. [6]

cue A stimulus that might indicate where (or what) a subsequent stimulus will be. Cues can be valid (giving correct information), invalid (incorrect), or neutral (uninformative). [7]

cultural relativism In sensation and perception, the idea that basic perceptual experiences (e.g., color perception) may be determined in part by the cultural environment. [5]

cycle For a grating, a pair consisting of one dark bar and one bright bar. [3]

cycles per degree The number of grating cycles per degree of visual angle. [3]

Cyclopean Referring to stimuli that are defined by binocular disparity alone. Named after the one-eyed Cyclops of Homer's *Odyssey*. [6]

D

decay The part of a sound during which amplitude decreases (offset). [10]

decibel (dB) A unit of measure for the physical intensity of sound. Decibels define the difference between two sounds as the ratio between two sound pressures. Each 10:1 sound pressure ratio equals 20 dB, and a 100:1 ratio equals 40 dB. [9]

decoding The process of determining the nature of a stimulus from the pattern of responses measured in the brain or, potentially, in an artificial system like a computer network. The stimulus could be a sensory stimulus or it could be an internal state (e.g., the contents of a dream). [4]

deep neural network (DNN) A type of "machine learning" in artificial intelligence in which a computer is programmed to learn something (here, object recognition). These are artificial neural networks that have a large number of layers of nodes with millions of connections. First, the network is "trained" using input for which the answer is known ("That is a cow"). Subsequently, the network can provide answers from input that it has never seen before. [1, 4]

dermis The inner of two major layers of skin, consisting of nutritive and connective tissues, within which lie the mechanoreceptors. [13]

deuteranope An individual who suffers from color-blindness that is caused by the absence of M-cones. [5]

dichoptic Referring to the presentation of two different stimuli, one to each eye. Different from *binocular* presentation, which could involve both eyes looking at a single stimulus. [6]

diffuse bipolar cell A bipolar retinal cell whose processes are spread out to receive input from multiple cones. [2]

diopter A unit of measurement of the optical power of a lens. It is equal to the reciprocal of the focal length, in meters. A 2-diopter lens will bring parallel rays of light into focus at 0.5 meter (50 centimeters). [2]

diplopia Double vision. If visible in both eyes, stimuli falling outside of Panum's fusional area will appear diplopic. [6]

direction The line one moves along (or faces), with reference to the point or region one is moving toward (or facing). [12]

directional transfer function (DTF) A measure that describes how the pinna, ear canal, head, and torso change the intensity of sounds with different frequencies that arrive at each ear from different locations in space (azimuth and elevation). [10]

discriminative touch Relies on mechanical and thermal sensations for information about surfaces and objects with which we are in contact. [13]

distractor In a visual search, any stimulus other than the target. [7]

divergence The ability of the two eyes to turn outward, often used to place the two images of a feature in the world on corresponding locations in the two retinal images (typically on the fovea of each eye). Divergence reduces the disparity of that feature to zero (or nearly zero). [6]

dizziness A commonly used lay term that nonspecifically indicates any form of perceived spatial disorientation, with or without instability. [12]

doctrine of specific nerve energies A doctrine, formulated by Johannes Müller, stating that the nature of a sensation depends on *which* sensory fibers are stimulated, rather than *how* they are stimulated. [1]

dorsal column–medial lemniscal (DCML) pathway The route from the spinal cord to the brain that carries signals from skin, muscles, tendons, and joints. [13]

dorsal horn A region at the rear of the spinal cord that receives inputs from receptors in the skin. [13]

double dissociation The phenomenon in which one of two functions, such as first- and second-order motion, can be damaged without harm to the other, and vice versa. [8]

duplex In reference to the retina, consisting of two parts: the rods and cones, which operate under different conditions. [2]

E

ear canal The canal that conducts sound vibrations from the pinna to the tympanic membrane and prevents damage to the tympanic membrane. [9]

eccentricity 1. The distance between the retinal image and the fovea. 2. The angular distance from the fovea (the region of highest visual acuity). [2, 3]

efference copy or corollary discharge signal 1. The phenomenon in which outgoing (efferent) signals from the motor cortex are copied as they exit the brain and are rerouted to other areas in the sensory cortices. 2. A neural copy of an efferent command sent from the central nervous system to the periphery. One example pertinent to spatial orientation is a copy of the efferent command sent to muscles; this muscle efferent copy transmits information about expected motion resulting from the anticipated muscle activation. [8, 12]

efferent commands Information flowing outward from the central nervous system to the periphery. A common example is motor commands that regulate muscle contraction. The copy of such motor commands is often called an efferent copy. [12]

efferent fiber A neuron that carries information from the central nervous system to the periphery. [9]

efficient coding models Theoretical and/or computational models that explain neural processing by assuming that sensory systems become tuned to predictability in natural environments in ways that economically encode predictable sensory inputs while highlighting inputs that are less predictable. [1]

egocenter The center of a reference frame used to represent locations relative to the body. [13]

electroencephalography (EEG) A technique that, using many electrodes on the scalp, measures electrical activity from populations of many neurons in the brain. [1]

electromotility The ability of outer hair cells to extend and contract, which changes the stiffness and sensitivity of the cochlear partition. [9]

emmetropia The condition in which there is no refractive error, because the refractive power of the eye is perfectly matched to the length of the eyeball. [2]

end stopping The process by which a cell in the cortex increases its firing rate as the length of a bar increases until the bar fills up its receptive field, and then it decreases its firing rate as the bar is lengthened further. [3]

endogenous cue In directing attention, a cue that is located in (*endo*) or near the current location of attention. [7]

endogenous opiate A chemical released by the body that blocks the release or uptake of neurotransmitters necessary to transmit pain sensations to the brain. [13]

ensemble statistics The average and distribution of properties like orientation or color over a set of objects or over a region in a scene. [7]

entorhinal cortex A phylogenetically old cortical region that provides the major sensory association input into the hippocampus. The entorhinal cortex also receives direct projections from olfactory regions. [14]

entry-level category For an object, the label that comes to mind most quickly when we identify it (e.g., "bird"). At the subordinate level, the object might be more specifically named (e.g., "eagle"); at the superordinate level, it might be more generally named (e.g., "animal"). [4]

epidermis The outer of two major layers of skin. [13]

equal-loudness curve A graph plotting sound pressure level against the frequency for which a listener perceives constant loudness. [9]

esotropia Strabismus in which one eye deviates inward. [6]

event-related potential (ERP) A measure of electrical activity from a subpopulation of neurons in response to particular stimuli that requires averaging many electroencephalography recordings. [1]

exogenous In reference to spatial attention, a form of bottom-up (stimulus-driven) attention reflexively (involuntarily) directed toward the site at which a stimulus has abruptly appeared. [7]

exogenous cue In directing attention, a cue that is located out (*exo*) at the desired final location of attention. [7]

exotropia Strabismus in which one eye deviates outward. [6]

exploratory procedure A stereotyped hand movement pattern used to touch objects in order to perceive their properties. Each procedure is best for determining one or more object properties. [13]

extinction In reference to visual attention, the inability to perceive a stimulus to one side of the point of fixation (e.g., to the right) in the presence of another stimulus, typically in a comparable position in the other visual field (e.g., on the left side). [7]

extrastriate body area (EBA) A region of extrastriate visual cortex in humans that is specifically and reliably activated by images of the body other than the face. [4]

extrastriate cortex The region of cortex bordering the primary visual cortex and containing multiple areas involved in visual processing. [4]

F

facial (VII) nerves The seventh pair of cranial nerves, which innervate the tongue, soft palate, facial muscles, salivary glands, and tear glands. [1]

familiar size A depth cue based on knowledge of the typical sizes of objects, such as humans or pennies. [6]

feature integration theory Anne Treisman's theory of visual attention, which holds that a limited set of basic features can be processed in parallel preattentively, but other properties, including the correct binding of features to objects, require attention. [7]

feature search Visual search for a target defined by a single attribute, such as a salient color or orientation. [7]

Fechner's law A principle describing the relationship between stimulus and resulting sensation that says the magnitude of subjective sensation increases proportionally to the logarithm of the stimulus intensity. [1]

feed-forward process A process that carries out a computation (e.g., object recognition) one neural step after another, without need for feedback from a later stage to an earlier stage. [4]

figure-ground assignment The process of determining that some regions of an image belong to a foreground object (figure) and other regions are part of the background (ground). [4]

filiform papillae Small structures on the tongue that provide most of the bumpy appearance. Filiform papillae have no taste function. [15]

filter An acoustic, electrical, electronic, or optical device, instrument, computer program, or neuron that allows the passage of some range of parameters (e.g., orientations, frequencies) and blocks the passage of others. [2, 3]

first-order motion The motion of an object that is defined by changes in luminance (reflected light). [8]

flavor Sensation evoked when volatiles released from foods in the mouth are forced up into the nose through the retronasal space by chewing and swallowing. Technical term, retronasal olfaction. [15]

focal distance The distance between the lens (or mirror) and the viewed object, in meters. [2]

focus of expansion The point in the center of the horizon from which, when we're in motion (e.g., driving on the highway), all points in the perspective image seem to emanate. The focus of expansion is one aspect of optic flow. [8]

foliate papillae Folds of tissue containing taste buds. Foliate papillae are located on the rear of the tongue lateral to the circumvallate papillae, where the tongue attaches to the mouth. [15]

formant A resonance of the vocal tract. Formants are specified by their center frequency and are denoted by integers that increase with relative frequency. [11]

Fourier analysis A mathematical procedure by which any signal can be separated into component sine waves at different frequencies. Combining the sine waves (Fourier synthesis) will reproduce the original signal. [3, 12]

fovea A small pit located near the center of the macula and containing the highest concentration of cones and no rods. It is the portion of the retina that produces the highest visual acuity and serves as the point of fixation. [2]

frame of reference The coordinate system used to define locations in space. [13]

free fusion The technique of converging (crossing) or diverging the eyes in order to view a stereogram without a stereoscope. [6]

free nerve ending The terminus of a neural fiber without a specialized ending. [13]

frequency In reference to sound, the number of times per second that a pattern of pressure change repeats. Frequency is perceived as *pitch*. [9]

frontal eye fields Brain regions in both frontal lobes that help to coordinate visual selective attention with the movements of the eyes. [7]

functional magnetic resonance imaging (fMRI) A variant of magnetic resonance imaging that makes it possible to measure localized patterns of activity in the brain. Activated neurons provoke increased blood flow, which can be quantified by measuring changes in the response of oxygenated and deoxygenated blood to strong magnetic fields. [1]

fundamental frequency The lowest-frequency component of a complex periodic sound. [9, 10]

fundus The back layer of the retina: what the eye doctor sees through an ophthalmoscope. [2]

fungiform papillae Mushroom-shaped structures (maximum diameter 1 millimeter) that are distributed most densely on the edges of the tongue, especially the tip. Taste buds (an average of six per papilla) are buried in the surface. [15]

fusiform face area (FFA) A region of extrastriate visual cortex in humans that is specifically and reliably activated by human faces. [4, 7]

G

G protein–coupled receptor Any of a class of receptors that are present on the cilia of olfactory sensory neurons. All G protein–coupled receptors are characterized by a common structural feature of seven membrane-spanning helices. Binding of a substrate molecule to the receptor transmits a signal across the membrane to a G protein, which then initiates a cascade of biochemical events. [14]

ganglion cell A retinal cell that receives visual information from photoreceptors via two intermediate neuron types (bipolar cells and amacrine cells) and transmits information to the brain and midbrain. [2]

gate control theory A description of the pain-transmitting system that incorporates modulating signals from the brain. [13]

geon In Biederman's recognition-by-components model, any of the "geometric ions" out of which perceptual objects are built. [4]

Gestalt In German, literally "form." In reference to perception, a school of thought stressing that the perceptual whole can be greater than the apparent sum of the parts. [4]

Gestalt grouping rules A set of rules describing which elements in an image will appear to group together. The original list was assembled by members of the Gestalt school of thought. [4]

gist The essential or primary character of a scene. In vision, gist typically refers to information that can be gleaned in a very brief glimpse, without voluntary eye movements. [7]

glabrous In reference to skin, lacking hair. [13]

global superiority effect The finding in various experiments that the properties of the whole object take precedence over the properties of parts of the object. [4]

glomerulus (pl. glomeruli) Any of the spherical conglomerates containing the incoming axons of the olfactory sensory neurons. Each olfactory sensory neuron converges onto two glomeruli (one medial, one lateral). [14]

glossopharyngeal (IX) nerves The ninth pair of cranial nerves, which innervate the tongue, tonsils, pharynx, and pharyngeal muscles. [1]

good continuation 1. A Gestalt grouping rule stating that two elements will tend to group together if they seem to lie on the same contour. For example, sounds will tend to group together as continuous if they seem to share a common path, similar to a shared contour for vision. [4, 10]

graded potential An electrical potential that can vary continuously in amplitude. [2]

granular cells Like mitral cells, granular cells are at the deepest level of the olfactory bulb. They comprise an extensive network of inhibitory neurons that integrate input from all the earlier projections and are thought to be the basis of specific odorant identification. [14]

graviception The physiological structures and processes that sense the relative orientation of gravity with respect to the organism. [12]

gravity A force that attracts a body toward the center of the Earth. [12]

guided search Search in which attention can be restricted to a subset of possible items on the basis of information about the target item's basic features (e.g., its color). [7]

gustation The sense of taste. [14]

H

hair cell Any cell that has stereocilia for transducing mechanical movement in the inner ear into neural activity sent to the brain. Some hair cells also receive inputs from the brain. [9, 12]

haptic perception Knowledge of the world that is derived from sensory receptors in skin, muscles, tendons, and joints, usually involving active exploration. [13]

harmonic spectrum The spectrum of a complex sound in which energy is at integer multiples of the fundamental frequency. [9, 10]

haze or aerial perspective A depth cue based on the implicit understanding that light is scattered by the atmosphere. More light is scattered when we look through more atmosphere. Thus, more distant objects are subject to more scatter and appear fainter, bluer, and less distinct. [6]

helicotrema The opening that connects the tympanic and vestibular canals at the apex of the cochlea. [9]

hertz (Hz) A unit of measure for frequency; 1 hertz equals 1 cycle per second. [9]

heterodimer A chain of two molecules (a *dimer*) that are different from each other (hence *hetero*). [15]

heuristic A mental shortcut. [4]

high-spontaneous fiber An auditory nerve fiber that has a high rate (more than 30 spikes per second) of spontaneous firing. High-spontaneous fibers increase their firing rate in response to relatively low levels of sound. [9]

hippocampus A region of the brain involved in spatial mapping, associative learning and memory, and processing olfactory information. It is adjacent to the amygdala, which processes emotion. [14]

holistic processing Processing based on analysis of the entire object or scene and not on adding together a set of smaller parts or features. [4]

homologous regions Brain regions that appear to have the same function in different species. [4]

homunculus A maplike representation of regions of the body in the brain. [13]

horizontal cell A specialized retinal cell that contacts both photoreceptor and bipolar cells. [2]

horopter The location of objects whose images lie on corresponding points. The surface of zero disparity. [6]

hue The perceptual attribute of colors that enables them to be classed as similar to red, green, or blue, or something in between. [2]

hyperalgesia An increased or heightened response to a normally painful stimulus. [13]

hypercolumn A 1-millimeter block of striate cortex containing two sets of columns, each covering every possible orientation (0–180 degrees), with one set preferring input from the left eye and one set preferring input from the right eye. [3]

hyperopia Farsightedness, a common condition in which light entering the eye is focused behind the retina and accommodation is required to see near objects clearly. [2]

hyperpolarization A change in membrane potential such that the inner membrane surface becomes more negative than the outer membrane surface. [2]

I

illuminant The light that illuminates a surface. [5]

illusory conjunction An erroneous combination of two features in a visual scene—for example, seeing a red *X* when the display contains red letters and *X*s but no red *X*s. [7]

illusory contour A contour that is perceived even though nothing changes from one side of it to the other in an image. [4]

image A picture or likeness. [2]

inattentional blindness A failure to notice—or at least to report—a stimulus that would be easily reportable if it were attended. [7]

inattentional deafness The failure to notice a fully audible, but unexpected sound because attention was engaged on auditory stream. [10]

imbalance Lack of balance; unsteadiness; nearly falling over. [12]

incus The middle of the three ossicles, connecting the malleus and the stapes. [9]

inferior colliculus A midbrain nucleus in the auditory pathway. [9]

inferotemporal (IT) cortex Part of the cerebral cortex in the lower portion of the temporal lobe, important in object recognition. [4]

inhibition of return The relative difficulty in getting attention (or the eyes) to move back to a recently attended (or fixated) location. [7]

inner ear A hollow cavity in the temporal bone of the skull and the structures within this cavity: the cochlea and the semicircular canals of the vestibular system. [9]

inner segment The part of a photoreceptor that lies between the outer segment and the cell nucleus. [2]

insula A cortical area lying beneath the surface of the brain, which plays a role in regulating the body and linking sensory to emotional systems. [13]

insular cortex The primary cortical processing area for taste—the part of the cortex that first receives taste information. Also called the *insula* or the *gustatory cortex*. [15]

interaural level difference (ILD) The difference between levels (intensities) of sound at one ear versus the other. [10]

interaural time difference (ITD) The difference in time between arrivals of sound at one ear versus the other. [10]

interoception The sense (or senses) of the internal state of the body. [1, 13]

interocular transfer The transfer of an effect (such as adaptation) from one eye to the other. [8]

intersensory integration The use of information from multiple senses to arrive at a single perceptual estimate. [13]

inverse-square law A principle stating that as distance from a source increases, intensity decreases faster such that decrease in intensity is equal to the distance squared. This general law also applies to optics and other forms of energy. [10]

ipsilateral Referring to the same side of the body (or brain). [3, 14]

ipsilesional field The visual field on the same side as a brain lesion. [7]

iris The colored part of the eye, consisting of a muscular diaphragm surrounding the pupil and regulating the light entering the eye by expanding and contracting the pupil. [2]

isointensity curve A map plotting the firing rate of an auditory nerve fiber against varying frequencies at varying intensities. [9]

J

just noticeable difference (JND) or difference threshold The smallest detectable difference between two stimuli, or the minimum change in a stimulus that enables it to be correctly judged as different from a reference stimulus. [1]

juxtaglomerular neurons The first layer of cells surrounding the glomeruli. They are a mixture of excitatory and inhibitory cells and respond to a wide range of odorants. The selectivity of neurons to specific odorants increases in a gradient from the surface of the olfactory bulb to the deeper layers. [14]

K

kinesthesia Perception of the position and movement of our limbs in space. [12, 13]

kinesthetic Referring to perception involving sensory mechanoreceptors in muscles, tendons, and joints. [13]

koniocellular Referring to cells in the koniocellular layer of the lateral geniculate nucleus of the thalamus. *Konio* from the Greek for "dust" refers to the appearance of the cells. [5]

koniocellular cell A neuron located between the magnocellular and parvocellular layers of the lateral geniculate nucleus. This layer is known as the koniocellular layer. [2, 3]

L

L-cone A cone that is preferentially sensitive to long wavelengths, colloquially (but not entirely accurately) known as a "red cone." [5]

labeled lines A theory of sensory coding in which each nerve fiber carries a particular stimulus quality. For example, a theory of taste coding in which each taste nerve fiber carries a particular taste quality. Thus, a fiber that responds best to sucrose but also responds with small responses to other stimuli mediates only sweet sensations. [13, 15]

lateral geniculate nucleus (LGN) A structure in the thalamus, part of the midbrain, that receives input from the retinal ganglion cells and has input and output connections to the visual cortex. [3, 5]

lateral inhibition Antagonistic neural interaction between adjacent regions of the retina. [2]

lateral interparietal area A brain region, present in both parietal lobes, that serves an important role in the control of visual attention. [7]

lateral superior olive (LSO) A relay station in the brainstem where inputs from both ears contribute to detection of the interaural level difference. [10]

learned taste aversion The avoidance of a novel flavor after it has been paired with gastric illness. The smell, not the taste, of the substance is key for the learned aversion response in humans. [14]

lens The structure inside the eye that enables the changing of focus. [2]

lesion In reference to neurophysiology, 1. (n) A region of damaged brain. 2. (v) To destroy a section of the brain. [4]

limbic system The group of neural structures that includes the olfactory cortex, the amygdala, the hippocampus, the piriform cortex, and the entorhinal cortex. The limbic system is involved in many aspects of emotion and memory. Olfaction is unique among the senses for its direct connection to the limbic system. [14]

linear acceleration The rate of change of linear velocity. Mathematically, the integral of linear acceleration is linear velocity, and the integral of linear velocity is linear displacement, which is also referred to as translation. Linear acceleration, linear velocity, and linear displacement all mathematically represent linear motion. [12]

linear motion Translational motion like the predominant movement of a train car or bobblehead doll. [12]

linear perspective A depth cue based on the fact that lines that are parallel in the three-dimensional world will appear to converge in a two-dimensional image. [6]

loudness The psychological aspect of sound related to perceived intensity (amplitude). [9]

low-spontaneous fiber An auditory nerve fiber that has a low rate (less than 10 spikes per second) of spontaneous firing. Low-spontaneous fibers require relatively intense sound before they will fire at higher rates. [9]

luminance-defined object An object that is delineated by differences in reflected light. [8]

M

M-cone A cone that is preferentially sensitive to middle wavelengths, colloquially (but not entirely accurately) known as a "green cone." [5]

M ganglion cell A ganglion cell resembling a little umbrella that receives excitatory input from diffuse bipolar cells and feeds the magnocellular layer of the lateral geniculate nucleus. [2]

macula 1. In reference to vision, the pigmented region with a diameter of about 5.5 millimeters near the center of the retina. It is sometimes referred to as the macula lutea (from the Latin) because of its yellow appearance. 2. In reference to the vestibular system, any of the specialized detectors of linear acceleration and gravity found in each otolith organ. [2, 12]

magnetic resonance imaging (MRI) An imaging technology that uses the responses of atoms to strong magnetic fields to form images of structures like the brain. The method can be adapted to measure activity in the brain as well. [1]

magnetoencephalography (MEG) A technique, similar to electroencephalography, that measures changes in magnetic activity across populations of many neurons in the brain. [1]

magnitude estimation A psychophysical method in which the participant assigns values according to perceived magnitudes of the stimuli. [1]

magnocellular layer Either of the bottom two neuron-containing layers of the lateral geniculate nucleus, the cells of which are physically larger than those in the top four layers. [3]

main olfactory bulb (MOB) The rounded extension of the brain just above the nose that is the first region of the brain where smells are processed. In humans, we refer simply to olfactory bulb(s); in nonhuman animals with accessory olfactory bulbs, we distinguish between main and accessory. [14]

malleus The most exterior of the three ossicles. The malleus receives vibration from the tympanic membrane and is attached to the incus. [9]

masking Using a second sound, frequently noise, to make the detection of another sound more difficult. [9]

mathematical integration Computing an integral—one of the two main operations in calculus (the other, the inverse operation, is differentiation). Velocity is the integral of acceleration. Change of position is the integral of velocity. [12]

mathematical model The use of mathematical language and equations to describe psychological and/or neural processes. [1]

mechanoreceptor A sensory receptor that responds to mechanical stimulation (pressure, vibration, or movement). [12, 13]

medial geniculate nucleus The part of the thalamus that relays auditory signals to the temporal cortex and receives input from the auditory cortex. [9]

medial superior olive (MSO) A relay station in the brainstem where inputs from both ears contribute to detection of the interaural time difference. [10]

Meissner corpuscle A specialized nerve ending associated with fast-adapting (FA I) fibers that have small receptive fields. [13]

melanopsin A photopigment that is sensitive to ambient light. [2]

melody A sequence of notes or chords perceived as a single coherent structure. [11]

Merkel disc A specialized nerve ending associated with slowly adapting (SA I) fibers that have small receptive fields (also known as Merkel cell neurite complex). [13]

metabolic hearing loss Hearing loss caused by degraded ability of the stria vascularis to provide sufficient nutrients and ions to the cochlear partition. [9]

metamers Different mixtures of wavelengths that look identical, or more generally, any pair of stimuli that are perceived as identical despite physical differences. [5]

method of adjustment A method of limits in which the participant controls the change in the stimulus. [1]

method of constant stimuli A psychophysical method in which many stimuli, ranging from rarely to almost always perceivable (or rarely to almost always perceivably different from a reference stimulus), are presented one at a time. Participants respond to each presentation: "yes/no," "same/different," and so on. [1]

method of limits A psychophysical method in which the particular dimension of a stimulus, or the difference between two stimuli, is varied incrementally until the participant responds differently. [1]

metrical depth cue A depth cue that provides quantitative information about distance in the third dimension. [6]

microsaccade An involuntary, small, jerky eye movement. [8]

microvilli Slender projections of the cell membrane on the tips of some taste bud cells that extend into the taste pore. [15]

middle canal One of three fluid-filled passages in the cochlea. The middle canal is sandwiched between the tympanic and vestibular canals and contains the cochlear partition. Also called *scala media*. [9]

middle ear An air-filled chamber containing the middle bones, or ossicles. The middle ear conveys and amplifies vibration from the tympanic membrane to the oval window. [9]

middle temporal area (MT) (V5) An area of the brain thought to be important in the perception of motion. Also called V5 in humans. [8]

midget bipolar cell A small bipolar cell in the central retina that receives input from a single cone. [2]

midlevel (or middle) vision A loosely defined stage of visual processing that comes after basic features have been extracted from the image (low-level, or early, vision) and before object recognition and scene understanding (high-level vision). [4]

mid-spontaneous fiber An auditory nerve fiber that has a medium rate (10–30 spikes per second) of spontaneous firing. The characteristics of mid-spontaneous fibers are intermediate between those of low- and high-spontaneous fibers. [9]

mitral cells The deepest layer of neurons in the olfactory bulb. Each mitral cell responds to only a few specific odorants. [14]

monocular Referring to one eye. [6]

monocular depth cue A depth cue that is available even when the world is viewed with one eye alone. [6]

monosodium glutamate (MSG) The sodium salt of glutamic acid (an amino acid). [15]

motion aftereffect (MAE) The illusion of motion of a stationary object that occurs after prolonged exposure to a moving object. [8]

motion parallax An important depth cue that is based on head movement. The geometric information obtained from an eye in two different positions at two different times is similar to the information from two eyes in different positions in the head at the same time. [6]

myopia Nearsightedness, a common condition in which light entering the eye is focused in front of the retina and distant objects cannot be seen sharply. [2]

N

nasal dominance The asymmetry characterizing the intake of air by the two nostrils, which leads to differing sensitivity to odorants between the two nostrils. Nasal dominance alternates nostrils throughout the day, but there is no predictability for when the nostrils alternate. [14]

Necker cube An outline that is perceptually bi-stable. Unlike the situation with most stimuli, two interpretations continually battle for perceptual dominance. [4]

negative afterimage An afterimage whose polarity is the opposite of the original stimulus. Light stimuli produce dark negative afterimages. Colors are complementary; for example, red produces green afterimages, and yellow produces blue. [5]

neglect In reference to a neurological symptom, in visual attention: 1. The inability to attend or respond to stimuli in the contralesional visual field (typically, the left field after right parietal damage). 2. Ignoring half of the body or half of an object. [7]

neural plasticity The ability of neural circuits to undergo changes in function or organization as a result of previous activity. [13]

neuroimaging A set of methods that generate images of the structure and/or function of the brain. In many cases, these methods allow us to examine the brain in living, behaving humans. [1]

neuron The fundamental type of cell in the nervous system, collecting signals from sense organs, transmitting signals to muscles, and performing the mental operations in between. [1]

neurotransmitter A chemical substance used in neuronal communication at synapses. [1]

neutral point The point at which an opponent color mechanism is generating no signal. If red-green and blue-yellow mechanisms are at their neutral points, a stimulus will appear achromatic. (The black-white process has no neutral point.) [15]

nocebo effect Increasing pain sensation when people expect pain. [13]

nociceptor A sensory receptor that responds to painful input, such as extreme heat or pressure. [13]

nonaccidental feature A feature of an object that is not dependent on the exact (or accidental) viewing position of the observer. [4]

nonmetrical depth cue A depth cue that provides information about the depth order (relative depth) but not depth magnitude (e.g., his nose is in front of his face). [6]

nontaster (of PTC/PROP) An individual born with two recessive alleles for the *TAS2R38* gene who experiences little or no taste from the compounds phenylthiocarbamide (PTC) and propylthiouracil (PROP). [15]

O

occlusion A cue to relative depth order in which, for example, one object obstructs the view of part of another object. [6]

octave The interval between two sound frequencies having a ratio of 2:1. [11]

ocular dominance The property of the receptive fields of striate cortex neurons by which they demonstrate a preference, responding somewhat more rapidly when a stimulus is presented in one eye than when it is presented in the other. [3]

oculomotor (III) nerves The third pair of cranial nerves, which innervate all the extrinsic muscles of the eye except the lateral rectus and the superior oblique muscles, and which innervate the elevator muscle of the upper eyelid, the ciliary muscle, and the sphincter muscle of the pupil. [1]

odor The translation of a chemical stimulus into the sensation of an odor percept. For example, "The cake has a chocolate odor." [14]

odor hedonics The liking dimension of odor perception, typically measured by ratings of an odor's perceived pleasantness, familiarity, and intensity. [14]

odorant A molecule that is defined by its physicochemical characteristics and that can be translated by the central nervous system into the perception of a smell. For example, "The odorant methyl salicylate smells like wintergreen mint." [14]

odorant receptor (OR) The region in the cilia of olfactory sensory neurons where odorant molecules bind. [14]

OFF bipolar cell A bipolar cell that hyperpolarizes in response to an increase in light captured by the cones. [2]

OFF-center cell A cell that increases firing in response to a decrease in light intensity in its receptive-field center. [2]

olfaction The sense of smell. [14]

olfactory bulb (OB) A blueberry-sized extension of the forebrain just above the nose, where olfactory information is first processed. There are two olfactory bulbs, one in each brain hemisphere, corresponding to the right and left nostrils. [14]

olfactory cleft A narrow space at the back of the nose into which air flows and where the olfactory epithelium is located. It can vary in size. [14]

olfactory epithelium A secretory mucous membrane in the nose whose primary function is to detect odorants in inhaled air. Located on both sides of the upper portion of the nasal cavity and the olfactory clefts, the olfactory epithelium contains three types of cells: sustentacular cells, basal cells, and olfactory sensory neurons. [14]

olfactory nerve The first cranial nerve. The axons of the olfactory sensory neurons bundle together after passing through the cribriform plate to form the olfactory nerve, which conducts impulses from the olfactory epithelium in the nose to the olfactory bulb. Also called *cranial nerve I*. [14]

olfactory (I) nerves The first pair of cranial nerves. The axons of the olfactory sensory neurons bundle together after passing through the cribriform plate to form the olfactory nerve, which conducts impulses from the olfactory epithelia in the nose to the olfactory bulb. [1, 14]

olfactory sensory neuron (OSN) Principal of the three cell types in the olfactory epithelium. OSNs are small neurons located within a mucous layer in the epithelium. Cilia on the OSN dendrites contain receptor sites for odorant molecules. [14]

olfactory tract The bundle of axons of the mitral and tufted cells within the olfactory bulb that sends odor information to the primary olfactory cortex. [14]

olfactory white The olfactory equivalent of white noise or the color white. When at least 30 odorants of equal intensity that span olfactory physiochemical and psychological (perceptual) space are mixed, they produce a resultant odor perception that is the same as that of every other mixture of 30 odorants meeting the same span and equivalent intensity criteria, even though the various mixtures do not share any common odorants. [14]

ON bipolar cell A bipolar cell that depolarizes in response to an increase in light captured by the cones. [2]

ON-center cell A cell that increases firing in response to an increase in light intensity in its receptive-field center. [2]

opponent color theory The theory that perception of color is based on the output of three mechanisms, each of them resulting from an opponency between two colors: red-green, blue-yellow, and black-white. [5]

optic array The collection of light rays that interact with objects in the world that are in front of a viewer. The term was coined by J. J. Gibson. [8]

optic flow 1. The pattern of apparent motion of objects in a visual scene produced by the relative motion between the observer and the scene. 2. The changing angular positions of points in a perspective image that we experience as we move through the world. [6, 8]

optic (II) nerves The second pair of cranial nerves, which arise from the retina and carry visual information to the thalamus and other parts of the brain. [1]

optokinetic nystagmus A reflexive eye movement in which the eyes will involuntarily track a continually moving object. [8]

orbitofrontal cortex (OFC) The part of the frontal lobe of the cortex that lies behind the bone (orbit) containing the eyes. The OFC is responsible for the conscious experience of olfaction, as well as the integration of pleasure and displeasure from food. The OFC is also involved in many other functions, and it is critical for assigning affective value to stimuli—in other words, determining hedonic meaning. It is also referred to as the *secondary olfactory cortex* and the *secondary taste cortex*. [14, 15]

organ of Corti A structure on the basilar membrane of the cochlea that is composed of hair cells and dendrites of auditory nerve fibers. [9]

orientation tuning The tendency of neurons in striate cortex to respond optimally to certain orientations and less to others. [3]

orthonasal olfaction Sniffing in and perceiving odors through our nostrils, which occurs when we are smelling something that is in the air. [14]

oscillatory Referring to back-and-forth movement that has a constant rhythm. [12]

ossicle Any of three tiny bones of the middle ear: malleus, incus, and stapes. [9]

otitis media Inflammation of the middle ear, common in children as a result of infection. [9]

otoconia Tiny calcium carbonate stones in the ear that provide inertial mass for the otolith organs, enabling them to sense gravity and linear acceleration. [12]

otolith organ Either of two mechanical structures (utricle and saccule) in the vestibular system that sense both linear acceleration and gravity. [12]

otosclerosis Abnormal growth of the middle-ear bones that causes hearing loss. [9]

outer ear The external sound-gathering portion of the ear, consisting of the pinna and the ear canal. [9]

outer segment The part of a photoreceptor that contains photopigment molecules. [2]

oval window The flexible opening to the cochlea through which the stapes transmits vibration to the fluid inside. [9]

P

P ganglion cell A small ganglion cell that receives excitatory input from single midget bipolar cells in the central retina and feeds the parvocellular layer of the lateral geniculate nucleus. [2]

Pacinian corpuscle A specialized nerve ending associated with fast-adapting (FA II) fibers that have large receptive fields. [13]

Panum's fusional area The region of space, in front of and behind the horopter, within which binocular single vision is possible. [6]

papilla (pl. papillae) Any of multiple structures that give the tongue its bumpy appearance. From smallest to largest, the papilla types that contain taste buds are fungiform, foliate, and circumvallate. Filiform papillae are the smallest and most numerous but do not contain taste buds. [15]

parabelt area A region of cortex, lateral and adjacent to the belt area, where neurons respond to more complex characteristics of sounds, as well as to input from other senses. [9]

parahippocampal place area (PPA) A region of extrastriate visual cortex in humans that is specifically and reliably activated more by images of places than by other stimuli. [4, 7]

parallel search Visual search in which multiple stimuli are processed at the same time. [7]

parallelism A rule for figure-ground assignment stating that parallel contours are likely to belong to the same figure. [4]

parietal lobe In each cerebral hemisphere, a lobe that lies toward the top of the brain between the frontal and occipital lobes. [7]

parvocellular Referring to cells in the parvocellular layers of the lateral geniculate nucleus of the thalamus. *Parvo* from the Greek for "small" refers to the size of the cells. [5]

parvocellular layer Any of the top four neuron-containing layers of the lateral geniculate nucleus, the cells of which are physically smaller than those in the bottom two layers. [3]

perception The act of giving meaning to a detected sensation. [1]

peripersonal space That part of the world that is near your body—especially, your hands. [7]

phantom limb Sensation perceived from a physically amputated limb of the body. [13]

phase The position of a grating relative to a fixed position measured in degrees, where one complete cycle is 360 degrees. [3]

phase locking Firing of a single neuron at one distinct point in the period (cycle) of a sound wave at a given frequency. (The neuron need not fire on every cycle, but each firing will occur at the same point in the cycle.) [9]

pheromone A chemical emitted by one member of a species that triggers a physiological or behavioral response in another member of the same species. Pheromones are signals for chemical communication and may or may not have any smell. [14]

phonation The process through which vocal folds are made to vibrate when air pushes out of the lungs. [11]

photoactivation Activation by light. [2]

photon A quantum of visible light or other form of electromagnetic radiation demonstrating both particle and wave properties. [2]

photopic Referring to light intensities that are bright enough to stimulate the cone receptors and bright enough to "saturate" the rod receptors, that is, drive them to their maximum responses. [5]

photoreceptor A light-sensitive receptor in the retina. [2]

pictorial depth cue A cue to distance or depth used by artists to depict three-dimensional depth in two-dimensional pictures. [6]

pinna (pl. pinnae) The outer, funnel-like part of the ear. [9]

piriform cortex (the primary olfactory cortex) The neural area where olfactory information is first processed. It comprises the amygdala, parahippocampal gyrus, and interconnected areas, and it interacts closely with the entorhinal cortex. [14]

pitch The psychological aspect of sound related mainly to the perceived frequency. [9, 11]

place code Tuning of different parts of the cochlea to different frequencies, in which information about the particular frequency of an incoming sound wave is coded by the place along the cochlear partition that has the greatest mechanical displacement. [9]

placebo effect Decreasing pain sensation when people think they're taking an analgesic drug but actually are not. [13]

polysensory Referring to blending multiple sensory systems. [1]

positivism A philosophical position arguing that all we really have to go on is the evidence of the senses, so the world might be nothing more than an elaborate hallucination. An adherent of positivism is a positivist. [6]

positron emission tomography (PET) An imaging technology that enables us to define locations in the brain where neurons are especially active by measuring the metabolism of brain cells using safe radioactive isotopes. [1]

preattentive stage The processing of a stimulus that occurs before selective attention is deployed to that stimulus. [7]

presbycusis Age-related hearing loss. [9]

presbyopia Literally "old sight"; the age-related loss of accommodation, which makes it difficult to focus on near objects. [2]

primary auditory cortex (A1) The first area within the temporal lobes of the brain responsible for processing acoustic information. [9]

primary visual cortex (V1), area 17, or striate cortex The area of the cerebral cortex of the brain that receives direct inputs from the lateral geniculate nucleus, as well as feedback from other brain areas. [3]

prime A stimulus that might make it easier or faster to respond to a subsequent stimulus. If you are primed by the word "cat," you will respond more quickly to the word "mouse" than to "broom" or some other unrelated word. [7]

primer pheromone A pheromone that triggers a physiological (often hormonal) change among conspecifics. This effect usually involves prolonged pheromone exposure. [14]

principle of univariance The fact that an infinite set of different wavelength-intensity combinations can elicit exactly the same response from a single type of photoreceptor. One photoreceptor type cannot make color discriminations based on wavelength. [5]

priority map A hypothetical neural representation of visual space in which the activity at each point reflects how much that location (or object) will attract attention. [7]

probability summation The increased detection probability based on the statistical advantage of having two (or more) detectors rather than one. [6]

projective geometry For purposes of studying perception of the three-dimensional world, the geometry that describes the transformations that occur when the three-dimensional world is projected onto a two-dimensional surface. For example, parallel lines do not converge in the real world, but they do in the two-dimensional projection of that world. [6]

proprioception Perception mediated by kinesthetic and internal receptors. [13]

prosopagnosia An inability to recognize faces. [4]

protanope An individual who suffers from color-blindness that is caused by the absence of L-cones. [5]

proto-object A term used to refer to object-like stimuli before they are attended and recognized. [7]

proximity A Gestalt grouping rule stating that the tendency of two features to group together will increase as the distance between them decreases. [4]

pruriceptor A neural fiber that carries the sensation of itchiness. [13]

psychoacoustics The branch of psychophysics that studies the psychological correlates of the physical dimensions of acoustics in order to understand how the auditory system operates. [9]

psychophysics The science of defining quantitative relationships between physical and psychological (subjective, perceptual) events. [1, 14]

pupil The dark, circular opening at the center of the iris in the eye, where light enters the eye. [2]

Q

qualia (sing. quale) In reference to philosophy, private conscious experiences of sensation or perception. [5]

R

random dot stereogram (RDS) A stereogram made of a large number (often in the thousands) of randomly placed dots. Random dot stereograms contain no monocular cues to depth. Stimuli visible stereoscopically in random dot stereograms are Cyclopean stimuli. [6]

rapid serial visual presentation (RSVP) An experimental procedure in which stimuli appear in a stream at one location (typically the point of fixation) at a rapid rate (typically about 8 per second). [7]

rate-intensity function A graph plotting the firing rate of an auditory nerve fiber in response to a sound of constant frequency at increasing intensities. [9]

rate saturation The point at which a nerve fiber is firing as rapidly as possible and further stimulation is incapable of increasing the firing rate. [9]

reachspace A region of visual space that is within arm's reach: bigger than most objects, smaller than a typical scene, and critically positioned where the arms can reach. [7]

reaction time (RT) A measure of the time from the onset of a stimulus to a response. [7]

realism A philosophical position arguing that there is a real world to sense. [6]

receiver operating characteristic (ROC) curve In reference to studies of signal detection, the graphical plot of the hit rate as a function of the false-alarm rate. If these are the same, points fall on the diagonal, indicating that the observer cannot tell the difference between the presence and absence of the signal. As the observer's sensitivity increases, the curve bows upward toward the upper left corner. That point represents a perfect ability to distinguish signal from noise (100% hits, 0% false alarms). [1]

receptive field The region on the retina in which visual stimuli influence a neuron's firing rate. [2]

receptor adaptation The biochemical phenomenon that occurs after continual exposure to an odorant, whereby receptors are no longer available to respond to the odorant and detection ceases. [14]

receptor potential A change in voltage across the membrane of a sensory receptor cell (in the vestibular system, a hair cell) in response to stimulation. [12]

recognition-by-components model Biederman's model of object recognition, which holds that objects are recognized by the identities and relationships of their component parts. [4]

reflect To redirect something that strikes a surface—especially light, sound, or heat—usually back toward its point of origin. [2]

reflectance The percentage of light hitting a surface that is reflected and not absorbed into the surface. Typically, reflectance is given as a function of wavelength. [5]

reflexive eye movement A movement of the eye that is automatic and involuntary. [8]

refract 1. To alter the course of a wave of energy that passes into something from another medium, as water does to light entering it from the air. 2. To measure the degree of refraction in a lens or eye. [2]

refractive error A very common disorder in which the image of the world is not clearly focused on the retina. The most common refractive errors are myopia, hyperopia, astigmatism, and presbyopia. [2]

Reissner's membrane A thin sheath of tissue separating the vestibular and middle canals in the cochlea. [9]

relatability The degree to which two line segments appear to be part of the same contour. [4]

related color A color, such as brown or gray, that is seen only in relation to other colors. For example, a "gray" patch in complete darkness appears white. [5]

relative disparity The difference in the absolute disparities of two objects. [6]

relative height As a depth cue, the observation that objects at different distances from the viewer on the ground plane will form images at different heights in the retinal image. Objects farther away will be seen as higher in the image. [6]

relative metrical depth cue A depth cue that could specify, for example, that object A is twice as far away as object B without providing information about the absolute distance to either A or B. [6]

relative size A comparison of size between items without knowing the absolute size of either one. [6]

releaser pheromone A pheromone that triggers an immediate behavioral response among conspecifics. [14]

resonator Most objects such as musical instruments and vocal tracts are resonators because, as a result of their shape, they increase amplitude at some frequencies, called resonant frequencies, compared to other frequencies. [11]

response enhancement An effect of attention on the response of a neuron in which the neuron responding to an attended stimulus gives a bigger response. [7]

retina A light-sensitive membrane in the back of the eye that contains photoreceptors and other cell types that transduce light into electrochemical signals and transmit them to the brain through the optic nerve. [2]

retinitis pigmentosa A progressive degeneration of the retina that affects night vision and peripheral vision. It commonly runs in families and can be caused by defects in a number of different genes that have recently been identified. [2]

retronasal olfaction Perceiving odors through the mouth while breathing and chewing. This is what gives us the experience of flavor. [14]

retronasal olfactory sensation The sensation of an odorant that is perceived when chewing and swallowing force that odorant in the mouth up behind the palate into the nose. Such odor sensations are perceived as originating from the mouth, even though the actual contact of odorant and receptor occurs at the olfactory mucosa. [15]

reverse-hierarchy theory A theory that fast, feed-forward processes can give you crude information about objects and scenes based on activity in high-level parts of the visual cortex. You become aware of details when activity flows back down the hierarchy of visual areas to lower-level areas where the detailed information is preserved. [4]

rhodopsin The visual pigment found in rods. [2]

rhythm A repeated pattern of sounds composed of strong and weak elements. [11]

rod A photoreceptor specialized for night vision. [2]

rod monochromat An individual with no cones of any type. In addition to being truly color-blind, rod monochromats are badly visually impaired in bright light. [5]

round window A soft area of tissue at the base of the tympanic canal that releases excess pressure remaining from extremely intense sounds. [9]

Ruffini ending A specialized nerve ending associated with slowly adapting (SA II) fibers that have large receptive fields. [13]

S

S-cone A cone that is preferentially sensitive to short wavelengths, colloquially (but not entirely accurately) known as a "blue cone." [5]

saccade A type of eye movement made both voluntarily and involuntarily, in which the eyes rapidly change fixation from one object or location to another. [8]

saccadic suppression The reduction of visual sensitivity that occurs when we make saccadic eye movements. Saccadic suppression eliminates the smear from retinal image motion during an eye movement. [8]

saccule One of the two otolith organs. A saclike structure that contains the saccular macula. Also called *sacculus*. [12]

salience The vividness of a stimulus relative to its neighbors. [7]

salty One of the four basic tastes; the taste quality produced by the cations of salts (e.g., the sodium in sodium chloride produces the salty taste). Some cations also produce other taste qualities (e.g., potassium tastes bitter as well as salty). The purest salty taste is produced by sodium chloride (NaCl), common table salt. [15]

satisfaction of search A type of error that occurs when detection of one target makes an observer less likely to find a second target in the same display or scene. [7]

scatter To disperse something—such as light—in an irregular fashion. [2]

scene-based guidance Information in our understanding of scenes that helps us find specific objects in scenes (e.g., objects do not float in air, faucets are found near sinks). [7]

scene grammar A set of implicit rules about what can be where that allow you to understand a scene, just as linguistic grammar allows you to understand language. [7]

scene semantics In language, semantics refers to the meaning of an utterance. In scenes, it refers to the meaning of the scene. [7]

scene syntax In language, syntax refers to the structure of sentences. In scenes, it refers to what is normal in the structure of the world. [7]

scotopic Referring to light intensities that are bright enough to stimulate the rod receptors but too dim to stimulate the cone receptors. [5]

second-order motion The motion of an object that is defined by changes in contrast or texture, but not by luminance. [8]

selective attention The form of attention involved when processing is restricted to a subset of the possible stimuli. [7]

semicircular canal Any of three toroidal tubes in the vestibular system that sense angular motion. [12]

sensation The ability to detect a stimulus and, perhaps, to turn that detection into a private experience. [1]

sense of angular motion The perceptual modality that senses rotation. [12]

sense of linear motion The perceptual modality that senses translation. [12]

sense of tilt The perceptual modality that senses head inclination with respect to gravity. [12]

sensitivity 1. The ability to perceive via the sense organs. 2. Extreme responsiveness to radiation, especially to light of a specific wavelength. 3. The ability to respond to transmitted signals. 4. In reference to signal detection theory, a measure that defines the ease with which an observer can tell the difference between the presence and absence of a stimulus or the difference between stimulus 1 and stimulus 2. [1, 2]

sensorineural hearing loss Hearing loss caused by defects in the cochlea or auditory nerve. [9]

sensory conflict Sensory discrepancies that arise when sensory systems provide conflicting information. For example, vision may indicate that you are stationary while the vestibular system tells you that you are moving (or vice versa). [12]

sensory integration or multisensory integration The process of combining different sensory signals. The senses typically work together to learn about the world and to guide behavior. Typically, combining several signals yields more accurate and/or more precise information than can be obtained from individual sensory signals. This is *different from* the mathematical process of integration learned in calculus (e.g., the integral of acceleration is velocity). [1, 12]

sensory exafference Change in afference caused by external stimuli. For the vestibular system, vestibular afference evoked by passive head motion would yield sensory exafference. [12]

sensory reafference Change in afference caused by self-generated activity. For the vestibular system, vestibular afference evoked by an active self-generated head motion would yield sensory reafference. [12]

serial self-terminating search A search from item to item, ending when a target is found. [7]

set size The number of items in a visual display. [7]

shape-pattern theory The current dominant biochemical theory for how chemicals come to be perceived as specific odors. Shape-pattern theory contends that different scents—as a function of the fit between odorant shape and olfactory receptor shape—activate different arrays of olfactory receptors in the olfactory epithelia. These various arrays produce specific firing patterns of neurons in the olfactory bulbs, which then determine the particular scent we perceive. [14]

sharper tuning An effect of attention on the response of a neuron in which the neuron responding to an attended stimulus responds more precisely. For example, a neuron that responds to lines with orientations from −20 degrees to +20 degrees might come to respond to ±10-degree lines. [7]

signal detection theory A psychophysical theory that quantifies the response of an observer to the presentation of a signal in the presence of noise. Measures obtained from a series of presentations are sensitivity (d') and criterion of the observer. [1]

similarity A Gestalt grouping rule stating that the tendency of two features to group together will increase as the similarity between them increases. For example, in hearing, the tendency of two sounds to group together will increase as the acoustic similarity between them increases. [4, 10]

simple cell A cortical neuron whose receptive field has clearly defined excitatory and inhibitory regions. [3]

sine wave or pure tone The single waveform for which variation as a function of time is a sine function. In hearing research, this is sometimes referred to as a pure tone. [9]

sine wave grating A grating with a sinusoidal luminance profile as shown in Figure 3.4A. [3]

sinusoidal Referring to any oscillation, such as a sound wave or rotational motion, whose waveform is that of a sine curve. The period of a sinusoidal oscillation is the time that it takes for one full back-and-forth cycle of the motion to occur. The frequency of a sinusoidal oscillation is defined as the numeral 1 divided by the period. [12]

smooth pursuit A type of voluntary eye movement in which the eyes move smoothly to follow a moving object. [8]

somatosensation Collectively, sensory signals from the skin, muscles, tendons, joints, and internal receptors. [13]

somatosensory area 1 (S1) The primary receiving area for touch in the cortex. [13]

somatosensory area 2 (S2) The secondary receiving area for touch in the cortex. [13]

somatotopic Referring to spatial mapping in the somatosensory cortex in correspondence to spatial events on the skin. [13]

sour One of the four basic tastes; the taste quality produced by the hydrogen ion in acids. [15]

spatial disorientation Any impairment of spatial orientation. More specifically, any impairment of our sense of linear motion, angular motion, or tilt. [12]

spatial frequency The number of grating cycles (e.g., changes in light and dark) per unit of visual angle (usually specified in degree) in a given unit of space. [3]

spatial-frequency channel A pattern analyzer, implemented by an ensemble of cortical neurons, in which each set of neurons is tuned to a limited range of spatial frequencies. [3]

spatial layout The description of the structure of a scene (e.g., enclosed, open, rough, smooth) without reference to the identity of specific objects in the scene. [7]

spatial orientation A sense consisting of three interacting modalities: perception of linear motion, angular motion, and tilt. [12]

specific anosmia The inability to smell one specific compound amid otherwise normal smell perception. [14]

specific hungers theory The idea that deficiency of a given nutrient produces craving (a specific hunger) for that nutrient. Curt Richter first proposed this theory and demonstrated that cravings for salty or for sweet are associated with deficiencies in those substances. However, the idea proved wrong for other nutrients (e.g., vitamins). [15]

spectral power distribution The physical energy in a light as a function of wavelength. [5]

spectral reflectance function The percentage of a particular wavelength that is reflected from a surface. [5]

spectral sensitivity The sensitivity of a cell or a device to different wavelengths on the electromagnetic spectrum. [5]

spectrogram In reference to sound analysis, a three-dimensional display that plots time on the horizontal axis, frequency on the vertical axis, and amplitude (intensity) on a color or gray scale. [11]

spectrum A representation of the relative energy (intensity) present at each frequency. [9]

specular reflections Bright spots produced by some light bouncing off an object. [4]

spinothalamic pathway The route from the spinal cord to the brain that carries most of the information about skin temperature and pain. [13]

staircase method A psychophysical method for determining the concentration of a stimulus required for detection at the threshold level. The staircase method is an example of a *method of limits*. A stimulus (e.g., odorant) is presented in an ascending concentration sequence until detection is indicated, and then the concentration is shifted to a descending sequence until the response changes to "no detection." This ascending and descending sequence is typically repeated several times, and the concentrations at which reversals occur are averaged to determine the threshold detection level of that odorant for a given individual. Also called *reverse staircase method*. [14]

stapedius The muscle attached to the stapes. Tensing the stapedius decreases vibration. [9]

stapes The most interior of the three ossicles. Connected to the incus on one end, the stapes presses against the oval window of the cochlea on the other end. [9]

statistical optimization model A computational account describing how a perceptual system uses the statistics of past experience to improve its current performance, for example, by minimizing the processing load or making the best use of multiple sources of information. [1]

stereoacuity A measure of the smallest binocular disparity that can generate a sensation of depth. [6]

stereoblindness An inability to make use of binocular disparity as a depth cue. This term is typically used to describe individuals with vision in both eyes. Someone who has lost one or both eyes is not typically described as "stereoblind." [6]

stereocilium Any of the hairlike extensions on the tips of hair cells in the cochlea that, when flexed, initiate the release of neurotransmitters. [9]

stereoisomers Isomers (molecules that can exist in different structural forms) in which the spatial arrangements of the atoms are mirror-image rotations of one another, like a right and left hand. [14]

stereopsis The ability to use binocular disparity as a cue to depth. [6]

stereoscope A device for simultaneously presenting one image to one eye and another image to the other eye. Stereoscopes can be used to present dichoptic stimuli for stereopsis and binocular rivalry. [6]

Stevens's power law A principle describing the relationship between stimulus and resulting sensation that says the magnitude of subjective sensation is proportional to the stimulus magnitude raised to an exponent. [1]

stimulus onset asynchrony (SOA) The time between the onset of one stimulus and the onset of another. [7]

strabismus A misalignment of the two eyes such that a single object in space is imaged on the fovea of one eye and on a nonfoveal area of the other (turned) eye. [3, 6]

stria vascularis Specialized tissue lines one side of the middle canal and maintains the right balance of charged ions in the endolymph to keep hair cells working at their best. [9]

structural description A description of an object in terms of the nature of its constituent parts and the relationships between those parts. [4]

structuralism In reference to perception, a school of thought that believed that complex objects or perceptions could be understood by analysis of the components. Adherents are known as *structuralists* [4]

submodality of touch A specialized domain of psychological functions, such as perceptual discrimination, social-emotional consequences, perceived unpleasantness, and interoception. [13]

substantia gelatinosa A region of interconnecting neurons in the dorsal horn of the spinal cord. [13]

subsurface scatter An event that occurs when some light gets into an object and bounces around before escaping, thus causing the object to appear translucent. [4]

subtraction method In functional magnetic resonance imaging, comparison of brain activity measured in two conditions: one with and one without the involvement of the mental process of interest. The difference between the images for the two conditions may show regions of brain specifically activated by that mental process. [4]

subtractive color mixture A mixture of pigments. If pigments A and B mix, some of the light shining on the surface will be subtracted by A and some by B. Only the remainder will contribute to the perception of color. [5]

superior colliculus A structure in the midbrain that is important in initiating and guiding eye movements. [8]

superior olive An early brainstem region in the auditory pathway where inputs from both ears converge. [9]

supertasters Those individuals whose perception of taste sensations is the most intense. A variety of factors may contribute to this heightened perception, including density of fungiform papillae. [15]

suppression In reference to vision, the inhibition of an unwanted image. Suppression occurs frequently in people with strabismus. [6]

surroundedness A rule for figure-ground assignment stating that if one region is entirely surrounded by another, it is likely that the surrounded region is the figure. [4]

sustentacular or supporting cell One of the three types of cells in the olfactory epithelium. Sustentacular cells provide metabolic and physical support for the olfactory sensory neurons. [14]

sweet One of the four basic tastes; the taste quality produced by some sugars, such as glucose, fructose, and sucrose. These three sugars are particularly biologically useful to us, and our sweet receptors are tuned to them. Some other compounds (e.g., saccharin, cyclamate, aspartame) are also sweet. [15]

symmetry A rule for figure-ground assignment stating that symmetrical regions are more likely to be seen as figure. [4]

synapse The junction between neurons that permits information transfer. [1]

synaptic terminal The location where axons terminate at the synapse for transmission of information by the release of a chemical transmitter. [2]

syncopation Any deviation from a regular rhythm. [11]

synesthesia The perceptual experience (e.g., a color) elicited by a stimulus (e.g., a letter) that does not typically produce that experience, while the stimulus (e.g., wavelength information) that does normally produce the experience is absent. [5]

synthesis An ability to put local bits of information together into recognizable objects. [4]

T

tactile Referring to the result of mechanical interactions with the skin. [13]

tactile agnosia The inability to identify objects by touch. [13]

target The goal of a visual search. [7]

tastant Any stimulus that can be tasted. [15]

taste Sensations evoked by solutions in the mouth that contact receptors on the tongue and the roof of the mouth that then connect to axons in cranial nerves VII, IX, and X. [15]

taste bud A globular cluster of cells that has the function of creating neural signals conveyed to the brain by the taste nerves. Some of the cells in a taste bud (receptor cells) have specialized sites on their apical projections that interact with taste stimuli. Receptor cells that mediate sourness form synapses with taste nerve fibers. Receptor cells that mediate sweetness and bitterness do not form synapses; rather, they communicate with nearby taste fibers chemically. [15]

taste receptor cell A cell within the taste bud that contains sites on its apical projections (microvilli) that can interact with taste stimuli. These sites fall into two major categories: those interacting with charged particles (e.g., sodium and hydrogen ions) and G protein–coupled receptors that interact with sweet and bitter stimuli. [15]

taster (of PTC/PROP) An individual born with one or two dominant alleles for the *TAS2R38* gene and able to taste the compounds phenylthiocarbamide (PTC) and propylthiouracil (PROP). PTC/PROP tasters who also have a high density of fungiform papillae tend to be PROP supertasters. [15]

tau (τ) Information in the optic flow that could signal time to collision (TTC) without the necessity of estimating either absolute distances or rates. The ratio of the retinal image size at any moment to the rate at which the image is expanding is tau, and TTC is proportional to tau. [8]

tectorial membrane A gelatinous structure, attached on one end, that extends into the middle canal of the cochlea, floating above inner hair cells and touching outer hair cells. [9]

template The internal representation of a stimulus that is used to recognize the stimulus in the world. Unlike its use in, for example, making a key, a mental template is not expected to look like the stimulus that it matches. [4]

tempo The perceived speed of the presentation of sounds. [11]

temporal code Tuning of different parts of the cochlea to different frequencies, in which information about the particular frequency of an incoming sound wave is coded by the timing of neural firing as it relates to the period of the sound. [9]

temporal integration The process by which a sound at a constant level is perceived as being louder when it is of greater duration. The term also applies to perceived brightness, which depends on the duration of light. [9]

tensor tympani The muscle attached to the malleus. Tensing the tensor tympani decreases vibration. [9]

tetrachromatic Referring to the rare situation (in humans, at least) where the color of any light is defined by the relationships of four numbers—the outputs of those four receptor types. [5]

texture-defined object or contrast-defined object An object that is defined by differences in contrast or texture, but not by luminance. [8]

texture gradient A depth cue based on the geometric fact that items of the same size form smaller images when they are farther away. An array of items that change in size smoothly across the image will appear to form a surface tilted in depth. [6]

texture segmentation Carving an image into regions of common texture properties. [4]

thermoreceptor A sensory receptor that signals information about changes in skin temperature. [13]

thermoTRP channel Thermally sensitive transient receptor potential ion channel found in sensory neurons. [13]

threshold tuning curve A graph plotting the thresholds of a neuron in response to sine waves with varying frequencies at the lowest intensity that will give rise to a response. [9]

tilt To attain a sloped position like that of the Leaning Tower of Pisa. [12]

tilt aftereffect The perceptual illusion of tilt, produced by adaptation to a pattern of a given orientation. [3, 6]

timbre The psychological sensation by which a listener can judge that two sounds with the same loudness and pitch are dissimilar. Timbre quality is conveyed by harmonics and other high frequencies. [9, 10]

time to collision (TTC) The time required for a moving object (such as a cricket ball) to hit a stationary object (such as a batsman's head). TTC = distance/rate. [8]

tip link A tiny filament that stretches from the tip of a stereocilium to the side of its neighbor. [9]

tip-of-the-nose phenomenon The inability to name an odor, even though it is very familiar. Contrary to the tip-of-the-tongue phenomenon, one has no lexical access to the name of the odor, such as first letter, rhyme, number of syllables, and so on, when in the tip-of-the-nose state. This is an example of how language and olfactory perception are deeply disconnected. [14]

tone chroma A sound quality shared by tones that have the same octave interval. [11]

tone height A sound quality corresponding to the level of pitch. Tone height is monotonically related to frequency. [11]

tonotopic organization An arrangement in which neurons that respond to different frequencies are organized anatomically in order of frequency. [9]

topographical mapping The orderly mapping of the world in the lateral geniculate nucleus and the visual cortex. [3]

touch The sensations caused by stimulation of the skin, muscles, tendons, and joints. [13]

transduce To convert from one form of energy to another (e.g., from light to neural electrical energy, or from mechanical movement to neural electrical energy). Neurons use electrical signals in their communication. [2, 12]

transduction The conversion of a physical stimulus, such as light or sound, into a neural response through the activity of sensory receptors. [1]

transmit To convey something (e.g., light) from one place or thing to another. [2]

transparent Referring to the characteristic of a material that allows light to pass through it with no interruption such that objects on the other side can be clearly seen. [2]

triangle test A test in which a participant is given three odorants to smell, of which two are the same and one is different. The participant is required to state which is the odd odor out. Typically, the order in which the three odorants are given (e.g., same, same, different; different, same, same; same, different, same) is manipulated and the test is repeated several times for greater accuracy. [14]

triangulation In vision, this refers to the triangle formed by the two eyes and the point on which they fixate in the three-dimensional world. The angles of that triangle are related to the location of the fixated point in depth. [6]

trichromacy or trichromatic theory of color vision The theory that the color of any light is defined in our visual system by the relationships of three numbers—the outputs of three receptor types now known to be the three cones. Also called the *Young-Helmholtz theory*. [5]

trigeminal nerve The fifth cranial nerve, which transmits information about the "feel" of an odorant (e.g., mint feels cool, cinnamon feels warm), as well as pain and irritation sensations (e.g., ammonia feels burning). Also called *cranial nerve V*. [14]

tritanope An individual who suffers from color-blindness that is caused by the absence of S-cones. [5]

trochlear (IV) nerves The fourth pair of cranial nerves, which innervate the superior oblique muscles of the eyeballs. [1]

tufted cells The next layer of cells after the juxtaglomerular neurons. They respond to fewer odorants than the juxtaglomerular neurons, but more than neurons at the deepest layer of cells. [14]

turbinates Curled bony protrusions inside the nasal cavity. The small ridges of the turbinates create turbulence to incoming air, causing a small puff of each breath to rise and pass through the olfactory cleft, facilitating the ability to detect odorants. [14]

two-point touch threshold The minimum distance at which two stimuli (e.g., two simultaneous touches) are just perceptible as separate. [13]

two-tone suppression A decrease in the response (firing rate) of one auditory nerve fiber to one tone when a second tone is presented at the same time. [9]

tympanic canal One of three fluid-filled passages in the cochlea. The tympanic canal extends from the round window at the base of the cochlea to the helicotrema at the apex. Also called *scala tympani*. [9]

tympanic membrane The eardrum; a thin sheet of skin at the end of the outer ear canal. The tympanic membrane vibrates in response to sound. [9]

U

umami The taste sensation produced by monosodium glutamate. [15]

uncrossed disparity The sign of disparity created by objects behind the plane of fixation (the horopter). The term *uncrossed* is used because images of objects located behind the horopter will appear to be displaced to the right in the right eye and to the left in the left eye. [6]

unique hue In the context of opponent color theory, any of four colors that can be described with only a single color term: red, yellow, green, blue. Other colors (e.g., purple or orange) can also be described as compounds (reddish blue, reddish yellow). [5]

uniqueness constraint In reference to stereopsis, the observation that a feature in the world is represented exactly once in each retinal image. This constraint simplifies the correspondence problem. [6]

unrelated color A color that can be experienced in isolation. [5]

utricle One of the two otolith organs. A saclike structure that contains the utricular macula. Also called *utriculus*. [12]

V

vagus (X) nerves The tenth pair of cranial nerves, which innervate the heart, lungs, gastrointestinal tract, bronchi, trachea, and larynx. [1]

vanishing point The apparent point at which parallel lines receding in depth converge. [6]

vection An illusory sense of self-motion caused by moving visual cues when one is not, in fact, actually moving. [12]

velocity The speed and direction in which something moves. Mathematically, velocity is the temporal derivative of position. In words, linear velocity is distance divided by time to traverse that distance; angular velocity is rotation angle divided by time to traverse that angle. [12]

velocity storage Prolongation of a rotational response by the brain beyond the duration of the rotational signal provided to the brain by the semicircular canals, typically yielding responses that are nearer the actual rotational motion than the signal provided by the canals. [12]

vergence A type of eye movement in which the two eyes move in opposite directions; for example, both eyes turn toward the nose (convergence) or away from the nose (divergence). [6, 8]

vergence angle The angle formed by lines from each eye to the current object of fixation. A larger vergence angle implies a closer object. [6]

vertigo A sensation of rotation or spinning. The term is often used more generally to mean any form of dizziness. [12]

vestibular canal One of three fluid-filled passages in the cochlea. The vestibular canal extends from the oval window at the base of the cochlea to the helicotrema at the apex. Also called *scala vestibuli*. [9]

vestibular organs The set of five sense organs located in each inner ear that sense head motion and head orientation with respect to gravity. [12]

vestibular system The vestibular organs as well as the vestibular neurons in cranial nerve VIII and the central neurons that contribute to the functional roles that the vestibular system participates in. [12]

vestibulocochlear (VIII) nerves The eighth pair of cranial nerves, which connect the inner ear with the brain, transmitting impulses concerned with hearing and spatial orientation. The vestibulocochlear nerve is composed of the cochlear nerve branch and the vestibular nerve branch. [1]

vestibulo-ocular reflex (VOR) A short-latency reflex that helps stabilize vision by counterrotating the eyes when the vestibular system senses head movement. [12]

vibration theory An alternative to shape-pattern theory for describing how olfaction works. Vibration theory proposes that every odorant has a different vibrational frequency and that molecules that produce the same vibrational frequencies will smell the same. [14]

Vieth-Müller circle The location of objects whose images fall on geometrically corresponding points in the two retinas. If life were simple, this circle would be the horopter, but life is not simple. [6]

visual acuity A measure of the finest detail that can be resolved by the eyes. [2]

visual angle The angle that an object subtends at the eye (retina). [2, 3]

visual crowding The deleterious effect of clutter on peripheral object recognition. [3]

visual-field defect A portion of the visual field with no vision or with abnormal vision, typically resulting from damage to the visual nervous system. [7]

visual search A search for a target in a display containing distracting elements. [7]

visual word form area (VWFA) A region of extrastriate visual cortex in humans that is specifically and reliably activated more by images of written words than by other stimuli. [4]

vitreous humor The transparent fluid that fills the vitreous chamber in the posterior part of the eye. [2]

vocal folds The pair of elastic tissues that vibrate as a result of airflow generated by lungs, depending on how close or apart and how tense or lax they are. [11]

vocal tract The airway above the larynx used for the production of speech. The vocal tract includes the oral tract and nasal tract. [11]

volatile A molecule that is buoyant in air and therefore can be inhaled. Odorants are volatile molecules. [14]

volley principle The idea that multiple neurons can provide a temporal code for frequency if each neuron fires at a distinct point in the period of a sound wave but does not fire on every period. [9]

vomeronasal organ (VNO) Found in nonhuman animals, it is a chemical-sensing organ at the base of the nasal cavity with a curved tubular shape. The VNO evolved to detect chemicals that cannot be processed by olfactory receptors, such as large and/or aqueous molecules, the types of molecules that constitute pheromones. Also called *Jacobson's organ*. [14]

W

warmth fiber A sensory nerve fiber that fires when skin temperature increases. [13]

wave An oscillation that travels through a medium by transferring energy from one particle or point to another without causing any permanent displacement of the medium. [2]

Weber fraction The constant of proportionality in Weber's law. [1]

Weber's law The principle describing the relationship between stimulus and resulting sensation that says the just noticeable difference is a constant fraction of the comparison stimulus. [11]

white noise Noise consisting of all audible frequencies in equal amounts. White noise in hearing is analogous to white light in vision, for which all wavelengths are present. [9]

References

A

Abraira, V. E., and Ginty, D. D. (2013). The sensory neurons of touch. *Neuron* 79: 618–639.

Abrams, J., Nizam, A., and Carrasco, M. (2012). Isoeccentric locations are not equivalent: The extent of the vertical meridian asymmetry. *Vision Res* 52: 70–78.

Accolla, R., Bathellier, B., Petersen, C. C. H., and Carleton, A. (2007). Differential spatial representation of taste modalities in the rat gustatory cortex. *J Neurosci* 27: 1396–1404. https://doi.org/10.1523/jneurosci.5188-06.2007.

Ackerman, D. (1990). *A Natural History of the Senses*. New York: Random House.

Addams, R. (1834). An account of a peculiar optical phenomenon seen after having looked at a moving body, etc. *Lond Edinb Philos Mag J Sci* 5: 373–374.

Adelson, E. H., and Bergen, J. R. (1985). Spatiotemporal energy models perception of motion. *J Opt Soc Am A* 2: 284–299.

Agrawal, Y., Carey, J. P., Della Santina, C. C., Schubert, M. C., and Minor, L. B. (2009). Disorders of balance and vestibular function in US adults: Data from the National Health and Nutrition Examination Survey, 2001–2004. *Arch Intern Med* 169(10): 938–944.

Aguirre M., A., Couderc A., Epinat-Duclos, J., and Mascaro, O. (2019). Infants discriminate the source of social touch at stroking speeds eliciting maximal firing rates in CT-fibers. *Dev Cogn Neurosci* 36: 100639.

Ahissar, M., and Hochstein, S. (2004). The reverse hierarchy theory of visual perceptual learning. *Trends Cogn Sci* 8: 457–464.

Al Aïn, S., Poupon, D., Hétu, S., Mercier, N., Steffener, J., and Frasnelli, J. (2019). Smell training improves olfactory function and alters brain structure. *NeuroImage* 189: 45–54. https://doi.org/10.1016/j.neuroimage.2019.01.008.

Alais, D., and Blake, R. (2005). *Binocular Rivalry and Perceptual Ambiguity*. Cambridge, MA: MIT Press.

Alberti, L. B. (1970). *On Painting* Translated with introduction and notes by John R. Spencer. New Haven, CT: Yale University Press.

Alexander, J. M. (2016). Nonlinear frequency compression: Influence of start frequency and input bandwidth on consonant and vowel recognition. *J Acoust Soc Am* 139: 938–957. https://doi.org/10.1121/1.4941916.

Alpern, M., Kitahara, K., and Krantz, D. H. (1983). Classical tritanopia. *J Physiol* 335: 655–681.

Alvarez, G. A. (2011). Representing multiple objects as an ensemble enhances visual cognition. *Trends Cogn Sci* 15: 122–131.

American Lung Association. (2018). *How Your Lungs Get the Job Done* https://www.lung.org/about-us/blog/2017/07/how-your-lungs-work.html.

American Standards Association. (1960). *Acoustical Terminology SI, 1–1960*. New York: American Standards Association.

Andersen, T. S., Tiippana, K., and Sams, M. (2004). Factors influencing audiovisual fission and fusion illusions. *Brain Res Cog Brain Res* 21: 301–308. https://doi.org/10.1016/j.cogbrainres.2004.06.004.

Anderson, B. L. (2020). Mid-level vision. *Curr Biol* 30(3): R105–R109. https://doi.org/10.1016/j.cub.2019.11.088.

Anderson, J. S., Lampl, I., Gillespie, D. C., and Ferster, D. (2000). Contribution of noise to contrast invariance of orientation tuning in cat visual cortex. *Science* 290: 1968–1972.

Anderson, P. W., and Zahorik, P. (2014). Auditory/visual distance estimation: Accuracy and variability. *Front Psychol* 5: 1097.

Andrew, D., and Craig, A. D. (2001). Spinothalamic lamina I neurons selectively sensitive to histamine: A central neural pathway for itch. *Nat Neurosci 4*, 72–77.

Anzai, A., Chowdhury, S. A., and DeAngelis, G. C. (2011). Coding of stereoscopic depth information in visual areas V3 and V3A. *J Neurosci 31*(28): 10270–10282. doi: 10.1523/jneurosci.5956-10.2011

Angelaki, D., McHenry, M., Dickman, J. D., Newlands, S., and Hess, B. (1999). Computation of inertial motion: Neural strategies to resolve ambiguous otolith information. *J Neurosci* 19: 316–327.

Anzai, A., and DeAngelis, G. C. (2010). Neural computations underlying depth perception. *Curr Opin Neurobiol* 20: 367–375.

Archie, P., Bruera, E., and Cohen, L. (2013). Music-based interventions in palliative cancer care: A review of quantitative studies and neurobiological literature. *Support Care Cancer* 21: 2609–2624.

Ardila, D., Kiraly, A. P., Bharadwaj, S., Choi, B., Reicher, J. J., Peng, L., et al. (2019). End-to-end lung cancer screening with three-dimensional deep learning on low-dose chest computed tomography. *Nat Med* 25: 954–961. https://doi.org/10.1038/s41591-019-0447-x.

Arena, E., & Hamburger, K. (2023). Olfactory and visual vs. multimodal landmark processing in human wayfinding: a virtual reality experiment. *Journal of Cognitive Psychology*, 35(6-7), 688–709.

Arend, L., and Reeves, A. (1986). Simultaneous color constancy. *J Opt Soc Am A* 3: 1743–1751.

Arshamian, A., Gerkin, R. C., Kruspe, N., Wnuk, E., Floyd, S., O'Meara, C., Rodriguez, G. G., et al. (2022). The perception of odor pleasantness is shared across cultures. *Curr Biol* 32(9): 2061–2066.

Arshamian, A., Iannilli, E., Gerber, J. C., Willander, J., Persson, J., Seo, H.-S., Hummel, T., and Larsson, M. (2013). The functional neuroanatomy of odor-evoked autobiographical memories cued by odors and words. *Neuropsychologia* 51: 123–131.

Arshamian, A., Iravani, B., Majid, A., and Lundström, J. N. (2018). Respiration modulates olfactory memory consolidation in humans. *J Neurosci* 38: 10286–10294. https://doi.org/10.1523/jneurosci.3360-17.2018.

Arzi, A., Holtzman, Y., Samnon, P., Eshel, N., Harel, E., and Sobel, N. (2014). Olfactory aversive conditioning during sleep reduces cigarette-smoking behavior. *J Neurosci* 34: 15382–15393.

Arzi, A., Rozenkrantz, L., Gorodisky, L., Rozenkrantz, D., Holtzman, Y., Ravia, A., Bekinschtein,T. A., et al. (2020). Olfactory sniffing signals consciousness in unresponsive patients with brain injuries. Nature 581(7809): 428–433.

Aschenbrenner, K., Hummel, C., Teszmer, K., Krone, F., Ishimaru, T., Seo, H. S., and Hummel, T. (2008). The influence of olfactory loss on dietary behaviors. *Laryngoscope* 118: 135–144.

Ashar, Y. K., Gordon, A., Schubiner, H., Uipi, C., Knight, K., Anderson, Z., Carlisle, J., et al. (2022). Effect of pain reprocessing therapy vs placebo and usual care for patients with chronic back pain: A randomized clinical trial. *JAMA Psychiatry* 79(1): 13–23. https://doi.org/10.1001/jamapsychiatry.2021.2669.

Athos, E. A., Levinson, B., Kistler, A., Zemansky, J., Bostrom, A., and Freimer, N. (2007). Dichotomy and perceptual distortions in absolute pitch ability. *Proc Nat Acad Sci USA* 104: 14795–14800.

Attneave, F. (1954). Some informational aspects of visual perception. *Psychol Rev* 61: 183–193.

Attneave, F., and Olson, R. K. (1971). Pitch as a medium: A new approach to psychophysical scaling. *Am J Psychol* 84: 147–166.

Au, R., Joung, P., Nicholas, M., Obler, L. K., Kass, R., and Albert, M. L. (1995). Naming ability across the adult life span. *Aging Neuropsychol Cogn* 2: 300–311.

Aubert, H. (1886). Die Bewegungsempfindung. *Arch Ges Physiol* 39: 347–370.

Awh, E., Belopolsky, A. V., and Theeuwes, J. (2012). Top-down versus bottom-up attentional control: A failed theoretical dichotomy. *Trends Cog Sci* 16: 437–443. https://doi.org/10.1016/j.tics.2012.06.010.

Ayabe-Kanamura, S., Schicker, I., Laska, M., Hudson, R., Distel, H., Kobayakawa, T., and Saito, S. (1998). Differences in perception of everyday odors: A Japanese-German cross-cultural study. *Chem Senses* 23: 31–38.

B

Babadi, B., Casti, A., Xiao, Y., Kaplan, E., and Paninski, L. (2010). A generalized linear model of the impact of direct and indirect inputs to the lateral geniculate nucleus. *J Vis* 10: 22.

Bach-y-Rita, P., Collins, C. C., Saunders, F. A., White, B., and Scadden, L. (1969). Vision substitution by tactile image projection. *Nature* 221: 963–964.

Bahill, A. T., and Stark, L. (1979). The trajectories of saccadic eye movements. *Sci Am* 240: 108–117.

Bai, L., Mesgarzadeh, S., Ramesh, K. S., Huey, E. L., Liu, Y., Gray, L. A., Aitken T. J., et al. (2019). Genetic identification of vagal sensory neurons that control feeding. *Cell* 179(5): 1129–1143.e23. https://doi.org/10.1016/j.cell.2019.10.031.

Bainbridge, W. A. (2017). The memorability of people: Intrinsic memorability across transformations of a person's face. *J Exp Psychol Learn Mem Cogn* 43(5): 706–716. https://doi.org/10.1037/xlm0000339.

Baldauf, D., and Desimone, R. (2014). Neural mechanisms of object-based attention. *Science* 344: 424–427.

Baloh, R., and Halmagyi, G. M. (Eds.). (1996). *Disorders of the Vestibular System*. Oxford: Oxford University Press.

Banks, M. S., Aslin, R. N., and Letson, R. D. (1975). Sensitive period for the development of human binocular vision. *Science* 190: 675–677.

Barclay, C. D., Cutting, J. E., and Kozlowski, L. T. (1978). Temporal and spatial factors in gait perception that influence gender recognition. *Percept Psychophys* 23: 145–152.

Baringa, M. (2002). How the brain's clock gets daily enlightenment. *Science* 295: 955–957.

Barlow, H. B. (1961). Possible principles underlying the transformations of sensory messages. In W. A. Rosenblith (Ed.), *Sensory Communication* (pp. 53–85). Cambridge, MA: MIT Press; and New York: Wiley.

Barlow, H. B. (1972). Single units and sensation: A neuron doctrine for perceptual psychology. *Perception* 1: 371–394.

Barlow, H. B. (1995). The neuron doctrine in perception. In M. S. Gazzaniga (Ed.), *The Cognitive Neurosciences* (pp. 415–435). Cambridge, MA: MIT Press.

Barlow, H. B. (2001). Redundancy reduction revisited. *Netw Comput Neural Syst* 12: 241–253.

Barlow, H. B., Blakemore, C., and Pettigrew, J. D. (1967). The neural mechanism of binocular depth discrimination. *J Physiol* 193: 327–342.

Barlow, H. B., and Levick, W. R. (1965). The mechanism of directionally selective units in rabbit's retina. *J Physiol* 178: 477–504.

Barnett-Cowan, M., and Harris, L. R. (2009). Perceived timing of vestibular stimulation relative to touch, light and sound. *Exp Brain Res* 198(2–3): 221–231. https://doi.org/10.1007/s00221-009-1779-4.

Barr, C. C., Schultheis, L. W., and Robinson, D. A. (1976). Voluntary, non-visual control of the human vestibulo-ocular reflex. *Acta Otolaryngol* 81: 365–375.

Barry, S. R. (2009). *Fixing My Gaze*. New York: Basic Books.

Bartoshuk, L. M. (1978). History of taste research. In E. C. Carterette and M. P. Friedman (Eds.), *Tasting and Smelling* (vol. VI.A, pp. 3–18). New York: Academic Press.

Bartoshuk, L. M. (1979). Bitter taste of saccharin: Related to the genetic ability to taste the bitter substance 6-*n*-propylthiouracil (PROP). *Science* 205: 934–935.

Bartoshuk, L. M. (1991). Taste, smell and pleasure. In R. C. Bolles (Ed.), *The Hedonics of Taste* (pp. 15–28). Hillsdale, NJ: Erlbaum.

Bartoshuk, L. M., Cartalanotto, J. A., Hoffman, H. J., Logan, H. L., and Snyder, D. J. (2012). Taste damage (otitis media, tonsillectomy and head and neck cancer) can intensify oral sensations. *Physiol Behav* 107: 516–526.

Bartoshuk, L. M., Fast, K., and Snyder, D. (2005). Differences in our sensory worlds: Invalid comparisons with labeled scales. *Curr Dir Psychol Sci* 14: 122–125.

Bartoshuk, L. M., Marino, S., Snyder, D. J., and Stamps, J. (2013). Head trauma, taste damage and weight gain. *Chem Senses* 38: 626.

Bartoshuk, L. M., and Wolfe, J. M. (1990). Conditioned taste aversions in humans: Are they olfactory aversions? *Chem Senses* 15: 551.

Basson, M. D., Bartoshuk, L. M., Dichello, S. Z., Weiffenbach, J., and Duffy, V. B. (2003). Colon cancer and genetic variation in taste. *Chem Senses* 28: 109.

Bates, L. A., Sayialel, K. N., Njiraini, N. W., Moss, C. J., Poole, J. H., and Byrne, R. W. (2007). Elephants classify human ethnic groups by odor and garment color. *Current Biology* 17(22): 1938–1942.

Baus, O., and Bouchard, S. (2017). Exposure to an unpleasant odour increases the sense of presence in virtual reality. *Virtual Reality* 21(2): 59–74.

Bautista, D. M., Siemens, J., Glazer, J. M., Tsuruda, P. R., Basbaum, A. I., Stucky, C. L., Jordt, S. E., and Julius, D. (2007). The menthol receptor TRPM8 is the principal detector of environmental cold. *Nature* 448: 204–208.

Beck, J. (1982). Textural segmentation. In J. Beck (Ed.), *Organization and Representation in Perception* (pp. 285–317). Hillsdale, NJ: Erlbaum.

Behrmann, M., and Avidan, G. (2005). Congenital prosopagnosia: Face-blind from birth. *Trends Cogn Sci* 9: 180–187.

Behrmann, M., and Plaut, D. C. (2020). Hemispheric organization for visual object recognition: A theoretical account and empirical evidence. *Perception* 49: 374–404. https://doi.org/10.1177/0301006619899049.

Bensmaia, S. J., Denchev, P. V., Dammann, J. F., 3rd, Craig, J. C., and Hsiao, S. S. (2008). The representation of stimulus orientation in the early stages of somatosensory processing. *J Neurosci* 28(3): 776–786. https://doi.org/10.1523/JNEUROSCI.4162-07.2008.

Benson, P. J., Beedie, S. A., Shephard, E., Giegling, I., Rujescu, D., and St. Clair, D. (2012). Simple viewing tests can detect eye movement abnormalities that distinguish schizophrenia cases from controls with exceptional accuracy. *Biol Psychiatry* 72: 716–724.

Bentham, J. (1876). *An Introduction to the Principles of Morals and Legislation*. Oxford: Clarendon Press.

Berbaum, K. S., Franken, E. A., Caldwell, R. T., Shartz, K., and Madsen, M. (2019). Satisfaction of search in radiology. In E. Samei and E. A. Krupinski (Eds.), *The Handbook of Medical Image Perception and Techniques* (2nd ed., pp. 121–166). Cambridge: Cambridge University Press.

Bergen, J. R., and Adelson, E. H. (1988). Early vision and texture perception. *Nature* 333: 363–364.

Berger, A., Henderson, M., Nadoolman, W., Duffy, V. B., Cooper, D., Saberski, L., and Bartoshuk, L. (1995). Oral capsaicin provides temporary relief for oral mucositis pain secondary to chemotherapy/radiation therapy. *J Pain Symptom Manage* 10: 243–248.

Berlin, B., and Kay, P. (1969). *Basic Color Terms: Their Universality and Evolution*. Berkeley: University of California Press.

Bermúdez Rey, M. C., Clark, T. K., Wang, W., Leeder, T., Bian, Y., and Merfeld, D. M. (2016). Vestibular perceptual thresholds increase above the age of 40. *Front Neurol* 7: 162.

Bernstein, I. L. (1978). Learned taste aversions in children receiving chemotherapy. *Science* 200: 1302–1303.

Berntson, G. G., and Khalsa, S. S. (2021). Neural circuits of interoception. *Trends Neurosci* 44(1): 17–28. https://doi.org/10.1016/j.tins.2020.09.011.

Berry, M. H., Holt, A., Salari, A., Veit, J., Visel, M., Levitz, J., Aghi, K., et al. (2019). Restoration of high-sensitivity and adapting vision with a cone opsin. *Nat Commun* 10: 1221. https://doi.org/10.1038/s41467-019-09124-x.

Berthoz, A., Israel, I., Georges-Francois, P., Grasso, R., and Tsuzuku, T. (1995). Spatial memory of body linear displacement: What is being stored? *Science* 269: 95–98.

Bertino, M., Beauchamp, G. K., and Engelman, K. (1982). Long-term reduction in dietary sodium alters the taste of salt. *Am J Clin Nutr* 36: 1134–1144.

Bertolini, G., Ramat, S., Laurens, J., Bockisch, C. J., Marti, S., Straumann, D., and Palla, A. (2011). Velocity storage contribution to vestibular self-motion perception in healthy human subjects. *J Neurophysiol* 105: 209–223.

Best, C. T., McRoberts, G. W., and Sithole, N. T. (1988). Examination of perceptual reorganization for non-native speech contrasts: Zulu click discrimination by English-speaking adults and infants*J Exp Psychol Hum Percept Perform.* 14: 345–360.

Bharadwaj, H. M., Verhulst, S., Shaheen L., Liberman, M. C., and Shinn-Cunningham, B. G. (2014). Cochlear neuropathy and the coding of supra-threshold sound. *Front Syst Neurosci* 8: 26. https://doi.org/10.3389/fnsys.2014.00026.

Bhutani, S., Gottfried, J., and Kahnt, T. (2017). *Central olfactory mechanisms underlying sleep-dependent changes in food processing.* Paper presented at the Cognitive Neuroscience Society Annual Meeting, San Francisco, CA, March 27, 2017.

Bhutani, S., Howard, J. D., Reynolds, R., Zee, P. C., Gottfried, J., and Kahnt, T. (2019). Olfactory connectivity mediates sleep-dependent food choices in humans. *eLife* 8: e49053. https://doi.org/10.7554/eLife.49053.

Bialystok, E., and Hakuta, K. (1994). *In Other Words: The Science and Psychology of Second-Language Acquisition.* New York: Basic Books.

Biederman, I. (1987). Recognition-by-components: A theory of human image understanding. *Psychol Rev* 94: 115–147.

Bigelow, R. T., and Agrawal, Y. (2015). Vestibular involvement in cognition: Visuospatial ability, attention, executive function, and memory. *Journal of Vestibular Research* 25: 73–89. doi: 10.3233/VES-150544.

Birch, E., and Petrig, B. (1996). FPL and VEP measures of fusion, stereopsis and stereoacuity in normal infants. *Vision Res* 36: 1321–1326.

Birznieks, I., Macefield, V. G., Westling, G., and Johansson, R. S. (2009). Slowly adapting mechanoreceptors in the borders of the human fingernail encode fingertip forces. *J Neurosci* 29: 9370–9379.

Bisley, J. W., and Mirpour, K. (2019). The neural instantiation of a priority map. *Curr Opin Psychol* 29: 108–112. https://doi.org/10.1016/j.copsyc.2019.01.002.

Björnsdotter, M., Löken, L., Olausson, H., Vallbo, A., and Wessberg, J. (2009). Somatotopic organization of gentle touch processing in the posterior insular cortex. *J Neurosci* 29: 9314–9320.

Blackshaw, L. A., Brookes, S. J., Grundy, D., and Schemann, M. (2007). Sensory transmission in the gastrointestinal tract. *Neurogastroenterol Motil* 19(1 Suppl): 1–19. https://doi.org/10.1111/j.1365-2982.2006.00871.x.

Blake, A., and Bulthoff, H. (1990). Does the brain know the physics of specular reflection? *Nature* 343(6254): 165–168.

Blake, R. (1988). Cat spatial vision. *Trends Neurosci* 11: 78–83.

Blake, R., and Logothetis, N. K. (2002). Visual competition. *Nat Rev Neurosci* 3: 13–21.

Blake, R., Sloane, M., and Fox, R. (1981). Further developments in binocular summation. *Percept Psychophys* 30: 266–276.

Blake, R., and Wilson, H. (2011). Binocular vision. *Vision Research 51*(7): 754–770. doi: 10.1016/j.visres.2010.10.009

Blakemore, C., and Campbell, F. W. (1969). On the existence of neurons in the human visual system selectively sensitive to the orientation and size of images. *J Physiol* 203: 237–260.

Blakemore, S.-J., Wolpert, D. M., and Frith, C. D. (1998). Central cancellation of self-produced tickle sensation. *Nat Neurosci* 1: 635–640.

Blakeslee, A.F. and Fox, A. L. (1932). Our different taste worlds. *J Heredity* 23: 97–107.

Blasdel, G. G., and Salama, G. (1986). Voltage-sensitive dyes reveal a modular organization in monkey striate cortex. *Nature* 321: 579–585.

Block, E., Jang, S., Matsunami, H., Sekharan, S., Dethier, B., Ertem, M. Z., Gundala, S., et al. (2015). Implausibility of the vibrational theory of olfaction. *Proc Natl Acad Sci USA* 112: E2766–E2774.

Blood, A. J., and Zatorre, R. J. (2001). Intensely pleasurable responses to music correlate with activity in brain regions implicated in reward and emotion. *Proc Natl Acad Sci USA* 98: 11818–11823.

Blundell, J., and Hill, A. J. (1986). Paradoxical effects of an intense sweetener (aspartame) on appetite. *Lancet* 1: 1092–1093.

Boesveldt, S., Lindau, S. T., McClintock, M. K., Hummel, T., and Lundstrom, J. N. (2011). Gustatory and olfactory dysfunction in older adults: A national probability study. *Rhinology* 49: 324–330.

Bolton, T. L. (1894). Rhythm. *Am J Psychol* 6: 145–238.

Bompas, A., Kendall, G., and Sumner, P. (2013). Spotting fruit versus picking fruit as the selective advantage of human colour vision. *i-Perception* 4: 84–94.

Bonneh, Y. S., Cooperman, A., and Sagi, D. (2001). Motion-induced blindness in normal observers. *Nature* 411: 798–801. https://doi.org/10.1038/35081073.

Bonnen, K., Matthis, J. S., Gibaldi, A., Banks, M. S., Levi, D. M., and Hayhoe, M. (2021). Binocular vision and the control of foot placement during walking in natural terrain. *Sci Rep* 11(1): 20881. https://doi.org/10.1038/s41598-021-99846-0.

Boothe, R. G., Dobson, V., and Teller, D. Y. (1985). Postnatal development of vision in human and non-human primates. *Annu Rev Neurosci* 8: 495–545.

Boring, E. G. (1942). *Sensation and Perception in the History of Experimental Psychology.* New York: Appleton-Century-Crofts.

Borstelmann, S. M. (2020). Machine learning principles for radiology investigators. *Acad Radiol* 27: 13–25. https://doi.org/10.1016/j.acra.2019.07.030.

Bortolami, S. B., Pierobon, A., DiZio, P., and Lackner, J. R. (2006). Localization of the subjective vertical during roll, pitch, and recumbent yaw body tilt. *Exp Brain Res* 173: 364–373.

Boshra, R., and Kastner, S. (2022). Attention control in the primate brain. *Curr Opin Neurobiol* 76: 102605. https://doi.org/10.1016/j.conb.2022.102605.

Bosmans, J., Jorissen, C., Gilles, A., Mertens, G., Engelborghs, S., Cras, P., Van Ombergen, A., et al. (2021). Vestibular function in older adults with cognitive impairment: A systematic review. *Ear and Hearing* 42: 1119–1126. doi: 10.1097/AUD.0000000000001040

Brady, T. F., Konkle, T., Alvarez, G. A., and Oliva, A. (2008). Visual long-term memory has a massive storage capacity for object details. *Proc Natl Acad Sci USA* 105: 14325–14329.

Brainard, D. H. (2019). Color, pattern, and the retinal cone mosaic. *Curr Opin Behav Sci* 30: 41–47. https://doi.org/10.1016/j.cobeha.2019.05.005.

Brainard, D. H., and Hurlbert, A. C. (2015). Colour vision: Understanding #TheDress. *Curr Biol* 25: R551–R554.

Bramble D. M., and Lieberman, D. E. (2004). Endurance running and the evolution of *Homo. Nature* 432: 345–352.

Brandt, T., et al. (2005). Vestibular loss causes hippocampal atrophy and impaired spatial memory in humans. *Brain* 128(11): 2732–2741.

Brann, D. H., Tsukahara, T., Weinreb, C., Lipovsek, M., Van den Berge, K., Gong, B., Chance, R., et al. (2020). Non-neuronal expression of SARS-CoV-2 entry genes in the olfactory system suggests mechanisms underlying COVID-19-associated anosmia. *Sci Adv* 6(31): eabc5801.

Brefczynski, J. A., and DeYoe, E. A. (1999). A physiological correlate of the "spotlight" of visual attention. *Nat Neurosci* 2: 370–374.

Bremner, E. A., Mainland, J. D., Khan, R. M., and Sobel, N. (2003). The prevalence of androstenone anosmia. *Chem Senses* 28: 423–432.

Bressler, S., Masud, S., Bharadwaj, H., and Shinn-Cunningham, B. (2014). Bottom-up influences of voice continuity in focusing selective auditory attention. *Psych Res* 78: 349–360.

Breuer, J. (1874). Ueber die Funktion der Bogengänge des Ohrlabyrinths [About the functions of the semicircular canals of the ear labyrinth]. *Med Jahrbücher* 2nd series 4: 72–124.

Bridgeman, B. (2014). Restoring adult stereopsis: A vision researcher's personal experience. *Optom Vis Sci* 91: e135–139.

Brown, A. C. (1874). The sense of rotation and the anatomy and physiology of the semicircular canals of the internal ear. *J Anat Physiol* 8: 327–331.

Brown, A. M. (1990). Development of visual sensitivity to light and color vision in human infants: a critical review. *Vision Res* 30(8): 1159–1188. doi: 10.1016/0042-6989(90)90173-i.

Brownell, W. E. (2017). What is electromotility? The history of its discovery and its relevance to acoustics. *Acoustics Today* 13: 20–27.

Brugge, J. F., and Howard, M. A. (2002). Hearing. In V. S. Ramachandran (Ed.), *Encyclopedia of the Human Brain* (pp. 429–448). New York: Academic Press.

Brughera, A., Dunai, L., and Hartman, W. M. (2013). Human interaural time difference thresholds for sine tones: The high-frequency limit. *J Acoust Soc Am* 133: 2839–2855.

Brungart, D. S., Durlach, N. I., and Rabinowitz, W. M. (1999). Auditory localization of nearby sources. II. Localization of a broadband source. *J Acoust Soc Am* 106: 1956–1968.

Buchsbaum, G. (1980). A spatial processor model for object colour perception. *J Franklin Inst* 310: 1–26.

Buchsbaum, G., and Gottschalk, A. (1983). Trichromacy, opponent colours coding, and optimum colour information transmission in the retina. *Proc R Soc Lond B Biol Sci* 220: 89–113.

Buck, L., and Axel, R. (1991). A novel multigene family may encode odorant receptors: A molecular basis for odor recognition. *Cell* 65: 175–187.

Buck, S. (2015). Brown. *Curr Biol* 25: R536–R537.

Buetti, S., Cronin, D. A., Madison, A. M., Wang, Z., and Lleras, A. (2016). Towards a better understanding of parallel visual processing in human vision: Evidence for exhaustive analysis of visual information. *J Exp Psychol Gen* 145(6): 672–707. https://doi.org/10.1037/xge0000163.

Burgess, A. (2018a). Signal detection in radiology. In E. Samei and E. A. Krupinski (Eds.), *The Handbook of Medical Image Perception and Techniques* (2nd ed., pp. 49–75). Cambridge: Cambridge University Press.

Burgess, A. (2018b). Signal detection theory: A brief history. In E. Samei and E. A. Krupinski (Eds.), *The Handbook of Medical Image Perception and Techniques* (2nd ed., pp. 28–48). Cambridge: Cambridge University Press.

Burton, A. M. (2013). Why has research in face recognition progressed so slowly? The importance of variability. *Q J Exp Psychol* 66: 1467–1485.

Burzynska, J., Wang, Q. J., Spence, C., and Bastian, S. E. P. (2019). Taste the bass: Low frequencies increase the perception of body and aromatic intensity in red wine. *Multisensory Res* 32: 429–254. https://doi.org/10.1163/22134808-20191406.

Bushnell, B. N., Harding, P. J., Kosai, Y., and Pasupathy, A. (2011). Partial occlusion modulates contour-based shape encoding in primate area V4. *J Neurosci* 31: 4012–4024.

Butowt, R., and von Bartheld, C. S. (2021). Anosmia in COVID-19: Underlying mechanisms and assessment of an olfactory route to brain infection. Neuroscientist 27(6): 582–603.

Bylinskii, Z., Isola, P., Bainbridge, C., Torralba, A., and Oliva, A. (2015). Intrinsic and extrinsic effects on image memorability. *Vision Res* 116(Pt B): 165–178.

C

Cadiou, H., Aoudé, I., Tazir, B., Molinas, A., Fenech, C., Meunier, N., and Grosmaitre, X. (2014). Postnatal odorant exposure induces peripheral olfactory plasticity at the cellular level. *J Neurosci* 34: 4857–4870.

Cahill, L., Babinsky, R., Markowitsch, H. J., and McGaugh, J. L. (1995). The amygdala and emotional memory. *Nature* 377: 295–296.

Cain, W. S., and Engen, T. (1969). Olfactory adaptation and the scaling of odor intensity. In C. Pfaffmann (Ed.), *Olfaction and Taste III* (pp. 127–141). New York: Rockefeller University Press.

Cain, W. S., and Johnson, F., Jr. (1978). Lability of odor pleasantness: Influence of mere exposure. *Perception* 7: 459–465.

Cameron, E. L. (2007). Measures of human olfactory perception during pregnancy. *Chem Senses* 32: 775–782.

Campbell, F. W., and Green, D. G. (1965). Optical and retinal factors affecting visual resolution. *J Physiol* 181: 576–593.

Campbell, F. W., and Robson, J. G. (1968). Application of Fourier analysis to the visibility of gratings. *J Physiol* 197: 551–556.

Campbell, R., Pascalis, O., Coleman, M., Wallace, B., and Benson, P. J. (1997). Are faces of different species perceived categorically by human observers? *Proc R Soc Lond B Biol Sci* 264: 1429–1434.

Cannon, W. B. (1939). *The Wisdom of the Body.* New York: Norton.

Canzoneri, E., Ubaldi, S., Rastelli, V., Finisguerra, A., Bassolino, M., and Serino, A. (2013). Tool use reshapes the boundaries of body and peripersonal space representations. *Exp Brain Res* 228: 25–42.

Capaldi, E. D., Hunter, M. J., and Privitera, G. J. (2004). Odor of taste stimuli in conditioned "taste" aversion learning. *Behav Neurosci* 118: 1400–1408.

Carriot, J., Cian, C., Paillard, A., Denise, P., Lackner, J. R., et al. (2011). Influence of multisensory graviceptive information on the apparent zenith. *Exp Brain Res* 208(4): 569–579.

Carskadon, M., and Herz, R. S. (2004). Minimal olfactory perception during sleep: Why odor alarms will not work for humans. *Sleep* 27: 402–405.

Carskadon, M. A., Wyatt, J., Etgen, G., and Rosekind, M. R. (1989). Nonvisual sensory experiences in dreams of college students. *Sleep Res* 18: 159.

Casagrande, V. A., Yazar, F., Jones, K. D., and Ding, Y. (2007). The morphology of the koniocellular axon pathway in the macaque monkey. *Cereb Cortex* 17: 2334–2345.

Cascio, C. J., Moore, D., and McGlone, F. (2019). Social touch and human development. *Dev Cogn Neurosci* 35: 5–11. https://doi.org/10.1016/j.dcn.2018.04.009.

Case, L. K., Laubacher, C. M., Olausson, H., Wang, B., Spagnolo, P. A., and Bushnell, M. C. (2016). Encoding of touch intensity but not pleasantness in human primary somatosensory cortex. *J Neurosci* 36: 5850–5860.

Castelhano, M. S., and Krzyś, K. (2020). Rethinking space: A review of perception, attention, and memory in scene processing. *Annu Rev Vis Sci* 6: 563–586. https://doi.org/10.1146/annurev-vision-121219-081745.

Castet, E., Jeanjean, S., and Masson, G. S. (2001). "Saccadic suppression": No need for an active extra-retinal mechanism. *Trends Neurosci* 24: 316–318.

Castro, J. B., Ramanathan, A., and Chennubhotla, C. S. (2013). Categorical dimensions of human odor descriptor space revealed by non-negative matrix factorization. *PLOS ONE* 8: e73289.

Caval-Holme, F., Zhang, Y., and Feller, M. B. (2019). Gap junction coupling shapes the encoding of light in the developing retina. *Curr Biol* 29: 4024–4035. https://doi.org/10.1016/j.cub.2019.10.025.

Cavanagh, P., Hunt, A. R., Afraz, A., and Rolfs, M. (2010). Visual stability based on remapping of attention pointers. *Trends Cogn Sci* 14: 147–153.

Cavdan, K. M., Doerschner, K., and Drewing, K. (2021). Task and material properties interactively affect softness explorations along different dimensions. *IEEE Trans Haptics* 14(3): 603–614. https://doi.org/10.1109/TOH.2021.3069626.

Cave, K. R., and Bichot, N. P. (1999). Visuospatial attention: Beyond a spotlight model. *Psychon Bull Rev* 6: 204–223.

Caves, E. M., Green, P. A., Zipple, M. N., Peters, S., Johnsen, S., and Nowicki, S. (2018). Categorical perception of colour signals in a songbird. *Nature* 560: 365–367. https://doi.org/10.1038/s41586-018-0377-7.

Chabris, C. F., and Simons, D. J. (2011). You do not talk about Fight Club if you do not notice Fight Club: Inattentional blindness for a simulated real-world assault. *i-Perception* 2. https://i-perception.perceptionweb.com.

Chae, H., Banerjee, A., Dussauze, M., and Albeanu, D. F. (2022). Long-range functional loops in the mouse olfactory system and their roles in computing odor identity. *Neuron* 110(23): 3970–3985.

Champagne, F. A. (2008). Epigenetic mechanisms and the transgenerational effects of maternal care. *Front Neuroendocrinol* 29: 386–397.

Chang, E. F., Rieger, J. W., Johnson, K., Berger, M. S., Barbaro, N. M., and Knight, R. T. (2010). Categorical speech representation in human superior temporal gyrus. *Nat Neurosci* 13: 1428–1432.

Chang, L., and Tsao, D. Y. (2017). The code for facial identity in the primate brain. *Cell* 169: 1013–1028 e1014. https://doi.org/10.1016/j.cell.2017.05.011.

Changizi, M. A., Zhang, Q., and Shimojo, S. (2006). Bare skin, blood, and the evolution of primate colour vision. *Biol Lett* 2: 217–221.

Chapuis, J., Messaoudi, B., Ferreira, G., and Ravel, N. (2007). Importance of retronasal and orthonasal olfaction for odor aversion memory in rats. *Behav Neurosci* 121: 1383–1392.

Chen. J., Zhou, W., and Chen, D. (2012). Binaral rivalry in the presence of visual perceptual and semantic influences. *PLOS ONE* 7(10): e47317. https://doi.org/10.1371/journal.pone.0047317.

Chen, K., Kogan, J. F., and Fontanini, A. (2021). Spatially distributed representation of taste quality in the gustatory insular cortex of behaving mice. *Curr Biol* 31: 247–256.

Chen, Z., and Padmanabhan, K. (2022). Top-down feedback enables flexible coding strategies in the olfactory cortex. *Cell Rep* 38(12): 110545.

Cheung, C., Hamilton, L. S., Johnson, K., and Chang, E. H. (2016). The auditory representation of speech sounds in human motor cortex. *eLife* 5: e12577.

Chino, Y. M., Smith, E. L., III, Hatta, S., and Cheng, H. (1997). Postnatal development of binocular disparity sensitivity in neurons of the primate visual cortex. *J Neurosci* 17: 296–307.

Choi, J. S., Jang, S. S., Kim, J., Hur, K., Ference, E., and Wrobel, B. (2021). Association between olfactory dysfunction and mortality in US adults. *JAMA Otolaryngol Head Neck Surg* 147(1): 49–55.

Chong, S. C., and Treisman, A. (2003). Representation of statistical properties. *Vision Res* 43: 393–404.

Chopin, A., Levi, D., Knill, D., and Bavelier, D. (2016). The absolute disparity anomaly and the mechanism of relative disparities. *J Vision* 16: 2. https://doi.org/10.1167/16.8.2.

Chu, S., and Downes, J. J. (2000). Long live Proust: The odour-cued autobiographical memory bump. *Cognition* 75: B41–B50.

Chubb, C., and Landy, M. S. (1994). Orthogonal distribution analysis: A new approach to the study of texture perception. In M. S. Landy and J. A. Movshon (Eds.), *Computational Models of Visual Processing* (pp. 291–301). Cambridge, MA: MIT Press.

Chun, M. M., Golomb, J. D., and Turk-Browne, N. B. (2011). A taxonomy of external and internal attention. *Annu Rev Psychol* 62: 73–101.

Chun, M. M., and Potter, M. C. (1995). A two-stage model for multiple target detection in RSVP. *J Exp Psychol Hum Percept Perform* 21: 109–127.

Cimmino, R. L., Spitoni, G., Serino, A., Antonucci, G., Catagni, M., Camagni, M., Haggard, P., et al. (2013). Plasticity of body representations after surgical arm elongation in an achondroplasic patient. *Restor Neurol Neurosci* 31: 287–298.

Clark, F. J., and Horch, K. W. (1986). Kinesthesia. In K. R. Boff, L. Kaufman, and J. P. Thomas (Eds.), *Handbook of Perception and Human Performance*, Vol. 1: *Sensory Processes and Perception* (pp. 13–1 to 13–62). New York: Wiley.

Classen, C., Howes, D., and Synnott, A. (1994). *Aroma: The Cultural History of Smell.* London: Routledge.

Cleary, A. M., Konkel, K. E., Nomi, J. S., and McCabe, D. P. (2010). Odor recognition without identification. *Mem Cognit* 38: 452–460.

Clifford, C. W. G. (2009). Binocular rivalry. *Curr Biol* 19: R1022–R1023.

Coan, J. A., Schaefer, H. S., and Davidson, R. J. (2006). Lending a hand: Social regulation of the natural response to threat. *Psychol Sci* 17: 1032–1039.

Cohen, M. A., Dennett, D. C., and Kanwisher, N. (2016). What is the bandwidth of perceptual experience? *Trends Cogn Sci* 20: 324–335.

Cohen, M. R., and Maunsell, J. H. (2009). Attention improves performance primarily by reducing interneuronal correlations. *Nat Neurosci* 12: 1594–1600.

Cong, X., Ludington-Hoe, S. M., Hussain, N., Cusson, R. M., Walsh, S., Vazquez, V., Briere, C. E., et al. (2015). Parental oxytocin responses during skin-to-skin contact in pre-term infants. *Early Hum Dev* 91: 401–406.

Conway, B. R. (2014). Color signals through dorsal and ventral visual pathways. *Vis Neurosci* 31 (Special Issue 02): 197–209.

Conway, B. R., Kitaoka, A., Yazdanbakhsh, A., Pack, C. C., and Livingstone, M. S. (2005). Neural basis for a powerful static motion illusion. *J Neurosci* 25: 5651–5656.

Conway, B. R., Moeller, S., and Tsao, D. Y. (2007). Specialized color modules in macaque extrastriate cortex. *Neuron* 56: 560–573.

Corbett, J. E., and Munneke, J. (2018). "It's not a tumor": A framework for capitalizing on individual diversity to boost target detection. *Psych Sci* 29: 1692–1705. https://doi.org/10.1177/0956797618784887.

Corbett, J. E., Utochkin, I., and Hochstein, S. (2023). *The Pervasiveness of Ensemble Perception: Not Just Your Average Review.* Cambridge: Cambridge University Press.

Cormack, L. K., Czuba, T. B., Knoll, J., and Huk, A. C. (2017). Binocular mechanisms of 3D motion processing. *Annu Rev Vis Sci* 3: 297–318. https://doi.org/10.1146/annurev-vision-102016-061259.

Cornell Kärnekull, S., Arshamian, A., Nilsson, M. E., and Larsson, M. (2016). From perception to metacognition: Auditory and olfactory functions in early blind, late blind, and sighted individuals. *Front Psychol* 7: 1450. https://doi.org/10.3389/fpsyg.2016.01450.

Cornell Kärnekull, S., Gerdfeldter, B., Larsson, M., and Arshamian, A. (2021). Verbally induced olfactory illusions are not caused by visual processing: Evidence from early and late blindness. *i-Perception* 12(3): 20416695211016483.

Cornsweet, T. (2017). *Seeing: How Light Tells Us About the World.* Oakland: University of California Press.

Coss, R. G., Gusé, K. L., Poran, N. S., and Smith, D. (1993). Development of antisnake defense in California ground squirrels (*Spermophilus beecheyi*). II. Microevolutionary effects of relaxed selection from rattlesnakes. *Behavior* 124: 137–165.

Courtiol, E., and Wilson, D. A. (2017). The olfactory mosaic: Bringing an olfactory network together for odor perception. *Perception* 46: 320–332. https://doi.org10.1177/0301006616663216.

Craig, J. C., and Johnson, K. O. (2000). The two-point threshold: Not a measure of tactile spatial resolution. *Curr Dir Psychol Sci* 9: 29–32.

Crick, F. (1984). Function of the thalamic reticular complex: The searchlight hypothesis. *Proc Natl Acad Sci USA* 81: 4586–4590.

Cronin, T. W., Jarvilehto, M., Weckstrom, M., and Lall, A. B. (2000). Tuning of photoreceptor spectral sensitivity in fireflies (Coleoptera: Lampyridae). *J Comp Physiol A* 186: 1–12.

Croy, I., Fairhurst, M. T., and McGlone, F. (2022). The role of C-tactile nerve fibers in human social development. *Curr Opin Behav Sci* 43: 20–26. https://doi.org/10.1016/j.cobeha.2021.06.010.

Croy, I., Luong, A., Triscoli, C., Hofmann, E., Olausson, H., and Sailer, U. (2016). Interpersonal stroking touch is targeted to C tactile afferent activation. *Behav Brain Res* 297: 37–40.

Cuevas, I., Plaza, P., Rombaux, P., Collignon, O., De Volder, A. G., and Renier, L. (2010). Do people who became blind early in life develop a better sense of smell? A psychophysical study. *J Visual Impairment Blindness*

104: 369–379. https://doi.org/10.1177/01454 82X1010400607.

Culham, J. C., Dukelow, S. P., Vilis, T., Hassard, F. A., Gati, J. S., Menon, R. S., and Goodale, M. A. (1999). Recovery of fMRI activation in motion area MT following storage of the motion aftereffect. *J Neurophysiol* 81: 388–393. https://doi.org/10.1152/jn.1999.81.1.388.

Cullen, K. E. (2011). The neural encoding of self-motion. *Curr Opin Neurobiol* 21: 587–595.

Curthoys, I., Blanks, R., and Markham, C. (1977). Semicircular canal functional anatomy in cat, guinea pig, and man. *Acta Otolaryngol* 83: 258–265.

Curwen, C. (2018). Music-colour synaesthesia: Concept, context and qualia. *Conscious Cogn* 61: 94–106. https://doi.org/10.1016/j.concog.2018.04.005.

D

Dahmani, L., Patel, R. M., Yang, Y., Chakravarty, M. M., Fellows, L. K., and Bohbot, V. D. (2018). An intrinsic association between olfactory identification and spatial memory in humans. *Nature Commun* 9: 4162. https://doi.org/10.1038/s41467-018-06569-4.

Dai, M., Cohen, B., Cho, C., Shin, S., and Yakushin, S. B, (2017). Treatment of the mal de debarquement syndrome: A 1-year follow-up. *Front Neurol* 8: 175.

Dalton, P. (1996). Odor perception and beliefs about risk. *Chem Senses* 21: 447–458.

Dalton, P. (2002). Olfaction. In H. Pashler, S. Yantis, D. Medin, R. Gallistel, and J. Wixted (Eds.), *Stevens' Handbook of Experimental Psychology* (3rd ed.), Vol. 1: *Sensation and Perception* (pp. 691–746). New York: Wiley.

Dalton, P., Doolittle, N., and Breslin, P. A. S. (2002). Gender-specific induction of enhanced sensitivity to odors. *Nat Neurosci* 5: 199–200.

Dalton, P., Wysocki, C. J., Brody, M. J., and Lawley, H. J. (1997). Perceived odor, irritation and health symptoms following short-term exposure to acetone. *Am J Ind Med* 31: 558–569.

Damasio, A. R., Damasio, H., and Van Hoesen, G. W. (1982). Prosopagnosia. *Neurology* 32: 331.

Davidoff, J., Davies, I., and Roberson, D. (1999). Is colour categorisation universal? New evidence from a stone-age culture. *Nature* 398: 203–204.

Davidson, R. J. (1984). Affect, cognition, and hemispheric specialization. In S. E. Izard, J. Kagan, and R. Zajonc (Eds.), *Emotions, Cognition and Behavior* (pp. 320–365). Cambridge: Cambridge University Press.

Davidson, R. J., Putnam, K. M., and Larson, C. L. (2000). Dysfunction in the neural circuitry of emotion regulation—A possible prelude to violence. *Science* 289: 591–594.

Davidson, S., Zhang, X., Khasabov, S. G., Simone D. A., and Giesler, G. J., Jr. (2009). Relief of itch by scratching: State-dependent inhibition of primate spinothalamic tract neurons. *Nat Neurosci* 12: 544–546.

Davidson, T. L., and Swithers, S. E. (2004). A Pavlovian approach to the problem of obesity. *Int J Obes Relat Metab Disord* 28: 933–935.

Davis, C. M. (1928). Self selection of diet by newly weaned infants: An experimental study. *Am J Dis Child* 36: 651–679.

Davis, M. (2006). Neural systems involved in fear and anxiety measured with fear-potentiated startle. *Am Psych* 61: 741–756.

De Araujo, I. E., Rolls, E. T., Velazco, M. I., Margot, C., and Cayeux, I. (2005). Cognitive modulation of olfactory processing. *Neuron* 46: 671–679. https://doi.org/10.1016/j.neuron.2005.04.021

de Bruijn, M. J., and Bender, M. (2018). Olfactory cues are more effective than visual cues in experimentally triggering autobiographical memories. *Memory* 26: 547–558. https://doi.org/10.1080/09658211.2017.1381744.

De Casper, A. J., and Fifer, W. P. (1980). Of human bonding: Newborns prefer their mother's voices. *Science* 208: 1174–1176.

DeCasper, A. J., and Spence, M. J. (1986). Prenatal maternal speech influences newborns' perception of speech sounds. *Infant Behav Dev* 9: 133–150.

De Gelder, B., Teunisse, J. P., and Benson, P. J. (1997). Categorical perception of facial expressions: Categories and their internal structure. *Cogn Emot* 11: 1–23.

de Haan, E. H., and Cowey, A. (2011). On the usefulness of "what" and "where" pathways in vision. *Trends Cogn Sci* 15(10): 460–466. https://doi.org/10.1016/j.tics.2011.08.005.

de Haas, B., Cecere, R., Cullen, H., Driver, J., and Romei, V. (2013). Duration of a co-occurring sound modulates visual detection performance in humans. *PLOS ONE* 8: e54789. https://doi.org/10.1371/journal.pone.0054789.

Dekker, T. M., Ban, H., van der Velde, B., Sereno, M. I., Welchman, A. E., and Nardini, M. (2015). Late development of cue integration is linked to sensory fusion in cortex. *Curr Biol 25*(21): 2856–2861. doi: 10.1016/j.cub.2015.09.043

de March, C. A., Matsunami, H., Abe, M., Cobb, M., and Hoover, K. C. (2023). Genetic and functional odorant receptor variation in the Homo lineage. *Iscience* 26(1): 105908.

Descartes, R. (1664). *Le Monde.* Paris: Jacques Le Gras.

DeSimone, J. A., Phan, T.-H. T., Heck, G. L., Ren, Z., Coleman, J., Mummalaneni, S., Melone, P., et al. (2011). Involvement of NADPH-dependent and cAMP-PKA sensitive H^+ channels in the chorda tympani nerve responses to strong acids. *Chem Senses* 36: 389–403.

Deutsch, D. (2013). Absolute pitch. In D. Deutsch (Ed.) *The Psychology of Music* (2nd ed., pp. 141–182). San Diego: Academic Press.

Deutsch, D., Le, J., Shen, J., and Li, X. (2011). Large-scale direct-test study reveals unexpected characteristics of absolute pitch. *J Acoust Soc Am* 130: 2398.

De Valois, R. L., Abramov, I., and Jacobs, G. H. (1966). Analysis of response patterns of LGN cells. *J Opt Soc Am A* 56: 966–977.

De Valois, R. L., Albrecht, D. G., and Thorell, L. G. (1982). Spatial frequency selectivity of cells in macaque visual cortex. *Vision Res* 22: 545–559.

De Valois, R. L., Yund, E. W., and Hepler, N. (1982). The orientation and direction selectivity of cells in macaque visual cortex. *Vision Res* 22: 531–544.

DeWitt, L. A., and Samuel, A. G. (1990). The role of knowledge-based expectations in music perception: Evidence from musical restoration. *J Exp Psychol Gen* 119: 123–144.

Diamond, J., Dalton, P., Doolittle, N., and Breslin, P. A. (2005). Gender-specific olfactory sensitization: Hormonal and cognitive influences. *Chem Senses* Suppl. 1: i224–i225.

DiCarlo, J. J., Johnson, K. O., and Hsiao, S. S. (1998). Structure of receptive fields in area 3b of primary somatosensory cortex in the alert monkey. *J Neurosci* 18: 2626–2645.

Dick, F. K., Lehet, M. I., Callaghan, M. F., Keller, T. A., Sereno, M. I., and Holt, L. L. (2017). Extensive tonotopic mapping across auditory cortex is recapitulated by spectrally directed attention and systematically related to cortical myeloarchitecture. *J Neurosci 37*(50): 12187–12201. https://doi.org/10.1523/JNEUROSCI.1436-17.2017.

Dieterich, M., and Brandt, T. (2008). Functional brain imaging of peripheral and central vestibular disorders. *Brain* 131(Pt. 10): 2538–2552.

Dijksterhuis, G. B., Møller, P., Bredie, W. L., Rasmussen, G., and Martens, M. (2002). Gender and handedness effects on hedonicity of laterally presented odours. *Brain Cogn* 50: 272–281. https://doi.org/10.1016/s0278-2626(02)00511-0.

Dilks, D. D., Dalton, P., and Beauchamp, G. K. (1999). Cross-cultural variation in responses to malodors. *Chem Senses* 24: 599.

Di Lollo, V. (2012). The feature-binding problem is an ill-posed problem. *Trends Cogn Sci 16*(6): 317–321.

Di Lollo, V., Enns, J. T., and Rensink, R. A. (2000). Competition for consciousness among visual events: The psychophysics of reentrant visual processes. *J Exp Psychol Gen* 129: 481–507. https://doi.org/10.1037//0096-3445.129.4.481.

Di Lollo, V., Kawahara, J., Shahab Ghorashi, S. M., and Enns, J. T. (2005). The attentional blink: Resource depletion or temporary loss of control? *Psychol Res* 69: 191–200.

Di Lorenzo, P. M. (2021). Neural coding of food is a multisensory, sensorimotor function. *Nutrients*, 13(2): 398–407.

Ding, J., and Levi, D. M. (2011). Recovery of stereopsis through perceptual learning in human adults with abnormal binocular vision. *Proc Natl Acad Sci USA* 108: e733–741.

Dittman, A., and Quinn, T. (1996). Homing in Pacific salmon: Mechanisms and ecological basis. *J Exp Biol* 199(Pt. 1): 83–91.

Djordjevic, J., Zatorre, R. J., Petrides, M., Boyle, J. A., and Jones-Gotman, M. (2005). Functional neuroimaging of odor imagery. *Neuroimage* 24: 791–801.

Dong, W., and Olson, E. S. (2013). Detection of cochlear amplification and its activation. *Biophys J* 105: 1067–1078.

Doty, R. L. (2010). *The Great Pheromone Myth.* Baltimore: Johns Hopkins University Press.

Doty, R. L., and Bromely, S. M. (2004). Effects of drugs on olfaction and taste. *Otolaryngol Clin North Am* 37: 1229–1254.

Doty, R. L., and Cameron, E. L. (2009). Sex differences and reproductive hormone influences on human odor perception. *Physiol Behav* 97: 213–228.

Doty, R. L., Shaman, P., Applebaum, S. L., Giberson, R, Siksorski, L., and Rosenberg, L. (1984). Smell identification ability: Changes with age. *Science* 226: 1441–1443.

Doty, R. L., Shaman, P., and Dann, M. (1984). Development of the University of Pennsylvania Smell Identification Test: A standardized microencapsulated test of olfactory function. *Physiol Behav* 32: 489–502.

Doty, R. L., Snyder, P., Huggins, G., and Lowry, L. D. (1981). Endocrine, cardiovascular and psychological correlates of olfactory sensitivity changes during the human menstrual cycle. *J Comp Physiol Psychol* 95: 45–60.

Dougherty, K., Cox, M. A., Westerberg, J. A., and Maier, A. (2019). Binocular modulation of monocular V1 neurons. *Curr Biol* 29: 381–391. https://doi.org/10.1016/j.cub.2018.12.004.

Downing, P. and Kanwisher, N. (1999). Where do cortical modules come from? Poster presented at the annual meeting of the Cognitive Neuroscience Society, Washington, DC.

Drew, T., Vo, M. L.-H., and Wolfe, J. M. (2013). The invisible gorilla strikes again: Sustained inattentional blindness in expert observers. *Psychol Sci* 24: 1848–1853.

Driscoll, M. A., Edwards, R. R., Becker, W. C., Kaptchuk, T. J., and Kerns, R. D. (2021). Psychological interventions for the treatment of chronic pain in adults. *Psychol Sci Public Interest* 22(2): 52–95. https://doi.org/10.1177/15291006211008157.

Driver, J. (1998). The neuropsychology of spatial attention. In H. Pashler (Ed.), *Attention* (pp. 297–340). Hove, East Sussex, UK: Psychology Press.

Dubin, M. W., and Cleland, B. G. (1977). Organization of visual inputs to interneurons of lateral geniculate nucleus of the cat. *J Neurophysiol* 40: 410–427.

Dubno, J. R., Eckert, M. A., Lee, F. S., Matthews, L. J., and Schmiedt, R. A. (2013). Classifying human audiometric phenotypes of age-related hearing loss from animal models. *J Assoc Res Otolaryngol* 14: 687–701. https://doi.org/10.1007/s10162-013-0396-x.

Duchaine, B., and Yovel, G. (2015). A revised neural framework for face processing. *Annu Rev Vis Sci* 1: 393–416.

Duffy, V. B., Bartoshuk, L. M., Striegel-Moore, R., and Rodin, J. (1998). Taste changes across pregnancy. In C. Murphy (Ed.), *Olfaction and Taste XIX: An International Symposium* (Vol. 855, pp. 805–809). New York: Annals of the New York Academy of Sciences.

Duffy, V. B., Davidson, A. C., Kidd, J. R., Kidd, K. K., Speed, W. C., Pakstis, A. J., Reed, D. R., et al. (2004). Bitter receptor gene (TAS2R38), 6-*n*-propylthiouracil (PROP) bitterness and alcohol intake. *Alcohol Clin Exp Res* 28: 1629–1637.

Duffy, V. B., Lanier, S. A., Hutchins, H. L., Pescatello, L. S., Johnson, M. K., and Bartoshuk, L. M. (2007). Food preference questionnaire as a screening tool for assessing dietary risk of cardiovascular disease within health risk appraisals. *J Am Diet Assoc* 107: 237–245.

Duhamel, J. R., Colby, C. L., and Goldberg, M. E. (1992). The updating of the representation of visual space in parietal cortex by intended eye movements. *Science* 255: 90–92.

Durgin, F. H., Proffitt, D. R., Olson, T. J., and Reinke, K. S. (1995). Comparing depth from motion with depth from binocular disparity. *J Exp Psychol Hum Percept Perform* 21: 679–699.

E

Eggermont, Jos. J. (2017). *Hearing Loss: Causes, Prevention, and Treatment.* United Kingdom: Elsevier Science.

Ehinger, K. A., Hidalgo-Sotelo, B., Torralba, A., and Oliva, A. (2009). Modelling search for people in 900 scenes: A combined source model of eye guidance. *Vis Cogn* 17: 945–978.

Eich, E. (1995). Mood as a mediator of place dependent memory. *J Exp Psychol* 124: 293–308.

Eippert, F., Finsterbusch, J., Bingel, U., and Büchel, C. (2009). Direct evidence for spinal cord involvement in placebo analgesia. *Science* 326: 404.

Elias, L. J., and Abdus-Saboor, I.(2022). Bridging skin, brain, and behavior to understand pleasurable social touch. *Curr Opin Neurobiol* 73: 102527. https://doi.org/10.1016/j.conb.2022.102527.

Ellingsen, D-M., Wessberg, J., Eikemo, M., Liljencrantz, J., Endestad, T., Olausson, H., and Leknes, S. (2013). Placebo improves pleasure and pain through opposite modulation of sensory processing. *Proc Nat Acad Sci USA* 110: 17993–17998.

Eliezer, M., Hamel, A. L., Houdart, E., Herman, P., Housset, J., Jourdaine, C., Eliot, C., Verillaud, B., and Hautefort, C. (2020). Loss of smell in patients with COVID-19: MRI data reveal a transient edema of the olfactory clefts. *Neurology* 95(23): e3145–e3152.

Endevelt-Shapira, Y., Shushan, S., Roth, Y., and Sobel, N. (2014). Disinhibition of olfaction: Human olfactory performance improves following low levels of alcohol, *Behav Brain Res* 272: 66–74.

Engbert, R., and Kliegl, R. (2003). Microsaccades uncover the orientation of covert attention. *Vision Res* 9: 1035–1045. https://doi.org/10.1016/s0042-6989(03)00084-1.

Engen, T. (1972). The effect of expectation on judgments of odor. *Acta Psychol* 36: 450–458.

Engen, T. (1982). *The Perception of Odors.* Toronto: Academic Press.

Engen, T. (1991). *Odor Sensation and Memory.* New York: Praeger.

Engen, T., and Engen, E. A. 1997. Relationship between development of odor perception and language. *Enfance* 50: 125–140.

Engen, T., Kuisma, J. E., and Eimas, P. D. (1973). Short-term memory of odors. *J Exp Psychol* 99: 222–225.

Engen, T., and Ross, B. M. (1973). Long-term memory odours with and without verbal descriptions. *J Exp Psychol* 100: 221–227.

Enns, J. T., and Rensink, R. A. (1990). Scene based properties influence visual search. *Science* 247: 721–723.

Enroth-Cugell, C., and Robson, J. G. (1984). Functional characteristics and diversity of cat retinal ganglion cells: Basic characteristics and quantitative description. *Invest Ophthalmol Vis Sci* 25: 250–267.

Ephron, N. (1983). *Heartburn.* New York: Vintage Books, Random House.

Epple, G., and Herz, R. S. (1999). Ambient odors associated to failure influence cognitive performance in children. *Developmental Psychobiology: The Journal of the International Society for Developmental Psychobiology* 35(2): 103–107.

Epstein, R., Harris, A., Stanley, D., and Kanwisher, N. (1999). The parahippocampal place area: Recognition, navigation, or encoding? *Neuron* 23: 115–125.

Epstein, R., and Kanwisher, N. (1998). A cortical representation of the local visual environment. *Nature* 392: 598–601.

Eriksen, C. W., and Yeh, Y. Y. (1985). Allocation of attention in the visual field. *J Exp Psychol Hum Percept Perform* 11: 583–597.

Ernst, M. O., and Banks, M. S. (2002). Humans integrate visual and haptic information in a statistically optimal fashion. *Nature* 415: 429–433.

Eskew, R. T., Jr. (2008). Chromatic detection and discrimination. In R. H. Masland and T. D. Albright (Eds.), *The Senses: A Comprehensive Reference*, Vol. 2: *Vision II* (pp. 101–117). New York: Academic Press.

Exner, S. (1875). "Über das Sehen von Bewegungen und die Theorie des zusammengesetzten Auges in". *Sitzungsberichte der Mathematisch-Naturwissenschaftlichen Classe der Kaiserlichen Akademie der Wissenschaften. V.71-72*: 363. Retrieved 12 December 2020. via HathiTrust.

F

Fahle, M. (1982). Binocular rivalry: Suppression depends on orientation and spatial frequency. *Vision Res* 22: 787–800.

Fain G. L. (2022). Vision: Life on the dark side. *Curr Biol* 32(13): R741–R743. https://doi.org/10.1016/j.cub.2022.06.001.

Fairhurst, M. T., Loken, L., and Grossmann, T. (2014). Physiological and behavioral responses reveal 9-month-old infants' sensitivity to pleasant touch. *Psychol Sci* 25: 1124–1131.

Fantz, R. L. (1963). Pattern vision in newborn infants. *Science* 140: 296–297. https://doi.org/10.1126/science.140.3564.296.

Farris, H. (2017). Perception drives the evolution of observable traits. *Science* 355: 25–26.

Fast, K. (2004). *Developing a Scale to Measure Just About Anything: Comparisons across Groups and Individuals*. New Haven, CT: Yale University School of Medicine.

Federer, F., Ichida, J. M., Jeffs, J., Schiessl, I., McLoughlin, N., and Angelucci, A. (2009). Four projection streams from primate V1 to the cytochrome oxidase stripes of V2. *J Neurosci* 29: 15455–15471.

Feldman, H. M., and Reiff, M. I. (2014). Attention deficit-hyperactivity disorder in children and adolescents. *N Engl J Med* 370: 838–846.

Feng, J., Luo, J., Yang, P., Du, J., Kim, B. S., and Hu, H. (2018). Piezo2 channel–Merkel cell signaling modulates the conversion of touch to itch. *Science* 360: 530–533.

Feord, R. C., Sumner, M. E., Pusdekar, S., Kalra, L., Gonzalez-Bellido, P. T., and Wardill, T. J. (2020). Cuttlefish use stereopsis to strike at prey. *Science Advances* 6: eaay6036. https://doi.org/10.1126/sciadv.aay6036.

Ferdenzi, C., Coureaud, G., Camos, V., and Schaal, B. (2010). Attitudes toward everyday odors for children with visual impairments: A pilot study. *J Visual Impairment Blindness* 104: 55–59. https://doi.org/10.1177/0145482X1010400109.

Fernandez, C., and Goldberg, J. (1971). Physiology of peripheral neurons innervating semicircular canals of the squirrel monkey. II. Response to sinusoidal stimulation and dynamics of peripheral vestibular system. *J Neurophysiol* 34: 661–675.

Fernandez, J. M., and Farell, B. (2005). Seeing motion in depth using interocular velocity differences. *Vision Res* 45: 2786–2798. https://doi.org/10.1016/j.visres.2005.05.021.

Ferrandiz-Huertas, C., Mathivanan, S., Wolf, C. J., Devesa, I., and Ferrer-Montiel, A. (2014). Trafficking of thermo TRP channels. *Membranes* 4: 525–564.

Fettiplace, R., and Hackney, C. M. (2006). The sensory and motor roles of auditory hair cells. *Nature* 7: 19–29.

Field, D. J. (1987). Relations between the statistics of natural images and the response properties of cortical cells. *J Opt Soc Am A* 4: 2379–2394. https://doi.org/10.1364/JOSAA.4.002379.

Field, D. J., Hayes, A., and Hess, R. F. (1992). Contour integration by the human visual system: Evidence for a local "association field." *Vision Res* 33: 173–193.

Fielder, A. R., and Moseley, M. J. (1996). Does stereopsis matter in humans? *Eye* 10: 233–238.

Firestein, S. (2001). How the olfactory system makes sense of scents. *Nature* 413: 211–218.

Fischer, R., and Griffin, F. (1964). Pharmacogenetic aspects of gustation. *Drug Res* 14: 673–686.

Fisher, S. K., and Ciuffreda, K. J. (1988). Accommodation and apparent distance. *Perception* 17: 609–621.

Fishman, M. C., and Michael, P. (1973). Integration of auditory information in the cat's visual cortex. *Vision Res* 13: 1415–1419. https://doi.org/10.1016/0042-6989(73)90002-3.

Fleming, R. W. (2022). Visual perception: Colour brings shape into stark relief. *Curr Biol* 32(6): R272–R273. https://doi.org/https://doi.org/10.1016/j.cub.2022.01.077.

Flesher, S. N., Downey, J. E., Weiss, J. M., Hughes, C. L., Herrera, A. J., Tyler-Kabara, E. C., Boninger, M. L., et al. (2021). A brain-computer interface that evokes tactile sensations improves robotic arm control. *Science* 372(6544): 831–836. https://doi.org/10.1126/science.abd0380.

Fletcher, H. (1940). Auditory patterns. *Rev Mod Phys* 12: 47–65.

Florida Atlantic University. (2017, July 20). "Sound" research shows slower boats may cause manatees more harm than good: Manatee alerting device research points to better solution. *ScienceDaily*. Retrieved from https://www.sciencedaily.com/releases/2017/07/170720095358.htm.

Fornazieri, M. A., Prina, D. M. C., Favoreto, J. P. M., Rodrigues e Silva, K., Ueda, D. M., de Rezende Pinna, F., Voegels, R. L., et al. (2019). Olfaction during pregnancy and postpartum period. *Chemosens Percep* 12: 125–134. https://doi.org/10.1007/s12078-019-09259-7.

Forster, S., and Spence, C. (2018). "What smell?" Temporarily loading visual attention induces a prolonged loss of olfactory awareness. *Psychol Sci* 29: 1642–1652. https://doi.org/10.1177/0956797618781325.

Foster, D. H. (2011). Color constancy. *Vision Res* 51: 674–700.

Fox, A. L. (1931). Six in ten "tasteblind" to bitter chemical. *Sci News Lett* 9: 249.

Fox, R., and Blake, R. R. (1971). Stereoscopic vision in the cat. *Nature* 233: 55–56.

Fracasso, A., Targher, S., Zampini, M., and Melcher, D. (2013). Fooling the eyes: The influence of a sound-induced visual motion illusion on eye movements. *PLOS ONE* 8(4): e62131. https://doi.org/10.1371/journal.pone.0062131.

Francis, D., Diorio, J., Liu, D., and Meaney, M. J. (1999). Nongenomic transmission across generations of maternal behavior and stress responses in the rat. *Science* 286: 1155–1158.

Francis, S. T., Rolls, E. T., Bowtell, R., McGlone, F., O'Doherty, J. O., Browning, A., Clare, S., et al. (1999). The representation of pleasant touch in the brain and its relationship with taste and olfactory areas. *Neuroreport* 10: 453–459.

Franco, M. I., Turin, L., Mershin, A., and Skoulakis, E. M. C. (2011). Molecular vibration sensing component in *Drosophila melanogaster* olfaction. *Proc Natl Acad Sci USA* 108: 3797–3802.

Freedman, D. J., Riesenhuber, M., Poggio, T., and Miller, E. K. (2001). Categorical perception of visual stimuli in the primate prefrontal cortex. *Science* 291: 312–316.

Freire, A., Lewis, T. L., Maurer, D., and Blake, R. (2006). The development of sensitivity to biological motion in noise. *Perception* 35: 647–657.

Frenzel, H., Bohlender, J., Pinsker, K., Wohlleben, B., Tank, J., Lechner, S. G., Schiska, D., et al. (2012). A genetic basis for mechanosensory traits in humans. *PLOS Biol* 10: e1001318.

Frey, S. H., Bogdanov, S., Smith, J. C., Watrous, S., and Breidenbach, W. C. (2008). Chronically deafferented sensory cortex recovers a grossly typical organization after allogenic hand transplantation. *Curr Biol* 18: 1530–1534.

Frisby, J. P. (1980). *Seeing, Illusion, Brain, and Mind*. Oxford: Oxford University Press.

Fuentes, C. T., Longo, M. R., and Haggard, P. (2013). Body image distortions in healthy adults. *Acta Psychol (Amst)* 144: 344–351.

Fulton, A. (1988). The development of scotopic retinal function in human infants. *Doc Ophthalmol* 69(2): 101–9. doi: 10.1007/BF00153690.

G

Gadziola, M. A., Stetzik, L. A., Wright, K. N., Milton, A. J., Arakawa, K., del Mar Cortijo, M., & Wesson, D. W. (2020). A neural system that represents the association of odors with rewarded outcomes and promotes behavioral engagement. *Cell Reports*, 32(3). https://doi.org/10.1016/j.celrep.2020.107919

Galef, B. G., and Wigmore, S. W. (1983). Transfer of information concerning distant foods: A laboratory investigation of the "information-centre" hypothesis. *Anim Behav* 31: 748–758.

Gallant, J. L., Braun, B., and Van Essen, D. C. (1993). Selectivity for polar, hyperbolic, and cartesian gratings in macaque visual cortex. *Science* 259: 100–103.

Gandhi, S. P., Heeger, D. J., and Boynton, G. M. (1998). Spatial attention affects brain activity in human primary visual cortex. *Proc Natl Acad Sci USA* 96: 3314–3319.

Gangrade, A. (2012). The effect of music on the production of neurotransmitters, hormones, cytokines, and peptides: A review. *Music Med* 4(1): 40–43. https://doi.org/10.1177/1943862111415117.

Gauthier, I., Williams, P., Tarr, M. J., and Tanaka, J. (1998). Training "greeble" experts: A framework for studying expert object recognition processes. *Vision Res* 38: 2401–2428.

Gegenfurtner, K. R. (2016). The interaction between vision and eye movements. *Perception* 45: 1333–1357.

Gegenfurtner, K. R., Bloj, M., and Toscani, M. (2015). The many colours of "the dress." *Curr Biol* 25: R543–R544.

Geisler, W. S. (2011). Contributions of ideal observer theory to vision research. *Vision Res* 51: 771–781. https://doi.org/10.1016/j.visres.2010.09.027.

Geisler, W. S., and Perry, J. S. (2009). Contour statistics in natural images: Grouping across occlusions. *Vis Neurosci* 26: 109–121.

Geldard, F. A. (1972). *The Human Senses* (2nd ed.). New York: Wiley.

Gelstein, S., Yeshurun, Y., Rozenkrantz, L., Shushan, S., Frumin, I., Roth, Y., and Sobel, N. (2011). Human tears contain chemosignal. *Science* 331: 226–230.

George, J. A., Kluger, D. T., Davis, T. S., Wendelken, S. M., Okorokova, E. V., He, Q., Duncan, C. C., et al. (2019). Biomimetic sensory feedback through peripheral nerve stimulation improves dexterous use of a bionic hand. *Sci Robot* 4: eaax2352.

Gerbino, W. (2020). Perception and past experience 50 years after Kanizsa's (im)possible experiment. *Perception* 49(3): 247–267. https://doi.org/10.1177/0301006619899005.

Gerkin, R. C., and Castro, J. B. (2015). The number of olfactory stimuli that humans can discriminate is still unknown. *Elife* 4: e08127.

Gerstein, E. R. (2002). Manatees, bioacoustics, and boats: Hearing tests, environmental measurements, and acoustic phenomena may together explain why boats and animals collide. *Am Sci* 90: 154–156.

Gescheider, G. A. (1974). *Temporal Relations in Cutaneous Stimulation* (Conference on Cutaneous Communication Systems and Devices). Oxford: Psychonomic Society.

Giaschi, D., Lo, R., Narasimhan, S., Lyons, C., and Wilcox, L. M. (2013). Sparing of coarse stereopsis in stereodeficient children with a history of amblyopia. *J Vis* 13: 17.

Gibson, J. J. (1957). Optical motions and transformations as stimuli for visual perception. *Psychol Rev* 64: 288–295.

Gibson, J. J. (1966). *The Senses Considered as Perceptual Systems*. Boston: Houghton Mifflin.

Gillam, B. (1980). Geometrical illusions. *Sci Am* 242: 102–111.

Gisladottir, R. S., Ivarsdottir, E. V., Helgason, A., Jonsson, L., Hannesdottir, N. K., Rutsdottir, G., et al. (2020). Sequence variants in TAAR5 and other loci affect human odor perception and naming. *Current Biology* 30(23): 4643–4653.

Gittinger, J. M., Jimenez, E. S., Holswade, E. A., and Nunna, R. S. (2017). Novel data visualizations of X-ray data for aviation security applications using the open threat assessment platform (OTAP). *43rd Review of Progress in Quantitative Nondestructive Evaluation*. American Institute of Physics Conference Proceedings 1806: 130006. https://doi.org/10.1063/1.4974715.

Glasauer, S., Amorim, M.-A., Viaud-Delmon, I., and Berthoz, A. (2002). Differential effects of labyrinthine dysfunction on distance and direction during blindfolded walking of a triangular path. *Exp Brain Res* 145: 489–497. doi: 10.1007/s00221-002-1146-1.

Glasser, D. M., Tsui, J. M. G., Pack, C. C., and Tadin, D. (2011). Perceptual and neural consequences of rapid motion adaptation. *Proc Nat Acad Sci USA* 108: E1080–E1088.

Gloriani, A. H., and Schütz, A. C. (2019). Humans trust central vision more than peripheral vision even in the dark. *Curr Biol* 29: 1206–1210.e4. https://doi.org/10.1016/j.cub.2019.02.023.

Goff, S. A., and Klee, H. J. (2006). Plant volatile compounds: Sensory cues for health and nutritional value? *Science* 311: 815–819.

Goldberg, J. M., and Fernandez, C. (1971). Physiology of peripheral neurons innervating semicircular canals of the squirrel monkey, Parts 1, 2, 3. *J Neurophysiol* 34: 635–684.

Goldberg, J. M., and Fernandez, C. (1976). Physiology of peripheral neurons innervating otolith organs of the squirrel monkey, Parts 1, 2, 3. *J Neurophysiol* 39: 970–1008.

Gómez-Robledo, L., Valero, E. M., Huertas, R., Martínez-Domingo, M. A., and Hernández-Andrés, J. (2018). Do EnChroma glasses improve color vision for colorblind subjects? *Opt Express* 26: 28693–28703. https://doi.org/10.1364/OE.26.028693.

Goncalves, N. R., and Welchman, A. E. (2017). "What not" detectors help the brain see in depth. *Curr Biol* 27: 1403–1412.

Gorea, A. (2015). A refresher of the original Bloch's law paper (Bloch, July 1885). *i-Perception* 6(4): 2041669515593043. https://doi.org/10.1177/2041669515593043C.

Govardovskii, V. I. (1983). On the role of oil drops in colour vision. *Vision Res* 23: 1739–1740.

Grabherr, L., Nicoucar, K., Mast, F. W., and Merfeld, D. M. (2008). Direction detection thresholds for yaw rotation about an earth-vertical axis as a function of frequency. *Exp Brain Res* 186: 677–681.

Grabherr, L., et al. (2011). Mental transformation abilities in patients with unilateral and bilateral vestibular loss. Experimental Brain Research 209(2): 205–214.

Graham, N., and Nachmias, J. (1971). Detection of grating patterns containing two spatial frequencies: A comparison of single-channel and multiple-channel models. *Vision Res* 11: 251–259.

Grant, S., and Moseley, M. J. (2011). Amblyopia and real-world visuomotor tasks. *Strabismus* 19: 119–128.

Grassi, M., and Casco, C. (2010). Audiovisual bounce-inducing effect: When sound congruence affects grouping in vision. *Attn Percept Psychophys* 72: 378–386. https://doi.org/10.3758/APP.72.2.378.

Graziano, M., and Gross, C. G. (1994). The representation of extrapersonal space: A possible role for bimodal, visual-tactile neurons. In M. S. Gazzaniga (Ed.), *The Cognitive Neurosciences* (pp. 1021–1034). Cambridge, MA: MIT Press.

Green, B. G. (1993). Evidence that removal of capsaicin accelerates desensitization on the tongue. *Neurosci Lett* 150: 44–48.

Green, B. G. (2005). Lingual heat and cold sensitivity following exposure to capsaicin or menthol. *Chem Senses* 30(Suppl 1): i201–i202. https://doi.org/10.1093/chemse/bjh184.

Green, C. S., and Bavelier, D. (2003). Action video game modifies visual attention. *Nature* 423: 534–537.

Green, D. M., and Swets, J. (1966). *Signal Detection Theory and Psychophysics*. New York: Wiley.

Greene, M. R., and Oliva, A. (2009). The briefest of glances: The time course of natural scene understanding. *Psychol Sci* 20: 464–472.

Gregory, R. L. (1966). *Eye and Brain*. New York: World University Library.

Gregory, R. L. (1970). *The Intelligent Eye*. London: Weidenfeld & Nicolson.

Grill-Spector, K., and Kanwisher, N. (2005). Visual recognition: As soon as you know it is there, you know what it is. *Psychol Sci* 16(2): 152–160.

Grill-Spector, K., and Malach, R. (2004). The human visual cortex. *Annu Rev Neurosci* 27: 649–677.

Grimaldi, P., Saleem, K., and Tsao, D. (2016). Anatomical connections of the functionally defined "face patches" in the macaque monkey. *Neuron* 90: 1325–1342. https://doi.org/10.1016/j.neuron.2016.05.009.

Groh, A. (2016). Culture, language and thought: Field studies on colour concepts. *J Cogn Cult* 16(1–2): 83–106. https://doi.org/https://doi.org/10.1163/15685373-12342169.

Gross, C. G., Rocha-Miranda, C. E., and Bender, D. B. (1972). Visual properties of neurons in inferotemporal cortex of the macaque. *J Neurophysiol* 35: 96–111.

Grushka, M., and Bartoshuk, L. M. (2000). Burning mouth syndrome and oral dysesthesias. *Can J Diagn* 17: 99–109.

Grusser, O.-J. (1983). Multimodal structure of the extrapersonal space. In A. Hein and M. Jeannerod (Eds.), *Spatially Oriented Behavior*. New York: Springer-Verlag.

Guducu, C., Oniz, A., Ikiz, A. O., and Ozgoren, M. (2016). Chemosensory function in congenitally blind or deaf teenagers. *Chemosens Percep* 9: 8–13. https://doi.org/10.1007/s12078-015-9199-2.

Guedry, F. (1974). Psychophysics of vestibular sensation. In H. H. Kornhuber (Ed.), *Vestibular System* (*Handbook of Sensory Physiology*, vol. 6) (pp. 1–154). New York: Springer.

Guinness World Records (50th anniv. ed.). (2005). New York: Guiness World Records.

Gurnsey, R., and Browse, R. A. (1987). Micropattern properties and presentation conditions influencing visual texture discrimination. *Percept Psychophys* 41: 239–252.

H

Habib, A. M., Okorokov, A. L., Hill, M. N., Bras, J. T., Lee, M.–C., Li, S., Gossage, S. J., et al. (2019). Microdeletion in a FAAH pseudogene identified in a patient with high anandamide concentrations and pain insensitivity. *Br J Anaesth* 123: e249–e253. https://doi.org/10.1016/j.bja.2019.02.019.

Habig, K., Schänzer, A., Schirner, W., Lautenschläger, G., Dassinger, B., Olausson, H., Birklein, F., et al. (2017). Low threshold unmyelinated mechanoafferents can modulate pain. *BMC Neurol* 17: 184. https://doi.org/10.1186/s12883-017-0963-6.

Hadad, B., Schwartz, S., Maurer, D., and Lewis, T. L. (2015). Motion perception: A review of developmental changes and the role of early visual experience. *Front Integr Neurosci* 9: 49. https://doi.org/10.3389/fnint.2015.00049.

Haenny, P. E., and Schiller, P. H. (1988). State dependent activity in monkey visual cortex. I. Single cell activity in V1 and V4 on visual tasks. *Exp Brain Res* 69: 225–244.

Haerazi, H. (2016). Principles of second language acquisition in children. *Journal of English Language Teaching* 3: 1–14.

Hafed, Z.M. and Clark, J. J. (2002). Microsaccades as an overt measure of covert attention shifts. *Vision Res* 42(22): 2533–45. doi: 10.1016/s0042-6989(02)00263-8.

Hafri, A., Wadhwa, S., and Bonner, M. F. (2022). Perceived distance alters memory for scene boundaries. *Psychol Sci* 33(12): 2040–2058. https://doi.org/10.1177/09567976221093575.

Haggard, P., Newman, C., Blundell, J., and Andrew, H. (2000). The perceived position of the hand in space. *Percept Psychophys* 68: 363–377.

Haller, R., Rummel, C., Henneberg, S., Pollmer, U., and Koster, E. P. (1999). The influence of early experience with vanillin on food preference in later life. *Chem Senses* 24: 465–467.

Hamburger, K., and Knauff, M. (2019). Odors can serve as landmarks in human wayfinding. *Cogn Sci* 43(11): e12798.

Hamer, R. D. and Schneck, M. E. (1984). Spatial summation in dark-adapted human infants. *Vision Res.* 24(1): 77–85. doi: 10.1016/0042-6989(84)90146-9.

Han, P., Stiller-Stut, F. P., Fjaeldstad, A., and Hummel, T. (2020). Greater hippocampal gray matter volume in subjective hyperosmia: A voxel-based morphometry study. *Sci Rep* 10(1): 1–10.

Handel, S. (1989). *Listening: An Introduction to the Perception of Auditory Events*. Cambridge, MA: MIT Press.

Handel, S., and Oshinsky, J. S. (1981). The meter of syncopated auditory polyrhythms. *Percept Psychophys* 30: 1–9.

Handelman, G. S., Kok, H. K., Chandra, R. V., Razavi, A. H., Huang, S., Brooks, M., et al. (2018). Peering into the black box of artificial intelligence: Evaluation metrics of machine learning methods. *Am J Roentgen* 212: 38–43. https://doi.org/10.2214/AJR.18.20224.

Hänig, D. (1901). Zur Psychophysik des Geschmackssinnes. *Philosophische Studien* 17: 576–623.

Harb, E. N., and Wildsoet, C. F. (2019). Origins of refractive errors: Environmental and genetic factors. *Annu Rev Vis Sci* 5: 47–72. https://doi.org/10.1146/annurev-vision-091718-015027.

Hare, R. M., Schlatter, S., Rhodes, G., and Simmons, L. W. (2017). Putative sex-specific human pheromones do not affect gender perception, attractiveness ratings or unfaithfulness judgements of opposite sex faces. *Roy Soc Open Sci* 4: 160831.

Harkness, L. (1977). Chameleons use accommodation cues to judge distance. *Nature* 267: 346–349.

Hartline, H. K. (1940). The nerve messages in the fibers of the visual pathway. *J Opt Soc Am* 30: 239–247.

Hartmann, M., and Müller, P. (2023). Illusory perception of visual patterns in pure noise is associated with COVID-19 conspiracy beliefs. *i-Perception* 14(1): 20416695221144732. https://doi.org/10.1177/20416695221144732.

Hautus, M. J., Macmillan, N. A., and Creelman, C. D. (2021). *Detection Theory*. New York: Routledge.

Haxby, J. V., Hoffman, E. A., and Gobbini, M. I. (2000). The distributed human neural system for face perception. *Trends Cogn Sci* 4: 223–233.

He, S., Liu, H., Jiang, Y., Chen, C., Gong, Q., and Weng, X. (2009). Transforming a left lateral fusiform region into VWFA through training in illiterate adults. *J Vision* 9: 853–853. https://doi.org/10.1167/9.8.853.

Hecht, S., Shlaer, S., and Pirenne, M. H. (1942). Energy, quanta, and vision. *J Gen Physiology* 25: 819–840.

Hedger, S. C., Heald, S. L. M., and Nusbaum, H. C. (2013). Absolute pitch may not be so absolute. *J Acoust Soc Am* 24(8): 1496–1502.

Hedner, M., Larsson, M., Arnold, N., Zucco, G. M., and Hummel, T. (2010). Cognitive factors in odor detection, odor discrimination, and odor identification tasks. *J Clin Exp Neuropsychol* 32: 1062–1067. https://doi.org/10.1080/13803391003683070.

Heider, E. R. (1972). Universals in color naming and memory. *J Exp Psychol* 93: 10–20.

Heiser, C., Baja, J., Lenz, F. Sommer, J. U., Hormann, K., Herr, R. M., and Stuck, B. A. (2012). Effects of an artificial smoke on arousals during human sleep. *Chemosens Percept* 5: 274–279.

Held, R. T., Cooper, E. A., and Banks, M. S. (2012). Blur and disparity are complementary cues to depth. *Curr Biol* 22: 426–431.

Held, R. T., Cooper, E. A., O'Brien, J. F., and Banks, M. S. (2010). Using blur to affect perceived distance and size. *ACM Trans Graph* 29(2): 19. https://doi.org/10.1145/1731047.1731057.

Held, R., Ostrovsky, Y., deGelder, B., Gandhi, T., Ganesh, S., Mathur, M., and Sinha, P. (2011). Newly sighted cannot match seen with felt. *Nat Neurosci* 14: 551–553.

Henderson, J. M., and Hayes, T. R. (2018). Meaning guides attention in real-world scene images: Evidence from eye movements and meaning maps. *J Vision* 18(6): 1–10. https://doi.org/10.1167/18.6.10

Henderson, M., Vo, V., Chunharas, C., Sprague, T., and Serences, J. (2019). Multivariate analysis of BOLD activation patterns recovers graded depth representations in human visual and parietal cortex. *eNeuro* 6(4). doi: 10.1523/eneuro.0362-18.2019

Hendry, S. H., and Reid, R. C. (2000). The koniocellular pathway in primate vision. *Annu Rev Neurosci* 23: 127–153.

Hense, M., Badde, S., and Röder, B. (2019). Tactile motion biases visual motion perception in binocular rivalry. *Atten Percept Psychophysics* 81: 1715–1724. https://doi.org/10.3758/s13414-019-01692-w.

Hering, E. (1878). *Zur Lehre vom Lichtsinn*. Vienna: Gerold.

Herz, R. S. (1997). Emotion experienced during encoding enhances odor retrieval cue effectiveness. *Am J Psychol* 110: 489–505.

Herz, R. S. (1998). Are odors the best cues to memory? A cross-modal comparison of associative memory stimuli. *Ann NY Acad Sci* 855: 670–674.

Herz, R. S. (2000). Scents of time. *The Sciences* 40: 34–39.

Herz, R. S. (2001). Ah, sweet skunk: Why we like or dislike what we smell. *Cerebrum* 3: 31–47.

Herz, R. S. (2004). A comparison of autobiographical memories triggered by olfactory, visual, and auditory stimuli. *Chem Senses* 29: 217–224.

Herz, R. S. (2006). I know what I like: Understanding odor preferences. In Jim Drobnick (ed.), *The Smell Culture Reader* (pp. 190–203). Oxford: Berg.

Herz, R. (2007). *The Scent of Desire: Discovering Our Enigmatic Sense of Smell*. New York: Morrow.

Herz, R. S. (2009). Aromatherapy facts and fictions: A scientific analysis of olfactory effects on mood, physiology and behavior. *Int J Neurosci* 119: 263–290.

Herz, R. S. (2016). The role of odor-evoked memory in psychological and physiological health. *Brain Sci* 6: 22.

Herz, R. S. (2021a). Scent perception and its therapeutic potential for pain management. *Int J Prof Holistic Aromather*, 10(1), 17–22.

Herz, R. S. (2021b). Olfaction and health. In *Olfaction: An Interdisciplinary Perspective from Philosophy to Life Sciences* (pp. 193–211). Cham: Springer International Publishing.

Herz, R. S., and Bajec, M. R. (2022). Your money or your sense of smell? A comparative analysis of the sensory and psychological value of olfaction. *Brain Sciences* 12(3): 299.

Herz, R. S., Beland, S. L., and Hellerstein, M. (2004). Changing odor hedonic perception through emotional associations in humans. *Int J Comp Psychol* 17: 315–339.

Herz, R. S., and Cupchik, G. C. (1992). An experimental characterization of odor-evoked memories in humans. *Chem Senses* 17: 519–528.

Herz, R. S., and Cupchik, G. C. (1995). The emotional distinctiveness of odor-evoked memories. *Chem Senses* 20: 517–528.

Herz, R. S., Eliassen, J. C., Beland, S. L., and Souza, T. (2004). Neuroimaging evidence for the emotional potency of odor-evoked memory. *Neuropsychologia* 42: 371–378.

Herz, R. S., Larsson, M., Trujillo, R., Casola, M. C., Ahmed, F. K., Lipe, S., and Brashear, M. E. (2022). A three-factor benefits framework for understanding consumer preference for scented household products: Psychological interactions and implications for future development. *Cognitive Research: Principles and Implications* 7(1): 1–20.

Herz, R. S., McCall, C., and Cahill, L. (1999). Hemispheric lateralization in the processing of odor pleasantness versus odor names. *Chem Senses* 24(6): 691–695. https://doi.org/10.1093/chemse/24.6.691.

Herz, R. S., Schankler, C., and Beland, S. (2004). Olfaction, emotion and associative learning: effects on motivated behavior. *Motivation and emotion* 28: 363–383.

Herz, R. S., and Schooler, J. W. (2002). A naturalistic study of autobiographical memories evoked by olfactory and visual cues: Testing the Proustian hypothesis. *Am J Psychol* 115: 21–32.

Herz, R. S., Van Reen, E., Barker, D., Bartz, A., and Carskadon, M. A. (2018a). Olfactory sensitivity declines with number of hours awake. *Chem Senses* 43: e110. https://doi.org/10.1093/chemse/bjy003.

Herz, R. S., Van Reen, E., Barker, D., and Carskadon, M. A. (2018b). The influence of circadian timing on odor detection. *Chem Senses* 43: 45–51. https://doi.org/10.1093/chemse/bjx067.

Herz, R. S., and von Clef, J. (2001). The influence of verbal labeling on the perception of odors: Evidence for olfactory illusions? *Perception* 30: 381–391. https://doi.org/10.1068/p3179.

Hillis, J. M., Watt, S. J., Landy, M. S., and Banks, M. S. (2004). Slant from texture and disparity cues: Optimal cue combination. *J Vis* 4: 9s67–992. https://doi.org/10.1167/4.12.1.

Hinton, P. B., and Henley, T. B. (1993). Cognitive and affective components of stimuli presented in three modes. *Bull Psychonomic Soc* 31: 595–598.

Hochstein, S., and Ahissar, M. (2002). View from the top: Hierarchies and reverse hierarchies in the visual system. *Neuron* 36: 791–804.

Hofer, M. K., Collins, H. K., Whillans, A. V., and Chen, F. S. (2018). Olfactory cues from romantic partners and strangers influence women's responses to stress. *J Personality Soc Psychol* 114: 1–9. https://doi.org/10.1037/pspa0000110.

Hoffman, D. D., and Richards, W. A. (1984). Parts of recognition. *Cognition* 18: 65–96.

Hoffman, D. M., and Banks, M. S. (2010). Focus information is used to interpret binocular images. *J Vis* 10: 13. https://doi.org/10.1167/10.5.13.

Hofman, P. M., Van Riswick, J. G. A., and Van Opsal, A. J. (1998). Relearning sound localization with new ears. *Nat Neurosci* 1: 417–421.

Hohmann A., and Creutzfeldt, O. D. (1975). Squint and the development of binocularity in humans. *Nature* 254: 613–614.

Holler, J., and Levinson, S. C. (2019). Multimodal language processing in human communication. *Trends Cog Sci* 23: 639–652. https://doi.org/10.1016/j.tics.2019.05.006.

Hollins, M. (2002). Touch and haptics. In H. Pashler and S. Yantis (Eds.), *Stevens Handbook of Experimental Psychology* (3rd ed.), Vol. 1: *Sensation and Perception* (pp. 585–618). New York: Wiley.

Holt, L. L., and Lotto, A. J. (2002). Behavioral examinations of the neural mechanisms of speech context effects. *Hear Res*, 167, 156–169.

Holt, L. L., and Lotto, A. J. (2010). Speech perception as categorization. *Attent Percept Psychophys* 72(5): 1218–1227. https://doi.org/10.3758/APP.72.5.1218.

Holt, L.L., Peelle, J. E., Coffin, A. B., Popper, A. N., and Fay, R. R. (2022). *Speech Perception*. Springer: Cham. https://doi.org/10.1007/978-3-030-81542-4.

Horak, F., Nashner, L., and Diener, H. (1990). Postural strategies associated with somatosensory and vestibular loss. *Exp Brain Res* 82: 167–177.

Horii, A., Russell, N. A., Smith, P. F., Darlington, C. L., and Bilkey, D. K. (2004). Vestibular influences on CA1 neurons in the rat hippocampus: An electrophysiological study in vivo. *Exp Brain Res* 155: 245–250.

Horikawa, T., Tamaki, M., Miyawaki, Y., and Kamitani, Y. (2013). Neural decoding of visual imagery during sleep. *Science* 340: 639–642.

Horton, J. C., and Hocking, D. R. (1996). An adult-like pattern of ocular dominance columns in striate cortex of newborn monkeys prior to visual experience. *J Neurosci* 16: 1791–1807.

Horton, J. C., and Trobe, J. D. (1999). Akinetopsia from nefazodone toxicity. *Am J Ophthalmol* 128: 530–531.

Howard, I. P., and Rogers, B. J. (1995). *Binocular Vision and Stereopsis*. New York: Oxford University Press.

Howard, I. P., and Rogers, B. J. (2001). *Seeing in Depth*. Toronto: Porteous.

Howard, J. D., Plailly, J., Grueschow, M., Hayens, J.-D., and Gottfried, J. A. (2009). Odor quality coding and categorization in human posterior piriform cortex. *Nat Neurosci* 12: 932–938.

Hubel, D. H. (1982). Exploration of the primary visual cortex, 1955–78. *Nature* 299: 515–524. https://doi.org/10.1038/299515a0.

Hubel, D., and Wiesel, T. N. (1961). Integrative action in the cat's lateral geniculate body. *J Physiol* 155: 385–398.

Hubel, D. H., and Wiesel, T. N. (1962). Receptive fields, binocular interaction and functional architecture in the cat's visual cortex. *J Physiol* 160: 106–154.

Hubel, D. H., and Wiesel, T. N. (1973). A reexamination of stereoscopic mechanisms in area 17 of the cat. *J Physiol* 232: 29P–30P.

Hubel, D. H., and Wiesel, T. N. (1979). Brain mechanisms of vision. *Sci Am* 241: 150–162. https://doi.org/10.1038/scientificamerican0979-150.

Hubel, D. H., Wiesel, T. N., and Stryker, M. P. (1978). Anatomical demonstration of orientation columns in macaque monkey. *J Comp Neurol* 177: 361–380.

Hudspeth, A. J. (1997). How hearing happens. *Neuron* 19: 947–950.

Hughes, A. (1977). The topography of vision in mammals of contrasting life styles: Comparative optics and retinal organization. In F. Crescitelli (Ed.), *Handbook of Sensory Physiology* (Vol. VII/5 The Visual System in Vertebrates). NY: Springer Verlag.

Huk, A. C., Ress, D., and Heeger, D. J. (2001). Neuronal basis of the motion aftereffect reconsidered. *Neuron* 32: 161–172.

Hummel, T., Futschik, T., Frasnelli, J., and Huttenbring, K. B. (2003). Effects of olfactory function, age and gender on trigeminally mediated sensations: A study based on the lateralization of chemosensory stimuli. *Toxicol Lett* 140: 273–280.

Hummel, T., Kobel, G., Gudziol, H., and Mackay-Sim, A. (2007). Normative data for the "Sniffin' Sticks" including tests of odor identification, odor discrimination, and olfactory thresholds: An upgrade based on a group of more than 3,000 subjects. *Eur Arch Otorhinolaryngol* 264: 237–243.

Hummel, T., von Mering, R., Huch, R., and Kolble, N. (2002). Olfactory modulation of nausea during early pregnancy? *BJOG* 109: 1394–1397.

Hung, C. P., Kreiman, G., Poggio, T., and DiCarlo, J. J. (2005). Fast readout of object identity from macaque inferior temporal cortex. *Science* 310: 863–866. https://doi.org/10.1126/science.1117593.

Hurvich, L., and Jameson, D. (1957). An opponent process theory of color vision. *Psychol Rev* 64: 384–404.

Hutchison, R. M., Culham, J. C., Everling, S., Flanagan, J. R., and Gallivan, J. P. (2014). Distinct and distributed functional connectivity patterns across cortex reflect the domain-specific constraints of object, face, scene, body, and tool category-selective modules in the ventral visual pathway. *Neuroimage* 96: 216–236.

Huterer, M., and Cullen, K. E. (2002). Vestibuloocular reflex dynamics during high-frequency and high-acceleration rotations of the head on body in rhesus monkey. *J Neurophysiol* 88: 13–28.

Hutmacher, F., and Kuhbandner, C. (2018). Long-term memory for haptically explored objects: Fidelity, durability, incidental encoding, and cross-modal transfer. *Psychol Sci* 29: 2031–2038. https://doi.org/10.1177/0956797618803644.

I

Ilg, U. J. (2008). The role of areas MT and MST in coding of visual motion underlying the execution of smooth pursuit. *Vision Res* 48: 2062–2069. https://doi.org/10.1016/j.visres.2008.04.015.

Imai, S., Flege, J., and Wayland, R. (2002). Perception of cross-language vowel differences: A longitudinal study of native Spanish learners of English. *J Acoust Soc Am* 111: 2364–2364.

Irwin, D. E., Zacks, J. L., and Brown, J. S. (1990). Visual memory and the perception of a stable visual environment. *Percept Psychophys* 47: 35–46.

Ishiyama, S., and Brecht, M. (2016). Neural correlates of ticklishness in the rat somatosensory cortex. *Science* 354: 757–760.

Itatani, N., and Klump, G. M. (2017). Animal models for auditory streaming. *Philos Trans R Soc Lond B Biol Sci* 372: 1–11.

Itti, L., Koch, C., and Niebur, E. (1998). A model of saliency-based visual attention for rapid scene analysis. *IEEE Trans Pattern Anal Machine Intelligence* 20: 1254–1259.

Iversen, K. D., Ptito, M., Møller, P., and Kupers, R. (2015). Enhanced chemosensory detection of negative emotions in congenital blindness. *Neural Plasticity* 2015: 469750(2). https://doi.org/10.1155/2015/469750.

Ivory, R., Kane, R., and Diaz, R. C. (2014). Noise-induced hearing loss: A recreational noise perspective. *Curr Opin Otolaryngol Head Neck Surg* 5: 394–398.

J

Jacob, S., Hayreh, D. J. S, and McClintock, M. (2001). Context-dependent effects of steroid chemosignals on human physiology and mood. *Physiol Behav* 74: 15–27.

Jacobs, L. F., Arter, J., Cook, A., and Sulloway, F. J. (2015). Olfactory orientation and navigation in humans. *PLOS ONE* 10: e0129387.

Jacoby, N., and McDermott, J. H. (2017). Integer ratio priors on musical rhythm revealed cross-culturally by iterated reproduction. *Curr Biol* 27: 359–370.

Jacoby, N., Undurraga, E. A., McPherson, J. V., Ossandón, T., and McDermott, J. H. (2019). Universal and non-universal features of musical pitch perception revealed by singing. *Curr Biol* 29: 3229–3243. https://doi.org/10.1016/j.cub.2019.08.020.

Jakubiak, B. K., and Feeney, B. C. (2017). Affectionate touch to promote relational, psychological, and physical well-being in adulthood. *Pers Soc Psychol Rev* 21: 228–252.

James, W. (1890). *The Principles of Psychology* (2 vols.). New York: Holt.

Jarocka, E., Pruszynski, A., and Johansson, R. S. (2021). Human touch receptors are sensitive to spatial details on the scale of single fingerprint ridges. *J Neurosci* 41(16): 3622–3634.

Jeffress, L. A. (1948). A place theory of sound localization. *J Comp Physiol Psychol* 41: 35–39.

Jeon, T.-I., Zhu, B., Larson, J. L., and Osborne, T. F. (2008). SREBP-2 regulates gut peptide secretion through intestinal bitter taste receptor signaling in mice. *J Clin Invest* 118: 3693–3700.

Ji, Y., Gupta, P., Shah, P., Tiwari, K., Gandhi, T., Ganesh, S., Phillips, F., et al. (2021). Resilience of temporal processing to early and extended visual deprivation. *Vision Res* 186: 80–86. https://doi.org/10.1016/j.visres.2021.05.004.

Jiang, R. S., Twu, C. W., and Liang, K. L. (2017). The effect of olfactory training on the odor threshold in patients with traumatic anosmia. *Am J Rhinol Allergy* 31: 317–322. https://doi.org/10.1002/alr.22409.

Johansson, G. (1975). Visual motion perception. *Sci Am* 232: 76–88.

Johnson, K. O. (2002). Neural basis of haptic perception. In H. Pashler and S. Yantis (Eds.), *Stevens Handbook of Experimental Psychology* (3rd ed.), Vol. 1: *Sensation and Perception* (pp. 537–583). New York: Wiley.

Johnsrude, I. S., Mackey, A., Hakyemez, H., Alexander, E., Trang, H. P., and Carlyon, R. P. (2013). Swinging at a cocktail party: Voice familiarity aids speech perception in the presence of a competing voice. *Psychol Sci* 24(10): 1995–2004. https://doi.org/10.1177/0956797613482467.

Johnston, E. B., Cumming, B. G., and Parker, A. J. (1993). Integration of depth modules: Stereopsis and texture. *Vis Res* 33: 813–826. https://doi.org/10.1016/0042-6989(93)90200-g.

Jolicoeur, P., Gluck, M. A., and Kosslyn, S. M. (1984). Pictures and names: Making the connection. *Cogn Psychol* 16: 243–275.

Jones, B., and Mishkin, M. (1972). Limbic lesions and the problem of stimulus–reinforcement associations. *Exp Neurol* 36: 362–377.

Jones, L. A. (1999). Somatic senses 3: Proprioception. In H. Cohen (Ed.), *Neuroscience for Rehabilitation* (2nd ed., pp. 111–130). Philadelphia: Lippincott.

Jones, M., and Love, B. C. (2011). Bayesian fundamentalism or Enlightenment? On the explanatory status and theoretical contributions of Bayesian models of cognition. *Behav Brain Sci* 34: 169–188.

Jones, R. K., and Lee, D. N. (1981). Why two eyes are better than one: The two views of binocular vision. *J Exp Psychol Hum Percept Perform* 7: 30–40.

Jordan, G., and Mollon, J. (2019). Tetrachromacy: The mysterious case of extra-ordinary color vision. *Curr Opin Behav Sci* 30: 130–134. https://doi.org/https://doi.org/10.1016/j.cobeha.2019.08.002.

Joris, P. X., Smith, P. H., and Yin, T. C. T. (1998). Coincidence detection in the auditory system: 50 years after Jeffress. *Neuron* 21: 1235–1238.

Joris, P., and van der Heijden, M. (2019). Early binaural hearing: The comparison of temporal differences at the two ears. *Annu Rev Neurosci* 42: 433–457. https://doi.org/10.1146/annurev-neuro-080317-061925.

Josephs, E. L., and Konkle, T. (2019). Perceptual dissociations among views of objects, scenes, and reachable spaces. *J Exp Psychol Hum Percept Perform* 45: 715–728. https://doi.org/10.1037/xhp0000626.

Joussain, P., Thevenet, M., Rouby, C., and Bensafi, M. (2013). Effect of aging on hedonic appreciation of pleasant and unpleasant odors. *PLOS ONE* 8(4): e61376. https://doi.org/10.1371/journal.pone.0061376.

Julesz, B. (1964). Binocular depth perception without familiarity cues. *Science* 45: 356–362.

Julesz, B. (1971). *Foundations of Cyclopean Perception*. Chicago: University of Chicago Press.

Julius, D. (2013). TRP channels and pain. *Annu Rev Cell Dev Biol* 29: 355–384.

K

Kadohisa, M., and Wilson, D. A. (2006). Olfactory cortical adaptation facilitates detection of odors against background. *J Neurophysiol* 95: 1888–1896.

Kaim, L., and Drewing, K. (2009). *Finger force of exploratory movements is adapted to the compliance of deformable objects*. Paper presented at the IEEE World Haptics Conference 2009, 565–569.

Kanow, M. A., Giamarco, M. M., Jankowski, C. S. Tsantilas, K., Engel, A. L., Du, J., Linton, J. D., et al. (2017). Biochemical adaptations of the retina and retinal pigment epithelium support a metabolic ecosystem in the vertebrate eye. *eLife* 6 pii: e28899. https://doi.org/10.7554/eLife.28899.

Kantono, K., Nazimah, H., Shepherd, D., Yoo, M. J. Y., Grazioli, G., and Carr, B.T. (2016). Listening to music can influence hedonic and sensory perceptions of gelati. *Appetite* 100: 244–255.

Kanwisher, N. (2017). The quest for the FFA and where it led. *J Neurosci* 37: 1056–1061.

Kanwisher, N., and Dilks, D. D. (2013). The functional organization of the ventral visual pathway in humans. In L. M. Chalupa and J. S. Werner (Eds.), *The New Visual Neurosciences* (pp. 733–746). Cambridge, MA: MIT Press.

Kanwisher, N., McDermott, J., and Chun, M. M. (1997). The fusiform face area: A module in human extrastriate cortex specialized for face perception. *J Neurosci* 17: 4302–4311.

Kapfer, C., Seidl, A. H., Schweizer, H., and Grothe, B. (2002). Experience-dependent refinement of inhibitory inputs to auditory coincidence-detector neurons. *Nat Neurosci* 5: 247–253.

Kappers, S. (2007). Haptic space perception. *Can J Exp Psychol* 61: 208–218.

Kay, K. N., Naselaris, T., Prenger, R. J., and Gallant, J. L. (2008). Identifying natural images from human brain activity. *Nature* 452: 352–355.

Kay, L. M. (2022). COVID-19 and olfactory dysfunction: A looming wave of dementia? *J Neurophysiol.* 128(2): 436–444.

Kaya, E. M., and Elhilali, M. (2017). Modelling auditory attention. *Philos Trans R Soc Lond B Biol Sci* 372: 1–10.

Keller, A., Gerkin, R. C., Guan, Y., Dhurandhar, A., Turu, G., Szalai, B., Mainland, J. D., et al. (2017). Predicting human olfactory perception from chemical features of odor molecules. *Science* 355: 820–826.

Keller, A., and Vosshall, L. B. (2004). A psychophysical test of the vibration theory of olfaction. *Nat Neurosci* 7: 337–338.

Keller, A., and Vosshall, L. B. (2016). Olfactory perception of chemically diverse molecules. *BMC Neurosci* 17: 55.

Keller, A., Zhuang, H., Chi, Q., Vosshall, L. B., and Matsunami, H. (2007). Genetic variation in a human odorant receptor alters odour perception. *Nature* 449: 468–472.

Kellman, P. J., and Shipley, T. F. (1991). A theory of visual interpolation in object perception. *Cogn Psychol* 23: 141–221.

Kepecs, A., Uchida, N., and Mainen, Z. F. (2007). Rapid and precise control of sniffing during olfactory discrimination in rats. *J Neurophysiol* 98: 205–213.

Kern, R. C., Conley, D. B., Haines, G. K., and Robinson, A. M. (2004). Pathology of the olfactory mucosa: Implications for the treatment of olfactory dysfunction. *Laryngoscope* 114: 279–285.

Khosla, A., Raju, A. S., Torralba, A., and Oliva, A. (2015, 7–13 December). *Understanding and predicting image memorability at a large scale.* Paper presented at the 2015 IEEE International Conference on Computer Vision. Santiago, Chile, 2015, pp. 2390–2398.

Khosla, M., Ratan Murty, N. A., and Kanwisher, N. (2022). A highly selective response to food in human visual cortex revealed by hypothesis-free voxel decomposition. *Curr Biol* 32(19): 4159–4171. e4159. https://doi.org/10.1016/j.cub.2022.08.009.

Kiang, N. Y. S. (1965). *Discharge Patterns of Single Fibers in the Cat's Auditory Nerve.* Cambridge, MA: MIT Press.

Kikuta, S., Fletcher, M. L. Homma, R., Yamasoba, T., and Nagayama, S. (2013). Odorant response properties of individual neurons in an olfactory glomerular module. *Neuron* 77: 1122–1135.

Kim, I., Hong, S. W., Shevell, S. K., and Shim, W. M. (2020). Neural representations of perceptual color experience in the human ventral visual pathway. *Proc Natl Acad Sci USA* 117(23): 13145–13150. https://doi.org/10.1073/pnas.1911041117.

Kim, U. K., Jorgenson, E., Coon, H., Leppert, M., Risch, N., and Drayna, D. (2003). Positional cloning of the human quantitative trait locus underlying taste sensitivity to phenylthiocarbamide. *Science* 299: 1221–1225.

Kirchner, H., and Thorpe, S. J. (2006). Ultra-rapid object detection with saccadic eye movements: Visual processing speed revisited. *Vision Res* 46: 1762–1776.

Kirstine, W., Galbally, I., Ye, Y., and Hooper, M. (1998). Emissions of volatile organic compounds (primarily oxygenated species) from pasture. *Journal of Geophysical Research: Atmospheres* 103(D9): 10605–10619.

Klatzky, R. L., Lederman, S. J., and Matula, D. E. (1993). Haptic exploration in the presence of vision. *J Exp Psychol Human Percept Perform* 19: 726–743.

Klatzky, R. L., Lederman, S. J., and Metzger, V. (1985). Identifying objects by touch: An "expert system." *Percept Psychophys* 37: 299–302.

Klein, R. M. (2000). Inhibition of return. *Trends Cogn Sci* 4: 138–147.

Klein, R. M., and MacInnes, W. J. (1999). Inhibition of return is a foraging facilitator in visual search. *Psychol Sci* 10: 346–352.

Kluender, K. R., Diehl, R. L., and Killeen, P. R. (1987). Japanese quail can learn phonetic categories. *Science* 237: 1195–1197.

Kluender, K. R., and Jenison, R. L. (1992). Effects of glide slope, noise intensity, and noise duration on the extrapolation of FM glides through noise. *Percept Psychophys* 51: 231–238.

Kluender, K. R., Lotto, A. J., and Holt, L. L. (2005). Contributions of nonhuman animal models to understanding human speech perception. In S. Greenberg and W. Ainsworth (Eds.), *Listening to Speech: An Auditory Perspective* (pp. 203–220). Mahwah, NJ: Erlbaum.

Kluender, K. R., Lotto, A. J., Holt, L. L., and Bloedel, S. L. (1998). Role of experience for language-specific functional mapping of vowel sounds. *J Acoust Soc Am* 104: 3596–3582.

Kluender, K. R., Stilp, C. E., and Llanos, F. (2019). Long-standing problems in speech perception dissolve within an information-theoretic perspective. *Atten Percept Psychophys* 81: 861–883. https://doi.org/10.3758/s13414-019-01702-x.

Knaapila, A., and Tuorila, H. (2014). Experiences of environmental odors among self-reported hyperosmics: A pilot study. *J Health Psychol* 19(7): 897–906.

Knill, D. C., and Saunders, J. A. (2003). Do humans optimally integrate stereo and texture information for judgments of surface slant? *Vis Res* 43: 2539–2558. https://doi.org/10.1016/s0042-6989(03)00458-9.

Ko, H. K., Poletti, M., and Rucci, M. (2010). Microsaccades precisely relocate gaze in a high visual acuity task. *Nat Neurosci* 13: 1549–1553.

Koch, C. (1999). *Biophysics of Computation: Information Processing in Single Neurons.* Oxford: Oxford University Press.

Koenderink, J., van Doorn, A., Witzel, C., and Gegenfurtner, K. (2020). Hues of color afterimages. *i-Perception* 11(1): 2041669520903553. https://doi.org/10.1177/2041669520903553.

Kolarik, A. J., Moore, B. C. J., Zahorik, P., Cirstea, S., and Pardhan, S. (2016). Auditory distance perception in humans: A review of cues, development, neuronal bases, and effects of sensory loss. *Atten Percept Psychophys* 78: 373–395.

Kondo, H. M., van Loon, A. M., Kawahara, J.-I., and Moore, B. C. J. (2017). Auditory and visual scene analysis: An overview. *Philos Trans R Soc Lond B Biol Sci* 372: 1–6.

Konen, C. S., and Kastner, S. (2008). Two hierarchically organized neural systems for object information in human visual cortex. *Nat Neurosci* 11: 224–231.

Kontaris, I., East, B. S., and Wilson, D. A. (2020) Behavioral and neurobiological convergence of odor, mood, and emotion: A review. *Front Behav Neurosci* 14: 35. https://doi.org/10.3389/fnbeh.2020.00035.

Koreimann, S., Gula, B., and Vitouch, O. (2014). Inattentional deafness in music. *Psych Res* 78: 304–312.

Kosslyn, S. M., Thompson, W. L., Kim, I. J., and Alpert, A. M. (1995). Topographic representations of mental images in primary visual cortex. *Nature* 378: 496–498.

Koulakov, A. A., and Rinberg, D. (2011). Sparse incomplete representations: A potential role of olfactory granule cells. *Neuron* 72: 124–136.

Kovacs, I., and Julesz, B. (1993). A closed curve is much more than an incomplete one: Effect of closure in figure-ground segmentation. *Proc Natl Acad Sci USA* 90: 7495–7497.

Kowler, E., and Collewijn, H. (2010). The eye on the needle. *Nat Neurosci* 13: 1443–1444.

Krauskopf, J., Williams, D. R., and Heeley, D. W. (1982). Cardinal directions of color space. *Vision Res* 22: 1123–1131.

Krestel, D., Passe, D., Smith, J. C., and Jonsson, L. (1984). Behavioral determinants of olfactory thresholds to amyl acetate in dogs. *Neurosci Biobehav Rev* 8: 169–174.

Kriegeskorte, N. (2015). Deep neural networks: A new framework for modeling biological vision and brain information processing. *Annu Rev Vis Sci* 1: 417–446. https://doi.org/10.1146/annurev-vision-082114-035447.

Kriegeskorte, N., and Douglas, P. K. (2018). Cognitive computational neuroscience. *Nature Neurosci* 21: 1148–1160. https://doi.org/10.1038/s41593-018-0210-5.

Krizhevsky, A., Sutskever, I., and Hinton, G. E. (2012). ImageNet classification with deep convolutional neural networks. *Adv Neural Inf Process Syst* 25 (NIPS Proceedings 2012). 60, pp. 84–90.

Krusemark, E. A., Novak, L. R., Gitelman, D. R., and Li, W. (2013). When the sense of smell meets emotion: Anxiety state dependent olfactory processing and neural circuitry adaption. *J Neurosci* 33: 15324–15332.

Kuffler, S. W. (1953). Discharge patterns and functional organization of mammalian retina. *J Neurophysiol* 16: 37–68.

Kuhl, P. K. (1981). Discrimination of speech by nonhuman animals: Basic sensitivities conducive to the perception of speech sound categories. *J Acoust Soc Am* 70: 340–349.

Kuhl, P. K., and Miller, J. D. (1978). Speech perception by the chinchilla: Identification functions for synthetic VOT stimuli. *J Acoust Soc Am* 63: 905–917.

Kuhl, P. K., Williams, K. A., Lacerda, F., Stevens, K. N., and Lindblom, B. (1992). Linguistic experience alters phonetic perception in infants six months of age. *Science* 255: 606–608.

Kuhn, G., and Kingstone, A. (2009). Look away! Eyes and arrows engage oculomotor responses automatically. *Atten Percept Psychophys* 71: 314–327.

Kumagami, T., Zhang, B., Smith, E. L., III, and Chino, Y. M. (2000). Effect of onset age of strabismus on the binocular responses of neurons in the monkey visual cortex. *Invest Ophthalmol Vis Sci* 41: 948–954.

Kurz, J. (2008, December 26). Getting to the root of the great cilantro divide. *National Public Radio*. https://www.npr.org.

Kwok, R. H. M. (1968). Chinese-restaurant syndrome. *N Engl J Med* 278: 796.

L

Lacey, S., and Sathian, K. (2012). Representation of object form in vision and touch. In M. M. Murray and M. T. Wallace (Eds.), *The Neural Bases of Multisensory Processes*. Boca Raton, FL: CRC Press/Taylor & Francis.

Lafer-Sousa, R., Hermann, K. L., and Conway, B. R. (2015). Striking individual differences in color perception uncovered by "the dress" photograph. *Curr Biol* 25: R545–R546.

Laing, D. G., and Francis, G. W. (1989). The capacity of humans to identify odors in mixtures. *Physiol Behav* 46: 809–814.

Laing, D. G., and Glemarec, A. (1992). Selective attention and the perceptual analysis of odor mixtures. *Physiol Behav* 33: 309–319.

Lamb, T. D. (2016). Why rods and cones? *Eye (Lond)* 30(2): 179–185. https://doi.org/10.1038/eye.2015.236.

Lamb, T. D., Collin, S. P., and Pugh, E. N., Jr. (2007). Evolution of the vertebrate eye: Opsins, photoreceptors, retina and eye cup. *Nat Rev Neurosci* 12: 960–976. https://doi.org/10.1038/nrn2283.

LaMotte, R. H., and Srinivasan, M. A. (1991). Surface microgeometry: Tactile perception and neural encoding. In O. Franzen and J. Westman (Eds.), *Information Processing in the Somatosensory System* (pp. 49–58). London: Macmillan.

Land, E. H., and McCann, J. J. (1971). Lightness and retinex theory. *J Opt Soc Am* 61: 1–11.

Larsson, M., and Willander, J. (2009). Autobiographical odor memory. *Ann NY Acad Sci* 1170: 318–323.

Larsson, M., Willander, J., Karlsson, K., and Arshamian, A. (2014). Olfactory LOVER: Behavioral and neural correlates of autobiographical odor memory. *Front Psychol* 5: 312. https://doi.org/10.3389/fpsyg.2014.00312.

Laska, M., Koch, B., Heid, B., and Hudson, R. (1996). Failure to demonstrate systematic changes in olfactory perception in the course of pregnancy: A longitudinal study. *Chem Senses* 21: 567–571.

Laurienti, P. J., Burdette, J. H., Maldjian, J. A., and Wallace, M. T. (2006). Enhanced multisensory integration in older adults. *Neurobiol Aging* 27: 1155–1163. https://doi.org/10.1016/j.neurobiolaging.2005.05.024.

Lawless, H., and Engen, T. (1977). Associations to odors: Interference, mnemonics, and verbal labelling. *J Exp Psychol* 3: 52–59.

Lawo, V., and Koch, I. (2014). Dissociable effects of auditory attention switching and stimulus–response compatibility. *Psych Res* 78: 379–386.

Lecanuet, J. P., Granier-Deferre, C., Cohen, C., Le Houezec, R., and Busnel, M. C. (1986). Fetal responses to acoustic stimulation depend on heart rate variability pattern stimulus intensity and repetition. *Early Hum Dev* 13: 269–283.

Lederman, S. J., and Klatzky, R. L. (1987). Hand movements: A window into haptic object recognition. *Cogn Psychol* 19: 342–368.

Lederman, S. J., and Klatzky, R. L. (1997). Relative availability of surface and object properties during early haptic processing. *J Exp Psychol Hum Percept Perform* 23: 1680–1707.

Lederman, S. J., Klatzky, R., Chataway, C., and Summers, C. (1990). Visual mediation and the haptic recognition of two-dimensional pictures of common objects. *Percept Psychophys* 47: 54–64.

Ledgeway, T. (1994). Adaptation to second-order motion results in a motion aftereffect for directionally-ambiguous test stimuli. *Vision Res* 34: 2879–2889.

Ledgeway, T., and Smith, A. T. (1994). The duration of the motion aftereffect following adaptation to first-order and second-order motion. *Perception* 23: 1211–1219.

Lee, B. K., Mayhew, E. E., Sanchez-Lengeling, B., Wei, J. N., Qian, W. W., Little, K., et al. (2022). A principal odor map unifies diverse tasks in human olfactory perception. *bioRxiv*.

Lee, C.-Y., and Lee, Y.-F. (2010). Perception of musical pitch and lexical tones by Mandarin speaking musicians. *J Acoust Soc Am* 127: 481–490.

Lee, D. N. (1976). A theory of visual control of braking based on information about time-to-collision. *Perception* 5: 437–459.

Lee, D. S., Kim, A. J., and Anderson, B. A. (2022). The influence of reward history on goal-directed visual search. *Atten Percept Psychophys* 84(2): 325–331. https://doi.org/10.3758/s13414-021-02435-6.

Lee, R. J., Kofonow, J. M., Rosen, P. L., Siebert, A. P., Chen, B., Doghramji, L., et al. (2014). Bitter and sweet taste receptors regulate human upper respiratory innate immunity. *J Clin Invest* 124: 1393–1405. https://doi.org/10.1172/JCI72094.

Leed, J. E., Chinn, L. K., and Lockman, J. J. (2019). Reaching to the self: The development of infants' ability to localize targets on the body. *Psychol Sci* 30:1063–1073. https://doi.org/10.1177/0956797619850168.

Legge, G. E., Granquist, C., Lubet, A., Gage, R., and Xiong, Y. Z. (2019). Preserved tactile acuity in older pianists. *Atten Percept Psychophys* 8: 2619–2625. https://doi.org/10.3758/s13414-019-01844-y.

Legge, G. E., Madison, C., Vaughn, B. N., Cheong, A. M. Y., and Miller, J. C. (2008). Retention of high tactile acuity throughout the life span in blindness. *Percept Psychophys* 70: 1471–1488.

Leonard, M. K., Baud, M. O., Sjerps, M. J., and Chang, E. F. (2016). Perceptual restoration of masked speech in human cortex. *Nat Commun* 7: 13619. https://doi.org/10.1038/ncomms13619.

LeVay, S., Hubel, D. H., and Wiesel, T. N. (1975). The pattern of ocular dominance columns in macaque visual cortex revealed by a reduced silver stain. *J Comp Neurol* 159: 559–576.

Levi, D. M. (2008). Crowding—an essential bottleneck for object recognition: A mini-review. *Vision Res* 48: 635–654.

Levi, D. M. (2023). Applications and implications for extended reality to improve binocular vision and stereopsis. *J Vis* 23(1): 14. https://doi.org/10.1167/jov.23.1.14.

Levi, D. M., Klein, S. A., and Aitsebaomo, A. P. (1985). Vernier acuity, crowding, and cortical magnification. *Vision Res* 25: 963–977.

Levi, D. M., and Li, R. W. (2009). Perceptual learning as a potential treatment for amblyopia: A mini-review. *Vision Res* 49: 2535–2549.

Levin, D. T., and Beale, J. M. (2000). Categorical perception occurs in newly learned faces, other-race faces, and inverted faces. *Atten Percept Psychophys* 62: 386–401.

Levinson, S. C. (2000). Yeli Dnye and the theory of basic color terms. *J Linguist Anthropol* 10: 3–55.

Li, B., Peterson, M. R., and Freeman, R. D. (2003). Oblique effect: A neural basis in the visual cortex. *J Neurophysiol* 90: 204–217.

Li, F. F., VanRullen, R., Koch, C., and Perona, P. (2002). Rapid natural scene categorization in the near absence of attention. *Proc Natl Acad Sci USA* 99: 9596–9601.

Li, R. W., Ngo, C., Nguyen, J., and Levi, D. M. (2011). Videogame play induces plasticity in the visual system of adults with amblyopia. *PLOS Biol* 9: e1001135.

Li, W., Lopez, L., Osher, J., Howard, J. D., Parrish, T. B., and Gottfried, J. A. (2010). Right orbitofrontal cortex mediates conscious olfactory perception. *Psychol Sci* 21: 1454–1463.

Liberman, A. M., Cooper, F. S., Shankweiler, D. P., and Studdert Kennedy, M. (1967). Perception of the speech code. *Psychol Rev* 74: 431–461.

Liberman, A. M., Harris, K. S., Hoffman, H. S., and Griffith, B. C. (1957). The discrimination of speech sounds within and across phoneme boundaries. *J Exp Biol* 54: 358–368.

Liberman, A. M., and Mattingly, I. G. (1985). The motor theory of speech perception revised. *Cognition* 21: 1–36.

Lieberman, P. (1984). *The Biology and Evolution of Language*. Cambridge, MA: Harvard University Press.

Liem, D. G., and Mennella, J. A. (2003). Heightened sour preferences during childhood. *Chem Senses* 28: 173–180.

Lima, C. F., Krishnan, S., and Scott, S. K. (2016). Roles of supplementary motor areas in auditory processing and auditory imagery. *Trends Neurosci* 39: 527–542.

Lin, J. Y., Murray, S. O., and Boynton, G. M. (2009). Capture of attention to threatening stimuli without perceptual awareness. *Curr Biol* 19: 1118–1122.

Lindeman, H. H. (1973). Anatomy of the otolith organs. *Adv Otorhinolaryngol* 20: 404–433.

Lindsey, D. T., and Brown, A. M. (2006). Universality of color names. *Proc Natl Acad Sci USA* 103: 16608–16613.

Lindsey, D. T., and Brown, A. M. (2014). The color lexicon of American English. *J Vis* 14: 17.

Lindsey, D. T., and Brown, A. M. (2021). Lexical color categories. *Annu Rev Vision Sci* 7(1): 605–631. https://doi.org/10.1146/annurev-vision-093019-112420C.

Linhares, J. M. M., Pinto, P. D., and Nascimento, S. M. C. (2008). The number of discernible colors in natural scenes. *J Opt Soc Am A Opt Image Sci Vis* 25: 2918–2924.

Lisker, L. (1986). "Voicing" in English: A catalogue of acoustic features signaling /b/ versus /p/ in trochees. *Lang Speech* 29: 3–11.

Livingstone, M., and Hubel, D. (1988) Segregation of form, color, movement, and depth: Anatomy, physiology, and perception. *Science* 240: 740–749.

Löfvenberg, J., and Johansson, R. S. (1984). Regional differences and interindividual variability in sensitivity to vibration in the glabrous skin of the human hand. *Brain Res* 301: 65–72.

Logothetis, N. K., Pauls, J., and Poggio, T. (1995). Shape representation in the inferior temporal cortex of monkeys. *Curr Biol* 5: 552–563.

Logothetis, N. K., and Schall, J. D. (1989). Neuronal correlates of subjective visual perception. *Science* 245: 761–763.

Lombard, M., and Ditton, T. (1997). At the heart of it all: The concept of presence. *Journal of Computer-Mediated Communication* 3(2): JCMC321.

Loomis, J. M. (1981). On the tangibility of letters and braille. *Percept Psychophys* 29: 37–46.

Loomis, J. M. (1990). A model of character recognition and legibility. *J Exp Psychol Hum Percept Perform* 16: 106–120.

Lorenzen, A., Scholz-Hehn, D., Wiesner, C. D., Wolff, S., Bergmann, T. O., van Eimeren, T. et al. (2016). Chemosensory processing in children with attention deficit/hyperactivity disorder. *J Psychiat Res* 76: 121–127. https://doi.org/10.1016/j.jpsychires.2016.02.007.

Lorig, T. (1999). On the similarity of odor and language perception. *Neurosci Biobehav Rev* 23: 391–398.

Lotter, W., Diab, A. R., Haslam, B., Kim, J. G., Grisot, G., Wu, E., Wu, K., et al. (2021). Robust breast cancer detection in mammography and digital breast tomosynthesis using an annotation-efficient deep learning approach. *Nat Med* 27: 244–249. https://doi.org/10.1038/s41591-020-01174-9.

Lotto, A. J., Kluender, K. R., and Holt, L. L. (1997). Perceptual compensation for coarticulation by Japanese quail (*Coturnix coturnix japonica*). *J Acoust Soc Am* 102(2, Pt 1): 1134–1140. https://doi.org/10.1121/1.419865.

Lovell, P. G., Bloj, M., and Harris, J. M. (2012). Optimal integration of shading and binocular disparity for depth perception. *J Vis* 12: 1. https://doi.org/10.1167/12.1.1.

Lowe, D. G. (1985). *Perceptual Organization and Visual Recognition*. Boston: Kluwer.

Lu, Z.-L., and Dosher, B. A. (1998). External noise distinguishes attention mechanisms. *Vision Res* 38: 1183–1198.

Lunde, S. J., Vuust, P., Garza-Villareal, E. A., and Vase, L. (2019). Music-induced analgesia: How does music relieve pain? *Pain* 160(5): 989–993. https://doi.org/10.1097/j.pain.0000000000001452.

Lundstrom, J. N., and Olsson, M. J. (2005). Subthreshold amounts of a social odorant affect mood, but not behavior, in heterosexual women when tested by a male, but not a female experimenter. *Biol Psychol* 60: 197–204.

Lynch, M. P., and Eilers, R. E. (1990). Innateness, experience, and music perception. *Psychol Sci* 1: 272–276.

M

Ma, Q. (2010). Labeled lines meet and talk: Population coding of somatic sensations. *J Clin Invest* 120: 3773–3778.

Ma, W. J., Kording, K. P., and Goldreich, D. (2023). *Bayesian Models of Perception and Action: An Introduction*. Cambridge, MA: MIT Press.

Mach, E. (1875/2001). *Fundamentals of the Theory of Movement Perception* (republished with translations in 2001). New York: Kluwer/Plenum.

MacLeod, D. I., and Lennie, P. (1976). Red-green blindness confined to one eye. *Vision Res* 16: 691–702.

Maddieson, I. (1984). *Patterns of Sound*. Cambridge: Cambridge University Press.

Magri, C., Konkle, T., and Caramazza, A. (2021). The contribution of object size, manipulability, and stability on neural responses to inanimate objects. *NeuroImage* 237: 118098. https://doi.org/10.1016/j.neuroimage.2021.118098.

Mahon, B. Z., Anzellotti, S., Schwarzbach, J., Zampini, M., and Caramazza, A. (2009). Category-specific organization in the human brain does not require visual experience. *Neuron* 63(3): 397–405. https://doi.org/10.1016/j.neuron.2009.07.012.

Majid, A., and Burenhult, N. (2014). Odors are expressible in language, as long as you speak the right language. *Cognition* 130: 266–270.

Majid, A., and Kruspe, N. (2018). Hunter-gatherer olfaction is special. *Curr Biol* 28: 409–413. https://doi.org/10.1016/j.cub.2017.12.014.

Majid, A., Speed, L., Croijmans, I., and Arshamian, A. (2017). What makes a better smeller? *Perception* 46(3–4): 406–430.

Malik, J., and Perona, P. (1990). Preattentive texture discrimination with early vision mechanisms. *J Opt Soc Am A* 7: 923–932.

Maloney, L. T. (1986). Evaluation of linear models of surface spectral reflectance with small numbers of parameters. *J Opt Soc Am A* 3: 1673–1683.

Mancini, F., Bauleo, A., Cole, J., Lui, F., Porro, C. A., Haggard, P., and Iannetti, G. D. (2014). Whole-body mapping of spatial acuity for pain and touch. *Ann Neurol* 75: 917–924.

Maquet, P., Peters, J., Aerts, J., Delfiore, G., Degueldre, C., Luxen, A., and Franck, G. (1996). Functional neuroanatomy of human rapid-eye-movement sleep and dreaming. *Nature* 383: 163–166.

Maresh, A., Gil, D. R., Whitman, M. C., and Greer, C. A. (2008). Principles of glomerular organization in the human olfactory bulb: Implications for odor processing. *PLOS ONE* 3: 1–6.

Marks, L. E., Stevens, J. C., Bartoshuk, L. M., Gent, J. G., Rifkin, B., and Stone, V. K. (1988). Magnitude matching: The measurement of taste and smell. *Chem Senses* 13: 63–87.

Marlow, P. J., Gegenfurtner, K. R., and Anderson, B. L. (2022). The role of color in the perception of three-dimensional shape. *Curr Biol* 32(6): 1387–1394.e1383. https://doi.org/10.1016/j.cub.2022.01.026.

Marotta, A., Ferre. E. R., and Haggard, P. (2015). Transforming the thermal grill effect by crossing the fingers. *Curr Biol* 25: 1069–1073.

Marr, D., and Poggio, T. (1979). A computational theory of human stereo vision. *Proc R Soc Lond B Biol Sci* 204: 301–328.

Marshall, J., and Arikawa, K. (2014). Unconventional colour vision. *Curr Biol* 24: R1150–R1154.

Martínez-Domingo, M. A., Gómez-Robledo, L., Valero, E. M., Huertas, R., Hernández-Andrés, J., Ezpeleta, S., and Hita, E. (2019). Assessment of VINO filters for correcting red-green color vision deficiency. *Opt Express* 27: 17954–17967. https://doi.org/10.1364/OE.27.017954.

Martínez-Molina, N., Mas-Herrero, E., Rodríguez-Fornells, A., Zatorre, R. J., and Marco-Pallarés, J. (2019). White matter microstructure reflects individual differences in music reward sensitivity. *J Neurosci* 39: 5018–5027. https://doi.org/10.1523/jneurosci.2020-18.2019.

Martinez-Trujillo, J. (2022). Visual attention in the prefrontal cortex. *Annu Rev Vision Sci* 8(1), 407–425. https://doi.org/10.1146/annurev-vision-100720-031711.

Martinho, A., III, and Kacelnik, A. (2016). Ducklings imprint on the relational concept of "same or different." *Science* 353: 286–288. https://doi.org/10.1126/science.aaf4247.

Masland, R. H. (2017). Vision: Two speeds in the retina. *Curr Biol* 27: R303–R305.

Mather, G., and Murdoch, L. (1994). Gender discrimination in biological motion displays based on dynamic cues. *Proc R Soc Lond B Biol Sci* 258: 273–279.

Matin, L., Picoult, E., Stevens, J. K., Edwards, M. W., Jr., Young, D., and MacArthur, R. (1982). Oculoparalytic illusion: Visual-field dependent spatial mislocalizations by humans partially paralyzed with curare. *Science* 216: 198–201.

Matsunaga, M., Bai, Y., Yamakawa, K., Toyama, A., Kashiwagi, M., Fukuda, K., et al. (2013). Brain–immune interaction accompanying odor-evoked autobiographic memory. *PLoS One* 8(8): e72523.

Matsunaga, M., Isowa, T., Yamakawa, K., Kawanishi, Y., Tsuboi, H., Kaneko, H., and Ohira, H. (2011). Psychological and physiological responses to odor-evoked autobiographic memory. *Neuroendocrinology Letters* 32(6): 774–780.

Maurer, D., Lewis, T. L., Brent, H. P., and Levin, A. V. (1999). Rapid improvement in the acuity of infants after visual input. *Science* 286: 108–110.

Mavrogeni, P., Kanakopoulos, A., Maihoub, S., Maihoub, S., Krasznai, M., and Szirmai, A. (2016). Anosmia treatment by platelet rich plasma injection. *Int Tinnitus J 20*(2): 102–105.

Mayhew, E. J., Arayata, C. J., Gerkin, R. C., Lee, B. K., Magill, J. M., Snyder, L. L., et al. (2022). Transport features predict if a molecule is odorous. *Proceedings of the National Academy of Sciences* 119(15): e2116576119.

Mays, L. E., and Sparks, D. L. (1980) Dissociation of visual and saccade-related responses in superior colliculus neurons. *J Neurophysiol* 43: 207–232.

McCandliss, B. D., Cohen, L., and Dehaene, S. (2003). The visual word form area: Expertise for reading in the fusiform gyrus. *Trends Cogn Sci* 7: 293–299. https://doi.org/10.1016/s1364-6613(03)00134-7.

McClintock, M. K. (1971). Menstrual synchrony and suppression. *Nature* 229(5282): 244–245.

McConkie, G. W., and Currie, C. (1996). Visual stability across saccades while viewing complex pictures. *J Exp Psychol Hum Percept Perform* 22: 563–581.

McDermott, J. H., Schultz, A. F., Undurraga, E. A., and Godoy, R. A. (2016). Indifference to dissonance in native Amazonians reveals cultural variation in music perception. *Nature* 535: 547–550.

McDermott, J. H., Wroblewski, D., and Oxenham, A. J. (2011). Recovering sound sources from embedded repetition. *Proc Natl Acad Sci USA* 108: 1188–1193.

McGann, J. P. (2017). Poor human olfaction is a 19th-century myth. *Science* 356(6338): eaam7263.

McGlone, F., Vallbo, A. B., Olausson, H., Loken, L. S., and Wessberg, J. (2007). Discriminative touch and emotional touch. *Can J Exp Psychol* 61: 173–183.

McGlone, F., Wessberg, J., and Olausson, H. (2014). Discriminative and affective touch: Sensing and feeling. *Neuron* 82: 737–755. https://doi.org/10.1016/j.neuron.2014.05.001.

McGowan, P. O., Sasaki, A., D'Alessio, A. C., Dymov, S., Labonté, B., Szy, M., Turecki, G., et al. (2009). Epigenetic regulation of the glucocorticoid receptor in human brain associates with childhood abuse. *Nat Neurosci* 12: 342–348.

McGurk, H., and MacDonald, J. (1976). Hearing lips and seeing voices. *Nature* 264: 746–748.

McIntyre, S., Hauser, S. C., Kusztor, A., Boehme, R., Moungou, A., Isager, P. M., Homman, L., et al. (2022). The language of social touch is intuitive and quantifiable. *Psychol Sci* 33(9): 1477–1494. doi: 10.1177/09567976211059801.

McKee, S. P. (1983). The spatial requirements for fine stereoacuity. *Vision Res* 23: 191–198.

McKee, S. P., and Taylor, D. G. (2010). The precision of binocular and monocular depth judgments in natural settings. *J Vis* 10: 5.

McMains, S. A., and Somers, D. C. (2004). Multiple spotlights of attentional selection in human visual cortex. *Neuron* 42: 677–686.

McMullen, D. P., Thomas, T. M., Fifer, M. S., Candrea, D. N., Tenore, F. V., Nickl, R. W., Pohlmeyer, E. A., et al. (2021). Novel intraoperative online functional mapping of somatosensory finger representations for targeted stimulating electrode placement: technical note. *J Neurosurg* 26: 1–8. https://doi.org/10.3171/2020.9.JNS202675.

McRae, J. F., Jaeger, S. R., Bava, C. M., Beresford, M. K., Hunter, D., Jia, Y., Chheang, S. L., et al. (2013). Identification of regions associated with variation in sensitivity to food-related odors in the human genome. *Curr Biol* 23: 1596–600.

McWalter, R., and McDermott, J. H. (2019). Illusory sound texture reveals multi-second statistical completion in auditory scene analysis. *Nat Commun* 10: 5096. https://doi.org/10.1038/s41467-019-12893-0.

Mehler, J., Jusczyk, P., Lambertz, C., Halsted, N., Bertoncini, J., and Amiel-Tison, C. (1988). A precursor of language acquisition in young infants. *Cognition* 29: 143–178.

Melin, A. D., Kline, D. W., Hickey, C. M., and Fedigan, L. M. (2013). Food search through the eyes of a monkey: A functional substitution approach for assessing the ecology of primate color vision. *Vision Res* 86: 87–96.

Melzack, R., and Wall, P. D. (1988). *The Challenge of Pain* (2nd ed.). New York: Penguin.

Menashe, I., Man, O., Lancet, D., and Gilad, Y. (2003). Different noses for different people. *Nat Genet* 34: 143–144.

Mendelson, E. B. (2018). Artificial intelligence in breast imaging: Potentials and limitations. *Am J Roentgenol* 212: 293–299. https://doi.org/10.2214/AJR.18.20532.

Mennella, J. A., and Beauchamp, G. K. (1991). The transfer of alcohol to human milk: Effects on flavor and the infant's behavior. *N Engl J Med* 325: 981–985.

Mennella, J. A., and Beauchamp, G. K. (1993). The effects of repeated exposure to garlic-flavored milk on the nursling's behavior. *Pediatr Res* 34: 805–808.

Mennella, J. A., Johnson, A., and Beauchamp, G. K. (1995). Garlic ingestion by pregnant women alters the odor of amniotic fluid. *Chem Senses* 20: 207–209.

Mercado-Perez, A., and Beyder, A. (2022). Gut feelings: Mechanosensing in the gastrointestinal tract. *Nat Rev Gastroenterol Hepatol* 19: 283–296. https://doi.org/10.1038/s41575-021-00561-y.

Merfeld, D. M., Young, L., Oman, C., and Shelhamer, M. (1993). A multi-dimensional model of the effect of gravity on the spatial orientation of the monkey. *J Vestib Res* 3: 141–161.

Merfeld, D., Zupan, L., and Peterka, R. (1999). Humans use internal models to estimate gravity and linear acceleration. *Nature* 398: 615–618.

Mesgarani, N., Cheung, C., Johnson, K., and Chang, E. F. (2014). Phonetic feature encoding in human superior temporal gyrus. *Science* 343: 1006–1010.

Mesholam, R. I., Moberg, P. J., Mahr, R. N., and Doty, R. L. (1998). Olfaction in neurodegenerative disease: A meta-analysis of olfactory functioning in Alzheimer's and Parkinson's diseases. *Archives of Neurology* 55(1): 84–90.

Meyerhof, W., Batram, C., Kuhn, C., Brockhoff, A., Chudoba, E., Bufe, B., Appendino, G. and Behrens, M. (2010). The molecular receptive ranges of human TAS2R bitter taste receptors. *Chem Senses* 35: 157–170.

Miconi, T., Groomes, L., and Kreiman, G. (2016). There's Waldo! A normalization model of visual search predicts single-trial human fixations in an object search task. *Cerebral Cortex* 26: 3064–3082. https://doi.org/10.1093/cercor/bhv129.

Miller, G. A., and Heise, G. A. (1950). The trill threshold. *J Acoust Soc Am* 22: 637–638.

Miller, G., Tybur, J. M., and Jordan, B. D. (2007). Ovulatory cycle effects on tip earnings by lap dancers: Economic evidence for human estrus? *Evol Hum Behav* 28: 375–381.

Miller, L. E., Fabio, C., Ravenda, V., Bahmad, S., Koun, E., Salemme, R., Luauté, J., et al. (2019). Somatosensory cortex efficiently processes touch located beyond the body. *Curr Biol* 29: 4276–4283. https://doi.org/10.1016/j.cub.2019.10.043.

Miller, S. L., and Maner, J. K. (2010). Scent of a woman: Men's testosterone responses to olfactory ovulation cues. *Psychol Sci* 21: 276–283.

Milne, A. O., Orton, L., Black, C. H., Jones, G. C., Sullivan, M., and Grant, R. A. (2021). California sea lions employ task-specific strategies for active touch sensing. *J Exp Biol* 224(21): jeb243085. https://doi.org/10.1242/jeb.243085.

Ming, D., Ninomiya, Y., and Margolskee, R. F. (1999). Blocking taste receptor activation of gustducin inhibits gustatory responses to bitter compounds. *Proc Natl Acad Sci USA* 96: 9903–9908.

Miranda, M. I. (2012). Taste and odor recognition memory: The emotional flavor of life. *Rev Neuroscience* 23: 481–499.

Mishor, E., Amir, D., Weiss, T., Honigstein, D., Weissbrod, A., Livne, E., Gorodisky, L., et al. (2021). Sniffing the human body volatile hexadecanal blocks aggression in men but triggers aggression in women. *Sci Adv* 7(47): eabg1530.

Mollon, J. D. (1989). "Tho' she kneel'd in that place where they grew ... ": The uses and origins of primate colour vision. *J Exp Biol* 146: 21–38.

Mombaerts, P., Wang, F., Dulac, C., Chao, S. K., Nemes, A., Mendelsohn, M., Edmondson, J., et al. (1996). Visualizing an olfactory sensory map. *Cell* 87: 675–686.

Moncrieff, R. W. (1966). *Odour Preferences.* New York: Wiley.

Mondloch, C. J., Lewis, T. L., Budreau, D. R., Maurer, D., Dannemiller, J. L., Stephens, B. R., and Kleiner-Gathercoal, K. A. (1999). Face perception during early infancy. *Psychol Sci* 10: 419–422.

Moore, B. C. J. (2003). *An Introduction to the Psychology of Hearing* (5th ed.). London: Academic Press.

Moore, M. J., Milosevich, E., Mattingley, J. B., and Demeyere, N. (2023). The neuroanatomy of visuospatial neglect: A systematic review and analysis of lesion-mapping methodology. *Neuropsychologia* 180: 108470. https://doi.org/10.1016/j.neuropsychologia.2023.108470.

Moran, J., and Desimone, R. (1985). Selective attention gates visual processing in the extrastriate cortex. *Science* 229: 782–784.

Morrell, F. (1972). Visual system's view of acoustic space. *Nature* 238: 44–46.

Morris, A. P., and Krekelberg, B. (2019). A stable visual world in primate primary visual cortex. *Curr Biol* 29: 1471–1480.e6. https://doi.org/10.1016/j.cub.2019.03.069.

Moskowitz, H. R., Dravnieks, A., and Klarman, L. A. (1976). Odor intensity and pleasantness for a diverse set of odorants. *Percept Psychophys* 19: 122–128.

Motohashi, K., and Umino, M. (2001). Heterotopic painful stimulation decreases the late component of somatosensory evoked potentials induced by electrical tooth stimulation. *Brain Res Cogn Brain Res* 11: 39–46.

Mounts, J. R. (2000). Evidence for suppressive mechanisms in attentional selection: Feature singletons produce inhibitory surrounds. *Percept Psychophys* 62: 969–983.

Mullane, J. C., and Klein, R. M. (2008). Visual search by children with and without ADHD. *J Attention Disord* 12: 44–53.

Munyan III, B. G., Neer, S. M., Beidel, D. C., and Jentsch, F. (2016). Olfactory stimuli increase presence in virtual environments. *PLOS ONE* 11(6): e0157568.

Murphy, C., Cain, W. S., Gilmore, M. M., and Skinner, R. B. (1991). Sensory and semantic factors in recognition memory for odors and graphic stimuli: Elderly versus young persons. *Am J Psychol* 104: 161–192.

Murphy, S., and Dalton, P. (2016). Out of touch? Visual load induces inattentional numbness. *J Exp Psychol Hum Percept Perform* 42: 761–765.

Musiek, F. E. (2003). What can the acoustic startle reflex tell us? *Hear J* 56: 55.

Musilova, Z., Cortesi, F., Matschiner, M., Davies, W. I. L., Patel, J. S., Stieb, S. M., de Busserolles, F., et al. (2019). Vision using multiple distinct rod opsins in deep-sea fishes. *Science* 364: 588–592. https://doi.org/10.1126/science.aav4632.

N

Nachev, V., Stich, K. P., Winter, C., Bond, A., Kamil, A., and Winter, Y. (2017). Cognition-mediated evolution of low-quality floral nectars. *Science* 355: 75–78.

Nadler, J. W., Angelaki, D. E., and DeAngelis, G. C. (2008). A neural representation of depth from motion parallax in macaque visual cortex. *Nature* 452: 642–645.

Nardini, M., Bedford, R., and Mareschal, D. (2010). Fusion of visual cues is not mandatory in children. *Proc Natl Acad Sci U S A*, 107(39): 17041–17046. doi: 10.1073/pnas.1001699107

Nassi, J., and Callaway, E. M. (2009). Parallel processing strategies of the primate visual system. *Nat Rev Neurosci* 10: 360–372.

Nathans, J. (1986). Molecular genetics of inherited variation in human color vision. *Science* 232: 203–210.

Nathans, J., Thomas, D., and Hogness, D. S. (1986). Molecular genetics of human color vision: The genes encoding blue, green, and red pigments. *Science* 232: 193–202.

Navon, D. (1977). Forest before the trees: The precedence of global features in visual perception. *Cogn Psychol* 9: 353–383.

Negoias, S., Croy, I., Gerber, J., Puschmann, S., Petrowski, K., Joraschky, P., and Hummel, T. (2010). Reduced olfactory bulb volume and olfactory sensitivity in patients with acute major depression. *Neuroscience* 169: 415–421.

Neitz, J., Geist, T., and Jacobs, G. H. (1989). Color vision in the dog. *Vis Neurosci* 3: 119–125.

Nerger, J. L., Volbrecht, V. J., and Ayde, C. J. (1995). Unique hue judgments as a function of test size in the fovea and at 20-deg temporal eccentricity. *J Opt Soc Am A Opt Image Sci Vis* 12: 1225–1232.

Neri, P., Luu, J. Y., and Levi, D. M. (2006). Meaningful interactions can enhance visual discrimination of human agents. *Nat Neurosci* 9: 1186–1192.

Neri, P., Morrone, M. C., and Burr, D. C. (1998). Seeing biological motion. *Nature* 395: 894–896.

Newcombe, F., and de Haan, E. H. F. (1994). Category specificity in visual recognition. In M. J. Farah and G. Ratcliff (Eds.), *The Neuropsychology of High-Level Vision: Collected Tutorial Essays* (Carnegie Mellon Symposia on Cognition) (pp. 103–132). Hillsdale, NJ: Erlbaum.

Newell, F. N., and Bülthoff, H. H. (2002). Categorical perception of familiar objects. *Cognition* 85: 113–143.

Newsome, W. T., and Paré, E. B. (1988). A selective impairment of motion perception following lesions of the middle temporal visual area (MT). *J Neurosci* 8: 2201–2211.

Niechwiej-Szwedo, E., Colpa, L., and Wong, A. M. F. (2019). Visuomotor behaviour in amblyopia: Deficits and compensatory adaptations. *Neural Plast* 2019: 6817839. https://doi.org/10.1155/2019/6817839.

Niimura, Y., Matsui, A., and Touhara, K. (2014). Extreme expansion of the olfactory receptor gene repertoire in African elephants and evolutionary dynamics of orthologous gene groups in 13 placental mammals. *Genome Res* 24: 1485–1496.

Nityananda, V., Tarawneh, G., Jones, L., Busby, N., Herbert, W., Davies, R., and Read, J. C. A. (2015). The contrast sensitivity function of the praying mantis *Sphodromantis lineola*. *J Comp Physiol A* 201: 741–750.

Nityananda, V., Tarawneh, G., Rosner, R., Nicolas, J., Crichton, S., and Read, J. (2016). Insect stereopsis demonstrated using a 3D insect cinema. *Sci Rep* 6: 18718.

Nobre, A. C., and Kastner, S. (2014). *Oxford Handbook of Attention*. New York: Oxford University Press.

Nodine, C. F., Mello-Thoms, C., Kundel, H. L., and Weinstein, S. P. (2002). Time course of perception and decision making during mammographic interpretation. *Am J Roentgenol* 179: 917–923.

Noel, A. C., and Hu, D. L. (2018). Cats use hollow papillae to wick saliva into fur. *Proc Natl Acad Sci USA* 115: 12377–12382. https://doi.org/10.1073/pnas.1809544115.

Norcia, A. M., Gerhard, H. E., and Meredith, W. J. (2017). Development of relative disparity sensitivity in human visual cortex. *J Neurosci* 37(23): 5608–5619. https://doi.org/10.1523/JNEUROSCI.3570-16.2017.

Norcia, A. M., Tyler, C. W., and Hamer, R. D. (1990). Development of contrast sensitivity in the human infant. *Vision Res* 30: 1475–1486.

Norman-Haignere, S., Kanwisher, N. G., and McDermott, J. H. (2015). Distinct cortical pathways for music and speech revealed by hypothesis-free voxel decomposition. *Neuron* 88: 1281–1296.

Nummenmaa, L., Glerean, E., Hari, R., and Hietanen, J. K. (2014). Bodily maps of emotions. *Proc Natl Acad Sci USA* 111(2): 646–651. https://doi.org/10.1073/pnas.1321664111.

O

O'Callaghan, C. (2016). Objects for multisensory perception. *Philosoph Stud* 173: 1269–1289. https://doi.org/10.1007/s11098-015-0545-7.

O'Craven, K. M., and Kanwisher, N. (2000). Mental imagery of faces and places activates corresponding stimulus-specific brain regions. *J Cogn Neurosci* 12: 1013–1023.

O'Dell, C., and Boothe, R. G. (1997). The development of stereoacuity in infant rhesus monkeys. *Vision Res* 37: 2675–2684.

Ohzawa, I., and Freeman, R. D. (1986a). The binocular organization of simple cells in the cat's visual cortex. *J Neurophysiol* 56: 221–242.

Ohzawa, I., and Freeman, R. D. (1986b). The binocular organization of complex cells in the cat's visual cortex. *J Neurophysiol* 56: 243–259.

Okano, T., Fukada, Y., and Yoshizawa, T. (1995). Molecular basis for tetrachromatic color vision. *Comp Biochem Physiol B* 112: 405–414.

Olausson, H., Cole, J., Rylander, K., McGlone, F., Lamarre, Y., Wallin, B. G., Krämer H., et al. (2008). Functional role of unmyelinated tactile afferents in human hairy skin: Sympathetic response and perceptual localization. *Exp Brain Res* 184: 135–140.

Oliva, A., and Torralba, A. (2001). Modeling the shape of the scene: A holistic representation of the spatial envelope. *Int J Comput Vis* 42: 145–175.

Oliva, A., and Torralba, A. (2007). The role of context in object recognition. *Trends Cogn Sci* 11(12): 520–527. https://doi.org/10.1016/j.tics.2007.09.009.

Oliveira-Pinto, A. V., Santos, R. M., Coutinho, R. A., Oliveira, L. M., Santos, G. B., Alho, A. T., et al. (2014). Sexual dimorphism in the human olfactory bulb: Females have more neurons and glial cells than males. *PLOS ONE* 9(11): e111733. https://doi.org/10.1371/journal.pone.0111733.

Olivers, C. N., and Meeter, M. (2008). A boost and bounce theory of temporal attention. *Psychol Rev* 115: 836–863.

Olney, J. W., and Sharpe, L. G. (1969). Brain lesions in an infant rhesus monkey treated with monosodium glutamate. *Science* 166: 386–388.

Oman, C. (1990). Motion sickness: A synthesis and evaluation of the sensory conflict theory. *Can J Physiol Pharmacol* 68: 294–303.

Ooi, T., and He, Z. (1999). Binocular rivalry and visual awareness: The role of attention. *Perception* 28: 551–574.

Ooi, T. L., Wu, B., and He, Z. J. (2001). Distance determined by the angular declination below the horizon. *Nature* 414: 197–200.

Orefice, L. L., Zimmerman, A. L., Chirila, A. M., Sleboda, S. J., Head, J. P., and Ginty, D. D. (2016). Peripheral mechanosensory neuron dysfunction underlies tactile and behavioral deficits in mouse models of ASDs. *Cell* 166: 299–313.

O'Regan, K. (1992). Solving the "real" mysteries of visual perception: The world as an outside memory. *Can J Psychol* 46: 461–488.

Otte, R. J., Agterberg, M. J. H., Van Wanrooij, M. M., Snik, A. F. M., and Van Opstal, A. J. (2013). Age-related hearing loss and ear morphology affect vertical but not horizontal sound-localization performance. *J Assoc Res Otolaryngol* 14: 261–273.

Owens, D. A. (1987). Oculomotor information and perception of three-dimensional space. In H. Heuer and A. F. Sanders (Eds.), *Perspectives on Perception and Action* (pp. 215–248). Hillside, NJ: Erlbaum.

Oxbury, J. M., Oxbury, S. M., and Humphrey, N. K. (1969). Varieties of colour anomia. *Brain* 92: 847–860.

Oyster, C. W. (1999). *The Human Eye: Structure and Function*. Sunderland, MA: Sinauer.

P

Paik, S. B., and Ringach, D. L. (2011). Retinal origin of orientation maps in visual cortex. *Nat Neurosci* 14: 919–925.

Palmer, J. (1995). Attention in visual search: Distinguishing four causes of a set size effect. *Curr Dir Psychol Sci* 4: 118–123.

Palmer, S. E., Schloss, K. B., Xu, Z., and Prado-Leon, L. R. (2013). Music-color associations are mediated by emotion. *Proc Natl Acad Sci USA* 110(22): 8836–8841. https://doi.org/10.1073/pnas.1212562110.

Palmisano, S., Gillam, B., Govan, D. G., Allison, R. S., and Harris, J. M. (2010). Stereoscopic perception of real depths at large distances. *J Vis* 10: 19.

Palouzier-Paulignan, B., Lacroix, M. C., Aimé, P., Baly, C., Caillol, M., Congar, P., et al. (2012). Olfaction under metabolic influences. *Chem Senses* 37: 769–797. https://doi.org/10.1093/chemse/bjs059.

Pangborn, R. M., Simone, M. J., and Platou, E. H. (1957). Natural food flavor intensity: Apricot, peach, and pear nectars studied to determine the sweetness-acid-flavor relationship in a natural food product. California Agriculture, November, p. 10.

Panum, P. L. (1940). *Physiological Investigations Concerning Vision with Two Eyes* (translated from German by C. Hubscher). Hanover, NH: Dartmouth Eye Institute. (Original work published 1858)

Papoiu, A. D. P., Nattkemper, L. A., Sanders, K. M., Kraft, R. A., Chan, Y.-H., Coghill, R. C., and Yosipovitch, G. (2014). Brain's reward circuits mediate itch relief. A functional MRI study of active scratching. *PLOS ONE* 8: e82389. https://doi.org/10.1371/annotation/c58aebe3-8f01-4c14-991a-c229e35b8f74.

Parker, A. J., Smith, J. E., and Krug, K. (2016). Neural architectures for stereo vision. *Philos Trans R Soc Lond B Biol Sci* 19: 371(1697). https://doi.org/10.1098/rstb.2015.0261.

Parr, W. V., Heatherbell, D. A., and White, K. G. (2002). Demystifying wine expertise: Olfactory threshold, perceptual skill, and semantic memory in expert and novice wine judges. *Chem Senses* 27: 747–755.

Parrish, E. E., Giaschi, D. E., Boden, C., and Dougherty, R. (2005). The maturation of form and motion perception in school age children. *Vision Res* 45: 827–837.

Pascual-Leone, A., and Hamilton, R. (2001). The metamodal organization of the brain. *Prog Brain Res* 134: 427–445.

Pastor, A., Fernández-Aranda, F., Fitó, M., Jiménez-Murcia, S., Botella, C., Fernández-Real, J. M., Frühbeck, G., et al. (2016). A lower olfactory capacity is related to higher circulating concentrations of endocannabinoid 2-arachidonoylglycerol and higher body mass index in women. *PLOS ONE* 11: e0148734.

Patel, A. S. and Jones, R. W. (1968). Increment and decrement visual thresholds. *J Opt Soc Am* 58(5): 696–9. doi: 10.1364/josa.58.000696

Patterson, R. D., and Johnsrude, I. S. (2008). Functional imaging of the auditory processing applied to speech sounds. *Philos Trans R Soc B Biol Sci* 363: 1023–1035.

Patterson, S. S., Bembry, B. N., Mazzaferri, M. A., Neitz, M., Rieke, F., Soetedjo, R., and Neitz, J. (2022). Conserved circuits for direction selectivity in the primate retina.

Curr Biol 32(11): 2529–2538.e4. https://doi.org/10.1016/j.cub.2022.04.056.

Pawling, R., Cannon, P. R., McGlone, F. P., and Walker, S. C. (2017). C-tactile afferent stimulating touch carries a positive affective value. *PLOS ONE* 12: e0173457.

Pearce, M. (2018). Statistical learning and probabilistic prediction in music cognition: Mechanisms of stylistic enculturation: Enculturation: Statistical learning and prediction. *Ann NY Acad Sci* 1423(1): 378–395. https://doi.org/10.1111/nyas.13654.

Peirs, C., and Seal, R. P. (2016). Neural circuits for pain: Recent advances and current views. *Science* 354: 578–584.

Pelchat, M. L., Bykowski, C., Duke, F. F., and Reed, D. R. (2011). Excretion and perception of a characteristic odor in urine after asparagus ingestion: A psychophysical and genetic study. *Chem Senses* 36: 9–17.

Pennock, I. M. L., Racey, C., Allen, E. J., Wu, Y., Naselaris, T., Kay, K. N., Franklin, A., et al. (2023). Color-biased regions in the ventral visual pathway are food selective. *Curr Biol* 33(1): 134–146.e134. https://doi.org/10.1016/j.cub.2022.11.063.

Perini, I., Olausson, H., and Morrison, I. (2015). Seeking pleasant touch: Neural correlates of behavioral preferences for skin stroking. *Front Behav Neurosci* 9: 8.

Perlman, M., and Krumhansl, C. L. (1996). An experimental study of internal interval standards in Javanese and Western musicians. *Music Percept* 14: 95–116.

Peterhans, E., von der Heydt, R., Baumgartner, G., Pettigrew, J. D., Sanderson, K. J., and Levick, W. R. (1986). Neuronal responses to illusory contour stimuli reveal stages of visual cortical processing. In J. D. Pettigrew, K. J. Sanderson, and W. R. Levick (Eds.), *Visual Neuroscience* (pp. 343–351). Cambridge: Cambridge University Press.

Peterka, R. J. (2002). Sensorimotor integration in human postural control. *J Neurophysiol* 88: 1097–1118.

Petkov, C. I., O'Connor, K. N., and Sutter, M. L. (2003). Illusory sound perception in macaque monkeys. *J Neurosci* 23: 9155–9161.

Petkov, C. I., O'Connor, K. N., and Sutter, M. L. (2007). Encoding of illusory continuity in primary auditory cortex. *Neuron* 54: 153–165.

Pettigrew, J. D., Nikara, T., and Bishop, P. O. (1968). Binocular interaction on single units in cat striate cortex: Simultaneous stimulation by single moving slit with receptive fields in correspondence. *Exp Brain Res* 6: 391–410.

Pfaffmann, C. (1974a). The sensory coding of taste quality. *Chem Senses Flavor* 1: 5–8.

Pfaffmann, C. (1974b). Specificity of the sweet receptors of the squirrel monkey. *Chem Senses Flavor* 1: 61–67.

Pierce, J. D., Jr., Wysocki, C. J., Aronov, E. V., Webb, J. B., and Boden, R. M. (1996). The role of perceptual and structural similarity in cross-adaptation. *Chem Senses* 21: 223–237.

Pignatiello, M. F., Camp, C. J., and Rasar, L. A. (1986). Musical mood induction: An alternative to the Velten technique. *J Abnorm Psychol* 95: 295–297.

Pinto, J. M., Wroblewski, K. E., Kern, D. W., Schumm, L. P., and McClintock, M. K. (2014). Olfactory dysfunction predicts 5-year mortality in older adults. *PLOS ONE,* 9(10): e107541.

Plailly, J., Delon-Martin, C., and Royet, J.-P. (2012). Experience induces functional reorganization in brain regions involved in odor imagery in perfumers. *Hum Brain Mapp* 33: 224–234.

Plailly, J., Howard, J. D., Gitelman, D. R., and Gottfried, J. A. (2008). Attention to odor modulates thalamocortical connectivity in the human brain. *J Neurosci* 28: 5257–5267.

Plaisier, M. A., Bergmann Tiest, W. M., and Kappers, A. M. L. (2009). Salient features in 3D haptic shape perception. *Atten Percept Psychophys* 71: 421–430.

Plomp, R. (1976). *Aspects of Tone Sensation: A Psychophysical Study*. New York: Academic Press.

Plotkin, A., Sela, L., Weissbord, A., Kahana, R., Haviv, L., Yeshurun, Y., and Soroker, N. (2010). Sniffing enables communication and environmental control for the severely disabled. *Proc Natl Acad Sci USA* 107: 14413–14418.

Plotnik, J. M., Brubaker, D. L., Dale, R., Tiller, L. N., Mumby, H. S., and Clayton, N. S. (2019). Elephants have a nose for quantity. *Proc Natl Acad Sci USA* 116: 12566–12571. https://doi.org/10.1073/pnas.1818284116.

Poggio, G. F., and Talbot, W. H. (1981). Mechanisms of static and dynamic stereopsis in foveal cortex of the rhesus monkey. *J Physiol* 315: 469–492.

Pointer, M. R., and Attridge, G. G. (1998). The number of discernible colours. *Color Res Appl* 23: 52–54.

Poivet, E., Peterlin, Z., Tahirova, N., Xu, L., Altomare, C., Paria, A., Zou, D-J., et al. (2016). Applying medicinal chemistry strategies to understand odorant discrimination. *Nat Commun* 7: 11157. https://doi.org/10.1038/ncomms11157.

Poivet, E., Tahirova, N., Peterlin, Z., Xu, L., Zou, D. J., Acree, T., Firestein, S., et al. (2018). Functional odor classification through a medicinal chemistry approach. *Sci Adv* 4: eaao6086. https://doi.org/10.1126/sciadv.aao6086.

Polat, U., and Sagi, D. (1993). Lateral interactions between spatial channels: Suppression and facilitation revealed by lateral masking experiments. *Vision Res* 33: 993–999.

Poletti, M., Listorti, C., and Rucci, M. (2010). Stability of the visual world during eye drift. *J Neurosci* 30: 11143–11150.

Poletti, M., Listorti, C., and Rucci, M. (2013). Microscopic eye movements compensate for nonhomogeneous vision within the fovea. *Curr Biol* 23: 1691–1695.

Pollan, M. (2006). *The Omnivore's Dilemma: A Natural History of Four Meals.* New York: Penguin.

Poltoratski, S., Maier A., Newton, A. T., and Tong, F. (2019). Figure-ground modulation in the human lateral geniculate nucleus is distinguishable from top-down attention. *Curr Biol* 29: 2051–2057.e3. https://doi.org/10.1016/j.cub.2019.04.068.

Poran N. S., and Coss, R. G. (1990). Development of antisnake defenses in California ground squirrels (*Spermaphilus beecheyi*): I. Behavioral and immunological relationships. *Behavior* 112: 222–245.

Porter, J., Carven, B., Khan, R. M., Chang, S. J., Kang, I., Judkewicz, B., Volpe, J., et al. (2007). Mechanisms of scent-tracking in humans. *Nat Neurosci* 10: 27–29.

Posner, M. I. (1980). Orienting of attention. *Q J Exp Psychol* 32: 3–25.

Potter, M. C. (1976). Short-term conceptual memory for pictures. *J Exp Psychol Hum Learn Mem* 2: 509–522.

Potter, M. C., Wyble, B., Hagmann, C. E. H., and McCourt, E. (2014). Detecting meaning in RSVP at 13 ms per picture. *Atten Percept Psychophys* 76: 270–279.

Powers, M. K., Schneck, M. and Teller, D.Y. (1981). Spectral sensitivity of human infants at absolute visual threshold. *Vision Res* 21(7): 1005–16. doi: 10.1016/0042-6989(81)90004-3.

Prescott, J. (2004). Effects of added glutamate on liking for novel flavors. *Appetite* 42: 143–150.

Prescott, S. L., and Liberles, S. D. (2022). Internal senses of the vagus nerve. *Neuron* 110(4): 579–599. https://doi.org/10.1016/j.neuron.2021.12.020.

Preston, T. J., Li, S., Kourtzi, Z., and Welchman, A. E. (2008). Multivoxel pattern selectivity for perceptually relevant binocular disparities in the human brain. *J Neurosci* 28(44): 11315–11327. https://doi.org/10.1523/JNEUROSCI.2728-08.2008.

Price, D. D. (2000). Psychological and neural mechanisms of the affective dimension of pain. *Science* 288: 1769–1772.

Price, D. D., Wu, J. W., Dubner, R., and Gracely, R. H. (1977). Peripheral suppression of first pain and central summation of second pain evoked by noxious heat pulses. *Pain* 3: 57–68.

Prinzmetal, W., and Beck, D. M. (2001). The tilt-constancy theory of visual illusions. *J Exp Psychol Hum Percept Perform* 27: 206–217.

Prinzmetal, W., Shimamura, A. P., and Mikolinski, M. (2001). The Ponzo illusion and the perception of orientation. *Percept Psychophys* 63: 99–114.

Pritchard, T. C., Macaluso, D. A., and Eslinger, P. J. (1999). Taste perception in patients with insular cortex lesions. *Behav Neurosci* 113: 663–671.

Pritchard, T. C., and Norgren, R. (2004). Gustatory system. In G. Paxinos and J. K. Mai (Eds.), *The Human Nervous System* (2nd ed., pp. 1171–1196). Amsterdam: Elsevier.

Prochnow, A., Erlandsson, S., Hesse, V., and Wermke, K. (2019). Does a "musical" mother tongue influence cry melodies? A comparative study of Swedish and German newborns. *Musicae Scientae* 23(2): 143–156.

Proust, M. (1928). *Swann's Way*. Volume 1 of *In Search of Lost Time* (*À la recherche du temps perdu*). New York: Modern Library.

Pugh, M. C., Ringach, D. L., Shapley, R., and Shelley, M. J. (2000). Computational modeling of orientation tuning dynamics in monkey primary visual cortex. *J Comput Neurosci* 8: 143–159.

Q

Quiroga, R. Q., Reddy, L., Kreiman, G., Koch, C., and Fried, I. (2005). Invariant visual representation by single neurons in the human brain. *Nature* 435: 1102–1107.

R

Rabin, M. D., and Cain, W. S. (1984). Odor recognition, familiarity, identifiability and encoding consistency. *J Exp Psychol Learn Mem Cogn* 10: 316–325.

Rader, A. A., Oman, C. M., and Merfeld, D. M. (2011). Perceived tilt and translation during variable-radius swing motion with congruent or conflicting visual and vestibular cues. *Exp Brain Res* 210: 173–184.

Raichlen, D. A., and Gordon, A. D. (2011). Relationship between exercise capacity and brain size in mammals. *PLOS ONE* 6: e20601.

Rainville, P., Duncan, G. H., Price, D. D., Carrier, B., and Bushnell, M. C. (1997). Pain affect encoded in human anterior cingulate but not somatosensory cortex. *Science* 277: 968–971.

Ramachandran, R., and Lisberger, S. G. (2005). Normal performance and expression of learning in the vestibulo-ocular reflex (VOR) at high frequencies. *J Neurophysiol* 93: 2028–2038.

Ramachandran, V. S. (1988). Perceiving shape from shading. *Sci Am* 259(2): 76–83. https://doi.org/10.1038/scientificamerican0888-76.

Ramachandran, V. S., and Hubbard, E. M. (2001). Psychophysical investigations into the neural basis of synaesthesia. *Proc R Soc Lond B Biol Sci* 268: 979–983. https://doi.org/10.1098/rspb.2000.1576.

Raphan, T., Matsuo, V., and Cohen, B. (1977). A velocity storage mechanism responsible for optokinetic nystagmus (OKN), optokinetic after-nystagmus (OKAN) and vestibular nystagmus. In R. Baker and A. Berthoz (Eds.), *Control of Gaze by Brain Stem Neurons: Proceedings of the Symposium Held in the Abbaye de Royaumont, Paris, France on July 12–15, 1977* (Developments in Neuroscience, vol. 1) (pp. 37–47). Amsterdam: Elsevier/North Holland.

Rasch, R. A. (1978). The perception of simultaneous notes such as in polyphonic music. *Acustica* 40: 1–72.

Raudenbush, B., Corley, N., and Eppich, W. (2001). Enhancing athletic performance through the administration of peppermint odor. *J Sport Exerc Psychol* 23: 156–160.

Raudenbush, B., Grayhem, R., Sears, T., and Wilson, I. (2009). Effects of peppermint and cinnamon odor administration on simulated driving alertness, mood and workload. *N Am J Psychol* 11: 245–256.

Raymond, J. E. (1993). Complete interocular transfer of motion adaptation effects on motion coherence thresholds. *Vision Res* 33: 1865–1870.

Rayner, K. (1978). Eye movements in reading and information processing. *Psychol Bull* 85: 618–660.

Rayner, K., Liversedge, S. P., White, S. J., and Vergilino-Perez, D. (2003). Reading disappearing text: Cognitive control of eye movements. *Psychol Sci* 14: 385–388.

Reale, R. A., Calvert, G. A., Thesen, T., Jenison, R. L., Kawasaki, H., Oya, H., Howard, M. A., et al. (2007). Auditory-visual processing represented in the human superior temporal gyrus. *Neuroscience* 145: 162–184.

Reason, J., and Brand, J. (1975). *Motion Sickness*. London: Academic Press.

Reed, C. L., Caselli, R. J., and Farah, M. J. (1996). Tactile agnosia: Underlying impairment and implications for normal tactile object recognition. *Brain* 119: 875–888.

Reed, C. L., Klatzky, R. L., and Halgren, E. (2005). What versus where in touch: An fMRI study. *Neuroimage* 25: 718–726.

Reed, C. L., Shoham, S., and Halgren, E. (2004). Neural substrates of tactile object recognition: A fMRI study. *Hum Brain Mapp* 21: 236–246.

Reese, A., List, N. H., Kongsted, J., and Solov'yov, I. A. (2016). How far does a receptor influence vibrational properties of an odorant? *PLOS ONE* 11: e0152345.

Regal, D.M. (1981). Development of critical flicker frequency in human infants. *Vision Res* 21(4): 549–555. doi: 10.1016/0042-6989(81)90100-0.

Regan, B. C., Julliot, C., Simmen, B., Viénot, F., Charles-Dominique, P., and Mollon, J. D. (2001). Fruits, foliage, and the evolution of primate colour vision. *Phil Trans R Soc Lond B* 356: 229–283.

Regan, D. (1991). Depth from motion and motion in depth. In D. Regan (Ed.), *Binocular Vision* (pp. 137–169). London: Macmillan.

Reichardt, W. (1986). Processing of optical information by the visual system of the fly. *Vision Res* 26: 113–126.

Reichenthal, A., Ben-Tov, M., Ben-Shahar, O., and Segev, R. (2019). What pops out for you pops out for fish: The four basic visual features. *J Vision* 1: 1. https://doi.org/10.1167/19.1.1.

Reichenthal, A., Segev, R., and Ben-Shahar, O. (2020). Feature integration theory in non-humans: Spotlight on the archerfish. *Attn Percept Psychophys* 82: 752–774. https://doi.org/10.3758/s13414-019-01884-4.

Reichert J. L., and Schöpf, V. (2018). Olfactory loss and regain: Lessons for neuroplasticity. *Neuroscientist* 24: 22–35. https://doi.org/10.1177/1073858417703910.

Reid, V. M., Dunn, K., Young, R. J., Amu, J., Donovan, T., and Reissland, N. (2017). The human fetus preferentially engages with face-like visual stimuli. *Curr Biol* 27: 1825–1828.

Rekow, D., Baudouin, J. Y., Durand, K., and Leleu, A. (2022). Smell what you hardly see: Odors assist visual categorization in the human brain. *NeuroImage* 255: 119181.

Rensink, R. A., O'Regan, J. K., and Clark, J. J. (1997). To see or not to see: The need for attention to perceive changes in scenes. *Psychol Sci* 8: 368–373.

Reynolds, J. H., and Chelazzi, L. (2004). Attentional modulation of visual processing. *Annu Rev Neurosci* 27: 611–647.

Reynolds, J. H., and Heeger, D. J. (2009). The normalization model of attention. *Neuron* 61: 168–185.

Rich, A. N., Bradshaw, J. L., and Mattingley, J. B. (2005). A systematic, large-scale study of synaesthesia: Implications for the role of early experience in lexical-colour associations. *Cognition* 98: 53–84. https://doi.org/10.1016/j.cognition.2004.11.003.

Richard, M. C., Taylor, S. R., and Greer, C. A. (2010). Age-induced disruption of selective olfactory bulb synaptic circuits. *Proc Nat Acad Sci USA* 107: 15613–15618.

Riecke, L., Esposito, F., Bonte, M., and Formisano, E. (2009). Hearing illusory sounds in noise: The timing of sensory-perceptual transformations in auditory cortex. *Neuron* 64: 550–561.

Riecke, L., van Opstal, A. J., Goebel, R., and Formisano, E. (2007). Hearing illusory sounds in noise: Sensory-perceptual transformations in primary auditory cortex. *J Neurosci* 27(46): 12684–12689.

Rind, F. C., and Simmons, P. J. (1999). Seeing what is coming: Building collision-sensitive neurones. *Trends Neurosci* 22: 215–220.

Riva, G., and Waterworth, J. A. (2003). Presence and the self: A cognitive neuroscience approach. *Presence Connect* 3(3).

Riva, G., Mantovani, F., Capideville, C. S., Preziosa, A., Morganti, F., Villani, D., et al. (2007). Affective interactions using virtual reality: The link between presence and emotions. *Cyber Psychology & Behavior* 10(1): 45–56.

Robinson, D. (1977). Vestibular and optokinetic symbiosis: An example of explaining by modelling. In R. Baker and A. Berthoz (Eds.), *Control of Gaze by Brain Stem Neurons: Proceedings of the Symposium Held in the Abbaye de Royaumont, Paris, France on July 12–15, 1977* (Developments in Neuroscience, vol. 1) (pp. 49–58). Amsterdam: Elsevier/North Holland.

Robson, J., and Campbell, F. (1997). A quick demonstration of your own contrast sensitivity function. In D. G. Pelli and A. M.

Torres, *Thresholds: Limits of Perception.* New York: NY Arts Magazine.

Rock, I., and Victor, J. (1964). Vision and touch: An experimentally created conflict between the two senses. *Science* 143: 594–596.

Rodieck, R. W. (1998). *The First Steps in Seeing.* Sunderland, MA: Sinauer.

Roe, A. W., Chelazzi, L., Connor, C. E., Conway, B. R., Fujita, I., Gallant, J. L., Lu, H., et al. (2012). Toward a unified theory of visual area V4. *Neuron* 74: 12–29.

Rogers, B. J., and Collett, T. S. (1989). The appearance of surfaces specified by motion parallax and binocular disparity. *Q J Exp Psychol A* 41: 697–717.

Rolls, B. J. (1986). Sensory-specific satiety. *Nutr Rev* 44: 93–101.

Romanos, M., Renner, T. J., Schecklmann, M., Hummel, B., Roos, M., von Mering, C., Pauli, P., et al. (2008). Improved odor sensitivity in attention-deficit/hyperactivity disorder. *Biol Psychiatry* 64: 938–940. https://doi.org/10.1016/j.biopsych.2008.08.013.

Roorda, A., and Williams, D. R. (1999). The arrangement of the three cone classes in the living human eye. *Nature* 397: 520–522.

Roper, S. D., and Chaudhari, N. (2017). Taste buds: Cells, signals and synapses. *Nat Rev Neurosci* 18: 485–497.

Roper, S. D. (2021). Chemical and electrical synaptic interactions among taste bud cells. *Curr Opin Physiol* 20: 118–125.

Rosen, S., Wise, R. J. S., Chadha, S., Conway, E.-J., and Scott, S. K. (2011). Hemispheric asymmetries in speech perception: Sense, nonsense, and modulations. *PLOS ONE* 6: e24672.

Ross, J., Morrone, M. C., Goldberg, M. E., and Burr, D. C. (2001). Changes in visual perception at the time of saccades. *Trends Neurosci* 24: 113–121.

Ross, S E. (2011). Pain and itch: Insights into the neural circuits of aversive somatosensation in health and disease. *Curr Opin Neurobiol* 21: 880–887.

Rossetti, Y., Rode, G., and Boisson, D. (1995). Implicit processing of somaesthetic information: A dissociation between where and how? *Neuroreport* 15: 506–510.

Rowe, T. B., Macrinin, T. E., and Luo, Z.-X. (2011). Fossil evidence on origin of the mammalian brain. *Science* 332: 955–957.

Roy, M., Peretz, I., and Rainville, P. (2007). Emotional valence contributes to music-induced analgesia. *Pain* 1–2: 140–147.

Royden, C. S., Banks, M. S., and Crowell, J. A. (1992). The perception of heading during eye movements. *Nature* 360: 583–585.

Royet, J.-P., and Plailly, J. (2004). Lateralization of olfactory processes. *Chem Senses* 29: 731–745.

Rozin, E., and Rozin, P. (1981). Culinary themes and variations. *Natural History* 90: 6–14.

Rozin, P. (Ed.). (1967). *Thiamin-Specific Hunger* (Vol. 1). Washington, DC: American Physiological Society.

Rozin, P., Gruss, L., and Berk, G. (1979). The reversal of innate aversions: Attempts to induce a preference for chili peppers in rats. *J Comp Physiol Psychol* 93: 1001–1014.

Rozin, P., and Schiller, D. (1980). The nature and acquisition of a preference for chili pepper by humans. *Motiv Emot* 4: 77.

Rubin, D. C., Groth, E., and Goldsmith, D. J. (1984). Olfactory cuing of autobiographical memory. *Am J Psychol* 97: 493–507.

Ruan, Y., Zheng, X. Y., Zhang, H. L., Zhu, W., and Zhu, J. (2012). Olfactory dysfunctions in neurodegenerative disorders. *Journal of Neuroscience Research* 90(9): 1693–1700.

Rucci, M. and Victor, J.D. (2015). The unsteady eye: An information-processing stage, not a bug. *Trends Neurosci* 38(4): 195–206. doi: 10.1016/j.tins.2015.01.005.

Ruijschop, R. M. A. J., Boelrijk, A. E. M., de Ru, J. A., de Graaf, C., and Westerterp-Plantenga, M. S. (2008). Effects of retronasal aroma release on satiation. *Br J Nutr* 99: 1140–1148.

Rumelhart, D. E., McClelland, J. L., and PDP Research Group. (1986). *Parallel Distributed Processing: Explorations in the Microstructure of Cognition, Vol 1: Foundations.* Cambridge, MA: MIT Press.

Rupp, C. I., Kurz, M., Kemmler, G., Mair, D., Hausmann, A., Hinterhuber, H., and Fleischhacker, W. W. (2003). Reduced olfactory sensitivity, discrimination, and identification in patients with alcohol dependence. *Alcohol Clin Exp Res* 27: 432–439.

Rupp, K., Hect, J., Remick, M., Ghuman, A., Chandrasekaran, B., Holt, L. L., and Abel, T. J. (2021). Categorical encoding of voice in human superior temporal cortex. *PLoS Biology* 20(7): e3001675.

Rushton, W. (1972). Visual pigments in man. In H. Dartnall (Ed.), *Photochemistry of Vision* (Vol. VII/1, pp. 364–394). New York: Springer.

Rust, N. C., and Jannuzi, B. G. L. (2022). Identifying objects and remembering images: Insights from deep neural networks. *Curr Dir Psychol Sci* 31(4): 316–323. https://doi.org/10.1177/09637214221083663.

S

Saal, H. P., Wang, X., and Bensmaia, S. J. (2016). Importance of spike timing in touch: An analogy with hearing? *Curr Opin Neurobiol* 40: 142–149.

Sabesan, R., Schmidt, B. P., Tuten, W. S., and Roorda, A. (2016). The elementary representation of spatial and color vision in the human retina. *Sci Adv* 2: e1600797.

Sacks, O. (2006, June 19). A neurologist's notebook: "Stereo Sue." *New Yorker* 64.

Saffran, J. R. (2001). Words in a sea of sounds: The output of statistical learning. *Cognition* 81: 149–169.

Saffran, J. R. (2002). Constraints on statistical language learning. *J Mem Lang* 47: 172–196.

Saffran, J. R., Aslin, R. N., and Newport, E. L. (1996). Statistical learning by 8-month-old infants. *Science* 274: 1926–1928.

Saffran, J. R., Johnson, E. K., Aslin, R. N., and Newport, E. L. (1999). Statistical learning of tone sequences by human infants and adults. *Cognition* 70: 27–52.

Saffran, J. R., Loman, M. M., and Robertson, R. R. W. (2000). Infant memory for musical experiences. *Cognition* 77: B15–B23.

Safran, A. B., and Sanda, N. (2015). Color synesthesia: Insight into perception, emotion, and consciousness. *Curr Opin Neurol* 28: 36–44. https://doi.org/10.1097/WCO.0000000000000169.

Salzman, C. D., Britten, K. H., and Newsome, W. T. (1990). Cortical microstimulation influences perceptual judgements of motion direction. *Nature* 346: 174–177.

Sarrafchi, A., Odhammer, A. M., Salazar, L. T. H., and Laska, M. (2013). Olfactory sensitivity for six predator odorants in CD-1 mice, human subjects, and spider monkeys. *PLOS ONE* 8: e80621.

Sayette, M. A., Marchetti, M. A., Herz, R. S., Martin, L. M., and Bowdring, M. A. (2019). Pleasant olfactory cues can reduce cigarette craving. *J Abnorm Psychol* 128: 327–340. https://doi.org/10.1037/abn0000431.

Saygin, A. P., Wilson, S. M., Hagler, D. J., Jr., Bates, E., and Sereno, M. I. (2004). Point-light biological motion perception activates human premotor cortex. *J Neurosci* 24: 6181–6188. https://doi.org/10.1523/jneurosci.0504-04.2004.

Sayles, M., Fontaine, B., Smith, P. H., and Joris, P. X. (2017). *Inter-aural time sensitivity of superior-olivary-complex neurons is shaped by systematic cochlear disparities.* Paper presented at the 40th Annual MidWinter Meeting of the Association for Research in Otolaryngology, Baltimore, MD.

Sayles, M., and Heinz, M. G. (2017). Afferent coding and efferent control in the normal and impaired cochlea. In G. Manley, A. Gummer, R. R. Fay, and A. N. Popper (Eds.), *Understanding the Cochlea, Springer Handbook of Auditory Research (SHAR)* (pp. 215–252). New York: Springer.

Scangas, G. A., and Bleier, B. S. (2017). Anosmia: Differential diagnosis, evaluation, and management. *Am J Rhinol Allergy* 31: e3–e7. https://doi.org/10.2500/ajra.2017.31.4403.

Sceniak, M. P., Ringach, D. L., Hawken, M. J., and Shapley, R. (1999). Contrast's effect on spatial summation by macaque V1 neurons. *Nat Neurosci* 2: 733–739.

Schaal, B., Marlier, L., and Soussignan, R. (1995). Responsiveness to the odor of amniotic fluid in the human neonate. *Biol Neonate* 671: 397–406.

Schaal, B., Marlier, L., and Soussignan, R. (1998). Olfactory function in the human fetus: Evidence from selective neonatal responsiveness to the odor of amniotic fluid. *Behav Neurosci* 112: 1438–1449.

Schild, D., and Restrepo, D. (1998). Transduction mechanism in vertebrate olfactory receptor cells. *Physiol Rev* 37: 369–375.

Schiller, P. H., and Sandell, J. H. (1983). Interactions between visually and electrically elicited saccades before and after superior colliculus and frontal eye field ablations in the rhesus monkey. *Exp Brain Res* 49: 381–392.

Schirmer, A., and Gunter, T. C. (2017). The right touch: Stroking of CT-innervated skin promotes vocal emotion processing. *Cogn Affect Behav Neurosci* 17: 1129–1140. https://doi.org/10.3758/s13415-017-0537-5.

Schleidt, M., Hold, B., and Attila, G. (1981). A cross-cultural study on the attitude towards personal odors. *J Chem Ecol* 7: 19–31.

Schmelz, M., Schmidt, R., Bickel, A., Handwerker, H. O., and Torebjörk, H. E. (1997). Specific C-receptors for itch in human skin. *J Neurosci* 17: 8003–8008.

Schnapf, J. L., Kraft, T. W., and Baylor, D. A. (1987). Spectral sensitivity of human cone photoreceptors. *Nature* 325: 439–441.

Schneider, B. A., and Hamstra, S. J. (1999). Gap detection thresholds as a function of tonal duration for younger and older listeners. *J Acoust Soc Am* 106: 371–380.

Schütz, A. C., Braun, D. I., and Gegenfurtner, K. R. (2011). Eye movements and perception: a selective review. *J Vis* 11(5).

Sclafani, A. (1997). Learned controls of ingestive behaviour. *Appetite* 29: 153–158.

Seay, C. F. (1975). *First Thoughts on a Theology of Music from the Psalter*. Dallas, TX: Dallas Theological Seminary.

Seeba, F., and Klump, G. M. (2009). Stimulus familiarity affects perceptual restoration in the European starling (*Sturnus vulgaris*). *PLOS ONE* 4: e5974.

Selfridge, O. G. (1959). Pandemonium: A paradigm for learning. In D. V. Blake and A. M. Uttley (Eds.), *Proceedings of the Symposium on the Mechanisation of Thought Processes* (pp. 511–529). London: Her Majesty's Stationery Office.

Seo, H. S., Gudziol, V., Hähner, A., and Hummel, T. (2011). Background sound modulates the performance of odor discrimination task. *Exp Brain Res* 212(2): 305–314.

Serences, J. T., and Yantis, S. (2006). Selective visual attention and perceptual coherence. *Trends Cogn Sci* 10: 38–45.

Serre, T. (2019). Deep learning: The good, the bad, and the ugly. *Annu Rev Vis Sci* 5: 399–426. https://doi.org/10.1146/annurev-vision-091718-014951.

Shams, L., Kamitani, Y., and Shimojo, S. (2000). Illusions. What you see is what you hear. *Nature* 408: 788. https://doi.org/10.1038/35048669.

Shams, L., Kamitani, Y., and Shimojo, S. (2002). Visual illusion induced by sound. *Brain Res Cog Brain Res* 14: 147–152. https://doi.org/10.1016/s0926-6410(02)00069-1.

Shanahan, L. K., and Kahnt, T.(2022). On the state-dependent nature of odor perception. *Frontiers in Neuroscience* 16: 964742.

Shankar, M., Simons, C., Shiv, B., McClure, S., Levitan, C., and Spence, C. (2010). An expectations-based approach to explaining the cross-modal influence of color on orthonasal olfactory identification: The influence of the degree of discrepancy. *Atten Percept Psychophys* 72: 1981–1993. https://doi.org/10.3758/APP.72.7.1981.

Shannon, C. E. (1948). A mathematical theory of communication. *Bell Labs Tech J* 27: 379–423.

Shapiro, K. L. (1994). The attentional blink: The brain's eyeblink. *Curr Dir Psychol Sci* 3: 86–89.

Shapley, R., and Hawken, M. J. (2011). Color in the cortex: Single- and double-opponent cells. *Vision Res* 51: 701–717.

Shepard, R. N. (1967). Recognition memory for words, sentences, and pictures. *J Verbal Learn Verbal Behav* 6: 156–163.

Shepherd, G. M. (1994). Discrimination of molecular signals by the olfactory receptor neuron. *Neuron* 13(4): 771–790.

Sherrick, C., and Cholewiak, R. (1986). Cutaneous sensitivity. In K. R. Boff, L. Kaufman, and J. P. Thomas (Eds.), *Handbook of Perception and Human Performance* (Vol 1., pp. 12.1–12.58). New York: Wiley.

Shevell, S. K. (2003). Color appearance. In S. K. Shevell (Ed.), *The Science of Color* (2nd ed., pp. 149–190). Oxford: Elsevier.

Shevell, S. K., and Kingdom, F. A. (2008). Color in complex scenes. *Annu Rev Psychol* 59: 143–146. https://doi.org/10.1146/annurev.psych.59.103006.093619.

Shoup, M. L., Streeter, S. A., and McBurney, D. H. (2008). Olfactory comfort and attachment within relationships. *J Appl Soc Psychol* 38: 2954–2963. https://doi.org/10.1111/j.1559-1816.2008.00420.x.

Shusterman, R. (2019). Active sampling optimizes processing of fluctuations in odor concentration. Abstract 399.19, Society for Neuroscience, October.

Simons, D. J., and Chabris, C. F. (1999). Gorillas in our midst: Sustained inattentional blindness for dynamic events. *Perception* 28: 1059–1074.

Singer, W. (1999). Neuronal synchrony: A versatile code for the definition of relations? *Neuron* 24: 49–65.

Sinha, R., Hoon, M., Baudin, J., Okawa, H., Wong, R. O., and Rieke, F. (2017). Cellular and circuit mechanisms shaping the perceptual properties of the primate fovea. *Cell* 168: 413–426.

Sipiora, M. L., Murtaugh, M. A., Gregoire, M. B., and Duffy, V. B. (2000). Bitter taste perception and severe vomiting during pregnancy. *Physiol Behav* 69: 259–267.

Siuda-Krzywicka, K., Boros, M., Bartolomeo, P., and Witzel, C. (2019). The biological bases of colour categorisation: From goldfish to the human brain. Cortex, 118: 82–106. https://doi.org/10.1016/j.cortex.2019.04.010.

Skedung, L., Arvidsson, M., Chung, J. Y., Stafford, C. M., Berglund, B., and Rutland, M. W. (2013). Feeling small: Exploring the tactile perception limits. *Sci Rep* 3: 2617.

Sloboda, J. A. (1999). Music: Where cognition and emotion meet. *Psychologist* 12: 450–455.

Small, D. M. and Jones-Gotman, M. (2001). Neural substrates of taste/smell interactions and flavour in the human brain. *Chem Senses* 26: 1034

Smith, J. D., Kemler Nelson, D. G., Grohskopf, L. A., and Appleton, T. (1994). What child is this? What interval was that? Familiar tunes and music perception in novice listeners. *Cognition* 52: 23–54.

Smith, W. M., Davidson, T. M., and Murphy, C. (2009). Toxin-induced chemosensory dysfunction: A case series and review. *Am J Rhinol Allergy* 23: 578–581.

Snyder, D. J., Davidson, A. C., Kidd, J. R., Kidd, K. K., Speed, W. C., Pakstis, A. J., Cubells, J. F., et al. (2005). *Oral sensation influences tobacco use: Genetic and psychophysical evidence.* Paper presented at the Society for Research on Nicotine and Tobacco, Prague, Czech Republic.

Snyder, D. J., Dwivedi, N., Mramor, A., Bartoshuk, L. M., and Duffy, V. B. (2001). *Taste and touch may contribute to the localization of retronasal olfaction: Unilateral and bilateral anesthesia of cranial nerves V/VII.* Paper presented at the Society of Neuroscience Abstract, San Diego, CA.

Snyder, J. S., and Alain, C. (2007). Toward a neurophysiological theory of auditory stream segregation. *Psychol Bull* 133: 780–799.

Solbu, E. H., Jellestad, F. K., and Strætkvern, K. O. (1990). Children's sensitivity to odor of trimethylamine. *J Chem Ecol* 16: 1829–1840. https://doi.org/10.1007/BF01020497.

Sollberger, B., Reber, R., and Eckstein, D. (2003). Musical chords as affective priming context in a word-evaluation task. *Music Percept* 20: 263–283.

Solvi, C., Gutierrez al-Khudhairy, S., and Chittka, L. (2020). Bumble bees display cross-modal object recognition between visual and tactile senses. *Science* 367: 910–912. https://doi.org/10.1126/science.aay8064.

Soranzo, A., and Gilchrist, A. (2019). Layer and framework theories of lightness. *Atten Percept Psychophys* 81: 1179–1188. https://doi.org/10.3758/s13414-019-01736-1.

Soria-Gómez, E., Bellocchio, L., Reguero, L., Lepousez, G., Martin, C., Bendahmane, M., Ruehle, S., et al. (2014). The endocannabinoid system controls food intake via olfactory processes. *Nat Neurosci* 17: 407–415.

Sorokowska, A. (2016). Olfactory performance in a large sample of early-blind and late-blind individuals. *Chem Senses* 41: 703–709. https://doi.org/10.1093/chemse/bjw081.

Sorokowska, A., Drechsler, E., Karwowski, M., and Hummel, T. (2017). Effects of olfactory training: A meta-analysis. *Rhinology* 55: 17–26. https://doi.org/10.4193/Rhin16.195.

Sorokowska, A., Sorokowski, P., and Frackowiak, T. (2015). Determinants of human olfactory performance: A cross-cultural study.

Sci Total Environ 506: 196–200. https://doi.org/10.1016/j.scitotenv.2014.11.027.

Sorokowska, A., Sorokowski, P., Karwowski, M., Larsson, M., and Hummel, T. (2019). Olfactory perception and blindness: A systematic review and meta-analysis. *Psychol Res* 83(8): 1595–1611.

Soto-Faraco, S., Lyons, J., Gazzaniga, M., Spence, C., and Kingstone, A. (2002). The ventriloquist in motion: Illusory capture of dynamic information across sensory modalities. *Cogn Brain Res* 14: 139–146. https://doi.org/10.1016/s0926-6410(02)00068-x.

Spagnolli, A., and Gamberini, L. (2005). A Place for presence. Understanding the human involvement in mediated interactive environments. *PsychNology Journal* 3(1): 6–15.

Spence, C. (2020). Wine psychology: Basic and applied. *Cogn Res Princ Implic* 5: 22. https://doi.org/10.1186/s41235-020-00225-6.

Spence, C., and Ngo, M. K. (2012). Does attention or multisensory integration explain the crossmodal facilitation of masked visual target identification? In B. E. Stein (Ed.), *The New Handbook of Multisensory Processing* (pp. 345–358). Cambridge, MA: MIT Press.

Spence, C., Richards, L., Kjellin, E., Huhnt, A.-H., Daskal, V., Scheybeler, A., Velansco, C., et al. (2013). Looking for crossmodal correspondences between classical music and fine wine. *Flavour* 2: 29.

Sperling, G., and Weichselgartner, E. (1995). Episodic theory of the dynamics of spatial attention. *Psychol Rev* 102: 503–532.

Spinal Cord Injury Facts and Figures at a Glance. (2020). Birmingham: National Spinal Cord Injury Statistical Center, University of Alabama. https://www.nscisc.uab.edu/Public/Facts and Figures 2020.pdf

Spitschan, M., Jain, S., Brainard, D. H., and Aguirre, G. K. (2014). Opponent melanopsin and S-cone signals in the human pupillary light response. *Proc Natl Acad Sci USA* 111: 15568–15572. https://doi.org/10.1073/pnas.1400942111.

Spoor, F., Wood, B., and Zonneveld, F. (1994). Implications of early hominid labyrinthine morphology for evolution of human bipedal locomotion. *Nature* 369: 645–648.

Sreenivasan, V., Babinsky, E. E., Wu, Y., and Candy, T. R. (2016). Objective measurement of fusional vergence ranges and heterophoria in infants and preschool children. *Invest Ophthalmol Vis Sci* 57: 2678–2688.

Srinath, R., Emonds, A., Wang, Q., Lempel, A. A., Dunn-Weiss, E., Connor, C. E., et al. (2021). Early emergence of solid shape coding in natural and deep network vision. *Curr Biol* 31(1): 51–65.e55. https://doi.org/10.1016/j.cub.2020.09.076.

Stager, D. R., and Birch, E. (1986). Preferential-looking acuity and stereopsis in infantile esotropia. *J Pediatr Ophthalmol Strabismus* 23: 160–165.

Standing, L. (1973). Learning 10,000 pictures. *Q J Exp Psychol* 25: 207–222.

Standing, L., Conezio, J., and Haber, R. N. (1970). Perception and memory for pictures: Single trial learning of 2500 visual stimuli. *Psychon Sci* 19: 73–74.

Starling, E. H. (1923). *The Wisdom of the Body* (Harveian Oration). London: H. K. Lewis.

Stein, B. E., and Meredith, M. A. (1993). *The Merging of the Senses*. Cambridge, MA: MIT Press.

Stein, B. E., Stanford, T. R., and Rowland, B. A. (2014). Development of multisensory integration from the perspective of the individual neuron. *Nat Rev Neurosci* 15: 520–535. https://doi.org/10.1038/nrn3742.

Stein, M., Ottenberg, M. D., and Roulet, N. (1958). A study of the development of olfactory preferences. *Arch Neurol Psychiatry* 80: 264–266.

Steiner, J. E. (1973). The gustofacial response: Observation on normal and anencephalic newborn infants. In J. F. Bosma (Ed.), *Development in the Fetus and Infant* (pp. 254–278). Washington, DC: U.S. Government Printing Office.

Stellman, S. D., and Garkinkel, L. (1988). Patterns of artificial sweetener use and weight change in an American Cancer Society Prospective Study. *Appetite* 11: 85–91.

Steuer, J.(1992). Defining virtual reality: Dimensions determining telepresence. *Journal of Communication 42*(4): 73–93.

Stevens, J. C. (1959). Cross-modality validation of subjective scales for loudness, vibration, and electric shock. *J Exp Psychol* 57: 201–209.

Stevens, J. C., and Cain, W. S. (1987). Old-age deficits in the sense of smell as gauged by thresholds, magnitude matching and odor identification. *Psychol Aging* 2: 36–42.

Stevens, S. S. (1962). The surprising simplicity of sensory metrics. *Am Psychol* 17: 29–39.

Stevens, S. S. (1975). *Psychophysics*. New York: Academic Press.

Stevens, S. S., Carton, A. S., and Shickman, G. M. (1958). A scale of apparent intensity of electric shock. *J Exp Psychol* 56: 328–334.

Stevens, S. S., and Galanter, E. H. (1957). Ratio scales and category scales for a dozen perceptual continua. *J Exp Psychol* 54: 377–411.

Stilp, C. E., Donaldson, G., Oh, S., and Kong, Y.-Y. (2016). Influences of noise-interruption and information-bearing acoustic changes on understanding simulated electric-acoustic speech. *J Acoust Soc Am* 140: 3971–3979. https://doi.org/10.1121/1.4967445.

Stilp, C. E., and Kluender, K. R. (2010). Cochlea-scaled entropy, not consonants, vowels, or time, best predicts speech intelligibility. *Proc Natl Acad Sci USA* 107: 12387–12392.

Stockman, A., and Brainard, D. H. (2010). Color vision mechanisms. In M. Bass (Ed.), *OSA Handbook of Optics* (3rd ed., pp. 11.11–11.104). New York: McGraw–Hill.

Stryker, M. P., and Schiller, P. H. (1975). Eye and head movements evoked by electrical stimulation of monkey superior colliculus. *Exp Brain Res* 23: 103–112.

Sulmont, C., Issanchou, S., and Koster, E. P. (2002). Selection of odorants for memory tests on the basis of familiarity, perceived complexity, pleasantness, similarity and identification. *Chem Senses* 27: 307–317.

Sun, H.-C., Welchman, A. E., Chang, D. H. F., and Di Luca, M. (2016). Look but don't touch: Visual cues to surface structure drive somatosensory cortex. *NeuroImage* 128: 353–361.

Sun, P., Chubb, C., Wright, C. E., and Sperling, G. (2016). Human attention filters for single colors. *Proc Natl Acad Sci USA* 113: E6712–E6720.

Sun, Y.-G., Zhao, Z.-Q., Meng, X.-L., Yin, J., Liu, X.-Y., and Chen, Z.-F. (2009). Cellular basis of itch sensation. *Science* 325: 1531–1534.

Supple, J. A., Pinto-Benito, D., Khoo, C., Wardill, T. J., Fabian, S. T., Liu, M., and Pusdekar., S. (2020). Binocular encoding in the damselfly pre-motor target tracking system. *Curr Biol* 30(4): 645–656. https://doi.org/10.1016/j.cub.2019.12.031.

Suresh, A. K., Greenspon, C. M., He, Q., Rosenow, J. M., Miller, L. E., and Bensmaia, S. J. (2021). Sensory computations in the cuneate nucleus of macaques. *Proc Natl Acad Sci USA* 118(49): e2115772118. https://doi.org/10.1073/pnas.2115772118.

Suzuki, Y., and Takeshima, H. (2004). Equal-loudness-level contours for pure tones. *J Acoust Soc Am* 116: 918–933.

Svaetichin, G., and Macnichol, E. F., Jr. (1959). Retinal mechanisms for chromatic and achromatic vision. *Ann NY Acad Sci* 74: 385–404.

Szmajda, B. A., Grünert, U., and Martin, P. R. (2008). Retinal ganglion cell inputs to the koniocellular pathway. *J Comp Neurol* 510: 251–268.

T

Takamata, A., Mack, G. W., Gillen, C. M., and Nadel, E. R. (1994). Sodium appetite, thirst, and body fluid regulation in humans during rehydration without sodium replacement. *Am J Physiol* 266: R1493–R1502.

Takeuchi, A. H., and Hulse, S. H. (1993). Absolute pitch. *Psychol Bull* 113: 345–361.

Tanaka, Y., Bergmann Tiest, W. M., Kappers, A. M., and Sano, A. (2014). Contact force and scanning velocity during active roughness perception. *PLoS One* 9(3): e93363. doi: 10.1371/journal.pone.0093363.

Tang, Q., Guo, G., Zhang, Z., Zhang, B., and Wu, Y. (2020). Olfactory facilitation of takeover performance in highly automated driving. *Human Factors* 63(4): 553–564. https://doi.org/10.1177/0018720819893137.

Tarragon, E., and Moreno, J. J. (2019). Cannabinoids, chemical senses, and regulation of feeding behavior. *Chem Senses* 44: 73–89. https://doi.org/10.1093/chemse/bjy068.

Taube, J. S. (2007). The head direction signal: Origins and sensory-motor integration. *Annu Rev Neurosci* 30: 181–207.

Taylor-Phillips, S., Jenkinson, D., Stinton, C., Wallis, M. G., Dunn, J., and Clarke, A. (2018). Double reading in breast cancer screening: Cohort evaluation in the CO-OPS Trial. *Radiology* 287: 749–757. https://doi.org/10.1148/radiol.2018171010.

Teller, D. Y. and Bornstein, M. H. (1986). Infant color vision and color perception. In P. Salapatek and L. B. Cohen (Eds.), *Handbook of infant perception, Vol. 1: From Sensation to Perception* (pp. 185–236). Orlando, FL: Academic Press.

Teller, D. Y., and Movshon, J. A. (1986). Visual development. *Vision Res* 26: 1483–1506.

Thaler, L., Arnott, S. R., and Goodale, M. A. (2011). Neural correlates of natural human echolocation in early and late blind echolocation experts. *PLOS ONE* 6: e20162.

Thaler, L., and Goodale, M. A. (2016). Echolocation in humans: An overview. *WIREs Cogn Sci* 7: 382–393.

Theusch, E., and Gitschier, J. (2011). Absolute pitch twin study and segregation analysis. *Twin Res Hum Genet* 14: 173–178. https://doi.org/10.1375/twin.14.2.173.

Thompson, P. (1980). Margaret Thatcher: A new illusion. *Perception* 9: 482–484.

Thorpe, S., Fize, D., and Marlot, C. (1996). Speed of processing in the human visual system. *Nature* 381: 520–552.

Thuerauf, N., Gossler, A., Lunkenheimer, J., Lunkenheimer, B., Maihöfner, C., Bleich, S., Kornhuber, J., et al. (2008). Olfactory lateralization: Odor intensity but not the hedonic estimation is lateralized. *Neurosci Lett* 438: 228–232. https://doi.org/10.1016/j.neulet.2008.04.038.

Tieman, D., Bliss, P., McIntyre, L. M., Blandon-Ubeda, A., Bies, D., Odabasi, A. Z., Rodriguez, G. R., et al. (2012). The chemical interactions underlying tomato flavor preferences. *Curr Biol* 22: 1–5.

Tinnermann, A., Geuter, S., Sprenger, C., Finsterbusch, J., and Büchel, C. (2017). Interactions between brain and spinal cord mediate value effects in nocebo hyperalgesia. *Science* 358: 105–108.

Tinsley, J. N., Molodtsov, M. I., Prevedel, R., Wartmann, D., Espigulé-Pons, J., Lauwers, M., and Alipasha Vaziri, A. (2016). Direct detection of a single photon by humans. *Nat Comm* 7: Article 12172.

Tipper, S. P., and Behrmann, M. (1996). Object-centered not scene-based visual neglect. *J Exp Psychol Hum Percept Perform* 22: 1261–1278.

Tochitsky, I., Polosukhina, A., Degtyar, V. E., Gallerani, N., Smith, C. M., Friedman, A., Van Gelder, R. N., et al. (2014). Restoring visual function to blind mice with a photoswitch that exploits electrophysiological remodeling of retinal ganglion cells *Neuron* 81: 800–813.

Todd, A. J. (2010). Neuronal circuitry for pain processing in the dorsal horn. *Nat Rev Neurosci* 11: 823–836.

Todd, J. T., and Petrov, A. A. (2022). The many facets of shape. *J Vision* 22(1): 1–1. https://doi.org/10.1167/jov.22.1.1.

Tomchek, S. D., and Dunn, W. (2007). Sensory processing in children with and without autism: A comparative study using the short sensory profile. *Am. J. Occup Ther* 61: 190–200.

Tomko, D., Barbaro, N., and Ali, F. (1981). Effect of body tilt on receptive field orientation of simple visual cortical neurons in unanesthetized cats. *Exp Brain Res* 43: 309–314.

Tong, F., Meng, M., and Blake, R. (2006). Neural bases of binocular rivalry. *Trends Cogn Sci* 10: 502–511.

Tong, F., Nakayama, K., Vaughan, J. T., and Kanwisher, N. (1998). Binocular rivalry and visual awareness in human extrastriate cortex. *Neuron* 21(4): 753–9.

Torres, C. A., León, L., and Sánchez-Contreras, J. (2016). Spectral fingerprints during sun injury development on the tree in Granny Smith apples: A potential nondestructive prediction tool during the growth season. *Sci Hortic* 209: 165–172.

Treisman, A. (1986a). Features and objects in visual processing. *Sci Am* 255: 114–125.

Treisman, A. (1986b). Properties, parts, and objects. In K. R. Boff, L. Kaufmann, and J. P. Thomas (Eds.), *Handbook of Perception and Human Performance*, Vol. 2: *Cognitive Processes and Performance* (pp. 35.31–35.70). New York: Wiley.

Treisman, A. (1996). The binding problem. *Curr Opin Neurobiol* 6: 171–178.

Treisman, A., and Gelade, G. (1980). A feature-integration theory of attention. *Cogn Psychol* 12: 97–136.

Treisman, A. M., and Schmidt, H. (1982). Illusory conjunctions in the perception of objects. *Cogn Psychol* 14: 107–141.

Treisman, M. (1977). Motion sickness: An evolutionary hypothesis. *Science* 197: 493–495.

Tresilian, J. R. (1999). Visually timed action: Time-out for "tau"? *Trends Cogn Sci* 3: 301–310.

Treue, S., and Trujillo, J. C. M. (1999). Feature-based attention influences motion processing gain in macaque visual cortex. *Nature* 399: 575–579.

Trimmer, C., Keller, A., Murphy, N. R., Snyder, L. L., Willer, J. R., Nagai, M. H., Katsanis, N., et al. (2019). Genetic variation across the human olfactory receptor repertoire alters odor perception. *Proc Natl Acad Sci USA* 116: 9475–9480. https://doi.org/10.1073/pnas.1804106115.

Troscianko, T., Baddeley, R., Parraga, C. A., Leonards, U., and Troscianko, J. (2003). Visual encoding of green leaves in primate vision. *J Vis* 3: 137–137.

Tse, P. U. (1999). Volume completion. *Cogn Psychol* 39: 37–68.

Tsotsos, J. K. (1990). Analyzing vision at the complexity level. *Behav Brain Sci* 13: 423–469.

Tsukahara, T., Brann, D. H., Pashkovski, S. L., Guitchounts, G., Bozza, T., and Datta, S. R. (2021). A transcriptional rheostat couples past activity to future sensory responses. *Cell* 184(26): 6326–6343.

Tsuruhara, A., Corrow, S., Kanazawa, S., Yamaguchi, M. K., and Yonas, A. (2014). Measuring young infants' sensitivity to height-in-the-picture-plane by contrasting monocular and binocular preferential-looking. *Dev Psychobiol* 56: 109–116.

Turk, I., Dirjec, J., and Kavur, B. (1995). The oldest musical instrument in Europe discovered in Slovenia? Razprave 4. *Razreda Sazu* 36: 287–293.

Turin, L. (1996). A spectroscopic mechanism for primary olfactory reception. *Chem Senses* 21: 773–791.

Turin, L., Gane, S., Georganakis, D., Maniati, K., and Skoulakis, E. M. (2015). Plausibility of the vibrational theory of olfaction. *Proc Natl Acad Sci USA* 112: E3154.

Tyler, C. W. (1991). Cyclopean vision. In D. Regan (Ed.), *Binocular Vision* (Vol. 9, pp. 38–74). Boca Raton, FL: CRC Press.

U

Uddin, L. Q., Nomi, J. S., Hébert-Seropian, B., Ghaziri, J., and Boucher, O. (2017). Structure and function of the human insula. *J Clin Neurophysiol* 34(4): 300–306. https://doi.org/10.1097/WNP.0000000000000377.

Ungerleider, L. G., and Bell, A. H. (2011). Uncovering the visual "alphabet": Advances in our understanding of object perception. *Vision Res* 51: 782–799.

Ungerleider, L. G., and Mishkin, M. (1982). Two cortical visual systems. In D. J. Ingle, M. A. Goodale, and R. J. W. Mansfield (Eds.), *Analysis of Visual Behavior* (pp. 549–586). Cambridge, MA: MIT Press.

Uppenkamp, S., Johnsrude, I. S., Norris, D., Marslen-Wilson, W., and Patterson, R. D. (2006). Locating the initial stages of speech-sound processing in human temporal cortex. *Neuroimage* 31: 1284–1296.

V

Vaden, K. I., Jr., Matthews, L. J., Eckert, M. A., and Dubno, J. R. (2017). Longitudinal changes in audiometric phenotypes of age-related hearing loss. *J Assoc Res Otolaryngol* 18: 371–385. https://doi.org/10.1007/s10162-016-0596-2.

Vaina, L. M., and Cowey, A. (1996). Impairment of the perception of second-order motion but not first-order motion in a patient with unilateral focal brain damage. *Proc R Soc Lond B Biol Sci* 263: 1225–1232.

Vaina, L. M., Makris, N., Kennedy, D., and Cowey, A. (1998). The selective impairment of the perception of first-order motion by unilateral cortical brain damage. *Vis Neurosci* 15: 333–348.

Valko, Y., Lewis, R. F., Priesol, A. J., and Merfeld, D. M. (2012). Vestibular labyrinth contributions to human whole-body motion discrimination. *J Neurosci* 32: 13537–13542. https://doi.org/10.1523/jneurosci.2157-12.2012.

Van de Cruys, S., Van der Hallen, R., and Wagemans, J. (2017). Disentangling signal and noise in autism spectrum disorder. *Brain Cogn* 112: 78–83. https://doi.org/10.1016/j.bandc.2016.08.004.

Van Hedger, S. C., Heald, S. L. M., and Nusbaum, H. C. (2019). Absolute pitch can be learned by some adults. *PLOS ONE* 14(9): e0223047. https://doi.org/10.1371/journal.pone.0223047.

Varlamov, A. A., and Skorokhodov, I. V.(2022). Knismesis: The aversive facet of tickle. *Curr Opin Behav Sci* 43: 230–235. https://doi.org/10.1016/j.cobeha.2021.11.007.

Vedamurthy, I., Knill, D. C., Huang, S. J., Yung, A., Ding, J., Kwon, O-S., Bavelier, D., et al. (2016). Recovering stereo vision by squashing virtual bugs in a virtual reality environment. *Philos Trans R Soc Lond B Biol Sci* 371: 20150264. https://doi.org/10.1098/rstb.2015.0264.

Verhagen, J. V., Wesson, D. W., Netoff, T. I., White, J. A., and Wachowiak, M. (2007). Sniffing controls an adaptive filter of sensory input to the olfactory bulb. *Nat Neurosci* 10: 631–639.

Verhoef, B. E., Vogels, R., and Janssen, P. (2016). Binocular depth processing in the ventral visual pathway. *Philos Trans R Soc Lond B Biol Sci* 371(1697): 20150259. https://doi.org/10.1098/rstb.2015.0259.

Vermetten, E., Schmahl, C., Southwick, S. M., and Bremner, J. D. (2007). A positron tomographic emission study of olfactory induced emotional recall in veterans with and without combat-related posttraumatic stress disorder. *Psychopharmacol Bull* 40: 8–30.

Verrillo, R. T. (1963). Effect of contactor area on the vibrotactile threshold. *J Acoust Soc Am* 35: 1962–1966.

Vishwanath, D., Girshik, A. R., and Banks, M. (2005). Why pictures look right when viewed from the wrong place. *Nat Neurosci* 8: 1401–1410.

Vlasits, A. L., Euler, T., and Franke, K. (2019). Function first: Classifying cell types and circuits of the retina. *Curr Opin Neurobiol* 56: 8–15. https://doi.org/10.1016/j.conb.2018.10.011.

Võ, M. L.-H. (2021). The meaning and structure of scenes. *Vision Res* 181: 10–20. https://doi.org/10.1016/j.visres.2020.11.003.

Vo, M. L., Boettcher, S., and Draschkow, D. (2019). Reading scenes: How scene grammar guides attention and aids perception in real-world environments. *Curr Opin Psychol* 29: 205–210. https://doi.org/10.1016/j.copsyc.2019.03.009.

Vockely, J., and Ensenauer, R. (2006). Isovaleric acidemia: New aspects of genetic and phenotypic heterogeneity. *Am J Med Genet C Semin Med Genet* 142: 95–103.

Vodicka, J., and Kopal, A.(2016). New test of odor pleasantness in Parkinson's disease. *Functional Neurology* 31(3): 149.

Volkow, N. D., and Swanson, J. M. (2013). Adult attention deficit-hyperactivity disorder. *N Engl J Med* 369: 1935–1944.

von Helmholtz, H. (1863). On the Motions of the Human Eye. Heidelberg lecture. In: Koeningsberger, L. Hermann von Helmholtz. Dover Publications Inc. New York. Pp. 218.

von Helmholtz, H. (1924). *Helmholtz's Treatise on Physiological Optics* (translated from the 3rd German edition; J. P. C. Southall, Ed.). Rochester, NY: Optical Society of America.

von der Heydt, R., Peterhans, E., and Baumgartner, G. (1984). Illusory contours and cortical neuron responses. *Science* 224: 1260–1262.

Von Holst, E., and Mittelstaedt, H. (1950). Das Reafferenzprinzip (Wechselwirkungen zwischen Zentralnervensystem und Peripherie) [The principle of reafference]. *Naturwissenschaften* 37: 464–476.

Voskuil, P. (2013). Van Gogh's disease in the light of his correspondence. *Front Neurol Neurosci* 31: 116–125. https://doi.org/10.1159/000343265.

Voss, P., and Zatorre, R. J. (2012). Organization and reorganization of sensory-deprived cortex. *Curr Biol* 22: 168–173.

Vuong, Q. C., Domini, F., and Caudek, C. (2006). Disparity and shading cues cooperate for surface interpolation. *Perception* 35(2): 145–155. doi: 10.1068/p5315

W

Wade, N. J. (2000). William Charles Wells (1757–1817) and vestibular research before Purkinje and Flourens. *J Vestib Res* 10: 127–137.

Wagemans, J., Feldman, J., Gepshtein, S., Kimchi, R., Pomerantz, J. R., van der Helm, P. A., and van Leeuwen, C. (2012). A century of Gestalt psychology in visual perception: II. Conceptual and theoretical foundations. *Psychol Bull* 138: 1218–1252.

Walker, R., and Lupien, J. R. (2000). The safety evaluation of monosodium glutamate. *J Nutr* 130 (4S Suppl.): 1049S–1052S.

Wall, M. B., Lingnau, A., Ashida, H., and Smith, A. T. (2008). Selective visual responses to expansion and rotation in the human MT complex revealed by functional magnetic resonance imaging adaptation. *Eur J Neurosci* 27: 2747–2757. https://doi.org/10.1111/j.1460-9568.2008.06249.x.

Walla, P. (2008). Olfaction and its dynamic influence on word and face processing: Cross-modal integration. *Prog Neurobiol* 84: 192–209.

Walla, P., Hufnagl, B., Lehern, J., Mayer, D., Lindinger, G., Imhof, H., Deeke, L., et al. (2003). Olfaction and depth of word processing: A magnetoencephalographic study. *Neuroimage* 18: 104–116.

Wallisch, P. (2017). Illumination assumptions account for individual differences in the perceptual interpretation of a profoundly ambiguous stimulus in the color domain: "The dress." *J Vis* 17: 5.

Wallisch, P., and Movshon, J. A. (2008). Structure and function come unglued in the visual cortex. *Neuron* 60: 195–197. https://doi.org/10.1016/j.neuron.2008.10.008.

Wandell, B. A., and Winawer, J. (2011). Imaging retinotopic maps in the human brain. *Vision Res* 51: 718–737.

Wang, Q., and Spence, C. (2018). Assessing the influence of music on wine perception among wine professionals. *Food Sci Nutrit* 6: 295–301. https://doi.org/10.1002/fsn3.554.

Wang, Q. J., and Spence, C. (2019). Drinking through rosé-coloured glasses: Influence of wine colour on the perception of aroma and flavour in wine experts and novices. *Food Res Int* 126: 108678.

Wang, X., Liang, G., Zhang, Y., Blanton, H., Bessinger, Z., and Jacobs, N. (2020). Inconsistent performance of deep learning models on mammogram classification. *J Am College Radiol* 17(6): 796–803. https://doi.org/10.1016/j.jacr.2020.01.006.

Wang, Y., and Frost, B. J. (1992). Time to collision is signalled by neurons in the nucleus rotundus of pigeons. *Nature* 356: 236–238.

Ward, J., and Meijer, P. (2010). Visual experiences in the blind induced by an auditory sensory substitution device. *Conscious Cogn* 1: 492–500. https://doi.org/10.1016/j.concog.2009.10.006.

Ward, W. D. (1954). Subjective musical pitch. *J Acoust Soc Am* 26: 369–380.

Warren, R. M. (1984). Perceptual restoration of obliterated sounds. *Psychol Rev* 96: 371–385.

Warren, R. M., and Obusek, C. J. (1971). Speech perception and phonemic restorations. *Percept Psychophys* 9: 358–362.

Warren, W. H., Jr., and Hannon, D. J. (1990). Eye movements and optical flow. *J Opt Soc Am A* 7: 160–169.

Warren, W. H., Jr., Morris, M. W., and Kalish, M. (1988). Perception of translational heading from optical flow. *J Exp Psychol Hum Percept Perform* 14: 646–660.

Warren, W. H., Jr., and Verbrugge, R. R. (1984). Auditory perception of breaking and bouncing events: A case study in ecological acoustics. *J Exp Psychol Hum Percept Perform* 10: 704–712.

Webster, M. A. (2017). Color vision. In J. T. C. Wixted (Ed.), *The Stevens' Handbook of Experimental Psychology and Cognitive Neuroscience* (4th ed.). New York: Wiley.

Webster, M. A. (2020). Color vision: Glasses half full. *Curr Biol* 30(16): R952–R954. https://doi.org/10.1016/j.cub.2020.06.062.

Webster, M. A. (2020). The Verriest Lecture: Adventures in blue and yellow. *J Opt Soc Am A* 37(4): V1–V14. https://doi.org/10.1364/JOSAA.383625.

Weiland J. D., Cho, A. K., and Humayun, M. S. (2011). Retinal prostheses: Current clinical results and future needs. *Ophthalmology* 118: 2227–2237.

Weinstein, S. (1968). Intensive and extensive aspects of tactile sensitivity as a function of body part, sex, and laterality. In D. R. Kenshalo (Ed.), *The Skin Senses* (pp. 195–222). Springfield, IL: Thomas.

Weiss, T., Snitz, K., Yablonka, A., Khan, R. M., Gafsou, D., Schneidman, E., and Sobel, N. (2012). Perceptual convergence of multi-component mixtures in olfaction implies an olfactory white. *Proc Nat Acad Sci USA* 109: 19959–19964.

Weiss, T., Soroka, T., Gorodisky, L., Shushan, S., Snitz, K., Weissgross, R. et al. (2020). Human olfaction without apparent olfactory bulbs. *Neuron* 105: 35–45. https://doi.org/10.1016/j.neuron.2019.10.006.

Welch, R.B., DuttonHurt, L. D., and Warren, D. H. (1986). Contributions of audition and vision to temporal rate perception. *Percept Psychophys* 39: 294–300. https://doi.org/10.3758/bf03204939.

Wells, W. (1792). *An Essay upon Single Vision with Two Eyes: Together with Experiments and Observations on Several Other Subjects in Optics*. London: Cadell.

Werker, J. F., and Tees, R. C. (1984). Cross-language speech perception: Evidence for perceptual reorganization during the first year of life. *Infant Behavior & Development*, *7*(1): 49–63.

Werner, J. S. (1982). Development of scotopic sensitivity and the absorption spectrum of the human ocular media. *J Opt Soc Am* 72(2): 247–58. doi: 10.1364/josa.72.000247.

Werner, J. S., Marsh-Armstrong, B., and Knoblauch, K. (2020). Adaptive changes in color vision from long-term filter usage in anomalous but not normal trichromacy. *Curr Biol* 30(15): 3011–3015.e3014. https://doi.org/https://doi.org/10.1016/j.cub.2020.05.054.

Werner, J. S., Peterzell, D. H., and Scheetz, A. J. (1990). Light, vision, and aging. *Optom Vision Sci* 67: 214–229.

Wertheim, A. H., Mesland, B. S., and Bles, W. (2001). Cognitive suppression of tilt sensations during linear horizontal self-motion in the dark. *Perception* 30: 733–741.

Wessel, D. L. (1979). Timbre space as a musical control structure. *Comput Music J* 3: 45–52.

Westö, J., Martyniuk, N., Koskela, S., Turunen, T., Pentikäinen, S., and Ala-Laurila, P. (2022). Retinal OFF ganglion cells allow detection of quantal shadows at starlight. *Curr Biol* 32(13): 2848–2857.e6. https://doi.org/10.1016/j.cub.2022.04.092.

Westling, G., and Johansson, R. S. (1984). Factors influencing the force control during precision grip. *Exp Brain Res* 53: 277–284.

Wever, E. G. (1949). *Theory of Hearing*. New York: Wiley.

Wheatstone, C. (1852). Some remarkable and hitherto unobserved phenomena of binocular vision: Part two. *Philos Mag* 4: 504–523.

White, A. L., Boynton, G. M., and Yeatman, J. D. (2019). You can't recognize two words simultaneously. *Trends Cogn Sci* 23(10): 812–814. https://doi.org/https://doi.org/10.1016/j.tics.2019.07.001.

Whitney, D., and Levi, D. M. (2011). Visual crowding: A fundamental limit on conscious perception and object recognition. *Trends Cogn Sci* 15: 160–168.

Whitney, D., and Yamanashi Leib, A. (2018). Ensemble perception. *Annu Rev Psychol* 69: 105–129. https://doi.org/10.1146/annurev-psych-010416-044232.

Wiesel, T. N. (1982). Postnatal development of the visual cortex and the influence of environment. *Nature* 299: 583–591.

Wightman, F., and Kistler, D. (1998). Of Vulcan ears, human ears and "earprints." *Nat Neurosci* 1: 337–339.

Wijntjes, M. W. A., Sato, A., Hayward, V., and Kappers, A. M. L. (2009). Local surface orientation dominates haptic curvature discrimination. *IEEE Trans Haptics* 2: 94–102.

Wilkins, L., and Richter, C. P. (1940). A great craving for salt by a child with cortico-adrenal insufficiency. *J Am Med Assoc* 114: 866–868.

Willander, J., and Larsson, M. (2007). Olfaction and emotion: The case of auto-biographical memory. *Mem Cognit* 35: 1659–1663.

Willems, C., and Martens, S. (2016). Time to see the bigger picture: Individual differences in the attentional blink. *Psychon Bull Rev* 23: 1289–1299.

Williams, D. W. and Sekuler, R. (1984). Coherent global motion percepts from stochastic local motions. *Vision Res* 24(1): 55–62. doi: 10.1016/0042-6989(84)90144-5.

Willis, C. M., Church, S. M., Guest, C. M., Cook, W. A., McCarthy, N., Bransbury, A. J., Church, M. R. T., et al. (2004). Olfactory detection of human bladder cancer by dogs: Proof of principle study. *Br Med J* 329: 712–714.

Wilson, D. A., Best, A. R., and Sullivan, R. M. (2004). Plasticity in the olfactory system: Lessons for the neurobiology of memory. *Neuroscientist* 10: 513–524.

Wilson, F. A. W., and Rolls, E. T. (2005). The primate amygdala and reinforcement: A dissociation between rule-based and associatively-mediated memory revealed in neuronal activity. *Neuroscience* 133: 1061–1072.

Wilson, V. J., and Melvill Jones, G. (1979). *Mammalian Vestibular Physiology*. New York: Plenum.

Winberg, J., and Porter, R. H. (1998). Olfaction and human neonatal behaviour: Clinical implications. *Acta Paediatr* 87: 6–10.

Witthoft, N., and Winawer, J. (2013). Learning, memory, and synesthesia. *Psychol Sci* 24(3): 258–265. https://doi.org/10.1177/0956797612452573.

Witzel, C. (2019). Misconceptions about colour categories. *Rev Phil Psychol* 10(3): 499–540. https://doi.org/10.1007/s13164-018-0404-5.

Witzel, C., and Gegenfurtner, K. R. (2016). Categorical perception for red and brown. *J Exp Psychol Hum Percept Perform* 42: 540–570.

Witzel, C., and Gegenfurtner, K. R. (2018). Color perception: Objects, constancy, and categories. *Annu Rev Vision Sci* 4(1): 475–499. https://doi.org/10.1146/annurev-vision-091517-034231.

Witzel, C., O'Regan, J. K., and Hansmann-Roth, S. (2017). The dress and individual differences in the perception of surface properties. *Vision Res* 141: 76–94. https://doi.org/https://doi.org/10.1016/j.visres.2017.07.015.

Wixted, J. T. (2020). The forgotten history of signal detection theory. *J Exp Psychol: Learn Mem Cogn* 46: 201–233. https://doi.org/10.1037/xlm0000732.

Wixted, J. T., and Wells, G. L. (2017). The relationship between eyewitness confidence and identification accuracy: A new synthesis. *Psychol Sci Public Interest* 18(1): 10–65. https://doi.org/10.1177/1529100616686966.

Wolfe, J. M. (2021). Guided Search 6.0: An updated model of visual search. *Psych Bull Rev* 28: 1060–1092. https://doi.org/10.3758/s13423-020-01859-9.

Wolfe, J. M., and Bennett, S. C. (1997). Preattentive object files: Shapeless bundles of basic features. *Vision Res* 37: 25–43.

Wolfe, J. M., Cave, K. R., and Franzel, S. L. (1989). Guided search: An alternative to the feature integration model for visual search. *J Exp Psychol Hum Percept Perform* 15: 419–433.

Wolfe, J. M., and DiMase, J. S. (2003). Do intersections serve as basic features in visual search? *Perception* 32: 645–656.

Wolfe, J. M., and Held, R. (1981). A purely binocular mechanism in human vision. *Vision Res* 21: 1755–1759.

Wolfe, J. M., and Horowitz, T. S. (2017). Five factors that guide attention in visual search. [Review Article]. *Nat Hum Behav* 1: Article 0058. https://doi.org/10.1038/s41562-017-0058.

Wolfe, J. M., Vo, M. L.-H., Evans, K. K., and Greene, M. R. (2011). Visual search in scenes involves selective and non-selective pathways. *Trends Cogn Sci* 15: 77–84.

Womelsdorf, T., Anton-Erxleben, K., Pieper, F., and Treue, S. (2006). Dynamic shifts of visual receptive fields in cortical area MT by spatial attention. *Nat Neurosci* 9: 1156–1160.

Woo, S-H., Lumpkin, E. A., and Patapoutian, A. (2015). Merkel cells and neurons keep in touch. *Trends Cell Biol* 25(2): 74–81. https://doi.org/10.1016/j.tcb.2014.10.003.

Woodrow, H. (1909). A quantitative study of rhythm. *Arch Psychol* 14: 1–66.

Wrzesniewski, A., McCauley, C., and Rozin, P. (1999). Odor and affect: Individual differences in the impact of odor on liking for places, things and people. *Chem Senses* 24: 713–721.

Wu, Y., Chen, K., Ye, Y., Zhang, T., and Zhou, W.(2020). Humans navigate with stereo olfaction. *Proceedings of the National Academy of Sciences* 117(27): 16065–16071.

Wysocki, C. J., Dalton, P., Brody, M. J., and Lawley, H. J. (1997). Acetone odor and irritation thresholds obtained from acetone-exposed factory workers and from control (occupationally non-exposed) subjects. *Am Ind Hyg Assoc J* 58: 704–712.

Wysocki, C. J., Dorries, K. M., and Beauchamp, G. K. (1989). Ability to perceive androstenone can be acquired by ostensibly anosmic people. *Proc Natl Acad Sci USA* 86: 7976–7978.

X

Xiao, Y. (2014). Processing of the S-cone signals in the early visual cortex of primates. *Vis Neurosci* 31 (Special Issue 02): 189–195.

Xie, Y., Bigelow, R. T., Frankenthaler, S. F., Studenski, S. A., Moffat, S. D., and Agrawal, Y. (2017). Vestibular loss in older adults is associated with impaired spatial navigation: Data from the triangle completion task. *Frontiers in Neurology*, 173.

Xu, L., Li, W., Voleti, V., Hillman, E. M., and Firestein, S. (2020). Widespread receptor-driven modulation in peripheral olfactory coding. *Science* 368: eaaz5390. https://doi.org/10.1126/science.aaz5390.

Y

Yabuta, N. H., and Callaway, E. M. (1998). Functional streams and local connections of layer 4C neurons in primary visual cortex of the macaque monkey. *J Neurosci* 18: 9489–9499.

Yamin-Pasternak, S., Kliskey, A., Alessa, L., Pasternak, I., and Schweitzer, P. (2014). The rotten renaissance in the Bering Strait: Loving, loathing, and washing the smell of foods with a (re)acquired taste. *Curr Anthropol* 55: 619–646. https://doi.org/10.1086/678305.

Yan, C. H., Mundy, D. C., and Patel, Z. M. (2020). The use of platelet-rich plasma in treatment of olfactory dysfunction: A pilot study. *Laryngoscope Invest Otolaryngol* 5(2): 187–193. https://doi.org/10.1002/lio2.357.

Yantis, S. (1993). Stimulus-driven attentional capture. *Curr Dir Psychol Sci* 2: 156–161.

Yarbus, A. L. (1967). *Eye Movements and Vision*. New York: Plenum.

Yates, B., and Miller, A. (1998). Physiological evidence that the vestibular system participates in autonomic and respiratory control. *J Vestib Res* 8: 17–26.

Yates, B. J., Bolton, P. S., and Macefield, V. G. (2014). Vestibulo-sympathetic responses. *Compr Physiol* 4: 851–887.

Yeshurun, Y., Lapid, H., Dudai, Y., and Sobel, N. (2009). The privileged brain representation of first olfactory associations. *Curr Biol* 19: 1869–1874.

Yin, T. C., and Chan, J. C. (1990). Interaural time sensitivity in medial superior olive of cat. *J Neurophysiol* 65: 465–488.

Yonas, A., Craton, L. G., and Thompson, W. B. (1987). Relative motion: Kinetic information for the order of depth at an edge. *Percept Psychophys* 41: 53–59.

Yoshinaka, M., Ikebe, K., Uota, M., Ogawa, T., Okada, T., Inomata, C., et al. (2016). Age and sex differences in the taste sensitivity of young adult, young-old and old-old Japanese. *Geriatrics & Gerontology International* 16(12): 1281–1288.

Young, L. R. (1984). Perception of the body in space: Mechanisms. In I. Darian-Smith (Ed.), *Handbook of Physiology—The Nervous System* (Vol. 3[2], pp. 1023–1066). Bethesda, MD: American Physiological Society.

Young, L. R., Shelhamer, M., and Modestino, S. (1986). M.I.T./Canadian vestibular experiments on the Spacelab-1 mission. 2. Visual vestibular tilt interaction in weightlessness. *Exp Brain Res* 64: 299–307.

Yu, K., and Blake, R. (1992). Do recognizable figures enjoy an advantage in binocular rivalry? *J Exp Psychol Hum Percept Perform* 18: 1158–1173.

Yuille, A., and Kersten, D. (2006). Vision as Bayesian inference: Analysis by synthesis? *Trends Cogn Sci* 10: 301–308.

Yuodelis, C., and Hendrickson, A. (1986). A qualitative and quantitative analysis of the human fovea during development. *Vision Res* 26: 847–855.

Z

Zadra, A., Nielsen, T. A., and Donderi, D. C. (1998). Prevalence of auditory, olfactory, and gustatory experiences in home dreams. *Percept Mot Skills* 87: 819–826.

Zahorick, P., and Wightman, F. L. (2001). Loudness constancy with varying sound source distance. *Nat Neuro* 4: 78–83.

Zahorik, P. (2002). Assessing auditory distance perception using virtual acoustics. *J Acoust Soc Am* 111: 1832–1846.

Zaidi, Q. (1997). Decorrelation of L- and M-cone signals. *J Opt Soc Am A Opt Image Sci Vis* 14: 3430–3431.

Zaidi, Q., Ennis, R., Cao, D., and Lee, B. (2012). Neural locus of color afterimages. *Curr Biol* 22: 220–224.

Zapiec, B., Dieriks, B. V., Tan, S., Faull, R. L., Mombaerts, P., and Curtis, M. A. (2017). A ventral glomerular deficit in Parkinson's disease revealed by whole olfactory bulb reconstruction. *Brain* 140: 2722–2736. https://doi.org/10.1093/brain/awx208.

Zatorre, R. J. (2001). Do you see what I'm saying? Interactions between auditory and visual cortices in cochlear implant users. *Neuron* 1: 13–14.

Zeki, S. (1983a). Colour coding in the cerebral cortex: The reaction of cells in monkey visual-cortex to wavelengths and colours. *Neuroscience* 9: 741–765.

Zeki, S. (1983b). Colour coding in the cerebral cortex: The responses of wavelength-selective and colour-coded cells in monkey visual cortex to changes in wavelength composition. *Neuroscience* 9: 767–781.

Zelano, C., Bensafi, M., Porter, J., Mainland, J., Johnson, B., Bremner, E., Telles, C., et al. (2005). Attentional modulation in human primary olfactory cortex. *Nat Neurosci* 8: 114–120.

Zelano, C., Jiang, H., Zhou, G., Arora, N., Schuele, S., Rosenow, J., and Gottfried, J. A. (2016). Nasal respiration entrains human limbic oscillations and modulates cognitive function. *J Neurosci* 36: 12448–12467. https://doi.org/10.1523/jneurosci.2586-16.2016.

Zellner, D. A. (2013). Color-odor interactions: A review and model. *Chemosens Percept* 6: 155–169.

Zellner, D. A., Rozin, P., Aron, M., and Kulish, C. (1983). Conditioned enhancement of human's liking for flavor by pairing with sweetness. *Learn Motiv* 14: 338–350.

Zera, J., and Green, D. M. (1993). Detecting temporal onset and offset asynchrony in multicomponent complexes. *J Acoust Soc Am* 93: 1038–1052. https://doi.org/10.1121/1.405552.

Zhang, B., Zheng, J., Watanabe, I., Maruko, I., Bi, H., Smith, E. L., III, and Chino, Y. (2005). Delayed maturation of receptive field center/surround mechanisms in V2. *Proc Natl Acad Sci USA* 102: 5862–5867.

Zhao, G. Q., Zhang, Y., Hoon, M. A., Chandrashekar, J., Erlenbach, I., Ryba, N. J., and Zuker, C. S. (2003). The receptors for mammalian sweet and umami taste. *Cell* 115: 255–266.

Zheng, J., Zhang, B., Bi, H., Maruko, I., Watanabe, I., Nakatsuka, C., Smith, E. L., III, et al. (2007). Development of temporal response properties and contrast sensitivity of V1 and V2 neurons in macaque monkeys. *J Neurophysiol* 97: 3905–3916.

Zhou, B., Feng, G., Chen, W., and Zhou, W. (2018). Olfaction warps visual time perception. *Cereb Cortex* 28: 1718–1728. https://doi.org/10.1093/cercor/bhx068.

Zhou, F., Wong, V., and Sekuler, R. (2007). Multisensory integration of spatio-temporal segmentation cues: One plus one does not always equal two. *Exp Brain Res* 180: 641–654. https://doi.org/10.1007/s00221-007-0897-0.

Zhou, H., Friedman, H. S., and von der Heydt, R. (2000). Coding of border ownership in monkey visual cortex. *J Neurosci* 20: 6594–6611.

Zhou, W., and Chen, D. (2009). Binaral rivalry between the nostrils and the cortex. *Curr Biol* 19: 1561–1565.

Zimmerman, A., Bai, L., and Ginty, D. D.(2006). The gentle touch receptors of mammalian skin. *Science* 346(6212): 950–954. https://doi.org/10.1126/science.1254229.

Ziomkiewicz, A. (2006). Menstrual synchrony: Fact or artifact? *Human Nature*

17: 419–432. https://doi.org/10.1007/s12110-006-1004-0.

Zipser, K., Lamme, V. A., and Schiller, P. H. (1996). Contextual modulation in primary visual cortex. *J Neurosci* 16: 7376–7389.

Zirnsak, M., Steinmetz, N. A., Noudoost, B., Xu, K. Z., and Moore, T. (2014). Visual space is compressed in prefrontal cortex before eye movements. *Nature* 507: 504–507.

Zivony, A., and Lamy, D. (2022). What processes are disrupted during the attentional blink? An integrative review of event-related potential research. *Psychon Bull Rev* 29(2): 394–414. https://doi.org/10.3758/s13423-021-01973-2.

Zucco, G. M., Aiello, L., Turuani, L., and Köster, E. (2012). Odor-evoked autobiographical memories: Age and gender differences along the life span. *Chem Senses* 37: 179–189.

Credits

CHAPTER 1

[Ch 1 opener]© Oleg Shupliak art, p. 2; Figure 1.1: The Bold Bureau/Shutterstock, p. 4; Figure 1.7: Fast, K. (2004). *Developing a Scale to Measure Just About Anything: Comparisons across Groups and Individuals.* New Haven, CT: Yale University School of Medicine, p. 13; Figure 1.13A-B: A: pixbull/Shutterstock, B: Olive Merchandise/Shutterstock, p. 17; Figure 1.14: After Breedlove, S. M. and Watson, N. V. (2013). *Biological Psychology: An Introduction to Behavioral, Cognitive, and Clinical Neuroscience* (7th ed.). Sunderland, MA: Sinauer, p. 19; Figure 1.20C: After N. Y. S. Kiang. 1965. *Discharge Patterns of Single Fibers in the Cat's Auditory Nerve.* MIT Press: Cambridge, MA, p. 23; Figure 1.21A-C: A–C after S. M. Breedlove et al. 2010. *Biological Psychology: An Introduction to Behavioral, Cognitive, and Clinical Neuroscience*, 6th ed. Oxford University Press/Sinauer Associates: Sunderland, MA, p. 25; Figure 1.21D: Courtesy of Steven Luck, p. 25; Figure 1.22A-B: A:© Jim Thompson/Albuquerque Journal/ZumaPress, B: Courtesy of Daniel Baldauf, p. 26; Figure 1.23A-B: A: Amaka Umeh (Hamlet—Stratford Festival, 2020). Creative direction by Punch & Judy Inc. Photography by David Cooper, B: Courtesy of Geoff Young, MD, p. 26; Figure1.24A-B: A: Joseph Rahi/Shutterstock; Twin Design/Shutterstock; B_27/Shutterstock, B: Brain images courtesy of Emilie Josephs, p. 27; Figure 1.25A: Pawel Michalowski/Shutterstock, goldenjack/Shutterstock, p. 28.

CHAPTER 2

[Ch 2 opener]© Alicia Hunsicker, 2011, p. 32; Figure 2.2: After S. M. Breedlove and N. V. Watson. 2013. *Biological Psychology: An Introduction to Behavioral, Cognitive, and Clinical Neuroscience*, 7th ed., Oxford University Press/Sinauer: Sunderland, MA, p. 35; Figure 2.5A-D: After C. W. Oyster. 1999. *The Human Eye: Structure and Function.* Oxford University Press/Sinauer: Sunderland, MA, p. 38; Figure 2.6: karn684/Shutterstock, bestv/Shutterstock, p. 38; Figure 2.8: © iStock.com/olaaf, p. 39; Figure 2.10: © 2020 American Academy of Ophthalmology, p. 41; Figure 2.11: After R. W. Rodieck. 1998. *The First Steps in Seeing.* Oxford University Press/Sinauer: Sunderland, MA, p. 41; Figure 2.12: Graphs after C. W. Oyster. 1999. *The Human Eye: Structure and Function.* Oxford University Press/Sinauer: Sunderland, MA, Micrographs from C. A. Curcio et al. 1990. *J Comp Neurol* 292: 497–523, p. 42; Figure 2.14: After D. Purves et al. 2013. *Neuroscience*, 5th edition. Oxford University Press/Sinauer: Sunderland, MA, p. 44; Figure 2.16: © Diane Hirsch/Fundamental Photographs, NYC, p. 45; Figure 2.17: After J .D. Weiland et al. 2005. *Ann Rev Biomed Eng* 7: 361–401, p. 47; Figure 2.18: From A. Roorda and D. R. Williams 1999. *Nature* 397: 520–522; courtesy of Austin Roorda., p. 48; Figure 2.19: After R. W. Rodieck et al. 1985. *J Comp Neurol* 233: 115–132; and S. L. Polyak. 1941. *The Retina.* University of Chicago Press: Chicago, p. 50; Figure 2.20C-D: C,D after D. Hubel and T. N. Wiesel. 1961. *J Physiol* 155: 385–398.

CHAPTER 3

[Ch 3 opener]Courtesy of the artist, Iruka Maria Toro, © 2014, p. 56; Figure 3.1A-C: A after D. Purves et al. 2013. *Neuroscience*, 5th ed., Oxford University Press/Sinauer: Sunderland, MA, B after S. M. Breedlove and N. V. Watson. 2013. *Biological Psychology: An Introduction to Behavioral, Cognitive, and Clinical Neuroscience*, 7th ed., Oxford University Press/Sinauer: Sunderland, MA, C after M. R. Rosenzweig et al. 2002. *Biological Psychology*, 3rd ed., Oxford University Press/Sinauer: Sunderland, MA, p. 58; Figure 3.5: From D. Whitney and D. M. Levi. 2011. *Trends Cogn Sci* 15: 160–168, p. 61; Figure 3.9: Image by Izumi Ohzawa, with credit to John Robson and Fergus W. Campbell, p. 65; Figure 3.10A-C: A: Courtesy of Vladimir Sacek/telescope-optics.net, B: After J. G. Robson. 1966. *J Opt Soc Am* 56: 1141–1142, C: After F. Schieber. 1992. In *Handbook of Mental Health and Aging.* J. E. Birren et al. (Eds.), pp. 251–306. Academic Press: New York, p. 66; Figure 3.11: J. Ng and J. J. Goldberger. 2007. Understanding and interpreting dominant frequency analysis of AF electrograms. *Journal of Cardiovascular Electrophysiology* 18(6): 680–685, p. 67; Figure 3.14: BrainMaps: An Interactive Multiresolution Brain Atlas; http://brainmaps.org [retrieved on 14APR2020], p. 69; Figure 3.16: From D. H. Hubel. 1988. *Eye, Brain, and Vision.* Scientific American Library: New York, p. 71; Figure 3.17: After J. P. Frisby. 1980. *Seeing: Illusion, Brain and Mind.* Oxford University Press: Oxford, p. 72; Figure 3.18A-B: A after J. C. Horton and W. F. Hoyt. 1991. *Arch Ophthalmol* 109: 816–824; B from B. A. Wandell and J. Winawer. 2011. *Vision Res* 51: 718–737, p. 73; Figure 3.20A: Ira Wyman/Getty Images, p. 74; Figure 3.21: Receptive fields, binocular interaction and functional architecture in the cat's visual cortex. *J Physiol* 160: 106–154, p. 75; Figure 3.25A-B: From D. H. Hubel et al. 1978. *J Comp Neurol* 177: 361–379, p. 78; Figure 3.25C: From I. Nauhaus et al. 2008. *Neuron* 57: 673–679, p. 78; Figure 3.26: After S. M. Breedlove et al. 2007. *Biological Psychology: An Introduction to Behavioral, Cognitive, and Clinical Neuroscience*, 5th ed., Oxford University Press/Sinauer: Sunderland, MA, p. 79; Figure 3.27: From D. H. Hubel. 1988. *Eye, Brain, and Vision.* Scientific American Library: New York, p. 79 Figure 3.29: After J. M. Wolfe. 1984. *Vis Res* 24: 1959–1964, p. 82; Figure 3.30B-C: B, C courtesy of Izumi Ohzawa, with credit to John Robson and Fergus W. Campbell, p. 83; Figure 3.31A-B): A, B after C. Blakemore and F. Campbell. 1969. *J Physiol* 203: 237–260, p. 84; Figure 3.32: After N. Graham and J. Nachmias. 1971. *Vision Res* 11: 251–259, p. 84; Figure 3.33: Courtesy of David McIntyre, p. 85; Figure 3.34: From L. D. Harmon and B. Julesz. 1973. *Science* 180: 1194–1197, p. 85; Figure 3.35: After D. Bavelier and H. J. Neville. 2002. *Nat Rev Neurosci* 6: 443–452; based on F. Morrell. 1972. *Nature* 238: 44–46, p. 86; Figure 3.36C: After A. M. Norcia et al. 2015. *J Vis* 15: 1–46, p. 87; Figure 3.37: After A. M. Norcia and R. E. Manny. 2003. Development of vision in infancy. In *Adler's Physiology of the Eye*, 10th edition, Kaufman PL, Alm A (Eds.), pp. 531–551. Elsevier: London, p. 90.

CHAPTER 4

[Ch 4 opener]Marvin Oliver/Owen Oliver photo/www.alaskaeaglearts.com, p. 92; Figure 4.1: © Island Images/Alamy Stock Photo, p. 94; Figure 4.2: After J. Parker. 2007. *Nat Rev Neurosci* 8: 379–391, based on R. C. Reid. 1999. In *Fundamental Neuroscience*, L. R. Squire et al., eds., pp. 821–851. Academic Press: San Diego and T. D. Albright. 1993. In *Visual Motion and Its Role in the Stabilization of Gaze*, F. A. Miles and J. Wallman, eds., pp. 177–201. Elsevier Science, Amsterdam, p. 94; Figure 4.3: After P. Wallisch and J. A. Movshon. 2008. *Neuron* 60: 195–197, prepared in 1998 by John Maunsell. Based on data from D. J. Felleman and D. C. Van Essen. 1991. *Cereb Cortex* 1: 1–47 and P. Lennie. 1998. *Perception* 27: 889–935, p. 95; Figure 4.4: Courtesy of Sabine Kastner and Mike Arcaro, p. 95; Figure 4.6: Jennifer Aniston: Stills from Picture Perfect © 3 Art Entertainment, Jennifer Aniston and Brad Pitt: © Allstar Picture Library/Alamy Stock Photo, Laura Linney: Still from *The Truman Show* © Paramount Pictures, spider: © John Bell/Shutterstock.com, Sydney Opera House: Christian Mehlführer/CC BY 2.5, Leaning Tower: © iStock.com/Lawrence Sawyer, Eiffel Tower: © iStock.com/S. Greg Panosian, graphs: After R. Q. Quiroga et al. 2005. *Nature* 435: 1102–1107, p. 98; Figure 4.7: Reprinted from *Current Biology*, Volume 32, Issue 19, Meenakshi Khosla, N. Apurva Ratan Murty, Nancy Kanwisher, "A highly selective response to food in human visual cortex revealed by hypothesis-free voxel decomposition," pp. 4159–4171, 2022, with permission from Elsevier, p. 99; Figure 4.8: top row, left to right: Nortongo/Shutterstock, Jagodka/Shutterstock, Tiger Images/Shutterstock; middle row, left to right: Leoniek van der Vliet/Shutterstock, Tiger Images/Shutterstock, PCHT/Shutterstock; bottom row, left to right: Sergio33/Shutterstock, Joca de Jong/Shutterstock, Suradech Prapairat/Shutterstock, p. 100; Figure 4.9A-D: A: © Michael Potter11/Shutterstock, B: © Stefano Panzeri/Shutterstock, C: Mark William Penny/Shutterstock, D: Kengkbs/Shutterstock, p. 102; Figure 4.10A-B: A: Hanabusa Itchō, 1888, Public domain, via Wikimedia Commons, B: © Paula Joyce/Dreamstime.com, p. 103; Figure 4.11 photos: Tim UR/Shutterstock, Fotaw/Shutterstock, CoolR/Shutterstock, p. 104; Figure 4.14E-F: E: C. Coles Phillips (1880–1927), F: C. Coles Phillips (1880–1927), p. 106; Figure 4.15D-E: D after U. Polat and D. Sagi. 1993. *Vision Res* 33: 993–999, E after W. S. Geisler and J. S. Perry. 2009. *Vis Neurosci* 26: 109–121, p. 107; Figure 4.18A-B: A: © Laura Williams, B: Tse, P. U. (1998). Illusory volumes from conformation. *Perception* 27(8), 977–992, p. 108; Figure 4.19: Reprinted from *Trends in Cognitive Sciences*, 11(12), Oliva, A., & Torralba, A., "The role of context in object recognition," pp. 520–527, 2007, with permission from Elsevier, p. 109; Figure 4.23A-D: A: © Asther Lau Choon Siew/Shutterstock.com, B: © Asther Lau Choon Siew/Shutterstock.com, C: © Miles Boyer/Shutterstock.com, D: Courtesy of the Naval Historical Foundation, p. 111; Figure 4.25: Courtesy of Paul Philippon/The Duck-Rabbit Craft Brewery, p. 112; Figure 4.27A-D: A: © darios/123RF, B: © William Perugini/Shutterstock.com, C: © gorillaimages/Shutterstock.com, D: © D-VISIONS/Shutterstock.com, p. 113; Figure 4.31: After P. J. Kellman, 1998. In *Perception, Cognition, and Language: Essays in Honor of Henry and Lila Gleitman*, B. Landau et al. (Eds.), pp. 157–190. MIT Press: Cambridge, MA, p. 115; Figure 4.36A-B: A: From J. L. Gallant et al. 1993. *Science* 259: 100–103, B: Srinath, R. et al. 2021. *Current Biology*, 31(1), 51–65.e55., p. 118; Figure 4.37A: From A. Pasupathy and C. E. Connor. 2002. *Nat Neurosci* 5: 1332–1338, p. 119; Figure 4.38: After L. G. Ungerleider and A. H. Bell. 2011. *Vision Res* 51: 782–799, p. 119; Figure 4.42: cow grazing: © iStock.com/dschaef, cow with bell: © iStock.com/Augenblicke, cow tongue: © iStock.com/SebastianKnight, cow nose: © iStock.com/SebastianKnight, cow lying down: © iStock.com/danefromspain, Scottish cow: © iStock.com/dcookd, cow conversation: © iStock.com/esvetleishaya, cow on tightrope: © iStock.com/themacx, kissing calfs: © iStock.com/VeraOsco, p. 122; Figure 4.44: Images courtesy of Jim Todd, p. 123; Figure 4.46A-D: A: © William Leaman/Alamy Stock Photo, B: © SuperStock/Alamy Stock Photo, C: © Gerry Ellis/DigitalVision, D: © Gerry Ellis/DigitalVision, p. 125; Figure 4.47A-B: A: After P. Thompson. 1980. *Perception* 9: 482–484, B: After P. Thompson. 1980. *Perception* 9: 482–484, p. 126.

CHAPTER 5

[Ch 5 opener]Courtesy of Philip Wolfe, p. 130; Figure 5.1: Ground Picture/Shutterstock.com, p. 131; Figure 5.5: Ricardo Reitmeyer/Shutterstock, p. 134; Figure 5.7: After C. A. Torres et al. (2016). *Sci Hortic* 209: 165–172, p. 136; Figure 5.13: From R. Sabesan et al., 2016. *Sci Adv* 2: e1600797. DOI: 10.1126/sciadv.1600797. With permission from AAAS/CC BY-NC 4.0, p. 140; Figure 5.14: By kind permission of Ecilua Bleasdale, p. 141; Figure 5.17: From A. Stockman and D. H. Brainard, 2010. In *OSA Handbook of Optics*, 3rd ed., M. Bass [Ed.], pp. 11.11–11.104. McGraw–Hill: New York, p. 144; Figure 5.19: From A. Stockman and D. H. Brainard, 2010. In *OSA Handbook of Optics*, 3rd ed., M. Bass [Ed.], pp. 11.11–11.104. McGraw–Hill: New York, p. 146; Figure 5.20: From D. T. Lindsey and A. M. Brown. 2014. *J Vis* 14: 17, 1–25. https://doi.org/10.1167/14.2.17, p. 148; Figure 5.22: After C. Witzel and K. R. Gegenfurtner, 2016. *J Exp Psychol* 42: 540–570. Published by APA; reprinted with permission, p. 150; Figure 5.24: From A. Stockman and D. H. Brainard, 2010. In *OSA Handbook of Optics*, 3rd ed., M. Bass [Ed.], pp. 11.11–11.104. McGraw–Hill: New York, p. 154; Figure 5.25: Courtesy of David Novick, p. 155; Figure 5.26C-E: All photos courtesy of Jeremy Wolfe, p. 156; Figure 5.27: After H. E. Smithson. 2005. *Philos Trans R Soc Lond B Biol Soc* 360: 1329–1346, p. 157; Figure 5.28: Courtesy of Jeremy Wolfe, p. 159; Figure 5.29A-B: A: © Joerg Huettenhoelscher/123RF, B:© Pakhnyushchy/Shutterstock, p. 160; Figure 5.30: © Vphoto/Shutterstock, p. 160; Figure 5.31: After Q. J. Wang and C. Spence (2019). *Food Res Int* 126: 108678, p. 161; Figure 5.32A-C: A: © Vlad61/Shutterstock.com, B: © Marcel Mooij/Shutterstock.com, C: © Dynamic Graphics Group/Creatas/Alamy Stock Photo, p. 162; Figure 5.33A-B: A after Z. Musilova et al. (2019). *Science* 364: 588–592, B after Z. Musilova et al. (2019). *Science* 364: 588–592, p. 162; Figure 5.35: After P. Sun et al. 2016. *Proc Natl Acad Sci USA* 113: E6712–E6720. doi: 10.1073/pnas.1614062113, p. 164.

CHAPTER 6

[Ch 6 opener]"Clarity II" by Aaron Jasinski © 2015, p. 166; Figure 6.1: Ondrej Prosicky/Shutterstock, p. 168; Figure 6.5: M. C. Escher's "Relativity" © 2020 The M. C. Escher Company—The Netherlands. All rights reserved. www.mcescher.com, p. 171; Figure 6.7A-B: Courtesy of David McIntyre, p. 173; Figure 6.08: © iStock.com/GlobalP, p. 173; Figure 6.9: © iStock.com/GlobalP, p.174; Figure 6.10: © iStock.com/GlobalP, p. 174; Figure 6.11: © iStock.com/GlobalP, p. 175; Figure 6.14:

Courtesy of Jeremy Wolfe, p. 176; Figure 6.16: Francesco di Giorgio Martini—Architectural Veduta—Google Art Project, p. 177; Figure 6.17: Canaletto, "Bucentaur's return to the pier by the Palazzo Ducale," 1727–1729/Wikimedia, p. 177; Figure 6.18: Courtesy of Dhanraj Vishwanath and Martin S. Banks, p. 178; Figure 6.19: Hans Holbein the Younger, Jean de Dinteville and Georges de Selve ('The Ambassadors'), 1533 The National Gallery, London/Wikimedia, p. 178; Figure 6.20A-B: © Julian Beever, p. 179; Figure 6.23: Hafri A. et al. 2022. *Psychol Sci* 33(12): 2040–2058. Photos courtesy of Alon Hafri, p. 181; Figure 6.24: Permission granted by photographer, Adrian Borda, p. 182; Figure 6.32: After K. N. Ogle 1952. *AMA Arch Opthamol* 14: 50–60; L. M. Wilcox and R. S. Allison 2009. *Vis Res* 49: 2653–2665, p. 186; Figure 6.33: After C. Wheatstone. 1838. *Philos T R Soc B* 128: 371–394, p. 187; Figure 6.34A-B: A: © Pattarapong Kumlert/Shutterstock.com, B: Courtesy of the Library of Congress, p. 187; Figure 6.36: Courtesy of the Library of Congress, p. 190; Figure 6.38: From Goddard, 1951; Hearst Communications, Inc., reprinted with permission, p. 191; Figure 6.39: © Lai Seng Sin/ASSOCIATED PRESS, p. 192; Figure 6.44: From Preston, T. J. et al. 2008. *J Neurosci* 28(44): 11315–11327. https://www.jneurosci.org/content/28/44/11315/tab-figures-data, p. 196; Figure 6.45: From R. C. Feord et al. 2020. *Sci Adv* 6: eaay6036. DOI: 10.1126/sciadv.aay6036; with permission from AAAS/CC BY-NC 4.0, p. 197; Figure 6.46: From V. Nityananda et al., 2016. *Sci Rep* 6:18718/CC BY-4.0, p. 198; Figure 6.49: Photo by Jeremy Wolfe, p. 200; Figure 6.51: Courtesy of Akiyoshi Kitaoka, p. 201; Figure 6.52A: © iStock.com/Colonnade photo/xyno, p. 202; Figure 6.54A: © dpa picture alliance/Alamy Stock Photo, p. 203; Figure 6.57: All images from I. Kovacs et al. 1996. *Proc Natl Acad Sci USA* 93: 15508–15511. © 1996 National Academy of Sciences, U.S.A., p. 205; Figure 6.58: After E. E. Birch. 1993. In *Early Visual Development Normal and Abnormal*, K. Simons (Ed.), pp. 224–234. Oxford University Press: NY, p. 206; Figure 6.59: After E. E. Birch and B. Petrig. 1996. *Vision Res* 36: 1321–1326, p. 206; Figure 6.60: After Y. M. Chino et al. 1997. *J Neurosci* 17: 296–307. ©1997 Society for Neuroscience, p. 207; Figure 6.61: D. M. Levi. 2023. *Journal of Vision*, 23, 14, p. 209; Figure 6.63: After D. R. Stager and E. Birch. 1986. *J Pediatr Ophthalmol Strabismus* 23: 160–165, p. 210.

CHAPTER 7

[Ch 7 opener]Sergi Reboredo / Alamy Stock Photo, p. 212; Figure 7.2: Courtesy of Mary Griggs Burke Collection, Gift of the Mary and Jackson Burke Foundation, 2015. Metropolitan Museum of Art, p. 214; Figure 7.3: After M. I. Posner 1980. *Q J Exp Psychol* 32: 3–25, p. 215; Figure 7.4: After M. I. Posner 1980. *Q J Exp Psychol* 32: 3–25, p. 216; Figure 7.5: Courtesy of Philip Wolfe, p. 217; Figure 7.7: After J. T. Enns and R. A. Rensink. 1990. *Science* 247: 721–723, p. 219; Figure 7.9: Courtesy of Shai Gabay, Institute of Information Processing and Decision Making, Department of Psychology, University of Haifa, p. 221; Figure 7.10: After A. Reichenthal et al. 2020. *Atten Percept Psychophys* doi: 10.3758/s13414-019-01884-4, p. 222; Figure 7.11: © Sara Ryan/Alamy Stock Photo, p. 223; Figure 7.12: monkey puppet: © Hannah Gleghorn/Shutterstock.com, bowling ball: © Marusea Turcu/Dreamstime.com, figurine: © Rusu Ioana/Dreamstime.com, salt & pepper: © Tracy Decourcy/Dreamstime.com, monitor: © Aleks/Dreamstime.com, cooking oil: Courtesy of M. H. Siddall, binoculars: Courtesy of M. H. Siddall, cranes: Courtesy of M. H. Siddall, p. 223; Figure 7.13: kitchen: HamsterMan/Shutterstock.com, clown fish: Kitch Bain/Shutterstock.com, p. 224; Figure 7.16: After C. S. Green and D. Bavelier. 2003. *Nature* 423: 534–537, p. 227; Figure 7.18: From S. A. McMains and D. Somers. 2004. *Neuron* 42: 677–686, p. 229; Figure 7.19: © Sara Ryan/Alamy Stock Photo, p. 229; Figure 7.20: MRIs courtesy of Nancy Kanwisher, face: Courtesy of Jennifer Basil-Whitaker, house: Courtesy of Nancy and Marc Desrosiers., typewriter: Photo via Visualhunt, p. 230; Figure 7.21: left: From P. Downing, et al. 2001. *Neuropsychologia* 39:1329–1342. right: Courtesy of Jennifer Basil-Whitaker, p. 231; Figure 7.23: From T. Womelsdorf et al. 2006. *Nat Neurosci* 9: 1156–1160, p. 232; Figure 7.24: Images courtesy of Lynn Robertson and Krista Schendel, p. 233; Figure 7.27: After S. P. Tipper and M. Berhmann, 1996. *Exp Psychol Hum Percept Perform* 22: 1261–1278. Published by APA; reprinted with permission, p. 235; Figure 7.28: Courtesy of Jeremy and Philip Wolfe, p. 236; Figure 7.29A-C: After J. M. Wolfe et al. 2011. *Trends Cogn Sci* 15: 77–84, p. 237; Figure 7.29D: © HamsterMan/Shutterstock.com, p. 237; Figure 7.30: © CyberEak/Shutterstock.com, p. 238; Figure 7.31A-B: A: From T. F. Brady et al. 2017. *J Exp Psychol Hum Percept Perform* 43: 1160–1176. Published by APA, reprinted with permission, B: © iStock.com/kellyvandellen, p. 239; Figure 7.32: Courtesy of Aude Oliva, p. 240; Figure 7.33: bird: © iStock.com/webguzs, rice: © iStock.com/ibeirorocha, frog: © iStock.com/NajaShots, hiking boots: courtesy of M. H. Siddall, motorcycle: courtesy of M. H. Siddall, caterpillar: courtesy of M. H. Siddall, heron: Scott Bauer/USDA, rocket: NASA's Earth Observatory, sheep: USDA/ARS, camera: courtesy of M. H. Siddall, pinecone: courtesy of M. H. Siddall, scientists: Scott Bauer/USDA, shell: Courtesy of David McIntyre, stairway: Courtesy of Andrew D. Sinauer, strawberries: Kent Hammond/USDA, tractor: Jack Dykinga/USDA, p. 241; Figure 7.34: cacti: Courtesy of Andrew D. Sinauer, caterpillar: courtesy of M. H. Siddall, grain silos: Photosani/Shutterstock, flooded corn field: iStock.com/photosbyjim, hiking boots: courtesy of M. H. Siddall, lighthouse: courtesy of M. H. Siddall, motorcycle: courtesy of M. H. Siddall, pinecone: courtesy of M. H. Siddall, scientist-waders: courtesy of M. H. Siddall, castle: courtesy of M. H. Siddall, rabbit: Courtesy of David McIntyre, rocket: NASA, sheep: USDA, scientists: Scott Bauer/USDA, vegetables: Scott Bauer/USDA, heron: Scott Bauer/USDA, p. 242; Figure 7.35: Bylinskii, Z. (2015). Intrinsic and extrinsic effects on image memorability. *Vision Research*, V. 116, Part B: 165–178, p. 243; Figure 7.36A-B: Both images courtesy of David McIntyre, p. 243 Figure 7.37: Both images courtesy of David McIntyre, p. 244; Figure 7.38: © iStock.com/ivansmuk, p. 244; Figure 7.39A-B: A: © iStock.com/ivansmuk, B: © iStock.com/ivansmuk, p. 245; Figure 7.40: From T. Drew et al. 2013. *Psychological Sci* 24: 1848–1853, p. 246.

CHAPTER 8

[Ch 8 opener]Albert Beukhof/Shutterstock, p. 248; Figure 8.2: © David Robertson/Alamy Stock Photo, p. 250; Figure 8.4: From the Looney Tunes animation Yankee Doodle Daffy, p. 254; Figure 8.8: After D. Heeger. 2006. *Visual motion perception*. Lecture notes. New York University, Department of Psychology, p. 257; Figure 8.9: After W. T. Newsome and E. B. Paré. 1988. *J Neurosci* 8: 2201–2211, p. 257; Figure 8.12: After W. H. Warren Jr. and J. A. Saunders. 1995. *Perception* 24: 315–331, p. 260; Figure 8.13: © Rick Rycoft/Associated Press, p. 261; Figure 8.14A-B: A: © Neale Cousland/Shutterstock.com, B: After

R. H. Wurtz, 2008. *Vision Res* 48: 2070–2089, p. 262; Figure 8.17: From A. L. Yarbus, 1967. *Eye Movements and Vision.* New York: Plenum (now Springer). DOI 10.1007/978-1-4899-5379-7, p. 267; Figure 8.19: Courtesy of Andrew D. Sinauer, p. 269; Figure 8.20: After V. Nityananda et al. 2015. *J Comp Physiol A Neuroethol Sens Neural Behav Physiol* 201: 741–750/CC BY 4.0, p. 270

CHAPTER 9

[Ch 9 opener]Sounds Like Infinity © Micah Ofstedahl Arts, p. 272; Figure 9.7: human pinna: © iStock.com/PacoRomero, capybara: © John de la Bastide/Shutterstock.com, sea otter: © Menno Schaefer/Shutterstock.com, jackrabbit: © iStock.com/Heather Craig, bat ears: © iStock.com/GlobalP, elephant ear: Courtesy of Andrew D. Sinauer, fennec fox: © iStock.com/wrangel, p. 278; Figure 9.9b inset: Leonardo R. Andrade, Waitt Advanced Biophotonics Core BPHO., p. 280; Figure 9.11A: Courtesy of A. J. Hudspeth, p. 283; Figure 9.21: From J. F. Brugge and M. A. Howard. 2002. In *Encyclopedia of the Human Brain*, V. S. Ramachandran (Ed.), pp. 429–448. Academic Press: New York, p. 292; Figure 9.22: After Y. Suzuki and H. Takeshima. 2004. *J Acoust Soc Am* 116: 918–933, p. 293; Figure 9.23A-C: A: © iStock.com/NaluPhoto, B: After E. R. Gerstein. 2002. *Am Sci* 90: 154–156, C: After E. R. Gerstein. 2002. *Am Sci* 90: 154–156, p. 294; Figure 9.24B: B adapted from G. P. Schoonevelt and B. C. J. Moore. 1989. *J Acoust Soc Am* 85: 273–281; with the permission of the Acoustical Society of America, p. 296; Figure 9.25: From J. Wang and J-L Puel. 2020. *J Clin Med* 9: 218–240, p. 298; Figure 9.26A-B: A: Dutch National Archives/CC0 1.0, B: © Monika Wisniewska/Shutterstock.com, p. 299; Figure 9.27: After C. D. Geisler. 1998. *From Sound to Synapse: Physiology of the Mammalian Ear.* Oxford University Press: New York, with data from V. Pluvinage. 1994. In *Understanding Digitally Programmable Hearing Aids*, R. E. Sandlin (Ed.). Allyn & Bacon: Boston, MA and guidance from Professor Joshua M. Alexander, p. 299; Figure 9.28: All photos courtesy of Vijaya Prakash Krishnan Muthaiah, p. 301; Figure 9.29A: Courtesy of Cochlear®, p. 302.

CHAPTER 10

[Ch 10 opener]Courtesy of Studio Weave, www.studioweave.com, p. 304; Figure 10.3: Data from W. E. Fedderson et al. 1957. *J Acoust Soc Am* 29: 988–991, p. 307; Figure 10.6: Data from W. E. Fedderson et al. 1957. *J Acoust Soc Am* 29: 988–991, p. 310; Figure 10.7: B after F. Wightman and D. Kistler. 1998. *Nat Neurosci* 1: 337–339, p. 311; Figure 10.9: man's ear: © image100/Alamy Stock Photo, Rosemary Cole's ear: Courtesy of David McIntyre, David McIntyre's ear: Courtesy of David McIntyre, Alex Scudder's ear: Courtesy of David McIntyre, Richard Cole's ear: Courtesy of David McIntyre, Jennifer Basil's ear: Courtesy of David McIntyre, p. 312; Figure 10.10A-B: A from D. J. Kistler and F. L. Wightman. 1992. *J Acoust Soc Am* 91: 1637–1647, B from F. L. Wightman and D. J. Kistler, 1993. In *Springer Handbook of Auditory Research*, Vol. 3. W. A. Yost et al. (Eds.), pp. 155–192. Springer-Verlag: New York, p. 313; Figure 10.11A-C: A:© Great Pics-Ben Heine/Shutterstock.com, B: Alan Mothner/Associated Press, C:Atlaspix/Alamy Stock Photo, p. 315; Figure 10.14: From L. Thaler et al. 2011. *PLOS ONE* 6:e20162. CC BY, p. 318; Figure 10.15: After T. Kellner. 2014. *How Loud Is a Wind Turbine? GE Global Research and National Institute of Deafness and Other Communication Disorders.* Accessed via GE Reports archive: https://www.ge.com/news/reports/how-loud-is-a-wind-turbine, p. 319; Figure 10.16 inset: Courtesy of Jennifer Basil-Whitaker, p. 320; Figure 10.21E: Courtesy of Andrea Kluender, p. 324; Figure 10.25A-B: A from, B after, J. H. McDermott et al. 2011. *Proc Natl Acad Sci USA* 108: 1188–1193, p. 328; Figure 10.26: © Raymond Neil Farrimond/Shutterstock.com, p. 329; Figure 10.27: Courtesy of Rick L. Jenison and Richard A. Reale, p. 330; Figure 10.28: © Richard Saker/REX/Shutterstock.com.com, p. 331.

CHAPTER 11

[Ch 11 opener]Iryna Hramavataya / Alamy Stock Photo, p. 334; Figure 11.2: After Figure 5 in RCA Photophone, Inc. 1930. *Handbook for Projectionists*, 2nd ed. RCA Photophone, Inc.: New York. © 1927 National Association of Musical Instrument & Accessories Manufacturers, p. 337; Figure 11.5: From J. H. McDermott et al., 2016. *Nature* 535: 547–550, p. 339; Figure 11.8: Courtesy Library of Congress, p. 344; Figure 11.13: After H. Fletcher and R. H. Galt. 1950. *J Acoust Soc Am* 22: 89–151, p. 348; Figure 11.16A-B: A: Courtesy of Keith R. Kluender, B: Courtesy of David McIntyre, and Annie Huyler, Pioneer Valley Chinchillas, p. 351; Figure 11.17: After R. Campbell et al., 1997. *Proc R Soc Lond B Biol Sci* 264: 1429–1434. Monkey: © iStock.com/GlobalP, cow: © iStock.com/CreativeNature_nl, p. 351; Figure 11.20: After C. E. Stilp and K. R. Kluender. 2010. *Proc Natl Acad Sci USA* 107: 12387–12392, p. 354; Figure 11.21: Courtesy of Nancy Asai and Joanne Delphia, p. 356; Figure 11.22: After J. F. Werker and R. C. Tees. 1984. *Infant Behav Dev* 7: 49–63, p. 356; Figure 11.26: After S. Rosen et al., 2011. *PLOS ONE* 6: e24672, p. 360; Figure 11.27: After S. Rosen et al., 2011. *PLOS ONE* 6: e24672, p. 360.

CHAPTER 12

[Ch 12 opener]ILfoto/Shutterstock, p. 364; Figure 12.3A-B: A: © Reinhard Dirscherl/Minden Pictures, B: © Science Stock Photography/Science Source, p. 368; Figure 12.4: © David GABIS/Alamy Stock Photo, p. 370; Figure 12.14: After J. M. Goldberg and C. Fernandez. 1971. *J Neurophysiol* 34: 635–684, p. 370; Figure 12.15: After C. Fernandez and J. Goldberg. 1971. *J Neurophysiol* 34: 661–675, p. 371; Figure 12.16C: © MicroScan/Medical Images, p. 371; Figure 12.17: After J. M. Goldberg and C. Fernandez. 1976. *J Neurophysiol* 39: 970–1008, p. 372; Figure 12.18: After L. R. Young. 1984. In *Handbook of Physiology—The Nervous System*, I. Darian-Smith (Ed.), Vol. 3[2], pp. 1023–1066. American Physiological Society: Bethesda, MD, p. 385; Figure 12.19: After L. Grabherr et al. 2008. *Exp Brain Res* 186: 677–681, p. 387; Figure 12.20A-C: illustrations: After S. B. Bortolami et al. 2006. *Exp Brain Res* 173: 364–373, graphs: After S. B. Bortolami et al. 2006. *Exp Brain Res* 173: 364–373, p. 388; Figure 12.21: After L. R. Young et al. 1986. *Exp Brain Res* 64: 299–307, p. 391; Figure 12.22B-C: B, C after K. E. Cullen. 2011. *Curr Opin Neurobiol* 21: 587–595, p. 393; Figure 12.27: After B. Yates and A. Miller. 1998. *J Vestib Res* 8: 17–26, p. 398; Figure 12.28A: Courtesy of M. H. Siddall, p. 399; Figure 12.29A-B: A: After R. J. Peterka. 2002. *J Neurophysiol* 88: 1097–1118, B: After R. J. Peterka. 2002. *J Neurophysiol* 88: 1097–1118, p. 400; Figure 12.30: After F. Netter. 1983. *Nervous System: Anatomy and Physiology.* CIBA Pharmaceutical Company: West Caldwell, NJ, p. 401; Figure 12.31: Brain images from M. Dieterich and T. Brandt. 2008. *Brain* 131: 2538–2552; courtesy of Marianne Dieterich, p. 403; Figure 12.33: After M. C. Bermúdez Rey et al., 2016. *Front Neurol* 7: 162. CC BY 4.0, p. 405; Figure 12.34: © iStock.com/umdash9, p. 406.

CHAPTER 13

[Ch 13 opener]Abaporu 1928 Tarsila do Amaral. Museo de Arte Latinoamericano, Buenos Aires; Album / Alamy Stock Photo, p. 408; Figure 13.1: courtesy of M. H. Siddall, p. 410; Figure 13.2: After M. R. Rosenzweig et al. 2005. *Biological Psychology: An Introduction to Behavioral and Cognitive Neuroscience*, 4th ed. Sinauer Associates: Massachusetts, p. 411; Figure 13.3: After F. McGlone et al. 2014. *Neuron* 82: 737–755, p. 412; Figure 13.4: After A. Zimmerman et al. 2014. *Science* 346: 950–954, p. 414; Figure 13.5: E. Jarocka et al., *Journal of Neuroscience* 21 April 2021, 41 (16) 3622–3634. https://www.jneurosci.org/content/41/16/3622/tab-figures-data, p. 414; Figure 13.7: After A. C. Guyton. 1991. *Textbook of Medical Physiology*, 8th ed. Saunders: Philadelphia, p. 416; Figure 13.8: From R. Latorre et al., 2009. *Q Rev Biophys* 42: 210–246; after C. Ferrandiz-Huertas et al., 2014. *Membranes* 4: 525–564, p. 417; Figure 13.9: After A. J. Todd et al., 2010. *Nat Rev Neurosci* 11: 823–836, p. 419; Figure 13.10: After M W. Levine. 2000. *Levine & Shefner's Fundamentals of Sensation and Perception* (3rd ed.). Oxford University Press: Oxford, UK, p. 420; Figure 13.12B: B after W. Penfield and T. Rasmussen. 1950. *The Cerebral Cortex of Man: A Clinical Study of Localization of Function.* Macmillan: New York, p. 422; Figure 13.13: After S. M. Breedlove and N. V. Watson. 2023. *Behavioral Neuroscience* 10th ed. Oxford University Press. New York, p. 423; Figure 13.14A-B: A: After L. K. Case et al. 2016. *J Neurosci* 36: 5850–5860/CC BY 4.0, photo courtesy of M. H. Siddall, B: After L. K. Case et al. 2016. *J Neurosci* 36: 5850–5860/CC BY 4.0, p. 424; Figure 13.16: After V. S. Ramachandran. 1993. *Proc Natl Acad Sci USA* 90: 10413–10420. © 1993. National Academy of Sciences, U.S.A., p. 425; Figure 13.17B: photo: From J. A. George et al., 2019. *Science Robotics* 4: eaax2352, illustration: From J. A. George et al., 2019. *Sci Robot* 4: eaax2352, p. 426; Figure 13.18: After C. T. Fuentes et al. 2013. *Acta Psychol (Amst)* 144: 344–351/CC BY 3.0, p. 426; Figure 13.19: After E. Canzoneri et al., 2013. *Exp Brain Res* 228: 25–42, p. 427; Figure 13.20: After J. Löfvenberg and R. Johansson. 1984. *Brain Res* 301: 65–72, p. 428; Figure 13.22: After F. Mancini et al., 2014. *Ann Neurol* 75: 917–924, p. 429; Figure 13.23: After G. E. Legge et al., 2008. *Percept Psychophys* 70: 1471–1488, p. 431; Figure 13.24: illustration: After M. T. Fairhurst et al., 2014. *Psychol Sci* 25: 1124–1131, graph: After M. T. Fairhurst et al., 2014. *Psychol Sci* 25: 1124–1131, p. 433; Figure 13.25: McIntyre, S. et al. 2022. The language of social touch is intuitive and quantifiable. *Psychol Sci* 33(9): 1477–1494. Available through Open Access and Open Data, p. 434; Figure 13.26: After C. Peirs and R. P. Seal. 2016. *Science* 354: 578–584, p. 435; Figure 13.27: After Q. Ma. 2010. *J Clin Invest* 120: 3773–3778, p. 437; Figure 13.28A-B: A: Albina Gavrilovic/Shutterstock.com, B: Oleksii Synelnykov/Shutterstock.com, p. 439; Figure 13.29: From L. Nummenmaa. 2014. *Proc Natl Acad Sci* 111: 646-651, p. 440; Figure 13.30: After R. S. Johansson and G. Westling. 1984. *Exp Brain Res* 56: 550–564, p. 441; Figure 13.31: SA after Lederman, S. J. and Klatzky, R. L. (1987). Hand movements: A window into haptic object recognition. *Cogn Psychol* 19: 342–368, p. 442; Figure 13.32A: From A. O. Milne et al, 2021. *J Experimental Biology* 224, 224,jeb243085.doi:10.1242/jeb.243085, p. 443; Figure 13.33A-D: A, D after, and B, C from H. P. Saal et al., 2016. *Curr Opin Neurobiol* 40: 142–149, p. 444; Figure 13.34: After J. M. Loomis et al. (1991). Similarity of tactual and visual picture recognition with limited field of view. *Perception*, 20(2), 167–177, p. 445. Figure 13.35: After M. W. A. Wijntjes et al. 2009. *IEEE Trans Haptics* 2: 94–102, p. 446; Figure 13.36A-C: A after T. Moore et al. 1991. *Behav Res Methods Instrum Comput* 23: 27–35, B after S. J. Lederman and R. L. Klatzky. 1997. *J Exp Psychol Hum Percept Perform* 23: 1680–1707. Published by APA; reprinted with permission. C after M. A. Plaisier et al., 2009. *Atten Percept Psychophys* 71: 421–430, p. 447; Figure 13.37: After J. M. Loomis. 1990. *J Exp Psychol Hum Percept Perform* 16: 106–120. Published by APA; reprinted with permission, p. 447; Figure 13.38: After P. Haggard et al. 2000. *Percept Psychophys* 68: 363–377, p. 448; Figure 13.39A-B: A: From J. E. Leed et al. 2019. *Psychol Sci* 7: 1063–1073, B after J. E. Leed et al. 2019. *Psychol Sci* 7: 1063–1073, p. 449; Figure 13.40: After M. O. Ernst and M. S. Banks. 2002. *Nature* 415: 429–433, p. 450; Figure 13.41A-B: A: From S. N. Flesher et al. *Science* 2021 May 21; 372(6544): 831–836. doi:10.1126/science.abd0380, B: From S. N. Flesher et al. *Science* 2021 May 21; 372(6544): 831–836. doi:10.1126/science.abd0380, p. 451.

CHAPTER 14

[Ch 14 opener]© Stephen Hanson 2017 www.intheredpress.com, p. 454; Figure 14.04A-B: A: Courtesy of C. Balmer and A. LaMantia, B: After an illustration by Dr. Nicolas Thiebaud, p. 458; Figure 14.05: After J. Porter et al. 2007. *Nat Neurosci* 10: 27–29, p. 462; Figure 14.06: Adapted from Hamburger, K., & Knauff, M. (2011). SQUARELAND: A virtual environment for investigating cognitive processes in human wayfinding. *PsychNology Journal*, 9, 137–163. https://psycnet.apa.org/record/2012-04030-003, p. 463; Figure 14.07A-B: A from J. P. McGann. 2017. *Science* 356: 6338, B after, J. P. McGann. 2017. *Science* 356: 6338, p. 464; Figure 14.10: After Y. Niimura et al. 2014. *Genome Res* 9: 1485–1496, p. 468; Figure 14.11B: Sergei Kozak/Getty Images, p. 470; Figure 14.13A-B: A: © iStock.com/Savany, B: © suwat wongkham/123RF, p. 473; Figure 14.14: Pornsawan Baipakdee/Shutterstock, p. 473; Figure 14.17: photo: © Africa Studio/Shutterstock.com, graph: After A. Brunning. 2014. *Why Does Bacon Smell So Good?—The Aroma of Bacon.* Compound Interest: Cambridge, UK. Online: https://www.compoundchem.com/2014/04/16/why-does-bacon-smell-so-good-the-aroma-of-bacon/. Based on data from M. L. Timón et al. 2004. *J Sci Food Agric* 84: 825–831, p. 476; Figure 14.18: After A. Arshamian et al. 2018. *J Neurosci* 38:10286–10294/CC BY 4.0, p. 477; Figure 14.19: From T. Engen and B. M. Ross. 1973. *J Exp Psychol* 100: 221–227. Published by APA; reprinted with permission, p. 480; Figure 14.21: After R. L. Doty et al. 1984. *Science* 226: 1441–1443, p. 484; Figure 14.22: After K. Pospichalova. et al. 2016. *Funct Neurol* 31: 149–155, p. 485; Figure 14.23: Courtesy of David McIntyre, p. 488; Figure 14.25: Courtesy of David McIntyre, p. 493; Figure 14.26: Courtesy of Sveta Yamin-Pasternak, in memory of Mary-Ann Noongwook of Little Diomede and Savoonga, Alaska, p. 493; Figure 14.27A-B: A inset: Courtesy of Hey Paul, Flickr. Licensed under a Creative Commons Attribution 2.0 license, creativecommons.org/licenses/by/2.0/. Cropped from original., B: © John Bell/Shutterstock.com, p. 494; Figure 14.28: Adapted from De March, C. A., Matsunami, H., Abe, M., Cobb, M., & Hoover, K. C. (2023). Genetic and functional odorant receptor variation in the Homo lineage. *iScience*, 26, 105908. doi.org/10.1016/j.isci.2022.105908, p. 495; Figure 14.29: After an illustration by Dr. Michael Meredith; © Michael Meredith and Florida State University Program in Neuroscience, p. 497.

CHAPTER 15

[Ch 15 opener]© Illustration by Jing J - 2014, p. 506; Figure 15.2A-C: A: blanche/Shutterstock.com, B: Courtesy of Harry Klee, C: C after T. A. Colquhoun et al. 2015. *Chem Senses* 40: 622, p. 510; Figure 15.4: Courtesy of Linda Bartoshuk and the Bartoshuk Lab, p. 513; Figure 15.5A-C: A: E. G. Boring. 1942. *Sensation and Perception in the History of Experimental Psychology*. Appleton-Century-Crofts: New York. Data from D. Hänig. 1901. *Philosophische Studien* 17: 576–623. In the public domain., B: Hänig, David (1901). "Zur Psychophysik des Geschmackssinnes." *Philosophische Studien* 17: 576–623, C: Hoon, M. A., Adler, E., Lindemeier, J., Battey, J. F., Ryba, N. J., & Zuker, C. S. (1999). Putative mammalian taste receptors: A class of taste-specific GPCRs with distinct topographic selectivity. *Cell*, 96(4), 541–551, p. 514; Figure 15.6: Roper, S. D., & Chaudhari, N. (2017). Taste buds: Cells, signals and synapses. *Nature Reviews Neuroscience*, 18, 485–497, p. 514; Figure 15.8: Chaudhari, N., & Roper, S. D. (2010). The cell biology of taste. *The Journal of Cell Biology*, 190(3), 285–296, p. 518; Figure 15.9: (1) Roper, SD (2020) Fig. 9 from *Microphysiology of Taste Buds*. In: B Meyerhof, Ed; Vol. 3, *Olfaction and Taste; The Senses: A Comprehensive Reference*; 2nd Edition; Editor-in-Chief Bernd Fritzsch, Elsevier, in press (doi.org/10.1016/B978-0-12-805408-6.24152-3). (2) A. Laffitte et al. L., 2014. Functional roles of the sweet taste receptor in oral and extraoral tissues. *Current Opinion in Clinical Nutrition and Metabolic Care*, 17(4), p. 379. Data sources: Sucrose, glucose, sucralose (Y. Nie et al. *Curr Biol* 15: 1948–1952); Aspartame, neotame (H. Xu et al. *Proc Natl Acad Sci* 101: 14258–14263); Neoculin (A. Koizumi et al. *Biochem Biophys Res Commun* 358: 585–589); Cyclamate (P. Jiang et al. *J Biol Chem* 280: 34296e34305 and H. Xu et al. 2004. *Proc Natl Acad Sci USA* 101: 14258e14263); Neohesperidin (M. Winnig et al. 2007. *BMC Struct Biol* 7: 66); Lactisole (P. Jiang et al. 2005. J Biol Chem 280: 15238e15246 and H. Xu et al. 2004. *Proc Natl Acad Sci USA* 101: 14258e14263); Saccharin, inhibitor @ high conc (V. Galindo-Cuspinera et al. 2006. *Nature* 441: 354); Brazzein (F. M. Assadi-Porter et al. 2010. *J Mol Biol* 398: 584–599 and P. Jiang et al. 2004. *J Biol Chem* 279: 45068e45075); S819 (S. K. Kim et al. 2017. *Proc Natl Acad Sci* 114: 2568–2573). p. 520; Figure 15.10: Bartoshuk, L. M. (1975). Taste mixtures: Is mixture suppression related to compression? *Physiology & Behavior*, 14(5), 643-649, p. 524; Figure 15.11A-B: A: Mcimage/Shutterstock.com, B: vitmark/Shutterstock.com, p. 528; Figure 15.12: Courtesy of David McIntyre, p. 529; Figure 15.13: Courtesy of David McIntyre, p. 533.

Index

A

A-alpha fibers, 411
Abaporu (Amaral), 408*f*
abducens (VI) nerves, 19*f*, 20, 395*f*
A-beta fibers, 411–412, 415, 418–419, 435
absolute disparity, 19*f*, 183, 194
absolute metrical depth cue, 175, 181
absolute pitch (AP), 339–340
absolute threshold
  hearing and, 293
  sensory neuroscience and, 5*t*, 7–9, 16, 31
  vision and, 44*f*
absorption
  color and, 132, 133*f*, 136, 138, 162*f*, 165
  hearing and, 297, 316
  object recognition and, 103, 104*f*
  taste and, 515
  vision and, 33–38, 43, 45, 48, 54
acceleration
  angular, 369–370, 374, 386, 387*f*
  linear, 369–370, 374, 382–384, 386, 406–407
  sensory integration and, 21
  velocity as integral of, 21
  vestibular sensation and, 369–370, 374, 376, 380–387, 390, 406–407
accessory olfactory bulb (AOB), 497, 504
accidental tourist, 113*f*
accidental viewpoint
  object recognition and, 112–118
  space perception and, 172, 199
accommodation
  space perception and, 180–181, 188, 211
  vision and, 36–39
achromatopsia, 152
acoustic reflex, 279
acoustic startle reflex, 330
acquired anosmia, 461–462
action for perception, 441–444
active sensing, 368, 392
acuity
  attention and, 213
  color and, 152
  olfaction and, 469, 484–486
  space perception and, 192, 195, 206, 208
  touch and, 415, 427, 429–432, 447–448, 452
  vestibular sensation and, 394*f*
  vision and, 40, 43, 44*f*, 49*t*, 50, 53–54, 58–67, 71–74, 87*f*, 88–90, 152
  visual motion perception and, 263, 266
adaptation
  color and, 155–157
  light/dark, 44–46, 49*f*
  olfaction and, 478–490, 495*f*, 504
  selective, 80–86, 91
  Snellen test and, 62
  space perception and, 209
  taste and, 532
  vestibular sensation and, 404, 412–413, 442
  vision and, 44–46, 49*f*, 62, 65, 66*f*, 80–86, 91, 155–157
  visual motion perception and, 251–252
adapting stimulus, 80–82, 155
Addams, Robert, 250
additive color mixture, 138, 139*f*, 165
A-delta fibers, 411, 413*f*, 415–417
aerial perspective, 175
affective touch
  emotion and, 4, 410, 427, 432–434, 452
  tickling and, 438
afferent fibers, 284, 392
afferent signals, 368, 386, 392, 393*f*
afterimages, 155–156
age-related macular degeneration, 46, 55
agnosia
  object recognition and, 98, 127–128, 152
  olfaction and, 472, 480
  tactile, 422
  touch and, 422
akinetopsia, 258
Alberti, Leon Battista, 176
altered tuning, 231
amacrine cells
  vision and, 35*f*, 40–41, 47–50, 53
  visual motion perception and, 253
Amaral, Tarsila do, 408*f*
ambiguous figures, 112
amblyopia, 62, 88, 192, 210
American Association for the Advancement of Science, 523
Ames Room, 201–202
Amoore, John, 470
amplitude
  coding of, 283–284
  hearing and, 274–277, 283, 285*f*, 288–289, 292–293, 295, 302, 305, 320–322, 323*f*-324*f*
  intensity and, 274–275, 292, 295, 302, 346*f*
  music and, 345*f*, 346
  otolith organs and, 382–384
  semicircular canals and, 378–379
  speech perception and, 359–360
  striolae and, 382
  touch and, 428*f*
  vestibular sensation and, 370–371, 376, 378–382, 395–400, 407
  vision and, 37*f*, 48, 66–67
ampulla, 376, 377*f*, 379*f*
amygdala-hippocampal complex, 466, 494
analgesia, 436, 438
anamorphosis, 178–180
anchor objects, 224
angular acceleration, 369–370, 374, 386, 387*f*
angular motion
  modalities of, 369–373
  sensing, 369–370
  spatial orientation and, 365, 369–373, 376, 377*f*, 400, 407
anisometropia, 88–89
anosmia
  acquired, 461–462
  congenital, 461–462
  COVID-19 and, xxvi, 461
  dysfunctional effects of, 460
  olfaction and, 459–462, 472–473, 478–479, 483, 490, 503, 537–538, 540, 552
  as smell blindness, 459
  specific, 472–473, 478, 483
anterior cingulate cortex (ACC), 423, 424*f*, 435–438, 489
aperture, 36, 253–257, 271
aperture problem, 255–257, 271
apparent motion, 180, 244, 253, 254*f*, 259
aqueous humor, 35*f*, 36–38
Architectural View (Giorgio Martini), 176, 177*f*
Aristotle, 365–366, 507–508, 517
aromatherapy, 455, 496, 500–501, 504
articulation
  classifying sounds and, 346–348
  coarticulation and, 349, 352–353, 357, 362
  invariance and, 349, 353
  manner of, 347–348
  place of, 347
  spectral contrast and, 352–353
  speech perception and, 344–349, 352–353, 357, 361–362
  voicing and, 348
artificial neural networks, 29–30, 123
astigmatism, 38–39
attack, 321–322, 323*f*, 332

attention
acuity and, 213
altered tuning and, 231
anchor objects and, 224
apparent motion and, 244
Balint syndrome and, 236
Bayesian models and, 225
binding problem and, 225–226, 232
blindness and, 233, 243–247
cerebral cortex and, 230
change blindness and, 243–247
color and, 151, 159, 164
contralesional field and, 234–235
covert, 214–215
COVID-19 and, 526
cues and, 215–217, 229
disorders of, 233–236
distractors and, 218–222, 246
efficiency and, 218–223, 235, 246–247
ensemble statistics and, 238–239, 244–247
extinction and, 233–236
extrastriate cortex and, 93, 101
feature integration theory and, 225
feature searches and, 218–220, 223, 235
feedback and, 229
fovea and, 229*f*, 245
frequency and, 239, 240*f*
frontal eye fields and, 230
functional magnetic resonance imaging (fMRI) and, 229–230
fusiform face area (FFA) and, 230, 233
gist and, 237*f*, 238–240, 244, 245*f*, 247
guided search and, 220–222, 225, 230
hearing and, 305, 328, 330–333
hippocampus and, 230, 233
illusory conjunctions and, 226
inattentional blindness and, 245, 247, 479
inhibition of return and, 217
ipsilesional field and, 235
lateral interparietal area and, 230
lenses and, 217
lesions and, 233–237, 247
magnetic resonance imaging (MRI) and, 229–230, 233*f*
masking and, 238
memory and, 228, 233, 240–247
music and, 340, 343
neglect and, 233–237, 247
neural communication and, 232–233
neural enhancement and, 29
nonselective processing and, 217, 237–238, 244, 247
object recognition and, 96, 101
olfaction and, 460–461, 475, 479, 484, 489
overload and, 213
overt, 214
parahippocampal place area (PPA) and, 97, 230, 233
parallel search and, 219
parietal lobe and, 230, 233, 234*f*, 236, 247
peripersonal space and, 237
physiological basis of, 228–233
Posner on, 215–217, 229
preattentive stage and, 225
primary visual cortex (V1) and, 233
primes and, 223
priority map and, 229*f*, 230
proto-objects and, 238, 247
rapid serial visual presentation (RSVP) and, 226–228
rate-intensity functions and, 288
rate saturation and, 288
reachspace and, 236–237
reaction time (RT) and, 216, 218*f*, 246
receptive field and, 232, 247
retina and, 213, 237*f*, 245
saccades and, 217, 244
salience and, 216, 219
satisfaction of search and, 225–226
scene-based guidance and, 224
scene grammar and, 224
scene semantics and, 224
scene syntax and, 224
selective, 215, 217, 225, 230, 235, 237*f*-238*f*
sensitivity and, 232
serial-self-terminating search and, 220
set size and, 218–219
sharper tuning and, 230–232
similarity and, 221
sine waves and, 240
single cells and, 230–232
in space, 215–217
spatial frequency and, 239–240
speech perception and, 347
spotlight of, 217, 246
stimulus enhancement and, 229–230
stimulus onset asynchrony (SOA) and, 216
striate cortex and, 233, 249
suppression and, 217, 232
symmetry and, 221
targets and, 215*f*, 216–228, 246–247
taste and, 530
tilt and, 225, 238
in time, 226–228
touch and, 431, 434*f*, 446, 453
two pathways to, 237
use of term, 214
vestibular sensation and, 366–369
vision and, 37, 89
visual motion perception and, 251, 261, 266–269
visual search and, 217–227, 235, 246–247
waivers and, 8
attentional blink (AB), 226–228, 247
attention deficit hyperactivity disorder (ADHD), 235, 461
Aubert, Hermann Rudolf, 72, 387
audibility threshold, 293
auditory nerve (AN)
hearing and, 19*f*, 278*f*, 280*f*, 281, 283*f*, 284–290, 297, 301*f*, 302–303, 308, 320, 374*f*, 419
touch and, 419
vestibular sensation and, 374*f*
auditory scene analysis
acoustic environment and, 322–328
hearing and, 305, 322–328, 333
sound onsets and, 323*f*, 326, 327*f*, 332
auditory stream segregation, 324–325, 331, 333
auditory system. *See* hearing
autism spectrum, 432, 461
autonomic nervous system, 396–397, 410
azimuth, 307, 311*f*, 313–314, 332

B

Bach-y-Rita, P., 46
balance
hearing and, 280, 333
motor cortex and, 20*f*
vestibular sensation and, 19*f*, 365–368, 386, 392–393, 398–400, 401*f*, 404–407
vision and, 48
visual motion perception and, 250–251
balance system, 393, 398–400
Balint syndrome, 236
Banks, M. S., 181, 450
Barlow, Horace, 96
Barry, Susan, 189
basal cells, 457, 459
basic color terms, 148–150
basic tastes
bitterness, 5, 12, 13*f*, 343, 512–528, 531, 534–535
music and, 343
number of, 517–523, 527–528, 531, 534–535
saltiness, 5, 343, 513–518, 524, 527–535
sourness, 5, 343, 509, 513–519, 524, 527–528, 531–534
sweetness, 5, 343, 507–535
basilar membrane
hearing and, 280–286, 289, 291–292, 295–296, 305, 309
speech perception and, 354
Bayesian models
attention and, 225
color and, 159
computational models and, 5*t*
context and, 30
maximum-likelihood and, 29
object recognition and, 117–118, 128
pixel predictability and, 28*f*
space perception and, 199, 204
vision and, 159
Baylor, D. A., 137
Behrmann, Marlene, 234
belt area, 292, 326, 359
Bentham, Jeremy, 526–527
Beukhof, Albert, 248*f*
bifocal lenses, 37
binaral rivalry, 192, 475–476, 503
binding problem, 225–226, 232
binocular depth cue, 171, 211
binocular disparity
hearing and, 314
space perception and, 170, 182, 184–190, 195–198, 200, 206–207, 211
visual motion perception and, 262

binocular rivalry
color and, 147
olfaction and, 475–476
space perception and, 187*f*, 202–205, 210–211
vision and, 7, 147, 187*f*, 202–205, 210–211, 475–476
binocular summation, 170, 211
binocular vision
abnormal visual experience and, 208–210
absolute disparity and, 183
correspondence problem and, 192–194
corresponding retinal points and, 183–184
crossed disparity and, 184
development of, 205–210
diplopia and, 184
esotropia and, 209–210
fovea and, 180–188, 193, 209–210
horopter and, 184
monocular cues and, 171–178
Panum's fusional area and, 184
relative disparity and, 183
retina and, 167–175, 180–188, 192–199, 202, 204, 210–211
stereograms and, 187–193, 194*f*, 196*f*, 206*f*, 211
stereopsis and, 170–171, 178–198, 182–198, 205–211
suppression and, 202–205
triangulation cues and, 178–182
uncrossed disparity and, 184
use of term, 170
Vieth-Müller circle and, 184
biological motion, 262–263, 270
biomemetic feedback, 425
bipolar cells
convergence and, 49–50
divergence and, 49–50
vision and, 35*f*, 40, 43*t*, 47–53
bitterness
genetic variation of, 523–526
music and, 343
receptor cells and, 512
taste and, 5, 12, 13*f*, 343, 512–528, 531, 534–535
tasters and, 523–526
tongue map and, 513–515
Blakeslee, Albert, 523
blindness
attention and, 233, 243–247
Braille and, 413, 424, 431, 447–448
change, 243–247
color, 134, 151–152, 165, 472–473
hearing and, 317
light and, 35*f*, 39–40, 43, 46, 47*f*, 55
object recognition and, 101, 103*f*, 128
olfaction and, 459–460, 463, 472, 479, 484–485
sensory neuroscience and, 4
sensory substitution and, 46
space perception and, 188–190, 205–209
spatial vision and, 68*f*, 71, 88, 90
stereo, 188–190, 206, 209
taste and, 519
touch and, 409–410, 424, 426, 431, 450
vestibular sensation and, 367, 389, 404
visual motion perception and, 256, 263, 266–268
blind spot, 35*f*, 39–40
Bloch's law, 17
blood oxygen level-dependent (BOLD) signal, 27, 70, 72
blood pressure, 393, 397–398, 501
body image, 426–427
Bolivia, 339
Borda, Adrian, 181–182
border ownership, 94, 96*f*, 118–119, 196
bottom-up processes, 435
Braille, 413, 424, 431, 447–448
Bridgeman, Bruce, 189

C

cameras
hearing and, 314
object recognition and, 103, 113
space perception and, 173*f*, 180, 187–188, 191
vision and, 36, 39, 46, 52, 57, 60
Cameron, Joanne, 437
camouflage, 111*f*, 190, 260, 263
Campbell, Fergus, 64
cancer
attention and, 246
detecting, 6, 13–14, 16, 26*f*, 30–31
mammograms and, 6, 13, 125
music and, 336
object recognition and, 125
space perception and, 170
taste and, 517, 519, 521, 523, 525, 533, 535
X-rays and, xvi, 6, 13, 26*f*, 30
capsaicin, 532–533
Carroll, Lewis, 58
cataracts, 38, 88, 271
categorical perception, 349–352, 363
Caval-Holme, Franklin, 53
Census at Bethlehem (Reboredo), 212*f*
cerebral cortex
attention and, 230
hearing and, 291–292, 305
object recognition and, 96
olfaction and, 516
sensory neuroscience and, 20, 31
speech perception and, 358
touch and, 420*f*
vision and, 57, 70, 90
C fiber, 411, 418
Chang, E. F., 361
change blindness, 243–247
characteristic frequency (CF), 286–288, 396
chemosignals, 497–502, 505
chili peppers, 532–533
Chinese restaurant syndrome, 522
chorda tympani, 509, 512*f*, 515–516, 526, 531
chords
harmony and, 339
music and, 336, 338–340, 343, 362, 475*f*
pleasant, 336
chromophore, 48
cilia
hearing and, 280–283, 288–289, 302
olfaction and, 457*f*, 458–459, 465, 470*f*
space perception and, 188
taste and, 515
vestibular sensation and, 368*f*, 374–376, 377*f*, 379*f*, 382, 383*f*
vision and, 20, 35*f*, 36–37
circumvallate papillae, 512*f*, 513, 534
Clarity II (Jasinski), 166*f*
CMYK colors, 143
coarticulation, 349, 352–353, 357, 362
CO blobs, 79–80
cochlea, 19*f*, 20
AN fibers and, 286
coding of, 283–284
frequency and, 283–291, 297, 309*f*
hair cells and, 281–289, 297, 301, 303, 323, 419
left, 308*f*-309*f*, 310
localization and, 308*f*
organ of Corti and, 279–284
right, 308*f*-309*f*, 310
stapes and, 278*f*
tectorial membrane and, 281
tickling, 354
touch and, 419
unrolling of, 284, 285*f*
vestibular sensation and, 365–366, 374
cochlear canals, 279–281
cochlear implants, 301, 302*f*, 362
cochlear membrane, 279–281, 309
cochlear nucleus, 290–291, 308, 320
cochlear partition, 279–287, 297
cognitive habituation, 489, 504
cold fibers, 20, 415–417
color
absolute threshold and, 44*f*
absorption and, 132, 133*f*, 136, 138, 162*f*, 165
achromatopsi and, 152
acuity and, 152
adaptation and, 155–157
additive color mixture and, 138, 139*f*, 165
afterimages and, 155–156
appearance and, 141–147
attention and, 151, 159, 164
basic color terms and, 148–150
basic perception principles of, 131–132
Bayesian models and, 159
binocular rivalry and, 147
CMYK, 143
cones and, 132–143, 146–147, 151–152
cultural relativism and, 148
detection of, 132–133
deuteranopes and, 151
discrimination of, 133–140
The Dress and, 141
eccentricity and, 162
emotion and, 152–153
filters and, 138, 152, 159, 163–165
flavor and, 161
fovea and, 140, 152

frequency and, 148, 193–194, 207–208, 211
functional magnetic resonance imaging (fMRI) and, 147
ganglion cells and, 139
genetic differences in vision and, 151–152
HSB, 142–144
hue and, 137, 142–147, 155*f*, 164, 482
human range of, 131–132
illuminants and, 154, 157–159, 165
importance of seeing, 159–164
individual differences in perceiving, 147–153
language and, 147–153
lateral geniculate nucleus (LGN) and, 139–140
lesions and, 152
magnetic resonance imaging (MRI) and, 147
memory and, 150
metamers and, 135–138, 141, 151, 165, 474
negative afterimage and, 155–157
neutral point, 145*f*
opponent color theory and, 144–146, 151, 154, 156, 165
parvocellular layer and, 140
photons and, 153, 162
photopic illumination and, 132–133
photoreceptors and, 132–134, 137, 141, 151–152, 154, 161–165
picking, 142–143
primary visual cortex (V1) and, 152
principle of univariance and, 133–134
protanopes and, 152
proximity and, 154
qualia and, 151, 153
rainbows and, 33, 143–144
receptive field and, 93–97, 102, 103*f*, 139–140
related, 154–155
retina and, 133*f*, 137–141, 152, 155–156
RGB, 127, 142
rhodopsin and, 134
rods and, 132–134, 152, 162, 165
scotopic illumination and, 132–134, 165
sensitivity and, 132–134, 146*f*, 155, 157*f*, 162*f*, 163, 165
spectral power distribution and, 158
spectral reflectance function and, 158
spectral sensitivity and, 132, 163*f*
spectrum and, 131–132, 136*f*, 137, 141–144, 162*f*
subtractive color mixture and, 138, 165
synesthesia and, 152–153
targets and, 154, 164
tetrachromatic, 151, 162
transduction and, 134*f*
transmission and, 129, 138*f*
trichromacy and, 49*f*, 134–137, 143–144, 151, 160–161
tritanopes and, 152
unrelated, 154–155
visual acuity and, 89
visual cortex and, 146–147
wavelength and, 131–147, 151–159, 162*f*, 163–165
world of, 153–159
color assimilation, 154, 155*f*
color-blindness, 134, 151–152, 165, 472–473
color constancy, 154, 157–159, 165
color contrast, 154–155
color space, 141–143, 146–152
columns, 77–80, 91
common fate, 326
comparator, 261, 267–269
complex cells, 75–77, 123
computational models, 5*t*, 7, 27–31
Condillac, Étienne Bonnot de, 4
conductive hearing loss, 297
cone monochromat, 152
cone-opponent cells, 139–141, 146*f*, 165
cones, 288–289, 323
color and, 132–143, 146–147, 151–152
difference from rods, 43
energy use of, 43–44
L-cones, 48–49, 132, 135–140, 146, 151–152, 155, 157*f*, 163, 165
light and, 35*f*, 40–54
M-cones, 49, 132–140, 143, 146, 151–152, 160–161, 165
photoactivation and, 48
photopigment regeneration and, 45
protanopes and, 152
S-cones, 48, 51, 69, 132, 135–136, 139–140, 143, 151–152, 155, 158, 160
space perception and, 195
spatial vision and, 57–65, 69, 89–90
transduction and, 47–49
cones of confusion, 310–311, 312*f*
congenital anosmia, 461–462
congenital prosoaganosia, 128
conjunction search, 218*f*, 222–223, 225
connectionist models, 29
consonants
language and, 347–357, 361–362
learning words and, 357
native listeners and, 355–357
speech production and, 347–357, 361–362
contact lenses, 300
continuity constraint, 193–194
contralateral area, 70, 291, 308*f*, 310
contralesional field, 234–235
contrast
space perception and, 203, 207
speech perception and, 350, 352–353
touch and, 410
vision and, 39*f*, 46, 49–54, 58–60, 63–66, 74, 76, 82–85, 89–90
visual motion perception and, 258, 270–271
contrast-defined objects, 64, 258
contrast-sensitivity function (CSF), 64–65, 66*f*, 83*f*, 84, 89*f*
contrast threshold, 64, 65*f*, 83, 84*f*
convergence
bipolar cells and, 49–50
space perception and, 171, 178, 180–184, 188, 194, 206–207, 211
vestibular sensation and, 401–402, 430
vision and, 43*f*, 49–54
visual motion perception and, 266
cornea
astigmatism and, 38–39
image formation and, 35–39
light and, 35–39, 54
as protective barrier, 466
singe-photon sensitivity and, 54
vision and, 35–39, 54, 57, 466, 470*f*
corollary discharge signal, 268–269, 392, 393*f*
correspondence problem
space perception and, 192–194, 211
visual motion perception and, 253–255
corresponding retinal points, 183–184, 195, 202
cortical magnification, 71–73, 79, 422
COVID-19
anosmia and, xxvi, 461
conspiracy theories on, 109
olfaction and, 458, 460–461, 486, 491, 503
SARS-CoV-2 virus and, 458
taste and, 526
cranial nerves
abducens (VI) nerves, 19*f*, 20, 395*f*
chorda tympani, 509, 512*f*, 515, 526, 531, 540
facial nerves, 509, 512*f*, 515
forebrain and, 459
glossopharyngeal (IX) nerves, 19*f*, 20, 512*f*, 516, 526
gustatory experiences and, 417, 455
hearing and, 290
hyperglosal (XII) nerves, 19*f*
number of, 19–20
oculumotor (III) nerves, 20, 395*f*, 547
olfactory (I) nerves, 20, 417, 455, 459, 462, 464, 465*f*, 469–470, 496, 497*f*, 500, 503, 512, 530
optic (II) nerves, 18–19, 35*f*, 36, 39–40, 51, 54, 58*f*, 72, 418–419
spinal (XI) nerves, 19*f*
structure of, 19–20, 31
taste (VII) and, 507, 509, 512, 515–517, 525
trigeminal (V) nerves, 20, 455, 462, 469, 470*f*, 503, 509, 530
trochlear (IV) nerves, 19*f*, 20, 395*f*
vagus (X) nerves, 19*f*, 20, 416, 439–440, 512*f*
vestibular sensation and, 365, 374*f*, 395*f*
vestibulocochlear (VIII) nerves, 19*f*, 20, 290, 374*f*
cribriform plate, 20, 457*f*, 459, 464, 465*f*
cristae, 376, 377*f*, 464*f*
criterion
decision, 5*t*
response, 14*f*, 15–16, 428
signal detection theory and, 12
touch and, 428
critical bandwidth, 296
critical period, 88–89, 189, 208–211
cross-adaptation, 487–488, 532
crossed disparity, 185, 186*f*

cross-modality matching, 12, 13*f*, 524–525
C tactile (CT) afferent, 412*f*, 418, 432–433
cues
attention and, 215–217, 229
color and, 164
combining, 198–205
depth, 171–180, 195, 198–205
endogeneous, 216–217
exogenous, 216
head, 311–314
hearing and, 306, 309–317, 326, 349, 352–353, 361
illusions and, 200–202
McGurk effect and, 361, 390
metrical depth, 172, 175–176, 195
monocular, 88, 167, 170–178, 183, 188–193, 207–208, 211
multiple acoustic, 353
music and, 335–343
object recognition and, 104, 108*f*
olfaction and, 460, 463, 476, 484, 486, 498–501, 504
pictorial depth, 171, 178
Posner cueing diagram and, 215–217, 229
relative metrical depth, 175, 180
space perception and, 167, 170–208, 211
speech perception and, 343–364
taste and, 509, 529–533
touch and, 434*f*, 443*f*, 446
triangulation, 178–182
vestibular sensation and, 370, 385, 389–392, 398*f*-399*f*
visual, 62, 86
visual motion perception and, 249, 262–263
cultural relativism, 148
Cutting, James, 263
cycles
feedback, 29
hearing and, 274, 289*f*, 290
olfaction and, 477, 498–499
touch and, 413*t*
tuning curves and, 23
vestibular sensation and, 380–381, 386–387
vision and, 59–66, 75, 83, 84*f*, 87*f*, 89*f*
visual motion perception and, 270*f*
cycles per degree, 59, 64, 66
Cyclopean stimuli, 190

D

Dani of New Guinea, 148–150
Dayna, Dennis, 523
decay
hearing and, 321–322, 332
vestibular sensation and, 379–380, 385
decibel (dB) units
hearing and, 275, 288, 292–293, 316, 319*f*, 346
neural threshold and, 23
sound pressure and, 10
speech perception and, 346
taste and, 524
vibratory touch and, 428*f*
decoding, 120, 124
deep neural networks (DNNs), 30, 123–129
dermis, 411, 412*f*, 414
deuteranopes, 151
dichoptic stimuli, 187, 207
Dickinson, Emily, 336
difference threshold, 5*f*, 9, 10*f*, 31, 150
diffuse bipolar cells, 49–50, 53
diopter units, 36–37
diplopia, 184, 186*f*, 188, 210
direction
Cartesian coordinates and, 371–373
otolith organs and, 384
pitch angular velocity and, 372
roll angular velocity and, 372
semicircular canals and, 379
spatial orientation and, 379–396, 402, 405, 407
vestibular sensation and, 370–396, 402, 405, 407
directional transfer function (DTF), 313*f*, 314
discriminative touch, 409–410, 427, 434, 435*f*, 440, 452
distractors
attention and, 218–222, 246
hearing and, 328*f*
touch and, 442, 446, 447*f*
divergence
bipolar cells and, 49–50
space perception and, 180*f*, 181, 188
vestibular sensation and, 406
vision and, 49–50
visual motion perception and, 266
dizziness
Ménières syndrome and, 405–407
vestibular sensation and, 365–368, 386, 405–406
doctrine of specific nerve energies, 18, 20, 31
dorsal column-medial lemniscal (DCML) pathway, 420, 452
dorsal horn, 419–420, 435–438, 452
double dissociation, 259
Dress, The, 141
Duffy, Valerie, 525–527
duplex retinas, 41, 44–45

E

ear canal
auditory nerve and, 284–290
hearing and, 277–284, 293, 297, 299, 311, 314, 332
inner ear, 279–284
middle ear, 277–279
outer ear, 277
eccentricity
color and, 162
vision and, 40–41, 42*f*, 50, 53, 71–72, 73*f*
visual motion perception and, 263
efference copy, 268–269, 392, 393*f*
efferent commands, 368, 392
efferent fibers, 284
efficiency
attention and, 218–223, 235, 246–247
feature searches and, 219
hearing and, 311
method of limits and, 9
olfaction and, 485, 487
reaction time (RT) and, 218
touch and, 417, 442, 445–449
vision and, 43, 85
visual motion perception and, 263
visual search and, 219–220
efficient coding models, 29
egocenter, 448
electroencephalography (EEG)
olfaction and, 490, 499–501
speech perception and, 352
touch and, 423, 433
uses of, 24, 25*f*, 27, 31
electromotility, 286–287
emmetropia, 38
emotion
acoustic startle reflex and, 330
affective touch and, 4, 410, 427, 432–434
associative learning and, 495–496
color and, 152–153
language and, 474
music and, 152–153, 335–336
olfaction and, 455, 460, 462, 466, 474, 480, 484, 489–492, 495–504
tonotopic organization and, 440*f*
topographical mapping and, 440*f*
touch and, 409–410, 417–418, 423, 427, 433–437, 440, 452
vestibular sensation and, 386
endogeneous cues, 216–217
endogenous opiates, 436
end stopping, 76, 77*f*
Enroth-Cugell, Christina, 68
ensemble statistics, 238–239, 244–247
entorhinal cortex, 466
entry-level category, 125
epidermis, 411–415
epilepsy, 97, 330*f*, 360, 421
equal-loudness curve, 293
Escher, M. C., 171
esotropia, 209–210
event-related potentials (ERPs), 24
exogenous cues, 216
exotropia, 209
exploratory procedure, 441–445, 450, 453
extinction, 233–236
extrastriate body area (EBA), 97, 120
extrastriate cortex, 93, 101
eye movements. *See* saccades

F

FAAH gene, 437
facial recognition, 30, 126–128
facial (VII) nerves, 20, 509, 512*f*, 515
Fall Leaves (Wolfe), 130*f*
familiar size, 174–175, 199
Fantz, Robert, 86–87
feature integration theory, 225
feature searches, 218–220, 223, 235

Fechner, Gustav, 7, 9–13, 28, 31
feedback
  artificial neural networks and, 29–30, 123
  attention and, 229
  hearing and, 291, 314
  object recognition and, 95*f*, 101
  sensory neuroscience and, 29–30
  space perception and, 192
  taste and, 515
  touch and, 420, 425–426, 437, 450–452
  vestibular sensation and, 402
  vision and, 70, 77
feed-forward process, 70, 95*f*, 101
Feller, Marla, 53
figure-ground assignment, 114, 128
filiform papillae, 512, 534
filters
  color and, 138, 152, 159, 163–165
  hearing and, 303, 310, 313
  olfaction and, 456, 487
  space perception and, 194*f*
  speech perception and, 345, 355
  vision and, 52–53, 68–69, 75, 80, 85
  visual motion perception and, 253, 271
finger paints, 138
first-order motion, 258–259, 271
Fischer, Roland, 523
Fixing My Gaze (Barry), 189
flavor
  amacrine cells and, 49
  color and, 161
  olfaction and, 455, 460, 467, 469, 476, 492–495
  sensory neuroscience and, 6
  simple cells and, 75*f*
  taste and, 507–511, 517, 522, 525–530, 534
focal distance, 36–37
focus of expansion, 206
foliate papillae, 512*f*, 513, 534
formants, 345–353
Fourier analysis
  hearing and, 275
  sine waves and, 66–67, 275, 382
  vestibular sensation and, 380, 382
  vision and, 35*f*, 39*f*, 40–43, 48–50, 54, 61–63, 66, 67*f*, 71–73, 79, 85, 89
fovea
  attention and, 229*f*, 245
  color and, 140, 152
  space perception and, 180–188, 193, 209–210
  vision and, 35*f*, 39*f*, 40–43, 48–50, 54, 61–63, 71–73, 79, 89, 180–188, 193, 209–210, 306, 422
  visual motion perception and, 263, 266–267, 269
Fox, A. L., 523
frame of reference, 448–449
Franklin, Benjamin, 37
free fusion, 188
free nerve ending, 415–416
frequency
  attention and, 239, 240*f*
  cochlea and, 283–291, 297, 309*f*
  coding of, 283–284, 289–290
  color and, 148, 193–194, 207–208, 211
  fundamental, 276, 277*f*, 319–321, 322*f*, 332, 337, 345
  hearing and, 274–277, 283–305, 309–321, 325–326, 327*f*-328*f*, 332–333
  hertz (Hz), 23, 274, 292–293, 308, 313, 337, 380, 531
  music and, 336–339, 342
  octaves and, 337–342
  olfaction and, 468, 471–472, 483, 490, 501
  pitch and, 10 (*see also* pitch)
  sensory neuroscience and, 10, 23–24
  sound pressure and, 10
  speech perception and, 345–353, 359–360
  tempo and, 274, 340
  temporal code and, 289–290, 320
  tonotopic organization and, 292, 295, 303, 336
  touch and, 413, 428*f*, 429, 443–444, 453
  vestibular sensation and, 366, 380–382, 386–387, 396, 397*f*, 400*f*, 406
  vision and, 64–68, 75–77, 82–91
  visual motion perception and, 253, 270
fricatives, 348, 361
Friedman, H. S., 94
frontal eye fields, 230, 265, 269
functional magnetic resonance imaging (fMRI)
  attention and, 229–230
  color and, 147
  hearing and, 317, 318*f*
  object recognition and, 99, 119, 120*f*
  olfaction and, 478, 494
  sensory neuroscience and, 27, 31
  space perception and, 195, 196*f*, 204
  speech perception and, 359
  subtraction method and, 119
  touch and, 422–424, 436–437, 441
  vision and, 72–73, 99
  visual motion perception and, 251, 256
fundamental frequency
  hearing and, 276, 277*f*, 319–321, 322*f*, 332
  music and, 337
  speech perception and, 345
fundi, 39–40
fungiform papillae, 512–514, 523, 525, 533–535
fusiform face area (FFA)
  attention and, 230, 233
  object recognition and, 95*f*, 97, 99, 120, 126–127

G

ganglion cells
  center-surround receptive fields and, 51–53
  color and, 139
  communicating to the brain and, 50–51
  hearing and, 290
  intrinsically photo sensitive retinal ganglion cells (ipRGCs) and, 53
  Kuffler on, 51–52
  M, 50, 53, 69
  object recognition and, 102
  P, 50, 53, 69
  stripes and, 67–68
  vestibular sensation and, 378, 402
  vision and, 35*f*, 39–40, 41*f*, 45–54, 57, 58*f*, 61, 67–78, 89–90
  visual motion perception and, 253, 265
gate control theory, 435–437, 453
geons, 122–123
Gestalt grouping rules
  hearing and, 325–331
  object recognition and, 106–110, 117
Gestalt theory
  common fate and, 326
  good continuation and, 328–329
  hearing and, 305, 325–331
  object recognition and, 106–117, 128
  relatability and, 115, 117
Gibson, J. J., 260
Giorgio Martini, Francesco di, 176, 177*f*
gist
  attention and, 237*f*, 238–240, 244, 245*f*, 247
  hearing and, 287
  object recognition and, 108*f*
  sensory neuroscience and, 18
  vision and, 85
glabrous skin, 411–415, 423, 432, 434, 439
global superiority effect, 116
globs, 147
glomeruli
  olfaction and, 457*f*, 458, 464–466, 471
  taste and, 528
glossopharyngeal (IX) nerves, 19*f*, 20, 512*f*, 516, 526
Goddard, George W., 191–192
good continuation, 108, 115, 328–329
Google, 473
G protein-coupled receptor
  olfaction and, 458, 465, 486
  taste and, 512, 515, 518–521, 534
graded potential, 48
grandmother cells, 96–97, 123–124
granular cells, 465
graviception, 365, 368–369, 392
gravity
  object recognition and, 113
  vestibular sensation and, 365–374, 382–384, 390–391, 397–399, 400*f*, 407
Green, Dan, 64
guided search, 220–225, 230
gustation
  olfaction and, 455
  physiology of, 512–516
  taste and, 417, 512–516, 531

H

hair cells
  cochlea and, 281–289, 297, 301, 303, 323, 419
  electromotility and, 286–287
  hearing and, 280–289, 297–303, 305, 323, 326

as mechanoreceptors, 374–376
organ of Corti and, 279–284
rate saturation and, 287–289
receptor potential and, 375
striolae and, 382
touch and, 419
vestibular sensation and, 368*f*, 374–386, 407
Hänig, D. P., 513–514
Hanson, Stephen, 454*f*
haptic perception
action for perception and, 441–444
Braille and, 413, 424, 431, 447–448
curvature algorithm and, 445–446
localization and, 448–449
object recognition and, 444–448
pattern perception and, 447–448
perception for action and, 440–441
sea lions and, 442–443
search and, 446–447
touch and, 409, 440–451
vision and, 449–450
what/where pathways and, 444–452
harmonic spectrum, 276, 319–320, 345
haze, 175
hearing
absolute threshold and, 293
absorption and, 297, 316
acoustic reflex and, 279
acoustic startle reflex and, 330
afferent fibers and, 284
amplitude and, 274–277, 283, 285*f*, 288–289, 292–293, 295, 302, 305, 320–322, 323*f*-324*f*
attack and, 321–322, 323*f*, 332
attention and, 305, 328, 330–333
audibility threshold and, 293
auditory nerve (AN) and, 19*f*, 278*f*, 280*f*, 281, 283*f*, 284–290, 297, 301*f*, 302–303, 308, 320, 374*f*, 419
auditory scene analysis and, 305, 322–328, 333
auditory stream segregation and, 324–325, 331, 333
azimuth and, 307, 311*f*, 313–314, 332
balance and, 280, 333
basic structure of mammalian, 277–292
basilar membrane and, 280–286, 289, 291–292, 295–296, 305, 309
belt area and, 292, 326
binocular disparity and, 314
blindness and, 317
cameras and, 314
cerebral cortex and, 291–292, 305
characteristic frequency and, 286–288
cilia and, 280–283, 288–289, 302
cochlea and, 20 (*see also* cochlea)
complex sounds and, 319–322, 329–330
conductive hearing loss, 297
cones of confusion and, 310–311, 312*f*
cranial nerves and, 290
critical bandwidth and, 296
cues and, 306, 309–317, 326, 349, 352–353, 361
cycles and, 274, 289*f*, 290
decay and, 321–322, 332
decibel (dB) units and, 275, 288, 292–293, 316, 319*f*, 346
directional transfer function (DTF) and, 313*f*, 314
distance perception and, 314–317
distractors and, 328*f*
dominating vision, 326–327
ear canal and, 277–284, 293, 297, 299, 311, 314, 332
ear shape and, 312*f*, 315
efferent fibers and, 284
efficiency and, 311
electromotility and, 286–287
equal-loudness curve and, 293
familiar sounds and, 327–328
feedback and, 291, 314
filters and, 303, 310, 313
Fourier analysis and, 275
frequency and, 274–277, 283–305, 309–321, 325–326, 327*f*-328*f*, 332–333
functional magnetic resonance imaging (fMRI) and, 317, 318*f*
function of, 273
ganglion cells and, 290
Gestalt theory and, 305, 325–331
gist and, 287
good continuation and, 328–329
hair cells and, 280–289, 297–303, 305, 323, 326
harmonic spectrum and, 276, 319–320
heliotrema and, 279–281
high-spontaneous fiber and, 288, 289*f*
inattentional deafness and, 331
incus and, 277–279, 283
inferior colliculus and, 291
inner ear and, 277–281, 302, 306
interaural level difference (ILD) and, 309–310, 311*f*-312*f*
interaural time difference (ITD) and, 306–310, 311*f*-312*f*
inverse-square law and, 316, 318, 319*f*
isointensity curves and, 288
lateral superior olive (LSO) and, 308*f*, 310
loss of, 296–300, 296–30, 302*f*
loudness and, 273–276, 292–295, 299*f*, 302, 320–321, 524–525
low-spontaneous fibers and, 288, 289*f*
magnetic resonance imaging (MRI) and, 317, 318*f*
malleus and, 277–279, 283
masking and, 295–296, 329
medial superior olive (MSO) and, 308, 309*f*
metabolic loss of, 297
middle canal and, 279–283
middle ear and, 277–281, 297, 302–303, 305
mid-spontaneous fiber and, 288
music and, 335–343
neurotransmitters and, 281–284
occlusion and, 305
organ of Corti and, 279–284
ossicles and, 277–279, 297
otoconia and, 368*f*, 382–383
outer ear and, 277, 278*f*, 297, 302
oval window and, 277–284, 297
overtones and, 320, 326
parabelt area and, 292, 326, 359
phase and, 282*f*, 289–290, 302
pinnae and, 277, 278*f*, 282, 299, 305–306, 310*f*, 311–315, 332
pitch and, 273–276, 292, 295–296, 302, 320–321, 324–325, 332
place code and, 284, 289
presbycusis and, 298
primary auditory cortex (A1) and, 291*f*, 292, 295, 303, 326
primary visual cortex (V1) and, 292
psychoacoustics and, 292–296
psychophysics and, 293
rate saturation and, 287–289
refraction and, 290
Reissner's membrane and, 280
relative intensity and, 315–316
relative size and, 315–316
restoration effects and, 328–330
round window and, 278*f*, 279–281, 301–302
segregation and, 324–326
semicircular canals and, 279
sensitivity and, 282, 285*f*-286*f*, 287, 289, 293, 298*f*, 300
sensorineural loss of, 297–298
similarity and, 325, 333
sine waves and, 274–277, 286–292, 295, 319, 329
sound localization and, 305–318
sound onsets and, 290, 323*f*, 326
spatial, 317
spectrograms and, 327*f*
spectrum and, 275–277, 295–296, 319
speech perception and, 343–364
spinal cord and, 330
stapedius and, 278*f*, 279
stapes and, 277–283, 285*f*, 297
stria vascularis and, 280, 297, 303
superior olives and, 290–291, 308–310
suppression and, 287
symmetry and, 296, 310, 313
synapses and, 281–284, 288–292, 300, 301*f*, 308
targets and, 328*f*
tectorial membrane and, 280*f*, 281–283, 286, 289
tempo and, 274
temporal code and, 289–290, 320
temporal integration and, 293
tensor tympani and, 278*f*, 279
thresholds and, 275, 276*f*, 286–287, 293–300, 337*f*
threshold tuning curve and, 286–287
timbre and, 276–277, 320–326, 332–333, 444
tonotopic organization and, 292, 295, 303, 336
transduction and, 278*f*, 280–282, 283*f*, 287, 300
transmission and, 277–284, 301, 302*f*, 330
transparency and, 324*f*

two-tone suppression and, 287
tympanic canal and, 277–281
tympanic membrane and, 277–283, 297, 300, 313, 444
vestibular canal and, 279–283, 288
vestibulocochlear (VIII) nerves, 20, 290, 374*f*
volley principle and, 290, 297
wavelength and, 274–275, 289, 295, 310, 318–319
heart attacks, 527
Hecht, S., 54
helicotrema, 279–281
Helmholtz, Hermann von, 137
hertz (Hz), 23, 531
hearing and, 274, 292–293, 308, 313
music and, 337
vestibular sensations and, 380
heterodimer receptor, 520–521
heuristics
object recognition and, 115–117
sensory neuroscience and, 30
space perception and, 193
touch and, 445
visual motion perception and, 260
hidden hearing loss, 300, 301*f*
high-spontaneous fiber, 288, 289*f*
hippocampus
attention and, 230, 233
object recognition and, 97, 98*f*
olfaction and, 462, 466, 489, 494, 496, 497*f*, 500
vestibular sensation and, 388–389, 402
Hoffman, D. M., 181
Hogness, D. S., 137
holistic processing, 126
Homer, 190
homologous regions, 97
homunculus, 421, 422*f*, 425, 430, 449, 451
horizontal cells, 35*f*, 40, 47, 49, 52–53
horopter, 184–185, 186*f*, 195
Hramavataya, Iryna, 334*f*
HSB color space, 142–144
Hubel, David, 73–81, 88, 194, 208
hue
color and, 137, 142–147, 155*f*, 164, 482
rainbows and, 33, 143–144
unique, 145*f*, 146–147
vision and, 33
Hunsicker, Alicia, 32*f*
Hurvich, Leo, 144
hybrid sentences, 359, 360*f*
hyperacuity, 63–64
hyperalgesia, 438
hypercolumns, 77–80
hyperopia, 38–39
hyperpolarization, 48, 375*f*, 379*f*

I

illuminants, 154, 157–159, 165
illusions, 200–202
illusory conjunctions, 226
illusory contours, 105–106, 115, 118, 446*f*
image formation
cornea and, 35–39
light and, 35–44
pupil and, 35*f*, 36, 41, 44
retina and, 35–44
vision and, 35–44
imbalance
vestibular sensation and, 366–367, 386, 399*f*, 400, 404–406
visual motion perception and, 251
inattentional blindness, 245, 247, 479
inattentional deafness, 331
incus, 277–279, 283
induced motion, 251, 263, 266
infants
learning words and, 357–358
object recognition and, 128
olfaction and, 492
space perception and, 189, 205–210
speech perception and, 339, 342–343, 355–358, 363
taste and, 522, 528–530
touch and, 432–433, 449
vision and, 86–89
visual motion perception and, 266
word separation and, 357–358
inferior colliculus, 291
inferotemporal (IT) cortex, 96–97, 124, 196
inhibition of return, 217
inner ear
cochlea and, 20 (*see also* cochlea)
hair cells and, 279 (*see also* hair cells)
hearing and, 277–281, 302, 306
sensory neuroscience and, 20
vestibular sensation and, 365, 367*f*, 374–376, 377*f*, 406–407
inner segment, 41*f*-42*f*, 47
insula
olfaction and, 486
taste and, 512*f*, 516, 534
touch and, 423, 424*f*, 435, 437
insular cortex, 402, 403*f*, 516
intensity. *See* amplitude
interaural level difference (ILD), 309–310, 311*f*-312*f*, 314
interaural time difference (ITD), 306–310, 311*f*-312*f*, 314
interoception
sensory neuroscience and, 4, 19*f*, 20
touch and, 439–440, 452, 510–511
vestibular sensation and, 367, 391
interocular transfer
space perception and, 209
vision and, 83
visual motion perception and, 251
intersensory integration, 450
invariance, 349, 353
inverse-square law, 316, 318, 319*f*
ipsilateral area, 70, 310, 464, 466, 516, 534
ipsilesional field, 235
iris
light and, 35*f*, 36, 39, 45*f*
spatial vision and, 57
isointensity curves, 288
itchiness, 435–439

J

Jahai, 482
James, William, 86, 228
Jameson, Dorothea, 144
Japanese, 355–356
Jasinski, Aaron, 166*f*
Javanese scales, 339
Jenifer Aniston cell, 97, 98*f*
Jing J, 506*f*
Jolicoeur, Pierre, 125
Journal of Heredity, 523
Julesz, Bela, 190
just intonation, 337
just noticeable difference (JND), 9, 10*f*, 31, 150
juxtaglomerular neurons, 464–465

K

Kanizsa images, 105, 113
Kanwisher, Nancy, 18, 99–100, 230, 244, 359
Khosla, A., 99–100
kinesthesia, 367, 399*f*, 410
kinesthetic systems
touch and, 410, 415, 420, 424*f*, 439, 441
vestibular sensation and, 368, 399*f*
Koffka, Kurt, 106
Köhler, Wolfgang, 106
koniocellular cells, 50–51, 69
koniocellular layer, 140
Kraft, T. W., 137
Kuffler, Stephen, 51–52, 73

L

labeled lines, 419, 437*f*, 531–532
language
Arabic, 357
Chinese, 220, 357
color and, 147–153
consonants and, 347–357, 361–362
critical period and, 208
emotion and, 474
English, 7, 148–151, 159, 199, 267, 347–350, 355–358, 361, 447, 481, 521
fricatives and, 348, 361
German, 106, 355, 357, 513
grammar and, 224
Hindi, 356*f*, 361
hybrid sentences and, 359, 360*f*
Jahai and, 482
Japanese, 355–356
larynx and, 19*f*, 20, 344–345
learning words and, 357
mathematical, 27–28
native listeners and, 355–357
olfaction and, 474, 480–485
reading and, 267
Semaq Beri and, 482
sensory neuroscience and, 4, 27–28
Spanish, 7, 355, 357
speech perception and, 343–344, 348, 350, 354–363

Swedish, 355
touch and, 4
visual word form area (VWFA) and, 98
vowels and, 320–321, 322*f*, 345, 347–355, 357, 361–362
Zulu, 356
larynx, 19*f*, 20, 344–345
lateral geniculate nucleus (LGN)
color and, 139–140
object recognition and, 95*f*, 101, 120
vestibular sensation and, 402
vision and, 50–51, 58*f*, 69–70, 72*f*, 75
visual motion perception and, 251, 256
lateral inhibition, 49–52, 75, 84
lateral interparietal area, 230
lateral superior olive (LSO), 308*f*, 310
L-cones
color and, 132, 135–140, 146, 151–152, 155, 157*f*, 163, 165
light and, 48–49
protanopes and, 152
learned taste aversion, 465, 494
lenses
attention and, 217
bifocal, 37
camera, 314
contact, 300
distortion and, 450
light and, 35–39
space perception and, 180–181, 187–188, 198
spatial vision and, 57, 59, 88
zoom, 217
lesions
attention and, 233–237, 247
color and, 152
object recognition and, 98
taste and, 522, 533
vestibular sensation and, 398, 402
vision and, 69, 71, 72*f*-73*f*
visual motion perception and, 256–259
letter charts, 62, 73
Lettvin, Jerry, 96
Levi, Dennis M., 63–64
light
absorption and, 33–38, 43, 45, 48, 54
blindness and, 35*f*, 39–40, 43, 46, 47*f*, 55
color and, 131 (*see also* color)
electormagnetic spectrum and, 34*f*
focal distance and, 36–37
focusing, 37–39
hue and, 33 (*see also* hue)
image formation and, 35–44
intrinsically photo sensitive retinal ganglion cells (ipRGCs) and, 53
photons and, 33–36, 44–48, 54, 64, 103, 153, 162, 293
photopigment regeneration and, 45
physics of, 33–35
pupil size and, 44
reflectance and, 136, 158, 516
reflection and, 35–36, 54, 57, 64
refraction and, 35–39, 54, 62, 65, 88–89
retina and, 33–55
rods and, 35*f*, 40–50, 53–55
scatter and, 34–40, 54
scotopic illumination and, 43, 44*f*, 49, 66*f*, 132–134, 165
sensitivity and, 43*f*, 44–50, 54
spectral reflectance function and, 158
spectrum and, 33, 34*f*
transduction and, 36, 39–40, 47–49, 54
visual angle and, 41, 42*f*
wavelength and, 33–34, 43, 47–49, 456, 475*f*, 476
as waves, 33
limbic system, 466, 496, 504
linear acceleration
macula and, 382–384
vestibular sensation and, 369–370, 374, 382–384, 386, 406–407
linear motion, 365, 369–371, 374, 400, 407
linear perspective, 175–180, 201, 211
line cancellation test, 233–234
Lipstick (Hramavataya), 334*f*
Listening to the Sounds of the Sky (Studio Weave), 304*f*
London Medical and Physical Journal, 508
loudness
decibel (dB) units and, 275 (*see also* decibel (dB) units)
equal-loudness curve, 293
hearing and, 273–276, 292–295, 299*f*, 302, 320–321, 524–525
light and, 524
timbre and, 276–277, 320–321, 322*f*, 325–326, 332–333, 444
low-spontaneous fibers, 288, 289*f*
luminance defined object, 258, 271

M

machine learning (ML), 123, 473
maculae
degeneration of, 46, 55
fovea and, 40–43 (*see also* fovea)
linear acceleration and, 382–384
vestibular sensation and, 382–384
vision and, 40, 46, 55, 89
magnetic resonance imaging (MRI)
attention and, 229–230, 233*f*
color and, 147
hearing and, 317, 318*f*
object recognition and, 99, 119*f*, 120
olfaction and, 478, 494
sensory neuroscience and, 25–27, 31
space perception and, 195, 196*f*, 204
speech perception and, 359
touch and, 422
vision and, 72, 73*f*
visual motion perception and, 251, 256
magnetoencephalography (MEG)
sensory neuroscience and, 24–27, 31
vision and, 72
magnitude estimation, 5*t*, 11, 384–387
magnocellular layer, 50, 69, 256
main olfactory bulb (MOB), 497
mal de debarquement syndrome, 400, 404
malleus, 277–279, 283
mammograms, 6, 13, 125
Margolskee, Robert, 522
Marks, Lawrence, 524
masking
attention and, 238
hearing and, 295–296, 329
sensory neuroscience and, 5*t*, 17
visual motion perception and, 268
mathematical integration, 386
mathematical models, 27–28
Maxwell, James Clerk, 137–138
Mayans, 533
McClintock effect, 498
McGurk effect, 361, 390
M-cones
color and, 132–140, 143, 146, 151–152, 160–161, 165
deuteranopes and, 151
light and, 49
mechanoreceptors
hair cells and, 374–376
touch and, 411–416, 419–420, 423, 428*f*, 429, 439–443, 452–453
vestibular sensation and, 368*f*, 374, 407
medial geniculate nucleus, 70, 291
medial superior olive (MSO), 308, 309*f*
Meissner corpuscle, 412*f*, 413–415
melanopsin, 48
melody, 325*f*, 326, 329, 337–343
memory
attention and, 228, 233, 240–247
avian brain and, 90
change blindness and, 243–247
color and, 150
computers and, 30
inferotemporal (IT) cortex and, 97
object recognition and, 97, 101, 123, 127
olfaction and, 460, 462–463, 466, 477–480, 485, 494, 496, 500–501
picture, 241*f*-242*f*, 243, 247
taste and, 527
touch and, 445
vestibular sensation and, 388–389
Ménières syndrome, 405–407
Merkel disc, 413–414
metabolic hearing loss, 297
metamers, 135–138, 141, 151, 165, 474
method of adjustment, 9
method of constant stimuli, 7–9
method of limits, 9, 480
metrical depth cues, 172, 175–176, 195
M ganglion cells, 50, 53, 69
Michelson, Albert, 64–65
microsaccades, 266, 271
microvilli, 512, 514–515, 518, 534
middle canal, 279–283
middle ear
chorda tympani, 509, 512*f*, 515–516, 526, 531
hearing and, 277–281, 297, 302–303, 305
otosclerosis and, 297
taste and, 509, 526
vestibular sensation and, 374*f*
middle temporal area (MT), 196, 251, 256–258
midget bipolar cells, 50

midlevel vision
  committees and, 112–117, 125, 128
  finding edges and, 104–109
  object recognition and, 103–118, 128
  perceptual committees and, 112–117, 125, 128
  rules of evidence and, 106–107
  space perception and, 173
  specular reflections and, 103, 104*f*
  summarizing, 116–117
  texture segmentation and, 109–110, 117
mid-spontaneous fiber, 288
Milton, John, 121
mitral cells, 457*f*, 465
moderating, 436–437
Molyneux, William, 4
monocular cues
  space perception and, 167, 170–178, 183, 188–193, 207–208, 211
  vision and, 88
monocular depth cue, 171, 190
monosodium glutamate (MSG), 522, 534
Morris water maze, 389
motion aftereffect (MAE), 249–251, 258
motion-induced blindness, 263
motion parallax, 179–180, 194, 196, 249, 316
motor cortex, 20*f*
  speech perception and, 362
  touch and, 451
  visual motion perception and, 263, 268
Mozart, Wolfgang Amadeus, 340–343, 482
MSG, 522
Muhammad, Kenny, 344
Müller, Johannes, 18
multisensory integration
  sensory neuroscience and, 21
  spatial orientation and, 401–403
  speech perception and, 361*f*
  vestibular sensation and, 390–392, 404, 407
music
  absolute pitch (AP) and, 339–340
  amplitude and, 345*f*, 346
  attention and, 340, 343
  basic taste and, 343
  bitterness and, 343
  cancer and, 336
  chords and, 336, 338–340, 343, 362, 475*f*
  cultural differences and, 338–339
  emotion and, 152–153, 335–336
  frequency and, 336–339, 342
  hearing and, 335–343
  historical perspective on, 335–336
  Javanese scales and, 339
  just intonation and, 337
  making, 340–343
  melody and, 325*f*, 326, 329, 337–343
  Mozart and, 340–343, 482
  octaves and, 337–342
  overtones and, 320, 326
  pitch and, 336–341
  Pythagoras and, 335–336, 339
  resonators and, 335
  rhythm and, 341–343, 362
  syncopation and, 341–342
  taste and, 343
  tempo and, 340
  tone chroma and, 337–338, 362
  tone height and, 337–338, 339*f*, 362
  topographical mapping and, 336
  Tsimane' people and, 339
myopia, 38–39

N

Nadoolman, Wolffe, 533
nasal dominance, 457
Nathans, J., 137
native listeners, 355–357
Necker cube, 112–114
negative afterimage, 155–157
neglect
  attention and, 233–237, 247
  touch and, 418
neural plasticity, 88, 423–425
neuroimaging
  olfaction and, 478–479, 501
  sensory neuroscience and, 5*t*, 7, 24, 31
  space perception and, 196
neurons. *See also* specific type
  connections of, 21–22
  data acquisition and, 22–24
  firing of, 13
neurotransmitters
  action potentials and, 22
  hearing and, 281–284
  taste and, 515, 522
  touch and, 436
  vestibular sensation and, 375
  vision and, 48
neutral point, 145*f*
Newsome, W. T., 257
Next Generation (Oliver), 92
nocebo effect, 438
nociceptors
  olfaction and, 469
  touch and, 412*f*, 417–420, 435–438, 452
nonaccidental features, 116
nonmetrical depth cues, 172, 195
nonspatial cognition, 389–390
nontasters
  sensory neuroscience and, 12, 13*f*
  taste and, 12, 523, 526, 534–535
novelty, 94*f*

O

object recognition
  absorption and, 103, 104*f*
  accidental viewpoint and, 112–118
  agnosia and, 98, 127–128, 152
  ambiguous figures and, 112
  attention and, 96, 101
  Bayesian models and, 117–118, 128
  blindness and, 101, 103*f*, 128
  border ownership and, 94, 96*f*, 118–119, 196
  Braille and, 413, 424, 431, 447–448
  cameras and, 103, 113
  camouflage and, 111*f*, 190, 260, 263
  cerebral cortex and, 96
  color space and, 141–143, 146–152
  cues and, 104, 108*f*
  decoding and, 120, 124
  deep neural networks (DNNs) and, 30, 123–129
  extrastriate body area (EBA), 97, 120
  facial recognition and, 30, 126–128
  feedback and, 95*f*, 101
  feed-forward process and, 101
  figure-ground assignment and, 114, 128
  finding edges and, 104–109
  functional magnetic resonance imaging (fMRI) and, 99, 119, 120*f*
  fusiform face area (FFA) and, 95*f*, 97, 99, 120, 126–127
  ganglion cells and, 102
  geons and, 122–123
  Gestalt theory and, 106–117, 128
  gist and, 108*f*
  global superiority effect and, 116
  grandmother cells and, 96–97, 123–124
  gravity and, 113
  haptic perception and, 444–448
  heuristics and, 115–117
  hippocampus and, 97, 98*f*
  holistic processing and, 126
  homologous regions and, 97
  illusory contours and, 105–106, 115, 118, 446*f*
  infants and, 128
  inferotemporal (IT) cortex and, 96, 124
  Jenifer Aniston cell and, 97, 98*f*
  Kanizsa images and, 105, 113
  lateral geniculate nucleus (LGN) and, 95*f*, 101, 120
  lesions and, 98
  magnetic resonance imaging (MRI) and, 99, 119*f*, 120
  memory and, 97, 101, 123, 127
  midlevel vision and, 103–118, 128
  multiple committees and, 125–126
  Necker cube and, 112–114
  nonaccidental features and, 116
  novelty and, 94*f*
  occlusion and, 102, 105, 108*f*, 115–119, 128
  parahippocampal place area (PPA) and, 97
  parallelism and, 114, 117
  parietal lobe and, 94*f*, 96, 128
  perceptual committees and, 112–117, 125, 128
  phase and, 99
  photons and, 103
  primary visual cortex (V1) and, 93, 97, 128
  problems of, 101–103
  properties of objects and, 93–96
  prosopagnosia and, 98, 127–128
  proximity and, 110–112, 117
  Quiroga on, 97, 118
  recognition-by-components model and, 122, 123*f*

relatability and, 115, 117
relative size and, 95*f*
retina and, 101–102, 106, 112, 114, 116
reverse-hierarchy theory and, 101
rules of evidence and, 106–107
scatter and, 103–104
Selfridge model and, 120–123
sensitivity and, 118
similarity and, 110–112, 117, 122
simple cells and, 13, 102, 123
simple lines/edges and, 93–96
single cells and, 96–97, 102, 119*f*
specular reflections and, 103, 104*f*
striate cortex and, 93, 96, 101, 104, 128
strokes and, 98
structural description and, 122–123
structuralism and, 106
subsurface scatter and, 104
surroundedness and, 114
symmetry and, 114, 117
synapses and, 101
synthesis and, 104
templates and, 121–122, 129
texture segmentation and, 109–110, 117
tilt and, 94
touch and, 444–452
transmission and, 104
transparency and, 104, 108
visual motion perception and, 262–263
wavelength and, 103
what/where pathways and, 96–101, 118–119, 127–128, 444–452
occlusion
hearing and, 305
object recognition and, 102, 105, 108*f*, 115–119, 128
space perception and, 171–177, 199, 211
octaves, 337–342
ocular dominance
space perception and, 208
vision and, 74–80
oculomotor (III) nerves, 20, 395*f*, 547
odor, 122
odorant receptors (ORs), 458, 465, 467, 471
odorants
chemicals and, 470–478
hedonics and, 491–497
object recognition and, 122
olfaction and, 455–506
neurophysiology of, 464–470
physiology of, 455–464
psychophysics and, 478–490
taste and, 517, 530, 534
odor hedonics, 491–493, 496, 504
Odyssey (Homer), 190
OFF bipolar cells, 50
OFF-center cells, 52
Ofstedahl, Micah, 272*f*
olfaction
accessory olfactory bulb (AOB) and, 497, 504
acuity and, 469, 484–486
adaptation and, 478–490, 495*f*, 504
agnosia and, 472, 480
amygdala-hippocampal complex and, 466, 494
anosmia and, 459–462, 472–473, 478–479, 483, 490, 503, 537–538, 540, 552
aromatherapy and, 455, 496, 500–501, 504
attention and, 460–461, 475, 479, 484, 489
binocular rivalry and, 475–476
blindness and, 459–460, 463, 472, 479, 484–485
blood pressure and, 501
cerebral cortex and, 516
chemicals and, 470–478
chemosignals and, 497–502, 505
cilia and, 457*f*, 458–459, 465, 470*f*
cognitive habituation and, 489, 504
COVID-19 and, 458, 460–461, 486, 491, 503
cranial nerves and, 464, 465*f*, 469–470
cribriform plate and, 20, 457*f*, 459, 464, 465*f*
cross-adaptation and, 487–488, 532
cues and, 460, 463, 476, 484, 486, 498–501, 504
cycles and, 477, 498–499
declining, 483–484
detection and, 478–479
digitizing scent and, 502
discrimination and, 479–480
efficiency and, 485, 487
electroencephalography (EEG) and, 490, 499–501
emotion and, 455, 460, 462, 466, 474, 480, 484, 489–492, 495–504
entorhinal cortex and, 466
familiarity and, 491–492
filters and, 456, 487
flavor and, 455, 460, 467, 469, 476, 492–495
frequency and, 468, 471–472, 483, 490, 501
functional magnetic resonance imaging (fMRI) and, 478, 494
genetic basis of, 467–469
glomeruli and, 457*f*, 458, 464–466, 471
G protein-coupled receptor and, 458, 465, 486
granular cells and, 465
gustation and, 455
hedonics of, 491–497
hippocampus and, 462, 466, 489, 494, 496, 497*f*, 500
imagery and, 478
individual differences in, 483–486
infants and, 492
insula and, 486
intensity and, 491–492
juxtaglomerular neurons and, 464–465
language and, 474, 480–485
as learned affect, 530
learned taste aversion and, 465, 494
limbic system and, 466, 496, 504
magnetic resonance imaging (MRI) and, 478, 494
main olfactory bulb (MOB), 497
memory and, 460, 462–463, 466, 477–480, 485, 494, 496, 500–501
mitral cells and, 457*f*, 465
nasal dominance and, 457
nature/nurture debate and, 492–493
neuroimaging and, 478–479, 501
neurophysiology of, 464–470
nociceptors and, 469
orbitofrontal cortext (OFC) and, 462, 466, 474, 489
orthonasal, 455, 508*f*
oscillations and, 477
papillae and, 466
Parkinson's disease (PD) and, 461, 485
patterns and, 474–475
phase and, 486, 491, 499
pheromones and, 497–505
physiology of, 456–464
piroform cortex and, 466, 474–475, 478, 482, 486, 490, 496
pleasentness and, 491
primer pheromone and, 498
protein and, 458, 465*f*, 467, 485–486, 493
proximity and, 498
psychophysics and, 478–490
recognition and, 479–480
rhythm and, 486
sensitivity and, 455, 457, 461, 468–469, 472, 478–480, 483–489, 492, 495
shape-pattern theory and, 122, 471–473, 503
single cells and, 455
sourness and, 478
staircase method and, 480–481
stereoisomers and, 472–473
sustentacular cells and, 457–458
sweetness and, 472, 482–483, 493–496
symmetry and, 457
synapses and, 496, 500
synthesis and, 475, 477
synthetic/analytical perception and, 475–477
tactile response and, 500
targets and, 461, 469
taste buds and, 466
tasters and, 479
thresholds and, 478–481, 487, 489
tip-of-the nose phenomenon and, 481, 504
transduction and, 458, 487
transmission and, 458, 466*f*, 469, 471
triangle test and, 480–482
trigeminal nerves and, 20, 455, 462, 469, 470*f*, 483, 489–490, 496, 503
tufted cells and, 457*f*, 465–466, 471
turbinates and, 457, 457*f*
vibration theory and, 471–473, 503
virtual reality and, 463*f*, 502
visual search and, 446, 447*f*, 479
volatile molecules and, 456, 470*f*, 476, 487, 492, 496–497, 503
vomeronasal organ and, 497, 504
wavelength and, 456, 475*f*, 476

olfactor sensory neurons (OSNs), 20, 457–459, 464–465, 486, 497
olfactory bulb (OB), 457*f*-458*f*
  accessory olfactory bulb (AOB), 497, 504
  forebrain and, 459
  gender and, 483
  main olfactory bulb (MOB), 497
  neurological processing in, 470–471
  neurophysiology of, 464–467
  sensory neuroscience and, 20
  size of, 463
olfactory cleft, 457, 491
olfactory epithelium, 455–459, 464, 471, 508, 512
olfactory (I) nerves
  disgusting sensations and, 417
  forebrain and, 459
  neurophysiology of, 464, 465*f*
  smell and, 20, 417, 455, 459, 462, 464, 465*f*, 496, 497*f*, 500, 503, 512, 530
olfactory tract, 466
olfactory white, 476–477, 503
Oliver, Marvin, 92
Olney, John, 522
ominvore's dilemma, 526–527
ON bipolar cells, 50
ON-center cells, 51*f*, 52, 68
opponent color theory, 144–146, 151, 154, 156, 165
optic array, 260
optic flow, 180, 260–261
optic (II) nerves
  light and, 18–19, 35*f*, 36, 39–40, 51, 54, 418
  spatial vision and, 58*f*, 72
  vision and, 18–19, 35*f*, 36, 39–40, 51, 54, 58*f*, 72, 418–419
optokinetic nystagmus, 266, 270–271
orbitofrontal cortex (OFC)
  olfaction and, 462, 466, 474, 489
  taste and, 512*f*, 516, 534
  touch and, 423
organ of Corti, 279–284
orientation tuning, 74–78
orthonasal olfaction, 455, 508*f*
oscillations
  light and, 33
  olfaction and, 477
  touch and, 444
  vestibular sensation and, 380–382, 386–387, 396*f*
ossicles, 277–279, 297
otitis media, 297, 526
otoconia, 368*f*, 382–383
otolith organs
  amplitude and, 382–384
  direction and, 384
  striolae and, 382
  vestibular sensation and, 368*f*, 369–370, 374–376, 382–386, 390–391, 396, 402, 406–407
otosclerosis, 297
outer ear
  hearing and, 277, 278*f*, 297, 302
  pinnae and, 277
  vestibular sensation and, 374*f*
outer segment, 41*f*, 47–48, 89
oval window, 277–284, 297
overtones, 320, 326
Oxford Insight, xx

P

Pacinian corpuscles, 412*f*, 413, 440
pain
  levels of, 435–436
  moderating, 436–437
  submodality of, 435–439
  touch and, 435–439
Panum's fusional area, 184, 186, 200
papillae
  olfaction and, 466
  taste and, 512–514, 522–525, 533–535
  touch and, 412*f*, 414
parabelt area, 292, 326, 359
parahippocampal place area (PPA), 97, 230, 233
parallelism, 114, 117
parallel search, 219
Paré, E. B., 257
parietal lobe
  attention and, 230, 233, 234*f*, 236, 247
  object recognition and, 94*f*, 96, 128
  sensory neuroscience and, 20*f*
  touch and, 421, 452
  vestibular sensation and, 403*f*
Parkinson's disease (PD), 461, 485
parvocellular layer
  color and, 140
  vision and, 50, 58*f*, 69–70
pélog scales, 339
perception for action, 440–441
perceptual committees
  midlevel vision and, 112–117, 125, 128
  multiple, 125–126
  space perception and, 173, 198–200
peripersonal space, 237
P ganglion cells, 50, 53, 69
phantom limb, 425, 478, 517
phase
  hearing and, 282*f*, 289–290, 302
  object recognition and, 99
  olfaction and, 486, 491, 499
  sensory neuroscience and, 23*f*
  space perception and, 207–208
  touch and, 451*f*, 452
  vision and, 66–68, 76, 89
phase locking, 23*f*, 289–290
phenylthiocarbamide (PTC), 519, 523
pheromones
  chemosignals and, 497–502, 505
  olfaction and, 497–505
  primer, 498
  releaser, 498
  vomeronasal organ and, 497, 504
phonation, 345, 362
photoactivation, 48, 282
photons
  color and, 153, 162
  detecing a single, 54
  object recognition and, 103
  photopigment regeneration and, 45
  vision and, 33–36, 44–48, 54, 64, 293
photopic illumination
  color and, 132–133
  vision and, 43, 44*f*, 49, 66*f*
photoreceptors
  color and, 132–134, 137, 141, 151–152, 154, 161–165
  graded potentials and, 48
  inner segment and, 41*f*-42*f*, 47
  lateral inhibition and, 49
  outer segment and, 41*f*, 47–48, 89
  photoactivation and, 48
  retinal density and, 42*f*
  sensitivity and, 49–50
  space perception and, 195
  synaptic terminal and, 22*f*, 41*f*, 47–48
  vision and, 35*f*, 36, 39–57, 60, 62, 72, 76, 281–282, 422
photoswitch, 47
pictorial depth cues, 171, 178
picture memory, 241*f*-242*f*, 243, 247
pinnae
  head cues and, 311–314
  hearing and, 277, 278*f*, 282, 299, 305–306, 310*f*, 311–315, 332
  outer ear and, 277
Pirenne, M. H., 54
piriform cortex
  amygdala-hippocampal complex and, 466
  configural odor representation and, 474
  limbic system and, 466
  olfaction and, 466, 474–475, 478, 482, 486, 490, 496
pitch
  hearing and, 273–276, 292, 295–296, 302, 320–321, 324–325, 332
  music and, 336–341
  sensory neuroscience and, 10, 23
  speech perception and, 345, 350, 355, 362
  Tsimane' people and, 339
  vestibular sensation and, 369, 372–373, 379, 388*f*, 398
pitch angular velocity, 372
placebo effect, 436–438
place code, 284, 289
Polat, U., 107
Pollan, Michael, 526–527
polysensory systems, 21
Ponzo illusion, 201
Popular Mechanics magazine, 191–192
positivism, 167
positron emission tomography (PET), 27, 359, 403*f*
Posner cueing paradigm, 215–217, 229
preattentive stage, 225
prediction error, 29
preferential looking, 86–87
presbycusis, 298
presbyopia, 37–38, 188
primary auditory cortex (A1)
  hearing and, 291*f*, 292, 295, 303, 326
  speech perception and, 359

primary visual cortex (V1)
attention and, 233
color and, 152
hearing and, 292
object recognition and, 93, 97, 128
sensory neuroscience and, 23–24, 26*f*
space perception and, 105*f*, 194, 202, 207–208, 211
spatial vision and, 58*f*, 70, 90–91, 421
visual motion perception and, 249–251
primer pheromone, 498
primes, 223
principle of univariance, 133–134
priority map, 229*f*, 230
probability summation, 170
projective geometry, 172–173, 176, 182, 187
proprioception, 410–411, 423
propylthiouracil (PROP), 12, 13*f*, 523–525, 534
prosopagnosia, 98, 127–128
protanopes, 152
protein
crystallins, 37
olfaction and, 458, 465*f*, 467, 485–486, 493
taste and, 512, 515, 518–522, 534
umami and, 522
vision and, 37, 47
proto-objects, 238, 247
proximity
color and, 154
McClintock effect and, 498
object recognition and, 110–112, 117
olfaction and, 498
touch and, 409, 415, 423
pruiceptors, 417–418, 437
psychoacoustics, 292–296
psychophysics
hearing and, 293
olfaction and, 478–490
sensory neuroscience and, 7–18
taste and, 510–511
thresholds and, 7–18
touch and, 440
pupil
adaptability of, 44, 45*f*
image formation and, 35*f*, 36, 41, 44
light and, 35*f*, 36, 41, 44–45, 48
neural circuitry of, 46
sensory neuroscience and, 20
size of, 44, 45*f*
space perception and, 181
spatial vision and, 90
vestibular sensation and, 394
pure tone. *See* sine waves
Pythagoras, 335–336, 339

Q

qualia, 151, 153
Quiroga, R. Q., 97, 118

R

rainbows, 33, 143–144
random dot stereogram (RDS)
space perception and, 190–193, 196*f*, 206, 211
touch and, 450
visual motion perception and, 259
rapid serial visual presentation (RSVP), 226–228
Rasch, R. A., 326
Ratan Murty, N. A., 99–100
rate-intensity functions, 288
rate saturation, 287–289
Rayleigh scattering, 34
reachspace, 236–237
reaction time (RT)
attention and, 216, 218*f*, 246
efficiency and, 218*f*
sensory neuroscience and, 5*t*, 18
realism, 167
Reboredo, Sergi, 212*f*
receiver operating characteristic (ROC) curve, 16, 17*f*
receptive field
attention and, 232, 247
color and, 93–97, 102, 103*f*, 139–140
space perception and, 194, 195*f*, 208, 211
striate cortex and, 73–77
touch and, 412–415, 421, 429*f*, 430
vestibular sensation and, 368
vision and, 43*t*, 46, 49, 51–54, 68, 70, 73–77, 85–86, 90
visual motion perception and, 252–256, 263, 269, 271
receptor adaptation, 487, 489, 504
receptor potential
hair cells and, 375
touch and, 416
vestibular sensation and, 375–377, 382–384
recognition-by-components model, 122, 123*f*
reflectance, 136, 158, 516
reflection, 35–36, 54, 57, 64
reflexive eye movement, 266, 270, 395
refraction
hearing and, 290
vision and, 35–39, 54, 62, 65, 88–89
refractive error, 38, 62, 88–89
Reissner's membrane, 280
relatability, 115, 117
related color, 154–155
relative disparity, 183, 185*f*, 194–196, 208
relative height, 173–175, 198, 206
relative intensity, 315–316
relative metrical depth cues, 175, 180
relative size
hearing and, 315–316
object recognition and, 95*f*
space perception and, 172–175, 176*f*, 186*f*
Relativity (Escher), 171
releaser pheromone, 498
resonators, 335, 345–346
respiration, 344–345
response enhancement, 230–232
restoration effects, 328–330
retina
age-related macular degeneration and, 46
attention and, 213, 237*f*, 245
binocular vision and, 167–175, 180–188, 192–199, 202, 204, 210–211
blind spot and, 35*f*, 39–40
center-surround receptive fields and, 51–53
chromophore and, 48
color and, 133*f*, 137–141, 152, 155–156
cones and, 288–289 (*see also* cones)
correspondence problem and, 192–194
degeneration of, 300
duplex, 41, 44–45
focal distance and, 36–37
focusing light onto, 37–39
fovea and, 306 (*see also* fovea)
function of, 41–44
ganglion cells and, 290
geography of, 41–44
image formation and, 35–44
information processing by, 47–53
intrinsically photo sensitive retinal ganglion cells (ipRGCs) and, 53
Kuffler on, 51–52
lateral inhibition and, 49
light and, 33–55
object recognition and, 101–102, 106, 112, 114, 116
photoactivation and, 48
photoreceptors and, 42*f*, 132 (*see also* phororeceptors)
rods and, 323 (*see also* rods)
sensory neuroscience and, 18, 20
singe-photon sensitivity and, 54
somatotopy and, 419
space perception and, 167–175, 180–188, 192–199, 202, 204, 210–211
spatial vision and, 57–60, 63–78, 83, 88–90
transduction and, 39
vestibular sensation and, 366, 378, 392–395, 402
vestibulo-ocular reflex (VOR) and, 366, 367*f*
visual motion perception and, 251, 253, 260–271
retinal prostheses, 47
retinitis pigmentosa, 46–47, 55
retronasal olfaction. *See also* flavor
method of, 455
taste and, 508–511, 525–528, 534
reverse-hierarchy theory, 101
RGB, 127, 142
rhodopsin, 48, 87, 134
rhythm
music and, 341–343, 362
olfaction and, 486
sensory neuroscience and, 23
vestibular sensation and, 380
vision and, 48
Richter, Curt, 529
Roberson, Debi, 149
Robson, John, 68
rod monochrats, 152

rods
  color and, 132–134, 152, 162, 165
  difference from cones, 43
  energy use of, 43–44
  light and, 35*f*, 40–50, 53–55
  photoactivation and, 48
  photopigment regeneration and, 45
  space perception and, 187*f*
  spatial vision and, 57, 61, 87
  transduction and, 47–49
roll angular velocity, 372
Roorda, Austin, 137
rotation perception, 367*f*, 385–386, 396
round window, 278*f*, 279–281, 301–302
Rozin, Paul, 526
Ruffini endings, 413–414
rules of evidence, 106–107

S

saccades
  attention and, 217, 244
  comparators and, 261, 267–269
  compensation and, 269
  optokinetic nystagmus and, 265–266
  physiology of, 265–267
  reading and, 267
  smooth pursuit and, 264–271
  superior colliculus and, 265–266
  types of, 265–267
  vergence and, 266, 271
  visual motion perception and, 253, 261–271
saccadic suppression, 217, 261, 267–271
saccules, 369, 374*f*, 382–384, 407
Sacks, Oliver, 189
Sagi, D., 107
salience, 216, 219
  saltiness
  sensory neuroscience and, 5
  taste and, 5, 343, 513–518, 524, 527–535
  tongue map and, 513–515
satisfaction of search, 225–226
scaling, 5*t*, 6, 10–13, 385, 426*f*
scatter
  object recognition and, 103–104
  Rayleigh, 34
  space perception and, 172–175, 176*f*
  vision and, 34–40, 54, 77
scene-based guidance, 224
scene grammar, 224
scene perception
  disorders of, 233–236
  ensemble statistics and, 239*f*
  nonselective processing and, 217, 237–238, 244, 247
  overload and, 213
  physiological basis of, 228–233
  selective processing and, 215, 217, 225, 230, 235, 237–240, 244, 246–247
  in space, 215–217
  in time, 226–228
  two pathways to, 237
  understanding scenes and, 236–246
  visual search and, 217–226
scene semantics, 224
scene syntax, 224
Schade, Otto, 64
Schlaer, S., 54
Schnapf, J. L., 137
S-cones
  color and, 132, 135–136, 139–140, 143, 151–152, 155, 158, 160
  light and, 48, 51
  spatial vision and, 69
scotopic illumination, 43, 44*f*, 49, 66*f*, 132–134, 165
Scoville units, 533
sea lions, 442–443
second-order motion, 258–260, 271
selective adaptation
  effectual site and, 83
  as psychologist's electrode, 80–86
  spatial vision and, 80–86, 91
  visual motion perception and, 251
selective attention
  ADHD and, 235
  binding problem and, 225
  bottlenecks and, 237*f*
  direction of, 217
  ensembles and, 238
  frontal eye fields and, 230
  multiple stimuli and, 215
  processing of, 215, 217, 225, 230, 235, 237–240, 244, 246–247
  stimuli choice and, 215, 217
Self-Portrait under the Lime Trees (Shupliak), 2*f*
Selfridge, Oliver, 120–123
Semaq Beri, 482
semicircular canals
  amplitude and, 378–379
  direction and, 379
  dynamics of, 379–381
  hearing and, 279
  oscillatory motion and, 380
  push-pull relationship of, 379*f*
  sinusoidal motion and, 380–382, 387*f*, 396*f*
  vestibular sensation and, 369, 374, 376–382, 385–386, 390, 393–398, 402, 406–407
sense of angular motion, 369–372
sense of linear motion, 369–371, 400
sense of tilt, 365, 369–370
sensitivity
  attention and, 232
  color and, 132–134, 146*f*, 155, 157*f*, 162*f*, 163, 165
  hearing and, 282, 285*f*-286*f*, 287, 289, 293, 298*f*, 300
  light and, 43*f*, 44–50, 54
  object recognition and, 118
  olfaction and, 455, 457, 461, 468–469, 472, 478–480, 483–489, 492, 495
  photoreceptors and, 49–50
  sensory neuroscience and, 12, 15–16
  space perception and, 208, 210
  spatial vision and, 64–65, 66*f*, 74, 82–85, 89–90
  speech perception and, 349
  taste and, 514, 519
  touch and, 413*f*, 415, 427–432, 453
  vestibular sensation and, 369, 374, 378–384, 387
  visual motion perception and, 268, 270–271
sensorineural hearing loss, 297–298
sensory conflict, 370
sensory exafference, 392
sensory integration
  sensory neuroscience and, 21
  speech perception and, 361*f*
  touch and, 450
  vestibular sensation and, 390–392, 404, 407
sensory neuroscience
  cerebral cortex and, 20, 31
  context and, 30
  data recording and, 22–24
  experience and, 18–27
  feedback and, 29–30
  frequency and, 10, 23–24
  functional magnetic resonance imaging (fMRI) and, 27, 31
  gist and, 18
  heuristics and, 30
  inner ear and, 20
  interoception and, 4, 19*f*, 20
  just noticeable difference (JND) and, 9, 10*f*, 31, 150
  language and, 4, 27–28
  magnetic resonance imaging (MRI) and, 25–27, 31
  magnetoencephalography (MEG) and, 24–27, 31
  magnitude estimation and, 5*t*, 11, 384–387
  masking and, 5*t*, 17
  mathematical models and, 27–28
  method of adjustment and, 9
  method of constant stimuli and, 7–9
  method of limits and, 9, 480
  multisensory integration and, 21
  nerve energies and, 18–21
  neuroimaging and, 5*t*, 7, 24, 31
  nontasters and, 12, 13*f*
  olfactory bulb (OB) and, 20
  parietal lobe and, 20*f*
  perception and, 3–7
  phase and, 23*f*
  pitch and, 10, 23
  polysensory systems and, 21
  primary visual cortex (V1) and, 23–24, 26*f*
  prior knowledge and, 30
  probability and, 28–29
  psychophysics and, 7–18
  pupil and, 20
  reaction time (RT) and, 5*t*, 18
  receiver operating characteristic (ROC) curve and, 16, 17*f*
  retina and, 18, 20
  rhythm and, 23
  scaling and, 5*t*, 6, 10–13, 385, 426*f*
  sensitivity and, 12, 15–16
  sensory integration and, 21

signal detection theory and, 6, 9, 12–16, 21
similarity and, 12
sourness and, 5
spatial orientation and, 19*f*, 20
statistical optimization models and, 5*t*, 29
statistics and, 28–29
Steven's power law and, 11–12
stimulus onset asynchrony (SOA) and, 17*f*, 18
sweetness and, 5, 11–12
synapses and, 21*f*, 22, 29, 31
targets and, 5*t*, 17–18, 21*f*
tasters and, 11–12, 13*f*
thresholds and, 5*f*, 6–17, 23, 31
tilt and, 18, 23
time course of perception and, 5*t*, 6, 17–18
transduction and, 4
transmission and, 20–23, 29, 31
trigeminal nerve and, 19*f*, 20
vagus (X) nerves and, 19*f*, 20
velocity and, 21
Weber's law and, 10–12, 49*f*, 342
sensory reafference, 392
Ser Brunnellesco, Filippo di, 176
serial self-terminating search, 220
set size, 218–219
shape-pattern theory, 122, 471–473, 503
sharper tuning, 230–232
Shupliak, Oleg, 2*f*
signal detection theory, 6, 9, 12–16, 21
similarity
attention and, 221
hearing and, 325, 333
object recognition and, 110–112, 117, 122
sensory neuroscience and, 12
simple cells
object recognition and, 102, 123
striate cortex and, 75–77
vision and, 74–77
sine wave gratings, 60, 64–68, 207, 319
sine waves
attention and, 240
Fourier analysis and, 66–67, 275, 382
hearing and, 274–277, 286–292, 295, 319, 329
space perception and, 207
vestibular sensation and, 381
vision and, 60*f*, 64–68, 84
single cells
attention and, 230–232
object recognition and, 96–97, 102, 119*f*
olfaction and, 455
space perception and, 204
vision and, 35, 77
sinusoidal oscillation, 380–382, 387*f*, 396*f*
sléndro scales, 339
Small, Dana, 509
smooth pursuit
vestibular sensation and, 366
visual motion perception and, 264–271
Snellen, Herman, 62
Soba Love (Jing J), 506*f*
Sobel, Noam, 490
somatosensation
neural plasticity of, 423–426
taste and, 509, 521
touch and, 410–411, 418–424, 441, 444
vestibular sensation and, 367
somatosensory area 1 (S1), 421, 422*f*, 441
somatosensory area 2 (S2), 421, 422*f*, 441
somatotopic mapping, 419–422, 452
sonic seasoning, 343
sound onsets, 290, 323*f*, 326
Sounds Like Infinity (Ofstedahl), 272*f*
sourness
olfaction and, 478
sensory neuroscience and, 5
taste and, 5, 343, 509, 513–519, 524, 527–528, 531–534
tongue map and, 513–514, 517
space perception
absolute metrical depth cue and, 175, 181
accidental viewpoint and, 172, 199
accommodation and, 180–181, 188, 211
acuity and, 192, 195, 206, 208
adaptation and, 209
aerial perspective and, 175
anamorphosis and, 178–180
apparent motion and, 180
Bayesian models and, 199, 204
binocular depth cue and, 171, 211
binocular disparity and, 170, 182, 184–190, 195–198, 200, 206–207, 211
binocular rivalry and, 187*f*, 202–205, 210–211
binocular summation and, 170, 211
blindness and, 188–190, 205–209
cameras and, 173*f*, 180, 187–188, 191
camouflage and, 190
cilia and, 188
cones and, 195
continuity constraint and, 193–194
contrast and, 203, 207
convergence and, 171, 178, 180–184, 188, 194, 206–207, 211
correspondence problem and, 192–194, 211
corresponding retinal points and, 183–184, 195, 202
critical period and, 189, 208–211
crossed disparity and, 185, 186*f*
cues and, 167, 170–208, 211
Cyclopean stimuli and, 190
dichoptic stimuli and, 187, 207
diplopia and, 184, 186*f*, 188, 210
divergence and, 180*f*, 181, 188
esotropia and, 209–210
familiar size and, 174–175, 199
feedback and, 192
filters and, 194*f*
fovea and, 180–188, 193, 209–210
functional magnetic resonance imaging (fMRI) and, 195, 196*f*, 204
heuristics and, 193
horopter and, 184–185, 186*f*, 195
illusions and, 200–202
infants and, 189, 205–210
inferotemporal (IT) cortex and, 196
interocular transfer and, 209
lens and, 180–181, 187–188, 198
linear perspective and, 175–180, 201, 211
magnetic resonance imaging (MRI) and, 195, 196*f*, 204
middle temporal area (MT) and, 196
midlevel vision and, 173
monocular cues and, 167, 170–178, 183, 188–193, 207–208, 211
motion parallax and, 179–180, 194, 196, 316
neuroimaging and, 196
occlusion and, 171–177, 199, 211
ocular dominance and, 208
Panum's fusional area and, 184, 186, 200
perceptual committees and, 173, 198–200
phase and, 207–208
photoreceptors and, 195
positivism and, 167
primary visual cortex (V1) and, 105*f*, 194, 202, 207–208, 211
probability summation and, 170
projective geometry and, 172–173, 176, 182, 187
pupil and, 181
random dot stereogram (RDS) and, 190–193, 196*f*, 206, 211
realism and, 167
receptive field and, 194, 195*f*, 208, 211
relative disparity and, 183, 185*f*, 194–196, 208
relative height and, 173–175, 198, 206
relative size and, 172–175, 176*f*, 186*f*
retina and, 167–175, 180–188, 192–199, 202, 204, 210–211
rods and, 187*f*
scatter and, 172–175, 176*f*
scene perception and, 215–217
sensitivity and, 208, 210
sine waves and, 207
single cells and, 204
spatial frequency and, 193–194, 207–208, 211
stereoacuity and, 192, 195, 206, 208
stereograms and, 187–193, 194*f*, 196*f*, 206*f*, 211
stereopsis and, 170–171, 178–198, 182–198, 205–211
strabismus and, 189–190, 209–210
striate cortex and, 194, 195*f*
suppression and, 202, 208–210
targets and, 170, 191, 206
texture gradient and, 173, 174*f*
thresholds and, 186, 192, 195
tilt and, 173, 201, 209
triangulation and, 178–182
uncrossed disparity and, 185–186
understanding scenes and, 236–246
uniqueness constraint and, 193
vanishing point and, 177
velocity and, 207
vergence and, 209

Vieth-Müller circle and, 184
visual acuity and, 192
visual angle and, 175
visual search and, 191
wavelength and, 175
spatial cognition, 388–389
spatial disorientation
dizziness and, 365–368, 386, 405–406
vestibular sensation and, 366, 386, 392, 400, 404–406
spatial frequency
attention and, 239–240
space perception and, 193–194, 207–208, 211
speech perception and, 353
vision and, 64–68, 75–77, 82–85, 87*f*, 89*f*, 91
visual motion perception and, 253, 270*f*
spatial frequency channels, 83–84
spatial hearing, 317
spatial layout, 52, 239, 240*f*, 447
spatial navigation, 389
spatial orientation
active sensing and, 392
amplitude and, 370–371, 376, 378–382, 395–400, 407
angular motion and, 365, 369–373, 376, 377*f*, 400, 407
cognition and, 388–389
cortical influences and, 402–403
direction and, 379–396, 402, 405, 407
linear motion and, 365, 369–371, 374, 400, 407
modalities/qualities of, 369–373
multisensory cortex and, 401–403
perception of, 384–390
pitch angular velocity and, 372
roll angular velocity and, 372
rotation perception and, 367*f*, 385–386, 396
sensory neuroscience and, 19*f*, 20
thresholds and, 384–387
tilt and, 365–374, 381–391, 398–407
translation and, 386–387
vestibular sensation and, 365–392, 400–407
vision and, 66
spatial segregation, 324–326
spatial vision
adaptation and, 80–86, 91
cameras and, 57, 60
columns and, 77–80
contrast and, 58–60, 63–66, 74, 76, 82–85, 89–90
cycles and, 50–66, 75, 83, 84*f*, 86*f*, 89*f*
development of, 86–90
Fourier analysis and, 66, 67*f*, 85
ganglion cells and, 57, 58*f*, 61, 67–68, 89–90
lateral geniculate nucleus (LGN) and, 69–70
selective adaptation and, 80–86, 91
striate cortex and, 58*f*, 70–80, 83, 84*f*, 86
stripes and, 67–68
visual acuity and, 58–67
visual angle and, 59, 62, 64, 66, 71, 79
visual crowding and, 61
specific anosmia, 472–473, 478, 483
specific hungers theory, 529–530
spectral contrast, 352–353
spectral power distribution, 158
spectral reflectance function, 158
spectral segregation, 324–326
spectral sensitivity, 132, 163*f*
spectrograms
hearing and, 327*f*
speech perception and, 346, 349*f*-350*f*, 360*f*
touch and, 444
spectrum
autism, 432, 461
color and, 131–132, 136*f*, 137, 141–144, 162*f*
hearing and, 275–277, 295–296, 319
light and, 33, 34*f*
speech perception and, 345, 352*f*, 353
specular reflections, 103, 104*f*
speech perception
amplitude and, 359–360
articulation and, 344*f*, 345–349, 352–353, 357, 361–362
attention and, 347
basilar membrane and, 354
belt area and, 359
categorical perception and, 349–352, 363
cerebral cortex and, 358
coarticulation and, 349, 352–353, 357, 362
contrast and, 350, 352–353
cues and, 349, 352–353, 361
decibel (dB) units and, 346
electroencephalography (EEG) and, 352
filters and, 345, 355
formants and, 345–353
frequency and, 345–353, 359–360
functional magnetic resonance imaging (fMRI) and, 359
harmonic spectrum and, 345
hearing and, 343–364
infants and, 339, 342–343, 355–358, 363
language and, 343–344, 348, 350, 354–363
larynx and, 19*f*, 20, 344–345
learning to listen, 355–358
McGurk effect and, 361
magnetic resonance imaging (MRI) and, 359
parabelt area and, 359
phonation and, 344*f*, 345, 362
pitch and, 345, 350, 355, 362
primary auditory cortex (A1) and, 359
resonators and, 345–346
sensitivity and, 349
sensory integration and, 361*f*
spatial frequency and, 353
spatial orientation and, 361*f*
spectral contrast and, 352–353
spectrograms and, 346, 349*f*-350*f*, 360*f*
spectrum and, 345, 352*f*, 353
strokes and, 358
vocal folds and, 335, 344*f*, 345–348
vocal tract and, 335, 344–347, 351, 362
speech production. *See also* language
accents and, 341–342
articulation and, 344–349, 352–353, 357, 361–362
brain and, 358–362
categorical perception and, 349–352
classifying sounds and, 346–348
coarticulation and, 349, 352–353, 357, 362
consonants and, 347–357, 361–362
fluency and, 344
fricatives and, 348, 361
invariance and, 349, 353
Japanese, 355–356
larynx and, 19*f*, 20, 344–345
learning words and, 357
native listeners and, 355–357
phonation and, 344–345, 362
resonators and, 335, 345–346
respiration and, 344–345
spectral contrast and, 352–353
speed of, 348–349
vocal folds and, 335, 344–348
vocal tract and, 335, 344–347, 351, 362
vowels and, 320–321, 322*f*, 345, 347–355, 357, 361–362
word separation and, 357–358
Zulu, 356
spinal cord
brain-computer interface and, 451–452
hearing and, 330
injuries to, 451–452
sensory neuroscience and, 22
touch and, 409, 411, 418–421, 435–439, 451–453
vestibular sensation and, 399*f*-401*f*
spinothalamic pathway, 420, 452
Srinath, R., 118
staircase method, 480–481
stapedius, 278*f*, 279
stapes, 277–283, 285*f*, 297
Starling Murmuration (Beukhof), 248*f*
statistical optimization models, 5*t*, 29
stem cells, 457, 459
stereoacuity, 192, 195, 206, 208
stereoblindness, 188–190, 206, 209
stereograms
random dot (RDS), 190–193, 196*f*, 211, 259, 450
space perception and, 187–193, 194*f*, 196*f*, 206*f*, 211
stereoisomers, 472–473
stereopsis
absolute disparity and, 183
binocular vision and, 170–171, 178–198, 205–211
cats and, 190
correspondence problem and, 192–194
corresponding retinal points and, 183–184

crossed disparity and, 184
depth and, 182–183
development of, 205–210
diplopia and, 184
horopter and, 184
Panum's fusional area and, 184
physiological basis of, 194–198
praying mantis and, 198
recovering, 189
relative disparity and, 183
space perception and, 170–171, 178–198, 205–211
uncrossed disparity and, 184
using, 191–192
Vieth-Müller circle and, 184
vision and, 58, 88
"Stereo Sue" (Sacks), 189
steropsis, 205–210
Stevens, Joseph, 524
Stevens, S. S., 524
Steven's power law, 11–12, 524
stimulus onset asynchrony (SOA), 17*f*, 18, 216
strabismus
space perception and, 189–190, 209–210
vision and, 88–89, 424
striate cortex
attention and, 233, 249
CO blobs and, 79
complex cells and, 75–77
cortical magnification and, 71–73, 79
eccentricity and, 71–72
fMRI and, 72
hypercolumns and, 77–80
object recognition and, 93, 96, 101, 104, 128
orientation tuning and, 74–75
receptive fields in, 73–77
simple cells and, 75–77
space perception and, 194, 195*f*
spatial vision and, 58*f*, 70–80, 83, 84*f*, 86
topographical mapping of, 71
stria vascularis, 280, 297, 303
striolae, 382
strokes
object recognition and, 98
speech perception and, 358
taste and, 516
vestibular sensation and, 402
visual motion perception and, 258
structural description, 122–123
structuralism, 106
Studio Weave, 304*f*
submodality of touch, 410
substantia gelatinosa, 419*f*, 435
subsurface scatter, 104
subtraction method, 119
subtractive color mixture, 138, 165
Sunday Roast (Hanson), 454*f*
superior colliculus, 72, 86, 230, 265
superior olives, 290–291, 308–310
supertasters, 12, 13*f*, 513, 519, 523–525, 533–535
supporting cells, 457–458
suppression
attention and, 217, 232
hearing and, 287
space perception and, 202, 208–210
taste and, 511, 519
touch and, 423, 437
visual motion perception and, 261, 267–268, 271
surroundedness, 114
sustentacular cells, 457–458
sweetness
fructose and, 520
glucose and, 520
olfaction and, 472, 482–483, 493–496
sensory neuroscience and, 5, 11–12
taste and, 5, 343, 507–535
symmetry
attention and, 221
hearing and, 296, 310, 313
object recognition and, 114, 117
olfaction and, 457
vertical, 61
vestibular sensation and, 378
vision and, 61
visual motion perception and, 267
synapses
hearing and, 281–284, 288–292, 300, 301*f*, 308
object recognition and, 101
olfaction and, 496, 500
sensory neuroscience and, 21*f*, 22, 29, 31
taste and, 512–515
touch and, 414, 420–421, 435
vestibular sensation and, 375, 382, 392, 395, 400–402
vision and, 41, 47–50, 69
synaptic terminal, 22*f*, 41*f*, 47–48
syncopation, 341–342
synesthesia, 152–153
syntax, 224
synthesis
object recognition and, 104
olfaction and, 475, 477
taste and, 511
vision and, 66

T

tactile agnosia, 422
tactile response
olfaction and, 500
taste and, 509
touch and, 410–415, 418–423, 426–432, 435, 438–439, 441, 444–449
vision and, 46
targets
attention and, 215*f*, 216–228, 246–247
color and, 154, 164
hearing and, 328*f*
olfaction and, 461, 469
sensory neuroscience and, 5*t*, 17–18, 21*f*
space perception and, 170, 191, 206
touch and, 427*f*, 433, 442, 443*f*, 446–449
vestibular sensation and, 389, 394*f*, 402
vision and, 63, 65, 68–69, 74, 76
visual motion perception and, 263, 266, 269–270
tastants, 483, 515, 524*f*
taste, xvi
absorption and, 515
adaptation and, 532
attention and, 530
basic, 517–523, 527–528, 531, 534–535
bitterness, 5, 12, 13*f*, 343, 512–528, 531, 534–535
cancer and, 517, 519, 521, 523, 525, 533, 535
Chinese restaurant syndrome and, 522
chorda tympani and, 509, 512*f*, 515–516, 526, 531
cilia and, 515
circumvallate papillae and, 512*f*, 513, 534
cranial nerves and, 507, 509, 512, 515–517, 525
cross-modality matching and, 524–525
cues and, 509, 529–533
decibel (dB) units and, 524
fat and, 522–523
feedback and, 515
filiform papillae and, 512, 534
flavor and, 507–511, 517, 522, 525–530, 534
foliate papillae and, 512*f*, 513, 534
food preferences and, 527
fungiform papillae and, 512–514, 523, 525, 533–535
glabrous skin and, 411–415, 423, 432, 434, 439
glomeruli and, 528
G protein-coupled receptor and, 458, 512, 515, 518, 520–521, 534
gustation and, 417, 512–516, 531
health consequences and, 525–526
heart attacks and, 527
heterodimer and, 520–521
illusory contours and, 446*f*
infants and, 522, 528–530
insula and, 512*f*, 516, 534
learned taste aversion and, 465, 494
lesions and, 522, 533
localization of, 509–511
memory and, 527
microvilli and, 512, 514–515, 518, 534
middle ear and, 509, 526
monosodium glutamate (MSG) and, 522, 534
MSG and, 522
music and, 343
nature of qualities of, 531–533
neurotransmitters and, 515, 522
nontasters and, 12, 523, 526, 534–535
nutrient regulation and, 526–530
orbitofrontal cortex (OFC) and, 512*f*, 516, 534
papillae and, 512–514, 522–525, 533–535
phenylthiocarbamide (PTC) and, 519, 523
pleasure of burning sensation and, 532–533
propylthiouracil (PROP) and, 12, 13*f*, 523–525, 534
protein and, 512, 515, 518–522, 534
psychophysics and, 510–511

retronasal olfaction and, 508–511, 525–528, 534
saltiness, 5, 343, 513–518, 524, 527–535
sensitivity and, 514, 519
sensory neuroscience and, 6–7
somatosensation and, 509, 521
sourness, 343, 509, 513–519, 524, 527–528, 531–534
specific hungers theory and, 529–530
Steven's power law and, 524
strokes and, 516
supertasters and, 12, *13f*, 513, 519, 523–525, 533–535
suppression and, 511, 519
sweetness, 5, 343, 507–535
synapses and, 512–515
synthesis and, 511
tactile response and, 509
templates and, 513*f*
thresholds and, 513–514, 523–524
tongue map and, 513–514, 517
transduction and, 519
transmission and, 512*f*, 514*f*, 515, 522
trigeminal nerves and, 509, 530
umami, 517–518, 522, 534
vagus (X) nerves and, 512*f*
volatile molecules and, 508–511
taste blindness, 519
taste buds, 531
gustatory system and, 512–517
olfaction and, 466
papillae and, 512–514, 522–525, 533–535
taste receptor cells, 512, 514–515, 518*f*
tasters
bitterness and, 523–526
olfaction and, 479
sensory neuroscience and, 11–12, 13*f*
supertasters, 12, 13*f*, 513, 519, 523–525, 533–535
wine, 343
tau, 261–262
tectorial membrane, 280*f*, 281–283, 286, 289
templates, 121–122, 129, 513*f*
tempo, 274, 340
temporal code, 289–290, 320
temporal integration, 293
temporal segregation, 324–326
tensor tympani, 278*f*, 279
tetrachromatic color vision, 151, 162
texture-defined objects, 258
texture gradient, 173, 174*f*
texture segmentation, 109–110, 117
thermoreceptors, 415–417, 420, 440, 452
thermoTRP channel, 416–418
Thomas, D., 137
Thought Forms (Hunsicker), 32*f*
threshold models, 6
thresholds
difference, 5*f*, 9–10, 31
hearing and, 275, 276*f*, 286–287, 293–300, 337*f*
olfaction and, 478–481, 487, 489
sensory neuroscience and, 5*f*, 6–17, 23, 31
space perception and, 186, 192, 195
spatial orientation and, 384–387
taste and, 513–514, 523–524
touch and, 428–432, 436, 441*f*, 442, 448, 452
vestibular sensation and, 270, 384–387, 404–405, 407
vision and, 36, 44–45, 64–65, 83, 84*f*, ,87
threshold tuning curve, 286–287
tickling, 438–439
tilt
attention and, 225, 238
object recognition and, 94
orientation selectivity and, 73–74
sensory neuroscience and, 18, 23
space perception and, 173, 201, 209
spatial orientation and, 365–374, 381–391, 398–407
vestibular sensation and, 365–374, 382–391, 398–407
vision and, 73–74, 81–83
tilt aftereffect, 82–83, 209
timbre
loudness and, 276–277, 320–321, 322*f*, 325–326, 332–333, 444
psychological sensation of, 276
spectrum and, 277
touch and, 444
time course of perception, 5*t*, 6, 17–18
time to collision (TTC), 261
tip link, 282, 283*f*
tip-of-the nose phenomenon, 481, 504
Tipper, Steve, 234
Titchener, Edward Bradford, 106
tone chroma, 337–338, 362
tone height, 337–338, 339*f*, 362
tongue map, 513–514, 517
tonotopic organization, 292, 295, 303, 336
top-down processes, 30, 37, 433, 435, 453
topographical mapping, 70–71, 72*f*, 440*f*
Toro, Iruka Maria, 56*f*
touch
A-alpha fibers and, 411
A-beta fibers and, 411–412, 415, 418–419, 435
action for perception and, 441–444
acuity and, 415, 427, 429–432, 447–448, 452
A-delta fibers and, 411, 413*f*, 415–417
affective, 410, 427, 432–434, 452
agnosia and, 422
amplitude and, 428*f*
anterior cingulate cortex (ACC) and, 423, 424*f*, 435–438, 489
attention and, 431, 434*f*, 446, 453
auditory nerve (AN) and, 419
autonomic nervous system and, 410
blindness and, 409–410, 424, 426, 431, 450
body image and, 426–427
Braille and, 413, 424, 431, 447–448
cerebral cortex and, 420*f*
cochlea and, 419
contrast and, 410
criterion and, 428
cues and, 434*f*, 443*f*, 446
cycles and, 413*t*
DCML pathway and, 420, 452
decibel (dB) units and, 428*f*
dermis and, 411, 412*f*, 414
discriminative, 409–410, 427, 434, 435*f*, 440, 452
distractors and, 442, 446, 447*f*
dorsal horn and, 419–420, 435–438, 452
efficiency and, 417, 442, 445–449
egocenter and, 448
electroencephalography (EEG) and, 423, 433
emotion and, 409–410, 417–418, 423, 427, 433–437, 440, 452
endogenous opiates and, 436
epidermis and, 411–415
exploratory procedures and, 441–445, 450, 453
feedback and, 420, 425–426, 437, 450–452
frame of reference for, 448–449
free nerve endings and, 415–416
frequency and, 413, 428*f*, 429, 443–444, 453
functional magnetic resonance imaging (fMRI) and, 422–424, 436–437, 441
gate control theory and, 435–437, 453
hair cells and, 419
haptic perception and, 409, 440–451
heuristics and, 445
homunculus and, 421, 422*f*, 425, 430, 449, 451
hyperalgesia and, 438
infants and, 432–433, 449
insula and, 423, 424*f*, 435, 437
interoception and, 439–440, 452, 510–511
intersensory integration and, 450
itch and, 435–439
kinesthesia and, 410
kinesthetic systems and, 410, 415, 420, 424*f*, 439, 441
language and, 4
magnetic resonance imaging (MRI) and, 422
material vs. geometric properties and, 445
mechanical pressure and, 427–428
mechanoreceptors and, 411–416, 419–420, 423, 428*f*, 429, 439–443, 452–453
Meissner corpuscle and, 412*f*, 413–415
memory and, 445
Merkel disc and, 413–414
neglect and, 418
neural fibers and, 410–423
neural pathways of, 410–426
neural plasticity and, 88, 423–425
neurotransmitters and, 436
nocebo effect and, 438
nociceptors and, 412*f*, 417–420, 435–438, 452
object recognition and, 444–452
orbitofrontal context (OFC) and, 423
oscillations and, 444
Pacinian corpuscles and, 412*f*, 413, 440
pain and, 435–439

papillae and, 412*f*, 414
parietal lobe and, 421, 452
pattern perception and, 447–448
perception for action and, 440–441
phantom limb and, 425, 478, 517
phase and, 451*f*, 452
placebo effect and, 436–438
proprioception and, 410–411, 423
proximity and, 409, 415, 423
pruiceptors and, 417–418, 437
psychophysics and, 440
random dot stereogram (RDS) and, 450
receptive field and, 412–415, 421, 429*f*, 430
receptor adaptation and, 487, 489, 504
receptor potential and, 416
Ruffini endings and, 413–414
sensitivity and, 413*f*, 415, 427–432, 453
sensitivity differences and, 431–432
sensory integration and, 450
somatosensation and, 410–411, 418–424, 441, 444
somatosensory areas and, 421, 422*f*, 441
somatotopy and, 419
spatial details and, 429–430
spectrograms and, 444
spinal cord and, 409, 411, 418–421, 435–439, 451–453
stroking and, 409–410, 418, 423, 424*f*, 432–434, 437, 443, 452–453
submodalities of, 410, 427–440
substantia gelatinosa and, 419*f*, 435
suppression and, 423, 437
synapses and, 414, 420–421, 435
tactile response and, 410–415, 418–423, 426–432, 435, 438–439, 441, 444–449
targets and, 427*f*, 433, 442, 443*f*, 446–449
temporal details and, 430
thermoreceptors and, 415–417, 420, 440, 452
thermoTRP channel and, 416–418
thresholds and, 428–432, 436, 441*f*, 442, 448, 452
tickling and, 438–439
timbre and, 444
transduction and, 443
transmission and, 411, 413, 418–421, 426, 434–436, 437*f*
two-point touch threshold and, 429–430, 448
vagus (X) nerves and, 439–440
velocity and, 411*f*, 434*f*
vibratory thresholds and, 428*f*
visual acuity and, 429–430
warmth fibers and, 20, 415–416
what/where pathways and, 444–452
transduction
color and, 134*f*
cones and, 47–49
hearing and, 278*f*, 280–282, 283*f*, 287, 300
light and, 36, 39–40, 47–49, 54
olfaction and, 458, 487
rods and, 47–49
sensory neuroscience and, 4
taste and, 519
touch and, 443
vestibular sensation and, 369–370, 374–379, 382, 386, 406
vision and, 36, 39–40, 47, 54
transmission
color and, 129, 138*f*
hearing and, 277–284, 301, 302*f*, 330
object recognition and, 104
olfaction and, 458, 466*f*, 469, 471
sensory neuroscience and, 20–23, 29, 31
taste and, 512*f*, 514*f*, 515, 522
touch and, 411, 413, 418–421, 426, 434–436, 437*f*
vestibular sensation and, 375–376, 392, 395, 399*f*, 400
vision and, 34–36, 47–50, 54, 61
visual motion perception and, 252
transparency
hearing and, 324*f*
object recognition and, 104, 108
vestibular sensation and, 391*f*
vision and, 35–38, 41
visual motion perception and, 255
Tresilian, J. R., 262
triangle test, 480–482
triangulation, 178–182
trichromacy
color and, 49*f*, 134–137, 143–144, 151, 160–161
historical perspective on, 137–138
vision and, 49*f*, 134–137, 143–144, 151, 160–161
trigeminal (V) nerves
olfaction and, 20, 455, 462, 469, 470*f*, 483, 489–490, 496, 503
sensory neuroscience and, 19*f*, 20
taste and, 509, 530
tritanopes, 152
trochlear (IV) nerves, 19*f*, 20, 395*f*
tufted cells, 457*f*, 465–466, 471
turbinates, 457
two-point perspective, 177*f*
two-point touch threshold, 429–430, 448
two-tone suppression, 287
tympanic canal, 277–281
tympanic membrane
hearing and, 277–283, 297, 300, 313
malleus and, 277–279, 283

U

umami, 517–518, 522, 534
uncrossed disparity, 185–186
unique hue, 145*f*, 146–147
uniqueness constraint, 193
unrelated color, 154–155
utricle, 369, 374*f*, 382–384, 407

V

vagus (X) nerves, 19*f*, 20, 439–440, 512
Van Gogh, Vincent, 152–153
vanishing point, 177
vection, 390–391
velocity
sensory neuroscience and, 21
space perception and, 207
touch and, 411*f*, 434*f*
vestibular sensation and, 369–374, 378–380, 381*f*, 385–386, 387*f*, 390, 396, 402, 406
visual motion perception and, 250, 262, 270
velocity storage, 385–386, 396
vergence
space perception and, 209
vision and, 180*f*, 181–183, 195
visual motion perception and, 266, 271
vergence angle, 180*f*, 181, 183
Vernier, Pierre, 63
vertigo, 366, 402
vestibular aging, 405
vestibular canal, 279–283, 288
vestibular organs, 365, 367*f*, 401*f*, 403*f*
balance system and, 393
blood pressure and, 398
description of, 374–384, 407
graviception and, 368
human vertical canals and, 368–369
nuclei and, 395
vestibular sensation
acceleration and, 369–370, 374, 376, 380–387, 390, 406–407
active sensing and, 368, 392
acuity and, 394*f*
adaptation and, 404, 412–413, 442
afferent fibers and, 392
amplitude and, 370–371, 376, 378–382, 395–400, 407
angular motion and, 365, 369–373, 376, 377*f*, 400, 407
attention and, 366–369
balance and, 19*f*, 365–368, 386, 392–393, 398–400, 401*f*, 404–407
blindness and, 367, 389, 404
blood pressure and, 393, 397–398
characteristic frequency and, 396
cilia and, 368*f*, 374–376, 377*f*, 379*f*, 382, 383*f*
cochlea and, 365–366, 374
contributions to, 367–368
convergence and, 401–402, 430
cortical influences and, 402–403
cranial nerves and, 365, 374*f*, 395*f*
cues and, 370, 385, 389–392, 398*f*-399*f*
cycles and, 380–381, 386–387
decay and, 379–380, 385
development of, 368–369
direction and, 370–396, 402, 405, 407
divergence and, 406
dizziness and, 365–368, 386, 405–406
efferent commands and, 368, 392
emotion and, 386
failure of, 403–407
fall risk and, 404
feedback and, 402
Fourier analysis and, 380, 382
frequency and, 366, 380–382, 386–387, 396, 397*f*, 400*f*, 406
ganglion cells and, 378, 402
graviception and, 365, 368–369, 392

gravity and, 365–374, 382–384, 390–391, 397–399, 400*f*, 407
hair cells and, 368*f*, 374–386, 407
hippocampus and, 388–389, 402
hyperpolarization and, 375*f*, 379*f*
imbalance and, 366–367, 386, 399*f*, 400, 404–406
inner ear and, 365, 367*f*, 374–376, 377*f*, 406–407
interoception and, 367, 391
kinesthetic systems and, 368, 399*f*
lateral geniculate nucleus (LGN) and, 402
lesions and, 398, 402
linear acceleration and, 369–370, 374, 382–384, 386, 406–407
linear motion and, 365, 369–371, 374, 400, 407
McGurk effect and, 390
maculae and, 382–384
magnitdre estimation and, 384–387
mal de debarquement syndrome and, 400, 404
mathematical integration and, 386
mechanoreceptors and, 368*f*, 374, 407
memory and, 388–389
Ménières syndrome and, 405–407
middle ear and, 374*f*
modalities/qualities of, 369–373
multisensory integration and, 390–392, 404, 407
neurotransmitters and, 375
oscillations and, 380–382, 386–387, 396*f*
otolith organs and, 368*f*, 369–370, 374–376, 382–386, 390–391, 396, 402, 406–407
outer ear and, 374*f*
parietal lobe and, 403*f*
pitch and, 369, 372–373, 379, 388*f*, 398
pitch angular velocity and, 372
pupil and, 394
receptive field and, 368
receptor potential and, 375–377, 382–384
reflexive responses and, 392–401
reflexive eye movement and, 395
retina and, 366, 378, 392–395, 402
rhythm and, 380
roll angular velocity and, 372
rotation perception and, 367*f*, 385–386, 396
saccules and, 369, 374*f*, 382–384, 407
semicircular canals and, 369, 374, 376–382, 385–386, 390, 393–398, 402, 406–407
sense of angular motion and, 369–372
sense of linear motion and, 369–371, 400
sense of tilt and, 365, 369–370
sensitivity and, 369, 374, 378–384, 387
sensory conflict and, 370
sensory exafference and, 392
sensory integration and, 390–392, 404, 407
sensory reafference and, 392
sine waves and, 381
smooth pursuit and, 366
somatosensation and, 367
spatial disorientation and, 366, 386, 392, 400, 404–406
spatial orientation and, 365–392, 400–407
spinal cord and, 399*f*-401*f*
strokes and, 402
symmetry and, 378
synapses and, 375, 382, 392, 395, 400–402
targets and, 389, 394*f*, 402
thresholds and, 270, 384–387, 404–405, 407
tilt and, 365–374, 382–391, 398–407
transduction and, 369–370, 374–379, 382, 386, 406
transmission and, 375–376, 392, 395, 399*f*, 400
transparency and, 391*f*
trochlear (IV) nerves and, 20, 395*f*
utricle and, 369, 374*f*, 382–384, 407
vection and, 390–391
velocity and, 369–374, 378–380, 381*f*, 385–386, 387*f*, 390, 396, 402, 406
vertigo and, 366, 402
virtual reality and, 365, 370
visual acuity and, 394*f*
visual-vestibular, 390–391
vestibular thalamocortical pathways, 402
vestibulo-autonomic responses, 396–398
vestibulocochlear (VIII) nerves, 19*f*, 20, 290, 374*f*
vestibulo-ocular reflex (VOR)
reflex and, 392–393, 394*f*-397*f*, 407
retina and, 366, 367*f*
visual motion perception and, 266
vestibulo-ocular responses, 393–396
vestibulospinal responses, 398–401
vibration theory, 471–473, 503
vibratory thresholds, 428*f*
Vieth-Müller circle, 184
virtual reality, 365, 370, 463*f*, 502
vision
absolute threshold and, 44*f*
absorption and, 33–38, 43, 45, 48, 54
accommodation and, 36–39
acuity and, 40, 43, 44*f*, 49*t*, 50, 53–54, 58–67, 71–74, 87*f*, 88–90, 152
adaptation and, 44–46, 49*f*, 62, 65, 66*f*, 80–86, 91, 155–157
afferent signals and, 368, 386, 392, 393*f*
age-relatve macular degeneration and, 46, 55
amacrine cells and, 35*f*, 40–41, 47–50, 53
amblyopia and, 62, 88, 192, 210
amplitude and, 37*f*, 48, 66–67
ampulla and, 376, 377*f*, 379*f*
angular acceleration and, 369–370, 374, 386, 387*f*
anisometropia and, 88–89
aqueous humor and, 35*f*, 36–38
astigmatism and, 38–39
attention and, 37, 89
auditory nerve (AN) and, 374*f*
autonomic nervous system and, 396–397
balance and, 48
Bayesian models and, 159
binocular rivalry and, 7, 147, 187*f*, 202–205, 210–211, 475–476
bipolar cells and, 35*f*, 40, 43*t*, 47–53
blindness and, 39–40 (*see also* blindness)
BOLD signal and, 70, 72
cameras and, 36, 39, 46, 52, 57, 60
cataracts and, 37–38, 88, 271
cerebral cortex and, 57, 70, 90
chromophore and, 48
cilia and, 20, 35*f*, 36–37
CO blobs and, 79–80
color and, 131–165 (*see also* color)
columns and, 77–80, 91
comparator and, 261, 267–269
complex cells and, 75–77, 123
cones and, 57–65 (*see also* cones)
contrast and, 39*f*, 46, 49–54, 58–60, 63–66, 74, 76, 82–85, 89–90
contrast-defined objects and, 64
convergence and, 43*f*, 49–54
cornea and, 35–39, 54, 57, 466, 470*f*
cortical magnification and, 71–73, 79, 422
critical period and, 88–89
cues and, 62, 86, 164
cycles and, 59–66, 75, 83, 84*f*, 87*f*, 89*f*
development of, 86–90
dichoptic stimuli and, 187, 207
diffuse bipolar cells and, 49–50, 53
diopter units and, 36–37
diplopia and, 184, 186*f*, 188, 210
divergence and, 49–50
duplex retinas and, 41, 44–45
eccentricity and, 40–41, 42*f*, 50, 53, 71–72, 73*f*
efficiency and, 43, 85
emmetropia and, 38
end stopping and, 76, 77*f*
esotropia and, 209–210
feedback and, 70, 77
feed-forward process and, 70, 95*f*, 101
filters and, 52–53, 68–69, 75, 80, 85
focal distance and, 36–37
Fourier analysis and, 35*f*, 39*f*, 40–43, 48–50, 54, 61–63, 66, 67*f*, 71–73, 79, 85, 89
fovea and, 180–188, 193, 209–210, 306, 422
free fusion and, 188
frequency and, 64–68, 75–77, 82–91
functional magnetic resonance imaging (fMRI) and, 72–73, 99
fundus and, 39–40
ganglion cells and, 35*f*, 39–40, 41*f*, 45–54, 57, 58*f*, 61, 67–78, 89–90
genetic differences in, 151–152
gist and, 85
graded potentials and, 48
haptic perception and, 449–450
hearing dominating, 326–327
horizontal cells and, 35*f*, 40, 47, 49, 52–53
hue and, 33
hyperopia and, 38–39
hyperpolarization and, 48
image formation and, 35–44
infants and, 86–89

inner segment and, 41*f*-42*f*, 47
interocular transfer and, 83
iris and, 35*f*, 36, 39, 45*f*, 57
kinesthesia and, 367, 399*f*
lateral geniculate nucleus (LGN) and, 50–51, 58*f*, 69–70, 72*f*, 75
lateral inhibition and, 49–52, 75, 84
lens and, 35–39, 57, 59, 88
lesions and, 69, 71, 72*f*-73*f*
light/dark adaptation and, 44–46, 49*f*
McGurk effect and, 361, 390
maculae and, 40, 46, 55, 89
magnetic resonance imaging (MRI) and, 72, 73*f*
magnetoencephalography (MEG) and, 72
magnocellular layer and, 50, 69, 256
melanopsin and, 48
microsaccades and, 266, 271
middle temporal area (MT) and, 251, 256, 257*f*
midget bipolar cells and, 50
midlevel, 103–118, 128
monocular cues and, 88
myopia and, 38–39
neurotransmitters and, 48
object recognition and, 93–129
ocular dominance and, 74–80
OFF bipolar cells and, 50
ON bipolar cells and, 50
ON-center cells and, 51*f*, 52, 68
optic nerves and, 18–19, 35*f*, 36, 39–40, 51, 54, 58*f*, 72, 418–419
optokinetic nystagmus and, 266, 270–271
orientation selectivity and, 73–74
orientation tuning and, 74–78
outer segment and, 41*f*, 47–48, 89
parvocellular layer and, 50, 58*f*, 69–70
phase and, 66–68, 76, 89
photoactivation and, 48, 282
photons and, 33–36, 44–48, 54, 64, 293
photopic illumination and, 43, 44*f*, 49, 66*f*
photoreceptors and, 35*f*, 36, 39–57, 60, 62, 72, 76, 281–282, 422
preferential looking and, 86–87
presbyopia and, 37–38, 188
primary visual cortex (V1) and, 58*f*, 70, 90–91, 421
protein and, 37, 47
pupil and, 35*f*, 36, 41, 44–45, 48, 90
receptive field and, 43*t*, 46, 49, 51–54, 68, 70, 73–77, 85–86, 90
refraction and, 35–39, 54, 62, 65, 88–89
retina and, 33–55 (*see also* retina)
rhodopsin and, 48, 87, 134
rhythm and, 48
rods and, 57, 87 (*see also* rods)
scatter and, 34–40, 54, 77
scotopic illumination and, 43, 44*f*, 49, 66*f*, 132–134, 165
sensitivity and, 43*f*, 44–50, 54, 64–65, 66*f*, 74, 82–85, 89–90
simple cells and, 74–77
sine waves and, 60*f*, 64–68, 84
singe-photon sensitivity and, 54
single cells and, 35, 77
sinusoidal oscillations and, 380–382, 387*f*, 396*f*
spatial frequency and, 64–68, 75–77, 82–85, 87*f*, 89*f*, 91
spatial orientation and, 66 (*see also* spatial orientation)
spectral reflectance function and, 158
stereopsis and, 58, 88
strabismus and, 88–89, 424
striate cortex and, 58*f*, 70–80, 83, 84*f*, 86
symmetry and, 61
synapses and, 41, 47–50, 69
synthesis and, 66
tactile response and, 46
targets and, 63, 65, 68–69, 74, 76
tetrachromatic, 151, 162
thresholds and, 36, 44–45, 64–65, 83, 84*f*, ,87
tilt and, 73–74, 81–83
topographical mapping and, 70–71, 72*f*, 440*f*
transduction and, 36, 39–40, 47, 54
transmission and, 34–36, 47–50, 54, 61
transparency and, 35–38, 41
trichromacy and, 49*f*, 134–137, 143–144, 151, 160–161
trochlear (IV) nerves and, 20, 395*f*
vergence and, 180*f*, 181–183, 195
vestibulo-ocular reflex (VOR) and, 366, 367*f*
vitreous humor and, 35*f*, 36–38, 57
visual acuity
amblyopia and, 88
color and, 89
constrast and, 74
convergence and, 50
cortical magnification and, 72
description of, 58–67
eccentricity and, 71
fovea and, 40
hyperacuity, 63–64
letter charts and, 62, 73
minimum discriminable, 62*f*, 63–64
minimum recognizable, 62–63
minimum resolvable, 62–63
Snellen chart and, 62
space perception and, 192
spatial vision and, 58–67
stripes and, 64–65
touch and, 429–430
types of, 62–65
Vernier and, 63
vestibular sensation and, 394*f*
visual motion perception and, 266
visual angle
light and, 41, 42*f*
space perception and, 175
spatial vision and, 59, 62, 64, 66, 71, 79
visual motion perception and, 261
visual crowding, 61, 267
visual-field defect, 71, 233
visual motion perception
acuity and, 263, 266
adaptation and, 251–252
akinetopsia and, 258
amacrine cells and, 253
aperture and, 36, 253–257, 271
apparent motion and, 253, 254*f*, 259
attention and, 251, 261, 266–269
balance and, 250–251
binocular disparity and, 262
blindness and, 256, 263, 266–268
camouflage and, 260, 263
computation of, 251–260
contrast and, 258, 270–271
contrast-defined objects and, 258
convergence and, 266
correspondence problem and, 253–255
cues and, 249, 262–263
cycles and, 270*f*
development of, 270–271
direction selectivity and, 253
divergence and, 266
double dissociation and, 259
eccentricity and, 263
efficiency and, 263
eye movements and, 263–269
filters and, 253, 271
first-order motion and, 258–259, 271
focus of expansion and, 206
fovea and, 263, 266–267, 269
frequency and, 253, 270
frontal eye fields and, 265, 269
functional magnetic resonance imaging (fMRI) and, 251, 256
ganglion cells and, 253, 265
heuristics and, 260
imbalance and, 251
infants and, 266
interocular transfer and, 251
lateral geniculate nucleus (LGN) and, 251, 256
lesions and, 256–259
magnetic resonance imaging (MRI) and, 251, 256
masking and, 268
middle temporal area (MT) and, 256–258
motion aftereffects (MAE) and, 249–251, 258
motion-induced blindness and, 263
motion parallax and, 249
navigation and, 260–261
object recognition and, 262–263
optokinetic nystagmus and, 266, 270–271
primary visual cortex (V1) and, 249–251
random dot stereogram (RDS) and, 259
reading and, 267
receptive field and, 252–256, 263, 269, 271
reflexive eye movement and, 266, 270
retina and, 251, 253, 260–271
saccades and, 253, 261–271
second-order motion and, 258–260, 271
selective adaptation and, 251
sensitivity and, 268, 270–271
smooth pursuit and, 264–271
spatial frequency and, 253, 270*f*
strokes and, 258
suppression and, 261, 267–268, 271
symmetry and, 267

targets and, 263, 266, 269–270
texture-defined objects and, 258
time to collision (TTC) and, 261
transmission and, 252
transparency and, 255
using information from, 260–263
velocity and, 250, 262, 270
vergence and, 266, 271
vestibulo-ocular reflex (VOR) and, 266
visual acuity and, 266
visual angle and, 261
visual search and, 267
visual search
attention and, 217–227, 235, 246–247
binding problem and, 225–226
conjunction search and, 218*f*, 222–223, 225
efficiency and, 219–220
fish and, 221
guided, 220–225, 230
olfaction and, 446, 447*f*, 479
primes and, 223
rapid visual representation and, 226–228
space perception and, 191
visual motion perception and, 267
visual word form area (VWFA), 98
vitreous humor, 35*f*, 36–38, 57
Vive Pro Eye, 209
vocal folds, 335, 344–348
vocal tract, 335, 344–347, 351, 362
volatile molecules
olfaction and, 456, 470*f*, 476, 487, 492, 496–497, 503
taste and, 508–511
volley principle, 290, 297
vomeronasal organ (VNO), 497, 504
von der Heydt, R., 94
von Frey, Max, 427
vowels
native listeners and, 355–357
speech production and, 320–321, 322*f*, 345, 347–357, 361–362

W

warmth fibers, 20, 415–416
wavelength
color and, 131–147, 151–159, 162*f*, 163–165
hearing and, 274–275, 289, 295, 310, 318–319
light and, 33–34, 43, 47–49, 456, 475*f*, 476
object recognition and, 103
olfaction and, 456, 475*f*, 476
space perception and, 175
Weber fractions, 10, 12
Weber's law, 10–12, 49*f*, 342
Weizmann Institute, 490
Wells, William Charles, 393
Wertheimer, Max, 106
what/where pathways
object recognition and, 96–101, 118–119, 127–128
touch and, 444–452
white noise, 28, 295–296, 476
Wiesel, Torsten, 73–81, 88, 194, 208, 210
Williams, David, 137
winds farms, 318, 31*f*
Wolfe, Philip, 130*f*
World Health Organization (WHO), 88
Wundt, Wilhelm, 106

X

X-rays, xvi, 6, 13, 26*f*, 30, 125

Y

Young, Thomas, 137
Your Soul Has Become an Invisible Bee (Toro), 56*f*

Z

Zatorre, R. J., 362
Zeki, Samir, 146–147
Zhou, H., 94
Zulu, 356

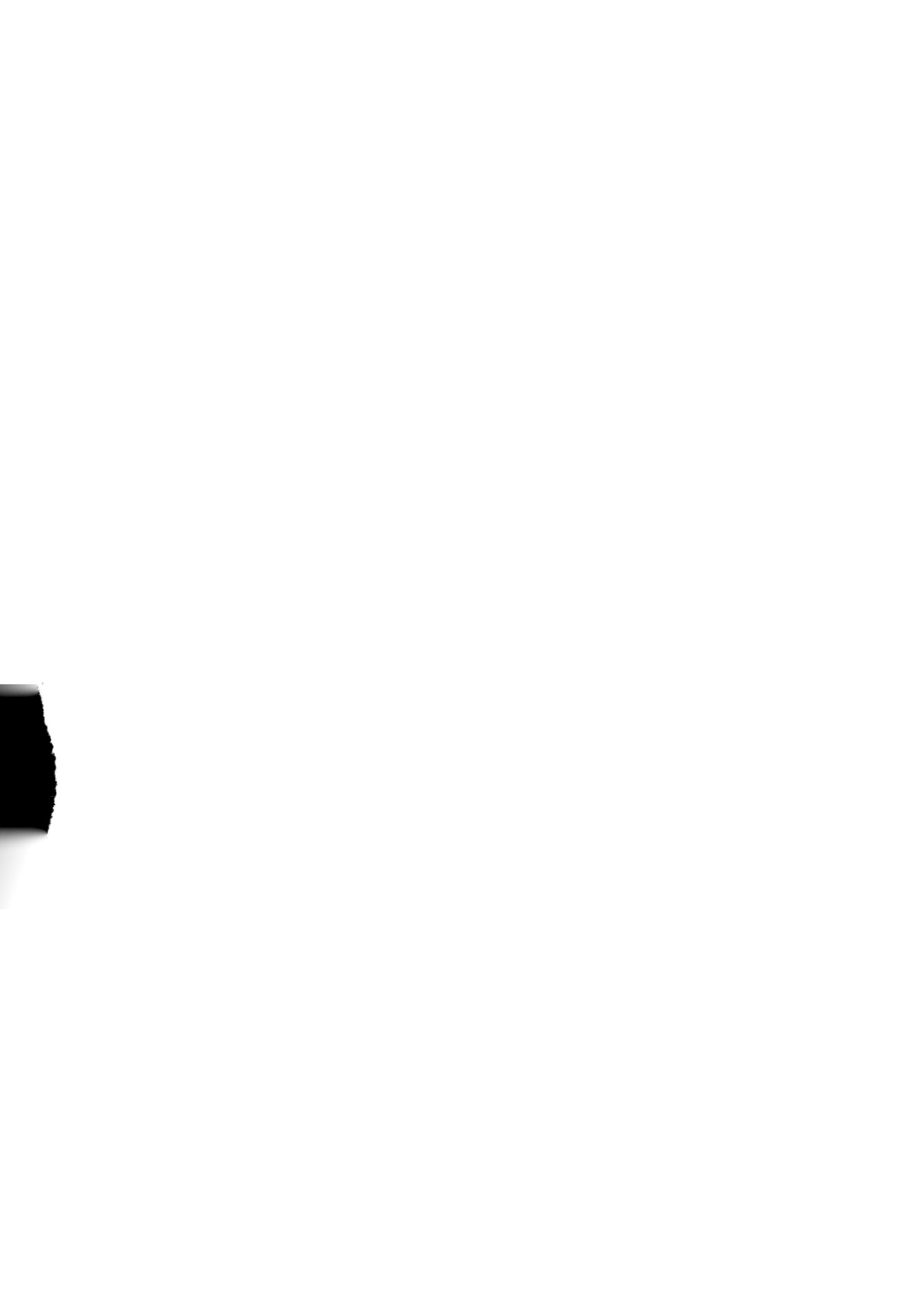